Shoulder and Elbow Injuries in Athletes: Prevention, Treatment, and Return to Sport

Shoulder and Elbow Injuries in Athletes:

Prevention, Treatment, and Return to Sport

Robert A. Arciero, MD
Professor
Department of Orthopaedic Surgery
University of Connecticut Health Center
Chief, Sports Medicine
Director, Orthopaedic Sports Medicine Fellowship
Team Physician, University of Connecticut
Farmington, Connecticut

Frank A. Cordasco, MD, MS
Professor of Orthopaedic Surgery
Weill Cornell Medical College
Attending Orthopaedic Surgeon
Sports Medicine and Shoulder Service
Senior Scientist, Research Division
Hospital for Special Surgery
New York, New York

Matthew T. Provencher, MD, CAPT, MC, USNR
Complex Shoulder Knee and Sports Surgery
The Steadman Clinic
Vail, Colorado

ELSEVIER

Mark D. Lazarus, MD
Professor, Department of Orthopaedic Surgery
The Rothman Institute
Sidney Kimmel Medical College
Thomas Jefferson University
Philadelphia, Pennsylvania

Brian Lee, MD
Orthopaedic Surgeon
Kerlan-Jobe Orthopaedic Clinic
Los Angeles, California

William N. Levine, MD
Frank E. Stinchfield Professor and Chairman
Chief, Shoulder Service
Co-Director, Center for Shoulder, Elbow and Sports Medicine
NYP/Columbia University Medical Center
New York, New York

Michael Levinson, BS
Clinical Supervisor
Sports Rehabilitation and Performance Center
Hospital for Special Surgery
New York, New York

Barrett A. Little, MD
Orthopaedic Sports Medicine and Shoulder Surgery
OrthoCarolina
Charlotte, North Carolina

C. Benjamin Ma, MD
Professor in residence
Chief, Sports Medicine and Shoulder Service
Department of Orthopedic Surgery
University of California
San Francisco, California

Peter MacDonald, BSc, MD, FRCS(C)
Professor and Head
Section of Orthopaedics
University of Manitoba
Winnipeg, Canada

Joshua W. Major, MD, MPH
Department of Orthopaedic Surgery
Naval Medical Center San Diego
San Diego, California

Joseph Marchese, MD
Department of Orthopaedic Surgery
University of Connecticut Health Center
Farmington, Connecticut

Keisuke Matsuki, MD, PhD
Shoulder and Elbow Service
Funabashi Orthopaedic Sports Medicine & Joint Center
Funabashi, Japan

Augustus D. Mazzocca, MS, MD
Professor and Chairman
Deparment of Orthopaedic Surgery
University of Connecticut Health Center
Farmington, Connecticut

Molly C. Meadows, MD
Division of Sports Medicine
Department of Orthopaedic Surgery
Rush University Medical Center
Chicago, Illinois

Giovanni Merolla, MD
Shoulder and Elbow Unit
"D. Cervesi" Hospital
Cattolica, Italy

Lucas S. McDonald, MD, MPH, LCDR MC USN
Assistant Professor of Surgery
Uniformed Services University of the Health Sciences
Division of Sports Medicine and Shoulder Surgery
Department of Orthopaedic Surgery
Naval Medical Center San Diego
San Diego, California

Micahel D. McKee, MD
Professor of Surgery
Department of Surgery, Division of Orthopaedics
St. Michael's Hospital
University of Toronto
Toronto, Canada

Karim A. Meijer, MD
Texas Sports Medicine and Orthopaedic Group
Dallas, Texas

Peter J. Millett, MD, MSC
Steadman Philippon Research Institute
The Steaman Clinic
Vail, Colorado

Antony Miniaci, MD, FRCSC
Department of Orthopaedic Surgery
Cleveland Clinic
Cleveland, Ohio

Philipp Moroder, MD
Department of Traumatology and Sports Injuries
Paracelus Medical University
Salzburg, Austria
Center for Musculoskeletal Surgery
Campus Virchow
Charité-Universitaetsmedizin
Berlin, Germany

Kevin R. Myers, MD
Orthopedic Surgeon and Sports Medicine
OrthoTexas
Dallas, Texas

Carl W. Nissen, MD
Physician
Elite Sports Medicine
Connecticut Children's Medical Center
Professor
Department of Orthopaedics
University of Connecticut
Farmington, Connecticut

Matthew P. Noyes, MD
Southern Oregon Orthopaedics
Medford, Oregon

Michael J. O'Brien, MD
Associate Professor
Department of Orthopaedics
Tulane University School of Medicine
New Orleans, Louisiana

Stephen J. O'Brien, MD, MBA
Attending Orthopaedic Surgeon
Sports Medicine Department
Hospital for Special Surgery
New York, New York

Kevin O'Donnell, MD
Department of Orthopedics
ThedaCare
Neenah, Wisconsin

Luke S. Oh, MD, MS
Fellowship Director, Harvard-MGH Sports Medicine Program
Department of Orthopaedic Surgery
Massachusetts General Hospital
Boston, Massachusetts

Brett D. Owens, MD
Professor of Orthopaedic Surgery
Warren Alpert Medical School
Brown University
Providence, Rhode Island

Ronak M. Patel, MD
The American Knee Institute
Hinsdale Orthopaedic Associates
Westmont, Illinois

Paolo Paladini, MD
Shoulder and Elbow Unit
"D. Cervesi" Hospital
Cattolica, Italy

Andrea Pelligrini, MD
Orthopedics and Traumatology Department
Parma University
Parma, Italy

Fabian Plachel, MD
Department of Traumatology and Sports Injuries
Paracelsus Medical University
Salzburg, Austria
Center for Musculoskeletal Surgery
Campus Virchow
Charité-Universitaetsmedizin
Berlin, Germany

Johannes E. Plath, MD
Alps Surgery Institute
Clinique Générale
Annecy, France

Kirsten L. Poehling-Monaghan, MD
Orthopaedic Sports Medicine
Precision Orthopedics and Sports Medicine
Washington, DC/Maryland

Jonas Pogorzelski, MD, MHBA
Department of Sport Orthopedics
Technical University of Munich
Steadman Philippon Research Institute
Vail, Colorado

Giuseppe Porcellini, MD
Chief of Shoulder and Elbow Unit
"D. Cervesi" Hospital
Cattolica, Italy

Matthew T. Provencher, MD, CAPT, MC, USNR
Complex Shoulder Knee and Sports Surgery
The Steadman Clinic
Vail, Colorado

Herbert Resch, MD
Department of Traumatology and Sports Injuries
Paracelus Medical University
Salzburg, Austria

Amy Resler, DPT, CMP, CSCS
Physical Therapy Supervisor
Naval Medical Center
San Diego, California

Dustin L. Richter, MD
Assistant Professor
Orthopaedic Surgery Sports Medicine
University of New Mexico
Albuquerque, New Mexico

Troy A. Roberson, MD
Steadman Hawkins Clinic of the Carolinas
Greenville Health System
Greenville, South Carolina

Anthony A. Romeo, MD
Professor, Department of Orthopaedic Surgery
Section Head, Shoulder and Elbow Surgery
Division of Sport Medicine
Rush University Medical Center
Team Physician, Chicago White Sox
Chicago, Illinois

David L. Rubenstein, MD
Associate Director, Sports Medicine Fellowship
Clinical Orthopedic Surgery Instructor
Thomas Jefferson University
Clinical Adjunct Assistant Professor
Philadelphia University
Philadelphia, Pennsylvania
Head of Sports Medicine
Lankenau Hospital
Wynnewood, Pennsylvania

Jessica Ryu, MD
Department of Orthopaedic Surgery
Stanford University Medical Center
Palo Alto, California

Richard Ryu, MD
The Ryu Hurvitz Orthopedic Clinic
Santa Barbara, California

Anthony Sanchez, BS
Research Assistant
Center for Outcomes-Based Orthopaedic Research
Department of Biomedical Engineering
Steadman Philippon Research Institute
Vail, Colorado

George Sanchez, BS
Research Assistant
Department of Biomedical Engineering
Steadman Philippon Research Institute
Vail, Colorado

Felix H. Savoie III, MD
Ray J. Haddad Professor and Chairman
Department of Orthopaedic Surgery
Tulane University School of Medicine
New Orleans, Louisiana

Katrina Schantz, PA-C
Massachusetts General Hospital
Boston, Massachusetts

Mark Schickendantz, MD
Director, Center for Sports Heath
Orthopaedic Surgery
Cleveland Clinic
Professor of Surgery
Cleveland Clinic Lerner College of Medicine at Case Western Reserve University
Head Team Physician, Cleveland Indians
Cleveland, Ohio

Emilie Schmidt, DPT, SCS, ATC, CSCS
Physical Therapist
United States Marine Corps Special Operations Command
Camp Lejeune, North Carolina

Terrance A. Sgroi, PT, DPT, SCS, MTC
Clinical Supervisor
Sports Rehabilitation and Performance
Hospital for Special Surgery
New York, New York

Seth L. Sherman, MD
Department of Orthopaedic Surgery
University of Missouri
Columbia, Missouri

Nathan Wm. Skelley, MD
Clinical Instructor
Harvard Medical School
Department of Orthopaedic Surgery
Massachusetts General Hospital
Boston, Massachusetts

Jarrod R. Smith, MD
President
Smith Orthopedics & Sports Medicine, PSC
Ashland, Kentucky
The Andrews Institute
Gulf Breeze, Florida

Patrick A. Smith, MD
Director Division of Sports Medicine
Head Team Physician, University of Missouri
Columbia Orthopaedic Group
Columbia, Missouri

Cory Stewart, MD
Department of Orthopaedic Surgery
Massachusetts General Hospital
Boston, Massachusetts

Derek Stokes
School of Medicine
University of Missouri
Columbia, Missouri

Hiroyuki Sugaya, MD
Shoulder and Elbow Service
Funabashi Orthopaedic Sports Medicine & Joint Center
Funabashi, Japan

Gautam Deepak Talawadekar, FRCS, MRCSEd, MS, DNB, MBBS
Consultant Shoulder and Elbow Surgeon
Furness General Hospital
Barrow in Furness, United Kingdom

Ettore Taverna, MD
Chirurgia della Spalla
IRCCS Istituto Ortopedico Galeazzi
Milano, Italy
Chirurgia Arto Superiore
Ospedale Beata Vergine
Mendrisio, Switzerland

Dean C. Taylor, MD
Professor of Orthopaedic Surgery
Duke University
Division of Sports Medicine and Shoulder Surgery
Department of Orthopaedic Surgery
Duke University Medical Center
Durham, North Carolina

Samuel A. Taylor, MD
Assistant Attending Surgeon
Orthopaedic Surgery
Hospital for Special Surgery
New York, New York
Assistant Professor
Orthopaedic Surgery
Weill Cornell Medical College
New York, New York

Jared Thomas, MD
Resident
Department of Orthopaedic Surgery
Univeristy of Michigan
Ann Arbor, Michigan

Robert J. Thorsness, MD
Division of Shoulder and Elbow Surgery
Hinsdale Orthpaedics
Hinsdale, Illinois

Jonathan B. Ticker, MD
Assistant Clinical Professor
Orthopaedic Surgery
College of Physicians & Surgeons of Columbia University
New York, New York
Orlin & Cohen Orthopaedic Group
Merrick, New York

Fotios P. Tjoumakaris, MD
Associate Professor
Orthopaedic Surgery
Sidney Kimmel College of Medicine
Jefferson Medical College
Rothman Institute Orthopaedics
Egg Harbor Township, New Jersey

John M. Tokish, MD
Steadman Hawkins Clinic of the Carolinas
Greenville Health System
Greenville, South Carolina

David P. Trofa, MD
Center for Shoulder, Elbow and Sports Medicine
NYP/Columbia University Medical Center
New York, New York

Jeremy N. Truntzer, MD
Department of Orthopaedic Surgery
Stanford University Medical Center
Palo Alto, California

Nikhil N. Verma, MD
Department of Orthopaedic Surgery
Rush University Medical Center
Chicago, Illinois

Patrick Vignona, MSPT, SCS, MDT
Clinical Specialist
Sports Rehab and Performance
Hospital for Special Surgery
New York, New York

Mandeep S. Virk, MD
Department of Orthopaedic Surgery
Division of Shoulder and Elbow
New York University Langone Medical Center and Hospital for Joint Diseases
New York, New York

Emil Stefan Vutescu, MD
Resident Department of Orthopaedic Surgery
Warren Alpert Medical School
Brown University
Providence, Rhode Island

Jon J.P. Warner, MD
Chief, The MGH Shoulder Service
Massachusetts General Hospital
Professor of Orthopaedic Surgery
Harvard Medical School
Co-Director, Boston Shoulder Institute
Boston, Massachusetts

Russell F. Warren, MD
Professor of Orthopedics
Weill Cornell Medical College
Ithaca, New York
Surgeon-in-Chief Emeritus
Hospital for Special Surgery
New York, New York

Paul E. Westgard, PT, DPT, OCS, SCS, CSCS
Physical Therapist
Howard Head Sports Medicine
Vail Valley Medical Center
Vail, Colorado

Taylor Wiley, MD
Department of Orthopaedic Surgery
University of Connecticut Health Center
Farmington, Connecticut

Kevin E. Wilk, PT, DPT, FAPTA
Associate Clinical Director
Champion Sports Medicine-Physiotherapy Associates
Birmingham, Alabama
Director of Rehabilitative Research
American Sports Medicine Institute
Birmingham, Alabama

Brian R. Wolf, MD, MS
John and Kim Callaghan Chair in Sports Medicine
Professor and Vice-Chairman
Department of Orthopaedics
University of Iowa
Head Team Physician
University of Iowa Athletics
Iowa City, Iowa

B. Israel Yahuaca, MD
Department of Orthopaedic Surgery
University of Missouri
Columbia, Missouri

Nobuyuki Yamamoto, MD, PhD
Assistant professor
Department of Orthopaedic Surgery
Tohoku University School of Medicine
Sendai, Japan

John Zajac, DPT, OCS, SCS, CSCS
Physical Therapist/Assistant Strength Coach
New York Mets Baseball Organization
New York, New York

Alan L. Zhang
Division of Sports Medicine and Shoulder Service
Department of Orthopaedic Surgery
University of California San Francisco Medical Center
San Francisco, California

Connor G. Ziegler, MD
Department of Orthopaedic Surgery
University of Connecticut Health Center
School of Medicine
Farmington, Connecticut

Foreword

There are many new books each year but rarely do we encounter one that is so inclusive and complete on its main theme of shoulder and elbow injuries in the athlete.

This is a book that clinicians will refer to and utilize for years to come.

The editors have brought together their skills and those of a superb array of researchers who are experts in their chosen areas. The depth of information provided is extraordinary and well presented. They have tackled different topics, such as bone loss and instability, providing information that allows a sound scientific approach. They have included many international contributors who have considerable experience in dealing with relatively uncommon issues.

The clinician who desires to be at the head of his or her class will benefit greatly from this book, which compiles in one place the information developed over decades of sports injuries. This book covers in detail shoulder instability, cuff tears, AC and SC joint injuries, and injuries of the elbow. It provides an understanding of the role for arthroscopic versus open procedures and AC joint stabilization as a combined approach. In treating athletes' injuries of the shoulder and elbow these past 40-odd years, I find the authors of this book have provided answers to a multitude of questions on management from both the nonoperative and the operative perspective.

The section on elbow issues is excellent in dealing with instability and ligament and tendon injuries as well as stress fractures and OCD lesions.

Throwing injuries of the shoulder are well addressed from a preventive point of view in addition to treatment programs.

Overall this edition will be a lasting book that we will all refer to and rely on for our different patient care issues. The editors have done all of us clinicians a great favor by bringing together a superb group of writers that have contributed so much to our understanding of these problems.

Russell F. Warren, MD

Preface

Shoulder and Elbow Injuries in Athletes is tailored to a multidisciplinary audience, including physician assistants, physical therapists, athletic trainers, physicians, residents, and fellows, and has been devised as a complete guide for the treatment of prevalent injuries of the shoulder and elbow in athletes of all ages and levels. From diagnosis to treatment to postoperative rehabilitation, this book provides a broad yet in-depth overview of how to get an athlete back to his or her sport following a shoulder or elbow injury. With contributions from internationally renowned experts, the latest treatments for shoulder and elbow injuries in athletes, including surgical techniques, are described in great detail to offer a comprehensive resource for any health professional.

This book is purposely designed to provide great detail not only in surgical technique and overall treatment but also on how the latest advancements in the field are relevant in the context of a highly active patient who regularly participates in sports. Their demand for a faster, more efficient return to sport makes highly active patients particularly difficult to treat. However, this comprehensive guide provides a resource that all health professionals can confidently use to maximize the probability of a safe and positive return to sport for their patients.

Made up of a total of eleven sections with thirty-three chapters, *Shoulder and Elbow Injuries in Athletes* successfully maintains its focus on operative treatment while also discussing preoperative and postoperative care. Through the use of many illustrations as well as listings of pearls and pitfalls, each surgical technique is presented in full with tips from experts in the field. In addition to surgical technique, experts contribute to and provide information on the latest methods of diagnosis and postoperative rehabilitation for each of the described conditions. Ultimately, treatment is given not just in the operating room but also in the clinic and the physical therapist's office. Therefore, as part of the summary of each condition, indications confirming treatment, preoperative physical examination, and postoperative management are all detailed. One of the notable features of this book is the excellent illustrations, step-by-step surgical descriptions, and accompanying videos.

We are tremendously indebted to the contributions of our authors, as this resource would not have been possible without their expertise. We believe this book given its extensive and wide-ranging scope across a variety of shoulder and elbow conditions, will be an invaluable asset to any health professional's toolbox. We hope health professionals who specialize in all points of care, regardless of their experience, use this resource to help them provide as effective care as possible to their highly active patients with shoulder and elbow injuries.

Robert A. Arciero
Frank A. Cordasco
Matthew T. Provencher

Contents

Video Table of Contents

PART 1

SHOULDER

PART OUTLINE

SECTION **I**

Shoulder Instability, Rehabilitation, and Return to Sport

SECTION OUTLINE

1 Anterior Shoulder Instability

1-1A EPIDEMIOLOGY, MECHANISM OF INJURY, HISTORY, PHYSICAL EXAMINATION, AND IMAGING FOR ANTERIOR INSTABILITY

LCDR JAMES R. BAILEY, MD, BARRETT A. LITTLE, MD, KEVIN M. DALE, MD, and DEAN C. TAYLOR, MD

Disclosures

The views expressed in this article are those of the author(s) and do not necessarily reflect the official policy or position of the Department of the Navy, Department of Defense, or the United States Government. Dr. Bailey is a military service member. This work was prepared as part of his official duties. Title 17, USC, §105 provides that 'Copyright protection under this title is not available for any work of the U.S. Government.' Title 17, USC, §101 defines a U.S. Government work as a work prepared by a military service member or employee of the U.S. Government as part of that person's official duties.

Imaging Introduction

- Anterior shoulder instability is most common in young active males.
- The position of the arm during a first-time dislocation is likely variable.
- The history should include the patient age, activity level, mechanism of injury, number of dislocations or subluxations, and symptoms. The history is the most important information to diagnose this condition and will guide treatment.
- Instability is a clinical diagnosis consisting of the symptom complex of pain, apprehension, the actual sensation or history of instability events, and reduced performance level.
- It is important to evaluate for multidirectional laxity and to recognize multidirectional instability to maximize treatment. It should be recognized that hyperlax patients and those with multidirectional laxity can sustain an injury and develop unidirectional instability.
- Physical examination should always start with the cervical spine and then move to the shoulder girdle. A systematic examination will ensure precise diagnoses.
- Although much can be assessed with the appropriate plain radiographs of the shoulder, advanced imaging to evaluate for glenoid and humeral head bone defects may be required to fully define the pathoanatomy contributing to the instability.

Epidemiology

The diverse spectrum of presentation contributes to the complexity of glenohumeral instability and leads to difficulties in diagnosis and management. It is important to distinguish between instability and laxity of the shoulder. Instability is characterized by the presence of symptoms in conjunction with abnormal laxity (Gaskill et al, 2011). Failure of static and dynamic glenohumeral stabilizers leads to instability, which can be unidirectional or multidirectional with the most common pattern being anterior unidirectional instability. Anterior unidirectional instability can be the result of repetitive microtrauma or a single macrotrauma as in an acute anterior shoulder dislocation.

The incidence of shoulder dislocations in the United States is 23.9 per 100,000 person-years with the overwhelming majority (89%–98%) being anterior shoulder dislocations (Zacchilli & Owens, 2010). This is consistent with data obtained by Nordqvist and Petersson (1995) on traumatic shoulder dislocations in Sweden. Put in perspective among other common orthopedic conditions presenting to emergency departments (EDs) in the United States, the incidence of shoulder dislocation is far less common than distal radius fractures, 62 per 100,000 person-years, and ankle sprains, 215 per 100,000 person-years (Zacchilli & Owens, 2010). However, the true incidence of anterior shoulder instability may be higher because of shoulders that spontaneously reduce and may never present to an ED. In a military epidemiologic study reviewing all U.S. Military Academy cadets who sustained a shoulder injury during one academic year, 85% of their instability events were subluxation with spontaneous reduction vs 15% dislocation (Owens et al, 2007).

Age is an important factor in shoulder instability because the mechanism of injury, pathoanatomy, and recurrence rate differ among age groups. Almost half of dislocations occur in individuals between the ages of 15 and 29 years (Zacchilli & Owens, 2010). Described by Bankart as the "essential lesion" of shoulder instability, the vast majority of this young population who sustain an anterior shoulder dislocation will have associated anterior capsulolabral tears (Arciero et al, 1994; Baker et al, 1990; Bankart, 1923; Norlin, 1993; Taylor & Arciero, 1997). Young age at the time of initial injury is the most consistent and significant factor for risk of recurrence.

The rate of recurrent instability ranges from 48% to 96% in this age group (McLaughlin & MacLellan, 1967; Rowe, 1956). Approximately 20% of all shoulder dislocations occur in individuals older than 60 years of age (Gumina & Postacchini, 1997). In those older than the age of 40 years, 35% to 86% will have an associated rotator cuff tear (Hawkins et al, 1986; Stayner et al, 2000). This age group has a much lower recurrence rate than younger individuals, with rates as low as 4% (Pevny et al, 1998).

Gender and activity level are two other epidemiologic conditions that influence the incidence of anterior shoulder instability. Overall, males account for more than 70% of dislocations and are 2.5 times more likely than females to sustain a shoulder dislocation (Zacchilli & Owens, 2010). In collegiate athletes at one institution, the highest incidence of shoulder instability occurred in football players and wrestlers (Owens et al, 2009). The majority of anterior shoulder instability occurs in active males, especially those who participate in contact sports.

Mechanism of Injury

The mechanism of injury in traumatic anterior shoulder instability can be repetitive microtrauma or, more commonly, a discrete traumatic event, leading to recurrent instability. In traumatic anterior unidirectional instability, the widely accepted position of the shoulder during a dislocation is abduction, extension, and external rotation (ER). This position is the point at which the anterior band of the inferior glenohumeral ligament (IGHL) is under maximum tension and is the primary restraint to anterior humeral translation (Blasier et al, 1992; O'Brien et al, 1995; Warner et al, 1992). The classic Bankart lesion is an avulsion of the IGHL complex from the anteroinferior glenoid, which likely occurs in this position when the humeral head is levered out of the glenoid. Tanaka et al (2012) evaluated the arm position of anterior shoulder dislocations under anesthesia in patients with recurrent dislocations and concluded that at 90 degrees of forward elevation in the scapular plane, anterior translation was maximal at 26 degrees of ER. Only one shoulder showed anterior translation at maximal ER. This study suggests that the position during initial injury is likely variable. Another factor that supports varying positions during subluxation or dislocation is anterior instability in boxers occurring when missing a punch as described by Owens et al (2007). The unexpected unopposed anterior momentum of the upper extremity leads to anterior subluxation or dislocation. Owens et al also reported the most common mechanisms of injury in the same population of students at the United States Military Academy to be falls (15%) and collisions (14.5%). The mechanism of complete anterior shoulder dislocation is most commonly a discrete traumatic event, but the position of the arm during injury may vary. A recent study by Di Giacomo et al (2016) used three-dimensional (3D) computed tomography (CT) scans to evaluate the position of Hill-Sachs lesions produced from dislocations of the shoulder in various degrees of abduction. They found that dislocations with the shoulder in a position of abduction greater than 60 degrees resulted in higher Hill-Sachs angles, or an angle more parallel to the anterior glenoid in a position of abduction, ER, placing the shoulder at a higher risk of engagement and recurrent dislocation. Shoulders that dislocated at lower abduction angles resulted in lower Hill-Sachs angles with less chance of engagement.

History

For anterior shoulder instability, the history is important for diagnosis and guiding treatment of the patient. Patient demographics are often the first part of the history that the clinician will obtain. The mechanism of injury should be investigated as to whether it was a traumatic injury or a spontaneous event. Symptoms at the time of injury should also be explored. Finally, history of instability of other joints or connective tissue diseases in the patient or family members should not be overlooked.

Patient age is often the first demographic information obtained upon meeting the patient. Whether the injured upper extremity is the patient's dominant arm is important. The history should not overlook if the patient sustained any other injuries at the time of the injury. If the anterior shoulder instability occurred during a sporting event, the patient's preferred sport, the time of the season, and the patient's goals for return to that sport or another sport should be investigated.

It is important to understand the mode of onset in evaluating a patient with shoulder instability. There are several key questions to ascertain:

1. Was there a specific single traumatic event that led to the recurrent instability?
2. Was it trivial? If so, this should make the examiner concerned that hyperlaxity is more the issue.
3. Was a radiograph taken showing the shoulder dislocated?
4. How long did it take for the patient to recover from the initial event? A complete traumatic dislocation will result in anteroinfero-capsulabral disruption and possible glenoid and humeral head injury and take several weeks to recover as opposed to a patient with multidirectional instability who can recover quickly.
5. What was the arm position at the time of dislocation? In the presence of a Hill-Sachs lesion, this may be able to predict on-track versus off-track lesions (Di Giacomo et al, 2016).
6. What is the arm position that the patient fears will reproduce symptoms (e.g., Abduction/External Rotation (ABD/ER); Adduction/Internal Rotation (ADD/IR))?
7. Does the patient have instability during sleep?
8. Does the patient require reduction for the recurrent instability events, or do they reduce spontaneously?
9. Has it become easier to provoke an instability episode? This can signify significant capsulolabral degeneration and bone loss.

Symptoms at the time of injury will help distinguish between an initial anterior instability event, recurrent anterior instability, and nonshoulder issues. Patients with a first-time anterior shoulder dislocation typically have severe shoulder pain until the humeral head is reduced into the glenoid. Also, they are unable to continue with the current sport or activity at the time of the injury. Patients with recurrent anterior instability will usually have less pain and may be able to reduce the dislocation themselves. It is possible for high-functioning athletes with recurrent anterior instability to return to sporting events after a recurrent instability event (Buss et al, 2004; Dickens et al, 2014). If neurologic symptoms of paresthesia or weakness after the shoulder has been reduced persist, then a workup of a neurologic injury is indicated. If a patient complains of swelling or symptoms provoked by temperature changes, then a vascular workup of the extremity is required.

For patients with recurrent anterior instability, it should be determined how the instability is affecting their activities of daily living along with their ability to compete athletically. Patients who continue with contact sports after an initial traumatic anterior instability event can go on to develop recurrent anterior instability after multiple dislocations and subluxations. On the other hand, patients should be evaluated for a family history of anterior instability or instability in multiple joints to determine connective tissue disorders (e.g., Ehlers-Danlos and Marfan syndromes). Patients with ligamentous laxity should not be ignored because they may develop acute anterior shoulder instability along with multidirectional laxity (Gerber & Nyffeler, 2002).

Physical Evaluation

A good history is instrumental in determining the diagnosis, and a well-performed physical examination will confirm the diagnosis and identify other conditions of the shoulder and the neck. Although most shoulder examination findings are imperfect in regards to sensitivity and specificity (Farber et al, 2006), a combination of thorough history, physical, and imaging findings will exponentially improve diagnostic accuracy. Because many shoulder examination findings lack absolute specificity, we prefer a systematic approach that involves observation, palpation, range of motion, strength testing, neurovascular examination, and provocative tests specific for the acromioclavicular joint, biceps, superior labrum, rotator cuff, and anterior, posterior, and inferior instability. Other tests can be included specific to the patient's symptoms (e.g., suprascapular nerve compression, thoracic outlet syndrome). It is important to always start with the cervical spine and then move on to the shoulder girdle because radiculopathy can often manifest as shoulder pain.

Multiple tests for anteroinferior shoulder instability have been described in the literature. Various described tests work imperfectly on different patient populations (multidirectional laxity vs traumatic unidirectional, thin female gymnast vs large football linebacker, acute vs chronic), so it is important to have several provocative tests specific for shoulder instability. It is also important to remember that in the acute setting; it is usually not possible to perform all these portions of a complete physical examination. In these cases, the practitioner will have to rely on a good history and imaging to make the diagnosis. A good examination still allows one to rule out other conditions because it is always possible to have multiple conditions at once in the shoulder. Instability can be associated with SLAP (superior labrum anterior and posterior) tears, axillary nerve injuries, multidirectional laxity with unidirectional instability, and scapular dyskinesia.

Specific tests to elicit anteroinferior shoulder instability (also see Video 1A.1) include the following.

Anterior load-and-shift testing (Silliman & Hawkins, 1993): This tests passive translation of the humeral head on the glenoid. The test can be performed with the patient standing, seated, or supine. The authors recommend having the patient in a supine position with the scapula stabilized by the examination table and the injured shoulder just coming off the bed. The arm is flexed in the plane of the scapula, the elbow is bent at 90 degrees, and various degrees of abduction should be tested (0, 45, and 90 degrees). One of the examiner's hands should be used to hold the elbow and apply a compressive load through the center of the humeral head into the glenoid as well as a posterior counterforce while the other hand is used to apply anterior (or posterior for posterior load-and-shift testing) force (Fig. 1A.1). Another variation of this maneuver is to have the patient lie on the examination table in the lateral position with the noninjured shoulder down. You can then kneel on the bed with your leg and thigh stabilizing the scapula and both hands free to manipulate the shoulder. The degree of translation should be graded on a 3-point scale. Grade 1 translation up to, but not over, the glenoid rim. Grade 2 anterior load and shift indicates that the humeral head can translate over the glenoid rim but reduces spontaneously. Grade 3 is when the humeral head translates over the glenoid rim and does not spontaneously reduce. The authors recommend against the use of "+" or "–" when using this grading scheme. Again, a differentiation between laxity and instability should be made at this point and depends on pain (Gaskill et al, 2011). As with all maneuvers, the other side should be examined to determine if this is a unilateral finding. It is important to note that the reproduction of symptoms is the most important part of load-and-shift testing in clinic. In the operating room under anesthesia, the amount of translation is most pertinent.

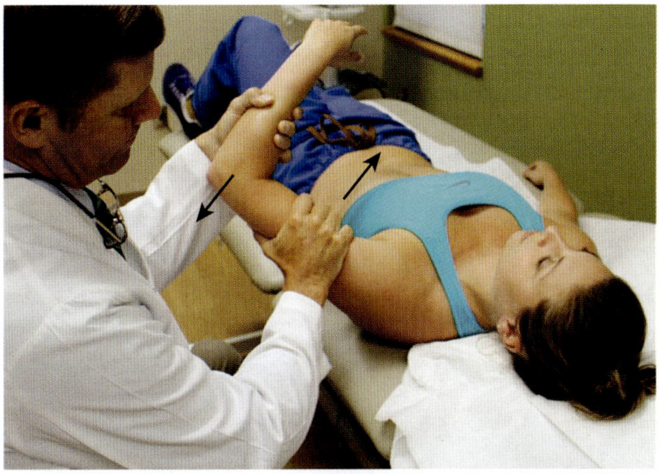

Fig. 1A.1 Anterior load-and-shift testing. The arm is flexed in the plane of the scapula, the elbow is bent at 90 degrees, and various degrees of abduction are tested (0, 45, and 90 degrees). One of the examiner's hands should be used to hold the elbow and apply a compressive load through the center of the humeral head into the glenoid as well as a posterior counterforce while the other hand is used to apply an anterior force.

Inferior sulcus sign testing: The inferior sulcus sign test should be performed with the patient in a seated position and relaxed with the arms at the side in neutral rotation. After ensuring that the patient is not guarding, a downward traction force is applied to the distal humerus or through a bent elbow while watching the lateral edge of the acromion (Fig. 1A.2). The amount of inferior sulcus is measured in centimeters from the inferior border of the acromion to the humeral head. Grade 1 is equivalent to 1cm; grade 2, 2 cm; and grade 3, 3 cm. Some believe that if this sulcus persists when performed in maximal ER that it is an indication of rotator interval and superior glenohumeral ligament incompetence; however, it has been our experience that most shoulders' sulcus signs persist in ER. Also, it is critical to note if symptoms are reproduced by the maneuver. Patients with multidirectional instability, whose hallmark feature is inferior patholaxity, often complain of pain

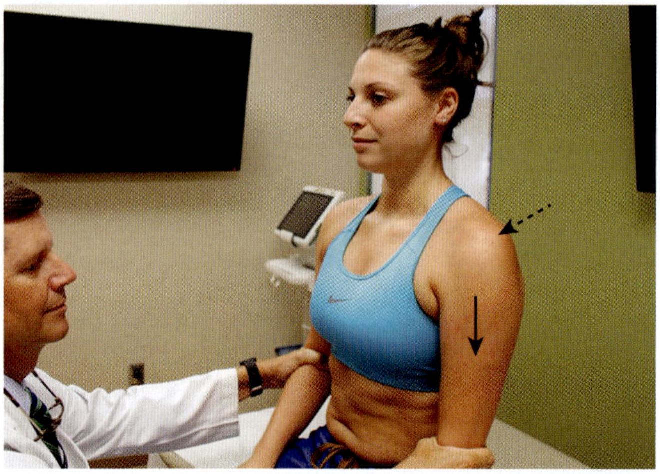

Fig. 1A.2 Inferior sulcus sign test. This test should be performed with the patient in seated position and relaxed with arms at the side in neutral rotation. A downward traction force is applied to the distal humerus or through a bent elbow *(solid arrow)* while watching the lateral edge of the acromion and looking for a dimple or sulcus formed between the humeral head and acromion *(dotted arrow)*.

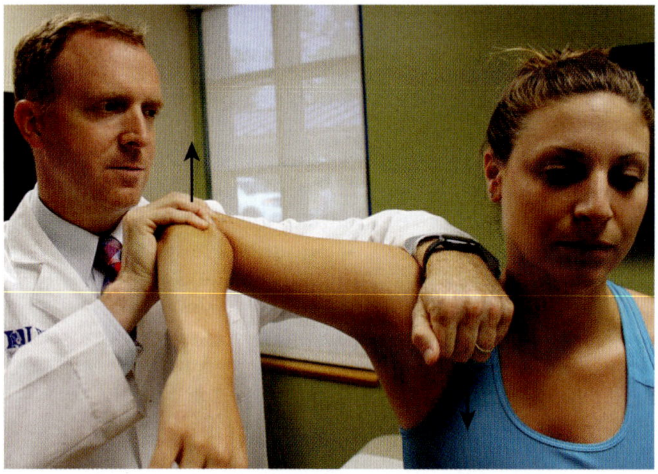

Fig. 1A.3 The Gagey hyperabduction test. This test is performed with the patient sitting comfortably with the arm in neutral rotation and at the side. The examiner stands behind the patient and with one hand stabilizes the upper shoulder while the other hand raises the elbow in pure abduction. The degree of abduction is measured.

and instability when there is an inferior directed load to the arm (carrying heavy objects at the side, for example)

The Gagey hyperabduction test: First described by Gagey and Gagey (2001), this test is used to assess the integrity of the inferior glenohumeral ligament. This test is performed with the patient sitting comfortably with the arm in neutral rotation and at the side. The examiner stands behind the patient and with one hand stabilizes the upper shoulder while the other hand raises the elbow in pure abduction (Fig. 1A.3). In their study, 85% of anesthetized patients with shoulder instability had passive abduction greater than 105 degrees.

The John Feagin test: First described in book chapter in 1984 (Rockwood, 1984), this maneuver has been often attributed to Dr. Feagin and can be particularly helpful when examining large, muscular patients. It is accomplished by placing the arm in internal rotation (IR) with

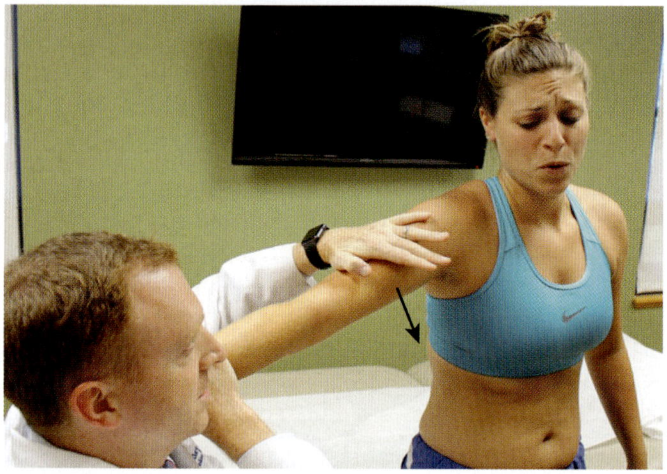

Fig. 1A.4 The John Feagin test. The maneuver is accomplished by placing the arm in internal rotation (IR) with the elbow fully extended on the examiner's shoulder. After the patient is appropriately calm and relaxed, one of the examiner's hands holds the patient's elbow in full extension while the other translates the humeral head anteroinferiorly on the glenoid. The amount of translation is measured, and it should be noted if this replicated the patient's symptoms.

elbow fully extended on examiner's shoulder. After the patient is appropriately calm and relaxed, one of the examiner's hands can hold the elbow in full extension while the other can translate the humeral head anteroinferiorly on the glenoid (Fig. 1A.4). This assesses the amount of anteroinferior translation of the humeral head on the glenoid and can be graded using the same grading scale as anterior load and shift. It should also be noted if this maneuver replicates the patient's symptoms. Similarly, inferior laxity can be tested with the abduction inferior stability (ABIS) test described by Itoi et al (1992, 1993), which places the patient in the same position while the examiner provides an inferior-only directed force. They describe this test as a way to study the effect of scapular inclination on inferior glenohumeral stability.

Apprehension test with or without Jobe's relocation: This test is best performed with the patient in a supine position of the edge of the bed with the scapula supported and the shoulder just off the table (Rowe, 1988). The arm should be at 90 degrees of abduction and ER with the elbow flexed to 90 degrees (throwing position). The humerus is held by the examiner with one hand while the other hand gently externally rotates the shoulder through the arm. Having apprehension, or the "feeling" that the shoulder is going to subluxate or dislocate, is a positive finding (Fig. 1A.5, *A*). Applying an anterior force to the humerus can augment the apprehension test. Positive findings in midrange apprehension (in a lower degree of abduction and ER) is a concerning sign for possible bone loss. The Jobe relocation test (Jobe et al, 1989) is then performed in the same position. Instead of an anteriorly directed force, a posteriorly directed force is applied to the humerus. If the patient is having a sense of instability, this posteriorly directed force should make the shoulder feel stable again and resolve any related pain (Fig. 1A.5, *B*). Resolution of pain and apprehension is a positive finding.

Finally, if treatment requires surgical intervention, it is important to always perform an examination under

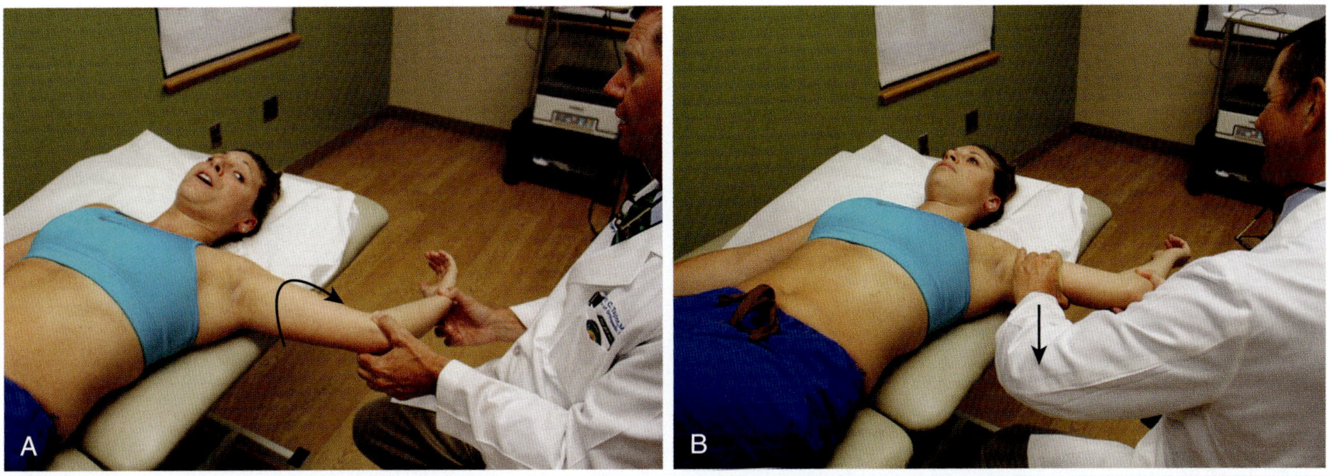

Fig. 1A.5 A, The apprehension test. This test is best performed with the patient in a supine position of the edge of the bed with the scapula supported and the shoulder just off the table. The arm should be at 90 degrees of abduction and external rotation with the elbow flexed to 90 degrees (throwing position). The humerus is held by the examiner with one hand while the other hand gently externally rotates the shoulder through the arm. Pain or apprehension that the shoulder is going to subluxate or dislocate is a positive finding. Applying an anterior force to the humerus can augment the apprehension test. **B,** The Jobe relocation test. This is performed after the apprehension test. A posteriorly directed force is applied to the humerus to simulate reduction of the joint. If the patient is having a sense of instability with the apprehension test, this posteriorly directed force should make the shoulder feel stable and resolve any related pain.

anesthesia after the patient is appropriately anesthetized. This should be performed on both arms and include forward flexion, abduction, abduction-ER, abduction-IR, anterior and posterior load shift testing, and inferior sulcus testing. The amount of translation should be noted. After surgical stabilization, this can be rechecked gently to assess for resolution of laxity.

Imaging

Plain radiographs should be obtained, at the time of injury and after reduction, to ensure the humeral head is actually reduced on the glenoid and to rule out any other bony abnormalities. The authors' normal shoulder series includes anteroposterior (AP), Grashey (true AP), Stryker notch view, and axillary or West Point modified axillary view. The Stryker notch view specifically helps to identify Hill-Sachs lesions, and the axillary views ensure the humeral head is reduced in the glenoid. The West Point view was developed to highlight the area of the anteroinferior glenoid, compared with the anterior glenoid highlighted in the axillary view. One can appreciate avulsion fractures, calcification, and anterior bone loss in the chronic setting. In a cadaveric study by Itoi et al (2003), good correlation of anteroinferior bone loss was noted between the West Point view and CT scans. If a large Hill-Sachs lesion is noted on plain radiographs, one should consider advanced imaging as larger Hill-Sachs lesions combined with glenoid bone loss can be a reason for recurrent instability after stabilization (Arciero et al, 2015). Indications for advanced imaging include revision, instability in sleep, seizure, midrange apprehension in physical examination, frequent instability events requiring manual reduction, and concerns for associated injuries. These indications are discussed further later.

Magnetic resonance imaging (MRI) is the standard for radiographic evaluation of the labrum and other soft tissue structures. An MR arthrogram can be helpful in visualizing the extent of labral tears, SLAP tears, and other possible soft tissue injuries such as a humeral avulsion of the glenohumeral ligament (HAGL) and anterior labroligamentous periosteal sleeve avulsion (ALPSA), which have both been associated with recurrent instability if not addressed (Bernhardson et al, 2014; Forsythe et al, 2015). ALPSA lesions are variants of the anteroinferior Bankart lesion where the labrum is displaced medially on the scapular neck. These should warn the surgeon to closely examine the amount of bone loss because they are associated with almost double the amount of bone loss compared with standard Bankart lesions (Bernhardson et al, 2014). It is important to note that there is some controversy on whether an MR arthrogram is needed for diagnosis of these lesions. In the acute setting, blood from the hemarthrosis is usually enough of a contrast medium to differentiate structures. It is the authors' preference to obtain an MR arthrogram when possible. However, if advanced imaging is unavailable, a study in West Point cadets found a 97% incidence of complete anterior capsuloligamentous detachment in patients with a first-time anterior shoulder dislocation requiring manual reduction by a health care professional (Taylor & Arciero, 1997). The capsuloligamentous lesions were observed during arthroscopic examination of these shoulders. Owens et al (2007) echoed these numbers with 93% of their patients who sustained an anterior shoulder dislocation had evidence on MRI of a soft tissue or bony Bankart lesion. More recently, his group looked at 27 military members who sustained a first-time, traumatic, anterior subluxation and found a 96% rate of Bankart lesions on MRI (Owens et al, 2010).

Computed tomography is a very helpful addition to preoperative workup, particularly in the setting of suspected bone loss, which is a known risk factor for recurrent instability (Boileau et al, 2006; Burkhart & De Beer, 2000; Forsythe et al, 2015; Lynch et al, 2009; Mologne et al, 2007; Rowe et al, 1984; Tauber et al, 2004). 3D

CT reconstructions are often very helpful in visualizing the extent of bone deficiency. Axial scans in the plane of the glenoid and three-dimensional rendered images help define the extent and orientation of glenoid bone loss as well as any concomitant humeral head bone loss or Hill-Sachs lesions (Chuang et al, 2008; Kodali et al, 2011; Kralinger et al, 2002; Lo et al, 2004; Provencher et al, 2010; Sugaya et al, 2003).

References

Arciero RA, Parrino A, Bernhardson AS, et al. The effect of a combined glenoid and Hill-Sachs defect on glenohumeral stability: a biomechanical cadaveric study using 3-dimensional modeling of 142 patients. *Am J Sports Med*. 2015;43(6):1422–1429.

Arciero RA, Wheeler JH, Ryan JB, McBride JT. Arthroscopic Bankart repair versus nonoperative treatment for acute, initial anterior shoulder dislocations. *Am J Sports Med*. 1994;22(5):589–594.

Baker CL, Uribe JW, Whitman C. Arthroscopic evaluation of acute initial anterior shoulder dislocations. *Am J Sports Med*. 1990;18(1):25–28.

Bankart AS. Recurrent or habitual dislocation of the shoulder-joint. *Br Med J*. 1923;2(3285):1132–1133.

Bernhardson AS, Bailey JR, Solomon DJ, Stanley M, Provencher MT. Glenoid bone loss in the setting of an anterior labroligamentous periosteal sleeve avulsion tear. *Am J Sports Med*. 2014;42(9):2136–2140.

Blasier RB, Guldberg RE, Rothman ED. Anterior shoulder stability: contributions of rotator cuff forces and the capsular ligaments in a cadaver model. *J Shoulder Elbow Surg*. 1992;1(3):140–150.

Boileau P, Villalba M, Hery JY, Balg F, Ahrens P, Neyton L. Risk factors for recurrence of shoulder instability after arthroscopic Bankart repair. *J Bone Joint Surg Am*. 2006;88(8):1755–1763.

Burkhart SS, De Beer JF. Traumatic glenohumeral bone defects and their relationship to failure of arthroscopic Bankart repairs: significance of the inverted-pear glenoid and the humeral engaging Hill-Sachs lesion. *Arthroscopy*. 2000;16(7):677–694.

Buss DD, Lynch GP, Meyer CP, Huber SM, Freehill MQ. Nonoperative management for in-season athletes with anterior shoulder instability. *Am J Sports Med*. 2004;32(6):1430–1433.

Chuang TY, Adams CR, Burkhart SS. Use of preoperative three-dimensional computed tomography to quantify glenoid bone loss in shoulder instability. *Arthroscopy*. 2008;24(4):376–382.

Di Giacomo G, Golijanin P, Sanchez G, Provencher MT. Radiographic analysis of the Hill-Sachs lesion in anteroinferior shoulder instability after first-time dislocations. *Arthroscopy*. 2016;32(8):1509–1514.

Dickens JF, Owens BD, Cameron KL, et al. Return to play and recurrent instability after in-season anterior shoulder instability: a prospective multicenter study. *Am J Sports Med*. 2014;42(12):2842–2850.

Farber AJ, Castillo R, Clough M, Bahk M, McFarland EG. Clinical assessment of three common tests for traumatic anterior shoulder instability. *J Bone Joint Surg Am*. 2006;88(7):1467–1474.

Forsythe B, Frank RM, Ahmed M, et al. Identification and treatment of existing copathology in anterior shoulder instability repair. *Arthroscopy*. 2015;31(1):154–166.

Gagey OJ, Gagey N. The hyperabduction test. *J Bone Joint Surg Br*. 2001;83(1):69–74.

Gaskill TR, Taylor DC, Millett PJ. Management of multidirectional instability of the shoulder. *J Am Acad Orthop Surg*. 2011;19(12):758–767.

Gerber C, Nyffeler RW. Classification of glenohumeral joint instability. *Clin Orthop Relat Res*. 2002;400:65–76.

Gumina S, Postacchini F. Anterior dislocation of the shoulder in elderly patients. *J Bone Joint Surg Br*. 1997;79(4):540–543.

Hawkins RJ, Bell RH, Hawkins RH, Koppert GJ. Anterior dislocation of the shoulder in the older patient. *Clin Orthop Relat Res*. 1986;206:192–195.

Itoi E, Lee SB, Amrami KK, Wenger DE, An KN. Quantitative assessment of classic anteroinferior bony Bankart lesions by radiography and computed tomography. *Am J Sports Med*. 2003;31(1):112–118.

Itoi E, Motzkin NE, Morrey BF, An KN. Scapular inclination and inferior stability of the shoulder. *J Shoulder Elbow Surg*. 1992;1(3):131–139.

Itoi E, Motzkin NE, Morrey BF, An KN. Bulk effect of rotator cuff on inferior glenohumeral stability as function of scapular inclination angle: a cadaver study. *Tohoku J Exp Med*. 1993;171(4):267–276.

Jobe FW, Kvitne RS, Giangarra CE. Shoulder pain in the overhand or throwing athlete. The relationship of anterior instability and rotator cuff impingement. *Orthop Rev*. 1989;18(9):963–975.

Kodali P, Jones MH, Polster J, Miniaci A, Fening SD. Accuracy of measurement of Hill-Sachs lesions with computed tomography. *J Shoulder Elbow Surg*. 2011;20(8):1328–1334.

Kralinger FS, Golser K, Wischatta R, Wambacher M, Sperner G. Predicting recurrence after primary anterior shoulder dislocation. *Am J Sports Med*. 2002;30(1):116–120.

Lo IK, Parten PM, Burkhart SS. The inverted pear glenoid: an indicator of significant glenoid bone loss. *Arthroscopy*. 2004;20(2):169–174.

Lynch JR, Clinton JM, Dewing CB, Warme WJ, Matsen FA 3rd. Treatment of osseous defects associated with anterior shoulder instability. *J Shoulder Elbow Surg*. 2009;18(2):317–328.

McLaughlin HL, MacLellan DI. Recurrent anterior dislocation of the shoulder. II. a comparative study. *J Trauma*. 1967;7(2):191–201.

Mologne TS, Provencher MT, Menzel KA, Vachon TA, Dewing CB. Arthroscopic stabilization in patients with an inverted pear glenoid: results in patients with bone loss of the anterior glenoid. *Am J Sports Med*. 2007;35(8):1276–1283.

Nordqvist A, Petersson CJ. Incidence and causes of shoulder girdle injuries in an urban population. *J Shoulder Elbow Surg*. 1995;4(2):107–112.

Norlin R. Intraarticular pathology in acute, first-time anterior shoulder dislocation: an arthroscopic study. *Arthroscopy*. 1993;9(5):546–549.

O'Brien SJ, Schwartz RS, Warren RF, Torzilli PA. Capsular restraints to anterior-posterior motion of the abducted shoulder: a biomechanical study. *J Shoulder Elbow Surg*. 1995;4(4):298–308.

Owens BD, Agel J, Mountcastle SB, Cameron KL, Nelson BJ. Incidence of glenohumeral instability in collegiate athletics. *Am J Sports Med*. 2009;37(9):1750–1754.

Owens BD, Duffey ML, Nelson BJ, DeBerardino TM, Taylor DC, Mountcastle SB. The incidence and characteristics of shoulder instability at the United States Military Academy. *Am J Sports Med*. 2007;35(7):1168–1173.

Pevny T, Hunter RE, Freeman JR. Primary traumatic anterior shoulder dislocation in patients 40 years of age and older. *Arthroscopy*. 1998;14(3):289–294.

Provencher MT, Bhatia S, Ghodadra NS, et al. Recurrent shoulder instability: current concepts for evaluation and management of glenoid bone loss. *J Bone Joint Surg Am*. 2010;92(suppl 2):133–151.

Rockwood C. Subluxations and dislocations about the shoulder. In: Rockwood CA Jr, Green DP, eds. *Fractures in Adults*. Philadelphia: Lippincott; 1984.

Rowe CR. Prognosis in dislocations of the shoulder. *J Bone Joint Surg Am*. 1956;38-A(5):957–977.

Rowe CR. Recurrent anterior transient subluxation of the shoulder. The "dead arm" syndrome. *Orthop Clin North Am*. 1988;19(4):767–772.

Rowe CR, Zarins B, Ciullo JV. Recurrent anterior dislocation of the shoulder after surgical repair. Apparent causes of failure and treatment. *J Bone Joint Surg Am*. 1984;66(2):159–168.

Silliman JF, Hawkins RJ. Classification and physical diagnosis of instability of the shoulder. *Clin Orthop Relat Res*. 1993;291:7–19.

Stayner LR, Cummings J, Andersen J, Jobe CM. Shoulder dislocations in patients older than 40 years of age. *Orthop Clin North Am*. 2000;31(2):231–239.

Sugaya H, Moriishi J, Dohi M, Kon Y, Tsuchiya A. Glenoid rim morphology in recurrent anterior glenohumeral instability. *J Bone Joint Surg Am*. 2003;85-A(5):878–884.

Tanaka M, Koizumi K, Kakiuchi M, Hayashida K. Evaluation of dislocation position in patients with recurrent anterior shoulder dislocation. *J Shoulder Elbow Surg*. 2012;21(11):1588–1592.

Tauber M, Resch H, Forstner R, Raffl M, Schauer J. Reasons for failure after surgical repair of anterior shoulder instability. *J Shoulder Elbow Surg*. 2004;13(3):279–285.

Taylor DC, Arciero RA. Pathologic changes associated with shoulder dislocations. Arthroscopic and physical examination findings in first-time, traumatic anterior dislocations. *Am J Sports Med*. 1997;25(3):306–311.

Warner JJ, Deng XH, Warren RF, Torzilli PA. Static capsuloligamentous restraints to superior-inferior translation of the glenohumeral joint. *Am J Sports Med*. 1992;20(6):675–685.

Zacchilli MA, Owens BD. Epidemiology of shoulder dislocations presenting to emergency departments in the United States. *J Bone Joint Surg Am*. 2010;92(3):542–549.

1-1B LATERAL DECUBITUS OR BEACH-CHAIR POSITIONING

MATTHEW T. PROVENCHER, MD, EMIL STEFAN VUTESCU, MD, and
GEORGE SANCHEZ, BS

Introduction

- Traumatic anterior shoulder dislocation may result in recurrent instability, ultimately leading to extensive soft tissue lesions, bone loss, and development of osteoarthritis (Hovelius & Saeboe, 2009).
- Several factors determine the outcome of an arthroscopic shoulder instability repair; one of the key factors is proper preoperative patient positioning.
- For a successful treatment outcome, a thorough understanding of the features of and differences between the beach-chair and lateral decubitus setup is essential.
- This chapter provides a comprehensive overview of both possible setups followed by a detailed description of the Bankart repair with key pearls when completed in the lateral decubitus position.

Lateral Decubitus versus Beach-Chair Position

Arthroscopic anterior shoulder stabilization can be performed in either the lateral decubitus or beach-chair position. Each option has several advantages and drawbacks.

LATERAL DECUBITUS POSITION

The lateral decubitus setup is preferred by many surgeons for its superior visualization potential, especially of the inferior aspect of the glenohumeral joint and subacromial space. It also provides enhanced instrumentation access to all areas (360 degrees) of the glenoid labrum. Detractors of this position stress the increased effort with conversion to an open procedure and the need for a more complex anesthesia airway management.

Setup Description

After operating room bed setup (Fig. 1B.1) and induction of general anesthesia, the patient is placed laterally on a standard surgical table. A large beanbag is the preferred option for support (Figs. 1B.2 and 1B.3), but a pegboard can also be used. Straps and braces can be used around the torso to secure the patient to the table. The operative shoulder is exposed vertically. An axillary roll is used to protect the brachial plexus (Fig. 1B.4). The patient is titled 20 to 30 degrees posteriorly to angle the glenoid parallel to the floor. A foam pad is used to keep the head in a neutral position, and the eyes are protected (Fig. 1B.5). The nonsurgical arm is placed onto an arm holder or arm board (Fig. 1B.6). The operative arm is positioned into a sleeve with the thumb directed upward and then connected to a traction system. The system uses pulleys with weights to adjust abduction and forward flexion of the shoulder. Ideal forward flexion is 20 to 30 degrees, and ideal abduction is 25 to 45 degrees (Fig. 1B.7). Anterior and posterior drapes cover the entire shoulder, and a lateral strap is used to improve visualization of the glenohumeral joint (Fig. 1B.8). An arthroscopy drape is used under the axilla to collect effluent. Incisions are done away from pustules or acne to avert *Propionibacterium* contamination.

Tips and Pearls

- Use a draw sheet on top of the deflated beanbag and underneath the patient's torso to enable maneuvering.
- Place patient supine on the deflated beanbag prior to start of anesthesia induction.
- Angle the nonoperative arm holder at 120 degrees to the table (Fig. 1B.9).
- After the lateral decubitus position is obtained, suction the beanbag while the patient is held in place at the legs and trunk (see Fig. 1B.2).
- Pad the legs appropriately to prevent common peroneal nerve injury or any leg compression injury (Fig. 1B.10).
- After the patient is secure, turn the operative table 90 degrees for easy access to both the anterior and posterior shoulder joint for final setup.
- The patient's shoulder joint should be held in traction through use of a balanced suspension.
- The posterior portal is linear with the lateral edge of the acromion and should be drawn after traction is in place.

Advantages

1. Ease of execution of instability repairs and superior labral anterior posterior repairs
2. Superior visualization of the glenohumeral joint and subacromial space

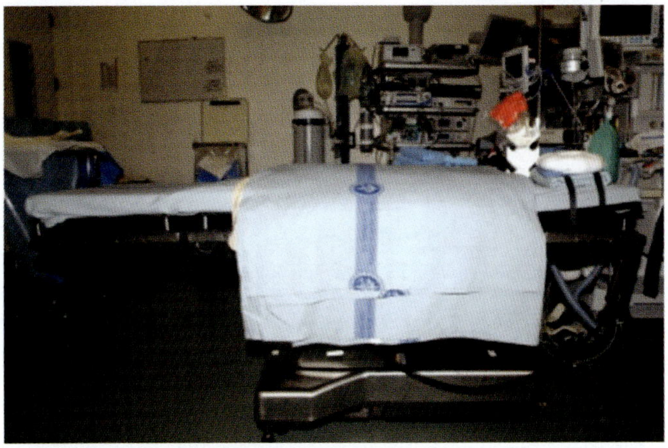

Fig. 1B.1 Setup of the operating room with beanbag and sheet prior to lateral decubitus positioning. (From Provencher MT, Romeo AA. *Shoulder Instability: A Comprehensive Approach*. Philadelphia: Saunders; 2012.)

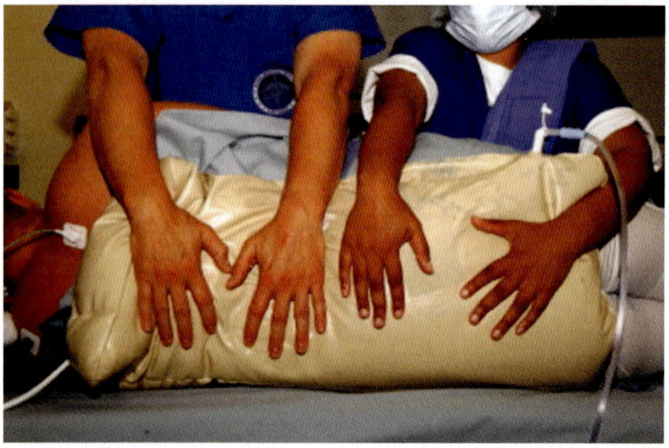

Fig. 1B.2 While vacuum suction is applied to the beanbag, the patient is held in place with the assistance of two individuals. (From Provencher MT, Romeo AA. *Shoulder Instability: A Comprehensive Approach*. Philadelphia: Saunders; 2012.)

3. Enhanced access to the anterior, posterior, and inferior areas of the shoulder joint
4. Decreased risk of cerebral desaturation events
5. Decreased surgeon fatigue because work is done near the waist level
6. Collection of cautery bubbles out of the field of view

Disadvantages

1. Nonanatomic orientation.
2. Conversion to an open procedure requires repositioning and may necessitate reprepping and redraping
3. Difficult to assess range of motion directly after repair
4. Potential increased risk of neurovascular injury caused by prolonged traction.

Complications

Intraoperative traction can cause excessive strain on the brachial plexus and may trigger transient nerve

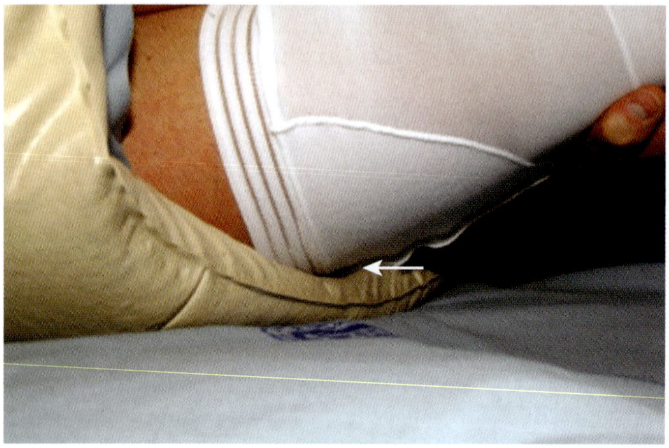

Fig. 1B.3 To avoid pressure sores, the edge of the beanbag where the edge of the bag meets the legs should be appropriately padded. (From Provencher MT, Romeo AA. *Shoulder Instability: A Comprehensive Approach*. Philadelphia: Saunders; 2012.)

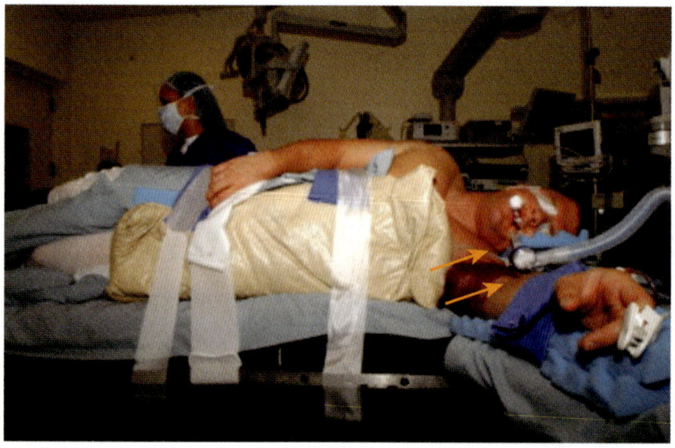

Fig. 1B.5 To protect the eyes and maintain the head in neutral position, a foam pad (indicated with *orange arrows*) is used. (From Provencher MT, Romeo AA. *Shoulder Instability: A Comprehensive Approach*. Philadelphia: Saunders; 2012.)

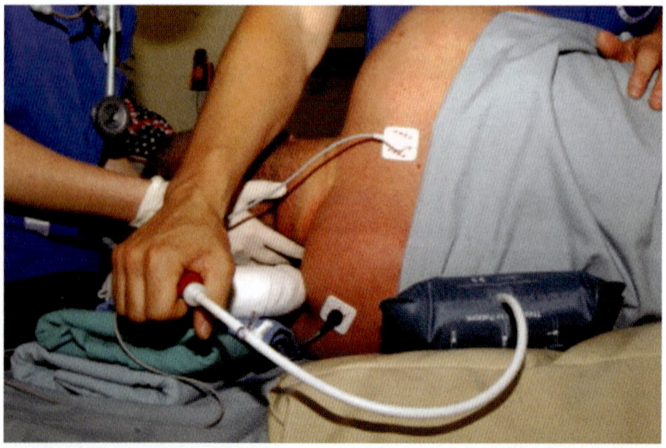

Fig. 1B.4 To avoid compression of the downside axilla, an axillary roll is used. This type is an inflatable axillary roll. (From Provencher MT, Romeo AA. *Shoulder Instability: A Comprehensive Approach*. Philadelphia: Saunders; 2012.)

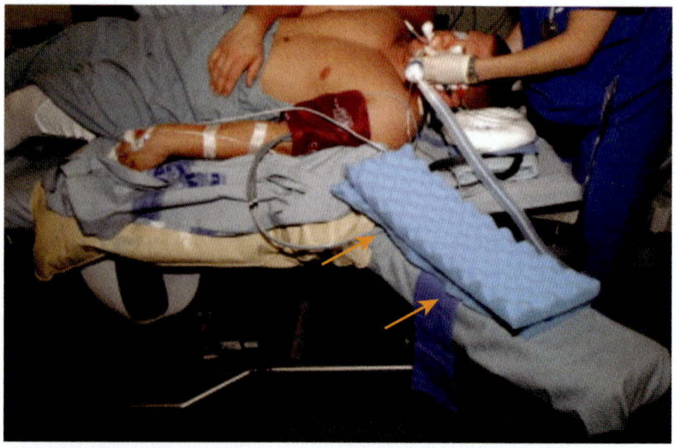

Fig. 1B.6 The nonsurgical arm is placed onto an arm holder or arm board. In this case, an arm board with foam pads and a strap (indicated with *orange arrows*) is used to maintain the nonsurgical arm in place. (From Provencher MT, Romeo AA. *Shoulder Instability: A Comprehensive Approach*. Philadelphia: Saunders; 2012.)

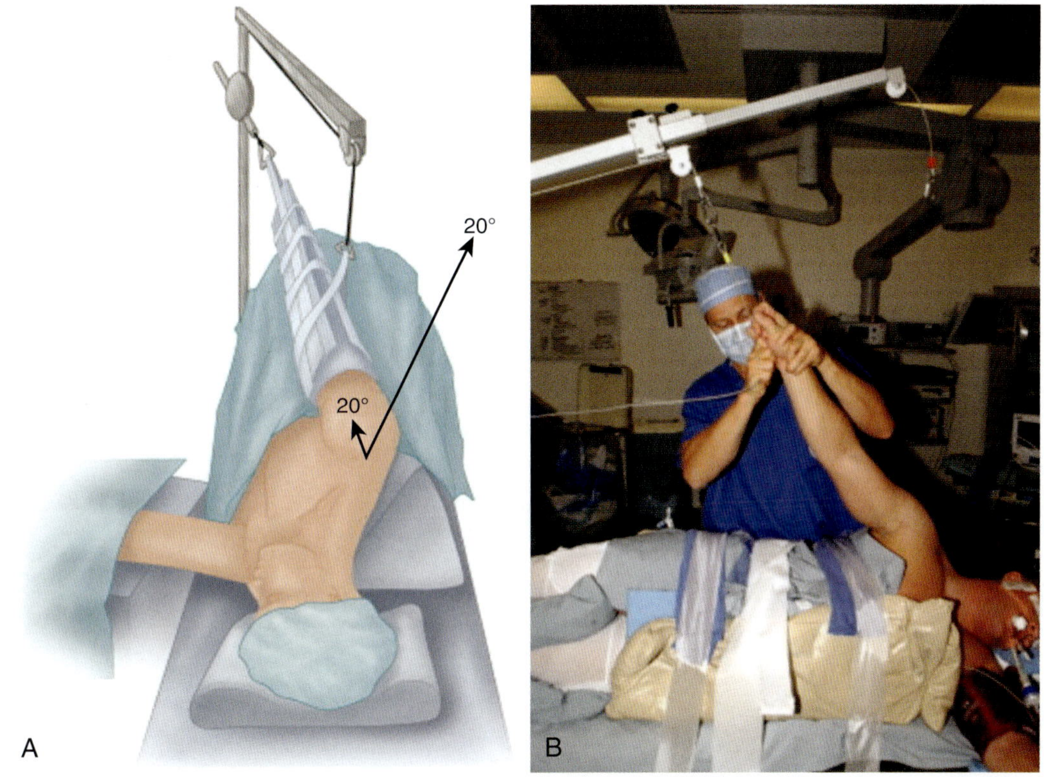

Fig. 1B.7 When positioning the surgical arm into place, forward flexion should be between 20 and 30 degrees (**A**), and abduction should be between 25 and 45 degrees (**B**). (From Provencher MT, Romeo AA. *Shoulder Instability: A Comprehensive Approach*. Philadelphia: Saunders; 2012.)

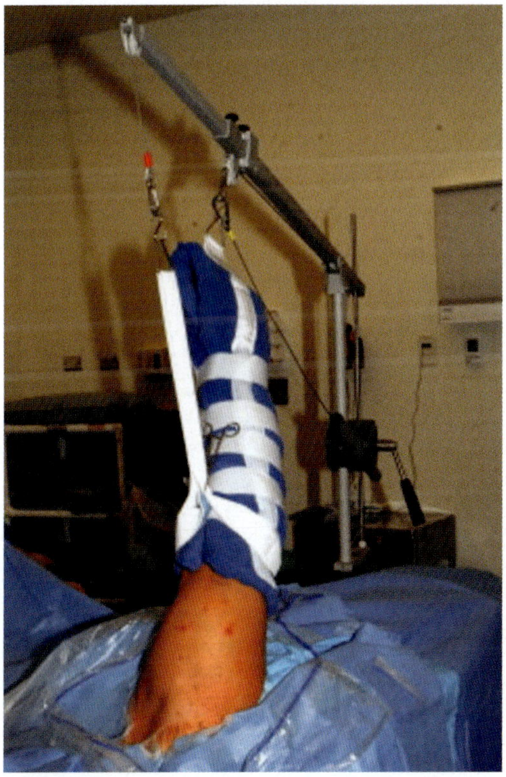

Fig. 1B.8 Final setup with the arm abducted about 50 degrees and a lateral strap for improved visualization of the glenohumeral joint. (From Provencher MT, Romeo AA. *Shoulder Instability: A Comprehensive Approach*. Philadelphia: Saunders; 2012.)

paresthesias (Skyhar et al, 1998). Of greater concern, permanent brachial plexus injuries have been reported (Weber et al, 2002). The current recommendation is to limit traction to 2 hours and use less than 7 lb of lateral traction and 12 lb of longitudinal traction.

Although the risk of thromboembolic events in shoulder arthroscopy is extremely low, there is an increased incidence of deep vein thrombosis and pulmonary embolism in the lateral decubitus position (Li et al, 2015).

BEACH-CHAIR POSITION

Advocates of the beach-chair position for shoulder arthroscopy reference its ease of conversion to an open procedure as the main advantage. Other benefits include flexibility of the anesthesia management, anatomic shoulder orientation, and greater freedom of shoulder motion during the procedure. Complications associated with the beach-chair position include a potential increase in risk of cerebral desaturation events (Salazar et al, 2013).

Setup Description

After anesthesia induction, the patient is placed on a standard or "beach-chair" table in the supine position (Fig. 1B.11). To get optimal visualization, the medial border of the scapular spine should be exposed. Therefore the patient is best situated close to the edge of the table or slightly off the table, depending on body habitus. Padding of all the bony prominences is then completed. The next portion of the technique is placing the table in 20 degrees reverse Trendelenburg, while the hip is flexed

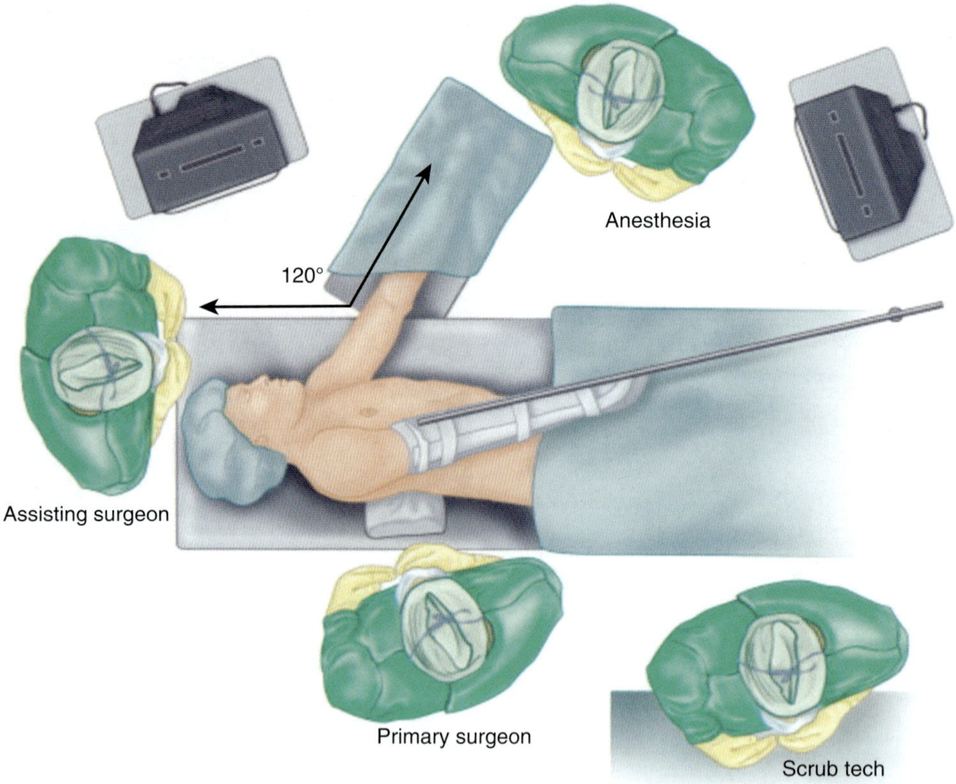

Fig. 1B.9 Overview of the lateral decubitus position at final setup. (From Provencher MT, Romeo AA. *Shoulder Instability: A Comprehensive Approach*. Philadelphia: Saunders; 2012.)

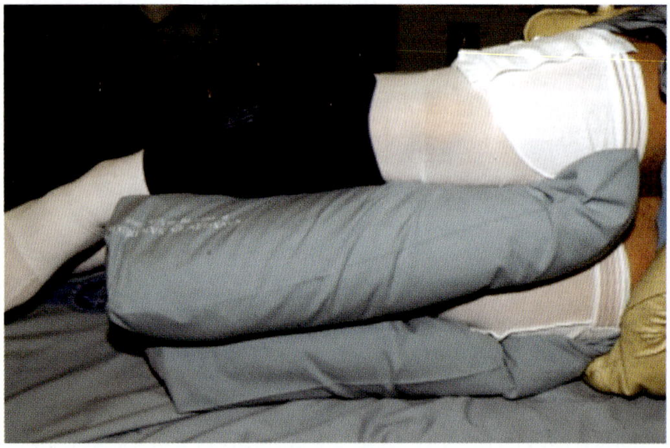

Fig. 1B.10 For prevention of leg compression injuries, a pillow under the bottom leg as well as a second pillow between the legs is used. (From Provencher MT, Romeo AA. *Shoulder Instability: A Comprehensive Approach*. Philadelphia: Saunders; 2012.)

45 to 60 degrees and knees are flexed to 30 degrees to ease the sciatic nerve through use of a leg positioner (Figs. 1B.12 and 1B.13). A well-padded head-holding device protects the head while covering the eyes during surgery (Fig. 1B.14). For stabilization of the scapula, one or two towels should be placed against the medial scapular border (Fig. 1B.15). The nonsurgical upper extremity can be positioned onto an arm holder, an arm board, or a sling or tucked at the side. The operative arm can be left free (an assistant will be needed to apply traction) or held in place through use of a commercially available sterile arm positioning device controlled by an assistant or placed on a well-padded Mayo stand (Fig. 1B.16). Drapes cover the entire shoulder both anteriorly and posteriorly. An arthroscopy drape can be used under the axilla to collect effluent. Incisions should be done away from pustules or acne to circumvent contamination with *Propionibacterium* spp.

Tips and Pearls

- Ensure the arm positioner is situated on the table before onset of the case.
- The table should be elevated to 60 to 80 degrees for shoulder arthroscopy.
- Avoid having the patient too inferior on the table because this may result in pressure ulcers and neuropraxia.
- A leg positioner can be used to maintain the pelvis level and against the back of the bed (see Fig. 1B.12).
- Various available head-holding devices with straps and gel foam can be used to ensure neutral head and neck position (Fig. 1B.17).
- A wedge pillow can be used under the thigh (placed all the way up to the buttocks) to prevent pressure sores.
- Place two towels posterior to the scapular spine against the table (see Fig. 1B.15).
- Table should be flexed to confirm that the legs are level.
- Pad the legs appropriately to prevent common peroneal nerve injury or any leg compression injury (see Fig. 1B.10).

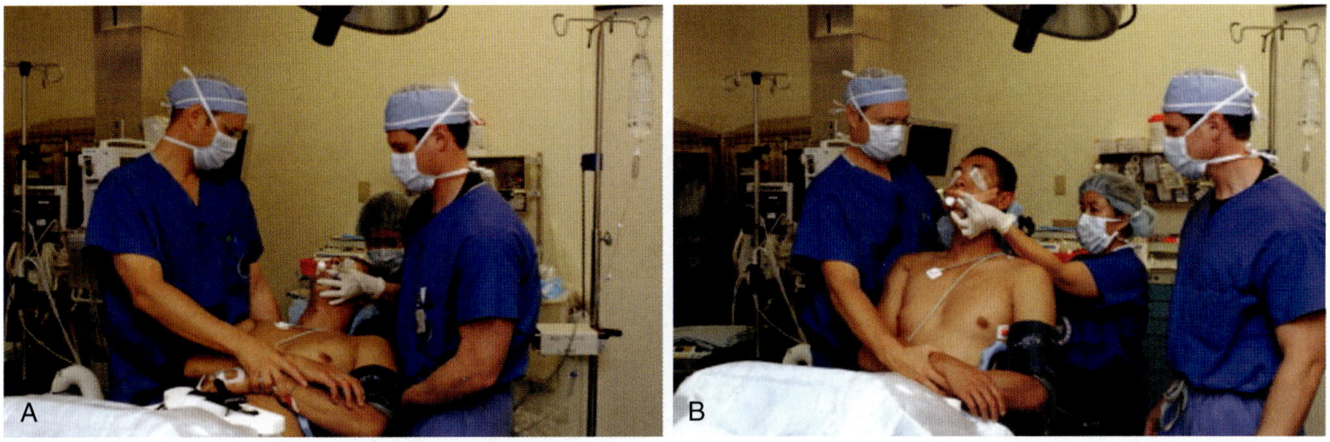

Fig. 1B.11 A, With the assistance of two individuals, the patient is placed into the beach-chair position. **B,** One person lifts up the patient while the other secures the head. (From Provencher MT, Romeo AA. *Shoulder Instability: A Comprehensive Approach*. Philadelphia: Saunders; 2012.)

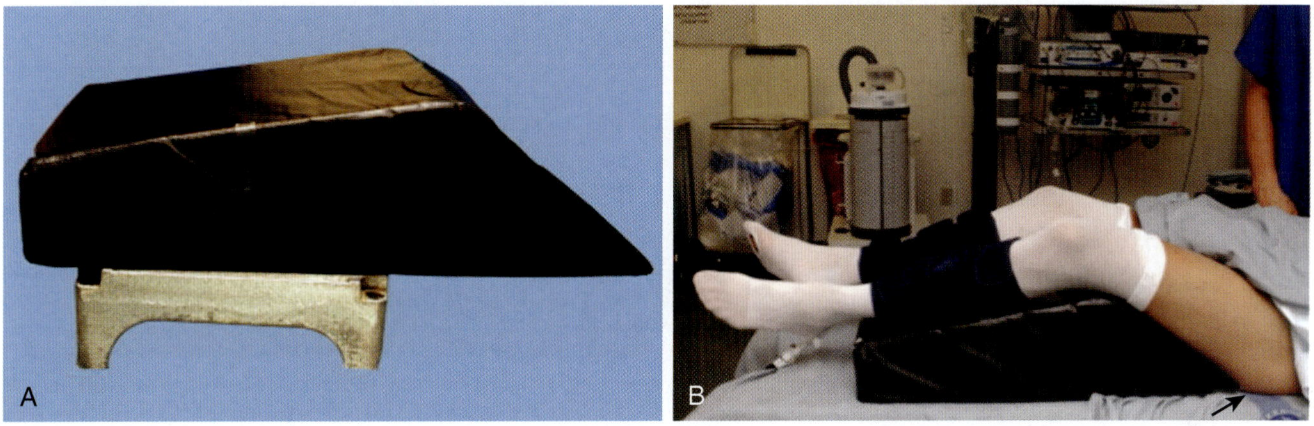

Fig. 1B.12 To ensure a comfortable position for the patient, a leg positioner is used (**A**) and will allow for the pelvis to be level and directly against the surgical table (**B**). (From Provencher MT, Romeo AA. *Shoulder Instability: A Comprehensive Approach*. Philadelphia: Saunders; 2012.)

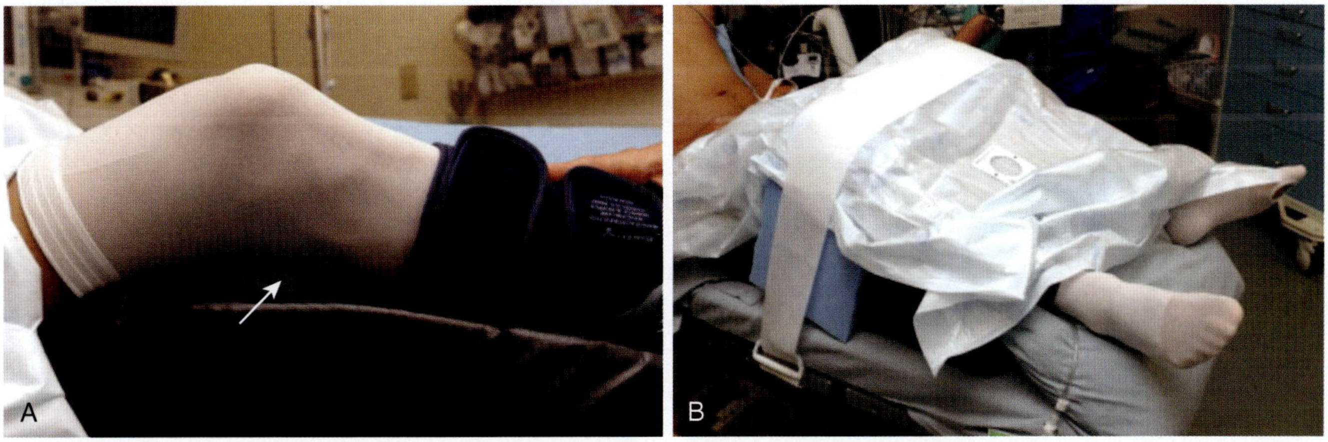

Fig. 1B.13 A, For final position, ensure that the leg pad is up against the buttocks and the buttocks and low back are not slumped. **B,** Ensure that no pressure is placed on the peroneal nerve at the knee. (From Provencher MT, Romeo AA. *Shoulder Instability: A Comprehensive Approach*. Philadelphia: Saunders; 2012.)

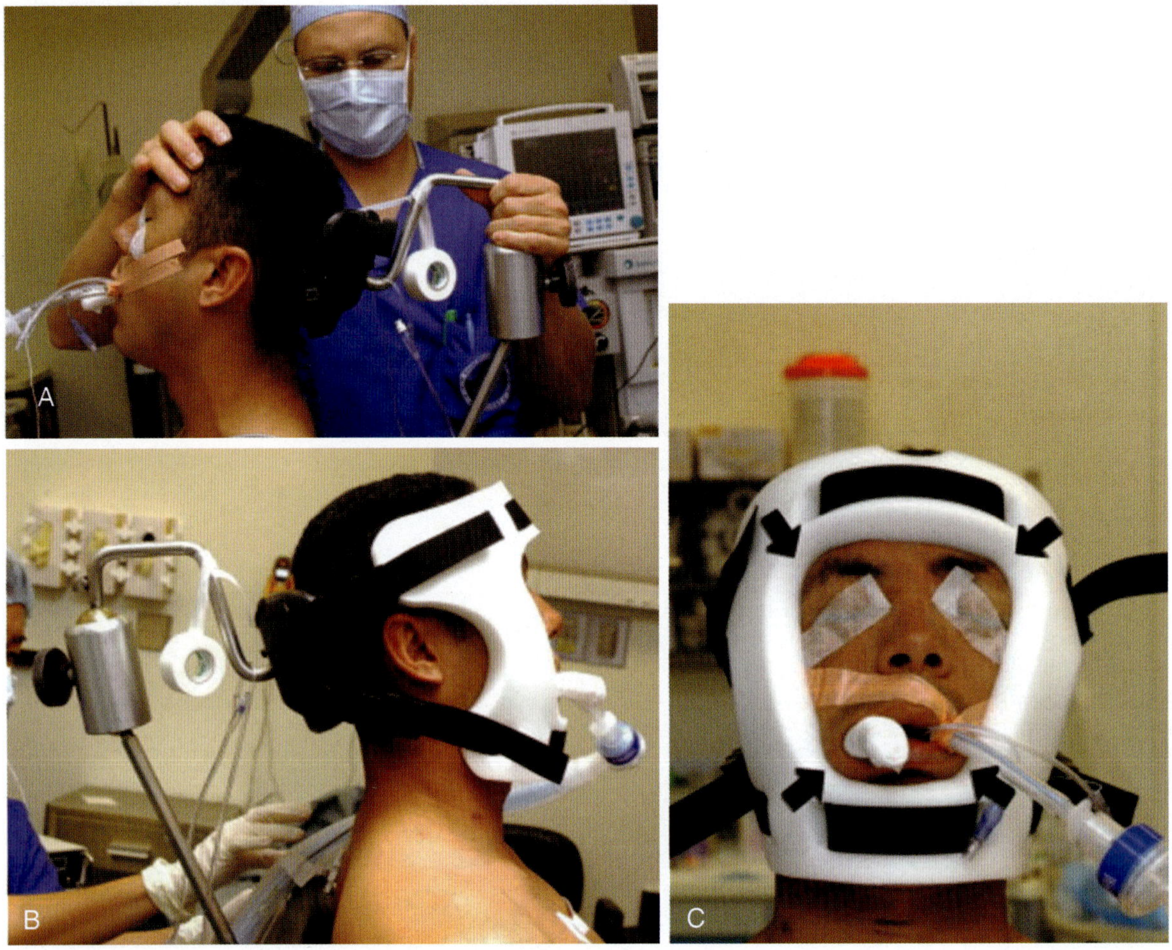

Fig. 1B.14 A and **B,** A foam facemask is used to secure the head. The neck should be positioned in a neutral position. **C,** The facemask should not cover any mucosal or sensitive areas. (From Provencher MT, Romeo AA. *Shoulder Instability: A Comprehensive Approach*. Philadelphia: Saunders; 2012.)

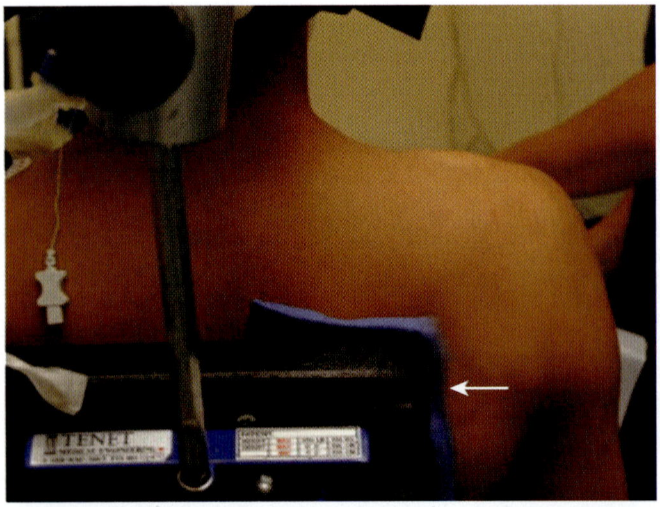

Fig. 1B.15 The back holder should have one to two towels placed against the medial scapular border for stabilization of the scapula during the procedure. (From Provencher MT, Romeo AA. *Shoulder Instability: A Comprehensive Approach*. Philadelphia: Saunders; 2012.)

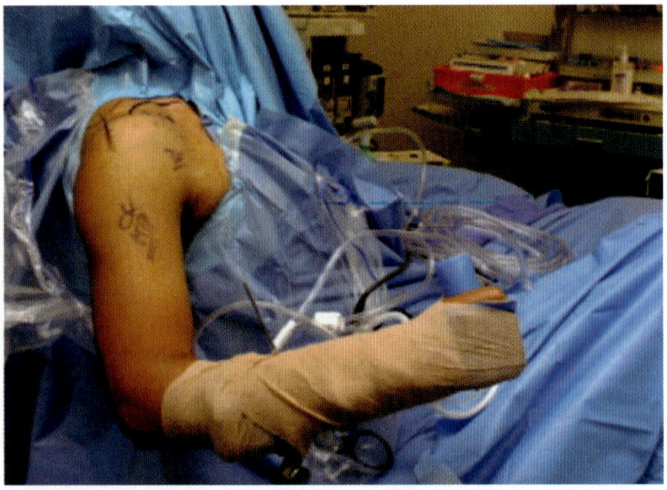

Fig. 1B.16 Final positioning with the arm reduced to a pneumatic arm positioner. (From Provencher MT, Romeo AA. *Shoulder Instability: A Comprehensive Approach*. Philadelphia: Saunders; 2012.)

- Maintain even shoulder height to prevent brachial plexus stretching.
- The operative arm should be in neutral position at the start of the arthroscopy and then manipulated as needed.
- Use cerebral oximetry in high-risk patients to identify potential cerebral hypoperfusion during surgery.

Advantages

1. Ease of conversion to open procedure
2. Upright, anatomic position of the glenohumeral joint—easier teaching and orientation
3. Ease of recognition of external shoulder landmarks allows increased precision in portal placement.
4. Potential decreased risk of nerve palsy (Rodeo et al, 1993)
5. Flexibility of anesthesia, whether regional or general
6. Easy airway access if complications arise during surgery
7. Superior anterior shoulder portal access
8. Increased range of motion of the operative arm

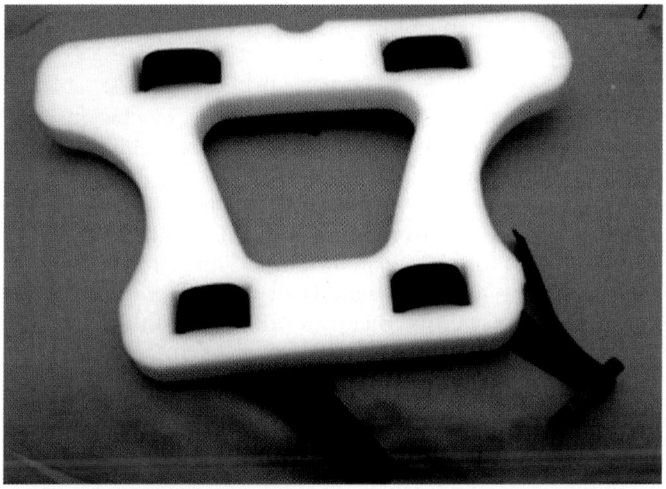

Fig. 1B.17 For securement of the head, a foam facemask may be used. (From Provencher MT, Romeo AA. *Shoulder Instability: A Comprehensive Approach*. Philadelphia: Saunders; 2012.)

Disadvantages

1. Increased risk for cardiovascular complications such as cerebral ischemia
2. Potential increased risk of air embolus
3. Head acts as a mechanical block for posterior and superior portals; a transrotator can be used during posterior Bankart repair (Costouros et al, 2006)
4. Collection of cautery bubbles can cloud the subacromial space
5. Challenging access to the inferior, superior, and posterior areas of the glenohumeral joint
6. Increased cost because of the beach-chair attachment and mechanical arm holder.

Complications

Cerebral ischemia during deliberate hypotensive anesthesia is a potential risk in the upright beach-chair position. Cerebral desaturation events have a higher incidence in the beach-chair position versus the lateral decubitus position (Murphy et al, 2010). Of note, the anesthesia literature recommends maintaining systolic blood pressure at above 90 mm Hg and mean arterial pressure (MAP) less than 20% to prevent cerebrovascular events (Gillespie et al, 2012).

Other reported complications include hypoglossal nerve palsy (Mullins et al, 1992) (attributed to repeated changes in neck position), greater auricular and lesser occipital palsy (Park and Kim, 2005) (caused by head holding device compression), and ventricular tachycardia (Cho et al, 2010).

Senior Author's Preferred Method: Bankart Repair Technique to Treat Recurrent Anterior Shoulder Instability in the Lateral Decubitus Position

An anterior shoulder dislocation even may result in a glenoid labrum avulsion known as a Bankart lesion (Fig. 1B.18).

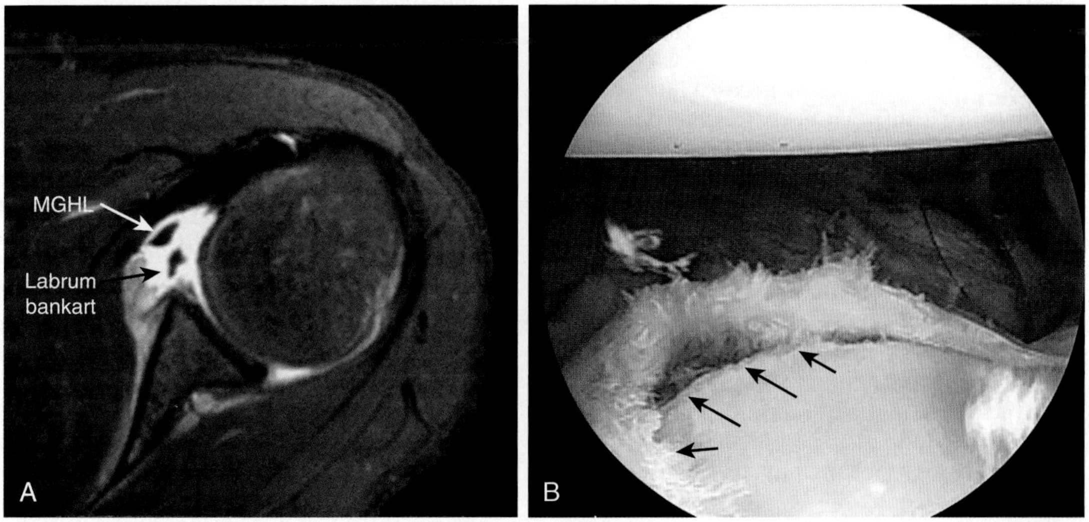

Fig. 1B.18 A, Axial view of a magnetic resonance arthrogram demonstrating a soft-tissue Bankart tear anteriorly. The black *arrow* points to the anteroinferior labrum. **B,** Corresponding arthroscopic image of the anterior Bankart tear indicated by *arrows*. *MGHL*, Middle Glenohumeral Ligament. (From Provencher MT, Ghodadra N, Romeo AA. Arthroscopic management of anterior instability: pearls, pitfalls, and lessons learned. *Orthop Clin North Am*. Philadelphia: Saunders; 2010 ; 41(3): 325–37.)

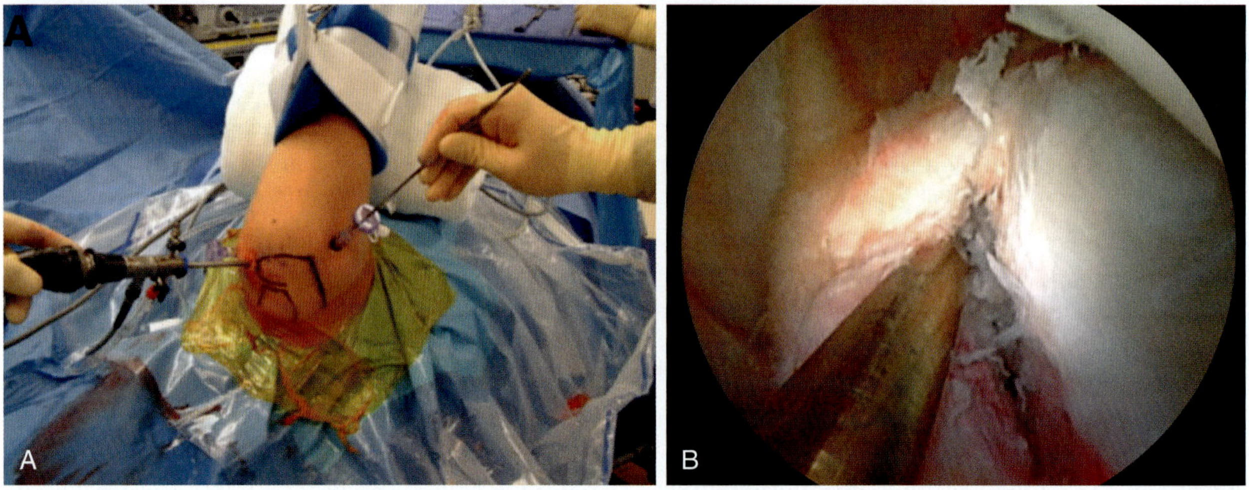

Fig. 1B.19 A, Outside view of shoulder demonstrating the arthroscope in the anterosuperior portal while the working portal is located at the anterior midglenoid portal and posterior portal. **B,** Corresponding arthroscopic view from anterosuperior portal demonstrating an anterior-inferior capsulolabral avulsion. (From Provencher MT, Romeo AA. *Shoulder Instability: A Comprehensive Approach*. Philadelphia: Saunders; 2012.)

The Bankart lesion causes an increase in anterior translation in all points of elevation, thereby generating recurrent instability (Speer et al, 1994). It is now widely agreed that the proper treatment for this type of shoulder pathology is surgical repair, either open or arthroscopic.

A recent meta-analysis suggests that the arthroscopic technique using modern suture anchor technique has similar outcomes to the open method (Harris et al, 2013). Previous reports indicate that the open technique has a lower recurrence rate, especially in young male patients (Mohtadi, 2014). This is controversial, but when using proper indications and excluding patients with significant bone loss, the arthroscopic technique can provide an excellent outcome with less surgical morbidity. Arthroscopic repair of the Bankart lesion can be performed through either lateral decubitus or beach-chair positioning as previously described.

The senior author prefers the lateral decubitus position because of the superior visualization of the capsulolabral complex and lower instability recurrence rates when compared with the beach-chair setup (Frank et al, 2014). Because of the greater exposure, particularly of the inferior aspects of the shoulder joint, the lateral decubitus position provides considerable instrumentation accessibility to the entire joint and labrum (360 degrees). In addition, this setup allows for lower suture anchor position on the glenoid, thus making the repair more easily secured.

BANKART REPAIR TECHNIQUE

1. Preoperative evaluation
   - Assessment of glenoid or humeral head bone loss
   - The most accurate method for measuring glenoid bone loss is a three-dimensional computed tomography scan with digital subtraction of the humeral head on sagittal oblique imaging. Magnetic resonance imaging or a magnetic resonance arthrogram may also be used.
2. Evaluation under anesthesia
   - Confirms the direction of instability
   - Indicates the amount of translation in the anterior, posterior and inferior directions
   - Helps demonstrate the amount of capsular plication to be performed
3. Patient positioning
   - Lateral decubitus position is preferred. Specific description of this setup is presented earlier in the chapter.
4. Portal placement
   - First two portals—anterosuperior and posterior—to assess injury pattern. The glenohumeral joint is inspected for chondral damage. The posterolateral side of the humeral head is examined for potential Hill-Sachs lesions. Biceps tendon, glenohumeral ligaments, rotator cuff and anterior, inferior and superior aspects of labrum are also inspected for pathology.
   - The standard posterior portal in the lateral decubitus setup is in line with the lateral edge of the acromion and 1 cm inferior to the posterior tip. Placing this portal more lateral than the typical beach-chair portal allows for slightly downward trajectory on the glenoid surface and provides satisfactory access to the posterior glenoid rim for anchor placement.
   - The anterosuperior portal is placed right at the anterior lateral edge of the acromion. This will be the principal visualization portal of the procedure.
   - After Bankart lesion detection, an anterior midglenoid portal is placed in line with the 3 o'clock glenoid. An 18-gauge needle just superior to the subscapularis tendon can aid with placement of this portal (Fig. 1B.19). The mid-glenoid portal with an 8-mm cannula acts as the working portal.
   - The last portal established is the posterolateral one. It is 4 cm inferior to the posterolateral border of the acromion, and its main role is to facilitate anchor placement in the inferior position of the shoulder.
   - Avoid the axillary nerve, which is 12 to 15 mm away from the articular margin of the glenoid, articular between the 5:30 and 6 o'clock positions.
5. Glenoid preparation
   - The arthroscope is placed in the anterosuperior portal.
   - An elevator tool (through the midglenoid portal) is used to complete soft tissue elevation from the glenoid.

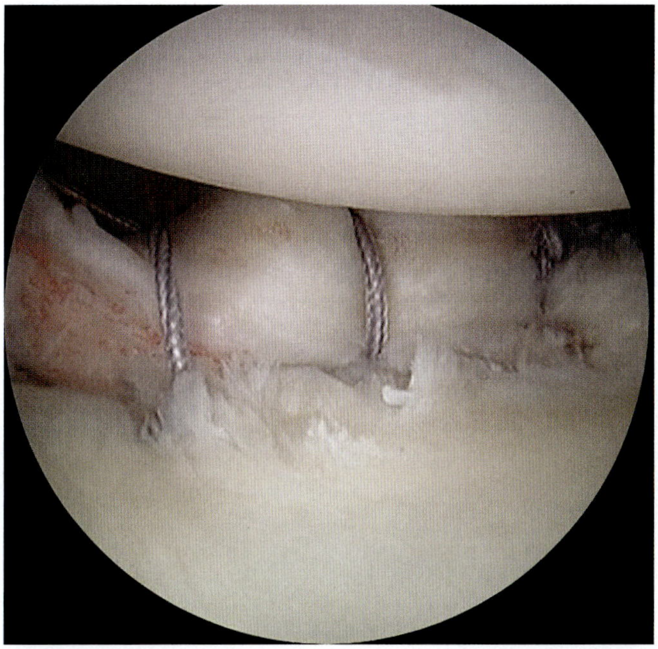

Fig. 1B.20 Arthroscopic view of an anatomic restoration of the labral-ligamentous complex following Bankart repair in the posterior viewing portal. (From Provencher MT, Ghodadra N, Romeo AA. Arthroscopic management of anterior instability: pearls, pitfalls, and lessons learned. *Orthop Clin North Am*. Philadelphia: Saunders; 2010.)

Attention is placed on maintaining the integrity of the circumferential fibers of the labrum.

- The labrum is peeled from the glenoid neck by using elevators and a small bone-cutting shaver.
- Bleeding bed of bone for healing should be present.
- Visualization of the posterior subscapularis muscle fibers indicates satisfactory glenoid preparation.
- The labrum and capsule should be freely mobile before repair.

6. Suture anchor placement and capsular plication
   - Anchor placement is always along the articular cartilage margin.
   - Anchors should be placed so that the sutures are perpendicular to the glenoid rim.
   - Standard repair consists of three or four anchors below the 3 o'clock position on the glenoid rim at a 45-degree angle to the glenoid surface (Fig. 1B.20). Additional anchors are placed 5 to 7 mm apart (depending on the extent of the defect).
   - The first suture anchor is completed via the posterolateral portal.
   - The remaining suture anchors are knotless and done with labral tape through the midglenoid portal.
   - Capsulolabral tensioning is ideal in slight external rotation.
   - Before knot tying, sutures are pulled to confirm sufficient capsular tissue has been integrated (see Fig. 1B.20).
7. Testing for stability
   - A gentle load-and-shift maneuver can be performed to be sure that patholaxity has been eliminated.
   - General range of motion is examined after portal closure and balance suspension removal. We check to be sure that there is at least 30 degrees of external rotation.
   - At the end of the procedure, the patient is placed in a padded abduction sling with a cold compression therapy device.

References

Cho SH, Yi JW, Kwack YH, Park SW, Kim MK, Rhee YG. Ventricular tachycardia during arthroscopic shoulder surgery: a report of two cases. *Arch Orthop Trauma Surg*. 2010;130(3):353–356.

Costouros JG, Clavert P, Warner JJ. Trans-cuff portal for arthroscopic posterior capsulorrhaphy. *Arthroscopy*. 2006;22(10):1138.e1–1138.e5.

Frank RM, Saccomanno MF, McDonald LS, Moric M, Romeo AA, Provencher MT. Outcomes of arthroscopic anterior shoulder instability in the beach chair versus lateral decubitus position: a systematic review and meta-regression analysis. *Arthroscopy*. 2014;30(10):1349–1365.

Gillespie R, Shishani Y, Streit J, et al. The safety of controlled hypotension for shoulder arthroscopy in the beach-chair position. *J Bone Joint Surg Am*. 2012;94(14):1284–1290.

Harris JD, Gupta AK, Mall NA, et al. Long-term outcomes after Bankart shoulder stabilization. *Arthroscopy*. 2013;29(5):920–933.

Hovelius L, Saeboe M. Arthropathy after primary anterior shoulder dislocation—223 shoulders prospectively followed up for twenty-five years. *J Shoulder Elbow Surg*. 2009;18(3):339–347.

Li X, Eichinger JK, Hartshorn T, Zhou H, Matzkin EG, Warner JP. A comparison of the lateral decubitus and beach-chair positions for shoulder surgery: advantages and complications. *J Am Acad Orthop Surg*. 2015;23(1):18–28.

Mohtadi NG, Chan DS, Hollinshead RM, Boorman RS, Hiemstra LA, Lo IK, Hannaford HN, Fredine J, Sasyniuk TM, Paolucci EO. A randomized clinical trial comparing open and arthroscopic stabilization for recurrent traumatic anterior shoulder instability: two-year follow-up with disease-specific quality-of-life outcomes.*J Bone Joint Surg Am*. 2014;96(5):353–60.

Mullins RC, Drez D Jr, Cooper J. Hypoglossal nerve palsy after arthroscopy of the shoulder and open operation with the patient in the beach-chair position. A case report. *J Bone Joint Surg Am*. 1992;74(1):137–139.

Murphy GS, Szokol JW, Marymont JH, et al. Cerebral oxygen desaturation events assessed by near-infrared spectroscopy during shoulder arthroscopy in the beach chair and lateral decubitus positions. *Anesth Analg*. 2010;111(2):496–505.

Park TS, Kim YS. Neuropraxia of the cutaneous nerve of the cervical plexus after shoulder arthroscopy. *Arthroscopy*. 2005;21(5):631.

Provencher MT, Ghodadra N, Romeo AA. Arthroscopic management of anterior instability: pearls, pitfalls, and lessons learned. *Orthop Clin North Am*. 2010;41(3):325–37.

Rodeo SA, Forster RA, Weiland AJ. Neurological complications due to arthroscopy. *J Bone Joint Surg Am*. 1993;75(6):917–926.

Salazar D, Sears BW, Andre J, Tonino P, Marra G. Cerebral desaturation during shoulder arthroscopy: a prospective observational study. *Clin Orthop Relat Res*. 2013;471(12)4027–4034.

Skyhar MJ, Altchek DW, Warren RF, Wickiewicz TL, O'Brien SJ. Shoulder arthroscopy with the patient in the beach-chair position. *Arthroscopy*. 1988;4(4):256–259.

Speer KP, Deng X, Borrero S, Torzilli PA, Altchek DA, Warren RF. Biomechanical evaluation of a simulated Bankart lesion. *J Bone Joint Surg Am*. 1994;76(12):1819–1826.

Weber SC, Abrams JS, Nottage WM. Complications associated with arthroscopic shoulder surgery. *Arthroscopy*. 2002;18(2 suppl 1):88–95.

1-1C ARTHROSCOPIC CAPSULOLABRAL REPAIR AND RECONSTRUCTION IN THE BEACH-CHAIR POSITION

PETER D. FABRICANT, MD, MPH, and FRANK A. CORDASCO, MD, MS

Introduction

- Primary arthroscopic anterior stabilization may be routinely performed for recurrent anterior instability and uncomplicated revision surgery without significant bone loss.
- Although the patient position in either the beach-chair (modified Fowler) or lateral decubitus position may be used to successfully treat glenohumeral instability arthroscopically, the beach-chair position offers some distinct advantages in some clinical scenarios. The use of an arm-holding traction device with a "bump" in the axilla facilitates access to the inferior aspect of the glenoid and capsule.
- The beach-chair position is advantageous in that it allows for an easy transition between arthroscopic and open approaches without patient repositioning.
- If a surgeon prefers the beach-chair position for rotator cuff repair, it may be advisable to use the same position for glenohumeral instability surgery, particularly in older patients in whom concomitant rotator cuff pathology frequently accompanies glenohumeral instability.

The use of arthroscopy for the treatment of shoulder instability has continued to increase as refined techniques have improved clinical outcomes. Arthroscopy provides several advantages in the treatment of glenohumeral instability, including improved visualization and clarification of pathoanatomy (Caspari & Geissler, 1993; McGlynn & Caspari, 1984), delineation and confirmation of preoperative imaging evaluation (Legan et al, 1991), and minimally invasive treatment of pathology. Although open stabilization continues to have a role in the surgical management of specific subtypes of glenohumeral instability (e.g., significant glenoid bone loss or bipolar lesions, poor tissue quality, extreme hypermobility, revision surgery), advanced arthroscopic techniques continue to offer expanded indications for arthroscopic stabilization (Fabricant et al, 2015). In addition to improved surgical visualization with minimal soft tissue dissection, there is a significant reduction in operative and hospitalization time and perioperative complications with arthroscopy compared with open surgery (Green & Christensen, 1993). Although both beach-chair (modified Fowler) and lateral decubitus positioning have been described extensively, this chapter focuses on glenohumeral arthroscopy in the beach-chair position, as popularized at the Hospital for Special Surgery (Skyhar et al, 1988). Open repair and reconstruction techniques are described in detail in the other chapters of this section. The epidemiology, pathoanatomy, patient evaluation, imaging, and surgical outcomes are also discussed elsewhere. The purpose of this chapter is to describe the indications and technique for arthroscopic capsulolabral repair in the beach-chair position.

Indications and Contraindications

The decision to use the beach-chair position for glenohumeral stabilization is based on the surgeon's preference and has similar indications to arthroscopy in the lateral decubitus position for many cases. However, there are certain clinical scenarios when the beach-chair position is preferable. If during preoperative planning the surgeon identifies pathology that may require conversion to an open approach (e.g., significant glenoid bone loss or bipolar lesions, poor capsulolabral tissue, HAGL [humeral avulsion of the glenohumeral ligament] lesion), this may be easily performed without patient repositioning, but an open deltopectoral approach is not readily performed in the lateral decubitus position and would require patient repositioning intraoperatively. Additionally, although either position is commonly used for treatment of glenohumeral instability, treatment of rotator cuff tears is more commonly addressed in the beach-chair position. If a surgeon prefers the beach-chair position for rotator cuff repair, it may be advisable to use the same position for glenohumeral instability surgery, particularly in older patients in whom concomitant rotator cuff pathology frequently accompanies glenohumeral instability (Snyder & Strafford, 1993).

With regard to indications for arthroscopic management of glenohumeral instability in general, many patients with glenohumeral instability expect arthroscopic stabilization. More important, therefore, is deciding which patients are not candidates for arthroscopic stabilization. Risk factors for failure include age younger than 20 years old, competitive overhead or contact athlete, shoulder capsular attenuation (caused by repetitive instability episodes, poor-quality capsulolabral tissue, or a genetic collagen disorder), significant bone loss on the glenoid or humeral sides, bipolar and engaging lesions, a Hill-Sachs lesion present on the anteroposterior (AP) radiograph in external rotation, and loss of the anteroinferior glenoid contour on the AP radiograph (Balg & Boileau, 2007; Castagna et al, 2012; Mohtadi et al, 2014; Porcellini et al, 2009; Voos et al, 2010; Waterman et al, 2014). These factors have been used to develop the instability severity index score (ISIS), which identifies patients who may be treated more effectively with open stabilization (Balg & Boileau, 2007). When the interval of time between the dislocation and reduction approaches 5 hours or more, stabilizations that address bone loss, such as the Latarjet reconstruction, should be considered (Denard et al, 2015). The number of formal reductions required after anterior dislocation has been shown to be directly correlated to failure after arthroscopic anterior stabilization and may warrant consideration for an open technique (Fabricant et al, 2015; Gerometta et al, 2016; Ozturk et al, 2013; Wasserstein et al, 2013). Recent literature indicates that more than one preoperative dislocation may increase the odds of failure of arthroscopic stabilization by 3.8 times (Gasparini et al, 2016; Shin et al, 2016).

We believe that patients with demonstrable bone loss from the glenoid or humeral head warranting bone augmentation or transfer (e.g., Latarjet procedure [Latarjet, 1954], Bristow procedure [Helfet, 1958], free allograft or autograft [Provencher et al, 2009]), patients with capsular injury, and patients requiring a revision stabilization who require an open approach should undergo diagnostic arthroscopy before open surgery to document all pathology (Cho et al, 2009; Sisto, 2007). In such cases or in the event the surgeon is unsure whether an arthroscopic or open approach is ideal, the beach-chair position is preferable because it allows for rapid conversion from arthroscopic to open surgery without patient repositioning if needed. This is important because arthroscopic examination may alter diagnoses in 40% of patients with atraumatic instability and in 8% of patients with traumatic anterior instability (Mok et al, 1990). Although capsular avulsions of the glenohumeral ligaments have been successfully repaired arthroscopically, many arthroscopic shoulder surgeons still consider anterior HAGL lesions a relative contraindication to an all-arthroscopic stabilization. In the senior author's practice, 80% of surgical cases of anterior instability are treated arthroscopically, 10% with open stabilization, and 10% with bone augmentation (majority Latarjet) reconstruction.

Surgical Technique of Capsulolabral Repair in the Beach-Chair Position

We perform primary arthroscopic anterior stabilization routinely for recurrent anterior instability and uncomplicated revision surgery without significant bone loss. We do not consider participation in contact or overhead athletics a contraindication to arthroscopic stabilization. We do counsel collision athletes that recurrence after stabilization depends on the repair type and on the activity level chosen after surgery. In general, we have been satisfied with our arthroscopic results (even in contact athletes) when the following conditions are met:

- The patient has unidirectional instability of traumatic origin consisting of anterior or isolated anteroinferior instability without more than 2+ sulcus sign on examination under anesthesia.
- Arthroscopic examination discloses a discrete Bankart lesion. The lesion in some cases has migrated and healed medially and inferiorly (ALPSA [anterior labroligamentous periosteal sleeve avulsion] lesion) (Neviaser, 1993). When the capsule and labrum have healed in the medialized position, the capsule and labrum must be elevated off the glenoid and brought to a functionally appropriate position on the anterior-inferior glenoid rim.
- There is no significant bone loss. Although historically, 20% to 25% glenoid bone loss was considered to be significant, Shaha et al (2015) reported that the critical level of bone loss may be lower and that in those with high level of mandatory activity, glenoid bone loss greater than 13.5% led to inferior clinical outcomes even without recurrent instability.
- The capsule is robust, and the Inferior Glenohumeral Ligament (IGHL) complex does not exhibit signs of attrition.
- No anterior HAGL is present.
- No off-track or engaging bony Bankart, Hill-Sachs, or combined lesion is contributing to instability within a functional range of motion. Arciero et al (2015) have recently shown that glenoid bone loss of as little as 2 to 4 mm (8%–15%) in the setting of a Hill-Sachs lesion could compromise isolated Bankart repair and may require concomitant additional procedures.

It is important to be prepared to convert to open surgery if examination under anesthesia and diagnostic arthroscopy reveal any of the aforementioned diagnoses not amenable to successful arthroscopic reconstruction. As mentioned earlier, the beach-chair position allows for an easy transition between approaches without patient repositioning.

Regional anesthesia with an interscalene block combined with general anesthesia is administered. The patient is placed in the beach-chair (modified Fowler) position. Arthroscopic landmarks are palpated and marked on the skin of the shoulder, including the acromion, acromioclavicular joint, clavicle, and coracoid.

An examination under anesthesia is performed to confirm the pattern of instability because the examination under anesthesia is more sensitive in determining both the degree and direction of instability. The load-and-shift test is conducted, and translation is noted in the anterior, inferior, and posterior directions. Grading reflects the degree of humeral head translation anterior and posterior to the glenoid rim. The grade is 1+ if the translation of the humeral head is to the edge of the glenoid, 2+ if the humeral head can be subluxated over the glenoid rim but reduces spontaneously, and 3+ if a frank dislocation of the humeral head over the glenoid rim does not reduce spontaneously.

The arm is positioned in a mechanical arm positioner. Supplementary local anesthesia with epinephrine is injected in the area of the posterior portal for analgesia and hemostasis. The arthroscope is introduced through the posterior portal 2 cm below and 1 cm medial to the posterolateral corner of the acromion. The anterior working portal less than 1 cm lateral to the coracoid is localized using a spinal needle and established with a 5.5-mm cannula. Diagnostic arthroscopy then confirms the presence of a Bankart lesion. It is important to rule out associated pathology, including rotator cuff tears, anterosuperior labral tears, and posterior labral tears. Before committing to an arthroscopic repair, it is vital to assess for the presence or absence of bone loss. The bare area of the glenoid has been advocated as a useful landmark to assess for bone loss (Burkhart et al, 2002) and while this technique may be utilized, it should be incoprorated in the overall assessment along with the preoperative imaging and Examination Under Anesthesia (EUA) because there have been recent publications demonstrating variability of this arthroscopic assessment tool (Bakshi et al, 2015; Barcia et al, 2013; Detterline et al, 2009). If there is an off-track or engaging lesion with less than a 20% anterior glenoid bone defect, an arthroscopic stabilization is performed in conjunction with remplissage (Di Giacomo et al, 2014); however, our threshold for moving to an open stabilization in this setting is low. Depending on the patient, sport, and position as well as the desired postoperative activity level, bipolar lesions with "subcritical" amounts of bone

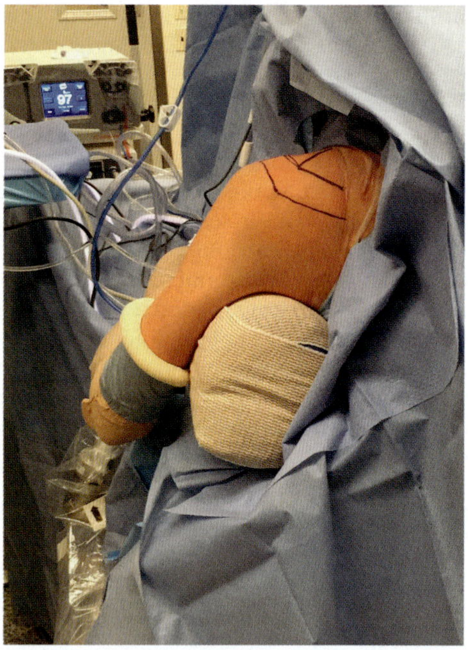

Fig. 1C.1 Axillary bump. An axillary "bump" is used in conjunction with a pneumatic arm-holding device in order to provide hands-free glenohumeral distraction and subsequent improved access and visualization of the inferior portion of the joint. (From Moran CJ, Fabricant PD, Kang R, Cordasco FA. Arthroscopic double-row anterior stabilization and Bankart repair for the "high-risk" athlete. *Arthrosc Tech.* 2014;3(1):65-71.)

loss have recently been shown to have inferior outcomes after isolated Bankart repair. Shaha et al (2015) noted that in patients engaged in high-level overhead activity, glenoid bone loss greater than 13.5% led to inferior Western Ontario Shoulder Instability (WOSI) scores despite the lack of frank recurrent instability. Furthermore, in the setting of bipolar lesions, Arciero et al (2015) reported that glenoid bone loss of as little as 2 to 4 mm (8%–15%) in the setting of a moderate-sized Hill-Sachs lesion could compromise isolated Bankart repair. To that end, we carefully consider level and type and engage in shared decision making with patients when devising a surgical plan, which has resulted in a lower threshold for advanced arthroscopic and open techniques in the setting of bipolar lesions in high-demand patients. If there is an off-track or engaging lesion with a greater than 20% anterior glenoid defect, an open Latarjet reconstruction is routinely performed.

After confirming that there is no significant bone loss involving the glenoid or an engaging Hill-Sachs lesion to prevent successful arthroscopic repair, a second anteroinferior portal is placed under direct vision using a spinal needle. The angle of approach of this portal is critical: Before inserting an 8.25-mm clear, twist-in cannula, we use the spinal needle to be certain that the direction afforded by the portal is both inferior enough to reach the 5:30 position on the glenoid with an anchor and lateral enough to place anchors on the face of the glenoid rather than on the glenoid neck. In addition, ensuring an appropriate distance between the two anterior portal skin incisions (2–3 cm) facilitates instrument and suture management. At this time, we have found that a "bump" in the axilla in conjunction with the arm holding device can provide improved access and visualization of the inferior portion of the glenohumeral joint (Fig. 1C.1).

After this second anterior portal is established, the labrum and capsule are mobilized from the glenoid using a combination of sharp elevator, dull elevator, and rasp. In an acute dislocation, the tissue is easily reducible, but in a chronic dislocator, the capsulolabral complex can be scarred down medially and inferiorly on the glenoid neck and must be mobilized for an anatomic repair. A 70-degree lens is helpful to visualize the anteroinferior and posteroinferior capsulolabral structures. The 70-degree lens is used for viewing via the posterior portal while elevating the labrum from the anterosuperior portal, especially when the labrum has healed in a medialized position. In this setting, we have found a sharp elevator (Fig. 1C.2) to be useful in elevating scarred tissue as a single flap. The arthroscope may be placed in the anterosuperior portal for additional visualization.

Proper mobilization of the tissue is critical for arthroscopic stabilization; the glenoid labrum and capsule complex should be elevated to the 6 o'clock position to ensure restoration of the tension of these structures and closure of the axillary pouch. A probe is used to assess the mobility of tissue before placing any anchors. Another indicator that the capsule and labrum have been mobilized sufficiently is visualization of the subscapularis muscle under the mobilized capsule and labrum. After satisfactory mobilization of the labral and capsular tissue, the labrum should float up to its near anatomic position. Next, a motorized shaver is used to gently decorticate the glenoid neck to prepare a bleeding bed to aid in healing. This maneuver should be performed without shaver suction to prevent damaging the soft tissues.

It is important to intraoperatively differentiate anterior glenohumeral instability that results in capsulolabral tear, capsuloligamentous deformation, or a combination of both phenomena. During a dislocation event, the capsuloligamentous structures (e.g., IGHL) may undergo plastic deformation before frank failure at the capsulolabral junction, glenoid–labrum interface, or glenoid. In the setting of a small Bankart lesion and a greater degree of capsular laxity, greater plication may be performed without formal takedown of the capsular attachment by creating pleats in the capsule itself (Kim et al, 2012; Sekiya et al, 2007; Wiley et al, 2005). The pleats are performed first by gently abrading the capsular tissue to encourage vascularity and promote healing followed by grasping capsular tissue with a curved suture passer in two locations and either securing it to a suture anchor to complete the plication or more commonly incorporating the pleat in a knotless mattress construct secured to a knotless anchor. Increasing the space between the capsular bites increases the degree of plication and may be easily controlled by the surgeon. When performed in conjunction with Bankart repair, both sites of pathology may be addressed in the setting of a combined lesion. This may also be performed when laxity persists after labral repair (Wiley et al, 2005).

It is quite common for the capsulolabral damage to extend into the posteroinferior zone (Song et al, 2015). When this is noted, we believe it is imperative to include this area in the repair and reconstruction by switching portals and viewing via the anterosuperior portal and reattaching the posteroinferior capsulolabral tissue. This in effect restores the posterior attachment of the "hammock." When we perform this associated repair, the anteroinferior sutures are not secured to the glenoid until the posteroinferior sutures have been placed.

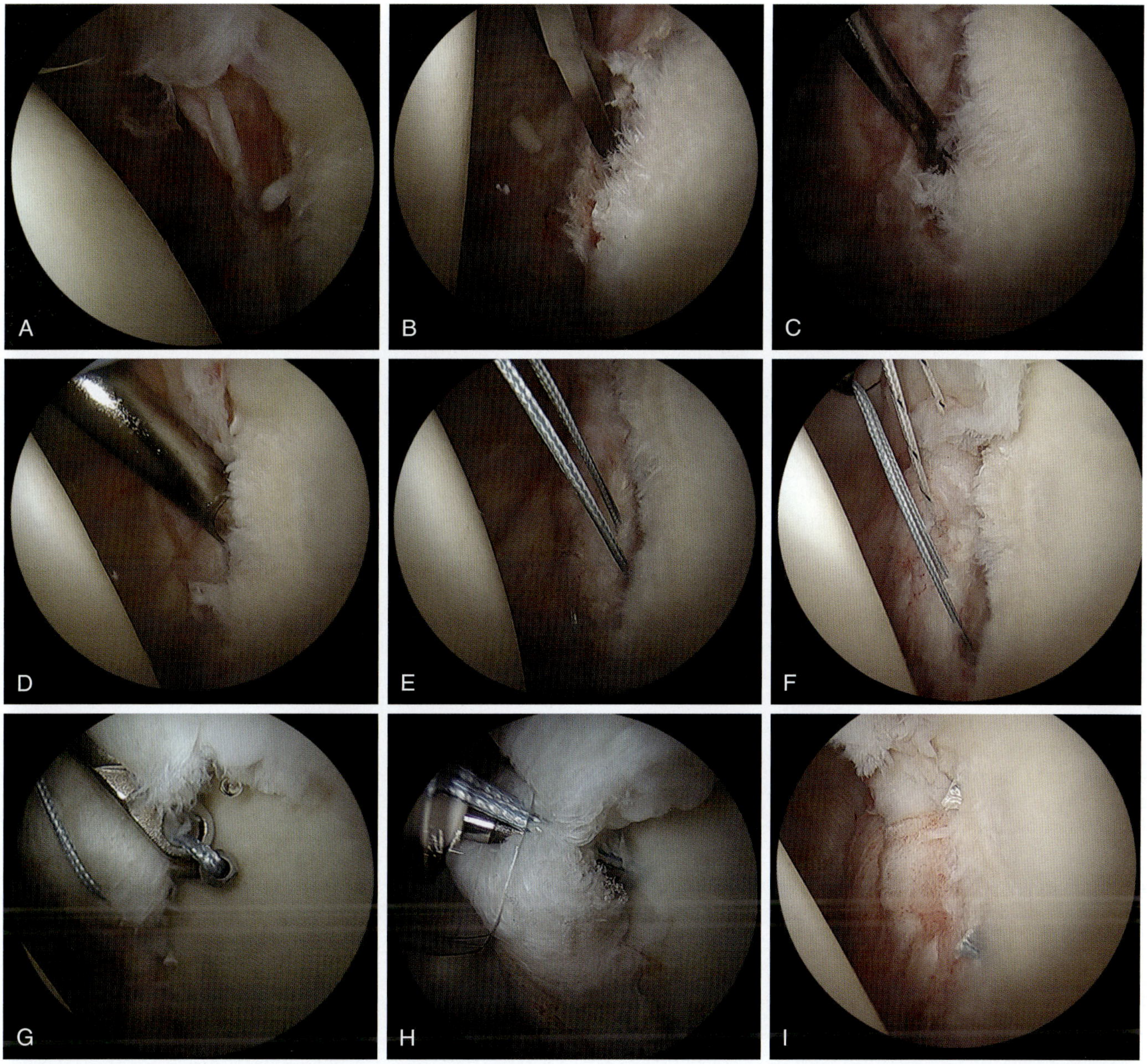

Fig. 1C.2 Single-row repair using a knotless mattress suture configuration. This patient was a 24-year-old NFL football player who sustained an acute traumatic anterior glenohumeral instability event. Evaluation with a 30-degree arthroscope from the posterior portal revealed an anterior capsulolabral avulsion (**A**). An arthroscopic blade (**B**) is used to sharply elevate and mobilize the retracted capsulolabral tissue off the anterior glenoid followed by preparation of the glenoid neck with a rasp (**C**) and shaver (**D**) to stimulate bony bleeding. Nonabsorbable mattress sutures are placed sequentially, starting at the anteroinferior glenoid (**E**) and progressing superiorly (**F** and **G**) while viewing from the posterior portal with a 70-degree arthroscope. Knotless anchors are sequentially deployed (**H**) in a superior progression with attached mattress suture construct. Completed mattress repair with three knotless suture anchors (**I**).

Multiple suture configurations and techniques have been described for the treatment of glenohumeral instability, including single row, double row, traditional (knotted), and knotless. In general, we prefer knotless techniques to minimize irritating suture abrading the joint surfaces and synovium. Whereas single-row repairs are excellent at providing powerful capsular shift, double-row techniques restore a broad footprint anatomy. Both are described next.

SINGLE-ROW REPAIR TECHNIQUE

We use a knotless anchor mattress technique (Fig. 1C.2). The 70-degree lens while viewing posteriorly is particularly helpful at this stage. Capsular plication to address capsular stretch should be performed (depending on the athlete being treated) with the arm in 30 degrees of abduction and in 30 to 40 degrees of external rotation to prevent overtightening the anterior structures. The amount of capsule plicated can be managed by varying the amount of tissue included in the shift much like a "pleat" can be used with garments (Fig. 1C.3). Suture-shuttling devices in the anteroinferior portal are used to pass stiff suture material through the capsule and into the defect between the labrum and the glenoid. The first suture is placed inferiorly. The limb is grasped and brought out through the anterosuperior portal. Without removing the shuttling device

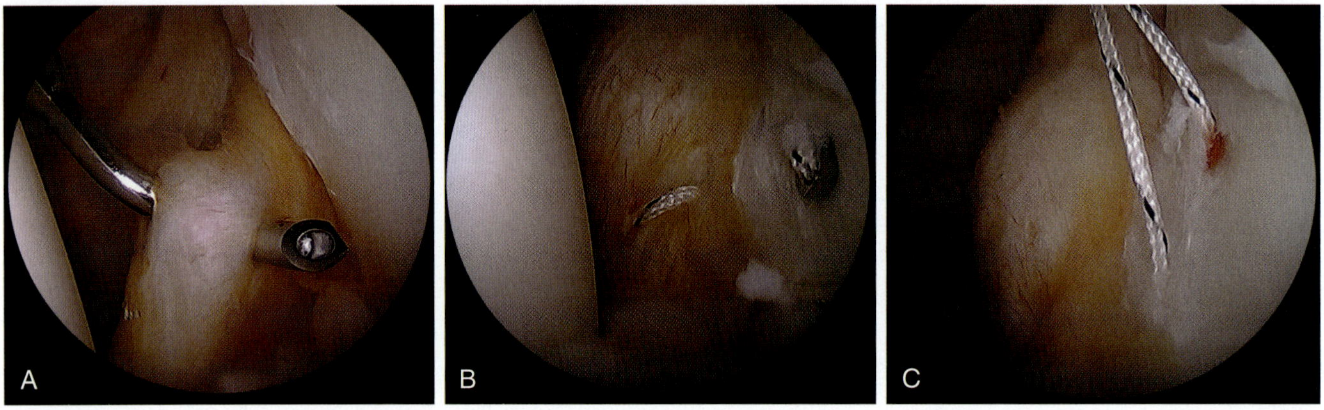

Fig. 1C.3 Plication without formal takedown of capsular attachment. A suture passing device is used to secure capsular tissue **(A)** followed by a second pass **(B)** to perform a plication. The amount of capsular tightening can be managed by varying the amount of tissue included in the plication. The suture is subsequently tightened **(C)** and then secured with an arthroscopic knot.

from the cannula, it is advanced through the capsule more superiorly and again advanced into the defect between the labrum and the glenoid. Here the suture is retrieved using a suture retriever and brought out through the anterosuperior portal. Before securing the suture to a knotless anchor, the next stitch is passed. Depending on the location of the capsulolabral injury, the repair can move from the most inferior 6 o'clock position as far superiorly as necessary. Care is taken to ensure that the suture anchors are placed 2 mm onto the glenoid face to prevent a medialized repair. Anchors placed more medial than this risk restoration of the glenoid labrum in a nonanatomic medialized position that will not restore the normal bumper effect of the anterior labrum. Conversely, if placed too far on the face of the glenoid, significant articular cartilage injury can occur.

DOUBLE-ROW REPAIR TECHNIQUE (Video 1C.1)

This technique is indicated for "high-risk" athletes (younger than 25 years of age, male, contact or forced overhead sports, higher levels of competition, more than two or three dislocations) and acute bony Bankart lesions that are amenable to arthroscopic repair (Fabricant et al, 2015; Moran et al, 2014). We use a percutaneous long needle while staying lateral to the conjoined tendon. A guidewire and cannulated drill are introduced. The correct location for medial row anchors 10 to 15 mm medial to articular surface of glenoid is identified. Each of two to four anchors (depending on the size of the lesion) are placed without removing the drill guide, progressing from inferior to superior. The anchor suture limbs are passed from the medial row using outside-in or inside-out technique. Sutures are prepared on knotless anchors for lateral-row fixation at the articular margin. After an arthroscopic Bankart repair is completed, anterior stability is reassessed. The subacromial space is inspected to evaluate the bursal surface of the rotator cuff and coracoacromial arch.

Conclusions

Improved instrumentation and understanding of the pathoanatomy and biomechanics of the shoulder have allowed surgeons to use advanced arthroscopic shoulder stabilization techniques in a larger fraction of patients with glenohumeral instability. Although patient position in either the beach-chair (modified Fowler) or lateral decubitus position may be used to successfully treat glenohumeral instability arthroscopically, the beach-chair position is preferred when the surgeon suspects pathology which may require conversion to an open approach (e.g., significant glenoid bone loss, poor capsulolabral tissue, HAGL lesion), which may be easily performed without patient repositioning.

References

Arciero RA, Parrino A, Bernhardson AS, et al. The effect of a combined glenoid and Hill-Sachs defect on glenohumeral stability: a biomechanical cadaveric study using 3-dimensional modeling of 142 patients. *Am J Sports Med*. 2015;43(6):1422–1429.

Bakshi NK, Patel I, Jacobson JA, Debski RE, Sekiya JK. Comparison of 3-dimensional computed tomography-based measurement of glenoid bone loss with arthroscopic defect size estimation in patients with anterior shoulder instability. *Arthroscopy*. 2015;31(10):1880–1885.

Balg F, Boileau P. The instability severity index score. A simple pre-operative score to select patients for arthroscopic or open shoulder stabilisation. *J Bone Joint Surg Br*. 2007;89(11):1470–1477.

Barcia AM, Rowles DJ, Bottoni CR, Dekker TJ, Tokish JM. Glenoid bare area: arthroscopic characterization and its implications on measurement of bone loss. *Arthroscopy*. 2013;29(10):1671–1675.

Burkhart SS, Debeer JF, Tehrany AM, Parten PM. Quantifying glenoid bone loss arthroscopically in shoulder instability. *Arthroscopy*. 2002;18(5):488–491.

Caspari RB, Geissler WB. Arthroscopic manifestations of shoulder subluxation and dislocation. *Clin Orthop Relat Res*. 1993;291:54–66.

Castagna A, Delle Rose G, Borroni M, et al. Arthroscopic stabilization of the shoulder in adolescent athletes participating in overhead or contact sports. *Arthroscopy*. 2012;28(3):309–315.

Cho NS, Yi JW, Lee BG, Rhee YG. Revision open Bankart surgery after arthroscopic repair for traumatic anterior shoulder instability. *Am J Sports Med*. 2009;37(11):2158–2164.

Denard PJ, Dai X, Burkhart SS. Increasing preoperative dislocations and total time of dislocation affect surgical management of anterior shoulder instability. *Int J Shoulder Surg*. 2015;9(1):1–5.

Detterline AJ, Provencher MT, Ghodadra N, Bach BR Jr, Romeo AA, Verma NN. A new arthroscopic technique to determine anterior-inferior glenoid bone loss: validation of the secant chord theory in a cadaveric model. *Arthroscopy*. 2009;25(11):1249–1256.

Di Giacomo G, Itoi E, Burkhart SS. Evolving concept of bipolar bone loss and the Hill-Sachs lesion: from "engaging/non-engaging" lesion to "on-track/off-track" lesion. *Arthroscopy*. 2014;30(1):90–98.

Fabricant PD, Taylor SA, McCarthy MM, et al. Open and arthroscopic anterior shoulder stabilization. *JBJS Rev*. 2015;3(2). 10.2106/JBJS.RVW.N.00060.

Gasparini G, De Benedetto M, Cundari A, et al. Predictors of functional outcomes and recurrent shoulder instability after arthroscopic anterior stabilization. *Knee Surg Sports Traumatol Arthrosc.* 2016;24(2):406–413.
Gerometta A, Rosso C, Klouche S, Hardy P. Arthroscopic Bankart shoulder stabilization in athletes: return to sports and functional outcomes. *Knee Surg Sports Traumatol Arthrosc.* 2016;24(6):1877–1883.
Green MR, Christensen KP. Arthroscopic versus open Bankart procedures: a comparison of early morbidity and complications. *Arthroscopy.* 1993;9(4):371–374.
Helfet AJ. Coracoid transplantation for recurring dislocation of the shoulder. *J Bone Joint Surg Br.* 1958;40-B(2):198–202.
Kim DW, Kim CK, Jung SW. An arthroscopic pleated capsular shift for recurrent anterior dislocation of the shoulder. *Knee Surg Sports Traumatol Arthrosc.* 2012;20(12):2579–2584.
Latarjet M. Treatment of recurrent dislocation of the shoulder. *Lyon Chir.* 1954;49(8):994–997.
Legan JM, Burkhard TK, Goff WB 2nd, et al. Tears of the glenoid labrum: MR imaging of 88 arthroscopically confirmed cases. *Radiology.* 1991;179(1):241–246.
McGlynn FJ, Caspari RB. Arthroscopic findings in the subluxating shoulder. *Clin Orthop Relat Res.* 1984;(183):173–178 (183).
Mohtadi NG, Chan DS, Hollinshead RM, et al. A randomized clinical trial comparing open and arthroscopic stabilization for recurrent traumatic anterior shoulder instability: two-year follow-up with disease-specific quality-of-life outcomes. *J Bone Joint Surg Am.* 2014;96(5):353–360.
Mok DW, Fogg AJ, Hokan R, Bayley JI. The diagnostic value of arthroscopy in glenohumeral instability. *J Bone Joint Surg Br.* 1990;72(4):698–700.
Moran CJ, Fabricant PD, Kang R, Cordasco FA. Arthroscopic double-row anterior stabilization and bankart repair for the "high-risk" athlete. *Arthrosc Tech.* 2014;3(1):e65–e71.
Neviaser TJ. The anterior labroligamentous periosteal sleeve avulsion lesion: a cause of anterior instability of the shoulder. *Arthroscopy.* 1993;9(1):17–21.
Ozturk BY, Maak TG, Fabricant P, et al. Return to sports after arthroscopic anterior stabilization in patients aged younger than 25 years. *Arthroscopy.* 2013;29(12):1922–1931.
Porcellini G, Campi F, Pegreffi F, Castagna A, Paladini P. Predisposing factors for recurrent shoulder dislocation after arthroscopic treatment. *J Bone Joint Surg Am.* 2009;91(11):2537–2542.
Provencher MT, Ghodadra N, LeClere L, Solomon DJ, Romeo AA. Anatomic osteochondral glenoid reconstruction for recurrent glenohumeral instability with glenoid deficiency using a distal tibia allograft. *Arthroscopy.* 2009;25(4):446–452.
Sekiya JK, Willobee JA, Miller MD, Hickman AJ, Willobee A. Arthroscopic multi-pleated capsular plication compared with open inferior capsular shift for reduction of shoulder volume in a cadaveric model. *Arthroscopy.* 2007;23(11):1145–1151.
Shaha JS, Cook JB, Song DJ, et al. Redefining "critical" bone loss in shoulder instability: Functional outcomes worsen with "subcritical" bone loss. *Am J Sports Med.* 2015;43(7):1719–1725.
Shin SJ, Ko YW, Lee J. Intra-articular lesions and their relation to arthroscopic stabilization failure in young patients with first-time and recurrent shoulder dislocations. *J Shoulder Elbow Surg.* 2016;25(11):1756–1763.
Sisto DJ. Revision of failed arthroscopic Bankart repairs. *Am J Sports Med.* 2007;35(4):537–541.
Skyhar MJ, Altchek DW, Warren RF, Wickiewicz TL, O'Brien SJ. Shoulder arthroscopy with the patient in the beach-chair position. *Arthroscopy.* 1988;4(4):256–259.
Snyder SJ, Strafford BB. Arthroscopic management of instability of the shoulder. *Orthopedics.* 1993;16(9):993–1002.
Song DJ, Cook JB, Krul KP, et al. High frequency of posterior and combined shoulder instability in young active patients. *J Shoulder Elbow Surg.* 2015;24(2):186–190.
Voos JE, Livermore RW, Feeley BT, et al. HSS Sports Medicine Service. Prospective evaluation of arthroscopic bankart repairs for anterior instability. *Am J Sports Med.* 2010;38(2):302–307.
Wasserstein D, Dwyer T, Veillette C, et al. Predictors of dislocation and revision after shoulder stabilization in Ontario, Canada, from 2003 to 2008. *Am J Sports Med.* 2013;41(9):2034–2040.
Waterman BR, Burns TC, McCriskin B, Kilcoyne K, Cameron KL, Owens BD. Outcomes after bankart repair in a military population: predictors for surgical revision and long-term disability. *Arthroscopy.* 2014;30(2):172–177.
Wiley WB, Goradia VK, Pearson SE. Arthroscopic capsular plication-shift. *Arthroscopy.* 2005;21(1):119–121.

1-1D OPEN STABILIZATION: BANKART AND CAPSULAR SHIFT AND HUMERAL AVULSION OF THE GLENOHUMERAL LIGAMENT REPAIR

TROY A. ROBERSON, MD, JARED C. BENTLEY, MD, and RICHARD J. HAWKINS, MD

Introduction

The open approach has long been considered the gold standard in addressing anterior shoulder instability (Rowe et al, 1978).

- Advances in arthroscopic technique over the past 2 decades have led to an increasing number of stabilization procedures being performed arthroscopically.
- Multiple authors (Malhotra et al, 2012; Owens et al, 2011; Zhang et al, 2014) have noted a dramatic increase in arthroscopic stabilizations, with Zhang et al most recently reporting an increase in arthroscopic repair from 71% in 2004 to 89% in 2009.
- In the United Kingdom, Malhotra et al (2012) reported an increase in the preferred stabilization approach from 16% arthroscopic in 2002 to 71% in 2009. This is particularly interesting given that the comfort level with arthroscopic stabilization versus open procedures may be fueling this trend.
- Considering much of these data were collected nearly a decade ago, the use of arthroscopic stabilization procedures may be considerably higher, especially among more recently trained surgeons who have had less exposure to open stabilization techniques.

Therefore it is reasonable to evaluate whether this increase is evidence based or simply an increased comfort level with the arthroscopic approach.

The controversy of open versus arthroscopic Bankart repair as evidenced by five previous meta-analyses (Freedman et al, 2004; Lenters et al, 2007, Mohtadi et al, 2005; Petrera et al, 2010; Wang et al, 2015).

- All found at least equivalent postoperative stability between arthroscopic and open repair.

- Four (Freedman et al, 2004; Lenters et al, 2007; Mohtadi et al, 2005; Wang et al, 2015) of five found evidence of lower recurrent instability with open repair.
- Three (Freedman et al, 2004; Lenters et al, 2007; Mohtadi et al, 2005) reported improved overall functional outcomes with open repair.
- One (Wang et al, 2015) found worse range of motion after open procedures.

There have been several retrospective comparative studies (Kim & Ha, 2002; Lützner et al, 2009; Mahiroğulları et al, 2010; Tjoumakaris et al, 2006, Zaffagnini et al, 2012) between open and arthroscopic treatment of anterior instability:

- All found generally comparable recurrence rates and outcomes between the two.
- The exceptions are one study (Lützner et al, 2009), which found a higher recurrence rate in arthroscopic repair but better range of motion versus open repair, and another reporting better postoperative functional outcomes after arthroscopic repair (Kim & Ha, 2002).

Two nonrandomized prospective studies (Cole et al, 2000; Karlsson et al, 2001) also report equivalent recurrence rates and outcomes.

- Cole et al, 2000 do state that the open repair group was chosen based on the degree of capsular laxity with an additional capsular shift performed, indicating a distinction not only of the pathology treated but the difference in the nuances of the procedure.

Finally, four level I randomized controlled trials exist comparing these techniques.

- Two (Bottoni et al, 2006; Fabbriciani et al, 2004) report slightly better postoperative external rotation with arthroscopic treatment.
- Two (Mohtadi et al, 2014; Sperber et al, 2001) report significant decreases in recurrence rates with open versus arthroscopic repair.
- The most recent study by Mohtadi et al (2014) reported a 23% recurrence rate in arthroscopic repair versus 11% in open repair with significant risk factors for recurrence being male gender under 25 years of age and significant preoperative Hill-Sachs lesion.

The totality of the presented literature suggests that open treatment of anterior shoulder instability may provide improved stability over arthroscopic treatment with the possible tradeoff of a modest decrease in range of motion in some cases.

There are some criticisms of open stabilization with presumed advantages of an arthroscopic approach.

- Ease of operation: Bottoni et al (2006) described operative time as an advantage of arthroscopic repair with open stabilization taking on average approximately 2.5 times longer. However, as we will show in the described technique, the open stabilization is not an onerous operation, and we believe this difference in operative time is more reflective of the previously mentioned lack of comfort with the open approach.
- Concern of subscapularis failure: This may be exaggerated because subscapularis failure has been scarcely reported (Greis et al, 1996; Rowe, 1978; Sachs et al, 2005; Scheibel et al, 2006).
  - Although Sachs et al (2005) found worse outcomes in patients with clinical signs of subscapularis insufficiency, only one of these patients had documentation by magnetic resonance imaging (MRI).
  - Scheibel et al (2006) reported MRI evidence of atrophy of the upper subscapularis after an inverted L-shaped tenotomy, while the lower subscapularis remained intact with some evidence of compensatory hypertrophy, but patient outcomes were not reported based on the presence of radiographic subscapularis abnormality.
  - Despite these findings, two studies have shown no difference in internal rotation strength after arthroscopic versus open stabilization (Hiemstra et al, 2008; Rhee et al, 2007).
  - Although it may be true that subscapularis dysfunction is a concern to some with the open approach, the available literature is inconclusive, and we have not found this to be a major concern in our practice.
- Another historical negative of open stabilization is the loss of some degree of external rotation.
  - More contemporary approaches value this concern and allow management of the capsule in such a way to minimize the loss of motion without compromising stability.
- An open approach allows uncomplicated treatment of the full pathology encountered including humeral avulsion of the glenohumeral ligament (HAGL) lesions, which are an uncommon but real cause of recurrent instability (Longo et al, 2016).

With these concerns mitigated and results that meet or exceed those of arthroscopic repair, we suggest that the trend toward arthroscopic stabilization is based more on comfort level than other factors, and open stabilization should not only remain a vital tool in the armamentarium of shoulder surgeons but in some cases may be the preferred technique. In the remainder of the chapter, we will discuss when this procedure may be particularly indicated or contraindicated, the key history and physical examination findings to promote success, and our preferred surgical technique.

Indications and Contraindications

Although successful surgery may be achieved in many instances with either an arthroscopic or open approach at discretion of the surgeon, certain situations may be indicated more strongly for open stabilization. Contact athletes provide one of the most challenging patient populations in shoulder instability treatment. Results of arthroscopic stabilization have generally been discouraging with failure rates ranging from 14% to 60% (Castagna et al, 2012; Cho et al, 2006; Hubbell et al, 2004; Rhee et al, 2006; Yamamoto et al, 2015). Hubbell et al (2004) found a 60% recurrence rate after arthroscopic stabilization versus 0% with open stabilization, and Rhee et al (2006) reported twice the risk of recurrence (25% vs 12.5%) with arthroscopic stabilization in this population. In contrast, Pagnani and Dome (2002) reported only a 3% recurrence rate among American football players with open stabilization. When taking age into consideration, open stabilization may be even more attractive. Only 57% of American Shoulder and Elbow Surgeon (ASES) member respondents chose arthroscopic stabilization as their preferred approach to the young contact athlete (Garcia et al, 2016). In this historically troublesome population, Hatch and Hennrikus (2016) recently reported no recurrences and good to excellent outcome scores in all patients at greater than 2-year follow-up with open stabilization.

Overlapping with the discussion of contact athletes, Burkhart and De Beer (2000) highlighted the importance of bone loss in recurrent instability, reporting a 89% failure rate in contact athletes with significant bone loss about the glenoid or humeral head and 67% recurrence in the overall group in the presence of bone loss with arthroscopic stabilization. With this concern over bone loss, the rate of bone block procedures has increased over the past 2 decades (Degen et al, 2016), and some have advocated for its place as a primary procedure in anterior instability (An et al, 2016; Bhatia et al, 2014). However, multiple authors have reported complication rates exceeding 20%, leaving understandable concern whether this should be considered a first-line treatment (Athwal et al, 2015; Degen et al, 2016; Shah et al, 2012). An option in between arthroscopic stabilization and bone block procedures may be open stabilization, but few studies have examined the results of open stabilization in the face of bone loss. In their classic study, Rowe et al (1978) found a slight decrease in recurrence with glenoid bone loss (3.5% vs 2%) and a slight increase in failure with moderate to severe Hill-Sachs lesions (3.5% vs 5%). Whereas Bigliani et al (1998) reported an overall 12% recurrence with varying degrees of glenoid rim defects with a technique that included capsular shift, while Gill et al (1997) found an increase in recurrence from 3% to 6% in the presence of a large Hill-Sachs lesion with open stabilization. More recently, Pagnani (2008) reported similar results with low recurrence rates in the face of glenoid or humeral head bone loss with open stabilization. These results suggest that the concerns over bone loss in arthroscopic stabilization may not be applicable to open stabilization, and we suggest open stabilization may be indicated and more advantageous in many instances when others propose bone block procedures.

Another instance in which open stabilization may be useful is in the situation of revision operations. Although arthroscopic procedures may be considered for revision surgeries, open stabilization has shown good results with recurrent instability reported from 0% to 22% (Cho et al, 2009; Levine et al, 2000; Rowe et al, 1984; Sisto, 2007; Zabinski et al, 1999). Most recently, Neviaser et al (2015) reported no recurrences with excellent patient reported outcomes and return to sport at a mean of over 10 years from revision open stabilization. In addition to those above, a primary failure of the subscapularis or concomitant HAGL lesion may be easily addressed with an open approach.

There are few contraindications to open stabilization with voluntary instability or psychological disease among them (Hattrup et al, 2001; Levine et al, 2000; Rowe et al, 1973). Large defects of the humeral head or glenoid may require bony augmentation, but as we have presented, most cases including bone loss may be successfully treated with a standard open stabilization. Finally, overhead throwing athletes are often preferentially treated with arthroscopic stabilization due to gravity of any issue with subscapularis dysfunction or loss of external rotation.

History

A thorough history and physical examination is the cornerstone of diagnosing and treating patients with shoulder instability. Among the key questions are age, handedness, initial or multiple events, number of previous events, amount of trauma required for instability, voluntary dislocation, position of the arm, whether Emergency Department (ED) reduction was required, whether it was painful, if there was dislocation during sleep, and what sport or recreational activities are desired. Of these, one of the most critical is age because it has been defined as one of the most important risk factors for higher recurrence with nonoperative management (Postacchini et al, 2000; Robinson et al, 2006; Wheeler et al, 1989). On the other end of the spectrum, patients older than 40 years of age have lower recurrence rates but should be closely scrutinized for a concomitant rotator cuff tear. Patients should be questioned to elicit signs of generalized ligamentous laxity and thus the possibility of multidirectional instability as opposed to isolated anterior instability. A first time dislocator or one who has had multiple dislocations requiring ED reduction is quite different from a patient who describes self-reduced events, but it is possible for a multidirectional lax individual to experience an isolated anterior instability event. The presence and distribution of pain should also be considered because neck pain or radiating arm pain may indicate cervical spine involvement or brachial plexus pathology. Pain in the subdeltoid region associated with worsening at night causes concern for rotator cuff involvement. A patient's desired activity level is one of the final important considerations, with contact athletes and overhead athletes getting special consideration. In the tertiary care setting, many patients present with a prior surgical history, which should be probed in detail with confirmation of previous medical records.

Physical Examination

Although a full examination of the shoulder should be performed to assess contour, range of motion, strength, and for the presence of neurovascular abnormalities, we provide a focused discussion of specific tests to aid in treatment decisions. The sulcus sign is assessed in the upright position with an inferiorly directed force on the arm with grade 1 being less than a 1-cm gap between the acromion and humeral head, grade 2 between 1 and 2 cm, and grade 3 more than 2 cm. It is critical to ask the patient whether this translation reproduces the symptoms or is simply a physiologic laxity. In the supine position, the anterior apprehension test, or fulcrum test, is performed in 90 degrees of abduction with gentle external rotation of the arm (Fig. 1D.1). As the arm is rotated, a positive test result is elicited with apprehension or feeling of a near instability event by the patient or examiner. A relocation test may be performed at this point with posteriorly directed force on the humeral head with a positive response being relief of the apprehension (Fig. 1D.2). Some

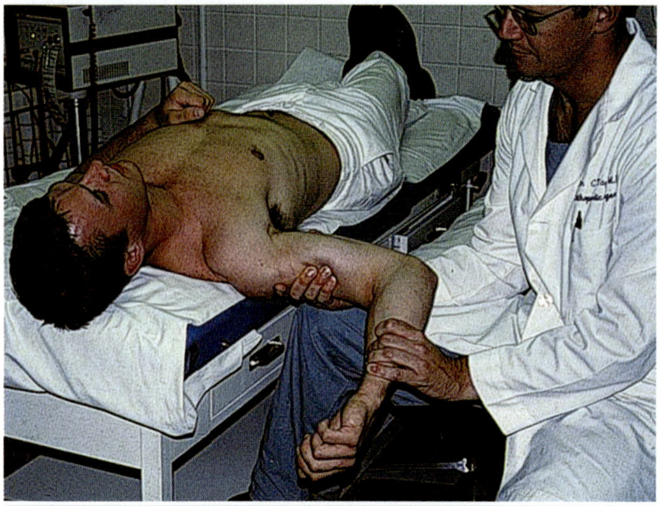

Fig. 1D.1 Performance of the anterior apprehension test. An examination result is positive when the patient expresses apprehension or the feeling of the shoulder slipping out of the socket when in this abducted externally rotated position. (Reprinted from Romeo A, Provencher M, eds. *Shoulder Instability: A Comprehensive Approach.* Philadelphia: Saunders; 2016.)

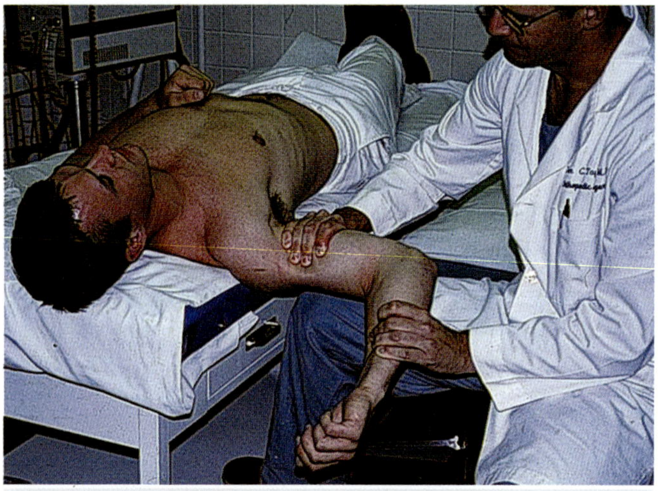

Fig. 1D.2 This clinical photograph shows the performance of the anterior relocation test. The addition of a posteriorly directed force to the anterior proximal arm results in relief of patient apprehension in the abducted, externally rotated position. (Reprinted from Romeo A, Provencher M, eds. *Shoulder Instability: A Comprehensive Approach.* Philadelphia: Saunders; 2016.)

may associate a relocation test as relief of pain with the same maneuver; however, this response is consistent with a diagnosis of internal impingement, not anterior instability. Although other tests may be performed for concomitant pathology, the final test specifically for instability is the load and shift (Fig. 1D.3). With an axial load, the humeral head is translated anterior with grade 1 being translation to the edge of the glenoid, grade 2 requiring translation over the glenoid rim but spontaneous reduction, and grade 3 involving translation beyond the glenoid rim that requires manual reduction (Fig. 1D.4). It is critical to assess whether these tests result in a reproduction of symptoms, and they combine to give a picture of the degree of instability and its correlation to symptoms.

Imaging

Plain radiographs remain the first-line imaging with standard anteroposterior (AP), scapular Y, and axillary views most commonly used. The scapular Y may be used to assess the position of the humeral head, but the axillary view is required to confirm position and reduction, especially in acute cases. The West Point view may be useful in evaluating the glenoid rim, and the Stryker notch view is helpful in assessing the extent of Hill-Sachs lesions (Engebretsen & Craig, 1993). In the case of a clear diagnosis of anterior instability without red flags for significant bone loss (i.e., plain radiograph findings, apprehension or instability at lower levels of abduction, low-energy dislocations), these plain radiographs may be sufficient. However, in many cases, advanced imaging such as computed tomography (CT) or MRI is advantageous in surgical planning. MRI has progressed to the point of excellent accuracy in confirming the diagnosis of injury to the capsulolabral complex (Flannigan et al, 1990; Gusmer et al, 1996). Although CT has generally been the modality of choice in assessing bone loss and three-dimensional CT at this point is considered the most reliable (Provencher et al, 2010), more recently, MRI has been shown to be an acceptable tool (Gyftopoulos et al, 2015; Owens et al, 2013; Stecco et al, 2013) for this purpose and may obviate the need for multiple three-dimensional scans.

Technique (Video 1D.1)

Every patient undergoing an instability procedure is routinely examined under anesthesia. The degree and direction of humeral translation as well as range of motion are objectively quantified and compared with the contralateral side. This step is vital to assisting in intraoperative decision making because the amount of capsular plication must take into consideration the degree of translation and size of the Bankart lesion (i.e., large translation on examination with small lesion present intraoperatively calls for a more substantial plication or shift). After the examination, the patient is placed in the beach-chair position with the head of the operating table raised 30 degrees. A bump is placed to stabilize the scapula, and the shoulder is prepped and draped with the arm free.

A vertical anterior axillary incision is used and can be identified preemptively by digitally pulling the skin vertically at the coracoid to identify an axillary crease. The incision is carried from directly inferior to the coracoid to the axillary margin. The incision can also be shifted inferiorly into the axilla in female patients for improved cosmesis but does require more superior retraction. Deeper dissection is carried through deltopectoral interval after identification of the cephalic vein, which is most often taken laterally with the deltoid. A Goelet or Richardson retractor is used to retract the deltoid laterally. The clavipectoral fascia is incised just lateral to the "red stripe" or muscular portion of the coracobrachialis and excised to permit visualization. In more muscular patients, the falciform fascial expansion of the pectoralis major tendon can be incised 1 cm inferiorly to assist in exposure. A Hohmann retractor is placed under coracoacromial ligament. Subacromial and subdeltoid

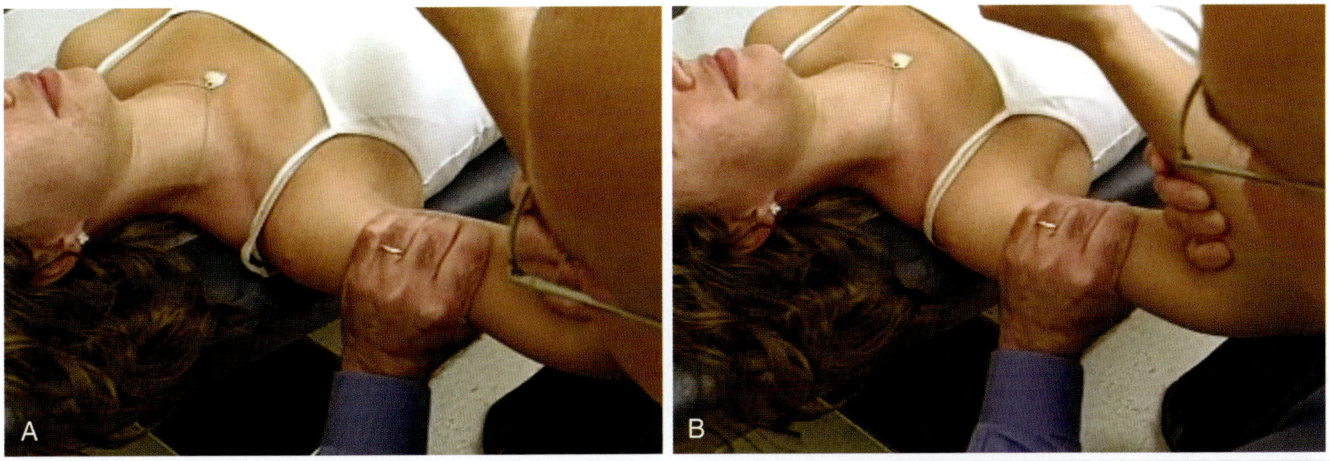

Fig. 1D.3 **A** and **B,** Clinical photographs showing the performance of the anterior load-shift examination. The examiner loads the humerus longitudinally into the glenoid socket and attempts to translate the humeral head over the glenoid rim in the anterior direction. This test also may be performed in the posterior and inferior directions. (Reprinted from Romeo A, Provencher M, eds. *Shoulder Instability: A Comprehensive Approach*. Philadelphia: Saunders; 2016.)

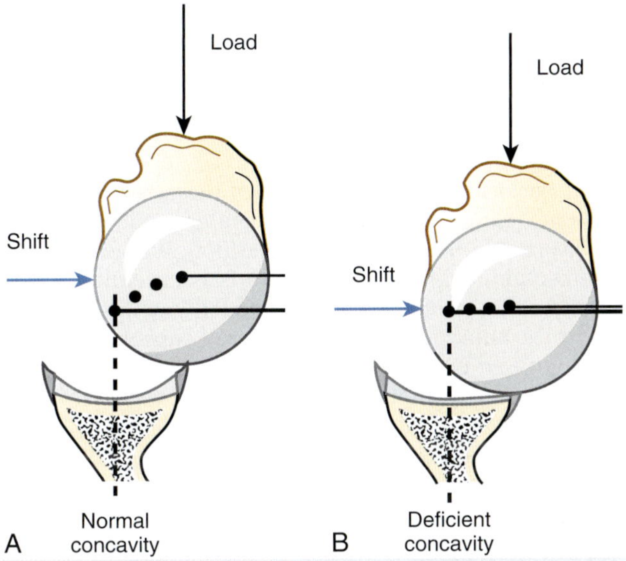

Fig. 1D.4 Load-and-shift test. The adequacy of the glenoid concavity in a given direction can be assessed by compressing the humeral head into the glenoid concavity and noting the amount of displacing force necessary to translate the head. **A** shows a normal concavity, and **B** shows a diminished concavity in the direction of texting. (From Matsen FA, III, et al: *Shoulder Surgery: Principles and Procedures*. Philadelphia: WB Saunders; 2004:113.)

tissue adhesions are freed using a Cobb elevator to facilitate placement of a Brown deltoid or self-retaining retractor. The short flexors and conjoined tendon are then freed digitally and then bluntly retracted, medially exposing the underlying subscapularis while being cognizant to limit prolonged forceful retraction distally because of the musculocutaneous nerve. The Coracoacromial (CA) ligament can be partially incised to assist in mobilizing the short flexors, further aiding visualization. The axillary and often the musculocutaneous nerves can be palpated on the undersurface of the conjoined tendon. The arm is externally rotated, fully exposing the subscapularis tendon. The biceps tendon and rotator interval are visually and palpably identified and serve as the barometer for preparation for the subscapularis tenotomy.

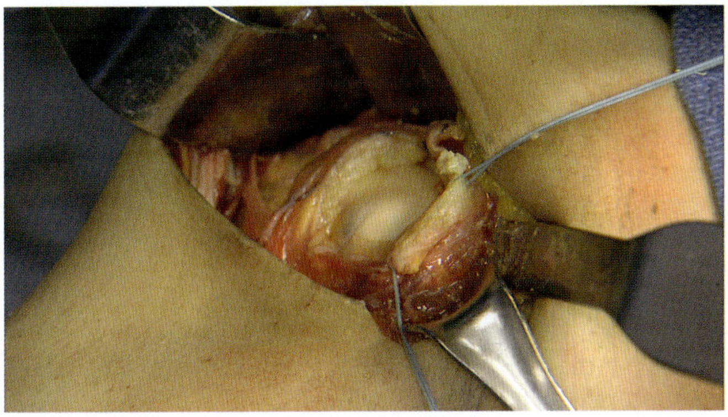

Fig. 1D.5 Cadaveric specimen, right shoulder. When an open Bankart repair is conducted without concomitant shift, the subscapularis and capsule are elevated as one and tagged with heavy nonabsorbable suture for retraction and later repair.

When an isolated Bankart repair is being performed, the subscapularis and underlying capsule are incised and elevated in continuity as one capsulotendinous unit (Fig. 1D.5). The tenotomy is performed beginning at the rotator interval superiorly and carried distally approximately 1.5 cm medial to the bicep tendon with the arm abducted and in external rotation to distance the tenotomy from the axillary nerve. It is important to leave a good cuff of tissue laterally on the greater tuberosity for later subscapularis repair. The lower third of the subscapularis is incised slightly more medially as the insertion becomes more muscular. Discrete branches of the circumflex vessels are coagulated with electrocautery or ligated with silk suture. Two heavy braided stay sutures are placed through the tendon and used for retraction as well as later repair (Fig. 1D.5). Metzenbaum scissors are used to incise the interval from lateral to medial. The humerus is translated laterally, and a Carter-Rowe or Fukuda humeral head retractor is then placed, exposing the glenoid and anterior capsulolabral structures. The blunt right-angled retractor previously used for retracting the conjoined tendon medially is replaced intra-articularly, reflecting the capsular-tendinous flap medially. The Bankart lesion is then clearly visualized and mobilized with a

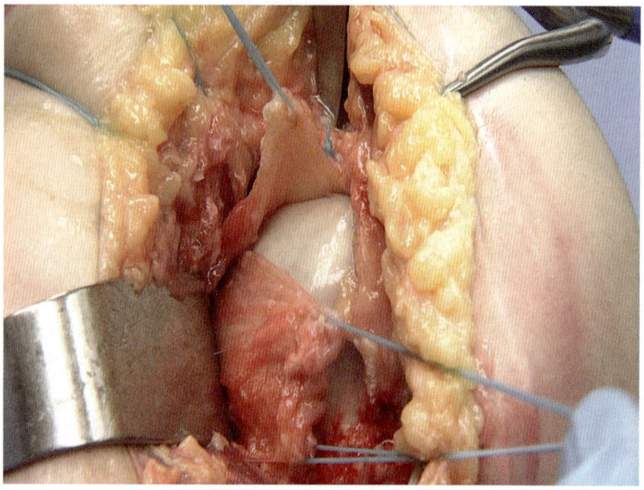

Fig. 1D.6 Cadaveric specimen, left shoulder. Inferior and superior leaflets of the laterally based T-capsulotomy are tagged in preparation for advancement of the inferior flap, obliterating the anterior inferior capsular redundancy.

series of elevators exposing the underlying anterior glenoid bone. The mobilization of the lesion is complete when the undersurface of the subscapularis is visible within the lesion medially. In larger lesions, a cleated anterior glenoid retractor can be placed inside the labral lesion to facilitate exposure of the bone bed. The bony anterior glenoid is then prepared biologically using manually powered rasps or curettage. In the typical Bankart lesion, three resorbable 3.0-mm single-loaded anchors with nonabsorbable stitch (SutureTak; Arthrex, Naples, FL) are placed beginning as low as the 5:30 or 6 o'clock position inferiorly. These anchors are placed directly onto the anterior margin glenoid face with attention paid to avoid medialization of the repair. Following anchor placement, the anterior glenoid retractor is removed. A tapered free needle or arthroscopic suture shuttle (Suture Lasso; Arthrex) is used to pass suture through the capsulolabral tissue. The amount of capsular tissue incorporated into the repair depends on the amount of instability present on examination, the quality of the capsular tissue, and the size of the labral tear. In general, a 5- to 7-mm capsular plication is performed; however, too-aggressive plication will place undue tension on the subscapularis repair later in the operation (Fig. 1D.6). Simple stitches are then tied, although one could consider mattress configuration by passing both limbs of the anchor through the capsule, thereby placing the knots extraarticular. This completes the Bankart repair. The subscapularis is then repaired using #5 braided nonabsorbable stitch in Mason Allen fashion from proximal to distal, typically using the two sutures that previously passed initially and o additional sutures. The degree of interval closure is titrated to the degree of stability gained and quality of tissue at the repair and is most often executed with two sutures incorporating 2 to 3 mm of interval and subscapularis tissue passed in figure-of-eight fashion. A standard layered interval and skin closure follows. Drains are typically not used.

In more complex anterior instability cases, including those involving glenoid bone loss of more than 10% to 15%, poor capsulolabral tissue, history of numerous dislocations, or patients with multidirectional laxity, an anterior capsular shift may be performed with Bankart repair. This repair represents two procedures with some concern for "overtightening" and increased potential for restricted motion. Performing a concomitant capsular shift requires several deviations from the described technique. After isolation of the subscapularis, but prior to tenotomy, the inferior lateral margin of the subscapularis is incised transversely, just superior to transverse humeral vessels. Metzenbaum scissors are then placed into the incision, under the subscapularis, and advanced superiorly into the interval bluntly separating capsule from subscapularis tendon. A tenotomy is then performed directly on top of the scissors allowing a sufficient lateral cuff of tissue for later tendinous repair. Nonabsorbable heavy braided retention stitches are used for retraction, and the subscapularis is carefully, bluntly dissected inferolaterally to superomedially with scissors.

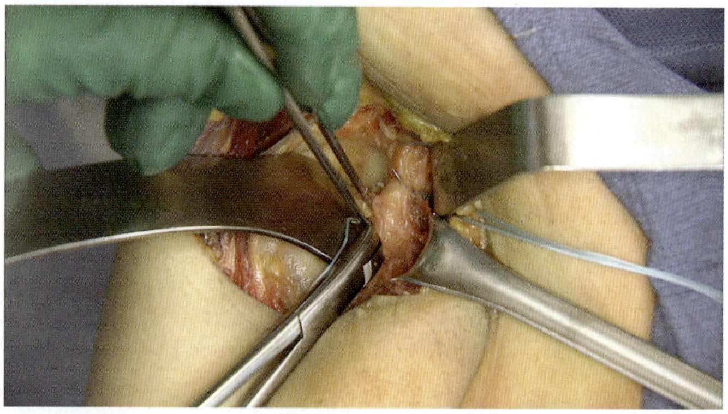

Fig. 1D.7 Cadaveric specimen, right shoulder. A capsulorrhaphy is incorporated into the labral repair and must be tailored to the patient.

With the subscapularis reflected and capsule exposed, a laterally based cruciate or "T" capsulotomy is performed. Laterally, the capsular incision is carried vertically to the rotator interval. The inferior leaflet is dissected off the humeral neck inferiorly to permit appropriate obliteration of the anterior-inferior pouch when advanced. The transverse limb of the cruciate capsular incision is made at the midglenoid level and extended medially to the labral margin. Superior and inferior leaflets are tagged laterally and retracted, and the Bankart repair is conducted as described earlier, with the "north–south" capsular shift performed after completion (see Fig. 1D.6). Adequate capsular release and mobilization of the leaflets can be appreciated palpably by placing a digit into the inferior pouch, which should collapse when the leaflet is advanced, or visibly as the exposed humeral articular surface should be nearly covered with simulated shift (Fig. 1D.7). The rotator interval is then closed laterally to form a firm foundation to base or "hang" the inferior shift. The inferior capsular leaflet is then mobilized superiorly. In preparation for capsular repair, the shoulder is placed in 30 degrees of abduction and external rotation. The first stitch is a corner stitch that will "set" the degree of shift and is followed by three additional mattress sutures inferiorly for additional security. The superior reconstruction is conducted by taking the superior leaflet inferiorly, over the top of the inferior flap, and securing it laterally with two sutures. Careful attention is paid not to suture the superior leaflet to its inferior counterpart because this can cause increased tension at the inferior capsular repair. The subscapularis is then repaired as described earlier.

Although less commonly encountered, HAGL lesions can be effectively managed using the traditional open techniques. An open, trans-subscapularis technique is used in cases of anterior lesions. The standard deltopectoral approach to expose the subscapularis is conducted as described earlier; however, the axillary incision can be made smaller using only the inferior 5 cm. Through this incision, the subcutaneous tissues are elevated from underlying fascia to increase mobility of the subcutaneous "window" as the interval outlined by the bicep tendon sheath laterally, subscapularis tendon medially, and pectoralis major tendon inferior is identified. Blunt dissection scissors are then used to establish a tissue plane between the capsule and subscapularis. This is done by penetrating the subscapularis in line with its fibers just superior and medial to the circumflex vessels, advancing the scissors superiorly approximately 2 cm, and then opening the blades creating a clear soft tissue plane. An L-shaped subscapularis tenotomy is performed, making a vertically subscapularis tendon incision 1.5 cm medial to the bicep tendon, and is directed from the midtendon inferiorly to just superior to the circumflex vessels. The incision is then taken from the inferior margin laterally to complete the "L." A stitch is placed in the subscapularis, allowing retraction and facilitating further separation from the underlying capsule. The humerus is then externally rotated and abducted to identify the avulsed capsule. The axillary nerve is identified medially by palpation and protected. After the lesion has been fully exposed, a direct repair is done using 3-mm anchors double loaded with braided nonabsorbable suture. Arthroscopic suture-passing instruments can be very helpful when working in the confined space of the axillary pouch. After repair, a standard tenotomy repair and closure is performed.

Rehabilitation

In general, patients undergoing open stabilization for anterior/inferior instability are placed in a sling secured anteriorly across the abdomen positioning the shoulder in neutral to slight internal rotation. Passive range of motion is initiated immediately, restricting supine external rotation to neutral for the first 2 weeks and then increasing to 30 degrees from postoperative weeks 2 to 4. After week 4, the sling is weaned, active range of motion is initiated, and external rotation is gradually increased to 45 degrees by week 8. Resistance training is initiated 6 weeks postoperatively, including internal and external rotation strengthening with bands and manual resistance scapular stabilization drills. Weeks 8 to 12 focus on regaining terminal external rotation and transitioning to restricted weight training. General restrictions focus on avoidance of anterior capsular stress and include keeping the hands within eyesight; keeping the elbows bent; and minimizing overhead activities such as military press, pull-downs, and so on. Conventional weight training commences at week 16. Reintroduction to sport generally begins at 4 months in both contact and overhead athletes with full return by 6 months.

Complications

Recurrent instability is of most concern, is well documented, and the most commonly cited complication after shoulder stabilization procedures. Recurrence after open repair is 5% or less in the vast majority of studies. Several series have shown similarly low rates of recurrence in collision athletes undergoing open procedures. Additionally, a meta-analysis including 18 studies reported a higher risk of recurrent instability (18% vs 8%) and reoperation Relative Risk ((RR), 2.32) in patients undergoing arthroscopic stabilization procedures compared with open (Freedman, 2004).

Subscapularis failure and secondary dysfunction are complications inherent to open stabilization procedures and a clear distinction from arthroscopic repairs. Rates of reoperation for subscapularis rupture after tenotomy for open stabilization have been reported as high as 4.5% (Greis et al, 1996, Hatch et al, 2016, Hiemstra et al, 2008, Mohtadi et al, 2014). However, numerous additional series do not report any revisions caused by postoperative subscapularis tendon disruption. Conversely, motion restriction and stiffness can occur. However, Pagnani (2008) reported no patient lost more than 15 degrees in a series of 58 professional athletes. The risks of postoperative subscapularis failure or stiffness highlight the importance of tailoring the capsulorrhaphy to the patient's clinical examination, meticulous surgical technique, and subscapularis repair as well as carefully monitored rehabilitation.

Damage to neurovascular structures and secondary dysfunction, although rare, have been reported. The axillary nerve must be identified and protected throughout the procedure. External rotation and abduction of the humerus during exposure and dissection increase the distance of the nerve from the surgical field. If self-retaining retractors are used on the conjoined tendon, they should be kept proximal avoiding excessive tension and prolonged placement to prevent undue traction on the musculocutaneous nerve. Wound complications are rare, and the vertical axillary incision, in our experience, has been cosmetically favorable.

Conclusion

Open Bankart repair and anterior stabilization procedures in the care of injured athletes' shoulders remains a powerful instrument in shoulder surgeons' toolbox. Their role is critically important in young collision athletes whose risk for recurrent instability and its implications are the highest. The literature supports open techniques for stabilization in contact athletes because the outcomes appear superior to arthroscopic techniques in this high-risk subset. Although complications inherent to open shoulder procedures exist, they can be mitigated with refined technique and appropriate rehabilitation. Despite arthroscopic advances, there lies a clear place for open capsulolabral reconstruction in the shoulder surgeons' armamentarium for management of anterior instability.

References

An VV, Sivakumar BS, Phan K, Trantalis J. A systematic review and meta-analysis of clinical and patient-reported outcomes following two procedures for recurrent traumatic anterior instability of the shoulder: latarjet procedure vs. Bankart repair. *J Shoulder Elbow Surg*. 2016;25(5):853–863.

Athwal GS, Meislin R, Getz C, Weinstein D, Favorito P. Short-term complications of the arthroscopic Latarjet procedure: a North American experience. *Arthroscopy*. 2016;32(10):1965–1970.

Bhatia S, Frank RM, Ghodadra NS, et al. The outcomes and surgical techniques of the Latarjet procedure. *Arthroscopy*. 2014;30(2):227–235.

Bigliani LU, Newton PM, Steinmann SP, Connor PM, McIlveen SJ. Glenoid rim lesions associated with recurrent anterior dislocation of the shoulder. *Am J Sports Med.* 1998;26(1):41–45.

Bottoni CR, Smith EL, Berkowitz MJ, Towle RB, Moore JH. Arthroscopic versus open shoulder stabilization for recurrent anterior instability: a prospective randomized clinical trial. *Am J Sports Med.* 2006;34(11):1730–1737.

Burkhart SS, De Beer JF. Traumatic glenohumeral bone defects and their relationship to failure of arthroscopic Bankart repairs: significance of the inverted-pear glenoid and the humeral engaging Hill-Sachs lesion. *Arthroscopy*. 2000;16(7):677–694.

Castagna A, Delle Rose G, Borroni M, et al. Arthroscopic stabilization of the shoulder in adolescent athletes participating in overhead or contact sports. *Arthroscopy*. 2012;28(3):309–315.

Cho NS, Hwang JC, Rhee YG. Arthroscopic stabilization in anterior shoulder instability: collision athletes versus noncollision athletes. *Arthroscopy*. 2006;22(9):947–953.

Cho NS, Yi JW, Lee BG, Rhee YG. Revision open Bankart surgery after arthroscopic repair for traumatic anterior shoulder instability. *Am J Sports Med.* 2009;37(11):2158–2164.

Cole BJ, L'Insalata J, Irrgang J, Warner JJ. Comparison of arthroscopic and open anterior shoulder stabilization. A two to six-year follow-up study. *J Bone Joint Surg Am.* 2000;82-A(8):1108–1114.

Degen RM, Camp CL, Werner BC, Dines DM, Dines JS. Trends in bone-block augmentation among recently trained orthopaedic surgeons treating anterior shoulder instability. *J Bone Joint Surg Am.* 2016;98(13):e56.

Engebretsen L, Craig EV. Radiologic features of shoulder instability. *Clin Orthop Relat Res.* 1993;291:29–44.

Fabbriciani C, Milano G, Demontis A, Fadda S, Ziranu F, Mulas PD. Arthroscopic versus open treatment of Bankart lesion of the shoulder: a prospective randomized study. *Arthroscopy*. 2004;20(5):456–462.

Flannigan B, Kursunoglu-Brahme S, Snyder S, Karzel R, Del Pizzo W, Resnick D. MR arthrography of the shoulder: comparison with conventional MR imaging. *AJR Am J Roentgenol.* 1990;155(4):829–832.

Freedman KB, Smith AP, Romeo AA, Cole BJ, Bach BR Jr. Open Bankart repair versus arthroscopic repair with transglenoid sutures or bioabsorbable tacks for recurrent anterior instability of the shoulder: a meta-analysis. *Am J Sports Med.* 2004;32(6):1520–1527.

Garcia GH, Taylor SA, Fabricant PD, Dines JS. Shoulder instability management: a survey of the American Shoulder and Elbow Surgeons. *Am J Orthop (Belle Mead NJ)*. 2016;45(3):E91–E97.

Gill TJ, Micheli LJ, Gebhard F, Binder C. Bankart repair for anterior instability of the shoulder. Long-term outcome. *J Bone Joint Surg Am.* 1997;79(6):850–857.

Greis PE, Dean M, Hawkins RJ. Subscapularis tendon disruption after Bankart reconstruction for anterior instability. *J Shoulder Elbow Surg.* 1996;5(3):219–222.

Gusmer PB, Potter HG, Schatz JA, et al. Labral injuries: accuracy of detection with unenhanced MR imaging of the shoulder. *Radiology*. 1996;200(2):519–524.

Gyftopoulos S, Beltran LS, Bookman J, Rokito A. MRI evaluation of bipolar bone loss using the on-track off-track method: a feasibility study. *AJR Am J Roentgenol.* 2015;205(4):848–852.

Hatch MD, Hennrikus WL. The open Bankart repair for traumatic anterior shoulder instability in teenage athletes. *J Pediatr Orthop.* 2016 Mar 3. [Epub ahead of print].

Hattrup SJ, Cofield RH, Weaver AL. Anterior shoulder reconstruction: prognostic variables. *J Shoulder Elbow Surg.* 2001;10(6):508–513.

Hiemstra LA, Sasyniuk TM, Mohtadi NG, Fick GH. Shoulder strength after open versus arthroscopic stabilization. *Am J Sports Med.* 2008;36(5):861–867.

Hubbell JD, Ahmad S, Bezenoff LS, Fond J, Pettrone FA. Comparison of shoulder stabilization using arthroscopic transglenoid sutures versus open capsulolabral repairs: a 5-year minimum follow-up. *Am J Sports Med.* 2004;32(3):650–654.

Karlsson J, Magnusson L, Ejerhed L, Hultenheim I, Lundin O, Kartus J. Comparison of open and arthroscopic stabilization for recurrent shoulder dislocation in patients with a Bankart lesion. *Am J Sports Med.* 2001;29(5):538–542.

Kim SH, Ha KI. Bankart repair in traumatic anterior shoulder instability: open versus arthroscopic technique. *Arthroscopy*. 2002;18(7):755–763.

Lenters TR, Franta AK, Wolf FM, Leopold SS, Matsen FA 3rd. Arthroscopic compared with open repairs for recurrent anterior shoulder instability. A systematic review and meta-analysis of the literature. *J Bone Joint Surg Am.* 2007;89(2):244–254.

Levine WN, Arroyo JS, Pollock RG, Flatow EL, Bigliani LU. Open revision stabilization surgery for recurrent anterior glenohumeral instability. *Am J Sports Med.* 2000;28(2):156–160.

Longo UG, Rizzello G, Ciuffreda M, et al. Humeral avulsion of the glenohumeral ligaments: a systematic review. *Arthroscopy*. 2016;32(9):1868–1876.

Lützner J, Krummenauer F, Lübke J, Kirschner S, Günther KP, Bottesi M. Functional outcome after open and arthroscopic Bankart repair for traumatic shoulder instability. *Eur J Med Res.* 2009;14(1):18–24.

Mahiroğulları M, Ozkan H, Akyüz M, Uğraş AA, Güney A, Kuşkucu M. Comparison between the results of open and arthroscopic repair of isolated traumatic anterior instability of the shoulder. *Acta Orthop Traumatol Turc.* 2010;44(3):180–185.

Malhotra A, Freudmann MS, Hay SM. Management of traumatic anterior shoulder dislocation in the 17- to 25-year age group: a dramatic evolution of practice. *J Shoulder Elbow Surg.* 2012;21(4):545–553.

Meehan RE, Petersen SA. Results and factors affecting outcome of revision surgery for shoulder instability. *J Shoulder Elbow Surg.* 2005;14(1):31–37.

Mohtadi NG, Bitar IJ, Sasyniuk TM, Hollinshead RM, Harper WP. Arthroscopic versus open repair for traumatic anterior shoulder instability: a meta-analysis. *Arthroscopy*. 2005;21(6):652–658.

Mohtadi NG, Chan DS, Hollinshead RM, et al. A randomized clinical trial comparing open and arthroscopic stabilization for recurrent traumatic anterior shoulder instability: two-year follow-up with disease-specific quality-of-life outcomes. *J Bone Joint Surg Am.* 2014;96(5):353–360.

Neviaser AS, Benke MT, Neviaser RJ. Open Bankart repair for revision of failed prior stabilization: outcome analysis at a mean of more than 10 years. *J Shoulder Elbow Surg.* 2015;24(6):897–901.

Owens BD, Burns TC, Campbell SE, Svoboda SJ, Cameron KL. Simple method of glenoid bone loss calculation using ipsilateral magnetic resonance imaging. *Am J Sports Med.* 2013;41(3):622–624.

Owens BD, Harrast JJ, Hurwitz SR, Thompson TL, Wolf JM. Surgical trends in Bankart repair: an analysis of data from the American Board of Orthopaedic Surgery certification examination. *Am J Sports Med.* 2011;39(9):1865–1869.

Pagnani MJ. Open capsular repair without bone block for recurrent anterior shoulder instability in patients with and without bony defects of the glenoid and/or humeral head. *Am J Sports Med.* 2008;36(9):1805–1812.

Pagnani MJ, Dome DC. Surgical treatment of traumatic anterior shoulder instability in American football players. *J Bone Joint Surg Am.* 2002;84-A(5):711–715.

Petrera M, Patella V, Patella S, Theodoropoulos J. A meta-analysis of open versus arthroscopic Bankart repair using suture anchors. *Knee Surg Sports Traumatol Arthrosc.* 2010;18(12):1742–1747.

Postacchini F, Gumina S, Cinotti G. Anterior shoulder dislocation in adolescents. *J Shoulder Elbow Surg.* 2000;9(6):470–474.

Provencher MT, Bhatia S, Ghodadra NS, et al. Recurrent shoulder instability: current concepts for evaluation and management of glenoid bone loss. *J Bone Joint Surg Am.* 2010;92(suppl 2):133–151.

Rhee YG, Ha JH, Cho NS. Anterior shoulder stabilization in collision athletes: arthroscopic versus open Bankart repair. *Am J Sports Med.* 2006;34(6):979–985.

Rhee YG, Lim CT, Cho NS. Muscle strength after anterior shoulder stabilization: arthroscopic versus open Bankart repair. *Am J Sports Med.* 2007;35(11):1859–1864.

Robinson CM, Howes J, Murdoch H, Will E, Graham C. Functional outcome and risk of recurrent instability after primary traumatic anterior shoulder dislocation in young patients. *J Bone Joint Surg Am.* 2006;88(11):2326–2336.

Rowe CR, Patel D, Southmayd WW. The Bankart procedure: a long-term end-result study. *J Bone Joint Surg Am.* 1978;60(1):1–16.

Rowe CR, Pierce DS, Clark JG. Voluntary dislocation of the shoulder. A preliminary report on a clinical, electromyographic, and psychiatric study of twenty-six patients. *J Bone Joint Surg Am.* 1973;55(3):445–460.

Rowe CR, Zarins B, Ciullo JV. Recurrent anterior dislocation of the shoulder after surgical repair. Apparent causes of failure and treatment. *J Bone Joint Surg Am.* 1984;66(2):159–168.

Sachs RA, Williams B, Stone ML, Paxton L, Kuney M. Open Bankart repair: correlation of results with postoperative subscapularis function. *Am J Sports Med.* 2005;33(10):1458–1462.

Scheibel M, Tsynman A, Magosch P, Schroeder RJ, Habermeyer P. Postoperative subscapularis muscle insufficiency after primary and revision open shoulder stabilization. *Am J Sports Med.* 2006;34(10):1586–1593.
Shah AA, Butler RB, Romanowski J, Goel D, Karadagli D, Warner JJ. Short-term complications of the Latarjet procedure. *J Bone Joint Surg Am.* 2012;94(6):495–501.
Sisto DJ. Revision of failed arthroscopic Bankart repairs. *Am J Sports Med.* 2007;35(4):537–541.
Sperber A, Hamberg P, Karlsson J, Swärd L, Wredmark T. Comparison of an arthroscopic and an open procedure for posttraumatic instability of the shoulder: a prospective, randomized multicenter study. *J Shoulder Elbow Surg.* 2001;10(2):105–108.
Stecco A, Guenzi E, Cascone T, et al. MRI can assess glenoid bone loss after shoulder luxation: inter- and intra-individual comparison with CT. *Radiol Med.* 2013;118(8):1335–1343.
Tjoumakaris FP, Abboud JA, Hasan SA, Ramsey ML, Williams GR. Arthroscopic and open Bankart repairs provide similar outcomes. *Clin Orthop Relat Res.* 2006;446:227–232.
Wang L, Liu Y1, Su X1, Liu S1. A meta-analysis of arthroscopic versus open repair for treatment of Bankart lesions in the shoulder. *Med Sci Monit.* 2015;21:3028–3035.
Wheeler JH, Ryan JB, Arciero RA, Molinari RN. Arthroscopic versus non-operative treatment of acute shoulder dislocations in young athletes. *Arthroscopy.* 1989;5(3):213–217.
Yamamoto N, Kijima H, Nagamoto H, et al. Outcome of Bankart repair in contact versus non-contact athletes. *Orthop Traumatol Surg Res.* 2015;101(4):415–419.
Zabinski SJ, Callaway GH, Cohen S, Warren RF. Revision shoulder stabilization: 2- to 10-year results. *J Shoulder Elbow Surg.* 1999;8(1):58–65.
Zaffagnini S, Marcheggiani Muccioli GM, et al. Long-term outcomes after repair of recurrent post-traumatic anterior shoulder instability: comparison of arthroscopic transglenoid suture and open Bankart reconstruction. *Knee Surg Sports Traumatol Arthrosc.* 2012;20(5):816–821.
Zhang AL, Montgomery SR, Ngo SS, Hame SL, Wang JC, Gamradt SC. Arthroscopic versus open shoulder stabilization: current practice patterns in the United States. *Arthroscopy.* 2014;30(4):436–443.

1-1E GLENOID BONE LOSS: OPEN LATARJET

MATTHEW T. PROVENCHER, MD, CAPT, MC, USNR, ANTHONY SANCHEZ, BS, GEORGE SANCHEZ, BS, and TISTIA GASTON, PA-C

Introduction

- Glenoid bone loss is a commonly encountered contributing pathology to recurrent anterior glenohumeral instability.
- The open Latarjet procedure is an established, validated technique that addresses this pathology via reconstruction of the bony defect and reinforcement of the surrounding associated supporting tissues, restoring stability.
- Proper execution of this technique starts with patient selection informed by physical examination and imaging studies and depends on appropriate coracoid process harvest, transfer, and fixation. Procedure outcomes are ensured by postoperative rehabilitation focused on graft union optimization.

Patient Selection

Indications

The Latarjet procedure is indicated for patients with recurrent anterior instability, significant loss in the glenoid or humeral bone, and failed prior Bankart repairs. In particular, the Bankart failure rate has been shown to increase from 4% to 67% with significant bone loss, specifically defined as greater than 25% loss of the inferior glenoid diameter giving an "inverted pear" appearance, wherein the inferior glenoid has a smaller diameter than the superior glenoid (de Beer & Roberts, 2010; Young et al, 2011). The incidence rates of bone defects in cases of chronic anterior shoulder instability have been radiographically identified to include a bony lesion rate, humeral or glenoid, of 95% with a humeral impaction fracture rate of 73.1% (Edwards et al, 2003). Patients with an inverted-pear glenoid have been previously reported to have a 67% failure rate after Bankart repair versus a 4.9% recurrence rate after open modified Latarjet.

Additionally, it is important to recognize the limitations of the Latarjet procedure and thus when it is contraindicated. When more than one third of the articular surface of the anterior glenoid is fractured or depleted, the coracoid is not sufficient. In these cases and after a failed Latarjet procedure, reconstruction is performed with an iliac crest bone graft or distal tibial allograft (Lunn et al, 2008; Provencher et al, 2009; Warner et al, 2006).

Physical Examination

As part of a standardized preoperative physical examination to rule out other pathologies, range of motion, rotator cuff, neurovascular status, and posterior instability are tested in addition to anterior stability. Using the Quality Assessment of Diagnostic Accuracy Studies (QUADAS) tool, the diagnostic accuracy of individual anterior instability physical examination tests was measured (Hegedus et al, 2008; Whiting et al, 2004). In descending order from high to low diagnostic accuracy the available tests for assessing anterior instability ranked as follows: relocation or Jobe relocation test (Farber et al, 2006; Lo et al, 2004a; Speer et al, 1994), Apprehension (Farber et al, 2006; Lo et al, 2004a), anterior release/surprise test (Gross & Distefano, 1997; Lo et al, 2004a), anterior drawer test (Farber et al, 2006), and anterior-superior instability with an anterior supraspinatus tear (SLAC lesion) tests (load and shift test, anterior-superior SLAP test, active compression or O'Brien test, Kibler test, and Whipple test [Savoie et al, 2001]).

Key Clues from History and Physical Examination That Suggest a Diagnosis of Glenoid Bone Loss

During assessment of a patient with recurrent anterior instability and possible glenoid bone loss, certain key clues will allude to a diagnosis of bone loss. These clues should be sought and considered for a definitive diagnosis. In regard to history, the patient should report a prolonged history of instability as well as a previous high-energy mechanism of injury. Most important, the patient should note most instability occurs in midrange of motion (20–60 degrees of abduction) because this highly suggests bone loss. During physical examination, shoulder apprehension should be very apparent in midranges of abduction (30–90 degrees) and less apparent in external rotation. Last, anterior translation of the humeral head over the glenoid rim should be reproducible (Provencher et al, 2010).

Preoperative Imaging and Arthroscopic Validation

The main method for detection of glenoid bone loss is the circle method on three dimensionally reconstructed computed tomography described by Sugaya et al (2003) This technique consists of performing imaging with three-dimensional (3D) computed tomography (CT) (Bishop et al, 2013; Rerko et al, 2013), which has been demonstrated to be the most reliable imaging modality, and subsequently using processing software to obtain the en face image of the glenoid fossa with the humeral head digitally subtracted in order to quantify bone loss. The area of the displayed osseous fragment or erosion traced by the particular software over the area of a best-fit circle based on the inferior two thirds glenoid contour from 3 to 9 o'clock is used to calculate total bone loss (Baudi et al, 2005; Sugaya et al, 2003). The glenoid bone loss quantification measure obtained by the circle method can then be reaffirmed arthroscopically. An arthroscope is used through the anterosuperior portal while a calibrated probe is inserted via the posterior portal to measure the distance from the anterior and posterior rims to the bare spot (Lo et al, 2004b). Despite questions as to bare spot landmark consistency, arthroscopic measurement is still well documented and is routine when planning an open Latarjet procedure (Kralinger et al, 2006).

Preferred Technique for Measurement of Glenoid Bone Loss

For measurement of glenoid bone loss, the senior author (MTP) prefers the use of the ratio method, which uses the intersection between the longitudinal axis and the widest anteroposterior diameter of the glenoid in an en face view of the glenoid on CT scan (Barchilon et al, 2008). With the bare area approximated, a best-fit circle is centered on the inferior two thirds of the glenoid. The distance from the bare spot to the edge of the defect is measured (d) as well as the radius of the best-fit circle (R). The ratio d/R is then inserted into the equation shown in Fig. 1E.1 for quantification of percent bone loss (Barchilon et al, 2008).

Preferred Surgical Technique

POSITIONING AND PREPARATION

After interscalene block placement and general anesthesia induction, the patient is placed in a modified beach-chair position with the head of the bed elevated 40 degrees (Arrington et al, 2011). Two folded towels are placed under the medial border of the ipsilateral scapula to flatten and stabilize the scapula. The arm is draped free to allow for intraoperative abduction and external rotation. To prevent the arm from dangling and shifting when not being manipulated, a pneumatic limb positioner (Smith & Nephew, Andover, MA) or a padded Mayo stand is used.

EXPOSURE AND APPROACH

An arthroscopic confirmation of diagnosis and extent of osseous deficiency is performed, and any concurrent intraarticular pathology may be treated at this point. An oblique 5- to 7-cm incision is made from the tip of the coracoid process and extending inferiorly down the deltopectoral groove to the superior portion of the axillary fold (Young & Walch, 2011). While maintaining hemostasis, a standard deltopectoral approach is used. The cephalic vein and its consistent medial branches are protected and gently retracted laterally with the deltoid musculature (Young

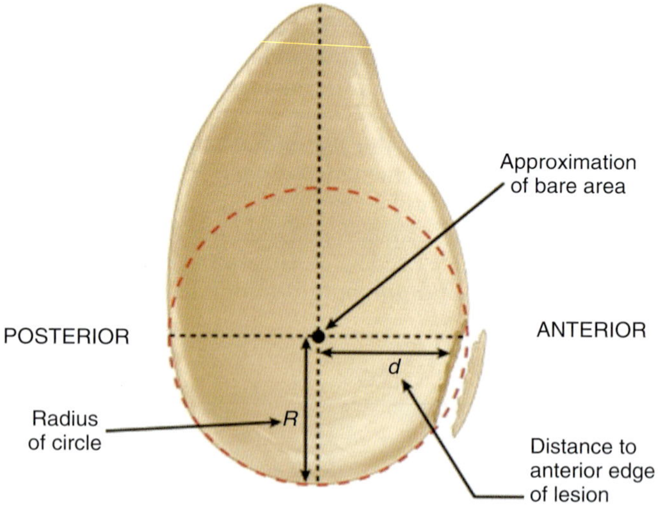

$$\text{Percent bone loss} = \frac{1}{\pi}\left(\cos^{-1}\left(\frac{d}{R}\right) - \left(\frac{d}{R}\sqrt{1-\left(\frac{d}{R}\right)^2}\right)\right)$$

Fig. 1E.1 Measurement of glenoid bone loss based on ratios. An en face view of the glenoid is acquired via computed tomography scan. At the intersection of the longitudinal axis and the widest anteroposterior diameter of the glenoid, the bare area is noted. A best-fit circle centered at the bare spot is then drawn about the inferior two thirds of the glenoid *(dashed red line)*. The distance to the anterior edge (d) is measured and compared with the radius (R). The ratio of d/R is entered into the equation shown for quantification of percent bone loss. (From Provencher MT, Romeo AA: *Shoulder Instability: A Comprehensive Approach.* Philadelphia: Saunders; 2012.)

et al, 2011). A self-retaining Kolbel retractor is placed between the pectoralis major and deltoid to maintain exposure. If more exposure is desired, a Hohmann retractor over the top of the coracoid may be used while the arm is in abduction and external rotation.

CORACOID GRAFT HARVEST

With proper coracoid exposure and the arm in external rotation and abduction, Mayo scissors are used to further expose the coracoid from its tip all the way to the insertion of the coracoclavicular ligaments at the coracoid base. The CA ligament is identified and sharply transected 1 cm laterally off its coracoid insertion (Fig. 1E.2). It is important to harvest 1 cm of this ligament so it can later be incorporated into the capsular repair to yield the bumper effect. To improve exposure on the medial side of the coracoid, the arm is now placed in adduction and internal rotation. The pectoralis minor is released directly from the coracoid by taking down its insertion sharply with an elevator, with care to protect the neurovascular structures inferiorly with a blunt retractor. The release should not continue past the tip of the coracoid to avoid risk to the graft blood supply. Using a periosteal elevator, excess soft tissue is removed from the undersurface of the coracoid. Palpation to identify and protect the axillary and musculocutaneous nerves is necessary throughout the coracoid exposure.

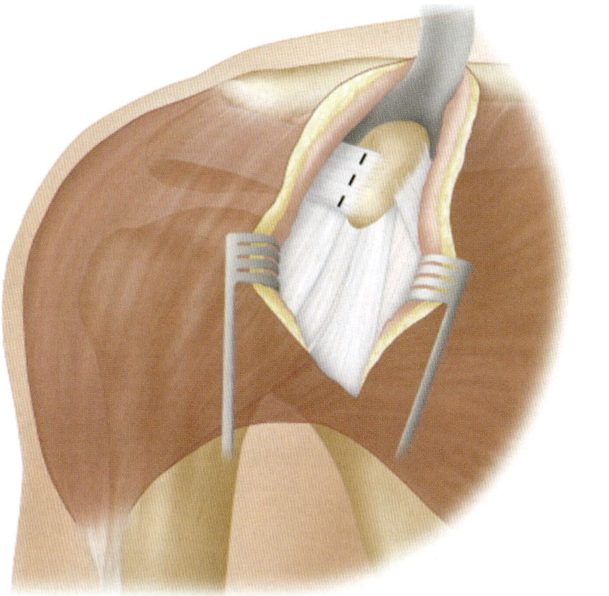

Fig. 1E.2 The coracoacromial ligament is incised 1 cm from the coracoid insertion (arm in externally rotated position). Note the position of the Hohmann retractor over the top of the coracoid process. (From Provencher MT, Romeo AA: *Shoulder Instability: A Comprehensive Approach*. Philadelphia: Saunders; 2012.)

Using a 90-degree oscillating saw blade, a medial-to-lateral osteotomy of the coracoid is created at a line just anterior to the coracoclavicular ligament insertion at the coracoid base (Young & Walch, 2011). Ensure that the coracoid graft will be 22 to 25 mm in length from the tip using a ruler (Fig. 1E.3). Make sure that the osteotomy is done perpendicular to the coracoid process to avoid accidentally extending it to the glenoid articular surface. An angled saw is used instead of a half-inch osteotome because the saw is less likely to cause iatrogenic glenoid fracture. Levering on the fragment with an osteotome can assist in completing the osteotomy but should be avoided if possible to avoid splitting the fragment. Chandler elevators are positioned inferior and medial to the coracoid to protect vital neurovascular structures. The blood supply to the graft enters the coracoid at the medial aspect of the insertion of the conjoined tendon; care is taken not to disturb it while performing the osteotomy. After the osteotomy, toothed grasping forceps are used to gently hold the graft at the level of the incision, and the coracohumeral ligament is released to liberate the coracoid.

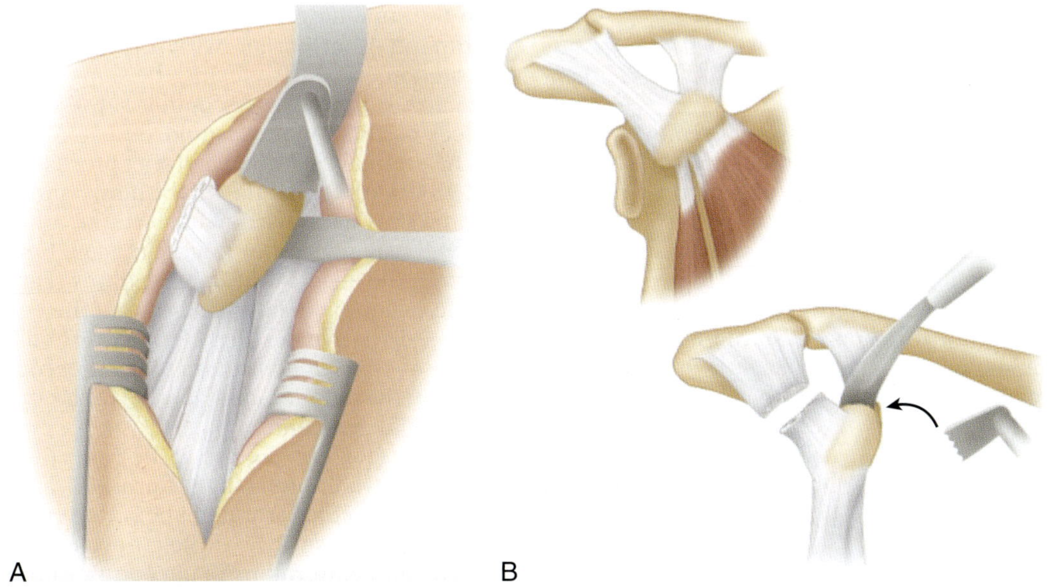

Fig. 1E.3 **A,** The coracoid is first exposed to carry out a successful osteotomy. **B,** After release of the pectoralis minor and preparation of the inferior aspect of the coracoid with a periosteal elevator, the osteotomy is performed at the "knee" of the coracoid (i.e., distal to the coracoclavicular ligaments) (arm in adducted, internally rotated position). (From Provencher MT, Romeo AA: *Shoulder Instability: A Comprehensive Approach*. Philadelphia: Saunders; 2012.)

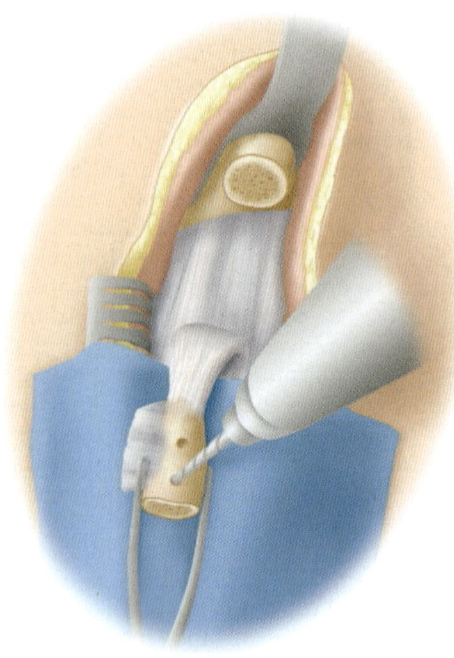

Fig. 1E.4 Preparation of the coracoid process. A gauze sponge is used to protect the skin. (From Provencher MT, Romeo AA: *Shoulder Instability: A Comprehensive Approach*. Philadelphia: Saunders; 2012.)

The musculocutaneous nerve is then identified and released from the posterior fascia of the conjoined tendon, just until it dives into muscle approximately 4 to 7 cm from the coracoid tip. The coracoid is brought out of the incision more than 1 to 2 cm to avoid any tension on the musculocutaneous nerve. It is paramount to completely release all soft tissue adhesion on the posterior aspect of the conjoint tendon to allow for ease of coracoid transfer. Moreover, the musculocutaneous nerve is also visualized and gently released until all tension is freed all the way up to the musculocutaneous nerve insertion into the muscle. The arm is now returned to the neutral position.

CORACOID GRAFT PREPARATION

Using a scalpel, any remaining soft tissue is removed from the deep surfaces of the graft, while making sure not to harm the blood supply or CA ligament stump. A microsagittal saw is then used to decorticate the medial coracoid surface and expose a broad, flat cancellous surface to optimize graft union. If the osteotomy resulted in a spike of bone (which means optimal length harvest), it is removed while making sure not to compromise the length of the graft. An osteotome is then placed beneath the coracoid, and a 3.2-mm drill is used to place two bicortical drill holes along the central longitudinal axis of the graft about 1 cm apart (Fig. 1E.4).

GLENOID EXPOSURE AND PREPARATION

The arm is externally rotated, putting the subscapularis on stretch. The subscapularis superior and inferior margins are identified, and the subscapularis split is performed with a #15 blade, 3 to 4 mm medial to the medial aspect of the biceps tendon. It is then divided medially up to the level of the coracoid but not farther because the subscapularis nerve supply enters the subscapularis about 1 to 1.5 cm medial to the coracoid. As first described by Walch and Boileau (2000), our preference is to split the subscapularis at the junction of the superior two thirds and inferior one third rather than detaching distally at the insertion. Then, by pushing the scissors as far as the capsule and opening them perpendicular to the direction of the muscle fibers, the plane between the upper subscapularis and anterior capsule is developed and better visualized. Next, a single-prong self-retaining Gelpi retractor is used to open the subscapularis split (Fig. 1E.5). The capsular cut is extended with a scalpel to the lesser tuberosity for exposure of the glenohumeral joint line and capsule. To preserve length, an L-shaped capsulotomy is performed—superior first at the superior glenoid and approximately 1 cm medial to the glenoid rim. A #2 high-strength suture is then used to tag the corner (superomedial) of the capsule for later repair. Electrocautery is next used to excise the anteroinferior labrum and periosteum off the region of the glenoid neck where the coracoid graft will sit. Last, a high-speed bur is used to lightly decorticate the anterior glenoid neck and create a flat, bleeding cancellous surface for graft placement. It is essential to form a bleeding bed of bone on the anterior glenoid and prepare the anterior aspect of the glenoid as perpendicular to the surface as possible.

CORACOID GRAFT FIXATION

Proper coracoid placement is arguably the most critical aspect of the Latarjet procedure. Allain et al (1998) noted that excessive lateral coracoid placement yields an elevated postoperative rate of degenerative changes. Additionally, failure to correct the recurrent anterior instability will occur if the graft is overly medialized. The graft should function as an extension of the previously deficient, inherent articular arc of the glenoid. A low-profile Fukuda retractor is inserted inside the joint to retract the humeral head. Exposure can be improved superiorly by placing a 4-mm Steinmann pin into the superior scapular neck, medially by replacing the Hohmann from earlier with the link Hohmann retractor, and inferiorly by placing the same Hohmann between the capsule and the subscapularis, thereby exposing the 6 o'clock position on the glenoid.

The original traditional Latarjet procedure first described in 1954 called for fixation of the horizontal limb of the coracoid process with a screw flush to the anteroinferior margin of the glenoid, after having made a horizontal incision through the fibers of the subscapularis (Latarjet, 1954). In this technique, the lateral surface of the coracoid becomes the face of the glenoid (Fig. 1E.6). Patte and Debeyre (1980) later proposed a modification to the procedure consisting of suturing the anterior joint capsule to the stump of the coracoacromial ligament.

de Beer et al first described the congruent-arc modification to the traditional Latarjet procedure. In this modification, the coracoid is rotated about its axis by 90 degrees to lay the inferior surface of the coracoid, which they found to be identical in radius of curvature to that of the native glenoid surface, parallel to the surface of the glenoid, thus eliminating the need to conform the graft with a bur (Fig. 1E.7) (de Beer et al, 2009; de Beer & Roberts, 2010). Essentially, this rotated position makes it so that the

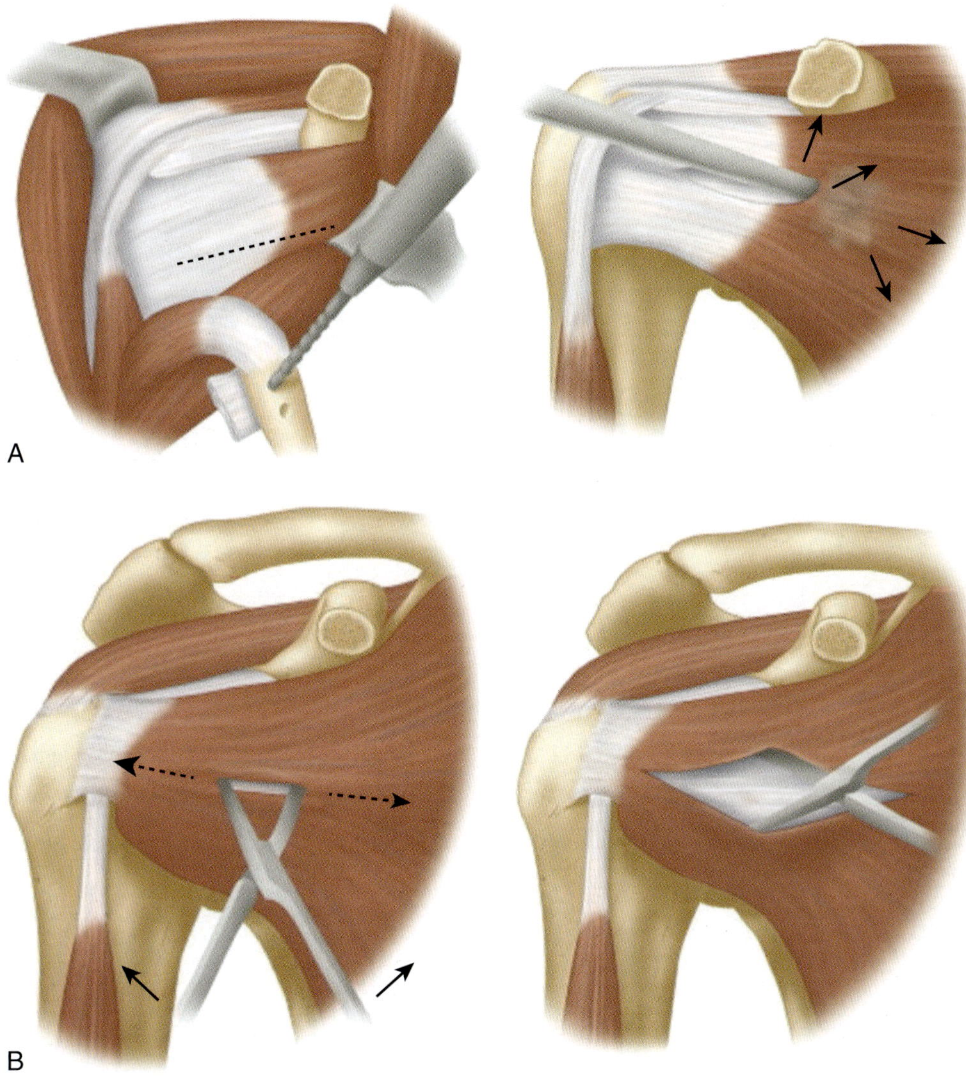

Fig. 1E.5 A, Division of the subscapularis at the junction of the upper two thirds and inferior one third. Arrows depict the extesnion of the subscapularis split to the level of the coracoid. **B,** The subscapularis is split in line with its fibers; then the scissors are oriented vertically to expose the underlying capsule, and a sponge is placed superomedially. Arrows depict opening of scissors to develop plane between capsule and subscapularis. (From Provencher MT, Romeo AA: *Shoulder Instability: A Comprehensive Approach.* Philadelphia: Saunders; 2012.)

inferior (deep) coracoid surface becomes contiguous with the glenoid surface (de Beer et al, 2009; de Beer & Roberts, 2010).

We recommend the congruent-arc technique. Ultimately, the inferior aspect of the coracoid becomes part of the glenoid face. After the ideal position (between 3 and 5 o'clock on the glenoid) is achieved, a 2.5-mm drill is used to create two bicortical anteroposterior holes parallel to the glenoid articular surface. For a successful technique, Kocher clamps on either side of the coracoid (one on the glenoid side and another on the alternative side) should be used during drilling with the 2.5-mm drill. The use of these clamps allows for a trajectory that will not compromise the bone. Alternatively, commercial devices are available that hold the coracoid while you drill. Fixation is achieved with two 3.5-mm cortical or 4.0-mm malleolar screws, typically 34 to 36 mm in length, and washers with preloaded Suture Washers (Arthrex, Naples, FL) (Fig. 1E.8). The screws should be snug but not overtightened. Any lateral overhang of the coracoid may be smoothed over with a high-speed bur.

CAPSULAR AND SUBSCAPULARIS REPAIR

A well-repaired capsule should allow the graft to function as an intraarticular platform and help protect the humeral head articular cartilage from the abrasive bone block (Boone & Arciero, 2010). Next, with the arm adducted to the side and placed in approximately 45 degrees of external rotation and the Fukada removed, the capsular repair is performed using the #2 FiberWires preloaded in the Suture Washers as well as with additional free high-strength #2 sutures to the capsule and the CA ligament. To allow for the imbrication of the capsular tissue, the sutures are placed in a figure-of-eight style. For further reinforcement, the CA ligament remnant on the coracoid graft is incorporated into the capsular repair. Finally, with the conjoined tendon exiting medially and anteriorly through the split, the subscapularis is repaired over the coracoid transfer with high-strength #2 suture. When repairing the lateral-most extent of the subscapularis split, care should be taken to avoid the long head of the biceps tendon. After copious irrigation, the wound is closed in a standard layered fashion.

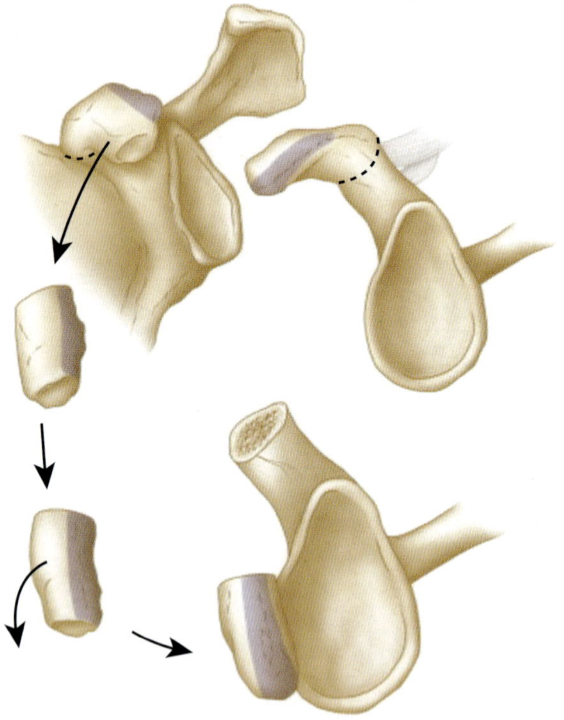

Fig. 1E.6 Removal of the coracoid process for coracoid graft harvest and placement of the graft with its inferior surface directly apposing the glenoid rim so that the lateral surface of the coracoid becomes the face of the glenoid as done in the traditional Latarjet procedure. (From Provencher MT, Romeo AA: *Shoulder Instability: A Comprehensive Approach*. Philadelphia: Saunders; 2012.)

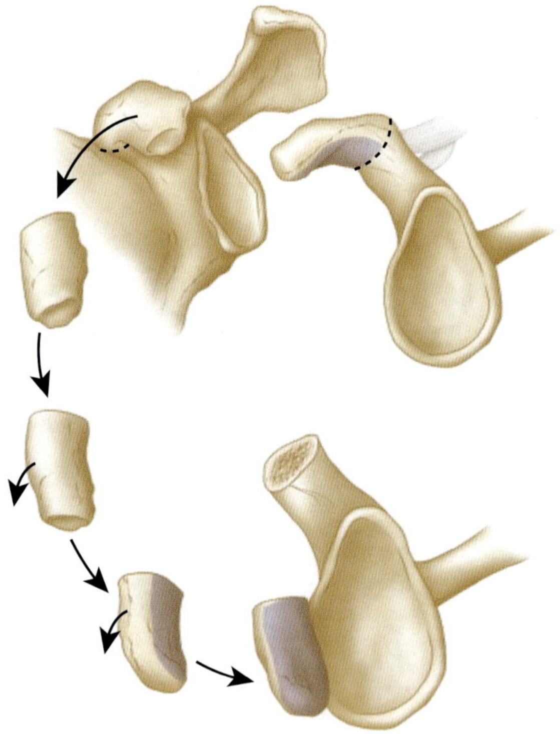

Fig. 1E.7 Removal of the coracoid process for coracoid graft harvest and placement of the graft with its lateral surface directly apposing the glenoid rim so that the inferior surface of the coracoid becomes the face of the glenoid as done in the congruent-arc technique of the Latarjet procedure. (From Provencher MT, Romeo AA: *Shoulder Instability: A Comprehensive Approach*. Philadelphia: Saunders; 2012.)

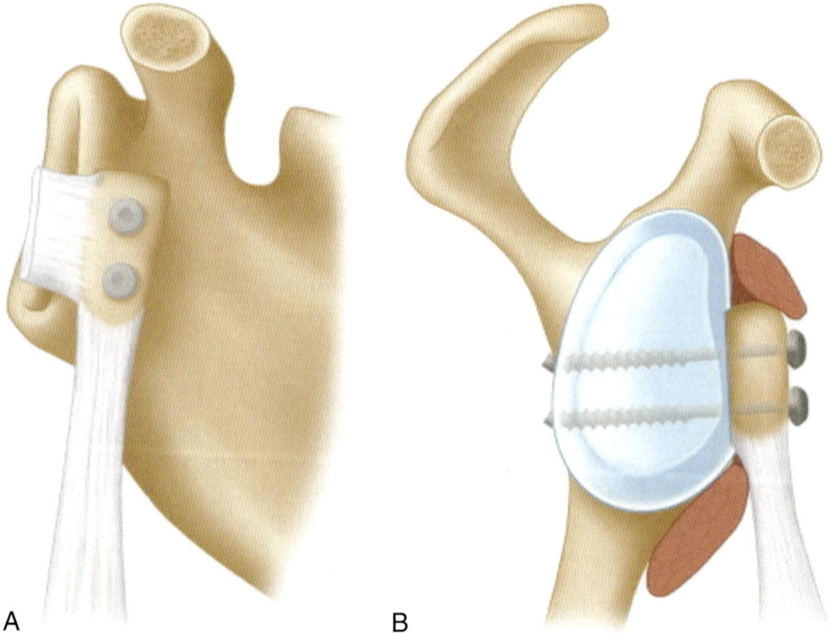

Fig. 1E.8 **A,** Coracoid graft securely fixed to glenoid with two screws with no lateral overhang. **B,** Lateral view of the reconstruction. (From Provencher MT, Romeo AA: *Shoulder Instability: A Comprehensive Approach*. Philadelphia: Saunders; 2012.)

Postoperative Management and Rehabilitation

The main goal of postoperative management and rehabilitation is to allow graft union. Because of the subscapularis split, a subscapularis protection protocol is usually not required. Moreover, a simple well-padded abduction sling is used to prevent strain, encourage rest, and reduce the risk of hematoma formation during the first 3 to 4 postoperative weeks. Gentle passive, active, and active-assisted shoulder ranges of motion in the scapular plane are permitted in this period, and motion of the fingers, hand, and elbow is encouraged. To reduce the risk of graft nonunion, no resisted elbow flexion is allowed for at least 6 weeks. Also, to optimize osseous healing, anti-inflammatory pain medications are avoided in the early postoperative period. After serial radiographic evaluation confirms continued maintenance of graft placement, patients are allowed to resume progressive strengthening and conditioning. At the 4-month mark, return to contact sports and heavy labor exertion is allowed. We typically obtain postoperative imaging, including radiographs as well as two-dimensional and 3D CT scans, at 4 to 6 months after surgery to assess for final coracoid union (Figs. 1E.9 and 1E.10).

Key Technical Pearls and Complications

Several steps have been proven to be crucial for efficacy and prevention of complications caused by technical error when performing the Latarjet procedure. First among these is performing a subscapularis split instead of a takedown or division. Full and partial takedowns of the subscapularis insertion require protection from passive external rotation for at least 6 weeks in addition to a graduated internal rotation strengthening program (Schroder et al, 2006). A split results in less morbidity while also having the added benefit of the sling effect (Schroder et al, 2006). Splitting is also done instead of dividing the subscapularis to avoid fatty infiltration of the subscapularis. Aside from less fatty degeneration, splitting has been shown to lead to significantly better Rowe and Walch-Duplay scores, which assess strength and functionality, respectively (Maynou et al, 2005). In particular, a subscapularis L-shaped tenotomy has been shown to lead to 28% less strength of the rotator cuff muscle at long-term follow-up compared with a subscapularis split (Paladini et al, 2012). Additionally, the decortication step is a key pearl that allows for improved graft union. Graft union is also promoted and graft lysis avoided by limiting pectoralis minor release to the tip of the coracoid process, thereby minimizing graft devascularization. Finally, extracapsular placement of the coracoid graft with suture anchors may theoretically soften the articulation contact pressures on the humerus, although this has not yet been clinically confirmed to result in a reduced incidence of degenerative arthritis.

Neurologic injury incidence after the Latarjet procedure has been reported to vary from 1.8% to 10.4% (Helfet, 1958; Shah et al, 2012; Young & Rockwood, 1991). Delaney et al (2014) using intraoperative neuromonitoring during the Latarjet procedure found that the axillary and musculocutaneous nerves are at particular risk, especially during glenoid exposure and graft insertion. Given these risks, be sure to identify and release the musculocutaneous nerve from the posterior fascia of the conjoined tendon. Thus, neuromonitoring may have a role in the future of the procedure, particularly in cases with extensive scar tissue and anatomic distortion (Delaney et al, 2014).

Open versus Arthroscopic Latarjet

The evolution of modern arthroscopic techniques has led to their application in a completely arthroscopic Latarjet procedure with reported benefits such as

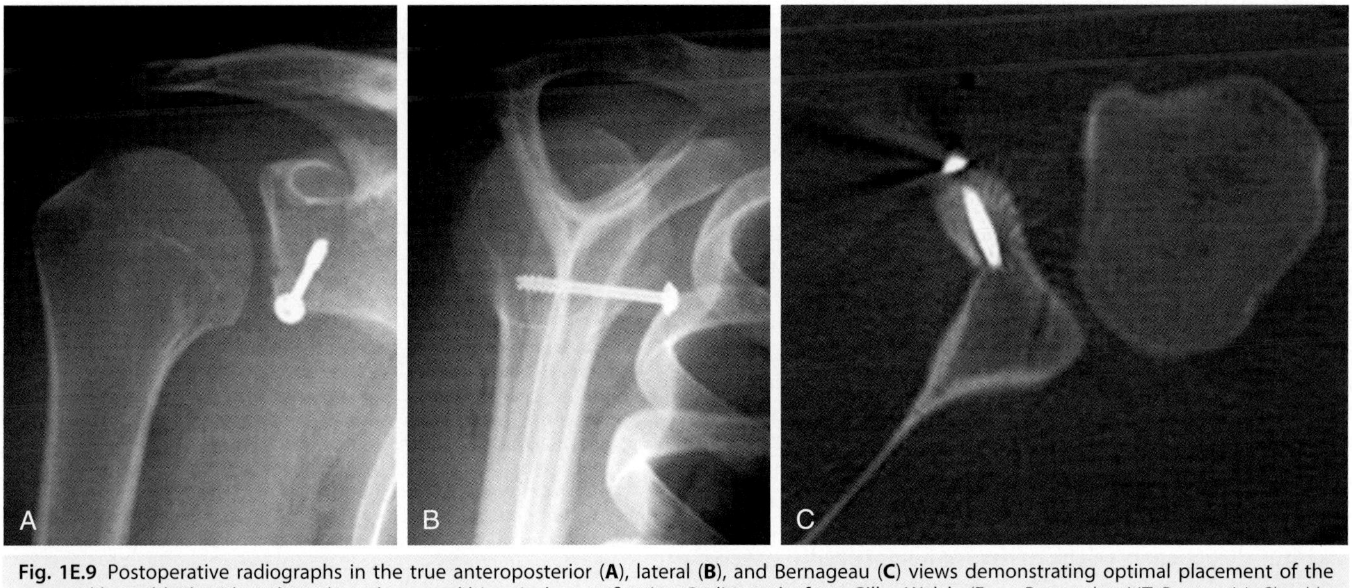

Fig. 1E.9 Postoperative radiographs in the true anteroposterior (**A**), lateral (**B**), and Bernageau (**C**) views demonstrating optimal placement of the coracoid bone block with no lateral overhang and bicortical screw fixation. Radiographs from Gilles Walch. (From Provencher MT, Romeo AA: *Shoulder Instability: A Comprehensive Approach*. Philadelphia: Saunders; 2012.)

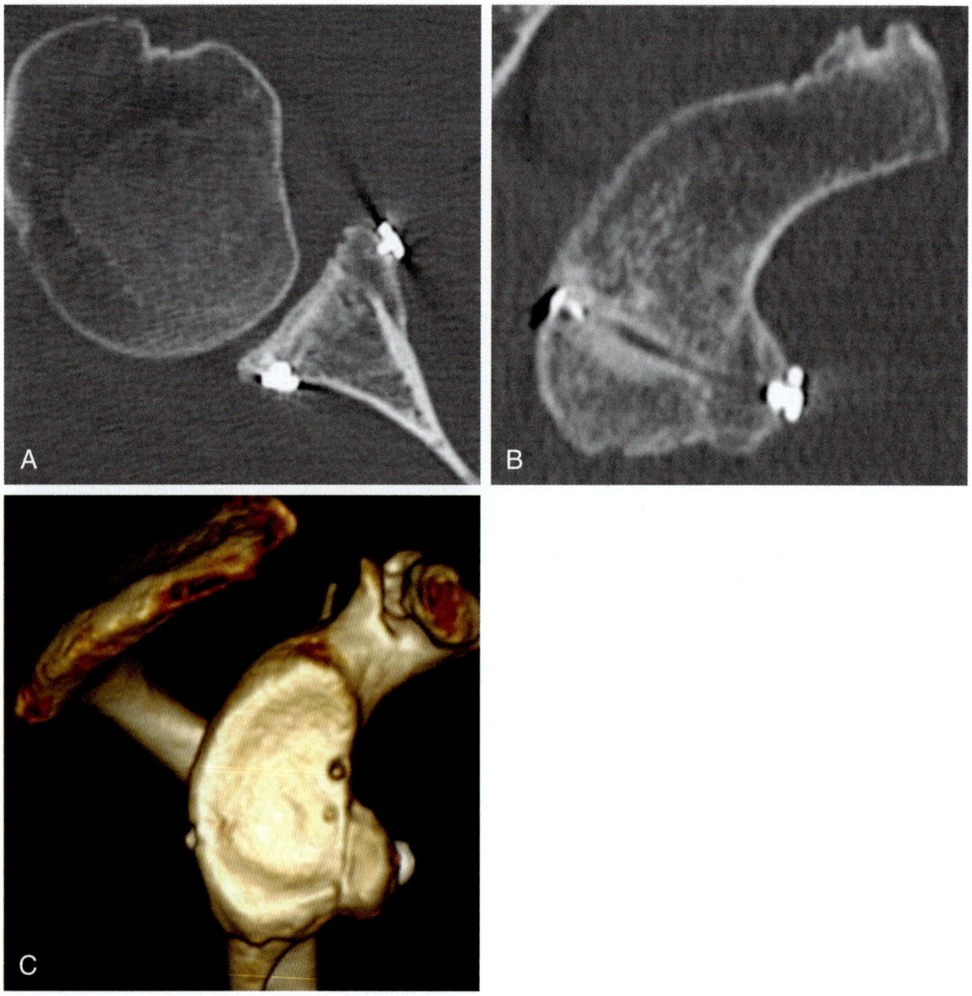

Fig. 1E.10 Example of axial view computed tomography (CT) (**A**), sagittal view CT (**B**), and three-dimensional CT (**C**) images at 6 months demonstrates a healed coracoid bone block (Latarjet). (From Gendre P, Thélu CE, D'Ollonne T, Trojani C, Gonzalez JF, Boileau P. Coracoid bone block fixation with cortical buttons: an alternative to screw fixation? *Orthop Traumatol Surg Res.* 2016;102(8):983-987).

decreased stiffness, quicker rehabilitation, and accelerated return-to-sport activities (Lafosse et al, 2007; Lafosse & Boyle, 2010). However, given the high complexity and required dexterity for this procedure, it is difficult to master and standardize (Boileau et al, 2014; Lafosse & Boyle, 2010). Such is the case that a comparative and learning curve analysis of the open versus all-arthroscopic Latarjet procedure found that 10 arthroscopic Latarjet procedures were needed to overcome the need for conversion to the open version and 20 procedures were necessary before an equal operating time to the open technique was achieved (Cunningham et al, 2016). Additionally, despite similar functional and patient satisfaction outcomes between both techniques, the arthroscopic cohort was measured as having higher incidence rates of complications, screw placement inaccuracy, persistent apprehension, and recurrences (Cunningham et al, 2016). A systematic review and cost analysis of open versus arthroscopic Latarjet evaluating 1317 patients found similar good outcomes between the two, but direct costs of the arthroscopic procedure were found to be double that of the open operation on average (Randelli et al, 2016).

References

Allain J, Goutallier D, Glorion C. Long-term results of the Latarjet procedure for the treatment of anterior instability of the shoulder. *J Bone Joint Surg Am.* 1998;80:841–852.

Arrington E, Parada S, Marchant B. Beach chair and lateral decubitus setup—pros and cons. In: Provencher MT, Romeo AA, eds. *Shoulder Instability: A Comprehensive Approach.* Philadelphia: Elsevier; 2011:33–42.

Barchilon VS, Kotz E, Barchilon Ben-Av M, Glazer E, Nyska M. A simple method for quantitative evaluation of the missing area of the anterior glenoid in anterior instability of the glenohumeral joint. *Skeletal Radiol.* 2008;37:731–736.

Baudi P, Righi P, Bolognesi D, et al. How to identify and calculate glenoid bone deficit. *Chir Organi Mov.* 2005;90:145–152.

Bishop JY, Jones GL, Rerko MA, Donaldson C. MOON Shoulder Group. 3-D CT is the most reliable imaging modality when quantifying glenoid bone loss. *Clin Orthop.* 2013;471:1251–1256.

Boileau P, Thélu C-É, Mercier N, et al. Arthroscopic Bristow-Latarjet combined with Bankart repair restores shoulder stability in patients with glenoid bone loss. *Clin Orthop.* 2014;472:2413–2424.

Boone JL, Arciero RA. Management of failed instability surgery: how to get it right the next time. *Orthop Clin North Am.* 2010;41:367–379.

Cunningham G, Benchouk S, Kherad O, Lädermann A. Comparison of arthroscopic and open Latarjet with a learning curve analysis. *Knee Surg Sports Traumatol Arthrosc.* 2016;24:540–545.

de Beer J, Burkhart SS, Roberts CP, et al. The congruent-arc Latarjet: tech. *Shoulder Elbow Surg.* 2009;10:62–67.

de Beer JF, Roberts C. Glenoid bone defects—open Latarjet with congruent arc modification. *Orthop Clin North Am.* 2010;41:407–415.
Delaney RA, Freehill MT, Janfaza DR, Vlassakov KV, Higgins LD, Warner JJ. 2014 Neer Award Paper: neuromonitoring the Latarjet procedure. *J Shoulder Elbow Surg.* 2014;Al(23):1473–1480.
Edwards TB, Boulahia A, Walch G. Radiographic analysis of bone defects in chronic anterior shoulder instability. *Arthroscopy.* 2003;19:732–739.
Farber AJ, Castillo R, Clough M, Bahk M, McFarland EG. Clinical assessment of three common tests for traumatic anterior shoulder instability. *J Bone Joint Surg Am.* 2006;88:1467–1474.
Gross ML, Distefano MC. Anterior release test. A new test for occult shoulder instability. *Clin Orthop.* 1997:105–108.
Hegedus EJ, Goode A, Campbell S, et al. Physical examination tests of the shoulder: a systematic review with meta-analysis of individual tests. *Br J Sports Med.* 2008;42:80–92. discussion 92.
Helfet AJ. Coracoid transplantation for recurring dislocation of the shoulder. *J Bone Joint Surg Br.* 1958;40-B:198–202.
Kralinger F, Aigner F, Longato S, Rieger M, Wambacher M. Is the bare spot a consistent landmark for shoulder arthroscopy? A study of 20 embalmed glenoids with 3-dimensional computed tomographic reconstruction. *Arthroscopy.* 2006;22:428–432.
Lafosse L, Boyle S. Arthroscopic Latarjet procedure. *J Shoulder Elbow Surg Am.* 2010;Al(19):2–12.
Lafosse L, Lejeune E, Bouchard A, Kakuda C, Gobezie R, Kochhar T. The arthroscopic Latarjet procedure for the treatment of anterior shoulder instability. *Arthroscopy.* 2007;23:1242.e1–1242.e5.
Latarjet M. Treatment of recurrent dislocation of the shoulder. *Lyon Chir.* 1954;49:994–997.
Lo IKY, Nonweiler B, Woolfrey M, Litchfield R, Kirkley A. An evaluation of the apprehension, relocation, and surprise tests for anterior shoulder instability. *Am J Sports Med.* 2004a;32:301–307.
Lo IKY, Parten PM, Burkhart SS. The inverted pear glenoid: an indicator of significant glenoid bone loss. *Arthroscopy.* 2004b;20:169–174.
Lunn JV, Castellano-Rosa J, Walch G. Recurrent anterior dislocation after the Latarjet procedure: outcome after revision using a modified Eden-Hybinette operation. *J Shoulder Elbow Surg Am.* 2008;17(5):744–750.
Maynou C, Cassagnaud X, Mestdagh H. Function of subscapularis after surgical treatment for recurrent instability of the shoulder using a bone-block procedure. *J Bone Joint Surg Br.* 2005;87:1096–1101.
Paladini P, Merolla G, De Santis E, Campi F, Porcellini G. Long-term subscapularis strength assessment after Bristow-Latarjet procedure: isometric study. *J Shoulder Elbow Surg Am.* 2012;21:42–47.
Patte D, Debeyre J. Luxations récidivantes de l'épaule. *Encycl Med Chir Paris Tech Chir Orthop.* 1980:44–265.
Provencher MT, Bhatia S, Ghodadra NS, et al. Recurrent shoulder instability: current concepts for evaluation and management of glenoid bone loss. *J Bone Joint Surg Am.* 2010;92(suppl 2):133–151.
Provencher MT, Ghodadra N, LeClere L, Solomon DJ, Romeo AA. Anatomic osteochondral glenoid reconstruction for recurrent glenohumeral instability with glenoid deficiency using a distal tibia allograft. *Arthroscopy.* 2009;25:446–452.
Randelli P, Fossati C, Stoppani C, Evola FR, De Girolamo L. Open Latarjet versus arthroscopic Latarjet: clinical results and cost analysis. *Knee Surg Sports Traumatol Arthrosc.* 2016;24:526–532.
Rerko MA, Pan X, Donaldson C, Jones GL, Bishop JY. Comparison of various imaging techniques to quantify glenoid bone loss in shoulder instability. *J Shoulder Elbow Surg Am.* 2013;22:528–534.
Savoie FH, Field LD, Atchinson S. Anterior superior instability with rotator cuff tearing: SLAC lesion. *Orthop Clin North Am.* 2001;32:457–461. ix.
Schroder DT, Provencher MT, Mologne TS, Muldoon MP, Cox JS. The modified Bristow procedure for anterior shoulder instability: 26-year outcomes in Naval Academy midshipmen. *Am J Sports Med.* 2006;34:778–786.
Shah AA, Butler RB, Romanowski J, Goel D, Karadagli D, Warner JJP. Short-term complications of the Latarjet procedure. *J Bone Joint Surg Am.* 2012;94:495–501.
Speer KP, Hannafin JA, Altchek DW, Warren RF. An evaluation of the shoulder relocation test. *Am J Sports Med.* 1994;22:177–183.
Sugaya H, Moriishi J, Dohi M, Kon Y, Tsuchiya A. Glenoid rim morphology in recurrent anterior glenohumeral instability. *J Bone Joint Surg Am.* 2003;85-A:878–884.
Walch G, Boileau P. Latarjet-Bristow procedure for recurrent anterior instability. *Tech Shoulder Elbow Surg.* 2000;1(4):256–261.
Warner JJP, Gill TJ, O'Hollerhan JD, Pathare N, Millett PJ. Anatomical glenoid reconstruction for recurrent anterior glenohumeral instability with glenoid deficiency using an autogenous tricortical iliac crest bone graft. *Am J Sports Med.* 2006;34:205–212.
Whiting P, Rutjes AWS, Dinnes J, Reitsma J, Bossuyt PMM, Kleijnen J. Development and validation of methods for assessing the quality of diagnostic accuracy studies. *Health Technol Assess.* 2004;8(25):iii, 1–234.
Young AA, Maia R, Berhouet J, Walch G. Open Latarjet procedure for management of bone loss in anterior instability of the glenohumeral joint. *J Shoulder Elbow Surg Am.* 2011;20:S61–S69.
Young AA, Walch G. Open bony augmentation of glenoid bone loss: the Latarjet and variants. In: Provencher MT, Romeo AA, eds. *Shoulder Instability: A Comprehensive Approach.* Philadelphia: Elsevier; 2011:197–208.
Young DC, Rockwood CA. Complications of a failed Bristow procedure and their management. *J Bone Joint Surg Am.* 1991;73:969–981.

1-1F GLENOID BONE LOSS: ARTHROSCOPIC LATARJET PROCEDURE

LAURENT LAFOSSE, MD and JOHANNES E. PLATH, MD

Introduction

- The arthroscopic Latarjet procedure is the evolution of the classic open technique, providing all benefits of arthroscopic surgery. The first all-arthroscopic Latarjet procedure was performed in 2003. Since then technique and instruments have continuously been refined over the years, most recently in 2016. The current technique is performed in eight defined surgical steps via seven portals. A conversion to an open Latarjet is possible during every step throughout the procedure. The instrumentation allows both open and arthroscopic techniques.
- The arthroscopic Latarjet procedure has shown excellent results through midterm follow-up, a low complication rate, and good graft positioning.
- The arthroscopic Latarjet procedure is an advanced arthroscopic technique requiring extraarticular soft tissue dissection in close proximity to the brachial plexus. A detailed knowledge of the anatomy and a high level of experience in arthroscopic shoulder surgery are mandatory to successfully perform this procedure.

Principles

The typical lesion after an anterior shoulder dislocation is the Bankart lesion, a detachment of the capsulolabral complex from the anterior glenoid. Arthroscopic suture anchor repair reconstitutes the capsulolabral anatomy by reattachment of the anterior soft tissue to the glenoid. Excellent clinical outcomes can be expected. Over the past decade, the arthroscopic Bankart repair has become the standard treatment method of shoulder instability for many surgeons.

However, in many cases, the surgeon is faced with more extensive soft tissue damage such as complex labral tears with disruption of the labral ring; anterior labroligamentous periosteal sleeve avulsion (ALPSA) lesions;, a torn, attenuated, or avulsed inferior glenohumeral ligament from the humerus (humeral avulsion of the glenohumeral ligament [HAGL] lesion); or even a combination of multiple lesions. These high-grade soft tissue defects make an anatomic repair of the capsulolabral complex impossible.

Moreover, bone loss at the anterior glenoid after shoulder dislocation caused by fracture and erosion adds to the complexity of shoulder instability. A glenoid defect of 20% to 25% of the glenoid diameter is usually referred to as the critical defect size for shoulder stability (Piasecki et al, 2009). However, isolated glenoid bone defects are rather the exception. Generally, we find additional humeral head impression fractures (Hill-Sachs lesion) that carry the risk of engagement and recurrence, especially if the "save arc" that the glenoid provides for humeral rotation is reduced (bipolar bone loss). The impact of glenohumeral bone loss on shoulder instability and failure of surgical treatment is well documented in the literature (Boileau et al, 2006; Burkhart & De Beer, 2000).

In our experience, bone loss is rather the rule than the exception in patients with chronic shoulder instability and is commonly underestimated. Sugaya et al (2003) investigated the incidence of glenoid rim lesions in 100 consecutive patients with recurrent anterior shoulder instability and found a glenoid defect in 90% of patients (50% bony Bankart lesion, 40% glenoid erosion).

In the complex situation of high-grade soft tissue and bony pathologies, a simple Bankart repair that reattaches the capsulolabral tissue to the glenoid cannot adequately address the complex underlying pathologies. Furthermore, a successful anatomical repair relies on good bone and soft tissue quality. However, tissue quality in patients with chronic shoulder instability is usually poor, and avulsed glenoid fragments are often subject to significant resorption and necrosis, which in principle prohibits an anatomic repair. The mentioned reasons may explain the significant number of persisting instabilities and recurrence in long-term follow-up studies of arthroscopic Bankart repair (Castagna et al, 2010; Plath et al, 2015).

Besides pathomorphologic findings, the patient's risk factors for failure as well as the individual patient expectation of surgery need to be taken into account. Within the literature, several authors have reported inferior outcomes and increased rates of recurrence after arthroscopic Bankart procedures in young patients, male patients, patients with general ligamentous laxity, patients with a high number of preoperative dislocations, and patients with participation in contact and overhead activities (Boileau et al, 2006; Randelli et al, 2012).

The Latarjet procedure involves the transfer of the coracoid with the attached conjoined tendon through a subscapularis split onto the anterior glenoid. In long-term studies, this procedure has proven its ability to reliably stabilize the shoulder joint, showing recurrent dislocation in fewer than 3% at 20 years of follow-up (Mizuno et al, 2014). The success of the Latarjet procedure is a result of several factors. First, the vascularized coracoid bone graft reconstructs the deficient anterior glenoid rim and enlarges the glenoid articular arc and therefore prevents a large Hill-Sachs lesion from engagement. Second, the intersection of the transferred conjoined tendon and the inferior subscapularis reinforce the insufficient inferior capsule and forms a dynamic sling system that creates dynamic tension as the shoulder moves into external rotation and abduction. Biomechanical studies clearly demonstrate the importance of the soft tissue sling to fully restore shoulder stability, with more than 50% of stability being attributed to the sling effect in external rotation, mostly when the arm is in 90 degrees of abduction (Wellmann et al, 2008; Yamamoto et al, 2013).

With a combination of bony and soft tissue grafting, the Latarjet procedure addresses a broad spectrum of various capsulolabral and osseous pathologies around the shoulder and allows the treatment even of complex pathomorphologic findings. The arthroscopic Latarjet procedure is the natural evolution of the classically open procedure, providing the following advantages over the open Latarjet procedure (Agneskirchner & Lafosse, 2014; Kany et al, 2016; Lafosse & Boyle, 2010):

- Accurate bone block placement under direct visualization from different perspectives
- Treatment of concomitant lesions (e.g., superior labrum anterior and posterior [SLAP], posterior Bankart, rotator cuff)
- General arthroscopic advantages because of the minimal invasiveness of surgery. These may include less postoperative pain, better cosmesis, less scarring and fewer deep adhesions, earlier mobility, fast rehabilitation and return to sports, and reduced risk for infection.
- Decision making for the Bankart or Latarjet procedure during diagnostic arthroscopy depends on Hill-Sachs engagement, extent of capsulolabral lesion and soft tissue quality, which is difficult to predict on preoperative imaging.

Indications

Indications include (Agneskirchner & Lafosse, 2014; Lafosse & Boyle, 2010):

- Significant glenoid bone loss (chronic Bankart fracture, glenoid erosion) as measured with three-dimensional (3D) computed tomography (CT)
- Bipolar bone loss with Hill-Sachs engagement
- Complex and irreparable capsulolabral lesions (labral ring disruption, destruction of labrum, ALPSA lesion, HAGL lesion, inferior glenohumeral ligament insufficiency)
- Activity in overhead and contact sport with high risk of recurrence
- Revision of failed soft tissue repair

Diagnostics

- Plain radiographs (true anteroposterior and lateral view, axial Bernageau view)
- 3D CT to assess bony deficiency

Surgical Technique

Seven standardized portals are needed for the arthroscopic Latarjet procedure (Agneskirchner & Lafosse; 2014; Lafosse et al, 2007; Lafosse & Boyle, 2010; Rosso et al, 2016) (Video 1F.1):

- **A portal:** Standard posterior portal at the soft spot of the posterior shoulder
- **D portal:** anterolateral portal in line with the superior border of the subscapularis tendon
- **E portal:** classic anterior instrument portal through the rotator interval
- **H portal:** This portal is the "high" portal, superior to the coracoid, used for coracoid preparation and osteotomy.
- **I portal:** Anterior viewing portal, "inferior" to the coracoid. The portal is located at the apex of the anterior axillary fold and established under direct vision with a spinal needle that is directed toward the coracoid.
- **J portal:** Additional anterior viewing portal used during graft shaping as well as graft transfer and fixation. The portal is located on an arc midway between the D and I portals.
- **M portal:** "Medial" to the conjoined tendon, this portal is located in line with the glenohumeral joint axis and midway between the inferior border of the pectoralis major and clavicle. The portal is used to insert the Double-barrel Cannula (DePuy Synthes Mitek, Raynham, MA).

The arthroscopic Latarjet procedure consists of eight defined key surgical steps:

1. **Joint evaluation and confirmation of indication:** The arthroscope is inserted in the A portal, and a thorough joint evaluation is performed. A probe may be introduced via the E portal. Rotator cuff tears, glenoid and humeral chondral defects, and labral and capsular lesions are noted. Particular attention is paid to the size and location of the Hill-Sachs lesions and anterior glenoid bone loss. Potential Hill-Sachs engagement is assessed with abduction and external rotation of the shoulder.
2. **Glenoid preparation and anterior exposure:** The anteroinferior labrum is resected between the 2 and 5 o'clock positions. The capsule is detached from the glenoid neck, and the 5 o'clock position is clearly marked (α-mark) with the electrocautery. It is mandatory to do this step now with the camera in the A portal and facing toward the glenoid to have a view with minimal optical distortion. At the upper border of the subscapularis, the rotator interval is opened. The clavipectoralis fascia is incised along the lateral border of the conjoined tendon, opening the space between the coracoid process and pectoralis major. The scope is moved to the D portal. With the instruments in the E portal, labral resection and capsular detachment are finalized, and the glenoid is flattened for graft placement.

   After sufficient working space between the conjoined tendon and pectoralis major has been created, the anteroinferior portals (I, M, and J portals) are placed. For M-portal placement, it is important to stay anterior to the pectoralis minor to avoid violating the plexus. Furthermore, the surgeon should be aware of the glenohumeral joint line. To determine the orientation of the glenoid, a switching stick or probe can be introduced in the A portal. Alternatively, the assistant may place her or his index finger at the A portal to guide the right direction.
3. **Coracoid preparation:** The scope is switched to the I portal. With the instrument in the M portal, the medial edge and, with the instrument in the J portal, the lateral edge of the coracoid can be accessed. For coracoid preparation, the arm rests in slight internal rotation. Medially, the interval between the conjoined tendon and pectoralis minor is dissected. Attention should be paid to avoid harming the musculocutaneous nerve. The interval is opened cautiously, and deep dissection is performed bluntly until the nerve has been located. Then the pectoralis minor tendon is detached. Laterally, the coracoacromial ligament is detached from the coracoid. Finally, all bursa and fat tissue is cleared from the superior and inferior aspects of the coracoid process, sparing the insertion site of the coracoclavicular ligaments. At this stage, the arm may be positioned in slight forward traction to expose the space lateral to the coracoid.
4. **Coracoid osteotomy:** The arm is in internal rotation without traction. The H-portal is determined with a needle and incised large enough to accommodate the Inline Coracoid Drill Guide (DePuy Synthes Mitek). The Coracoid Drill Guide is inserted and placed flush on the coracoid in its long axis between the middle and medial third of the width of the coracoid, leaving adequately room to the coracoid tip. The 7-mm offset pin of the guide can be used to facilitate placement. Two 1.5-mm K-wires are inserted bicortically. The α (distal) and the β (proximal) holes are drilled bicortically using the coracoid step drill, the holes tapped, and a "top hat" washer placed into each hole over a K-wire (Fig. 1F.1) Because there is always some resorption of the upper part of the graft, we like to countersink the superior β-screw in the graft. Accordingly, our preference is to only use a single washer at the α hole.

   Using a curved sharp osteotome, stress risers are created at the medial and lateral cortex at the desired level

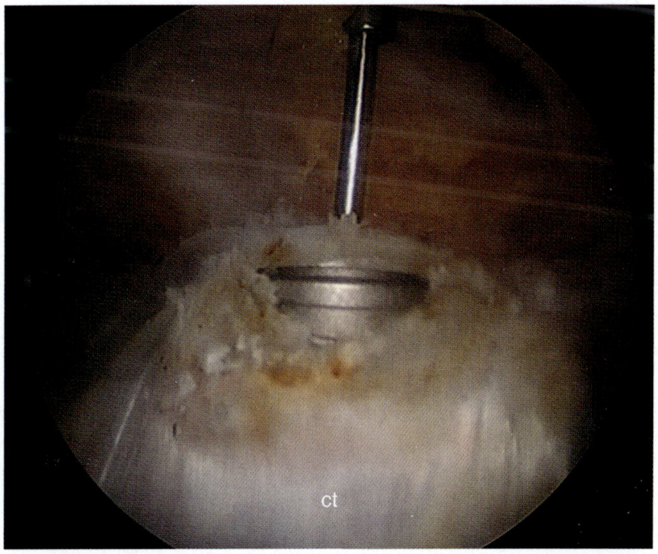

Fig. 1F.1 Coracoid preparation: view from the I portal. A "top-hat" washer has been placed in the α-coracoid hole. A cannulated drill is used to drill the β-coracoid hole. *ct*, Conjoined tendon.

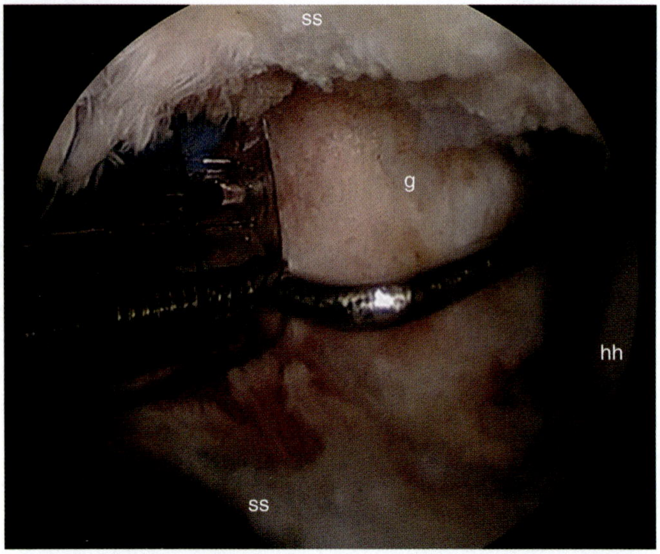

Fig. 1F.2 Glenoid tunnel placement: view from the I portal. A probe is inserted through the A portal and hooked onto the anterior glenoid at the α mark. The cannula is placed 5 mm medial to the cartilage (medial to the 5-mm probe tip), parallel to the glenoid (g). *hh,* Humeral head; *ss,* subscapularis.

of the osteotomy, anterior to the insertion site of the coracoclavicular ligaments. Finally, the osteotomy is completed between the two stress risers with the osteotome.

5. **Subscapularis split:** Before the subscapularis split, it is mandatory to expose the axillary nerve that crosses the subscapularis at the level of its myotendinous junction as well as the superior and inferior border of the subscapularis tendon. The subscapularis is split via the M portal between the inferior and the medial third of the tendon, starting lateral to the axillary nerve. A probe can be introduced through the H or the A portal (or both) to elevate the upper part of the tendon and facilitate this split. Laterally, special caution is required not to harm the cartilage of the humeral head. A subscapularis channeler is introduced through the M portal and placed at the future graft location. To fully achieve the subscapularis split at the level of the muscle, the arm is brought to maximum external rotation, with attention paid to avoid dislocating the shoulder.
6. **Screw-hole placement for graft fixation:** The screw holes can be placed using the Glenoid Guide (DePuy Synthes Mitek) or directly using the Double-barrel Cannula. For screw-hole placement, the table is tilted backward, which brings the scapular automatically in a position of scapular retraction. In addition, the shoulder is in internal rotation, and the elbow is in line with the scapula. This makes it easier to place the holes parallel to the joint axis. Two options are available to prepare the α hole:
   a. **Directly with the Double-barrel Cannula:** The cannula is introduced into the M portal. A probe with a 5-mm tip is inserted through the A portal, aligned parallel to the glenoid and hooked onto the anterior glenoid at the α-mark. The cannula is placed medial to the probe tip, parallel to the glenoid (Fig. 1F.2). The inferior coracoid screw is inserted into the cannula, and a K-wire is placed through the coracoid screw and at the level of the α-mark (accordingly 7 mm medial to the cartilage). When the guide is perfectly parallel to the inferior glenoid, the wire is introduced through the glenoid and through the skin of the posterior shoulder. A scaled tube is inserted from posterior over the K-wire. The α hole is drilled over the K-wire. After the second cortex is perforated by the drill, the tube is advanced anteriorly up to a stopper. The wire is removed while the tube remains in the glenoid and through the subscapularis split.
   b. **Glenoid guide**: The glenoid guide facilitates a parallel alignment of the graft screws to the glenoid and allows three offset options for graft placement (flush or 2 mm or 4 mm medialized to the articular surface). The guide is inserted into the M portal. A K-wire is inserted through the offset pin at the α-mark, advanced into the glenohumeral joint, and aligned parallel to the joint line. A second K-wire is placed in the appropriate cannula (0, 2, or 4) hole medially. As previously described, the K-wire is inserted into the glenoid and overdrilled, and a scaled tube is inserted posteriorly.

   Whatever technique is used, it is mandatory to control the correct position (vertical and horizontal introduction point and orientation) of the K-wire before drilling the hole, and the surgeons should not hesitate to repeat the wire placement to ensure accuracy.
7. **Coracoid placement:** The scope is moved to the J portal. With help of two 3.5-mm coracoid screws inserted through the cannula's α and β holes, the coracoid graft is firmly fixed to the cannula, but the tip of the cannulated coracoid screws should not extend past the far cortex. The coracoid is mobilized to ensure that there are no persisting soft tissue restrictions or fascial bands. A K-wire is inserted from anteriorly through the α-coracoid screw and inserted in the scaled glenoid tube. This connection between the cannula and glenoid stabilizes the graft during graft shaping. The coracoid graft that will meet the glenoid neck is now smoothened and shaped with a bur.

   The cannula is turned 90 degrees to orient the coracoid graft horizontally, and smoothly advanced through the subscapularis split along the K-wire pushing the scaled glenoid tube posteriorly. The graft is placed parallel and flush to the anterior glenoid. If necessary, the coracoid is removed back to the split and reshaped. When the coracoid fits perfectly, a second K-wire is drilled through the glenoid at the level of the β-coracoid screw to additionally fix the graft. It should be parallel to the first wire.
8. **Coracoid fixation:** The α-coracoid screw is unscrewed and removed, and the scaled tube is again advanced anteriorly up to the bone stopper. The required α screw length can be read directly off the scale. A screw of the right length is inserted, and the graft is fixed inferiorly. In the same way, the β hole is drilled and measured, and the β screw placed superiorly.

Finally, the graft and screw position is evaluated. If the graft is too proud, it can be smoothened with the bur (Fig. 1F.3).

Pearls and Pitfalls

- To improve working space: Place a switching stick in D portal to elevate the deltoid muscle and add slight forward flexion and traction during anterior dissection.

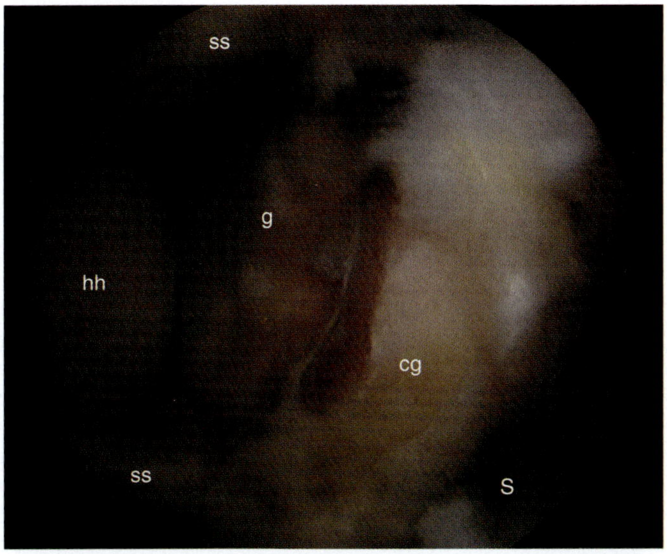

Fig. 1F.3 Final result: view from the I portal. The graft has been flattened to the level of the subchondral cartilage of the glenoid (g). The probe is left in the posterior portal to elevate the upper subscapularis (ss). *cg,* Coracoid graft; *hh,* humeral head; *S,* screw.

- To decrease fluid loss and improve visualization: Seal the portals with plastic stoppers or cover the portals with a finger.
- The arthroscopic Latarjet is "teamwork": Perfect collaboration between the anesthesiologist and the surgical team is mandatory to obtain perfect visualization (e.g., blood pressure vs pump pressure management).
- Partial superior graft osteolysis is a common finding after a Latarjet procedure (Di Giacomo et al, 2011). In our experience, this does not affect shoulder stability; however, the superior screw may get in contact with the subscapularis tendon. In cases with minor glenoid bone loss and expected partial graft resorption, respectively, we do not use a "top-hat" washer for the superior screw. This allows us to countersink the screw into the graft, so the head of the screw is less proud in case of resorption.
- Perform 6-month follow-up CT imaging and remove screws if necessary.
- If in doubt, you can always convert to an open Latarjet procedure. It is much better to convert and to manage a good open Latarjet procedure rather than performing a bad arthroscopic Latarjet procedure!

Rehabilitation and Follow-Up

- Return to daily activities and work immediately after surgery depending on postoperative pain; no restrictions of mobility
- Return to low-impact sports after 6 weeks to 3 months
- High-risk activities, including contact and overhead sports, at 4 to 6 months

Outcomes

The senior author and innovator of the technique has performed more than 700 cases of the arthroscopic Latarjet procedure to date. The longest systematically followed-up series (minimum follow-up, 5 years) was published in 2014, providing outcomes of 64 of the 89 shoulders operated before June 2008 (Dumont et al, 2014), representing early results during evolution of the technique and the innovator's own learning curve.

At a mean follow-up period of 6.4 years after surgery, the average Western Ontario Shoulder Instability Index (WOSII) was 90.6% ± 9.4%. One patient (1.6%) complained of persisting subluxations. No patient had a recurrent dislocation. Eight shoulders (12.5%) needed screw removal because of partial graft resorption, and one patient needed revision because of secondary graft dislocation. One patient underwent total shoulder replacement for dislocation arthropathy during follow-up. There were no neurovascular complications.

References

Agneskirchner JD, Lafosse L. Transfer of the coracoid process in recurrent anterior instability of the shoulder joint. *Orthop Traumatol.* 2014;26(3):296–306.

Burkhart SS, De Beer JF. Traumatic glenohumeral bone defects and their relationship to failure of arthroscopic Bankart repairs: significance of the inverted-pear glenoid and the humeral engaging Hill-Sachs lesion. *Arthroscopy.* 2000;16(7):677–694.

Boileau P, Villalba M, Héry JY, Balg F, Ahrens P, Neyton L. Risk factors for recurrence of shoulder instability after arthroscopic Bankart repair. *J Bone Joint Surg Am.* 2006;88(8):1755–1763.

Castagna A, Markopoulos N, Conti M, et al. Arthroscopic Bankart suture-anchor repair: radiological and clinical outcome at minimum 10 years of follow-up. *Am J Sports Med.* 2010;38(10):2012–2016.

Di Giacomo G, Constatini A, de Gasperis N, et al. Coracoid graft osteolysis after the Latarjet procedure for anteroinferior shoulder instability: a computed tomography scan study of twenty-six patients. *J Shoulder Elbow Surg.* 2011;20(6):989–995.

Dumont GD, Fogerty S, Rosso C, Lafosse L. The arthroscopic Latarjet procedure for anterior shoulder instability: 5-year minimum follow-up. *Am J Sports Med.* 2014;42(11):2560–2566.

Kany J, Flamand O, Grimberg J, et al. Arthroscopic Latarjet procedure: is optimal positioning of the bone block and screws possible? A prospective computed tomography scan analysis. *J Shoulder Elbow Surg.* 2016;25(1):69–77.

Lafosse L, Boyle S. Arthroscopic Latarjet procedure. *J Shoulder Elbow Surg.* 2010;19(suppl 2):2–12.

Lafosse L, Lejeune E, Bouchard A, Kakuda C, Gobezie R, Kochhar T. The arthroscopic Latarjet procedure for the treatment of anterior shoulder instability. *Arthroscopy.* 2007;23(11):1242.e1–1242.e5.

Mizuno N, Denard PJ, Raiss P, Melis B, Walch G. Long-term results of the Latarjet procedure for anterior instability of the shoulder. *J Shoulder Elbow Surg.* 2014;23(11):1691–1699.

Piasecki DP, Verma NN, Romeo AA, Levine WN, Bach BR, Provencher MT. Glenoid bone deficiency in recurrent anterior shoulder instability: diagnosis and management. *J Am Acad Orthop Surg.* 2009;17(8):482–493.

Plath JE, Aboalata M, Seppel G, et al. Prevalence of and risk factors for dislocation arthropathy: radiological long-term outcome of arthroscopic Bankart repair in 100 shoulders at an average 13-year follow-up. *Am J Sports Med.* 2015;43(5):1084–1090.

Randelli P, Ragone V, Carminati S, Cabitza P. Risk factors for recurrence after Bankart repair: a systematic review. *Knee Surg Sports Traumatol Arthrosc.* 2012;20(11):2129–2138.

Rosso C, Bongiorno V, Samitier G, Dumont GD, Szöllösy G, Lafosse L. Technical guide and tips on the all-arthroscopic Latarjet procedure. *Knee Surg Sports Traumatol Arthrosc.* 2016;24(2):564–572.

Sugaya H, Moriishi J, Dohi M, Kon Y, Tsuchiya A. Glenoid rim morphology in recurrent anterior glenohumeral instability. *J Bone Joint Surg Am.* 2003;85-A(5):878–884.

Wellmann M, Petersen W, Zantop T, et al. Open shoulder repair of osseous glenoid defects: biomechanical effectiveness of the Latarjet procedure versus a contoured structural bone graft. *Am J Sports Med.* 2008;37(1):87–94.

Yamamoto N, Muraki T, An K-N, et al. The stabilizing mechanism of the Latarjet procedure: a cadaveric study. *J Bone Joint Surg Am.* 2013;95(15):1390–1397.

1-1G GLENOID BONE LOSS: BONE GRAFT OPTIONS: ILIAC CREST AND DISTAL TIBIAL ALLOGRAFT

MATTHEW T. PROVENCHER, MD, ANTHONY SANCHEZ, BS, GEORGE SANCHEZ, BS, and KATRINA SCHANTZ, PA-C

Introduction

- Many argue that coracoid transfer techniques, namely the Bristow and Latarjet procedures, poorly reconstitute the glenoid arc and chondral surface; others claim these procedures significantly alter the native anatomy because of the placement of the conjoined tendon and the extraarticular capsulolabral repair.
- Although coracoid transfer techniques have been proven effective for treatment of glenoid bone loss, these procedures do fail as a result of graft resorption, graft malpositioning, and fixation screw loosening.
- Alternative bone graft augmentation procedures that may be implemented in the case of a failed Latarjet procedure include (1) anatomic glenoid reconstruction via fresh osteochondral distal tibial allograft (DTA) and (2) iliac crest bone autograft (ICBG).
- The indications, workup, surgical technique, pearls, and potential complications associated with each of these two bony augmentation techniques for treatment of recurrent shoulder instability with bone loss are reviewed in this chapter.

Indications and Preoperative Workup

The main indications for bone grafting using DTA or ICBG include a history of failed Latarjet procedure, an osseous deficiency, or fracture that involves more than one third of the glenoid. Post–Latarjet procedure breakage of fixation screws, coracoid graft resorption, and graft nonunion all warrant revision surgery featuring one of these two grafts (Young & Rockwood, 1991). It is difficult to state when these are the best options. Randomized trials are needed to expand the pool of patients that can be offered these techniques as a primary treatment. Early work described by Provencher et al (2001b) suggest that DTA may be a viable treatment option for postsurgical Latarjet failure.

The preoperative workup necessary for an anatomic glenoid bone reconstruction using DTA or ICBG closely resembles that of coracoid transfer techniques. Physical examination should evaluate anterior stability and ruling out of other possible pathologies contributing to the presenting sequelae. Imaging should include three-dimensional computed tomography (3D CT), imaging studies featuring the glenoid fossa circle method to quantify glenoid bone loss (Baudi et al, 2005; Sugaya et al, 2003), and arthroscopic bare spot landmark diameter-based measurement (Burkhart et al, 2002; Lo et al, 2004; Provencher et al, 2010a). All contribute to a comprehensive surgical plan before performing a glenoid bone reconstruction using DTA or ICBG.

The DTA offers multiple advantages as compared with ICBG. Along with the inferior aspect of the coracoid, the lateral DTA has been shown by cadaveric studies to have the best-match radius of curvature to reestablish the native glenoid (Dehaan et al, 2013). More clinical evidence is needed to confirm its validity with respect to long-term outcomes, but controlled laboratory studies have also shown that DTA exhibits improved joint congruity and lower peak forces within the glenohumeral joint compared with Latarjet reconstruction. Postoperative evaluation of patients with severe glenoid bone loss treated through DTA demonstrates positive outcomes, including significant improvements in American Shoulder and Elbow Society score, Western Ontario shoulder instability index, and single numerical assessment evaluation score (<0.01) at an average follow-up period of 45 months. Moreover, the healing rate of the allograft to the native glenoid was 89% with no cases of recurrent instability (Provencher et al, 2016). Tibial allografts are more readily available than fresh glenoid allografts because of greater graft contamination issues with tissues close to the gastrointestinal tract and lungs (Provencher et al, 2009). The distal tibia has weight-bearing bone with dense trabecular matrix, making it more accommodating for drilling while having the potential for improved bony incorporation (Provencher et al, 2009). In addition to the bony advantages, robust weight-bearing cartilage allows for a cartilaginous interface between the humerus and glenoid allograft, making the DTA a potentially ideal glenoid resurfacing graft (Provencher et al, 2009).

Evidence that can inform the decision when considering DTA versus inner table ICBG was found via cadaveric biomechanical studies in the context of posterior glenoid reconstruction. Similar contact mechanics were measured among the two (Frank et al, 2014). Cadaveric biomechanical studies in the context of posterior glenoid reconstruction provide similar evidence when comparing DTA and ICBG.

Patient Positioning and Surgical Approach

After anesthesia is induced (with an interscalene regional block if possible), the patient is placed in the beach-chair position with approximately 40 degrees of head elevation. Two towels are placed between the patient and the bed behind the medial border of the scapula to flatten, and more important, stabilize the glenoid and scapula, preventing unwanted anterior and internal rotation. Restricting anterior rotation of the glenoid ensures an optimal trajectory for working on the anterior aspect and allows for screw fixation of the graft with ease. The arm may be placed in a commercially available specialized arm holder or left free and controlled on either a padded Mayo stand or an adjustable operating room tray. A typical open Bankart incision of approximately 7 cm is made with a #10 scalpel, beginning from the tip of the coracoid process and extending directly inferiorly to the superior axillary fold.

After identifying the deltopectoral interval, the cephalic vein is preserved and gently retracted laterally. The fascia overlying the conjoined tendon is identified and incised with Metzenbaum scissors. Gelpi retractors are placed to expose the fascia, while mobilizing the subfascial plane of the deltoid. Next, the lateral aspect of the conjoined tendon is identified, incised just lateral to the muscle belly of the short head of the biceps, and retracted medially. The deltoid is retracted laterally with a Kolbel retractor placed between the deltoid and the conjoined tendon. Care should be taken to protect the musculocutaneous nerve by avoiding excessive medial retraction. The subscapularis is then identified and split in at the junction of the superior two thirds and middle third longitudinally in line with its fibers. A subscapularis takedown may be necessary in the revision setting, but subscapularis takedown or tenotomy should be avoided. When using the subscapularis splitting approach, caution should be taken to avoid splitting medial to the coracoid due to potential iatrogenic nerve injury (nerve supply to subscapularis). A subscapularis splitting approach should provide sufficient exposure to the glenoid neck. However, if needed, the superior two thirds and even the entire subscapularis may be taken off the humerus. A pointed retractor is placed in the split to gain access to the capsule, which is freed from the posterior aspect of the subscapularis. The glenohumeral joint capsule is more easily separated from the subscapularis medially.

After separating the capsule from the subscapularis medially, it is also separated laterally, which becomes difficult because of the close adherence of the subscapularis to the capsule laterally. A medial-based T-shaped capsulotomy is performed for exposure. To facilitate this, internal rotation, as well as gentle lateral traction may be used. Using a #15 scalpel, the capsule is elevated off the glenoid neck medially in a subperiosteal fashion. Subsequently, care is taken to protect the axillary nerve, the labral tissue is dissected and elevated medially because it will be repaired to the anterior aspect of the bone graft after fixation. In revision cases, anterior labral tissue may be deficient, not allowing repair. If in a Latarjet revision setting, hardware is now removed. An elevator and rongeur are used to debride the scar tissue and prior implants. A high-speed bur and rasp are used to establish a uniform, bleeding surface on the anterior glenoid rim as perpendicular as possible to the glenoid articular surface. Having identified the anterior glenoid, glenoid bone loss seen on the preoperative 3D CT scan is confirmed. Generally, a 25% to 30% loss indicates the need for approximately 8 to 9 mm of anterior glenoid bone augmentation (Provencher et al, 2009). Using the central bare spot as the landmark for assessing bone loss of the inferior glenoid provides custom dimensions of the allograft that is to be prepared. In addition, sizing blocks and preoperative measures are used to confirm the bone block size (Burkhart et al, 2002; Lo et al, 2004).

Distal Tibial Allograft Preparation

A fresh distal tibia is obtained from a donor cadaveric source (Decker et al, 2016). It is not necessary to size-match the DTA because it has a radius of curvature and sizing that has been shown to work well in the vast majority of cases (Dehaan et al, 2013; Provencher et al, 2009). Using the confirmed preoperative 3D CT scan and intraoperative bare spot measurements, the lateral third of the distal tibia is fashioned into a bone graft. After the distal tibia is marked (Fig. 1G.1), a 0.5-inch sagittal saw is used to cut while an assistant holds the graft in place with two towel clamps. While cutting, the allograft must be kept cool with irrigation. The allograft may be cut at various angles to accommodate any slope changes of the glenoid, but is usually 5 to 15 degrees angled. Typically, between 8 and 11 mm of tibial bone is used. Next, the superior- and inferior-most aspects of the allograft are rounded to the shape of the glenoid. Following pulsatile lavage, two 4.0-mm drill holes are drilled in the graft while the graft holder is used as a guide. To facilitate placement and positioning within the joint, two 1.6-mm K-wires are placed in the allograft bone at a 45-degree angle to the articular surface. The allograft is then placed in the position and orientation in which it will be fixed onto the native glenoid with a final assessment of fit, conformity, and angle relative to the articular surface.

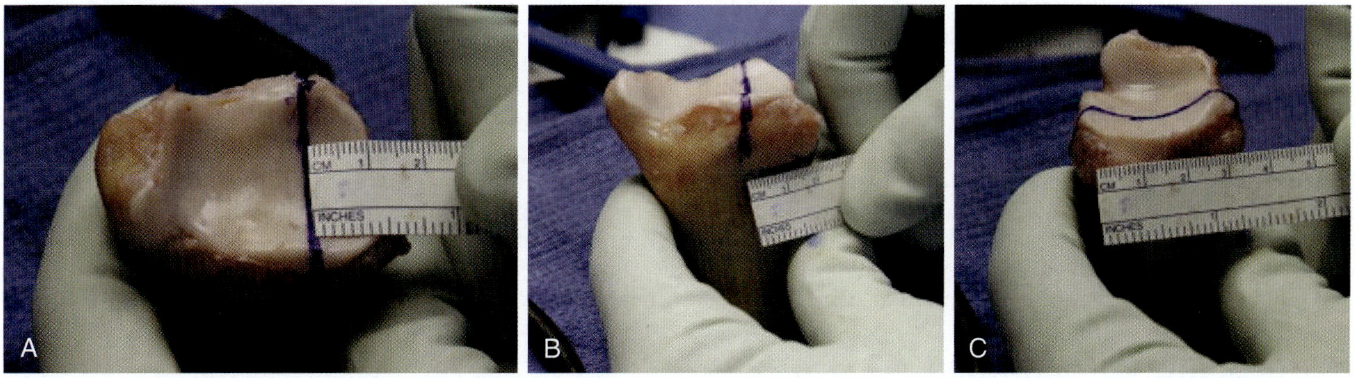

Fig. 1G.1 A, A surgical marker is used to mark a 10-mm measurement of the lateral chondral surface. **B,** An angular cut is marked at 5 to 10 degrees toward the medial tibia to retrovert the graft. **C,** Lateral view of the graft. (From Cole BJ, Sekiya JK: Surgical *Techniques of the Shoulder, Elbow, and Knee in Sports Medicine*. Philadelphia: Saunders; 2013.)

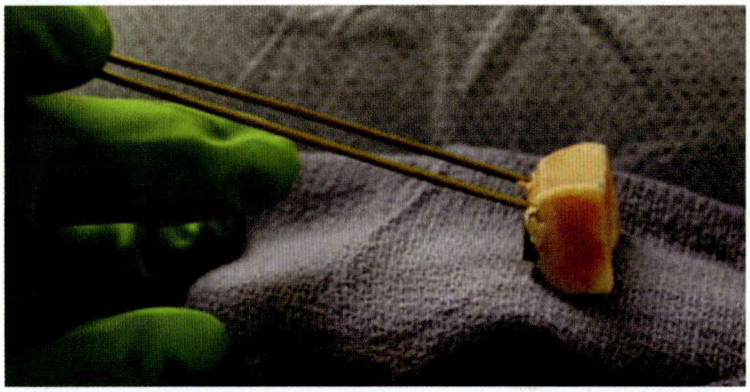

Fig. 1G.2 **Kirschner wires are placed at a 45-degree angle to facilitate placement of the graft.** (From Cole BJ, Sekiya JK: Surgical *Techniques of the Shoulder, Elbow, and Knee in Sports Medicine*. Philadelphia: Saunders; 2013.)

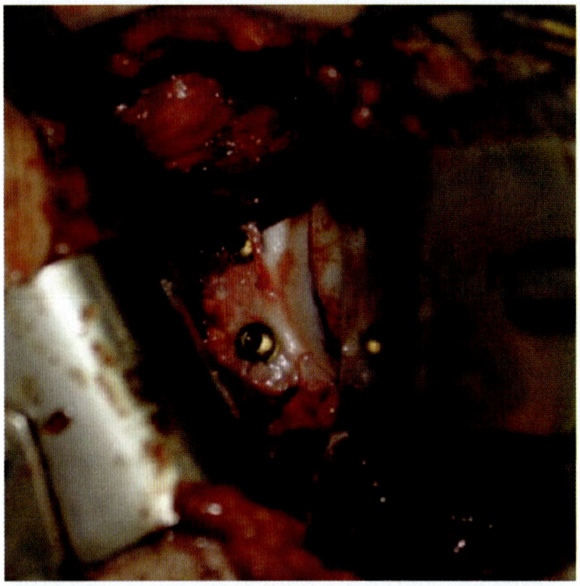

Fig. 1G.3 **Intraoperative photograph of the final anatomic glenoid bone reconstruction using distal tibial allograft.** (From Cole BJ, Sekiya JK: Surgical *Techniques of the Shoulder, Elbow, and Knee in Sports Medicine*. Philadelphia: Saunders; 2013.)

GLENOID PREPARATION AND GRAFT FIXATION

After any necessary adjustments, two small 1.6-mm K-wires are placed to temporarily hold the graft away from the future locations of screw placement (Fig. 1G.2). The graft is placed flush with the glenoid. The K-wires are measured to select the appropriate screw length, typically 32 to 38 mm. A cannulated drill is used over the K-wires, through the 4.0-mm holes drilled earlier in the graft, onto the glenoid. The graft is then fixed via a lag technique with two 3.75-mm noncannulated fully threaded cortical screws with Suture Washers (Arthrex, Naples, FL.) (Fig. 1G.3). After fixation, if the capsule and labrum are available for repair, they are repaired using the sutures from the Suture Washers. The subscapularis is then closed with multiple suture anchors. In our experience, a drain is not necessary if the deep wound remains dry. Pearls and pitfalls for this procedure are reviewed in Table 1G.1.

POSTOPERATIVE REHABILITATION

A padded abduction sling is to remain on at all times for the first 4 to 6 weeks postoperatively. Rehabilitation consists of six phases. The first phase is 2 weeks in duration and characterized by prohibition of biceps activation and aerobic exercises, including stationary bike and level surface walking capped by 30 minutes. In this first phase, 4 weekly passive range of motion routines are performed up to specific limits, as follows: 120 degrees of forward flexion, 120 degrees scapular plane, 30 degrees external rotation at side, and 90 degrees abduction. Active wrist and elbow range of motion are encouraged in phase 1.

Table 1G.1 Pearls and Pitfalls for a Successful Anatomic Glenoid Bone Reconstruction via Distal Tibial Allograft

Pearls	Pitfalls
Size-matching DTA using preoperative 3D CT and intraoperative bare spot measurements for optimal allograft size and dimensions	Radius of curvature mismatch or the dimensions of graft will not restore anatomy and biomechanics if measurement steps not taken
Limiting exposure via subscapularis split versus take-down or division when possible	Iatrogenic nerve damage if care is not taken
Protect the musculocutaneous nerve by avoiding excessive medial retraction.	
Protect the axillary nerve when dissecting and elevating labrum.	
Gentle neurolysis of the axillary nerve can be performed.	
Intraoperative neuromonitoring to ensure no iatrogenic injury is caused	
Irrigation and pulsatile lavage ensure minimal graft damage and clear marrow-free tunnels ready for placement.	
Before graft fixation, platelet-rich plasma can be used to improve the consolidation process.	

CT, Computed tomography; *DTA*, distal tibial allograft; *3D*, three dimensional.

In phase 2, typically weeks 2 to 4, the aerobic exercise limits are progressed to 45 to 60 minutes. Goals are set to improve passive range of motion: 150 degrees of forward flexion, 150 degrees scapular plane, 45 degrees of external rotation at the side, and 90 degrees of abduction. Isometric exercises are recommended for extension, abduction, and external and internal rotation. Deltoid isometric exercises are allowed at the 4-week mark.

The third phase, weeks 6 to 12, commences with discontinuing the ultra-sling. This period increases the passive benchmarks of forward flexion, scapular plane, external rotation at side, and abduction to 160, 160, 45, and 140 degrees, respectively.

Confirming successful graft incorporation using serial imaging (Fig. 1G.4), phase 4 adds an inclined treadmill to the rehabilitation plan. Passive range of motion exercises are transitioned to active-assisted and eventually, active range of motion.

From weeks 12 to 16, phase 5, strength training begins. The regimen consists of push-ups, plyometric exercise, and external and internal rotation at 90 degrees with a cable. Having met the goals set by the previous phase, the sixth phase begins typically after 16 weeks. Swimming, military press, and pull-downs are permitted. Finally, throwing is allowed and gradually increased in distance.

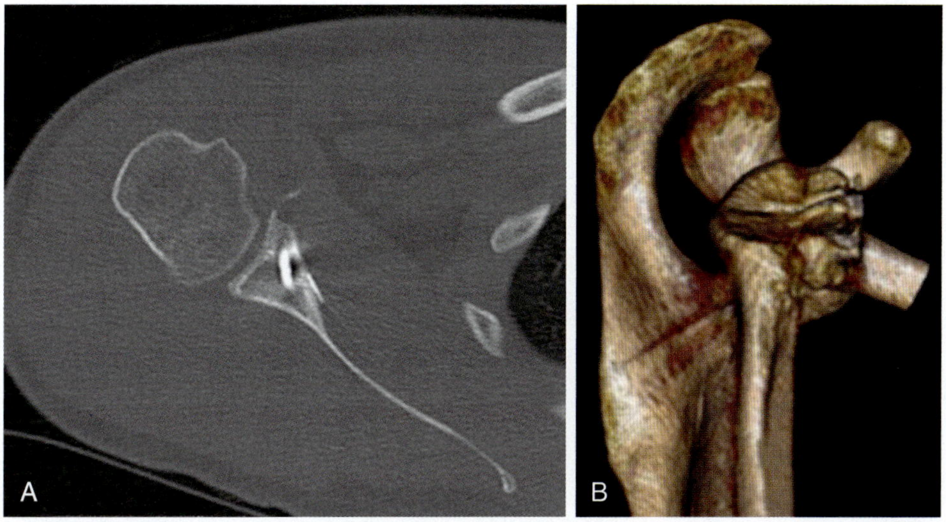

Fig. 1G.4 Two- (**A**) and three-dimensional (**B**) computed tomography images illustrating an excellent match of the radius of curvature between the distal tibial allograft and native glenoid. (From Provencher MT, Romeo AA: *Shoulder Instability: A Comprehensive Approach.* Philadelphia: Saunders; 2012.)

Iliac Crest Autograft

PATIENT POSITIONING

After anesthesia is induced (with a regional interscalene block if possible), the patient is positioned on a full-length beanbag with the head of the bed elevated to 30 degrees. Using the beanbag as support, the aim is to ensure mobility of the shoulder and exposure of the ipsilateral iliac crest. Degree and direction of instability is confirmed via reexamination under anesthesia. The shoulder, arm, and ipsilateral iliac crest are prepared and draped in the standard sterile orthopedic fashion.

SURGICAL APPROACH

The ICBG surgical approach is the same as that of the DTA procedure.

ILIAC CREST EXPOSURE AND AUTOGRAFT PREPARATION

A curvilinear incision posterior to the anterosuperior iliac spine is made. Electrocautery is then used to gain access to the fascial plane where the abdominal oblique and the tensor fascia lata muscles join. Care should be taken to leave the abductor insertion intact. After the superior iliac crest is exposed and blunt retractors are used to maintain exposure, a tricortical wedge-shaped graft is removed using an oscillating saw and osteotomes. This wedge-shaped graft should measure approximately 3 cm long by 2 cm wide (Fig. 1G.5). Using a small saw and bur, the graft is contoured in such a fashion that the concave inner table recreates the articulation. After harvest, the abdominal oblique muscle and tensor fascia lata are reattached followed by a layered closure, and finally the skin is approximated and closed with a running subcuticular stitch. To approximate the correct anatomic joint concavity, the graft-to-scapula interface angle is inclined. Care should be taken to not position the graft too acutely or horizontally to avoid possible impingement of the humeral head and failure to restore the glenoid concave depth, respectively. The inner table of the iliac crest is used as the glenoid face.

GLENOID PREPARATION AND GRAFT FIXATION

After adjustments to ensure anatomic approximation, two terminally threaded stainless steel 4.0-mm cannulated screw set K-wires with Suture Washers are used for fixation. To have the screw heads sit as far away medially from the humeral articular surface as possible, the wires are oriented medially and parallel to the joint surface. The transition between the autograft and native glenoid should be smooth visually and via palpation. A small bur is used to contour the transition if necessary. When the fixed graft is flush to the remaining glenoid (Fig. 1G.6), the humeral head retractor is removed and the humeral head is positioned on the newly reconstructed glenoid. Joint congruity and stability are confirmed by rotating the arm. Next, using sutures from the Suture Washers, as well as horizontal mattress sutures, the capsule-periosteal sleeve is repaired to the edge of the graft. Chronic bone loss can cause shortening of the capsule, limiting lateral capsule repair. If capsule reattachment to the humeral neck with at least 30 degrees of external rotation is not possible, the lateral subscapularis is used to extend the capsule (Warner et al, 2006). Using a #2 braided nonabsorbable horizontal mattress suture, the capsule is sewn into the undersurface of the lateral subscapularis so that the capsule becomes tensioned in external rotation (Warner et al, 2006). Through use of 2 braided nonabsorbable horizontal mattress sutures and direct fixation to bone with Suture Anchors, the subscapularis split is repaired. Incision closure is completed in layers with subcuticular resorbable 3-0 monofilament suture and Steri-Strips. The incision is then dressed, and the shoulder is placed into an immobilizer. Pearls and pitfalls for this procedure are reviewed in Table 1G.2.

POSTOPERATIVE REHABILITATION

A shoulder immobilizer is used for the first 4 postoperative weeks with pendulum exercises permitted after the first week. Supervised physical therapy to regain range of motion begins after week 4, along with permitted arm use in routine daily tasks. Gradually, with serial imaging confirmation of graft healing, active and passive assisted motion

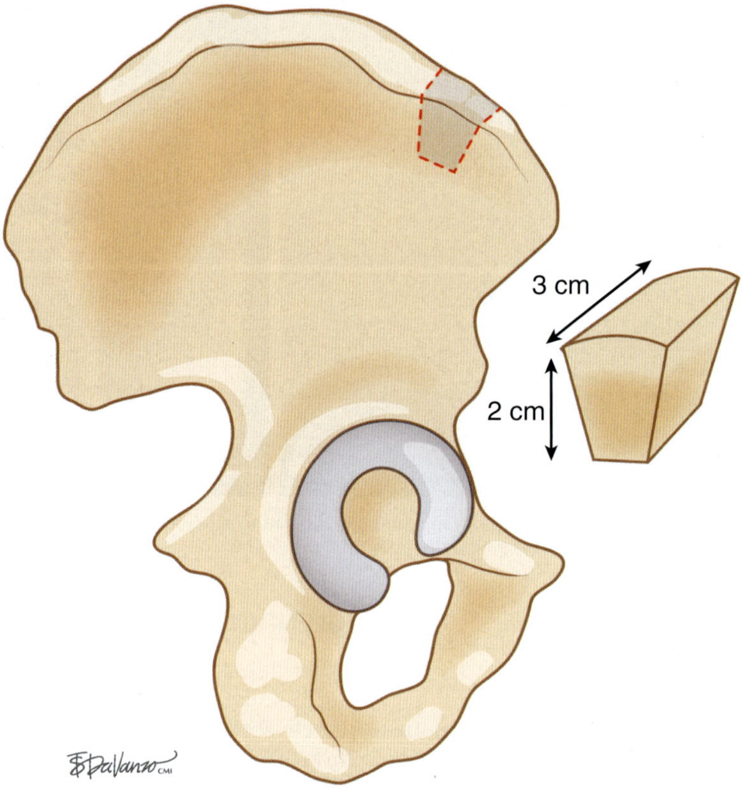

Fig. 1G.5 Illustration demonstrating harvest of the iliac crest autograft, approximately 3 cm long by 2 cm wide, from the greater pelvis. (From Provencher MT, Romeo AA: *Shoulder Instability: A Comprehensive Approach*. Philadelphia: Saunders; 2012.)

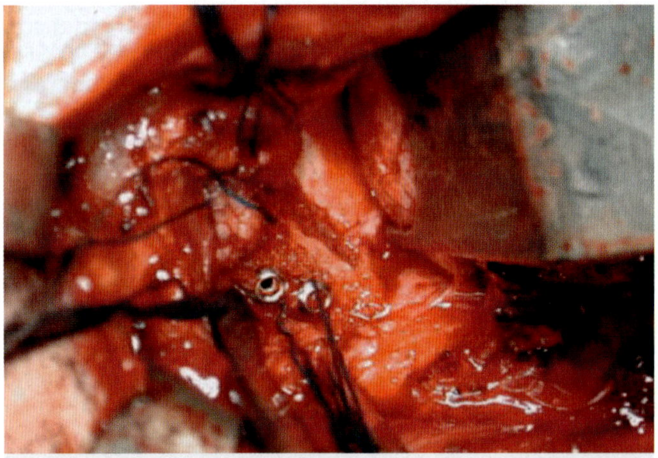

Fig. 1G.6 Intraoperative photograph of final anatomic glenoid bone reconstruction using iliac crest autograft. (From Provencher MT, Romeo AA: *Shoulder Instability: A Comprehensive Approach*. Philadelphia: Saunders; 2012.)

Table 1G.2 Pearls and Pitfalls for a Successful Anatomic Glenoid Bone Reconstruction via Iliac Crest Autograft

Pearl	Pitfalls
Preoperative and intraoperative measurements inform the fashioning of the graft	Nonanatomic glenoid bony reconstruction
Awareness and care of the neurovascular structures is necessary to prevent any possible damage. With neuromonitoring in extensive scar tissue revision setting when possible.	Iatrogenic neurovascular injury as a result of lack of awareness. This especially holds true in cases of revision surgery after failed Latarjet procedures.
Leave the abductor insertion intact.	
Conservative subscapularis management when possible.	
Do not position the graft with too acute so as to not risk impingement of the humeral head.	
Do not position the graft in a horizontally inclined interface angle to avoid risk of failing to restore glenoid concave depth.	

are added to therapy. Water therapy is also encouraged after at least 6 weeks. Strength training is allowed after 3 months. Noncontact overhead recreational sports are permitted after 4 months. After at least 8 months, collision and contact sports are allowed.

Complications

Potential complications associated with these two bony reconstruction procedures discussed are similar to those of coracoid transfer procedures. These include graft nonunion, resorption of the graft, loosening or breakage of the screws, neurovascular injury, and injury to the articular cartilage. Additional concerns include enlarged or torn capsules and latent residual lesions that were not treated at the time of graft procedure.

References

Baudi P, Righi P, Bolognesi D, et al. How to identify and calculate glenoid bone deficit. *Chir Organi Mov*. 2005;90(2):145–152.

Burkhart SS, Debeer JF, Tehrany AM, Parten PM. Quantifying glenoid bone loss arthroscopically in shoulder instability. *Arthroscopy*. 2002;18(5):488–491.

Decker MM, Strohmeyer GC, Wood JP. Distal tibia allograft for glenohumeral instability: does radius of curvature match? *J Shoulder Elbow Surg*. 2016;25(9):1542–1548.

Dehaan A, Munch J, Durkan M, Yoo J, Crawford D. Reconstruction of a bony Bankart lesion: best fit based on radius of curvature. *Am J Sports Med*. 2013;41(5):1140–1145.

Frank RM, Shin J, Saccomanno MF, et al. Comparison of glenohumeral contact pressures and contact areas after posterior glenoid reconstruction with an iliac crest bone graft or distal tibial osteochondral allograft. *Am J Sports Med*. 2014;42(11):2574–2582.

Lo IK, Parten PM, Burkhart SS. The inverted pear glenoid: an indicator of significant glenoid bone loss. *Arthroscopy*. 2004;20(2):169–174.

Provencher MT, Bhatia S, Ghodadra NS, et al. Recurrent shoulder instability: current concepts for evaluation and management of glenoid bone loss. *J Bone Joint Surg Am*. 2010a;92(suppl 2):133–151.

Provencher MT, Frank RM, Golijanin P, et al. Distal tibia allograft glenoid reconstruction in recurrent anterior shoulder instability: clinical radiographic outcomes. *Arthroscopy*. 2016. pii: S0749-8063 (16) 30789–7.

Provencher MT, Ghodadra N, LeClere L, Solomon DJ, Romeo AA. Anatomic osteochondral glenoid reconstruction for recurrent glenohumeral instability with glenoid deficiency using a distal tibia allograft. *Arthroscopy*. 2009;25(4):446–452.

Provencher MT, LeClere LE, Ghodadra N, Solomon DJ. Postsurgical glenohumeral anchor arthropathy treated with a fresh distal tibia allograft to the glenoid and a fresh allograft to the humeral head. *J Shoulder Elbow Surg*. 2010b;19(6):e6–e11.

Sugaya H, Moriishi J, Dohi M, Kon Y, Tsuchiya A. Glenoid rim morphology in recurrent anterior glenohumeral instability. *J Bone Joint Surg Am*. 2003;85-A(5):878–884.

Warner JJ, Gill TJ, O'Hollerhan JD, Pathare N, Millett PJ. Anatomical glenoid reconstruction for recurrent anterior glenohumeral instability with glenoid deficiency using an autogenous tricortical iliac crest bone graft. *Am J Sports Med*. 2006;34(2):205–212.

Young DC, Rockwood C. Complications of a failed Bristow procedure and their management. *J Bone Joint Surg Am*. 1991;73:969–981.

1-1H GLENOID BONE LOSS: BONE GRAFT OPTIONS DISTAL CLAVICLE

JOHN M. TOKISH, MD, ADAM KWAPISZ, MD, PhD, and W. STEPHEN CHOATE, MD

Introduction

- Bone loss has emerged as a critical issue in the treatment of glenohumeral instability (Burkhart & De Beer, 2000). Its presence is reported in 72% of instability cases and influences the outcome of arthroscopic treatment (Hunt et al, 2014; Mologne et al, 2007; Stevenson et al, 1991).
- Many studies have reported that the presence of significant bone loss results in higher failure rates and lower clinical outcomes than patients without bone loss (Balg & Boileau, 2007; Burkhart & De Beer, 2000; Shaha et al, 2015).
- The amount of glenoid bone loss that places an arthroscopic repair at risk has continued to evolve. Knowing that the glenoid diameter is 24 to 26 mm on average, a bone defect as small as 6 to 8 mm qualitatively translates into the "inverted pear" concept of Lo and Burkhart and is considered unacceptable by many (Lo et al, 2004).
- Traditionally, bone loss of up to 20% has been well tolerated, but greater amounts have been shown to affect biomechanical stability and clinical results (Hovelius et al, 2001; Itoi et al, 2000; Lo et al, 2004; Provencher, et al, 2010; Yang et al, 2016).

More recently, less bone loss, "subcritical bone loss" of 13.5%, has been shown to be detrimental to clinical outcomes (Shaha et al, 2015). It has also been shown in cadaveric study that less bone loss can compromise soft tissue repair (Yang et al, 2016).

Hill-Sachs Lesion

- Glenoid bone loss may also interact with the Hill-Sachs lesion of the humerus. Larger Hill-Sachs lesions may "engage" in functional positions and have also been shown to negatively affect arthroscopic results.
- Recently, these two bone loss conditions have been combined into an "on-track–off-track" concept (Burkhart & De Beer, 2000; Di Giacomo et al, 2014; Kurokawa et al, 2013; Yamamoto et al, 2007). This paradigm takes into account bipolar bone loss, recognizing that the individual lesions can affect one another, reducing the stability of the shoulder joint.
- This concept has been clinically validated, where applying the track concept was demonstrated to be highly predictive of outcome and more predictive than glenoid bone loss alone (Shaha et al, 2016).
- Furthermore, patients undergoing an arthroscopic repair for an off-track lesion demonstrated Western Ontario Shoulder Instability Index scores 450 points worse than those who were on track at the time of surgery.
- Thus, the recognition of the presence of bone loss is a critical aspect to the decision-making algorithm in the treatment of anterior shoulder instability (Shaha et al, 2015).

Measurement of Bone Loss

BACKGROUND

- Glenoid and humeral bone loss may be evaluated both pre- and intraoperatively. Although special x-ray evaluations have been shown to characterize both glenoid bone loss and Hill-Sachs lesions, three-dimensional computed tomography (3D CT) scans have become the gold standard (Gerber & Nyffeler, 2002; Stevens et al, 1999; Sugaya et al, 2003).

Table 1H.1 Comparison of Graft Types for Treatment of Glenoid Bone Loss in Shoulder Instability

	Distal Clavicular Autograft	Coracoid Transfer	Iliac Crest Transfer	Allograft
Cartilage source	Patient's own	None	None	Allograft only; tibial or glenoid
Versatility	Anterior or posterior	Anterior only	Anterior or posterior	Anterior or posterior
Graft rejection	None	None	None	Potentially
Cost	Free	Free	Free	Expensive give number if you can find a source
Availability	Readily	Readily	Readily	6–9 mo
Sling effect	None	Conjoint tendons, subscapularis	None	None

- Some authors suggest that magnetic resonance imaging (MRI) may be used to evaluate glenoid bone loss and that this evaluation can be as accurate as traditional methods (Owens et al, 2013; Shaha et al, 2015).

TECHNICAL NOTES

- Several methods of glenoid bone loss quantification have been proposed. Sugaya et al (2014) described a method based on the assumption that after humeral subtraction, the inferior two thirds of the glenoid approximates a perfect circle. The authors then calculated the lost area of this circle as bone loss.
- Barchilon et al (2008) calculated the distance from the glenoid diameter to the defect (d) and evaluated bone loss as a function of d/radius.
- Gerber measured the length of bone lesion (x) and the radius (r) of the glenoid and described that if $x > r$, there was less than 70% resistance to dislocation (Gerber & Nyffeler, 2002).
- Lo and Burkhart described an arthroscopic technique for measurement of bone loss based on the observation that the glenoid "bare area" is usually at its center. The glenoid bone loss may be calculated as the percentage of twice the intact radius (Lo et al, 2004).
- Barcia et al (2013) contradicted this, noting that the bare area is often not present, and when present, is rarely in the exact center of the glenoid. These authors recommended against using the arthroscopic bare area to calculate bone loss because it led to significant errors in measurement.

"ON-TRACK–OFF-TRACK" CONCEPT

- Di Giacomo et al (2014) recently described an on-track versus off-track concept of bipolar bone loss. In this setting, the authors compare glenoid track with the Hill-Sachs defect size. They note that when the Hill-Sachs lesion is larger than the glenoid track, the lesion is "off track" and is likely to engage.
- Shaha et al (2016) demonstrated that off-track patients sustained a 75% failure rate with arthroscopic stabilization compared with an 8% failure rate in on-track lesions.

Surgical Treatment Options

- There are number of options described to treat bone loss in shoulder instability. These include coracoid transfers such as the Latarjet and Bristow procedures, iliac crest bone grafting, and osteochondral allografts.
- Each approach has advantages and disadvantages unique to its application. Factors such as size of graft, whether it has an inherent cartilage source, immunocompatibility, availability, and cost are all considerations in decision making for graft selection, and are discussed later (Table 1H.1).
- The ideal graft should be such that it can restore the bone and cartilage loss seen in erosive glenoid bone loss with a source that is readily available, free, and without donor site morbidity.

Coracoid Bone Autograft

HISTORIC BACKGROUND

- In 1954, Latarjet described his technique of coracoid bone transfer as a treatment of recurrent dislocation of the shoulder (Latarjet, 1954). In 1958, Helfet described a coracoid tip transfer, and named it the Bristow technique (Helfet, 1958).
- Although it has been more than half a century, coracoid transfer is still considered the gold-standard technique of glenoid bone loss treatment.

ADVANTAGES

- Coracoid grafts have the advantage of restoring a significant amount of glenoid bone and provide what has become known as the "triple blocking effect" of bone restoration, capsular reconstruction, and the sling effect of myodesing the inferior subscapularis with the conjoined tendon.
- Biomechanical studies demonstrate that this procedure is quite effective in restoring shoulder stability, and clinical outcome studies have demonstrated low recurrence rates and excellent patient reported outcomes (Burkhart et al, 2007; Giles et al, 2013; Neyton et al, 2012; Yamamoto et al, 2013).

DISADVANTAGES

- The coracoid transfer is a nonanatomic approach, which may make future revision surgery more difficult, and its overall complication rate may reach 30% (Griesser et al, 2013).

- There is a limit to the amount of glenoid surface that can be restored. Paladini et al (2016) reported that this technique may be insufficient to restore defects exceeding 31%. Bueno et al (2012) described that in comparison to the traditional Latarjet technique, its modification, the congruent arc technique, may be used to reconstruct bone loss of an approximate size of 54%, but this modification results in a greater graft displacement and a lower clinical failure load.
- Other authors have shown that up to 60% of the graft may undergo osteolysis (Di Giacomo et al, 2011, 2014).
- Coracoid transfer lacks articular cartilage on the transferred graft. This has been cited as a potential reason for osteoarthritis development after Latarjet surgery, which is reported in up to 62% of cases (Allain et al, 1998).
- Unplanned reoperations have been reported at a higher rate than that of the traditional Bankart procedure, and the overall complication rate has been reported as high as 25% (Griesser et al, 2013; Shah et al, 2012).
- Delaney et al (2014) have reported that neuromonitoring during Latarjet surgery resulted in a nerve alert in 77% of patients and resulted in 21% of patients with a clinically detectable nerve deficit postoperatively.

Iliac Crest Bone Autograft

HISTORIC BACKGROUND

- The first reports of using bone block to restore glenoid deficiency were made by Eden (1918) and Hybinette (1932).
- In 2006, Warner et al reported autogenous tricortical iliac crest bone graft to be effective in treatment of recurrent instability in settings of glenoid bone loss.

ADVANTAGES

- This graft could restore defects up to 35 mm in length, which is significantly more surface than that of coracoid graft.
- There are excellent short-term results with a few complications in 4% of patients. The technique has the advantage of being readily available, essentially free, and is an autograft source of bone (Warner et al, 2006).

DISADVANTAGES

- The iliac crest is nonarticular and thus cannot restore the osteoarticular loss seen in the glenoid. This may lead to secondary osteoarthritis, which has been reported after this procedure (Bouju et al, 2014; Hovelius et al, 2006).
- There is the potential for donor site morbidity, from which persistent pain for longer than 1 year after surgery is described in up to 100% of cases.
- Local infection (14%) and anterior superior spine fracture (3%) incidences have been reported (Almaiman et al, 2013; Calori et al, 2014; Warner et al, 2006).
- The ICBG graft does not, in itself, address the soft tissue pathology that is frequently present in instability cases where it is used (Kleiner et al, 2016).

Distal Tibia Allograft

HISTORIC BACKGROUND

- Distal tibial allografts have recently been introduced as an osteochondral source for glenoid bone loss treatment.

ADVANTAGES

- It may provide equivalent biomechanical properties to the iliac crest bone graft, and the technique has been shown to produce a better articular pressure profile than the Latarjet.
- Glenoid arc articular conformity can be reproduced with this graft source (Frank et al, 2014; Provencher et al, 2009). Promising clinical outcomes have been presented but not yet published in the peer-reviewed literature.

DISADVANTAGES

- The distal tibia may be less congruous than originally reported.
- Decker et al (2016) reported that the chance of a random pairing of a distal tibial allograft matching the radius of curvature of a recipient glenoid was low. How precise a match is necessary to achieve optimal results remains to be studied.
- The possibility of graft resorption as well as immunologic response after this technique has not been investigated, but these concerns have plagued allograft usage in other transplant settings (Aponte-Tinao et al, 2016; Chapovsky & Kelly, 2005; Lozano-Calderon et al, 2016; Stevenson et al, 1991).
- The largest limitation to this method is its logistic application. The cost of a fresh osteochondral allograft can exceed tens of thousands of dollars, and there can be a significant wait time, which can exceed 6 months.
- Fresh allograft preparation requires a minimum of 14 days as quarantine for infectious disease, and chondrocyte viability has been shown to significantly drop after 28 days postmortem. This requires surgeons to perform transplantation in roughly a 2-week window, which can be a scheduling challenge for both the patient and surgeon in many facilities (Bolano & Kopta, 1991).

Distal Clavicle Osteochondral Autograft

HISTORIC BACKGROUND

- The distal clavicle provides a fresh, osteochondral autograft in the treatment of glenoid bone loss (Tokish et al, 2014) (Video 1H.1).

ADVANTAGES

- The distal clavicular autograft (DCA) is the first reported option that provides an autograft source of bone and cartilage to replace similar tissue loss on the glenoid.

- It is generally readily available and with minimal cost.
- It also can be placed arthroscopically as well as used in both anterior and posterior cases of bone loss.
- Although donor site morbidity has not been reported with this specific technique, graft harvest is similar to the Mumford technique, which has been reported to give excellent or good outcome in up to 85% of treated patients, with dissatisfaction correlated with clavicle over- or underresection. Researchers suggest excising 5 to 10 mm of a distal clavicle to be a safe method, which is similar to our technique (Strauss et al, 2010).
- Recent work by the authors demonstrated that the DCA may on average reproduce up to 44% of the glenoid radius, which compares favorably to a 31% restoration when a traditional coracoid transfer is used (Barcia et al, 2013).
- Petersen et al (2016) have reported supporting biomechanical data on this technique, describing that contact pressure differences between clavicular grafting and congruent arc coracoid transfer are favorable to the DCA.
- Moreover, the distal clavicle graft is capped with articular cartilage that is within 1 mm of native glenoid cartilage thickness. It is a fresh, unprocessed tissue source that is immediately transplanted, so concerns about chondrocyte viability, immunorejection, and infection are minimized (Kwapisz Tokish, 2017).

DISADVANTAGES

- Although promising anatomic results have been reported, there is a lack of clinical outcomes with this technique.
- It does not augment or address anterior capsular structures that are often a part of complex instability cases.

INDICATIONS

- It is the preference of the senior author to use the DCA in young patients who have glenoid bone loss as the primary reason for their instability, with defects from 15% to 30%, and relatively preserved soft tissue structures.

CONTRAINDICATIONS

- In cases of collagenopathies such as Ehlers-Danlos syndrome, previous thermal capsulorraphy, or multiply operated patients, we prefer an alternative technique that addresses these issues with soft tissue reinforcement.

Authors' Preferred Surgical Technique

PREOPERATIVE PREPARATION

Patients with glenohumeral instability should undergo a standard history and physical examination, as well as preoperative advanced imaging such as CT or MRI. Glenoid bone loss is calculated in every patient, and this calculation aids in determining the operative approach to the patient according to the "on-track–off-track" concept. As relative indications for bony augmentation of either anterior or posterior instability, bone loss of greater than 15% of the glenoid diameter or the existence of significant retroversion in the presence of posterior instability is considered. Other factors such as age, athletic status, capsular laxity, and patient preferences are weighed when deciding among different treatment options.

ARTHROSCOPIC PORTAL POSITIONING

After the induction of general anesthesia, examination under anesthesia to confirm the preoperative diagnosis is performed. The patient is positioned in the lateral decubitus position on a beanbag with a padded axillary roll, with the use of a padded arm sleeve (STAR sleeve; Arthrex, Naples, FL), with balanced suspension.

A standard posterior portal is established approximately 1 cm medial and 2 cm distal to the posterolateral acromial border. The arthroscope is introduced, and additional portals are established using an outside-in technique under direct visualization with the use of a switching stick. The anterosuperior portal is established first, approximately 1 cm inferior to the clavicle and lateral to the coracoid. The midglenoid portal is created just superior to the superior border of the subscapularis. In cases of posterior augmentation, a 7 o'clock portal is created approximately 4 cm off the posterolateral corner of the acromion, bisecting the angle created by the posterior and lateral borders of the acromion, respectively, under direct visualization. To allow efficient switching of the camera and instruments throughout the case, 8.25-mm cannulas are liberally used.

DIAGNOSTIC ARTHROSCOPY AND BIOLOGIC PREPARATION

After the diagnostic arthroscopy is performed with particular attention to the pathology, the arthroscope is switched to the anterosuperior portal, and a 3-mm graduated probe is placed to confirm our preoperative measurements of glenoid bone loss. Biologic preparation includes a wide release of the glenoid labrum to ensure its mobility for accurate reduction, especially when the bone block reconstitutes the glenoid shape. This is performed with arthroscopic liberators and ablators. The glenoid is also biologically prepared with either an arthroscopic rasp or high-speed cylindrical bur, with the goal to create a healthy bed of bleeding cancellous bone, as well as to create a flat surface perpendicular to the glenoid surface to ensure a flush fit with graft placement.

GRAFT HARVEST

A single 3-cm horizontal incision is made over the subcutaneous border of the acromioclavicular joint, along the midline of the clavicular axis. The skin and subcutaneous tissues are divided, and thick periosteal flap is raised to expose the joint and approximately 1 cm of the distal clavicle. A 1-cm-wide saw blade is used to remove the distal 1cm of clavicle, and soft tissue is cleaned from around the bone. The graft is placed on the back table, and the periosteal flap is closed with nonabsorbable #2 interrupted stitches. The remainder of the soft tissue is closed in two layers, and the wound is dressed at the completion of the case.

GRAFT PREPARATION

The distal clavicle is a versatile graft, with a variable amount of version and an articular surface that is generally 19 mm long 13 mm wide (Kwapisz Tokish, unpublished). The graft is evaluated based on its best fit and cut perpendicular to its articular surface to a width that matches the measurement of bone loss that was determined preoperatively and confirmed arthroscopically. In most cases, 7 to 8 mm of augmentation is normally sufficient to reconstruct up to 30% bone loss, and the graft is fashioned to anatomically fit and replace the loss. At this point, the method of fixation for the graft is chosen. If we decide on screw fixation, the graft is predrilled in a lag construct with pilot holes allowing compression of the autograft with the screw. Alternatively, we often use suture anchors to secure the graft; in these cases, three 1-mm holes are drilled in a triangular formation, with two drill holes, 1 mm in diameter, 3 to 4 mm off the articular surface, at the superior and inferior borders of the graft. The third hole is drilled medial with respect to the graft's final position on the glenoid.

DELIVERY AND FIXATION OF GRAFT

Screw Fixation

If the graft is to be fixed with screw fixation, it can be passed either freely into the joint or along a K-wire guide predrilled in the glenoid. The advantage of a free pass is that the graft may fit down a standard midglenoid cannula and, after it has been inserted, can be flipped 90 degrees and advanced through the rotator interval inferiorly to match its resting position at the anterior-inferior glenoid, where it can be held in place with a liberator introduced from the posterior portal for anterior bone augmentation. Trying to pass the graft down a K-wire will require a wider exposure through the subscapularis to obtain a proper position. Likewise, the graft can be introduced through a posterior cannula and held in place with a liberator from the midglenoid portal. When in place, a K-wire is placed through the pilot holes of the clavicle graft and advanced into the native glenoid. This is usually not difficult for posterior grafts, but with anterior screw placement, the standard midglenoid portal may not be sufficient to achieve the appropriate angle. In such situations, an additional 5 o'clock portal is established through the subscapularis to ensure the correct trajectory. Extreme care is taken to protect the axillary nerve, and if any doubt exists, it is dissected arthroscopically, visualized, and protected. After the graft is secured to the glenoid in the appropriate position with the K-wire, a cannulated drill is advanced into the glenoid to allow lag fixation of the graft, with a cannulated, titanium 3.75-mm screw (Arthrex). If the graft is too large to easily be delivered, the cannula can be removed, the portal expanded, and the graft delivered directly. If the proper trajectory cannot be achieved with wire provisional fixation, then one can consider using a suture anchor as an alternative or conversion to an open approach.

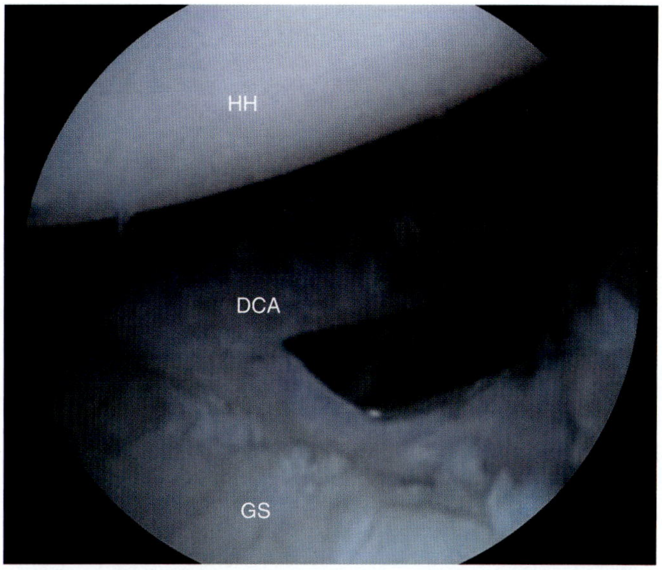

Fig. 1H.1 Distal clavicular osteochondral graft (DCA) after its placing on the glenoid ridge and fixing in a "double-row" fashion sutures. *GS,* Glenoid surface; *HH,* humeral head.

Suture Anchor Fixation

If suture anchor fixation is selected, the previously drilled holes in the graft are noted by their measurements from the articular sur face and from each other. From these measurements, two 3.0-mm BioComposite SutureTaks (Arthrex) are placed at the superior and inferior borders of the bone defect at the corresponding distances from the articular surface and each other, respectively. All limbs are delivered out of the working portal. One limb from each suture anchor is passed through the medial "conjoined" drill hole. The other two sutures are passed, one each, through the superior and inferior articular drill holes. These latter sutures are tied in a square-knot fashion over the intervening bone bridge with three stacked half-hitches. The excess suture is not cut. Graft delivery is then accomplished through the cannula by a "double-pulley" technique whereby the free limbs are pulled, which brings the graft to the suture anchor eyelets because of the knotted ends of the opposite limbs of suture. Either the graft can be assisted with a switching stick through a cannula or, if the graft is too large, the portal can be enlarged slightly, and the graft can be introduced with the assistance of a curved hemostat. After the slack is pulled out of the anchor system, an arthroscopic knot with three additional half-hitches is tied, and the graft is secured to the native glenoid across two bone bridges in a "double-row" fashion (Fig. 1H.1).

INCORPORATION OF NATIVE LABRUM INTO THE GRAFT

The remaining tails are passed through the native labrum to bring it up to the neoarticular surface with the aid of retrograde suture lassos and tied down with secondary similar knots (Fig. 1H.2). If screw fixation has been used, supplemental suture anchors can be placed either through grafts of larger size or at the superior and inferior borders of the graft if there is concern about there being enough accommodating graft. All arthroscopic instrumentation is removed, and the skin is closed and dressed sterilely.

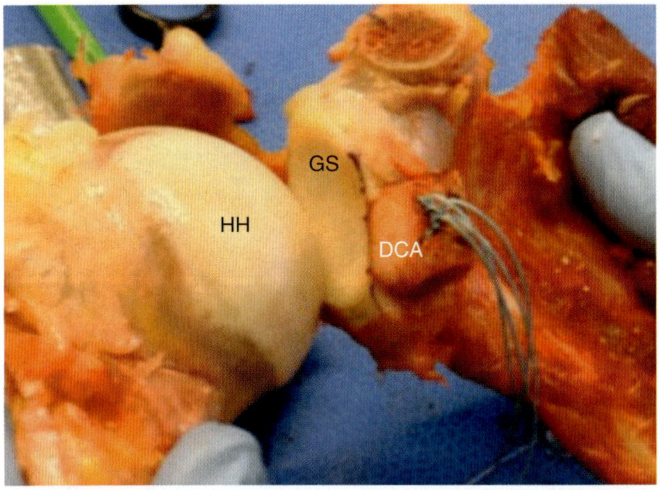

Fig. 1H.2 Distal clavicular osteochondral graft (DCA) after its fixation to the deficient glenoid. Sutures are tied in a "double-row" fashion, and the remaining tail can be used to reattach native labrum. *GS*, Glenoid surface; *HH*, humeral head.

POSTOPERATIVE REHABILITATION

The patient is placed in a neutral rotation sling for 6 weeks. Pendulums are allowed immediately, and passive motion is started at 3 weeks, with a goal to obtain full range of motion by 8 weeks. At 8 weeks' follow-up, imaging is obtained, and if the graft looks incorporated, active motion is begun. Strengthening is added at 4 months postoperatively, and return to full activity is assessed at 6 months. Final radiographs are obtained at this point to ensure graft incorporation.

Conclusion

- Glenoid bone loss can be addressed by a variety of different techniques.
- Each has unique advantages and limitations.
- This chapter has detailed the use of the distal clavicle osteochondral graft. This autograft provides a readily available and almost noncost method for anatomic reconstruction of glenoid bone loss.
- The graft restores both the radius of the native glenoid and comparable amount of its native cartilage thickness.
- It also compares favorably to the coracoid in terms of arc of restoration, providing a corticocancellous buttress for glenoid restoration.
- Although this graft provides promising theoretical, anatomic, and biomechanical promises, longer term clinical studies are necessary to validate its use in the clinical setting.

References

Allain J, Goutallier D, Glorion C. Long-term results of the Latarjet procedure for the treatment of anterior instability of the shoulder. *J Bone Joint Surg Am.* 1998;80(6):841–852.

Almaiman M, Al-Bargi HH, Manson P. Complication of anterior iliac bone graft harvesting in 372 adult patients from May 2006 to May 2011 and a literature review. *Cranio-maxillo-facial Trauma Reconstr.* 2013;6(4):257–266.

Aponte-Tinao LA, Ayerza MA, Muscolo DL, Farfalli GL. What are the risk factors and management options for infection after reconstruction with massive bone allografts? *Clin Orthop Relat Res.* 2016;474(3):669–673.

Balg F, Boileau P. The instability severity index score. A simple pre-operative score to select patients for arthroscopic or open shoulder stabilisation. *J Bone Joint Surg Br.* 2007;89(11):1470–1477.

Barchilon VS, Kotz E, Barchilon Ben-Av M, Glazer E, Nyska M. A simple method for quantitative evaluation of the missing area of the anterior glenoid in anterior instability of the glenohumeral joint. *Skeletal Radiol.* 2008;37(8):731–736.

Barcia AM, Rowles DJ, Bottoni CR, Dekker TJ, Tokish JM. Glenoid bare area: arthroscopic characterization and its implications on measurement of bone loss. *Arthroscopy.* 2013;29(10):1671–1675.

Bolano L, Kopta JA. The immunology of bone and cartilage transplantation. *Orthopedics.* 1991;14(9):987–996.

Bouju Y, Gadéa F, Stanovici J, Moubarak H2, Favard L. Shoulder stabilization by modified Latarjet-Patte procedure: results at a minimum 10 years' follow-up, and role in the prevention of osteoarthritis. *Orthop Traumatol Surg Res.* 2014;100(suppl 4):S213–S218.

Bueno RS, Ikemoto RY, Nascimento LG, Almeida LH, Strose E, Murachovsky J. Correlation of coracoid thickness and glenoid width: an anatomic morphometric analysis. *Am J Sports Med.* 2012;40(7):1664–1667.

Burkhart SS, De Beer JF. Traumatic glenohumeral bone defects and their relationship to failure of arthroscopic Bankart repairs: significance of the inverted-pear glenoid and the humeral engaging Hill-Sachs lesion. *Arthroscopy.* 2000;16(7):677–694.

Burkhart SS, De Beer JF, Barth JR, Cresswell T, Roberts C, Richards DP. Results of modified Latarjet reconstruction in patients with anteroinferior instability and significant bone loss. *Arthroscopy.* 2007;23(10):1033–1041.

Calori GM, Colombo M, Mazza EL, Mazzola S, Malagoli E, Mineo GV. Incidence of donor site morbidity following harvesting from iliac crest or RIA graft. *Injury.* 2014;45(suppl 6):S116–S120.

Chapovsky F, Kelly JDT. Osteochondral allograft transplantation for treatment of glenohumeral instability. *Arthroscopy.* 2005;21(8):1007.

Decker MM, Strohmeyer GC, Wood JP, et al. Distal tibia allograft for glenohumeral instability: does radius of curvature match? *J Shoulder Elbow Surg.* 2016;25(9):1542–1548.

Delaney RA, Freehill MT, Janfaza DR, Vlassakov KV, Higgins LD, Warner JJ. 2014 Neer Award paper: neuromonitoring the Latarjet procedure. *J Shoulder Elbow Surg.* 2014;23(10):1473–1480.

Di Giacomo G, Costantini A, de Gasperis N, et al. Coracoid graft osteolysis after the Latarjet procedure for anteroinferior shoulder instability: a computed tomography scan study of twenty-six patients. *J Shoulder Elbow Surg.* 2011;20(6):989–995.

Di Giacomo G, Itoi E, Burkhart SS. Evolving concept of bipolar bone loss and the Hill-Sachs lesion: from engaging/non-engaging lesion to on-track/off-track lesion. *Arthroscopy.* 2014;30(1):90–98.

Eden R. Zur Operation der habituellen Schulterluxation unter Mitteilung eines neuen Verfahrens bei Abriss am inneren Pfannenrande. *Langenbecks Arch Surg.* 1918;144(3):269–280.

Frank RM, Shin J, Saccomanno MF, et al. Comparison of glenohumeral contact pressures and contact areas after posterior glenoid reconstruction with an iliac crest bone graft or distal tibial osteochondral allograft. *Am J Sports Med.* 2014;42(11):2574–2582.

Gerber C, Nyffeler RW. Classification of glenohumeral joint instability. *Clin Orthop Relat Res.* 2002;400:65–76.

Giles JW, Boons HW, Elkinson I, et al. Does the dynamic sling effect of the Latarjet procedure improve shoulder stability? A biomechanical evaluation. *J Shoulder Elbow Surg.* 2013;22(6):821–827.

Griesser MJ, Harris JD, McCoy BW, et al. Complications and re-operations after Bristow-Latarjet shoulder stabilization: a systematic review. *J Shoulder Elbow Surg.* 2013;22(2):286–292.

Helfet AJ. Coracoid transplantation for recurring dislocation of the shoulder. *J Bone Joint Surg Br.* 1958;40-B(2):198–202.

Hovelius L, Sandstrom B, Saebo M. One hundred eighteen Bristow-Latarjet repairs for recurrent anterior dislocation of the shoulder prospectively followed for fifteen years: study II—the evolution of dislocation arthropathy. *J Shoulder Elbow Surg.* 2006;15(3):279–289.

Hovelius LK, Sandström BC, Rösmark DL, Saebö M, Sundgren KH, Malmqvist BG. Long-term results with the Bankart and Bristow-Latarjet procedures: recurrent shoulder instability and arthropathy. *J Shoulder Elbow Surg.* 2001;10(5):445–452.

Hunt HE, Sadr K, Deyoung AJ, Gortz S, Bugbee WD. The role of immunologic response in fresh osteochondral allografting of the knee. *Am J Sports Med.* 2014;42(4):886–891.

Hybinette S. De la transplantation d'un fragment osseux pour remédier aux luxations récidivantes de l'épaule: constatations et résultats opératoires. *Acta Chir Scand*. 1932;71:411–445.
Itoi E, Lee SB, Berglund LJ, Berge LL, An KN. The effect of a glenoid defect on anteroinferior stability of the shoulder after Bankart repair: a cadaveric study. *J Bone Joint Surg Am*. 2000;82(1):35–46.
Kleiner MT, Payne WB, McGarry MH, Tibone JE, Lee TQ. Biomechanical comparison of the Latarjet procedure with and without capsular repair. *Clin Orthop Surg*. 2016;8(1):84–91.
Kurokawa D, Yamamoto N, Nagamoto H, et al. The prevalence of a large Hill-Sachs lesion that needs to be treated. *J Shoulder Elbow Surg*. 2013;22(9):1285–1289.
Latarjet M. Treatment of recurrent dislocation of the shoulder. *Lyon Chir*. 1954;49(8):994–997.
Lo IK, Parten PM, Burkhart SS. The inverted pear glenoid: an indicator of significant glenoid bone loss. *Arthroscopy*. 2004;20(2):169–174.
Lozano-Calderón SA, Swaim SO, Federico A, Anderson ME, Gebhardt MC. Predictors of soft-tissue complications and deep infection in allograft reconstruction of the proximal tibia. *J Surg Oncol*. 2016;113(7):811–817.
Mologne TS, Provencher MT, Menzel KA, Vachon TA, Dewing CB. Arthroscopic stabilization in patients with an inverted pear glenoid: results in patients with bone loss of the anterior glenoid. *Am J Sports Med*. 2007;35(8):1276–1283.
Neyton L, Young A, Dawidziak B, et al. Surgical treatment of anterior instability in rugby union players: clinical and radiographic results of the Latarjet-Patte procedure with minimum 5-year follow-up. *J Shoulder Elbow Surg*. 2012;21(12):1721–1727.
Owens BD, Burns TC, Campbell SE, Svoboda SJ, Cameron KL. Simple method of glenoid bone loss calculation using ipsilateral magnetic resonance imaging. *Am J Sports Med*. 2013;41(3):622–624.
Paladini P, Singla R, Merolla G, Porcellini G. Latarjet procedure: is the coracoid enough to restore the glenoid surface? *Int Orthop*. 2016;40(8):1675–1681.
Petersen SA, Bernard JA, Langdale ER, Belkoff SM. Autologous distal clavicle versus autologous coracoid bone grafts for restoration of anterior-inferior glenoid bone loss: a biomechanical comparison. *J Shoulder Elbow Surg*. 2016;25(6):960–966.
Provencher MT, Bhatia S, Ghodadra NS, et al. Recurrent shoulder instability: current concepts for evaluation and management of glenoid bone loss. *J Bone Joint Surg Am*. 2010;92(suppl 2):133–151.
Provencher MT, Ghodadra N, LeClere L, Solomon DJ, Romeo AA. Anatomic osteochondral glenoid reconstruction for recurrent glenohumeral instability with glenoid deficiency using a distal tibia allograft. *Arthroscopy*. 2009;25(4):446–452.
Shah AA, Butler RB, Romanowski J, Goel D, Karadagli D, Warner JJ. Short-term complications of the Latarjet procedure. *J Bone Joint Surg Am*. 2012;94(6):495–501.
Shaha JS, Cook JB, Rowles DJ, Bottoni CR, Shaha SH, Tokish JM. Clinical validation of the on-track vs. off-track concept in anterior glenohumeral instability. *J Bone Joint Surg Am*. 2016;98(22):1918–1923.
Shaha JS, Cook JB, Song DJ, et al. Redefining critical bone loss in shoulder instability: functional outcomes worsen with subcritical bone loss. *Am J Sports Med*. 2015;43(7):1719–1725.
Stevens KJ, Preston BJ, Wallace WA, Kerslake RW. CT imaging and three-dimensional reconstructions of shoulders with anterior glenohumeral instability. *Clin Anat*. 1999;12(5):326–336.
Stevenson S, Li XQ, Martin B. The fate of cancellous and cortical bone after transplantation of fresh and frozen tissue-antigen-matched and mismatched osteochondral allografts in dogs. *J Bone Joint Surg Am*. 1991;73(8):1143–1156.
Strauss EJ, Barker JU, McGill K, Verma NN. The evaluation and management of failed distal clavicle excision. *Sports Med Arthrosc*. 2010;18(3):213–219.
Sugaya H. Techniques to evaluate glenoid bone loss. *Curr Rev Musculoskelet Med*. 2014;7(1):1–5.
Sugaya H, Moriishi J, Dohi M, Kon Y, Tsuchiya A. Glenoid rim morphology in recurrent anterior glenohumeral instability. *J Bone Joint Surg Am*. 2003;85-A(5):878–884.
Tokish JM, Fitzpatrick K, Cook JB, Mallon WJ. Arthroscopic distal clavicular autograft for treating shoulder instability with glenoid bone loss. *Arthrosc Tech*. 2014;3(4):e475–e481.
Warner JJ, Gill TJ, O'Hollerhan JD, Pathare N, Millett PJ. Anatomical glenoid reconstruction for recurrent anterior glenohumeral instability with glenoid deficiency using an autogenous tricortical iliac crest bone graft. *Am J Sports Med*. 2006;34(2):205–212.
Yamamoto N, Itoi E, Abe H, et al. Contact between the glenoid and the humeral head in abduction, external rotation, and horizontal extension: a new concept of glenoid track. *J Shoulder Elbow Surg*. 2007;16(5):649–656.
Yamamoto N, Muraki T, An KN, et al. The stabilizing mechanism of the Latarjet procedure: a cadaveric study. *J Bone Joint Surg Am*. 2013;95(15):1390–1397.
Yang JS, Mazzocca AD, Cote MP. Recurrent anterior shoulder instability with combined bone loss: treatment and results with the modified latarjet procefure. *Am J Sports Med*. 2016;44(4):922–932.

1-1I GLENOID BONE LOSS: ARTHROSCOPIC BONE BLOCK

ETTORE TAVERNA, MD and VINCENZO GUARRELLA

Introduction

- Shoulder dislocation can cause a variety of pathologic lesions. Patients with chronic anterior shoulder instability may present with recurrent dislocation, subluxation, or chronic shoulder pain (Provencher et al, 2010).
- Anteroinferior glenoid bone deficiency has been reported in 22% of initial traumatic anterior shoulder dislocations and in up to 90% of recurrent anteroinferior shoulder instability cases (Sayeg et al, 2014). Many different open and arthroscopic techniques have been described to address this pathology (Levy et al, 2016; Allain 1998; Burkhart 2007; Hill 1981; Hovelius 2004; Schroeder 2006; Taverna 2016).
- The benefits of using arthroscopic procedures for surgical stabilization of the shoulder include smaller incisions with less soft tissue dissection, better visualization of the joint, improved repair accessibility, and the best potential outcome for external rotation (Lafosse & Boyle, 2010).
- In 2005, we developed an arthroscopic technique that allows an accurate positioning of the bone graft (autograft or allograft) flush to the anteroinferior glenoid and a standard Bankart repair leaving the graft extraarticular. In November 2013, we made our last modification consisting in fixation using two arthroscopic EndoButtons (instead of two screws) placed through a guide; optimal compression is then obtained with a tensioning device (Anderl et al, 2012; Kraus et al, 2014; Scheibel et al, 2008; Warner et al, 2006). The guide permits parallel drilling of the two tunnels perpendicular to the glenoid neck, reducing the risk of graft resorption and nonunion (Taverna et al, 2014).

Other advantages include a quicker rehabilitation with early return to sport activities and a better cosmetic result. In our series, early clinical and radiologic results are promising.

Indications

Our indication to perform an arthroscopic bone-block procedure in the setting of recurrent anterior instability is young age (younger than 45 years old), maximum of five dislocations, first dislocation within 3 years, good radiologic quality of soft tissues, and glenoid bone deficit between 15% and 25% on preoperative computed tomography (CT) scans (according to Sugaya et al, 2003). Other indications include arthroscopic evidence of significant bone loss (Burkhart et al, 2002) or glenoid bone loss between 10% and 20% associated with a Bankart lesion or an instability severity index score (ISIS) (Balg & Boileau, 2007) between 3 and 6. Other indications include failure of previous isolated soft tissue repair or Bristow-Latarjet procedure. In our practice, indications for arthroscopic soft tissue repair are ISIS less than 3 and no glenoid bone loss, isolated bone loss of 10% or less, and a maximum of three dislocations. We prefer to perform Latarjet procedures in patients with ISIS greater than 6, more than five dislocations, chronic instability for more than 3 years, and glenoid bone loss greater than 25%.

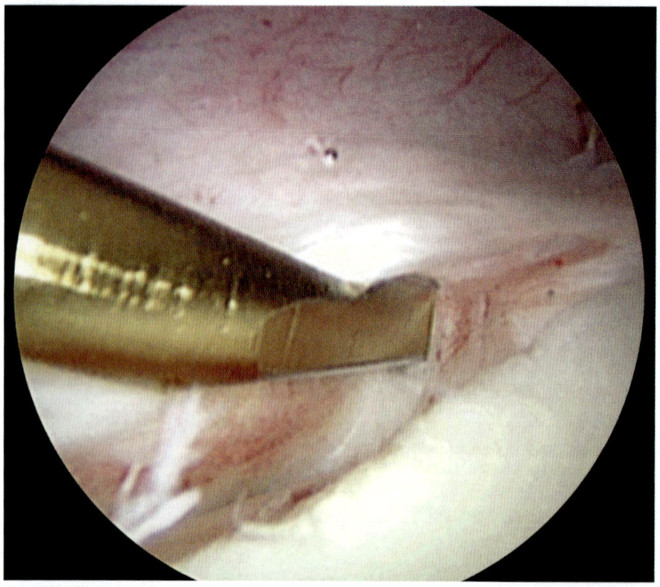

Fig. 1I.1 **Arthroscopic view from posterior portal. The labrum and capsule are elevated, and the anterior glenoid rim is decorticated to create a flat surface to accommodate the graft.** (From Taverna E, D'Ambrosi R, Perfetti C, et al. Arthroscopic bone graft procedure for anterior inferior glenohumeral instability. *Arthrosc Tech.* 2014;3(6):e653-660.)

Surgical Technique

PATIENT POSITIONING AND JOINT PREPARATION

Under general anesthesia and with the administration of perioperative antibiotics, the patient is placed in the beach-chair position. The scapula can be bolstered to rotate the glenoid externally.

A standard posterior portal is created for the insertion of the arthroscope. Viewing from the posterior portal, the surgeon creates an anterosuperior portal and midglenoid portal, and two 5.5-mm cannulas are introduced in the rotator interval. Initially, the labrum is accurately detached from the glenoid rim, and all soft tissues are removed from the anterior glenoid neck using a soft tissue shaver. We then introduce the arthroscope through the anterosuperior portal, and the anterior glenoid rim is further decorticated and flattened with a motorized bur to create a flat and bleeding bony surface to accommodate the graft (Fig. 1I.1). At this point, a spinal needle is inserted from posterior to anterior along, and perfectly parallel to, the face of the glenoid and centered on the anterior glenoid bone defect. Then a more posteromedial portal is made to provide access for the glenoid guide (Video 1I.1).

Glenoid Guide and Drill Pin Placement

The hook end of the glenoid guide is inserted through the posteromedial portal. The hook is passed along the glenoid parallel to the glenoid face to avoid damaging the articular surface, and then it is passed over the anterior edge (Fig. 1I.2, *A*). When sufficiently advanced, the guide is rotated to capture the anterior edge of the glenoid under the hook. The hook should be placed at the center of the anterior glenoid defect, usually between the 3 and 4 o' clock

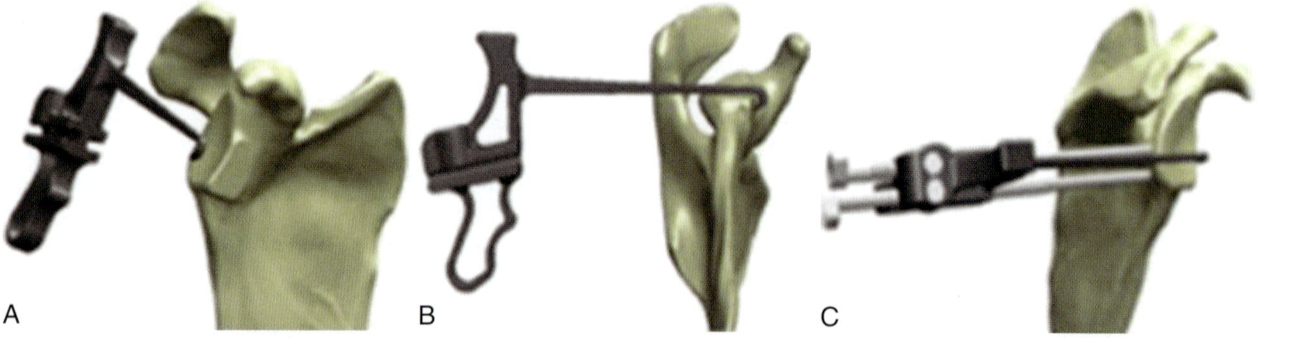

Fig. 1I.2 Glenoid guide and drill pin placement. **A,** Insertion of hook from posterior portal. **B,** Rotation of hook to capture glenoid rim. **C,** Insertion and advancement of bullet to posterior border of glenoid.

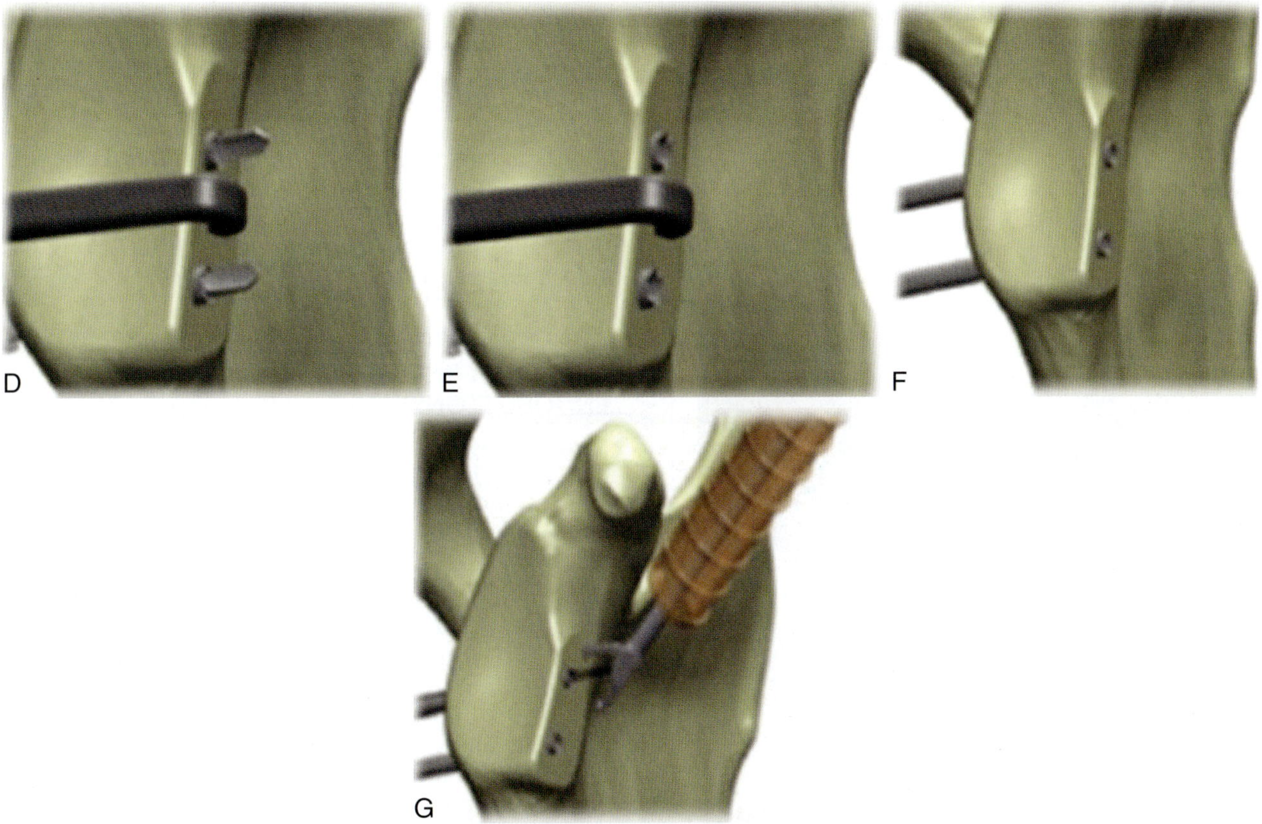

Fig. 11.2, cont'd D, Positioning and advancing of sleeves. **E,** Removal of inner drill. **F,** Removal of bullet. G, Introduction of 10-mm cannula through rotator interval and retrieval of wires. (From Taverna E, D'Ambrosi R, Perfetti C, et al. Arthroscopic bone graft procedure for anterior inferior glenohumeral instability. *Arthrosc Tech.* 2014;3(6):e653-660.)

positions (Fig. 11.2, *B*). It is mandatory that the glenoid guide is aligned with the posterior and anterior glenoid rim. After the guide is positioned, a bullet is placed in the inferior hole of the guide (Fig. 11.3). A small skin incision is made, and the bullet is advanced until it firmly contacts the posterior aspect of the glenoid neck (Fig. 11.4). The ratchet teeth of the bullet should be aligned with the screws adjacent to the guide handle. The process is repeated for the superior bullet (Fig. 11.2, *C*). A 2.8-mm sleeved drill is placed in each bullet and advanced under power until exiting from the anterior aspect of the glenoid. The drills are placed 5 mm on the center below the cortical edge of the glenoid face, parallel to one another and 10 mm apart (Fig. 11.2, *D*). The inner drill is removed, leaving the cannulated outer sleeve. Arthroscopic fluid exiting from the outer sleeve posteriorly confirms intraarticular positioning (Fig. 11.2, *E*).

After drilling is completed, the bullets can be removed by rotating each bullet to disengage the ratcheting teeth and extracting them posteriorly (Fig. 11.2, *F*). The guide can be removed at this stage. Care should be taken to ensure that the sleeves remain firmly positioned in the glenoid neck. Flexible looped guidewires are then introduced into the joint by passing one wire through each sleeve posterior to anterior (Fig. 11.5, *A*). Each guidewire is retrieved using a loop grasper, which is passed through the 10-mm cannula introduced through the rotator interval (Fig. 11.5, *B*). The wires are separated and stored. At this point, with the drill sleeves in place, drilling of anteroinferior glenoid rim should be performed for the placement of suture anchors for soft

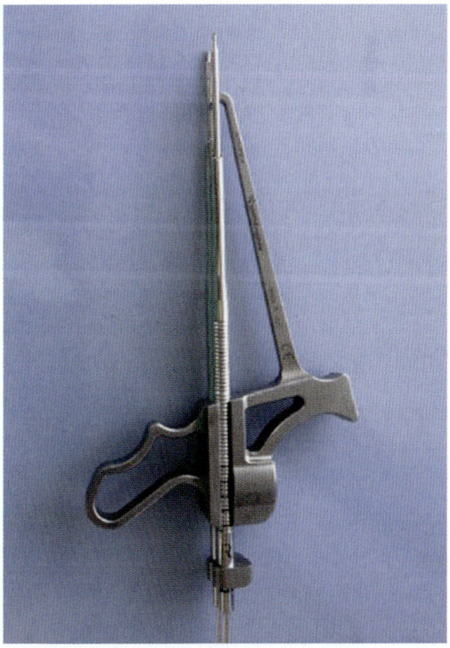

Fig. 11.3 Glenoid guide with special bullets used to create holes from posterior to anterior at level of glenoid rim and two 2.8-mm sleeves. (From Taverna E, D'Ambrosi R, Perfetti C, et al. Arthroscopic bone graft procedure for anterior inferior glenohumeral instability. *Arthrosc Tech.* 2014;3(6):e653-660.)

tissue Bankart repair (anchors will be inserted at the end of the procedure). The drill sleeves should be removed after this step is completed (Fig. 1I.2, *G*).

BONE-BLOCK PREPARATION

The tricortical bone graft is harvested from the ipsilateral anterior iliac crest. After a 4-cm skin incision has been made and splitting of the subcutaneous tissue has been performed, the inserting muscles are dissected from the iliac crest, and 2.5 to 3 cm of bone is marked with a fine-tip cautery while keeping a minimum safety distance of 4 cm posterior to the anterior superior iliac spine. The tricortical iliac crest bone block, measuring 20 mm × 8 mm × 8 mm, is fashioned using the graft master preparation board. Two 2.8-mm drill holes are made 10 mm apart and 5 mm from each edge. The drill enters through the cortex and exits the cancellous side of the bone block. The holes created correspond to the distance of the cannulated drill sleeves previously placed in the glenoid neck. With a marking pen, we color the superior aspect of the bone block.

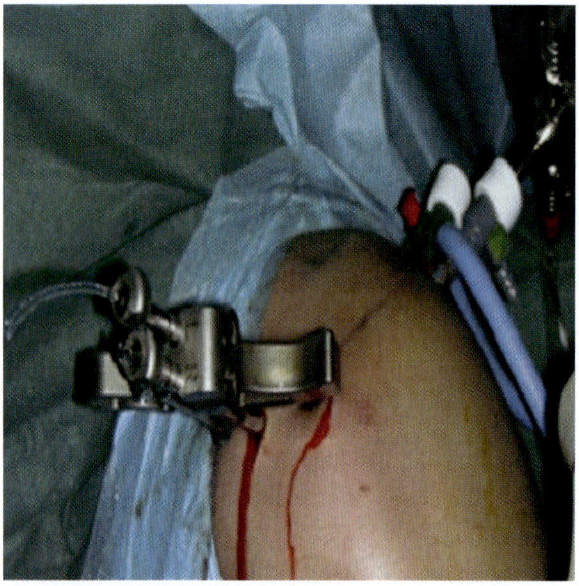

Fig. 1I.4 Outside view of proper positioning of glenoid guide and insertion of the bullet (right shoulder). (From Taverna E, D'Ambrosi R, Perfetti C, et al. Arthroscopic bone graft procedure for anterior inferior glenohumeral instability. *Arthrosc Tech.* 2014;3(6):e653-660.)

GRAFT PASSAGE AND LOADING OF IMPLANTS (ANTERIOR AND POSTERIOR ROUND ENDOBUTTONS)

Before loading the implant onto the guidewires, care is taken to ensure that the looped guidewires are not tangled within the joint. Each looped guidewire is fed through the prepared bone block and exits on the cortical side (Fig. 1I.6, *A*). The bone block is oriented so that the cancellous surface is facing the anterior neck of the glenoid. The anterior implant is fed with the preassembled suture through the end of the looped guidewire with a classic slip knot. This can be achieved by passing the lead suture through the looped guidewire and feeding the implant through the lead suture (Fig. 1I.6, *B*). The bone block is slid toward the end of the guidewires to lodge the implants. Anterior round EndoButtons (Smith & Nephew, London, England) (Fig. 1I.7) are advanced until they lie flat on the bone block. Sutures should be taut to allow smooth movement down the cannula (Fig. 1I.6, *C*). The bone block is tipped to be inserted into the 10-mm cannula, and care is taken to ensure that the superior end of the bone block enters the cannula first (Fig. 1I.6, *D*). The bone block is advanced by pulling the guidewires out posteriorly. Slight tension should be maintained on the sutures throughout this step (Fig. 1I.6, *E*). The sutures should advance the implant until the bone block sits flush on the anterior neck

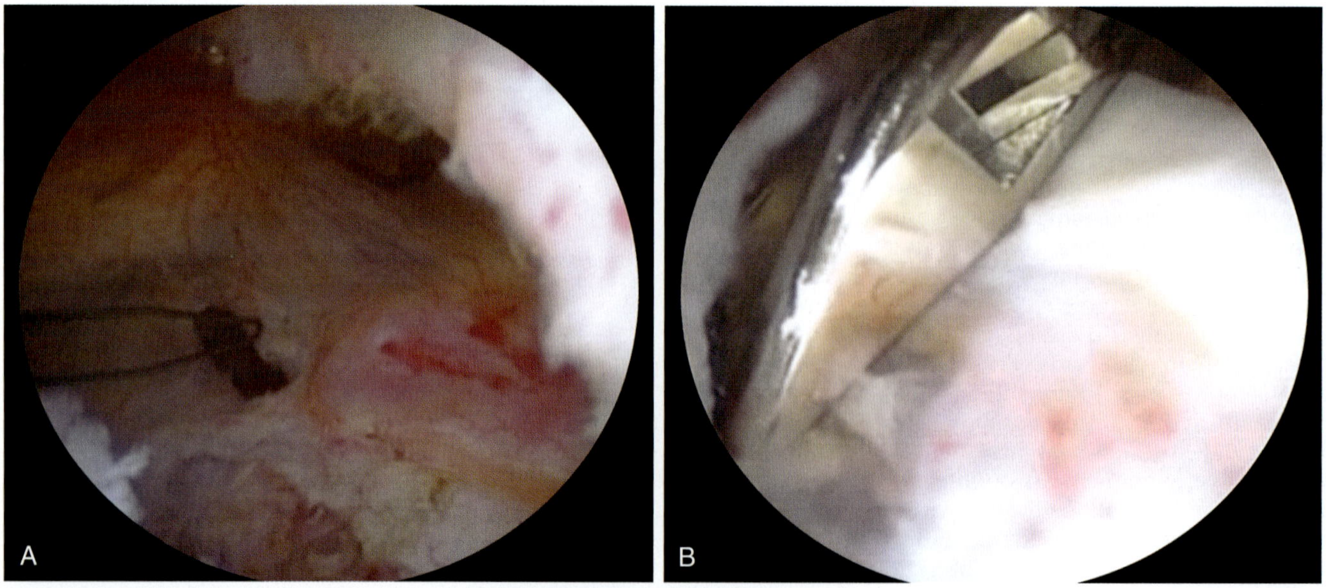

Fig. 1I.5 **A,** Arthroscopic view from the posterior portal of the flexible loop guidewires in the joint (Looped Guidewire). **B,** Arthroscopic view from posterior portal of loop grasper used to retrieve flexible loop (Loop Grasper). (From Taverna E, D'Ambrosi R, Perfetti C, et al. Arthroscopic bone graft procedure for anterior inferior glenohumeral instability. *Arthrosc Tech.* 2014;3(6):e653-60.)

of the glenoid, with each implant's lead suture exiting the skin posteriorly (Fig. 1I.6, *F*). The posterior implants are placed on the transporter by advancing the instrument through the eyelet of a posterior round EndoButton (Fig. 1I.6, *G*). The suture is passed through the transporter. The transporter is retracted to allow the suture to pass through the eyelet of the posterior round EndoButton. The same steps must be performed for the second eyelet with the other side of the suture (Fig. 1I.6, *H*). The posterior round EndoButtons are advanced until they sit flush against the posterior face of the glenoid. The knot pusher is used to secure the posterior round EndoButtons. The knot pusher will provide tactile feedback when the posterior round EndoButtons are properly seated (Fig. 1I.6, *I*).

NICE KNOT

The side of the suture that was cut with the remaining lead suture tails will serve as a post (Fig. 1I.8, *A*). With the post in hand, we create a figure-of-4 by placing the loop over the post (Fig. 1I.8, *B*). We then bring the loop underneath the post and through the figure-of-4. The loop is opened at the end of the thread (Fig. 1I.8, *C*). Then, we place the post through the open loop created previously (Fig. 1I.8, *D*). Finally, we build the knot behind the posterior implant by pulling tight on the loop (Fig. 1I.8, *E*). Care must be taken to ensure that the knot is fully taut before pulling the post and advancing the posterior implant (Fig. 1I.8, *F*).

SECURE NICE KNOT

We advance the Nice knot to the face of the posterior round EndoButton (Fig. 1I.9, *A*). At this point, we use a suture tensioner device (Fig. 1I.10) to secure the implant and to provide strong compression of the graft on the anterior glenoid neck. After the implant has been tensioned, we secure the posterior knots with half hitches, and we cut the remaining sutures using a blind knot cutter (Figs. 1I.9, *B* and *C* and 1I.11).

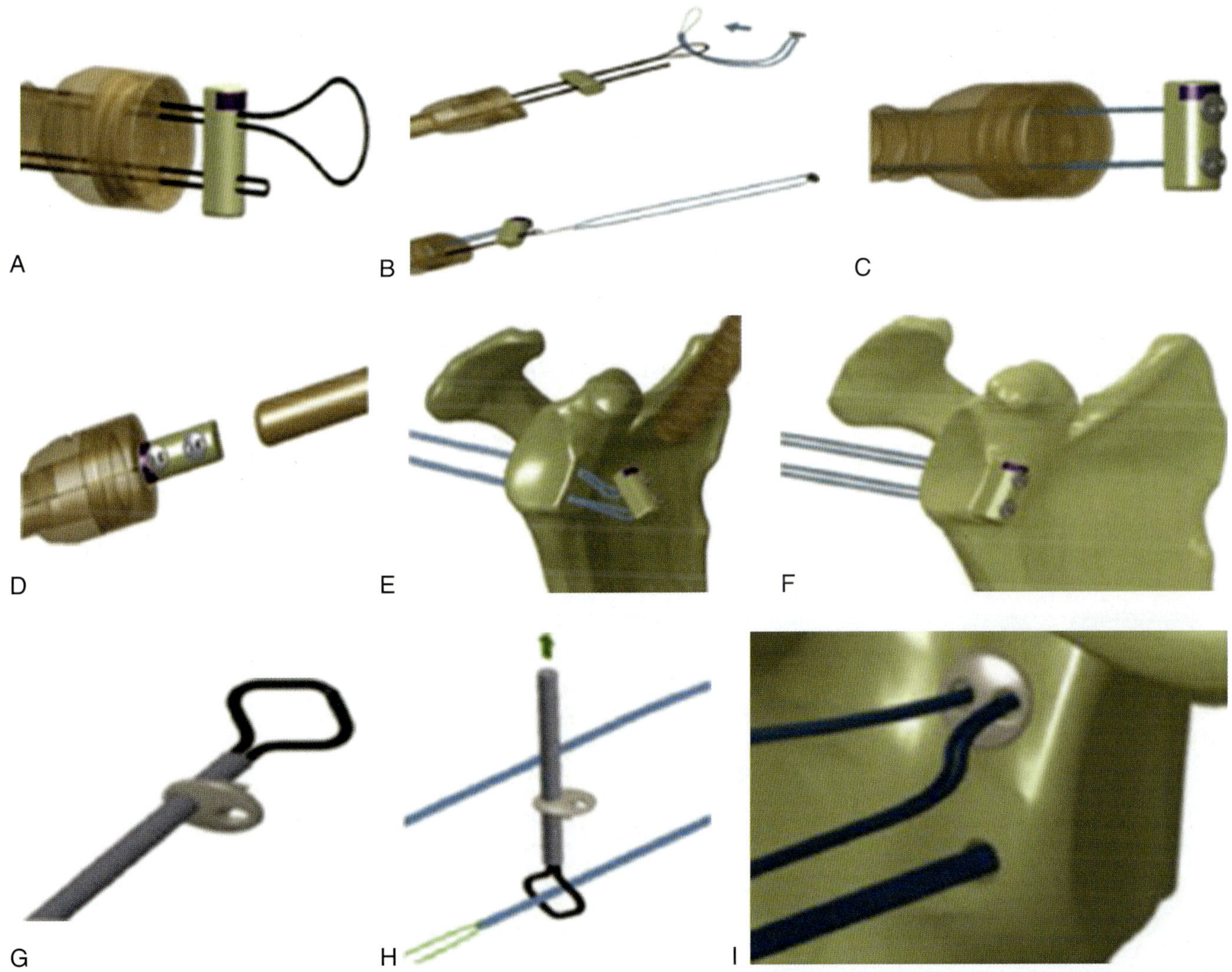

Fig. 1I.6 Graft passage and loading of implant. **A,** The implant is loaded onto the guidewires. Each guide is fed through the bone block. **B,** The implant is fed with the preassembled suture through the end of the looped guidewire with a classic slip knot. **C,** The bone block is slid toward the end of the guidewires to lodge the implants. **D,** The bone block is slid through the cannula up to the anterior glenoid rim. **E,** The bone block is advanced, pulling the suture from posterior. **F,** The bone block is made flush with the anterior glenoid rim. **G,** The implant is placed on the transporter. **H,** The suture is passed through the transporter. **I,** The posterior round EndoButton is advanced to sit flush against the posterior face of the glenoid. (From Taverna E, D'Ambrosi R, Perfetti C, et al. Arthroscopic bone graft procedure for anterior inferior glenohumeral instability. *Arthrosc Tech*. 2014;3(6):e653-660.)

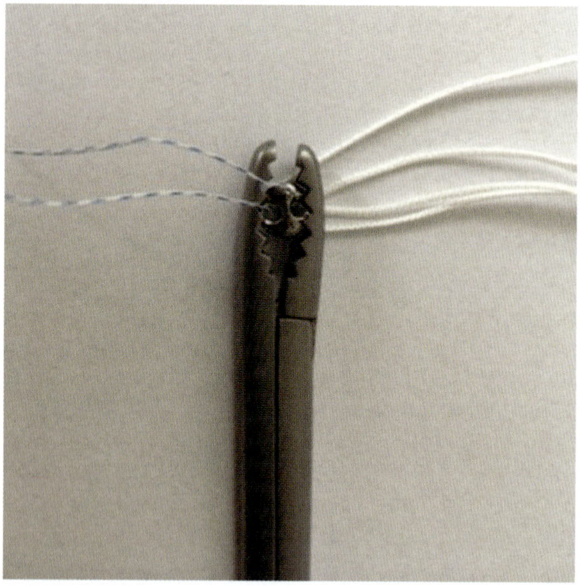

Fig. 1I.7 Round EndoButton used to fix the bone block to the anterior glenoid rim (Round EndoButton SS with No. 2 Suture Loop). (From Taverna E, D'Ambrosi R, Perfetti C, et al. Arthroscopic bone graft procedure for anterior inferior glenohumeral instability. *Arthrosc Tech.* 2014;3(6):e653-60.)

SOFT TISSUE REPAIR

The anterior labrum, capsule, and ligaments are repaired to the glenoid rim with suture anchors and a standard arthroscopic soft tissue repair technique (Fig. 1I.12).

REHABILITATION PROTOCOL

After surgery, the shoulder is immobilized in a brace at 10 degrees of abduction for 4 weeks. There are no limitations regarding passive movement after immobilization, and patients are subsequently allowed to regain full elevation and external rotation. After complete healing of the wound, pool exercises and return to work activities are authorized. Progressive stretching exercises are started after 6 to 8 weeks. Return to contact sports and overhead mobility is generally allowed 4 to 6 months after surgery (Figs. 1I.13 and 1I.14).

RISKS

The general risks related to our intervention can be compared with the risks that exist during an arthroscopic procedure for shoulder instability repair (Moen et al, 2014). Our procedure has some specific risks. If correct placement of the graft cannot be achieved, it is necessary to change to an open approach with consequent arthrotomy. This has

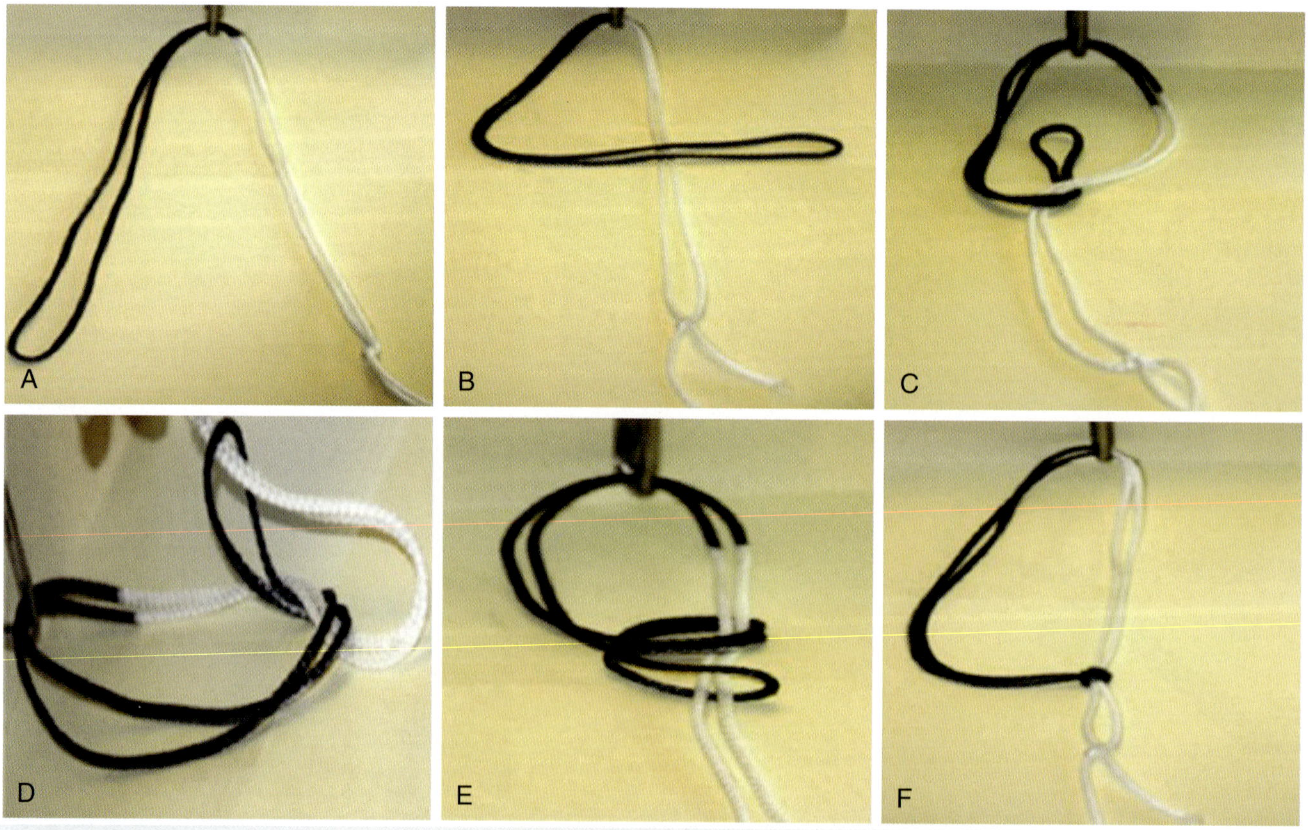

Fig. 1I.8 Nice knot. **A,** The side of the suture that was cut is the post. **B,** A figure-of-4 is created by placing the loop over the post. **C,** The loop is brought underneath the post, and the loop is opened at the end of the thread. **D,** The post is placed through the open loop created before. **E,** The knot is built behind the posterior implant by pulling tight on the loop. **F,** Care is taken to ensure that the knot is fully taut before pulling the post and advancing the implant. (From Taverna E, D'Ambrosi R, Perfetti C, et al. Arthroscopic bone graft procedure for anterior inferior glenohumeral instability. *Arthrosc Tech.* 2014;3(6):e653-660.)

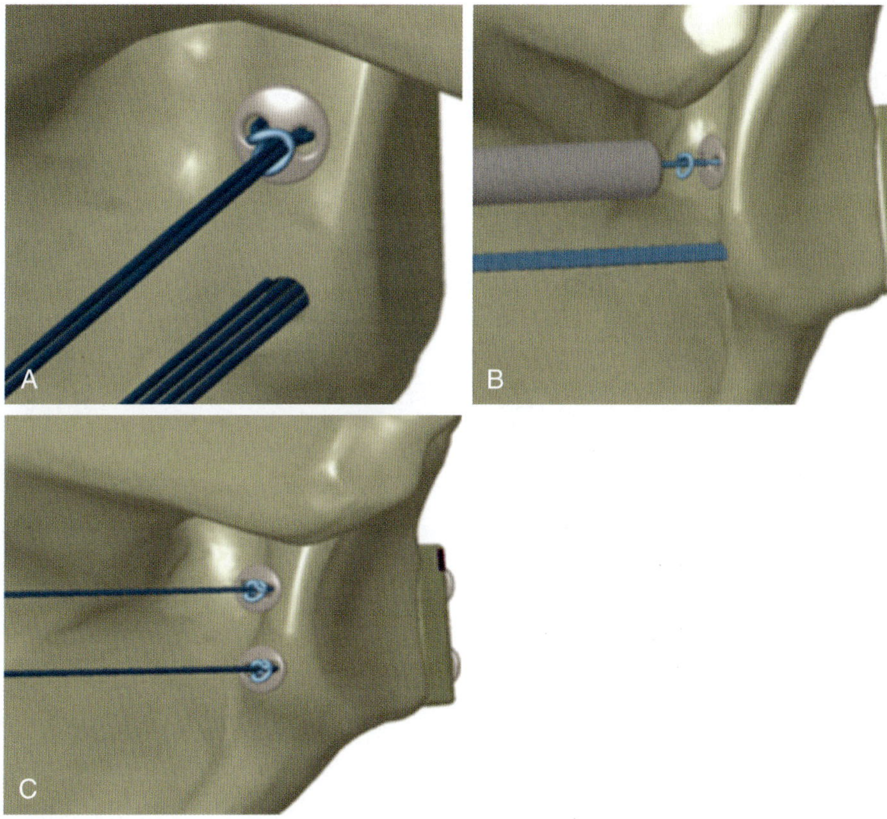

Fig. 1I.9 Secure Nice knot. **A,** The Nice knot is advanced up to the round button. **B,** The implant is secured with the tensioner, and the remaining suture is cut. **C,** The same steps are repeated for the inferior implant. (From Taverna E, D'Ambrosi R, Perfetti C, et al. Arthroscopic bone graft procedure for anterior inferior glenohumeral instability. *Arthrosc Tech.* 2014;3(6):e653-660.)

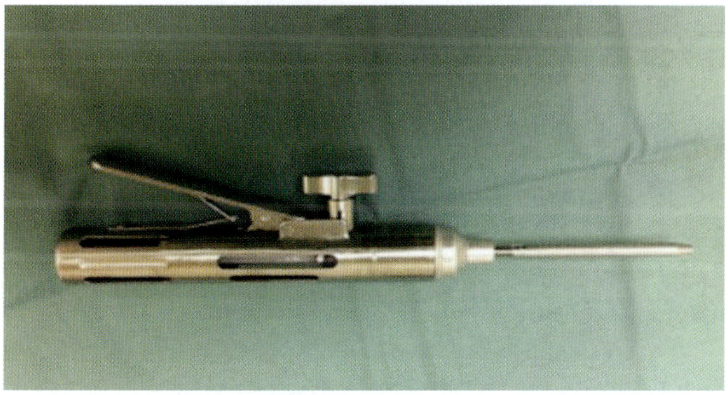

Fig. 1I.10 Tensioner device used to fix and secure implant (Suture Tensioner). (From Taverna E, D'Ambrosi R, Perfetti C, et al. Arthroscopic bone graft procedure for anterior inferior glenohumeral instability. *Arthrosc Tech.* 2014;3(6):e653-60.)

occurred twice with the previous technique of fixing the bone block with screws but to date has never occurred with the newly described procedure. To obtain perfect placement of the graft, it is mandatory to achieve perfect placement of the guide.

If the hook is not perfectly parallel to the glenoid face, there will be a bone graft offset greater than 5 mm, with final placement of the graft medial to the glenoid rim. The positioning of the anterior portals is performed at the level of the rotator interval, thereby avoiding possible nerve injuries. In the same manner, the glenoid guide is designed to maintain distance from the vascular or neural structures

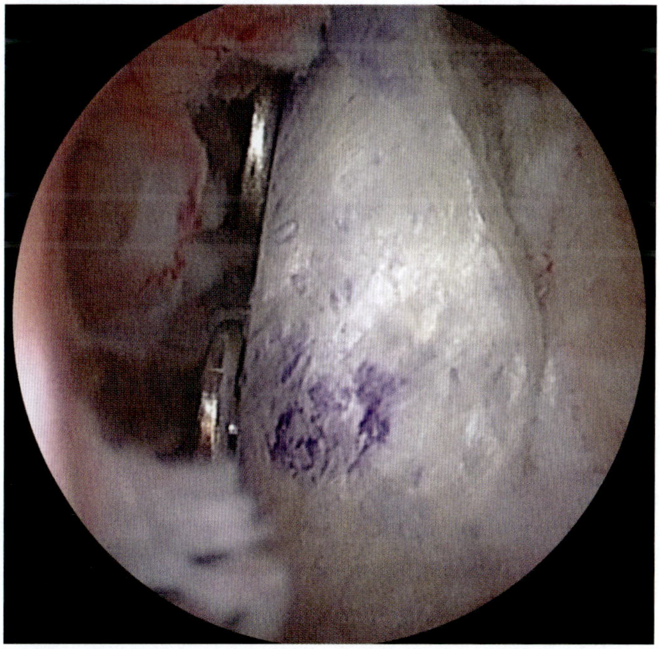

Fig. 1I.11 Arthroscopic view from the anterior portal. The bone block is perfectly flush with the anterior glenoid rim. (From Taverna E, D'Ambrosi R, Perfetti C, et al. Arthroscopic bone graft procedure for anterior inferior glenohumeral instability. *Arthrosc Tech.* 2014;3(6):e653-60.)

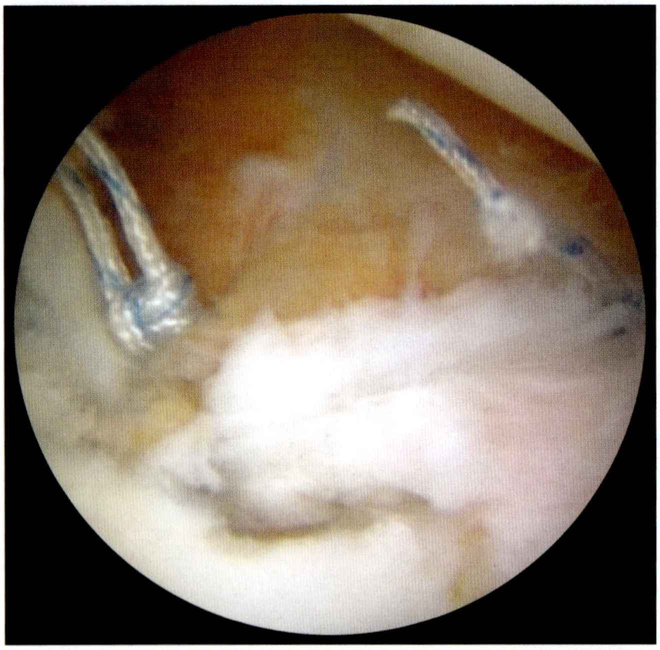

Fig. 1I.12 Arthroscopic view from the posterior portal. The anterior labrum and capsule are repaired to the glenoid rim with suture anchors and a standard Bankart repair technique. (From Taverna E, D'Ambrosi R, Perfetti C, et al. Arthroscopic bone graft procedure for anterior inferior glenohumeral instability. *Arthrosc Tech.* 2014;3(6):e653-660.)

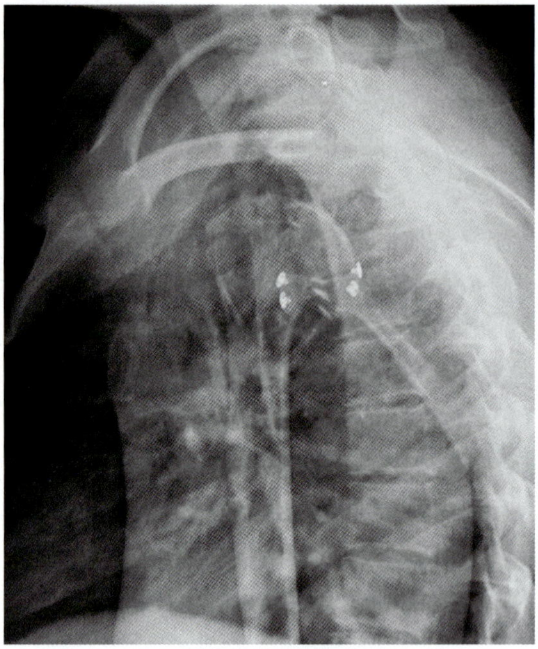

Fig. 1I.13 Lateral radiographic projection of a right shoulder the day after surgery. The bone block and buttons are correctly positioned. (From Taverna E, D'Ambrosi R, Perfetti C, et al. Arthroscopic bone graft procedure for anterior inferior glenohumeral instability. *Arthrosc Tech.* 2014;3(6):e653-660.)

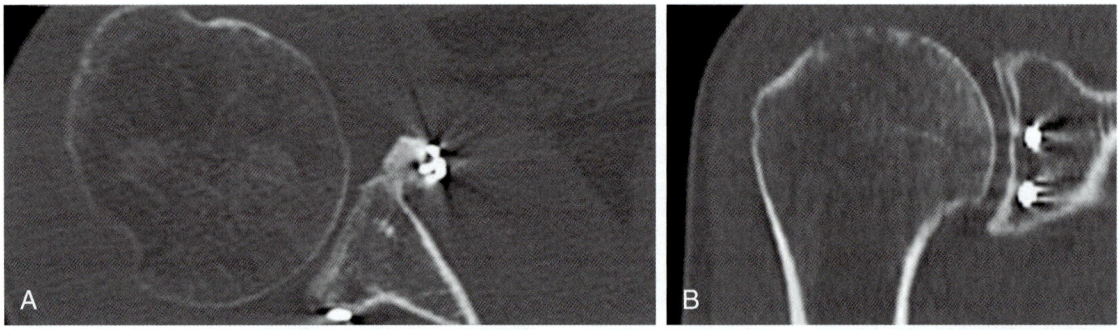

Fig. 1I.14 Computed tomography images showing bone graft healing and remodeling after 6 months in a right shoulder: axial (**A**) and coronal (**B**) views. (From Taverna E, D'Ambrosi R, Perfetti C, et al. Arthroscopic bone graft procedure for anterior inferior glenohumeral instability. *Arthrosc Tech.* 2014;3(6):e653-660.)

while positioning the sleeves. In case of mechanical inconsistency or absence of the soft tissues, it is possible to switch to an arthroscopically assisted Latarjet procedure that we have recently described (Taverna et al, 2013).

Clinical Results

Early results on a small series of 16 patients with an average of 20.6 months of follow-up (range, 13–30 months) are promising (Table 1I.1).

All patients had a pain-free shoulder in daily activities, 15 of the 16 patients had a stable shoulder without postoperative dislocations or subluxations, and 1 had a posterior dislocation caused by a new traumatic injury (ski fall). None had recurrent anterior dislocation or subluxation. At last clinical follow-up, 1 patient (6.25%) still had pain (visual analog scale score, 4) in abduction-external rotation with apprehension.

Table 1I.1 Functional Results

Scoring System	Value
Recurrence rate	0%
Walch-Duplay score (maximum, 100 points)	93.2 ± 7.76 SD (range, 75–100)
Rowe score (maximum, 100 points)	96.4 ± 6.45 SD (range, 75–100)
SSV (maximum, 100%)	87.36 ± 12.1 SD (range, 60–100)
Satisfaction grade	93.75% mostly or very satisfied

SD, Standard deviation; *SSV*, ***.

Excluding the patient with posterior dislocation, the average Rowe score was 96.4 (range, 75–100), the average Walch-Duplay score was 93.2 (range, 75–100), average and the SSV was 87.36 (range, 60–100).

Fourteen of 16 patients (87.5%) were mostly satisfied or very satisfied, and 15 (93.75%) would undergo the same procedure again if needed.

Average anterior flexion was 178 degrees (range, 160–180 degrees); average external rotation with elbow at side 61 degrees (range, 20–90 degrees) compared with 66 degrees (range, 30–90 degrees) on the contralateral side. Average loss of external rotation with elbow at side was 4.4 degrees, but no one was aware of it.

Eight of 12 patients returned to sport at preinjury level (67%) and 3 of 5 at a competitive level.

Two patients experienced a postoperative hematoma along the axillary fold and arm that resorbed spontaneously after 3 and 6 weeks. We did not detect any nerve injury.

In our series, although none of our patients experienced a recurrence of anterior instability, we are aware that the recurrence rate could increase over time.

Many authors emphasize the importance of the conjoined tendon sling (i.e., dynamic sling or seat belt effect) in stability outcomes after a Latarjet procedure (Collin et al, 2007; Giles et al, 2013; Latarjet, 1954; Patte & Debeyre, 1980; Walch & Boileau, 2000; Wellmann et al, 2012). The results of our technique (in which the conjoined tendon transfer is not performed) results in no sling effect. We therefore believe that the anatomic reinsertion of labrum and capsule and an anatomic reconstruction of glenoid bone deficiency addresses all components of pathoanatomy reducing instability and may theoretically reduce the risk of scapular dyskinesia (Carbone et al, 2016).

We believe that the capsulolabral repair is crucial in terms of shoulder stability (preventing subluxations (Collin et al, 2007; Yamashita et al, 2002) and proprioception tp provide a high rate of return to sport activity at preinjury level (Yamashita et al, 2002; Yoneda, 1999). Although several authors claimed that the anterior capsule regenerated after its resection (Lafosse & Boyle, 2010), it is well known that the fibrous scar tissue loses all proprioceptive capacity. A recent study by Hovelius et al (2012) reinforced this concept, showing better results for stability when the Bristow-Latarjet procedure was associated with a capsular repair using suture anchors.

The postoperative loss of external rotation has long been a major criticism of the Bristow-Latarjet procedure, leading some authors to contraindicate the procedure in overhead throwing athletes (Young & Rockwood, 1991; Zuckerman & Matsen, 1984). In our series, the loss of external rotation with the elbow at side was 4.4 degrees on average and was not a significant complaint in the overhead athletes. We believe that this range of movement results from some important intraoperative details, including the accurate placement of the graft flush to the articular surface and the soft tissue repair in an anatomic position. The restoration of stability and mobility has probably contributed to the high rate of return to sport at preinjury level (67%), also among competitive athletes.

Table 1I.2 Radiologic Results

Graft Positioning	Number of Shoulders
VERTICAL POSITION	
Under the equator	14 (87.5%)
High	2 (12.5%)
HORIZONTAL POSITION	
Flush	16 (100%)
Lateral	0
Too medial	0

Radiographic Findings

Twelve months after surgery, positioning and healing of the graft were assessed with a CT scan. On the sagittal plane, the bone graft was considered well placed in 14 patients (87.5%), 2 were judged high, and all cases were flush to the glenoid surface in the horizontal plane (Table 1I.2; see also Fig. 1I.15).

At a mean 20.6 months of follow-up, the bone block was healed in 14 patients (87.5%), there was one nonunion (6.5%), and one completely osteolysed. In none of the cases were the EndoButtons considered too lateral or migrated. Neither of the two patients with nonunion and osteolysis underwent revision surgery.

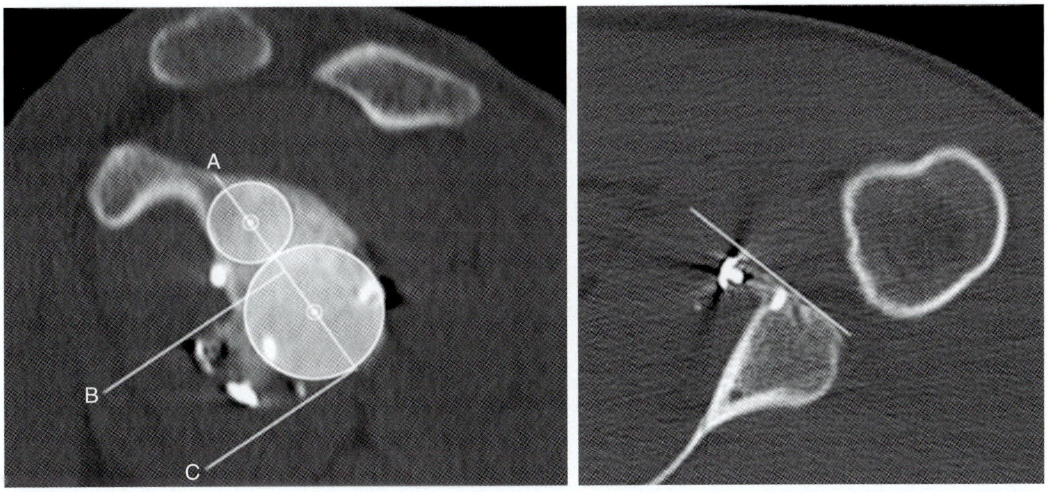

Fig. 1I.15 Computed tomography images showing bone graft healing and remodeling after 6 months. Graphic evaluation of graft positioning on sagittal and horizontal planes.

At last follow-up, 15 patients (93.75%) had no signs of osteoarthritis, and 1 patient had grade one (Samilson & Prieto, 1983) degenerative change but was not symptomatic to require further surgical treatment. No graft fracture or migration was detected. Our healing rate (87.5%) is better than the ones reported by Hovelius et al (2012) and Longo et al (2014) for the open Bristow-Latarjet and the open Eden-Hybinette procedures. This is likely because of the fixation with EndoButtons (instead of screws) of an arthroscopic guide and a tensioner device. EndoButtons avoid the risk of screw length errors, and the guide avoids excessive angulation (>25 degrees) of the tunnels (Patel et al, 2013; Walch, 1991). The tensioner device provides an optimal balanced tension between the two couples of EndoButtons.

Development of subsequent osteoarthritis after the Bristow-Latarjet and Eden-Hybinette procedures has been another major criticism of the bone grafting techniques (Young & Rockwood, 1991; Zuckerman & Matsen, 1984). In our series, 93.75% of patients had no glenohumeral osteoarthritis at last follow-up.

Arthroscopic visualization of the glenohumeral joint permits the Bankart repair and facilitates optimal positioning of the coracoid bone block in an extraarticular position. This prevents undesirable contact between the humeral head and the bone block, avoiding pain and the development of osteoarthritis. In the unlikely event of graft resorption, the use of EndoButtons avoids the risk of humeral head–screw contact, a major cause of cartilage injury.

Conclusion

Our results show that the arthroscopic bone-block grafting combined with a standard Bankart repair restores shoulder stability in patients with anteroinferior glenoid bone deficit. This procedure does not substantially limit external rotation and has a low incidence of secondary osteoarthritis at short-term follow-up.

The rate to return to sport activities was high even among competitive, overhead, and "at-risk" athletes. The direct visualization of the glenohumeral surface allows an optimal graft positioning and an anatomic labrum and soft tissue repair. The use of EndoButtons avoids common drawbacks of screw fixation (inappropriate length, screw breakage, screw pull-out, subscapularis impingement, humeral head contact), the aid of a guide allows the optimal positioning of the graft flush to the glenoid rim, avoiding excessive angulation of the tunnels, and the use of a tensioner device provides an optimal balanced compression of the two couples of EndoButtons. Last, an all-arthroscopic technique leads to a better cosmetic result.

References

Allain J, Goutallier D, Glorion C. Long-term results of the Latarjet procedure for the treatment of anterior instability of the shoulder. *J Bone Joint Surg Am*. 1998;80(6):841–852.

Anderl W, Kriegleder B, Heuberer PR. All-arthroscopic implant-free iliac crest bone grafting: new technique and case report. *Arthroscopy*. 2012;28:131–137.

Balg F, Boileau P. The instability severity index score. A simple preoperative score to select patients for arthroscopic or open shoulder stabilisation. *J Bone Joint Surg Br*. 2007;89(11):1470–1477.

Burkhart SS, De Beer JF, Barth JR, Cresswell T, Roberts C, Richards DP. Results of modified Latarjet reconstruction in patients with anteroinferior instability and significant bone loss. *Arthroscopy*. 2007;23(10):1033–1041.

Burkhart S.S, De Beer JF, Tehrany AM, Parten PM. Quantifying glenoid bone loss arthroscopically in shoulder instability. *Arthroscopy*. 2002;18(5):488–491.

Carbone S, Moroder P, Runer A, Resch H, Gumina S, Hertel R. Scapular dyskinesis after Latarjet procedure. *J Shoulder Elbow Surg*. 2016;25(3):422–427.

Collin P, Rochcongar P, Thomazeau H. [Treatment of chronic anterior shoulder instability using a coracoid bone block (Latarjet procedure): 74 cases] [in French]. *Rev Chir Orthop Reparatrice Appar Mot*. 2007;93:126–132.

Giles JW, Boons HW, Elkinson I, et al. Does the dynamic sling effect of the Latarjet procedure improve shoulder joint stability? A biomechanical evaluation. *J Shoulder Elbow Surg*. 2013;22:821–827.

Hill JA, Lombardo SJ, Kerlan RK, et al. The modification Bristow-Helfet procedure for recurrent anterior shoulder subluxations and dislocations. *Am J Sports Med*. 1981;9:283–287.

Hovelius L, Sandstrom B, Olofsson A, Svensson O, Rahme H. The effect of capsular repair, bone block healing, and position on the results of the Bristow-Latarjet procedure (study III): long-term follow-up in 319 shoulders. *J Shoulder Elbow Surg*. 2012;21(5):647–660.

Hovelius L, Sandstrom B, Sundgren K, Saebö M. One hundred eighteen Bristow-Latarjet repairs for recurrent anterior dislocation of the shoulder prospectively followed for fifteen years: study I—clinical results. *J Shoulder Elbow Surg*. 2004;13(5):509–516.

Kraus N, Amphansap T, Gerhardt C, Scheibel M. Arthroscopic anatomic glenoid reconstruction using an autologous iliac crest bone grafting technique. *J Shoulder Elbow Surg*. 2014;23(11):1700–1708.

Lafosse L, Boyle S. Arthroscopic Latarjet procedure. *J Shoulder Elbow Surg*. 2010;19:2–12.

Latarjet M. [Treatment of recurrent dislocation of the shoulder] [in French]. *Lyon Chirurg*. 1954;49:994–997.

Levy DM, Cole BJ, Bach BR Jr. *J Shoulder Elbow Surg*. 2016;25(6):e139. 50.

Longo UG, Loppini M, Rizzello G, Ciuffreda M, Maffulli N, Denaro V. Latarjet, Bristow, and Eden-Hybinette procedures for anterior shoulder dislocation: systematic review and quantitative synthesis of the literature. *Arthroscopy*. 2014;30(9):1184–1211.

Moen TC, Rudolph GH, Caswell K, Espinoza C, Burkhead WZ Jr, Krishnan SG. Complications of shoulder arthroscopy. *J Am Acad Orthop Surg*. 2014;22:410–419.

Patel RA, Wilson RF, Patel PA, Palmer RM. The effect of smoking on bone healing: a systematic review. *Bone Joint Res*. 2013;2:102–111.

Patte D, Debeyre J. Luxations recidivantes de l'epaule. Encycl Med Chir Paris [in French]. *Tech Chir Orthop*. 1980;44265. 4.4-02.

Provencher MT, Bhatia S, Ghodadra NS, et al. Recurrent shoulder instability: Current concepts for evaluation and management of glenoid bone loss. *J Bone Joint Surg Am*. 2010;92(suppl 2):133–151.

Samilson RL, Prieto V. Dislocation arthropathy of the shoulder. *J Bone Joint Surg Am*. 1983;65:456–460.

Sayegh ET, Mascarenhas R, Chalmers PN, Cole BJ, Verma NN, Romeo AA. Allograft reconstruction for glenoid bone loss in glenohumeral instability: a systematic review. *Arthroscopy*. 2014;30(12):1642–1649.

Scheibel M, Kraus N, Diederichs G, Haas NP. Arthroscopic reconstruction of chronic anteroinferior glenoid defect using an autologous tricortical iliac crest bone grafting technique. *Arch Orthop Trauma Surg*. 2008;128:1295–1300.

Schroder DT, Provencher MT, Mologne TS, Muldoon MP, Cox JS. The modified Bristow procedure for anterior shoulder instability: 26-year outcomes in Naval Academy midshipmen. *Am J Sports Med*. 2006;34(5):778–786.

Sugaya H, Moriishi J, Dohi M, Kon Y, Tsuchiya A. Glenoid rim morphology in recurrent anterior glenohumeral instability. *J Bone Joint Surg Am*. 2003;85-A(5):878–884.

Taverna E, D'Ambrosi R, Perfetti C, Garavaglia G. Arthroscopic bone graft procedure for anterior inferior glenohumeral instability. *Arthrosc Tech*. 2014;3(6):e653–e660.

Taverna E, Garavaglia G, Ufenast H, D'Ambrosi R. Arthroscopic treatment of glenoid bone loss. *Knee Surg Sports Traumatol Arthrosc*. 2016;24(2):546–556.

Taverna E, Ufenast H, Broffoni L, Garavaglia G. Arthroscopically assisted Latarjet procedure: a new surgical approach for accurate coracoid graft placement and compression. *Int J Shoulder Surg*. 2013;7:120–123.

Walch G. [Recurrent anterior shoulder instability] [in French]. *Rev Chir Orthop Reparatrice Appar Mot*. 1991;77:177–191.

Walch G, Boileau P. Latarjet-Bristow procedure for recurrent anterior instability. *Tech Shoulder Elbow Surg*. 2000;1:256–261.
Warner JJ, Gill TJ, O'Hollerhan JD, Pathare N, Millett PJ. Anatomical glenoid reconstruction for recurrent anterior glenohumeral instability with glenoid deficiency using an autogenous tricortical iliac crest bone graft. *Am J Sports Med*. 2006;34(2):205–212.
Wellmann M, de Ferrari H, Smith T, et al. Biomechanical investigation of the stabilization principle of the Latarjet procedure. *Arch Orthop Trauma Surg*. 2012;132:377–386.
Yamashita T, Okamura K, Hotta T, Wada T, Aoki M, Ishii S. Good clinical outcome of combined Bankart-Bristow procedure for recurrent shoulder instability: 126 patients followed for 2-6 years. *Acta Orthop Scand*. 2002;73:553–557.
Yoneda M, Hayashida K, Wakitani S, Nakagawa S, Fukushima S. Bankart procedure augmented by coracoid transfer for contact athletes with traumatic anterior shoulder instability. *Am J Sports Med*. 1999;27(1): 21–6.
Young DC, Rockwood CA. Complications of a failed Bristow procedure and their management. *J Bone Joint Surg Am*. 1991;73:969–981.
Zuckerman JD, Matsen FA. Complications about the glenohumeral joint related to the use of screws and staples. *J Bone Joint Surg Am*. 1984;66:175–180.

1-1J ARTHROSCOPIC REPAIR OF OSSEOUS BANKART LESIONS

KEISUKE MATSUKI, MD and HIROYUKI SUGAYA, MD

Introduction

- Osseous Bankart lesions are seen in approximately 50% of shoulders with traumatic anterior shoulder instability (Sugaya et al, 2003).
- The lesions are frequently found in male contact or collision athletes.
- Bony fragments are sometimes ignored or removed when the lesions are arthroscopically repaired (Bigliani et al, 1998; Burkhart & De Beer, 2000), and some studies have reported unfavorable outcomes after arthroscopic repair of Bankart lesion in shoulders with substantial glenoid bone loss (Burkhart & De Beer, 2000).
- Many surgeons prefer glenoid bone augmentation such as the Latarjet procedure for shoulders with substantial glenoid bone loss, regardless of the presence of a retained osseous fragment (Burkhart et al, 2007; Lafosse et al, 2007).
- We reported excellent outcomes after arthroscopic osseous Bankart repair without removing bony fragments in both short- and medium-term follow-ups (Kitayama et al, 2015; Sugaya et al, 2005).
- We introduce our evaluation and management for osseous Bankart lesions in this chapter.

Evaluation of Osseous Bankart Lesion

Precise evaluation of the size of bony fragments and glenoid bone loss is essential for preoperative planning. Based on the image evaluation, surgeons need to preoperatively decide how they manage the bone fragment, such as penetrating or passing around the fragment, and which augmentation procedures they should add.

RADIOGRAPHY

Radiographic images are helpful in detecting the bony lesions of the glenoid, but the ability of conventional anteroposterior images to detect the lesions should be limited (Edwards et al, 2003). However, Bernageau et al (1976) proposed an effective method for detection of the glenoid lesions with patients in the standing position. We have developed a modified Bernageau method with patients lying on their axilla in their most relaxed position, which we called the "TV-watching position" (Fig. 1J.1). We can acquire clear images to detect the anterior glenoid rim lesions with this method. This x-ray method may be useful as a screening at patients' first visit to clinics.

COMPUTED TOMOGRAPHY

Computed tomography (CT), especially three-dimensional (3D) CT, should be the gold standard for evaluation of the glenoid rim lesions at present. Several methods have been proposed to quantify bone loss and bony fragment of the glenoid using CT images in the sagittal plane. Width measurement is easy and reproducible but might be insufficient in terms of accuracy. Area measurements are more ideal to quantify the bone but need a longer time to precisely draw a region of interest on the edge of a fragment than to measure the width of a fragment. We simply evaluate bone loss and fragment size with width measurement because our recent study indicated that the bone loss measured with width and area were highly correlated (Kitayama et al, 2015). The size of Hill-Sachs lesions should be also evaluated using transverse and 3D reconstructed CT images and calculate if the lesion is on track or off track (Yamamoto et al, 2007). This is one of the factors to determine which augmentation procedures should be added.

MAGNETIC RESONANCE IMAGING

Magnetic resonance imaging (MRI) may be inappropriate for evaluation of bony fragments but is useful for assessment of soft tissue pathology. We usually perform MR arthrography with use of a diluted contrast agent because plain MRI does not provide much information in shoulders with instability. It is important for surgeons to preoperatively assess pathology other than Bankart lesions, such as rotator cuff tears, superior labrum anterior and posterior (SLAP) lesions, capsular tears, and humeral avulsion of the

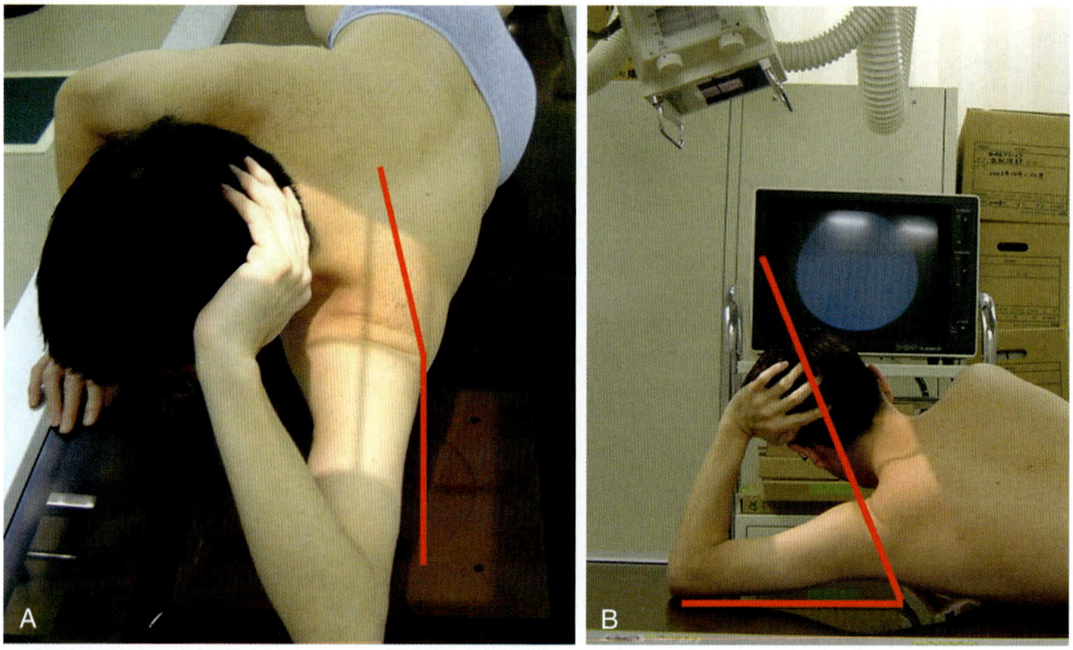

Fig. 1J.1 A modified Bernageau method. Patients lie on their axilla in their most relaxed position. In this position, the scapula needs to incline 5 degrees to the vertical line (**A**). Then the incident radiograph needs to be aimed craniocaudally with 70 to 75 degrees of inclination to the horizontal line (**B**). (Used with permission from Sugaya H. Instability with bone loss. In Angelo RA, Esch JE, Ryu RR, eds. *AANA Advanced Arthroscopy: The Shoulder*. Philadelphia: Elsevier; 2010:136–146.)

glenohumeral ligament (HAGL). We recommend obtaining both 3D CT and MR arthrography preoperatively for each patient if possible.

Surgical Management of Osseous Bankart Lesion

Several techniques for arthroscopic osseous Bankart repair have been proposed in the literature (Kim et al, 2009, 2014; Millett et al, 2009; Moran et al, 2014; Sugaya et al, 2005, 2016), and good clinical outcomes have been reported regardless of the repair techniques (Kim et al, 2009, 2014; Kitayama et al, 2015; Sugaya et al, 2005). Bony fragments have a high possibility to achieve bony union if the fragments are properly reduced and fixed (Sugaya et al, 2005). In addition, Kitayama et al (2015) have reported that the shape of the glenoid was restored to nearly normal to hypertrophic at 5- to 8-year follow-up. Regardless of the techniques, excellent fragment reduction and retensioning of the entire inferior glenohumeral ligament (IGHL) based on extensive labrum release may be keys to acquire favorable morphologic and clinical outcomes.

INDICATIONS

This procedure can be indicated to any shoulders with bone loss of less than 20% regardless of the size of bony fragments (Kitayama et al, 2015). For shoulders with bone loss of 20% or more, we generally indicate this procedure if the shoulder retains an osseous fragment of greater than 1% because even a small fragment can be expected to induce remodeling and restore glenoid shape (Kitayama et al, 2015). We add augmentation procedures, rotator interval closure, and/or Hill-Sachs remplissage, according to the risk of recurrence, including gender, age, joint laxity, sports activity, and the size of Hill-Sachs lesion. Bone grafting should be considered for shoulders with an osseous fragment of less than 1% and for shoulders with a fragment of less than 5% that is associated with medium to large Hill-Sachs defect, especially in young and active patients (Kitayama et al, 2015).

OUR SURGICAL TECHNIQUES (Video 1J.1)

Step 1: Settings

The patient is placed in the beach-chair position under general anesthesia with an interscalene block. Routine diagnostic arthroscopy is carried out through a standard posterior portal, and an anterior portal is then established just superior to the subscapularis and lateral to the conjoined tendon. Surgeries are performed using the posterior portal as a viewing portal and the anterior portal as a working portal. An anterosuperior portal is also established at the anterosuperior margin of the rotator interval. This portal is normally created after the labroligamentous complex release and mainly used as an additional working portal. The scope is occasionally introduced to the anterior portal when assessing the Bankart lesion during release and repair of the labroligamentous complex.

Step 2: Mobilization

The displaced osseous fragment with the labroligamentous complex is recognized and separated from the glenoid neck using a rasp introduced through the anterior portal. Mobilization of the labroligamentous complex together with the fragment is performed up to the 7 o'clock position (right shoulder) (Fig. 1J.2, *A*) The inferior labrum, even if it looks intact, needs to be released by arthroscopic scissors along with the border between the inferior glenoid and labrum.

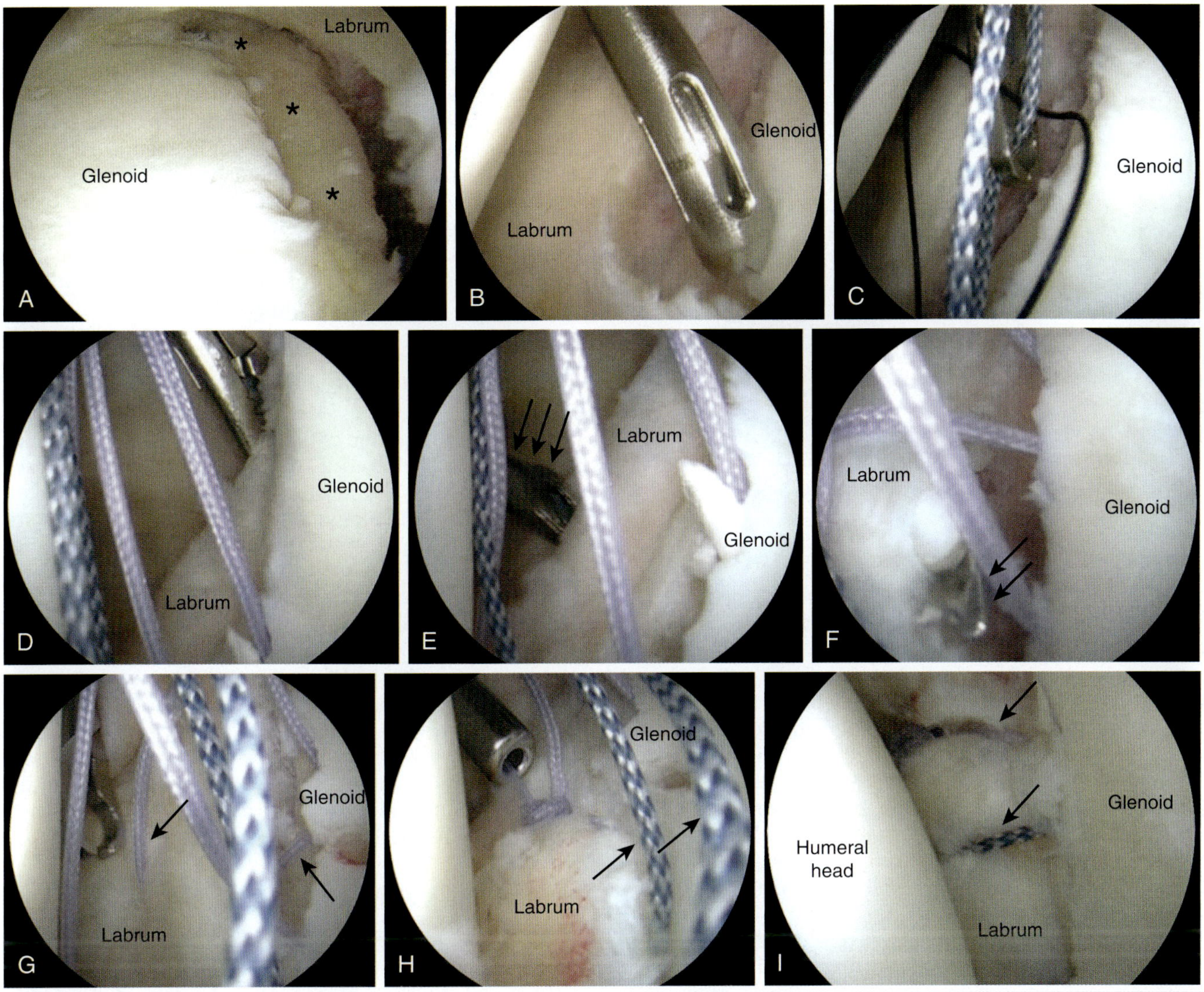

Fig. 1J.2 Arthroscopic views during surgery. **A,** Anterior view after mobilization of the labroligamentous complex. Mobilization of the labroligamentous complex together with the fragment is performed up to the 7 o'clock position (right shoulder). A small amount of articular cartilage at the face of the inferior glenoid from the 3 to 7 o'clock positions is removed to promote tissue healing after repair *(asterisks)*. **B,** Insertion of the 6 o'clock anchor. **C,** A looped nylon suture is placed through the inferior labrum at the 6:30 position using Caspari punch, and one limb of the 6 o'clock suture is retrieved through the loop. The suture is placed through the inferior labrum by pulling out the loop (intraarticular suture relay technique). **D,** The labrum, together with the fragment, is held and stabilized by a robust grasper introduced from the anterosuperior portal to facilitate the fragment management by a bone penetrator. **E,** A Bone Stitcher *(arrows)* is penetrating the labrum and osseous fragment. **F,** Osseous fragment is penetrated with the Bone Stitcher *(arrows)*. **G,** One limb of the 3:20 suture *(arrows)* is passed through the labrum and osseous fragment. **H,** Knot tying of the 4:40 suture. The blue suture of the 6:00 anchor *(arrows)* and the purple suture of the 3:20 suture *(arrowheads)* remain untied. **I,** Posterior view after fixation of bony fragment. The fragment is penetrated and fixed with sutures *(arrows)*.

This extensive labrum release enables excellent fragment reduction. In addition, a small amount of articular cartilage at the face of the inferior glenoid from 3 to 7 o'clock is removed to promote tissue healing after repair.

Step 3: Inferior Labrum Repair

One suture anchor loaded with a #2 high strength suture is inserted at the face of the anteroinferior glenoid (6 o'clock position) through a drill guide introduced from the anterior portal (Fig. 1J.2, *B*). One limb of a suture is placed through the labrum at 6:30 position with the intraarticular suture relay technique (Sugaya et al, 2004) using a 7-mm Caspari punch (Conmed Linvatec, Largo, FL) (Fig. 1J.2, *C*). Next, the second suture anchor is inserted at 4:40 position (right shoulder), and the one limb is placed to the anteroinferior labrum adjacent to the inferior side of the bony fragment using same technique. Knot tying is then performed from the suture of the 4:40 anchor using a cannula introduced from the anterior portal while reducing the labrum and fragment by pulling with a grasper introduced from the anterosuperior portal. After tying this suture, the grasper is removed, and the suture of the inferior anchor is tied. In case of a large bony fragment, suture placement to the bone fragment sometimes causes loosening of the inferior knots. Therefore, we recommend inserting the third anchor and placing the first fragment suture before proceeding to knot tying of the inferior labrum sutures.

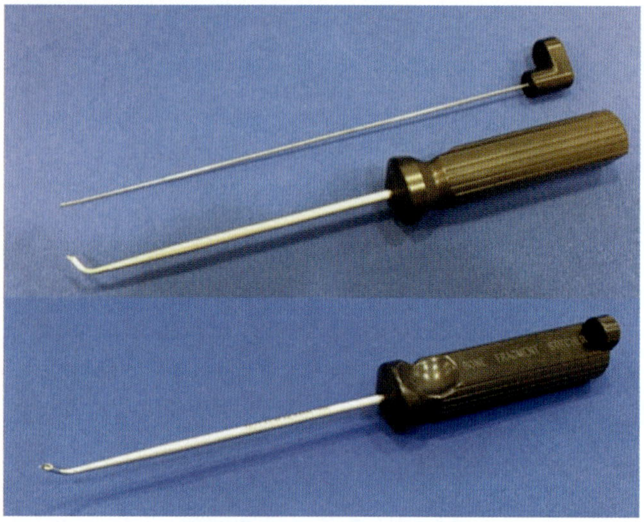

Fig. 1J.3 Bone Stitcher (Image courtesy of Smith & Nephew, Inc).

Step 4: Bony Fragment Fixation

The next step is the fixation of the osseous fragment, either by passing the suture through the fragment or around the fragment with use of a bone penetrator or Bone Stitcher (Smith & Nephew, Norwood, MA) (Fig. 1J.3). Two more suture anchors are used for the fragment and anterior labrum fixation. In this step, the labrum, together with the fragment, is held and stabilized by a robust grasper introduced from the anterosuperior portal to facilitate the fragment management by the bone penetrator, which is introduced from the anterior portal (Fig. 1J.2, *D*). The fragment is usually reattached to a higher position than the anatomic position as a result of retensioning of the entire IGHL.

The third suture anchor is inserted into the anterior glenoid face at the 3:20 position. Sutures are then retrieved from the anterosuperior portal. The bony fragment, which is stabilized by a large grasper introduced from the anterosuperior portal, is penetrated using a Bone Stitcher (Fig. 1J.2, *E*). After catching the fragment by the tip of the Bone Stitcher, the tip needs to be pushed with the fragment to the glenoid neck, and then the fragment can be penetrated (Fig. 1J.2, *F* and *G*). If surgeons believe it is too difficult to penetrate the fragment, they need to rotate the Bone Stitcher by pushing the tip and the fragment to the glenoid neck. In cases that fail to penetrate the fragment, the suture can be passed around the bony fragment.

In cases with the inferior sutures not tied in the previous step, these sutures should be tied before inserting the last anchor, starting from the suture of 4:40 anchor (Fig. 1J.2, *H*). Then another suture anchor is inserted to the edge of the anterior glenoid at the 2 o'clock position. If the fragment is large, a suture anchor loaded with two #2 high strength sutures is preferable. The bony fragment is penetrated with one limb of the sutures using the same manner described above, and the remaining suture is placed to the labrum superior to the fragment.

Finally, knot tying of fragment sutures is performed from the one suture from the last anchor that is placed to the bony fragment followed by the other suture from the last anchor, then the suture from the third anchor (Fig. 1J.2, *I*).

Fig. 1J.4 is a schematic showing anchor placement and relationship between bony fragments and suture placement. The key for successful suture placement is to penetrate an osseous fragment with a bone penetrator or Bone Stitcher while stabilizing the fragment with a large grasper. It will not become a serious problem if osseous fragment is cracked during suture placement because fragments are firmly attached to the labrum. Surgeons do not need to hesitate to strongly push fragments to the glenoid neck with a bone penetrator. As a grasper is introduced from the anterosuperior portal, we recommend using three portals with the posterior portal as a viewing portal.

Step 5: Range of Motion Evaluation After Repair

After completing the repair, the arm is freed and assessed to ensure that there is no restriction of normal external rotation. If external rotation with the arm at the side is restricted, this is normally due to a thick bite by the most superior suture. Therefore, the capsule next to the suture needs to be released with a radiofrequency device, and confirmation is required that the patient resumes normal external rotation.

Step 6: Augmentations

Augmentation procedures, such as rotator interval closure or Hill-Sachs remplissage, are often recommended to avoid postoperative early-stage failure before obtaining bone union, especially in potential noncompliant patients and collision and contact athletes. Rotator interval closure is the most frequently performed with the arm in more than 60 degrees of external rotation. Two or three suture anchors loaded with two #2 high strength sutures are used for Hill-Sachs remplissage, depending on the size of the Hill-Sachs lesion.

POSTOPERATIVE MANAGEMENT AND SPORTS RETURN

Postoperative management is exactly the same as for arthroscopic Bankart repair. After 3 weeks of immobilization using a sling immobilizer, passive and assisted-active exercises are initiated avoiding the provocation of pain. Three months after the surgery, patients are permitted to practice noncontact sports. Full return to throwing or contact sports is allowed after 6 months according to each individual's functional recovery.

Outcomes After Arthroscopic Osseous Bankart Repair

There have been several published papers on clinical outcomes after arthroscopic osseous Bankart repair (Kim et al, 2009, 2014; Kitayama et al, 2015; Sugaya et al, 2005). Kim et al (2009) reported six osseous Bankart lesions that repaired using three-point double-row technique. The mean postoperative Rowe score was 94.7 (range, 87–100), and there were no complications, including recurrence of dislocation and restriction of range of motion (ROM). Kim et al (2014) investigated 34 patients with small- or medium-sized osseous Bankart lesions who underwent arthroscopic repair using similar techniques with ours. Although two patients experienced recurrence of dislocation, Rowe score significantly improved postoperatively. There was no severe restriction of ROM.

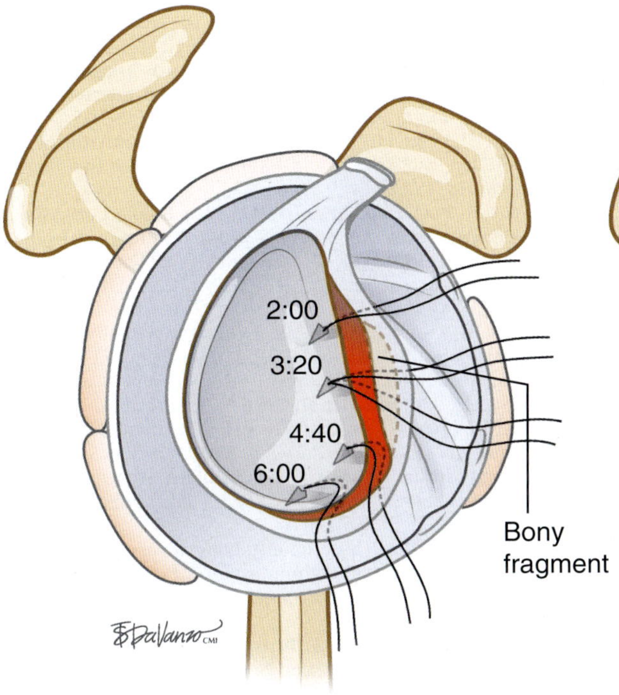

Fig. 1J.4 A schematic of arthroscopic osseous Bankart repair. Suture anchors are inserted at 2:00, 3:20, 4:40, and 6:00 positions. Two sutures are placed in the inferior labrum, and two sutures penetrate the fragment. After knot tying, the inferior glenohumeral ligament is retensioned, and the fragment is attached to the glenoid more superiorly than the anatomic position. The arrows demonstrate a superior shift of the fragment.

We also examined a consecutive series of 46 patients with osseous Bankart lesions who demonstrated more than 15% of glenoid bone loss regardless of the fragment size and underwent the index surgery during January 2005 through December 2006 (Kitayama et al, 2015). Thirty-eight patients (83%), including 34 male and 4 female patients with an average age of 23.4 years (range, 15–36) at the time of surgery, were available for final follow-up at 6.2 years (range, 5.0–8.1) after surgery. One patient sustained a redislocation during a traffic accident 5 months after surgery, which was deemed as an early-stage failure before obtaining a bony union. The rest of the patients demonstrated significant improvement of both Rowe score (Rowe et al, 1978) and the Western Ontario Shoulder Instability Index (Kirkley et al, 1998) postoperatively. Although the mean preoperative fragment size was measured as only 4.7%, the mean glenoid bone loss significantly improved from 20.4% preoperatively to −1.1% postoperatively. The shape of the glenoid was restored to nearly normal or slightly hypertrophic at the final follow-up. We presume that the restored mechanical tension of the IGHL, which is caused by extensive mobilization and superiorly positioned reattachment of the labroligamentous complex, might contribute to new bone formation and remodeling of the glenoid. Fig. 1J.5 shows an example of good glenoid remodeling after osseous Bankart repair.

Conclusions

Arthroscopic osseous Bankart repair yields successful outcomes regardless of repair techniques if the shoulder retains an osseous fragment. Although these techniques are technically demanding, most surgeons will be able to accomplish the surgery by securely performing each step as described

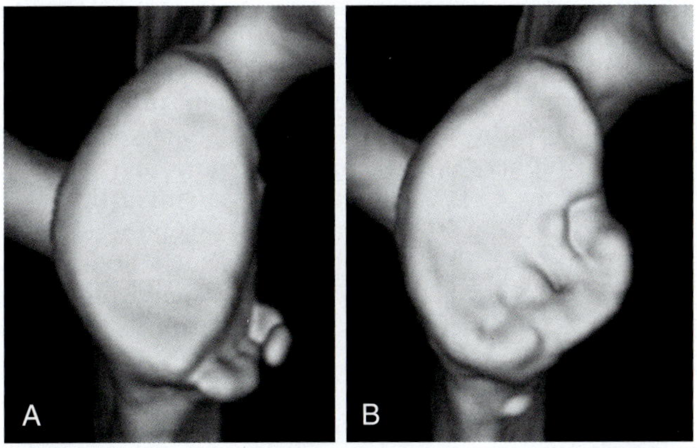

Fig. 1J.5 Three-dimensional computed tomography (CT) image of a 28-year-old man. **A,** Preoperative CT image. The glenoid had 19.0% of bone loss, and the fragment size was 4.0%. **B,** Postoperative CT image. The fragment was united to the glenoid, and the shape of the glenoid was remodeled. The bone loss improved to 5.1%.

in this chapter. We believe that the keys to achieve good clinical and morphologic outcomes are excellent fragment reduction and entire IGHL retensioning provided by extensive labrum release as described in this chapter.

References

Bigliani LU, Newton PM, Steinmann SP, Connor PM, McIlveen SJ. Glenoid rim lesions associated with recurrent anterior dislocation of the shoulder. *Am J Sports Med*. 1998;26(1):41–45.

Bernageau J, Patte D, Debeyre D, Ferrane J. Intérêt du profil glénoïdien dans les luxations récidivantes de l'épaule. *Rev Chir Orthop*. 1976;62:142–147.

Burkhart SS, De Beer JF. Traumatic glenohumeral bone defects and their relationship to failure of arthroscopic Bankart repairs: significance of the inverted-pear glenoid and the humeral engaging Hill-Sachs lesion. *Arthroscopy*. 2000;16(7):677–694.

Burkhart SS, De Beer JF, Barth JR, Cresswell T, Roberts C, Richards DP. Results of modified Latarjet reconstruction in patients with anteroinferior instability and significant bone loss. *Arthroscopy*. 2007;23(10):1033–1041.

Edwards TB, Boulahia A, Walch G. Radiographic analysis of bone defects in chronic anterior shoulder instability. *Arthroscopy*. 2003;19(7):732–739.

Kim KC, Rhee KJ, Shin HD. Arthroscopic three-point double-row repair for acute bony Bankart lesions. *Knee Surg Sports Traumatol Arthrosc*. 2009;17(1):102–106.

Kim YK, Cho SH, Son WS, Moon SH. Arthroscopic repair of small and medium-sized bony Bankart lesions. *Am J Sports Med*. 2014;42(1):86–94.

Kirkley A, Griffin S, McLintock H, Ng L. The development and evaluation of a disease-specific quality of life measurement tool for shoulder instability. The Western Ontario Shoulder Instability Index (WOSI). *Am J Sports Med*. 1998;26(6):764–772.

Kitayama S, Sugaya H, Takahashi N, et al. Clinical outcome and glenoid morphology after arthroscopic repair of chronic osseous Bankart lesions: a five to eight-year follow-up study. *J Bone Joint Surg Am*. 2015;97(22):1833–1843.

Lafosse L, Lejeune E, Bouchard A, Kakuda C, Gobezie R, Kochhar T. The arthroscopic Latarjet procedure for the treatment of anterior shoulder instability. *Arthroscopy*. 2007;23(11):1242. e1–e5.

Millett PJ, Braun S. The "bony Bankart bridge" procedure: a new arthroscopic technique for reduction and internal fixation of a bony Bankart lesion. *Arthroscopy*. 2009;25(1):102–105.

Moran CJ, Fabricant PD, Kang R, Cordasco FA. Arthroscopic double-row anterior stabilization and Bankart repair for the "high-risk" athlete. *Arthrosc Tech*. 2014;3(1):e65–e71.

Rowe CR, Patel D, Southmayd WW. The Bankart procedure: a long-term end result study. *J Bone Joint Surg Am*. 1978;60(1):1–16.

Sugaya H, Moriishi J, Dohi M, Kon Y, Tsuchiya A. Glenoid rim morphology in recurrent anterior glenohumeral instability. *J Bone Joint Surg Am*. 2003;85(5):878–884.

Sugaya H, Kon Y, Tsuchiya A. Arthroscopic Bankart repair in the beach-chair position: a cannulaless method using an intra-articular suture relay technique. *Arthroscopy*. 2004;20(suppl 1):116–120.

Sugaya H, Moriishi J, Kanisawa I, Tsuchiya A. Arthroscopic osseous Bankart repair for chronic recurrent traumatic anterior glenohumeral instability. *J Bone Joint Surg Am*. 2005;87(8):1752–1760.

Sugaya H. Instability with bone loss. In: RA, Angelo, JE, Esch, RR Ryu, eds. *AANA Advanced Arthroscopy: The Shoulder*. Philadelphia: Elsevier; 2010:136–146.

Sugaya H. Section 2: anterior instability: arthroscopic treatment of glenoid bone loss—surgical technique. In: MP, Provencher AR Romeo, eds. *Shoulder Instability: A Comprehensive Approach*. Philadelphia: Elsevier; 2011:186–196.

Sugaya H, Takahashi N. Arthroscopic osseous Bankart repair in the treatment of recurrent anterior glenohumeral instability. *JBJS Essent Surg Tech*. 2016;6(3):e26.

Yamamoto N, Itoi E, Abe H, et al. Contact between the glenoid and the humeral head in abduction, external rotation, and horizontal extension: a new concept of glenoid track. *J Shoulder Elbow Surg*. 2007;16(5):649–656.

1-1K HUMERAL HEAD BONE LOSS: SOFT TISSUE REMPLISSAGE

FELIX H. SAVOIE III, MD and JOHN T. HEFFERNAN, MD

Introduction

- A Hill-Sachs defect is a compression fracture of the humeral head associated with anterior shoulder dislocations.
- Arthroscopic capsulolabral repair of the unstable shoulder without addressing the Hill-Sachs defect may lead to higher rates of failure and recurrent instability.
- Management of the Hill-Sachs defect with arthroscopic suturing of the infraspinatus and posterior capsule into the defect, coined *remplissage* (French for "filling"), is an effective technique for management of the Hill-Sachs defect that can be performed at the time of capsulolabral repair.
- The surgical indication for remplissage is a moderate (<30%) or engaging Hill-Sachs defect with less than 20% glenoid bone loss. Assessment of combined glenoid and humeral bone loss is critical to achieve a satisfactory result; larger defects in the humeral head are best treated with open bone grafting, and glenoid bone loss of more than 20% may benefit from bone restoration.

Epidemiology and Pathoanatomy

The Hill-Sachs defect is a compression fracture of the posterolateral humeral head associated with anterior shoulder dislocations. First described by Hill and Sachs in 1940, the osseous defect results from the impaction of the soft cancellous bone of the humeral head onto the hard cortical rim of the glenoid. The posterolateral humeral head sustains the injury because the arm is characteristically in a position of abduction and external rotation during the initial anterior dislocation event.

The rate of occurrence of Hill-Sachs fractures is high with even a single dislocation and is present in nearly all shoulders with recurrent instability. Although the initial impression fracture may be small and easily missed on radiographs, the humeral defect tends to enlarge with each additional dislocation or with increased time spent in the dislocated position. Recurrent dislocation may lead to progressive bone loss of both the humerus and glenoid. Repeated dislocations result in attenuation of the static soft tissue restraints to glenohumeral translation. Over time this cycle of dislocation is thought to increase bone loss on both the humeral head and glenoid, resulting in an engaging Hill-Sachs defect and the "inverted pear" glenoid (Burkhart & De Beer, 2000). Bipolar bone loss allows dislocations to occur at lower arm abduction angles, and patients can experience symptomatic instability with activities of daily living. As a consequence, combined bone loss patients are at the greatest risk for recurrent instability after arthroscopic Bankart repair (Arciero et al, 2015; Boileau et al, 2006; Gottschalk et al, 2016).

The surgical treatment of glenoid bone loss is extensively described in the literature, but fewer series report outcomes of surgical management of humeral bone loss. Although Hill-Sachs defects are common in recurrent shoulder instability, not all are clinically significant. The most common criteria to determine the significance of a Hill-Sachs lesion are its size and location and whether it is an engaging lesion. A typical Hill-Sachs defect is located on the superior posterolateral humeral head. The engaging Hill-Sachs lesion occurs when the humeral head lesion engages the glenoid rim while the shoulder is in a position of athletic function (Burkhart & De Beer, 2000; Palmer & Widen, 1948). As the arm is brought into abduction and external rotation, the long axis of the defect aligns parallel to and engages with the glenoid, allowing the humeral head to lever forward on the glenoid. The recent concept of the glenoid track has helped to shed light on the significance of the Hill-Sachs lesion in combined bone loss (Itoi et al, 2013) The glenoid track concept by Itoi describes the path made by the humeral head on the glenoid during range of motion. Bone loss on either side can result in increased tendency to dislocation as the combined defects come in contact during certain ranges of motion. A bone defect sufficient to allow contact on either the humeral head or glenoid will necessitate treatment for a successful surgical result. Hill-Sachs lesions greater than 20% are often clinically significant, and those greater than 40% of the humeral head are typically responsible for instability (Flatow, 1998).

History of the Remplissage Procedure and Literature Review

Remplissage, French for "filling," is an arthroscopic technique to fill a Hill-Sachs lesion by suturing the local infraspinatus tendon and capsule into the defect. The transfer of tissue converts an intraarticular lesion of the humeral head to an extraarticular lesion. The Hill-Sachs is unable to engage the glenoid, thus neutralizing the contribution of the defect to glenohumeral instability. Connolly initially described the procedure in 1972 as a reverse McLaughlin procedure, adapting the surgery described by McLaughlin for posterior instability (and later modified by Neer) to assist with stabilization of anterior instability (Connolly 1972). Connolly's technique was an open procedure through a posterior approach with infraspinatus tenodesis and posterior capsulodesis. In 2008, Wolf and colleagues described their arthroscopic technique of the procedure using suture anchors to fill the defect with infraspinatus tendon and posterior capsule, a procedure they named "remplissage" (Purchase et al, 2008). Later, Koo et al (2009) described their modification of the technique using a double-pulley suture technique with two anchors to secure the infraspinatus tendon into the entire Hill-Sachs defect with a broader footprint of fixation.

Since Wolf described the arthroscopic technique, several studies have supported remplissage as an effective treatment option with low rates of recurrent instability. Recent studies by Park et al (2011) and McCabe et al (2014) showed excellent results in primary cases with remplissage, although Kelly et al noted an inability to return to throw in overhead athletes, and McCabe et al noted decreased success in revision situations (McCabe et al, 2014; Park et al, 2011). Similar or better results are consistently reported in the literature. Wolf & Arianjam's (2014) case series of 59 patients treated with arthroscopic remplissage for engaging Hill-Sachs lesion demonstrated 4.4% recurrent instability with 2- to 10-year follow-up. A systematic review by Buza et al (2014) highlights overall recurrence rates of 5.4% in 167 patients.

The remplissage procedure is an attractive option for management of moderate-sized Hill-Sachs lesions because it can be performed entirely arthroscopically at the time of Bankart repair, with less morbidity than an open approach or bone grafting procedures. Concern exists in the literature, however, for decreased postoperative range of motion as a consequence of remplissage and nonanatomic repair of the humeral osseous defect. Several studies have highlighted the effect of remplissage on postoperative range of motion, although the clinical significance of this is unclear (Elkinson et al, 2012). Boileau et al (2012) compared range of motion in the operated extremity to the unaffected side and found a difference of 8 degrees of external rotation with the arm at the side and 9 degrees of external rotation with the arm abducted. Despite this, 90% of athletes in their series returned to sport, and 70% returned to the same level of play (Boileau et al, 2012).

Patient History

Patients with humeral head bone loss report a history of shoulder instability. Important information for the examiner includes the details of the initial episode of instability, the mechanism and energy involved, the position of the arm during the injury, and whether reduction under sedation was required or the shoulder self-reduced. The examiner should ask about the number and frequency of instability events, as well as the ease with which they occur and reduce. Because repeated instability events lead to progressive bony defects, patients who complain of shoulder dislocations during activities of daily life and at lower arm angles are likely to have significant Hill-Sachs lesions, glenoid bone loss, or both. Additionally, acquiring any information about previous surgery performed on the unstable shoulder will inform the examiner about the cause of previous failures and future surgical options.

Clinical Examination

Physical examination of the shoulder begins with inspection. The examiner should note the overall resting posture

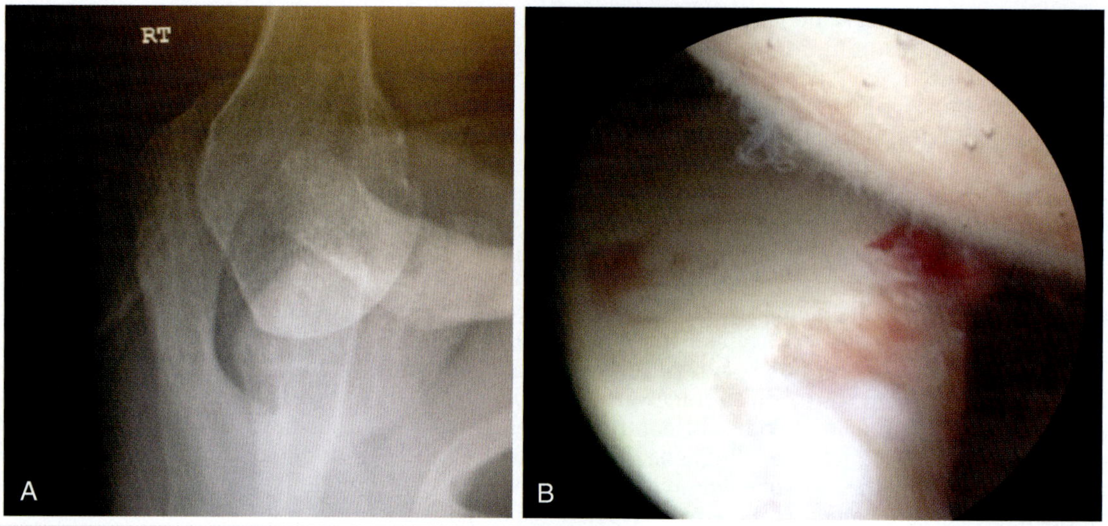

Fig. 1K.1 **A,** The Bernageau view of an unstable shoulder with bone loss demonstrates both glenoid and humeral bone loss. **B,** Bernageau view of the shoulder is optimal for demonstrating combined bone loss of the humeral head and the glenoid.

of the patient as well as if the shoulder and upper extremity are held in a position of protraction or retraction. Assessment should be made of the shape of the shoulder and any muscular atrophy noted, specifically the deltoid and supraspinatus fossa.

The shoulder should be palpated for any areas of tenderness. Both active and passive range of motion should be examined. Apprehension by the patient in positions of external rotation and abduction suggests instability. With the patient standing, the examiner uses one hand to stabilize the scapula while grasping the forearm with the other hand. The patient's arm is slowly brought away from her or his side and externally rotated while increasing the abduction angle. Apprehension by the patient suggests instability, and when it occurs at lower arm angles, it should raise the index of suspicion for glenohumeral bone loss from prior dislocations.

Strength of the rotator cuff must also be assessed because trauma from dislocation can cause subscapularis rupture or avulsion of the supraspinatus or infraspinatus. Examination of the biceps strength and provocative maneuvers may reveal concomitant biceps pathology.

Finally, provocative maneuvers are of vital importance in examination of the unstable shoulder. The anterior load and shift test can be performed with the patient in a supine or upright sitting position. Using the table (supine) or the examiner's hand (upright) to stabilize the scapula, the humeral head is translated in both anterior and posterior directions. Translation of the head across the glenohumeral joint implies anterior instability. Crepitus and pain reproduced with humeral head translation imply a glenoid labral tear. Posterior glenohumeral stability can be evaluated with the posterior load and shift as well as the jerk test. The apprehension and relocation tests are used to further confirm instability on exam. Valadie et al, 2000 series of apprehension, augmentation, and relocation is very effective in determining the position of apprehension, with lower levels of abduction and external rotation being indicative of disturbance of the glenoid track and the need for additional surgical options.

Imaging

Multiple modalities of imaging studies can be useful in the diagnosis of glenohumeral instability with bone loss. Imaging should always begin with the standard series of shoulder radiographs, which include the anteroposterior (AP) radiograph of the glenohumeral joint, the scapular Y view, the axillary view, and the Bernageau view. Glenoid loss on the anteroinferior rim is most evident on the axillary view. The Hill-Sachs defect on the posterolateral surface of the humeral head is best visualized on an internal rotation view of the AP radiograph of the shoulder. The Bernageau view may be the best plain radiographic means to determine combined bone loss (Fig. 1K.1). Certain specific radiographs are useful in the evaluation of bone loss. The Stryker notch view brings the posterolateral surface of the humeral head into view and hence is useful for visualizing the size and orientation of any Hill-Sachs defects. Any irregularity of the bony contours of the humeral head or glenoid visualized on plain radiographs should raise the suspicion of bone loss.

Computed tomography (CT) provides cross-sectional imaging and greatly facilitates evaluation of bone loss. Oblique, sagittal, and in particular three-dimensional CT help to quantify the size and location of bone loss and should be used for preoperative planning. Magnetic resonance imaging (MRI) and MR arthrography are important modalities for evaluating the soft tissue stabilizers (rotator cuff, labrum, ligaments) of the shoulder. Together these images help to determine the size of the defect and as such are invaluable in planning the surgical technique. Hill-Sachs defects that occupy less than 30% of the humeral head can be treated effectively with arthroscopic remplissage,but larger defects may require open bone grafting with humeral head allograft.

Indications

Indications for surgical stabilization of the shoulder include bone loss and instability with pain and loss of function after failing appropriate conservative therapy.

Table 1K.1 Algorithm for Surgical Decision Making for Remplissage

Pathology	Treatment
Glenoid bone loss <20% and Hill-Sachs lesion <30%	Perform arthroscopic Bankart repair and remplissage
Glenoid bone loss <20% and Hill-Sachs lesion >30%	Perform soft tissue Bankart repair and open bone grafting of Hill-Sachs lesion
Glenoid bone loss >20% and Hill-Sachs lesion >30%	Perform Latarjet or open bone grafting procedure

The decision to treat the Hill-Sachs lesion with remplissage depends on several factors, most notably the size of the defect and whether it engages the glenoid. Remplissage is performed in patients with moderate-sized Hill-Sachs defects with glenoid bone loss of less than 20%. Patients with Hill-Sachs defects larger than 30% may require conversion to an open bone grafting procedure, but glenoid defects greater than 20% may require conversion to an augmentation procedure. The algorithm for surgical decision making is provided in Table 1K.1.

Surgical Technique

PATIENT POSITIONING

The surgery can be performed either in the beach-chair or lateral decubitus position. The authors' preferred surgical technique is to perform surgery under general anesthesia in the lateral decubitus position on a beanbag, with the patient reclining 30 degrees posterior.

Before portal placement, an examination of the shoulder is performed with the patient under anesthesia. The examination allows the surgeon to identify instability in the anterior, posterior, and inferior directions. Note is also made if the Hill-Sachs lesion engages the glenoid rim, and if so, in what position of abduction and external rotation. Together these inform the surgical plan.

PORTALS

Standard arthroscopic portals are used. A standard posterior portal is placed first in the raphe of the infraspinatus. Anterior portals are localized using an outside-in technique with a spinal needle. Anterior-superior and anterior-inferior portals are created and used for the repair of the anterior labrum. An accessory posterolateral portal may be created, if necessary, for completion of the remplissage or bone grafting of the humeral head. Although the entry sites of the anterior portals are relatively close inside the shoulder joint, it is important to keep the skin incisions as far apart as possible. This creates more working space on the outside of the shoulder and limits collision of the arthroscopic instruments with the arthroscope.

With the arthroscope in the posterior portal, the anterior-inferior portal is created first. This portal's placement is the most critical because it is the primary portal used for repair of the glenoid labrum. Its position should be tested with a spinal needle to ensure access to the inferior glenoid and that the correct angle for anchor placement can be achieved. We recommend passing the needle through the subscapularis for accuracy, but the portal should be placed over the upper border of the subscapularis. The portal can be placed such that the cannula can lever the subscapularis inferiorly, allowing more exposure to the inferior glenoid. Appropriate placement of the anterior-inferior portal routinely allows access to the 5:30 o'clock position on the anterior-inferior glenoid for repair of the labrum.

An anterior-superior portal is established next, as the viewing portal for the arthroscope. This portal is established directly above the biceps tendon through the rotator interval just anterior to (but not through) the supraspinatus tendon and allows the surgeon to work on either side of the biceps. For the majority of cases, the arthroscope is placed in the anterior-superior portal. This allows full visualization of the entire glenohumeral joint, with access to both anterior and posterior compartments through one viewing portal. Cannulas are placed in the anterior-inferior and posterior portals for anchor placement, suture shuttling, and knot tying. Accessory portals may include posterior-inferior and posterior-superior placement for access to all of the shoulder joint.

Diagnostic Arthroscopy

Diagnostic arthroscopy begins with the arthroscope in the posterior portal. With every instability case, it is critical to evaluate the biceps tendon, biceps anchor, and superior labrum. The biceps anchor and superior labrum should be probed to evaluate for a superior labrum anterior and posterior (SLAP) tear. The subscapularis is assessed for tears, and a 70-degree arthroscope can be used if any concern exists for partial tearing. The supraspinatus and infraspinatus are also inspected from the posterior portal to assess for partial- or full-thickness tears. From this position, the Hill-Sachs defect will be visualized, and the size can be assessed (Fig. 1K.2, *A*).

The anterior shoulder capsuloligamentous area is carefully evaluated from all portals for pathology. Injuries can involve the labrum (Bankart or anterior labroligamentous periosteal sleeve avulsion [ALPSA]), midcapsule or humeral side (humeral avulsion of the glenohumeral ligament [HAGL]), or a combination of these. The glenoid labrum is closely inspected for the presence of a Bankart tear. The labrum can be probed to evaluate for instability. Each glenohumeral ligament (superior, middle, and inferior) can be inspected directly. The arthroscope is driven into the axillary pouch and assessed for the presence of loose bodies. The capsule is inspected for any tearing off the humerus. In this way, HAGL is diagnosed and can be addressed accordingly.

The Hill-Sachs defect is assessed to determine both the size and if the lesion is engaging or nonengaging. With the arthroscope in the posterior portal, the arm is taken out of traction and brought into the athletic position of abduction and external rotation. In the presence of a large Hill-Sachs lesion, the defect will engage the anterior glenoid rim, and the humeral head will fall off the track of the glenoid, subluxating anteriorly. This dynamic assessment confirms the presence of an engaging lesion, which must be addressed at the time of surgery for a successful outcome (Fig. 1K.1, *B*).

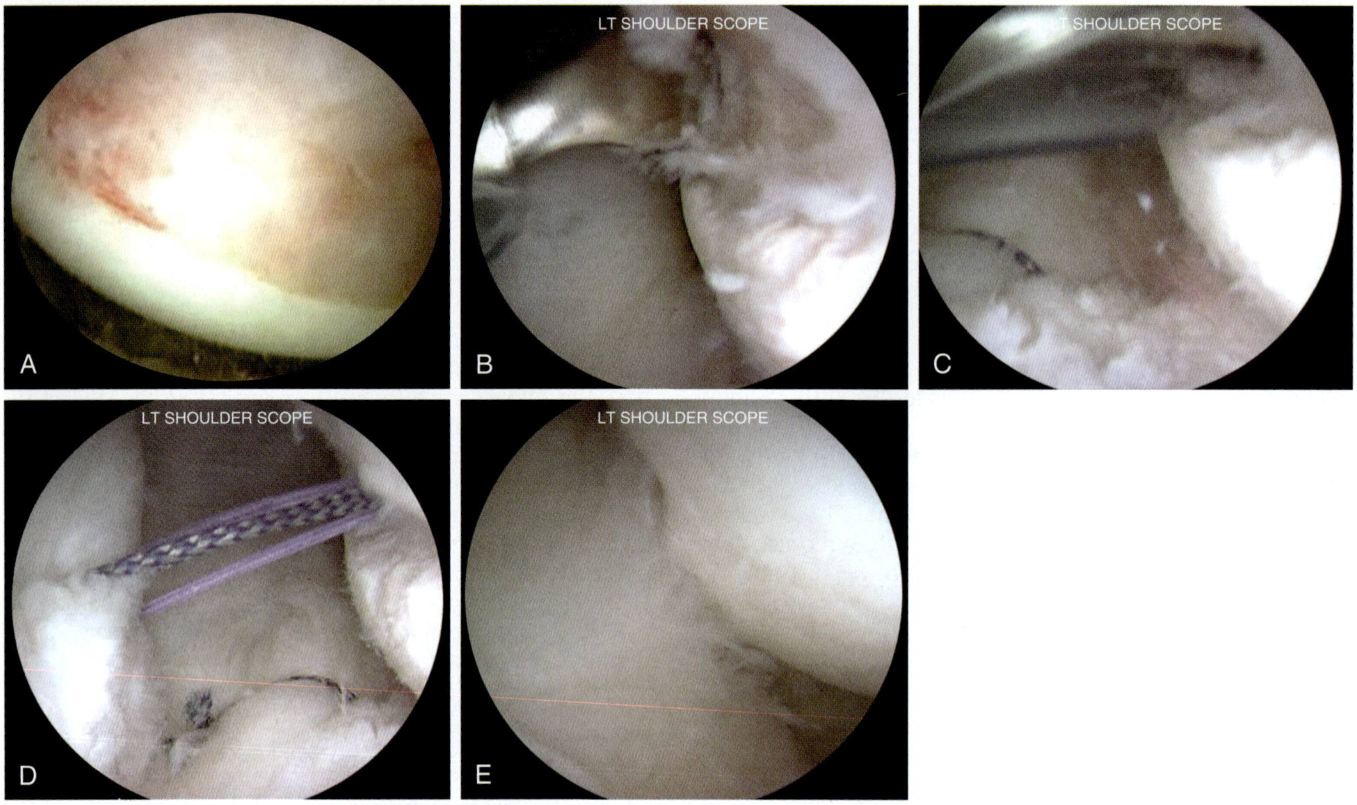

Fig. 1K.2 Arthroscopic images **A,** View from the posterior portal measuring bone loss in the humeral head. **B,** Viewing from the anterosuperior portal of the preparation of the Hill-Sachs with a shaver to abrade fibrous tissue. **C,** The awl is used to trephinate the defect bed to facilitate healing. **D,** The remplissage is completed by placement of a double-loaded suture anchor with retrieval in standard double-mattress suture technique. **E,** Arthroscopic appearance of completed remplissage.

The diagnostic arthroscopy is continued with the arthroscope in the anterior-superior portal. This provides the surgeon a 360-degree view of the glenohumeral joint. The anterior, posterior, and inferior labrum can be visualized and assessed for tearing and instability. The presence of glenoid bone loss can be assessed, and if significant anterior glenoid bone loss is present, the decision may be made to proceed with a bone grafting procedure.

Finally, the Hill-Sachs defect can again be visualized from the anterior-superior portal. Determining the presence of an engaging Hill-Sachs lesion can be performed while viewing from the posterior portal or the anterior-superior portal, depending on surgeon preference.

Step-By-Step Procedure: Arthroscopic Bankart Repair with Remplissage

(See Video 1K.1)

1. After completion of the diagnostic arthroscopy and identification of all pathology, the repair can be performed. The case begins with preparation of the glenoid labrum. With the arthroscope in the anterior-superior portal, an arthroscopic elevator is introduced through the anterior-inferior portal. The elevator is used to release the torn labrum from the medial glenoid neck. The labrum is elevated away from the bony attachment throughout the tear, down to and past the 6 o'clock position up to the attachment of the Posterior Inferior Glenohumeral Ligament [PIGHL]. It is important to elevate the labrum until the muscle fibers of the subscapularis are visualized, completely mobilizing the capsule–labral complex for repair. A motorized shaver is then introduced to remove all fibrous debris between the labrum and the bony glenoid. The hood of the shaver is placed against the labrum, protecting it from iatrogenic damage. The shaver is also used to prepare the medial glenoid neck and anterior glenoid rim. The bony surface is roughened before repair to facilitate healing of the labrum.
2. The first glenoid anchor is placed before addressing the Hill-Sachs defect. This facilitates reaching the inferior aspect of the glenoid. If the Hill-Sachs defect is addressed first and a remplissage is performed, the space inside the glenohumeral joint is reduced, and reaching the inferior glenoid for anchor placement can be challenging.

   The first glenoid anchor is placed, typically at the 5:30 to 6 o'clock position. Double-loaded suture anchors are used for the labral repair. The anterior-inferior cannula can be used to lever the subscapularis down to routinely reach the 5:30 to 6 o'clock position. Alternatively, the anchor drill guide can be placed either from a posterolateral portal while pushing the humeral head anteriorly or via a transtendon through the subscapularis to reach the 6 o'clock position. A percutaneous suture passer is used to pass both sutures in vertical mattress fashion. The first suture is placed at the 6:30 to 7 o'clock position posteriorly via a posterior inferior portal, and the second suture is placed at the 6:00 position. The sutures are retrieved and tied via the posterior portal to start the capsular shift. The second set of sutures is passed at the 6:00 and 5:30 positions to complete the inferior repair and begin the capsular shift. This is the most important part of the stabilization procedure and is always completed first.

3. The remplissage is performed at this portion of the procedure, before completing the Bankart repair. Completion of the Bankart repair before addressing the Hill-Sachs defect will tighten the glenohumeral joint and translate the humeral head posteriorly, making visualization of the Hill-Sachs defect difficult. This step begins with the preparation of the Hill-Sachs defect. The arthroscope remains in the anterior-superior portal and a motorized shaver is placed through the posterior portal. The base of the Hill-Sachs defect is prepared. The shaver is used to remove all fibrous tissue from the base of the defect until bleeding bone is encountered. We will also usually create multiple small trephination holes using a Steadman microfracture awl to maximize the healing potential (Figs. 1K.2, *B* and *C*).

   Placement of anchors: In a small defect, a single double-loaded anchor can be sufficient; in broader defects, two anchors can be placed. In each case, the anchor is placed into the most medial aspect of the defect adjacent to the articular cartilage. After one or two double-loaded rotator cuff anchors have been placed directly into the Hill-Sachs defect, the sutures are shuttled out the anterior portal.

   Next, the posterior cannula is slightly backed out into the subacromial space, so that the tip of the cannula lies just outside the posterior capsule and infraspinatus tendon. A percutaneous suture passer is used to retrieve the sutures through the posterior capsule and infraspinatus tendon. The area of penetration is in line or slightly lateral to the defect in the humeral head. The most inferior stitch is retrieved first and can be used to shift the inferior capsule if necessary. The matching stitch is retrieved slightly more superiorly and the suture can be tied blindly or the arthroscope placed into the subacromial area and the sutures retrieved and tied. Typically, two mattress sutures are placed for each anchor (Fig. 1K.2, *D*). Tying the sutures completes the transfer of the posterior capsule and infraspinatus tendon into the Hill-Sachs defect, converting the Hill-Sachs defect into a nonengaging lesion (Fig. 1K.2, *E*).

4. Complete the Bankart repair: The Bankart labral repair is completed using two more double-loaded anchors with mattress sutures placed to complete the repair and capsular shift.

Postoperative Care

Patients are placed into a shoulder abduction sling for the initial postoperative period. The sling is used for 4 weeks, and patients are allowed to remove the sling to shower, dress, and perform elbow range of motion exercises. Patients are instructed on posture training and periscapular exercises immediately. Home active range of motion exercises that do not involve external rotation are initiated at 2 to 3 weeks postoperatively. At 4 to 6 weeks after surgery, the abduction sling is discontinued and formal physical therapy initiated. Return to most activities begins at 4 months, and full return to sport is allowed at 6 months after surgery.

Results

Remplissage is an effective technique for treating Hill-Sachs defects arthroscopically at the time of capsulolabral repair. Rates of recurrent glenohumeral instability after remplissage are described in the literature ranging from 0% to 15%. Postoperative shoulder-specific scores after remplissage in multiple studies were good to excellent (Buza et al, 2014). Hill-Sachs remplissage is a nonanatomic repair, which has created concern about postoperative loss of shoulder mobility. Multiple studies have reported no significant loss in preoperative and postoperative range of motion and no significant difference in range of motion compared with Bankart repair alone. A recent study suggests recurrent glenohumeral instability may be higher in arthroscopic reconstruction with remplissage in the revision setting (McCabe et al, 2014). In a very recent study by Garcia et al (2016) with 5-year follow-up, the recurrence rate was 11.8%. Increased preoperative dislocations led to a greater risk of a postoperative dislocation, and higher postoperative dislocation rates were observed in patients who underwent revision. The rate of return to one or more sports was 95.5% of patients at an average of 7.0 months postoperatively; 81.0% returned to their previous intensity and level of sport. Of patients who played a throwing sport, 65.5% stated that they had problems throwing, and 58.6% thought that they could not normally wind up throwing a ball. Direct rates of return to overhead sports were volleyball, 100%; basketball, 69%; baseball, 50%; and football, 50%. The authors caution use of remplissage in throwing and overhead athletes (Garcia et al, 2016).

Complications

The most common complication after Hill-Sachs remplissage is recurrent glenohumeral instability. Patients may also experience postoperative posterolateral shoulder pain. Decreased postoperative range of motion, especially in internal and external rotation, is described in the literature, although the reported magnitude is small and the clinical significance unclear.

Conclusions

Hill-Sachs defects are compression fractures of the posterolateral humeral head resulting from anterior inferior shoulder dislocations. Unrecognized or untreated bone loss of either the humeral head or glenoid is a common cause of recurrent instability after arthroscopic soft tissue reconstruction surgery. It is paramount for the orthopedic surgeon to identify clinically significant osseous defects in the humeral head or glenoid and address them at the time of the index procedure. Arthroscopic remplissage is an effective technique for treating moderate-sized Hill-Sachs defects (<30%) that can be performed at the time of capsulolabral repair with low associated morbidity.

References

Arciero RA, Parrino A, Bernhardson AS, et al. The effect of a combined glenoid and Hill-Sachs defect on glenohumeral stability: a biomechanical cadaveric study using 3-dimensional modeling of 142 patients. *Am J Sports Med*. 2015;43(6):1422–1429.

Boileau P, Villaba M, Hery JY, Balg F, Ahrens P, Neyton L. Risk factors for recurrence of shoulder instability after arthroscopic Bankart repair. *J Bone Joint Surg Am*. 2006;88:1755–1763.

Boileau P, O'Shea K, Vargas P, Pinedo M, Old J, Zumstein M. Anatomical and functional results after arthroscopic Hill-Sachs remplissage. *J Bone Joint Surg Am*. 2012;94:618–626.

Burkhart SS, De Beer JF. Traumatic glenohumeral bone defects and their relationship to failure of arthroscopic Bankart repairs: significance of the inverted-pear glenoid and the humeral engaging Hill-Sachs lesion. *Arthroscopy*. 2000;16:677–694.

Buza JA, Jaicharan JI, Oke AA, Ahmad CS, Levine WN. Arthroscopic Hill-Sachs remplissage: a systematic review. *J Bone Joint Surg Am*. 2014;96(7):549–555.

Connolly JF. Humeral head defects associated with shoulder dislocation—their diagnostic and surgical significance. *Instr Course Lect*. 1972;21:42–54.

Elkinson I, Giles JW, Faber KJ, et al. The effect of the remplissage procedure on shoulder stability and range of motion. *J Bone Joint Surg Am*. 2012;94:1003–1012.

Flatow. 1998.

Garcia GH, Wu HH, Liu JN, Huffman GR, Kelly JD 4th. Outcomes of the remplissage procedure and its effects on return to sports: average 5-year follow-up. *Am J Sports Med*. 2016;44(5):1124–1130.

Gottschalk LJ 4th, Walia P, Patel RM, Kuklis M, Jones MH, Fening SD, Miniaci A. Influence of Combined Hill-Sachs and Bony Bankart Defects on Range of Motion in Anterior Stability of the Glenohumeral Joint With Combined Humeral Head and Glenoid Defects: A Cadaveric Study. *Am J Sports Med*. 2016;44(4):933–40.

Hill HA, Sachs MD. The grooved defect of the humeral head: a frequently unrecognized complication of dislocations of the shoulder joint. *Radiology*. 1940;35:690–700.

Itoi E, Yamamoto N, Kurokawa D, Sano H. Bone loss in anterior instability. *Curr Rev Musculoskelet Med*. 2013;6(1):88–94.

Koo SS, Burkart SS, Ochoa E. Arthroscopic double-pulley remplissage technique for engaging Hill-Sachs lesions in anterior shoulder instability repairs. *Arthroscopy*. 2009;25(11):1343–1348.

McCabe MP, Weinberg D, Field LD, O'Brien MJ, Hobgood ER, Savoie FH. Primary versus revision arthroscopic reconstruction with remplissage for shoulder instability with moderate bone loss. *Arthroscopy*. 2014;30(4):444–450.

Palmer I, Widen A. The bone block method for recurrent dislocation of the shoulder joint. *J Bone Joint Surg Br*. 1948;30(1):53–58.

Park MJ, Tjoumakaris FP, Garcia G, Patel A, Kelly JD. Arthroscopic remplissage with Bankart repair for the treatment of glenohumeral instability with Hill-Sachs defects. *Arthroscopy*. 2011;27(9):118711–118794.

Purchase RJ, Wolf EM, Hobgood ER, Pollock ME, Smalley CC. Hill-Sachs "remplissage": an arthroscopic solution for the engaging Hill-Sachs lesion. *Arthroscopy*. 2008;24(6):723–726.

Valadie AL 3rd, Jobe CM, Pink MM, Ekman EF, Jobe FW. Anatomy of provocative tests for impingement syndrome of the shoulder. *J Shoulder Elbow Surg*. 2000;9(1):36–46.

Wolf EM, Arianjam A. Hill-Sachs remplissage, an arthroscopic solution for the engaging Hill-Sachs lesion: 2- to 10-year follow-up and incidence of recurrence. *J Shoulder Elbow Surg*. 2014;23(6):814–820.

Recommended Reading List

1. Calandra JJ, Baker CL, Uribe J. The incidence of Hill-Sachs lesions in initial anterior shoulder dislocations. *Arthroscopy*. 1989;5(4):254–257.
2. Elkinson I, Giles JW, Faber KJ, et al. The shoulder remplissage procedure for Hill-Sachs defects: does technique matter? *J Shoulder Elbow Surg*. 2013;22(6):835–841.
3. Giles JW, Elkinson I, Ferreira LM, et al. Moderate to large engaging Hill-Sachs defects: an in vitro biomechanical comparison of the remplissage procedure, allograft humeral head reconstruction, and partial resurfacing arthroplasty. *J Shoulder Elbow Surg*. 2012;21(9):1142–1151.
4. Nourissat G, Kilinc AS, Werther JR, Doursounian L. A prospective, comparative radiological and clinical study of the influence of the "remplissage" procedure on shoulder range of motion after stabilization by arthroscopic Bankart repair. *Am J Sports Med*. 2011;39(8):2147–2152.
5. Ong CC, Meislin RJ. Addressing the Hill-Sachs lesion: humeral head bone loss and glenohumeral instability. *Bull Hosp Jt Dis (2013)*. 2015;73(2):109–115.
6. Provencher MT, Bhatia S, Ghodadra NS, et al. Recurrent shoulder instability: current concepts for evaluation and management of glenoid bone loss. *J Bone Joint Surg Am*. 2010;92(suppl 2):133–151.
7. Provencher MT, Frank RM, Leclere LE, et al. The Hill-Sachs lesion: diagnosis, classification, and management. *J Am Acad Orthop Surg*. 2012;20(4):242–252.
8. Taylor DC, Arciero RA. Pathologic changes associated with shoulder dislocations: arthroscopic and physical examination findings in first-time, traumatic anterior dislocations. *Am J Sports Med*. 1997;25(3):306–311.
9. Walia P, Patel RM, Gottschalk L, et al. The reduction in stability from combined humeral head and glenoid bony defects is influenced by arm position. *Am J Sports Med*. 2016;44(3):715–722.
10. Wolf EM, Arianja A. Hill-Sachs remplissage, an arthroscopic solution for the engaging Hill-Sachs lesion: 2- to 10-year follow-up and incidence of recurrence. *J Shoulder Elbow Surg*. 2014;23(6):814–820.
11. Yamamoto N, Itoi E, Abe H, et al. Contact between the glenoid and the humeral head in abduction, external rotation, and horizontal extension: a new concept of glenoid track. *J Shoulder Elbow Surg*. 2007;16(5):649–656.

1-1L HUMERAL HEAD BONE LOSS: GRAFT OPTIONS—HUMERAL HEAD ALLOGRAFT

ANTONY MINIACI, MD, FRCSC, RONAK M. PATEL, MD, and ASHRAF M. ELBANNA, MD

- Humeral head bone defects, also known as Hill-Sachs lesions, have been found to occur with an incidence between 32% and 51% at the time of initial anterior glenohumeral dislocation (Calandra et al, 1989).
- In shoulders sustaining a Hill-Sachs lesion during the initial dislocation, there exists a statistically significant association with recurrent dislocation (Hovelius et al, 1996).
- Rowe et al (1984) found a 76% incidence of Hill-Sachs lesions in patients evaluated for recurrent anterior dislocation of the shoulder after a variety of surgical procedures were performed and stated that "a Hill-Sachs lesion of the humeral head may play a role in the development of recurrent dislocation after surgical repair."

Engaging versus Nonengaging Lesions

Burkhart and De Beer (2000) introduced the concept of engaging Hill-Sachs defects. In an engaging Hill-Sachs lesion, the long axis of the defect is parallel to the anterior glenoid with the shoulder in a functional position of abduction and external rotation. This leads to the Hill-Sachs lesion engaging or catching the corner of the glenoid. Conversely, a nonengaging Hill-Sachs lesion is one that either fails to engage the glenoid in a functional arm position or engages the glenoid only in a nonfunctional arm position.

Although the failure of soft tissue repair alone in patients with unipolar (glenoid or humeral head) or bipolar bone loss in the setting of recurrent instability is well documented and well accepted, the direct treatment of humeral head bone loss has been less widely recognized. Furthermore, many studies on bone loss in recurrent shoulder instability have focused on unipolar bone loss, providing thresholds for reconstruction in an isolated setting. Gottschalk et al (2016) performed a cadaveric study demonstrating increased instability at lower bony thresholds in the setting of both glenoid and humeral head defects. Walia et al (2016) elaborated on this work and described the loss of rotational stability from humeral head defects with the arm in varying positions of abduction and external rotation. Last, Patel et al (2016) found that an anterior bone block procedure (i.e., Latarjet) in the setting of combined bony defects restores some translational stability but does not restore rotational stability with all humeral head defects. Thus, directly restoring the humeral head articular arc may be necessary to restore shoulder stability. The treatment of clinically significant anterior glenohumeral instability involving an engaging Hill-Sachs lesion can be accomplished with a technique of anatomic allograft reconstruction of the humeral head using a side- and size-matched humeral head osteoarticular allograft. This technique involves an anatomic reconstruction, which eliminates the structural pathology while maintaining the range of motion of the glenohumeral joint.

Indications and Contraindications

Indications for anatomic allograft reconstruction of the humeral head are:

1. A large engaging Hill-Sachs lesion, particularly in the setting of combined bony defects. Biomechanical data support the threshold of 31%; however, further analysis and clinical experience suggest that lesions involving more than 25% of the articular surface may be significant (Miniaci & Martineau, 2006; Patel et al, 2016).
2. Patients who have failed previous soft tissue stabilization procedures. These patients typically present with a large engaging Hill-Sachs lesion and persistent symptomatic anterior glenohumeral instability or painful clicking, catching, or popping.
3. Patients at high risk of redislocation (e.g., epilepsy, contact athletes with combined bony defects to the glenoid and humeral head).

Contraindications to this procedure include routine medical comorbidities precluding an elective surgical procedure with general anesthetic, existing infection, or presence of a nonengaging or functionally nonengaging Hill-Sachs lesion.

Preoperative Planning

All patients are initially evaluated with a complete history and physical examination, including assessing for any generalized laxity. Specifics of the history to obtain include mode of the initial injury; arm position and need for reduction; and details of present symptoms, including pain, frequency, instability, and level of function. Make special note of all prior surgical procedures performed on the extremity, and if possible, obtain operative reports.

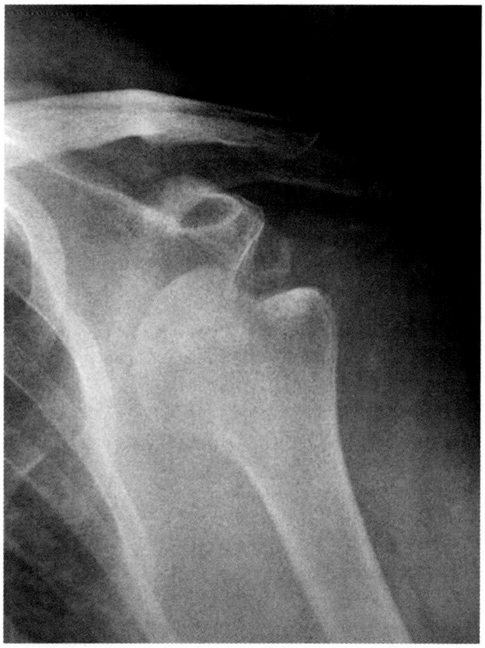

Fig. 1L.1 Anteroposterior radiograph demonstrating a large Hill-Sachs lesion.

Physical examination should focus on inspection for previous scars; a thorough determination of active and passive range of motion; evaluation of the integrity and strength of the rotator cuff; and a detailed examination for glenohumeral laxity in the anterior, posterior, and inferior directions. Examination for apprehension should be performed in varying levels of abduction because patients with large Hill-Sachs lesions usually exhibit apprehension with the arm in significantly less than 90 degrees of abduction and 90 degrees of external rotation.

Preoperative imaging includes a comprehensive plain film evaluation with anteroposterior (AP), true AP, axillary, and Stryker notch views of the involved shoulder (Fig. 1L.1).

All patients require a preoperative axial imaging study (computed tomography [CT] or magnetic resonance imaging [MRI]) to more fully define the bony architecture of the glenoid and humeral head. Three-dimensional reconstruction can be a useful tool to aid in more clearly defining the size and location of the defect and to provide an estimate of the amount of the articular surface involved.

A fresh-frozen cryopreserved osteoarticular humeral head allograft is obtained from a reputable, certified tissue bank. It is important to obtain a side- and size-matched graft because this allows for an optimal re-creation of the radius of curvature of the humeral head. Fresh-frozen grafts are preferred but can be difficult to obtain. Irradiated grafts are a less desirable alternative. In our series of 20 cases, the 2 cases involving irradiated grafts had partial collapse of the graft, which required reoperation and screw removal. Fortunately, this did not lead to recurrent instability. Proper allograft sizing of the humeral head requires the patient's imaging to be sent to the chosen bone bank for measurement. Plain radiographs are acceptable as long as calibration is performed with accepted magnification markers. CT or MR imaging of the proximal humerus allows for direct sizing as magnification is accounted for in the scan. The match from the tissue bank should have a side and size match within ± 2 mm. Clinically, we have found that this tolerance yields acceptable results for this procedure. Availability of a matched humeral allograft can be unpredictable. For time-sensitive cases, a nonmatched humeral head allograft can be used. Of note, femoral heads often have evidence of osteoarthritis, including loss of articular cartilage, and should be avoided if possible. If nonmatched humeral grafts are used, careful trimming and resection may be needed to match the curvature of the native humeral head.

Surgical Technique

The patient is positioned in a modified beach-chair position, inclined about 45 degrees, with the upper extremity draped free. An extended deltopectoral approach is used. The lateral border of the conjoined tendon is identified and gently retracted medially to expose the underlying subscapularis tendon. The entire tendon is transected vertically about 0.5 cm medial to its insertion onto the lesser tuberosity. Tag sutures are placed in the lateral aspect of the subscapularis tendon as it is released from the lesser tuberosity. The interval between the subscapularis and the anterior capsule is then carefully developed using sharp dissection, continuing medially to the neck of the glenoid. The inferior capsule is then further isolated using careful blunt dissection. A laterally based capsulotomy is made with the vertical limb in line with the subscapularis incision and continuing superiorly. The anteroinferior capsule is then released off the surgical neck of the humerus with intraarticular dissection using a periosteal elevator. A standard humeral head retractor is placed into the glenohumeral joint, allowing inspection of the glenoid and anteroinferior capsulolabral structures for any pathology. If a Bankart lesion is found, it is repaired in the usual fashion using either bony drill holes or suture anchors. The sutures can be left untied until completion of the allograft reconstruction.

The humeral head retractor is withdrawn, and the humerus is brought into maximal external rotation to expose the Hill-Sachs lesion. Unroof the synovial expansion of the supraspinatus to allow the humerus to be more fully externally rotated, allowing better visualization and access to the Hill-Sachs lesion. A flat, narrow retractor is then placed over the reflected undersurface of the subscapularis tendon and behind the neck of the humerus on the posterior rotator cuff to lever out the humeral head (Fig. 1L.2).

With the Hill-Sachs lesion adequately exposed, a microsagittal saw is used to smooth and reshape the defect into a chevron-type configuration (Fig. 1L.3, *A*).

The base and side of the defect can then be further smoothed using a hand rasp to achieve precise, flat surfaces. The base (*X*), height (*Y*), length (*Z*), and rough outside partial circumference (*C*) of the defect are then measured to the nearest millimeter (Fig. 1L.3, *B*).

A corresponding piece is cut from the matched humeral head allograft that is 2 to 3 mm larger in all dimensions than the measured defect. The allograft segment is then provisionally placed into the Hill-Sachs defect and resized in all three planes. Excess graft is then carefully trimmed with the microsagittal saw and is reshaped in the other two planes as well. Fine tuning of the graft size is then continued in one plane at a time until a perfect size match is achieved in all planes, including base (*X*), height (*Y*), length (*Z*), and outside partial circumference (*C*).

The allograft segment is placed into the defect and aligned so as to achieve a congruent articular surface.

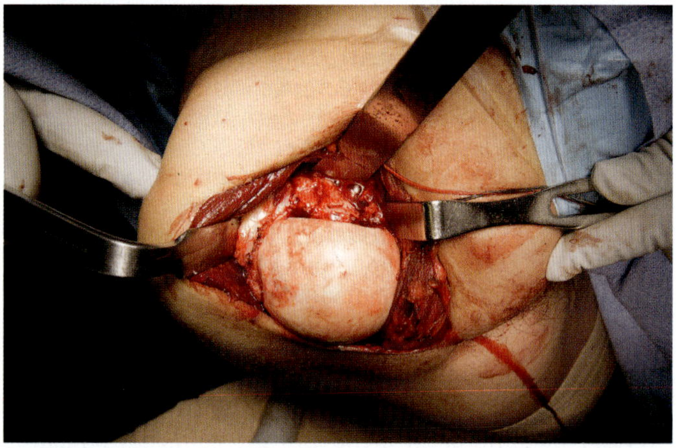

Fig. 1L.2 Intraoperative photograph demonstrating exposure of the humeral head.

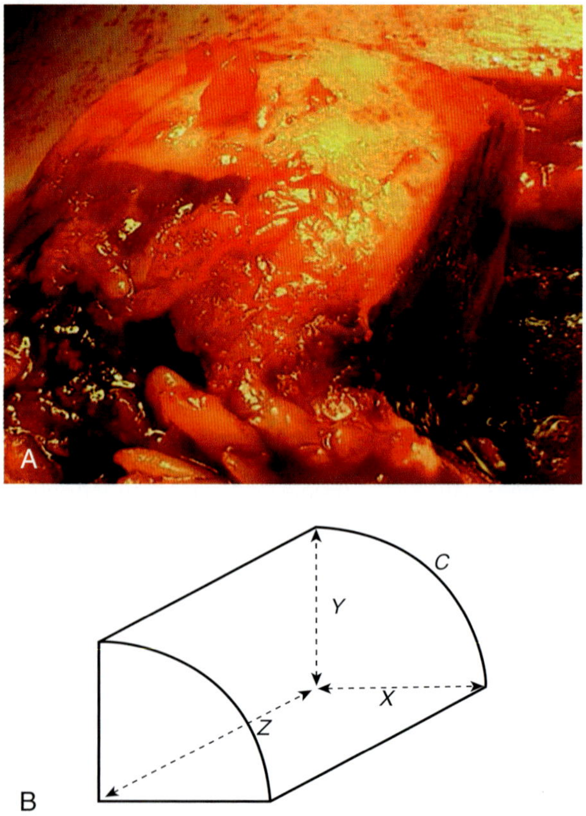

Fig. 1L.3 A, With the Hill-Sachs lesion adequately exposed, a microsagittal saw is used to smooth and reshape the defect into a chevron-type configuration. The base and side of the defect can then be further smoothed using a hand rasp to achieve precise, flat surfaces. **B,** The base *(X)*, height *(Y)*, length *(Z)*, and rough outside partial circumference *(C)* of the defect are then measured to the nearest millimeter.

It is provisionally secured in place with two or three smooth 0.045-inch Kirschner wires (Fig. 1L.4).

The wires are then sequentially replaced with 3.5-mm fully threaded cortical or 4.0-mm cancellous screws placed in a lag fashion (Fig. 1L.5).

Ensure that the screw heads are countersunk so that they are below the level of the articular surface. The joint is irrigated and taken through a range of motion to ensure that the reconstructed humeral head provides a smooth congruent articulating surface.

The capsulotomy is closed with absorbable suture, tying any previously placed sutures used to repair the capsulolabral pathology if present. The subscapularis tendon is then reapproximated to its stump anatomically, without shortening, using suture anchors or a soft tissue repair with nonabsorbable suture. Allow the conjoined tendon, deltoid, and pectoralis major muscles to return to their normal anatomic positions. A routine subcutaneous and skin closure is then performed. Sterile dressing is applied. The arm is placed into a shoulder immobilizer.

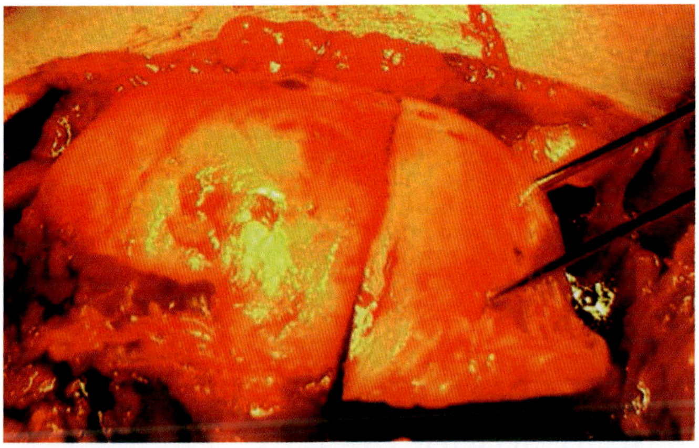

Fig. 1L.4 The allograft is provisionally secured into the defect with K-wires.

Complications

Complications that occurred in our series of humeral osteoarticular allograft reconstruction of the Hill-Sachs lesions included radiographic follow-up evidence of partial graft collapse in 2 of 18 patients, early evidence of osteoarthritis in 3 patients (marginal osteophytes), and 1 mild subluxation (posterior). Hardware complications developed in 2 patients who complained of pain with extreme external rotation. The screws were removed at approximately 2 years postoperatively in both patients, thereby relieving their symptoms.

Postoperative Care

After surgery, patients are given a sling for comfort and allowed full passive range of motion immediately as tolerated. Because of the subscapularis detachment, we protect against active and resisted internal rotation for 6 weeks. After the initial 6-week period, patients are allowed terminal stretching and strengthening exercises. The shoulders are imaged with repeat radiographs at 6 weeks and 6 months and with CT scans at 6 months to assess for consolidation and incorporation of the graft.

Outcomes

Between 1995 and 2001, we performed and reviewed this procedure in 18 patients who had failed previous attempts at surgical stabilization with an average follow-up of 50 months (range, 24–96 months) (Miniaci & Gish, 2004). Fifteen patients had a history of traumatic anterior glenohumeral instability related to sports, and three patients had instability related to seizures or other trauma. All had posterolateral humeral head defects (Hill-Sachs lesions) that represented greater than about 25% to 30% of the humeral head.

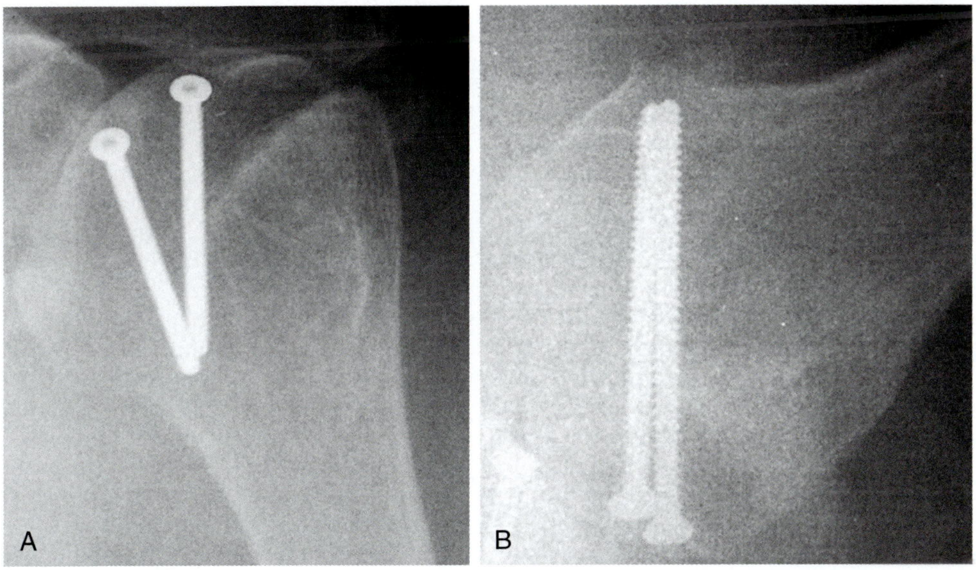

Fig. 1L.5 AP radiographs after screw fixation of the allograft. (From Miniaci A, Martineau PA. *Surgical Techniques in Sports Medicine.* 1st ed. 2006:189-194 Lippincott Williams and Wilkins, Philadelphia.)

One patient had both anterior and posterior humeral head defects from bidirectional shoulder instability sustained as a result of a seizure disorder. No patients had true multidirectional instability. Patients in the formal review were assessed preoperatively and postoperatively with: Radiographic evaluation (plain films and axial imaging [CT, MRI, or both]), validated clinical evaluation measures (Constant-Murley shoulder scale, Western Ontario Shoulder Instability Index [WOSII], and Short Form 36). Findings at the time of surgery included nine patients with recurrent Bankart lesions; nine patients with capsular redundancy only; no patients with subscapularis tears; one patient with posterior glenoid erosion; and three patients with anterior glenoid deficiency (<20%), which was not reconstructed. There were no episodes of recurrent instability. Sixteen of 18 (89%) patients returned to work.

The average Constant score postoperatively was 78.5. The WOSII, which is a validated quality-of-life scale specific to shoulder instability using a visual analog scale response format, decreased significantly, indicating improvement. Overall, this represents the first reported series of anatomic allograft reconstruction of Hill-Sachs defects for recurrent traumatic anterior instability after failed repairs.

Diklic et al (2010) treated 13 patients with fresh-frozen femoral head allograft reconstructions for Hill-Sachs lesions between 25% to 50% of the humeral head. At an average of 54 months postoperatively, the mean Constant score for the cohort was 86.8. Twelve patients had stable shoulders, and one patient had evidence of osteonecrosis. Although infrequently a cause for clinical concern, Hill-Sachs defects can be the source of significant disability and recurrent instability in a subset of patients. This technique has been shown to be effective for a difficult problem with few available treatment options.

One should consider anatomic allograft reconstruction of these defects as a viable treatment alternative.

References

Burkhart SS, De Beer JF. Traumatic glenohumeral bone defects and their relationship to failure of arthroscopic Bankart repairs: significance of the inverted-pear glenoid and the humeral engaging Hill-Sachs lesion. *Arthroscopy.* 2000;16(7):677–694.

Calandra JJ, Baker CL, Uribe J. The incidence of Hill-Sachs lesions in initial anterior shoulder dislocations. *Arthroscopy.* 1989;5:254–257.

Diklic ID, Ganic ZD, Blagojevic ZD, Nho SJ, Romeo AA. Treatment of locked chronic posterior dislocation of the shoulder by reconstruction of the defect in the humeral head with an allograft. *J Bone Joint Surg Br.* 2010;92(1):71–76.

Gottschalk LJ 4th, Walia P, Patel RM, et al. Stability of the glenohumeral joint with combined humeral head and glenoid defects: a cadaveric study. *Am J Sports Med.* 2016;44(4):933–940.

Hovelius L, Augustini BG, Fredin H, et al. Primary anterior dislocation of the shoulder in young patients: a ten-year prospective study. *J Bone Joint Surg Am.* 1996;78:1677–1684.

Miniaci A, Gish MW. Management of anterior glenohumeral instability associated with large Hill-Sachs defects. *Tech Shoulder Elbow Surg.* 2004;5(3):170–175.

Miniaci A, Martineau PA. *Surgical Techniques in Sports Medicine.* 1st ed. Philadelphia: Lippincott Williams and Wilkins; 2006:189–194.

Patel RM, Walia P, Gottschalk L, et al. The effects of latarjet reconstruction on glenohumeral kinematics in the presence of combined bony defects: a cadaveric model. *Am J Sports Med.* 2016;44(7):1818–1824.

Rowe CR, Zarins B, Ciullo JV. Recurrent anterior dislocation of the shoulder after surgical repair: apparent causes of failure and treatment. *J Bone Joint Surg Am.* 1984;66:159–168.

Walia P, Patel RM, Gottschalk L, et al. The reduction in stability from combined humeral head and glenoid bony defects is influenced by arm position. *Am J Sports Med.* 2016;44(3):715–722.

1-1M BIPOLAR LESIONS: PATHOMECHANICS, EVALUATION, AND SURGICAL APPROACHES

ALEX G. DUKAS, MD, MA and ROBERT A. ARCIERO, MD

Introduction

Bone loss in the setting of glenohumeral instability has classically focused on either glenoid *or* the humeral head defect. A bipolar lesion is the combination of glenoid and humeral head bone loss in the setting of glenohumeral instability. Arthroscopic Bankart repair of an unstable shoulder without addressing the bone loss of either the glenoid or the Hill-Sachs defect may lead to higher rates of failure and recurrent instability. Classically, glenoid bone loss of more than 20% to 25% has been treated with bone augmentation, and Hill-Sachs lesions of more than 30% to 40% have been addressed. Proper treatment of the bipolar lesion depends on detailed patient evaluation and imaging.

Background

The concept of concavity–compression describing the interplay of dynamic muscle compression from rotator cuff function, static forces of the capsulolabral structures, and bony articulation is necessary to keep the humeral head centered on the glenoid (Lippitt & Matsen, 1993). A disruption in any of these structures can result in glenohumeral instability. The geometry of the glenohumeral surface provides minimal static stabilization compared with other joints. This is mainly because of the smaller surface area and relatively shallow glenoid compared with the humeral head. Traumatic anterior dislocation often results in combined injury of soft tissue restraints in conjunction with bony defects on the glenoid fossa and humeral head, which can contribute to glenohumeral instability and predispose to increased failure rate with traditional arthroscopic Bankart repair. These combinations of injuries can manifest with great variability, making it extremely unlikely for one surgical treatment method to restore stability in all cases.

Bone loss in the setting of instability has either focused on the implications of isolated glenoid lesions or humeral head lesions. However, it has been increasingly recognized that neither of these lesions may be mutually exclusive and if so are exceedingly rare. During an anterior glenohumeral dislocation, the combined forces of external rotation and anterior translation overcome soft tissue restraints and result in a dislocation event. This event may also result in a compression fracture of the posterior and superolateral proximal humerus as it engages on the anterior rim of the glenoid or fracture of the glenoid rim itself. It is now recognized that recurrent instability is an interplay between both lesions, and treatment implications should take into consideration the contribution from each pathology.

Glenoid Bone Loss

Isolated glenoid defects are present in the setting of traumatic first time anterior dislocation 22% of the time (Taylor & Arciero, 1997; Calandra et al, 1989). Griffith and colleagues (2008) used computed tomography (CT) to analyze the prevalence of glenoid bone loss and found that it was present in 41% of patients with first-time unilateral dislocation and 86% of 137 patients with recurrent unilateral dislocation (Griffith et al, 2008). Recurrent instability often leads to attritional glenoid bone loss and bony fragment resorption from the inferior anterior glenoid. In the setting of associated bone loss, arthroscopic Bankart repair has an increased rate of recurrent instability (Arciero et al, 2015; Bollier & Arciero, 2010; Burkhart & De Beer, 2000; Garcia, 2015; Long et al, 2014; Nakagawa et al, 2015; Taylor & Arciero, 1997). Itoi and colleagues (2003) performed progressive osteotomies of the anteroinferior glenoid to represent progressive bone loss in the setting of Bankart repairs and found that stability to anterior translation and range of motion was significantly less with a bony glenoid defect greater than 21% of the diameter of the glenoid.

Humeral Head Compression Fracture (Hill-Sachs Lesions)

The countercoup to the Bankart lesion is a superolateral posterior compression defect in the humeral head, termed a "Hill-Sachs lesion." The incidence of Hill-Sachs lesions has been reported to be present in 40% to 90% of first-time dislocators and up to 100% in recurrent dislocators. Historically, the traditional approach has concluded that lesions involving less than 20% of the humeral head articular surface are rarely of clinical significance and rarely addressed, but lesions more than 30% to 40% of that surface are clinically significant and can be responsible for recurrent instability (Armitage et al, 2010; Provencher et al, 2012). Sekiya et al (2006) have shown that defects of as little as 12.5% of humeral head diameter can significantly decrease the distance of anterior translation before the humeral head engages the glenoid rim. Furthermore, Kaar and colleagues (2010) noted defects that were equal to five eighths of the humeral head radius or greater had decreased glenohumeral stability.

Combined Defects: Bipolar Lesions

A bipolar lesion occurs when bone loss is present on both the glenoid and humeral head. The prevalence of bipolar lesions has been reported anywhere from 33% to 70% in first-time dislocators and 61.8% to 84% in recurrent dislocators (Griffith et al, 2012; Nakagawa et al, 2015; Widjaja et al, 2006). Different mechanisms result in varying amounts of lesion on either the glenoid or humeral side. Glenoid rim avulsions are usually caused by low-energy mechanism as indirect traction of the capsulolabral tissue (Trivedi et al, 2014). Hill-Sachs lesions are seldom found in shoulders without dislocation, and it is suggested that engagement with the anterior glenoid rim at the time of complete dislocation is essential for their occurrence (Ozaki et al, 2014). Glenoid fractures are associated with high-energy traumatic dislocation more readily seen in collision athletes, male sex, frequent dislocation/subluxation, and joint tightness, among others (Nakagawa et al, 2014, 2015; Van Oostveen et al, 2014). In recurrent instability, glenoid defects are enlarged not only by the recurrent dislocation but also by recurrent subluxation without dislocation, and Hill-Sachs defects are enlarged with recurrent engagement (Calandra et al, 1989; Di Giacomo & Itoi, 2014; Di Giacomo et al, 2016; Griffith et al, 2012; Milano et al, 2011; Nakagawa et al, 2014, 2015; Streubel et al, 2014; Van Oostveen et al, 2014).

Arciero et al (2015) evaluated the additive negative effect bipolar lesions have on soft tissue Bankart repairs alone. Small- and medium-sized Hill-Sachs defects were created in a cadaveric model based on a consecutive series of anterior-instability patients. A three-dimensional (3D) printer was used to create a humeral head representing these defects from the 3D reconstructions of the CT images. These were then used to create humeral head defects in the cadaver. Glenoid defects of 2, 4, and 6 mm were also created, simulating a bipolar lesion. Despite a robust Bankart repair, there was a significant reduction in load to translation when a medium- and small-sized Hill-Sachs lesion was combined with 8% and 16% glenoid bone loss, respectively. This is well below the often quoted 21% that Itoi et al (2003) had shown to compromise soft tissue Bankart repair.

Burkhart and De Beer (2000) recognized that the presence of combined glenoid defect and Hill-Sachs lesions introduces a level of complexity that can compromise soft tissue repair. They introduced the concept of engaging Hill-Sachs defect and the "inverted pear" glenoid to represent critical glenoid bone loss. An engaging Hills-Sachs lesion is one that articulates with the glenoid rim particularly as the arm is brought into abduction and external rotation. This leads to symptoms of recurrent instability with little provocation and even during sleep. Larger defects engage the glenoid rim with less humeral external rotation and abduction. Reviewing 194 cases of traumatic anterior instability repaired with arthroscopic soft tissue Bankart procedures, patients with less than a 25% glenoid bone defect or engaging Hill-Sachs lesion showed a recurrence rate of 4%. Those with greater than 25% glenoid defect or engaging Hill-Sachs had a recurrence rate of 67%, and if they were contact athletes, the rate ballooned to 89%.

Balg and Boileau (2007) aimed to further identify patients at risk for recurrence after arthroscopic Bankart repair. They performed a prospective case series of 131 arthroscopic Bankart repairs in all patients. Looking at those who had recurrence at 31.2 months, they identified the following risk factors: patient aged younger than 20 years at the time of surgery, involvement in competitive

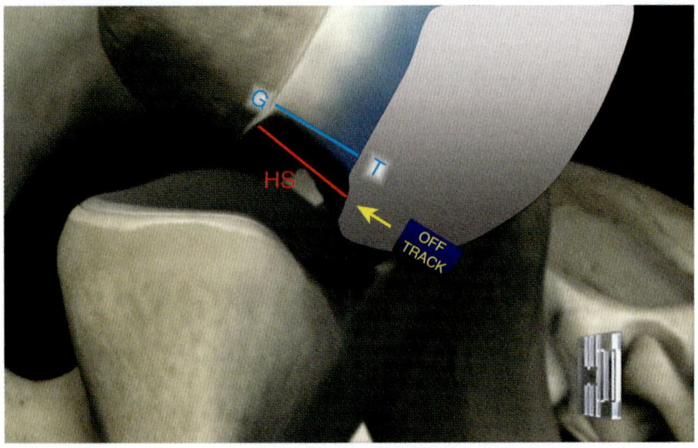

Fig. 1M.1 Example of an "off-track" lesion. Glenohumeral joint in abduction and external rotation illustrating engaging glenoid and humeral head defects. The Hill-Sachs (HS) lesion extends medial to the medial margin of the glenoid track. *G, lateral margin*; *T*, medial margin. (Adapted from Di Giacomo G, Itoi E, Burkhart SS. Evolving concept of bipolar bone loss and the Hill-Sachs lesion: from "engaging/non-engaging" lesion to "on-track/off-track" lesion. *Arthroscopy*. 2014;30(1):90-98.)

or contact sports or in sports involving vigorous overhead activity, shoulder hyperlaxity, and radiographically identifiable bone defects (anteroposterior [AP] radiograph of the shoulder in external rotation showing Hill-Sachs lesion and/or loss of the sclerotic inferior glenoid border). From these findings, they deduced an "instability severity index score" that viewed humeral and glenoid bone loss as a clear contraindication to arthroscopic treatment.

Yamamoto et al (2007) introduced the concept of the "glenoid track" in 2007. This concept serves to illustrate the dynamic of glenohumeral instability and interplay of bipolar lesions. Using a bipolar model, they examined the exact anatomic relation between the humeral head and the glenoid in varying degrees of abduction. They found that with an increase in arm elevation, the glenoid contact area shifted from the inferomedial to the superolateral portion of the posterior aspect of the humeral head, creating a zone of contact, the *glenoid track*. They further showed that if a Hill-Sachs lesion extends or is located beyond 18.4 mm medial to the rotator cuff footprint or 84% of the width on the inferior glenoid, the lesion will engage. Lesions that extended or were located medial to this threshold are "off track," and lesions lateral to this are "on track." They have advocated that off-track lesions treated with Bankart repair alone will have high failure rates. DiGiacomo and colleagues (2014) have suggested an algorithm for the treatment of on-track and off-track lesions with surgical strategies that may include remplissage, bone grafting of the glenoid, coracoid transfer, or humeral head allograft (Fig. 1M.1).

Diagnosis, History, and Physical Examination

The initial evaluation of a patient with anterior instability should include a complete history of the onset, including mechanism, position of arm at onset, recurrence, chronology, and frequency of dislocations. Other pertinent information includes whether the patient competes in collision or contact sports and any operative or nonoperative treatment to date. As the frequency and ease of instability episodes increase, the likelihood of significant bone defects is also increased. Subluxations or frank dislocations that occur over a short period of time, at increasing frequencies, with activities of daily living, or during slumber or dislocations with greater than 5 hours before reduction are all factors associated with bone loss (Boone & Arciero, 2010; Denard et al, 2015; Provencher et al, 2012; Wang & Arciero, 2008). Patients who have undergone failed instability procedures in the past are more likely to have significant bony defects. Patients with an engaging Hill-Sachs lesion may complain of pain, crepitus, or catching as the glenoid engages the Hill-Sachs lesion when the arm is externally rotated and abducted. Often patients with significant bipolar lesions require sedation or anesthesia for manual reduction.

Physical examination begins with an inspection of the shoulder contour, muscle symmetry, and active and passive range of motion. Assessment of laxity with translation tests and instability with apprehension tests is essential. Laxity can be elicited with the sulcus sign, and general laxity can be ascertained from Beighton criteria. Balg and Boileau (2007) argue that external rotation greater than 85 degrees is indicative of laxity. The load and shift test is another useful examination tool to assess glenohumeral laxity, and the examiner can assess anterior and posterior laxity of the humeral head on the glenoid in the plane of the scapula. Decreased resistance will be felt with a defect in the anterior glenoid rim, and any grinding or crepitus may indicate a bone defect. Translation can be graded by assessment of humeral head excursion over the glenoid: 1+ to the rim, 2+ over the rim with spontaneous reduction, and 3+ locked. The apprehension and relocation test will reproduce the patient's symptoms with the arm abducted and externally rotated. If there is apprehension at lower angles of abduction, or midrange apprehension, this is indicative of significant bone loss (Patel et al, 2014; Yamamoto et al, 2007).

Assessment of Bone Loss

Bone deficiency of the glenoid and the humeral head can be assessed with plain radiographs, CT scan, and at the time of arthroscopy. (Please refer to Table 1M.1 for a list of methods to quantify bone loss.)

Routine radiographs consist of an AP, transscapular lateral, and axillary views and may confirm the direction of dislocation, associated bone defects, or fracture. A modified axillary radiograph, the West Point view, specifically examines the anteroinferior aspect of the glenoid. Itoi and colleagues (2003) have reported that the West Point view demonstrates a high correlation with CT in estimating glenoid bone loss (Fig. 1M.2). The patient is positioned prone with the head turned to the contralateral side and the x-ray beam is angled 25 degrees from the midline and directed through the axilla.

The imaging modality of choice to evaluate bone deficiencies is CT. We have a low threshold to obtain CT with 3D reconstructions in the case of suspected bone loss. Although magnetic resonance imaging is valuable in assessing the location and degree of soft tissue injury and

Table 1M.1 Methods of Quantifying Bone Loss

Location	Method to Quantify Bone Loss	Measurement Type	Description
Glenoid	Arthroscopic	Bare spot	Using an arthroscopic probe, the distance in millimeters between the bare spot and the anterior glenoid rim is measured (A), as is the distance between the bare spot and the posterior glenoid rim (B). Bone loss = ([B+A]/[2XB]) X 100 = % of Remaining Glenoid
Glenoid	CT (en face view of the glenoid on 3D surface rendering with humeral head subtraction or 2D oblique sagittal reconstruction)	Best-fit circle	A perfect circle is fit to the inferior two thirds of the glenoid. The surface area of the anterior rim defect is measured digitally. The defect area is divided by the total area of the best-fit circle to obtain the percentage of anterior bone loss.
Glenoid	CT (en face view of the glenoid on 3D surface rendering)	Glenoid index	Ratio of the maximum diameter of the lower two thirds of the injured glenoid fossa compared with the maximum diameter of the contralateral uninjured glenoid fossa. A glenoid index of 0.75 indicates that the patient will benefit from an open Latarjet procedure.
Glenoid	CT (en face view of the glenoid on 2D oblique sagittal reconstruction)	Pico method	A best-fit circle is drawn on the uninjured side. An identical circle is drawn on the injured glenoid, and the missing part of the circle is measured. The defect is quantified as a percentage of the total area of the uninjured circle.
Glenoid	CT	Glenoid rim distances	Distances are measured in millimeters from the bare spot to both the anterior glenoid rim (distance A) and the posterior rim (distance B). Bone loss = ([B+A]/[2XB]) X 100 = % of Remaining Glenoid
Glenoid	CT (en face view of the glenoid on 3D surface rendering with humeral head subtraction or 2D oblique sagittal reconstruction)	Ratio method	Mathematical calculation. Percentage of the missing area is expressed as a function of the ratio between the distance from the center of the best-fit circle to the anterior glenoid rim and the radius of the circle.
Humeral head	Radiography	Hill-Sachs quotient	AP view of the shoulder in 60 degrees IR. Bernageau view (i.e., Neer lateral view with 30 degrees of cephalad tilt with the arm in maximum scapular plane elevation and 45 degrees ER). Maximum defect width and depth are measured on each view. Volume defect = (maximum defect width on AP view) · (maximum defect width on Bernageau view) · (maximum defect depth on either view)
Humeral head	CT (2D reconstructions in the axial, sagittal, and coronal planes)	Kodali et al	Axial, sagittal, and coronal reconstruction images depicting the maximum size of the Hill-Sachs lesion. A best-fit circle is drawn using the intact humeral head circumference. Edge-to-edge distances of the defect are measured in each plane. Depth of the defect is measured in each plane with regard to the periphery of the best-fit circle.

AP, Anteroposterior; *CT,* computed tomography; *ER, External Rotation*; *IR, Internal Rotation*; *3D,* three dimensional; *2D,* two dimensional.
Adapted from Streubel PN, Krych AJ, Simone JP, et al. Anterior glenohumeral instability: a pathology-based surgical treatment strategy. *J Am Acad Orthop Surg.* 2014;22(5):283-294.

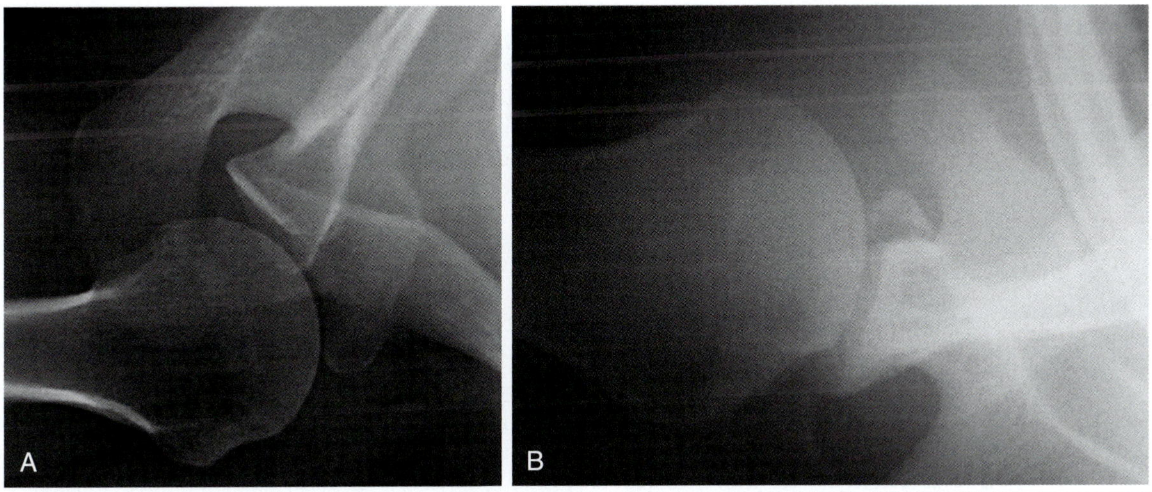

Fig. 1M.2 A, Example of a West Point axillary view of a left shoulder demonstrating a small bony Bankart lesion. **B,** An additional example of a West Point View axillary of a right shoulder demonstrating a bony Bankart lesion.

has been used to assess bone loss, it can often underestimate the degree of deficiency (Baudi et al, 2013; Friedman et al, 2014; Provencher et al, 2012). Our indications for obtaining a CT include significant midrange apprehension, instability with minimal provocation, multiple instability events, revision surgery, and any bone loss detected on plain radiographs. Many authors now advocate the use of 3D CT with digital subtraction of the humeral head. We advocate for calculating the presence of bone loss of the glenoid to use the methods previously established by Sugaya et al (2003) and humeral bone loss established by Cho et al (2011).

Significant glenohumeral bone loss can be identified at the time of arthroscopy as well. However, the authors prefer to have the surgical strategy to be well defined before going to the operating room. To check for engaging Hill-Sachs lesions, the arm can be removed from traction and brought to abduction and external rotation, and direct visualization of the Hill-Sachs articulating on the anterior glenoid can be made. The "'inverted-pear" glenoid (>25% loss of the inferior glenoid diameter) can be viewed from the anterosuperior portal (Lo et al, 2004). Burkhart and De Beer described their method of intraoperative measurement of the glenoid defect using a constant reference point of the bare area in the center of the glenoid face. Using an arthroscopic probe, the measured distance from the posterior rim to bare area is multiplied by 2, providing the estimation of the diameter of an intact glenoid. Then the distance from the posterior rim to the anterior remaining rim is measured. This ratio will represent the percentage of remaining glenoid and therefore provide the percentage of bone loss. This method, however, has been shown to be inconsistent, and we caution surgeons to have a thorough preoperative plan before the procedure (Barcia et al, 2013; Miyatake et al, 2014).

Table 1M.2 Instability Severity Index Score

Prognostic Factors	Points
AGE AT SURGERY (YR)	
<20	2
>20	0
DEGREE OF SPORT PARTICIPATION (PREOPERATIVELY)	
Competitive	2
Recreational or none	0
TYPE OF SPORT (PREOPERATIVELY)	
Contact or forced overhead	1
Other	0
SHOULDER HYPERLAXITY	
Shoulder hyperlaxity (anterior or inferior)	1
Normal laxity	0
HILL-SACHS ON AP RADIOGRAPH	
Visible in external rotation	2
Not visible in external rotation	0
GLENOID LOSS OF CONTOUR ON AP RADIOGRAPHS	
Loss of contour	2
No lesion	0
TOTAL POINTS	10

AP, Anteroposterior.

Reproduced with permission from Balg F, Boileau P. The instability severity index score. A simple pre-operative score to select patients for arthroscopic or open shoulder stabilization. *J Bone Joint Surg Br.* 2007;89(11):1470-1477.

Surgical Decision Making

Balg and Boileau (2007) attempted to preoperatively predict success or failure with arthroscopic soft tissue repair with development of the Instability Severity Index Score (ISIS) after review of their own case series (Table 1M.2). They found that patients with a score greater than 6 points had a recurrence rate of 70%, but those with less than 3 had only 5% with soft tissue repair alone. In a follow-up study, Boileau and colleagues (2007) found that arthroscopic Bankart repairs had a recurrent instability rate of 22%, but those stabilized with the Latarjet procedure had a 10% rate over a 6-year period. They therefore recommend the Latarjet procedure for patients with an ISIS score greater than 3 (Balg & Boileau, 2007; Bessière et al, 2014). Although this is a simple and concise algorithm, it is largely not validated (Weber, 2014).

The management of bipolar or combined humeral and glenoid bone loss in the context of shoulder instability is an evolving concept. The key factors are not only the degree of bone loss involved but also whether the humeral Hill-Sachs lesion engages or not. Burkhart and De Beer's concept of *engaging* versus *nonengaging* lesions has been refined by Itoi's concept of the "glenoid track" (Burkhart & De Beer 2000; Di Giacomo et al, 2014; Yamamoto et al, 2007). Few recent reports have attempted to clinically validate this concept. Metzger et al, (2013) performed exam under anesthesia (EUA) in 140 patients with recurrent instability. They classified patients with bipolar lesions into either off- or on-track groups. They found based on imaging that 13.4% of patients had off-track lesions and 84.5% of these patients had an engaging Hill-Sachs on EUA, but 12.4% of on-track lesions engaged.

DiGiacomo and colleagues have recently proposed a bipolar lesion treatment algorithm based on Hill-Sachs lesions and the glenoid track concept (Di Giacomo et al, 2016). If a Hill-Sachs lesion is off track, they recommend augmentation with remplissage and Bankart repair if glenoid bone loss is less than 20%. Glenoid bone augmentation is recommended when glenoid bone loss is more than 20% with the iliac crest, J-span (Tauber et al, 2004), or Latarjet (Di Giacomo et al, 2016; Tauber et al, 2004) procedure. This is likely acceptable in the majority of bipolar lesions; however, for larger Hill-Sachs lesions, this may fall short if the lesion is more than 30% (Patel et al, 2016; Provencher et al, 2009).

Authors' Preferred Approach

Numerous instability events (more than five dislocations), instability requiring reduction especially under anesthesia, failed prior stabilization, and instability in sleep all suggest clinically significant bone loss. This is further defined by imaging and specifically 3D CT reconstruction.

We prefer arthroscopic stabilization for patients with little or no bone loss (<10% on the glenoid and a nonengaging Hill-Sachs lesion), overhead athletes, primary dislocation, older patients, and noncollision athletes. Collision athletes, especially male patients younger than 25 years of age and those with 10% to 20% glenoid bone loss with small *nonengaging* Hill-Sachs lesions, we believe have unacceptably high rates of recurrent instability after arthroscopic repair, so we prefer the open Bankart procedure (Castagna et al, 2010; Ozturk et al, 2013; Plewa et al, 1998; Shaha et al, 2015; van der Linde et al, 2011; Voos et al, 2010). The open Bankart procedure has a long history of satisfactory results in patients with intermediate amounts of bone loss (Charalambous & Eastwood, 2014; Hovelius et al, 1996; Moroder et al, 2015; Pagnani et al, 2008; Rowe et al, 1984).

In patients with 20% to 30% glenoid bone loss and any sized Hill-Sachs defect, we prefer the Latarjet procedure. In patients with severe bipolar bone loss, Ranne et al (2013) described successfully combining an open Latarjet procedure and remplissage. This may be a reasonable option in those with more than 25% glenoid bone loss with engaging humeral defects. For very large glenoid bone defects (>30%) and in young patients, fresh osteochondral grafting using the distal tibia has had early favorable results (Provencher et al, 2008).

In the more unusual occurrence when significantsized Hill-Sachs lesions are present but there is little or no glenoid bone loss, the exam under anesthesia (EUA) and the arthroscopic examination are important. During the EUA, if the humeral head dislocates and "locks," requiring a manual reduction, this represents true engagement of these two articular components, and a Latarjet procedure is preferred. Engagement or the "off-track" nature of these lesions can be further validated by the arthroscopic exam.

Although the remplissage procedure has been popularized in the setting of engaging or large Hill-Sachs lesions and little or no glenoid bone loss, there have been recent reports of unfavorable outcomes in the athletes who require frequent overhead positioning of the arm (Weber, 2014) . There are reports of Hill-Sachs elevating humeralplasty in the acute setting with mixed results (Armitage et al, 2010; Garcia, 2015).

In patients with very large humeral head defects (>30%), direct treatment with osteochondral grafting of the humeral defect may be required (Patel et al, 2014). In patients older than 45 years of age, these large defects may require partial arthroplasty or resurfacing. These patients may also have significant rotator cuff lesions.

In rare instances, such as in neglected recurrent instability or seizure patients, there will be substantial bone defects involving the glenoid and humeral head, and both will require surgical attention. In this setting, the senior author prefers combined glenoid bone grafting with tricortical iliac crest graft and osteochondral grafting of the humeral head.

Anterior Bone Block Procedure (Video 1M.1)

In cases of significant, more than 20% glenoid bone loss, or an engaging Hill-Sachs defect with any glenoid bone loss, we prefer the Latarjet procedure with a modified Bankart capsular repair (Yang et al, 2016). This has become the procedure of choice in this situation and is very successful in restoring stability. In the senior author's experience, it is used 10% of the time to treat recurrent anterior shoulder instability. It does, however, have a steep learning curve, and complications are not insignificant (Griesser et al, 2013; Shaha et al, 2015; Yang et al, 2016). It has been shown to have a low recurrence rate, and if coracoid is placed flush with glenoid face, the rate of premature osteoarthritis is low (Hovelius et al, 2004). The beach-chair position provides the opportunity to easily convert to open surgery. An EUA is then performed. If the patient has 3+ anterior laxity with the load and shift test, has greater than 20% glenoid bone loss when viewing from the anterior superior arthroscopy portal, and demonstrates a dynamic engaging Hill-Sachs lesion, an open Latarjet procedure will be performed. We currently recommend the Latarjet procedure for an engaging Hill-Sachs, glenoid bone loss greater than 20%, and revision surgery, as well as for young collision athletes who are younger than 20 years of age with the previous mentioned bone loss.

The senior author's modified Latarjet technique involves the transfer of an approximately 2.5 cm portion of the coracoid with conjoined tendon attached through a subscapularis split and a capsular repair. A rolled towel is placed supporting the medial border of the scapula to prevent scapular protraction, which makes subsequent parallel drilling and screw fixation easier. After arthroscopy, the patient is returned to more of a supine position, and the arm is rested on a padded Mayo stand. Incision is placed from coracoid tip to axillary fold. The cephalic vein is taken laterally. The pectoralis minor tendon is released from the coracoid. The coracoid is then exposed. The coracoacromial ligament is incised, leaving as much tissue attached to the coracoid as possible for future capsular repair. The coracoid harvest is performed with a 90-degree sagittal saw at the base, just anterior to the coracoclavicular ligaments. The graft, along with the conjoined tendon, is gently dissected free from surrounding attachments. The musculocutaneous nerve is explored and freed so as to not have undue tension with coracoid fixation. A capsulotomy is made as medial as possible on the edge of the glenoid with the arm in external rotation. The inferior coracoid surface is decorticated. The glenoid rim is taken down to bleeding cancellous bone. The graft is secured flush to the glenoid surface using two 3.5-mm fully threaded cortical screws in a parallel fashion utilizing lag by technique (Fig. 1M3). Then two or three suture anchors are placed just posterior to the graft on the face of the glenoid. The sutures from the anchors are passed through the medial edge of the capsule and tied, repairing the medial edge of the capsule to the glenoid edge, representing a modified Bankart repair. With the previous capsulotomy being performed on the edge of the glenoid with the arm in external rotation, subsequent repair also with the arm in 30 to 45 degrees of external rotation ensures that the patient will not lose motion postoperatively. It should be noted that in repairing the capsule in this manner, the coracoid transfer is now extraarticular (Fig. 1M.4). Postoperatively, the patient's arm is kept in a sling for 4 weeks, but supine assisted forward flexion to 140 degrees and external rotation to 30 degrees are permitted soon after surgery. Rotator cuff and general shoulder strengthening are started at 8 weeks. Return to play for athletes is allowed at 3 to 6 months if evidence of bony union is seen on radiographs.

Approach to Significant Humeral Head Defect

Because of the loss of motion, we prefer to reserve remplissage for non-overhead athletes and older patients. If the

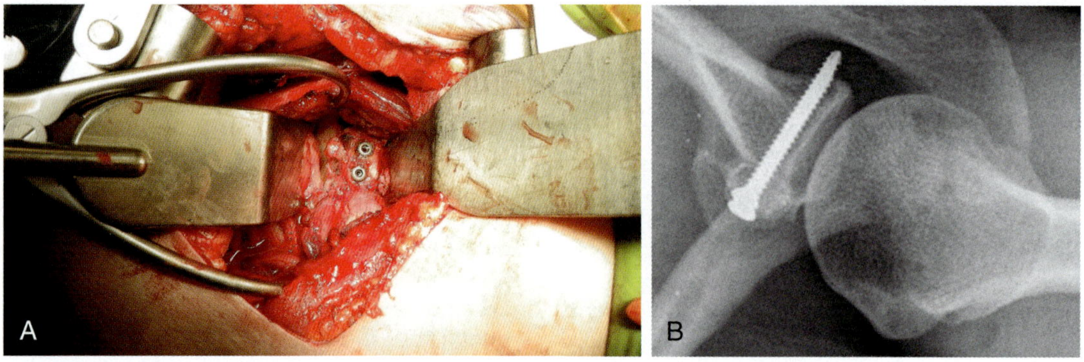

Fig. 1M.3 **A,** Intraoperative view of the correct position of the coracoid during the open Latarjet procedure. **B,** Postoperative imaging demonstrating the correct position of the transferred coracoid.

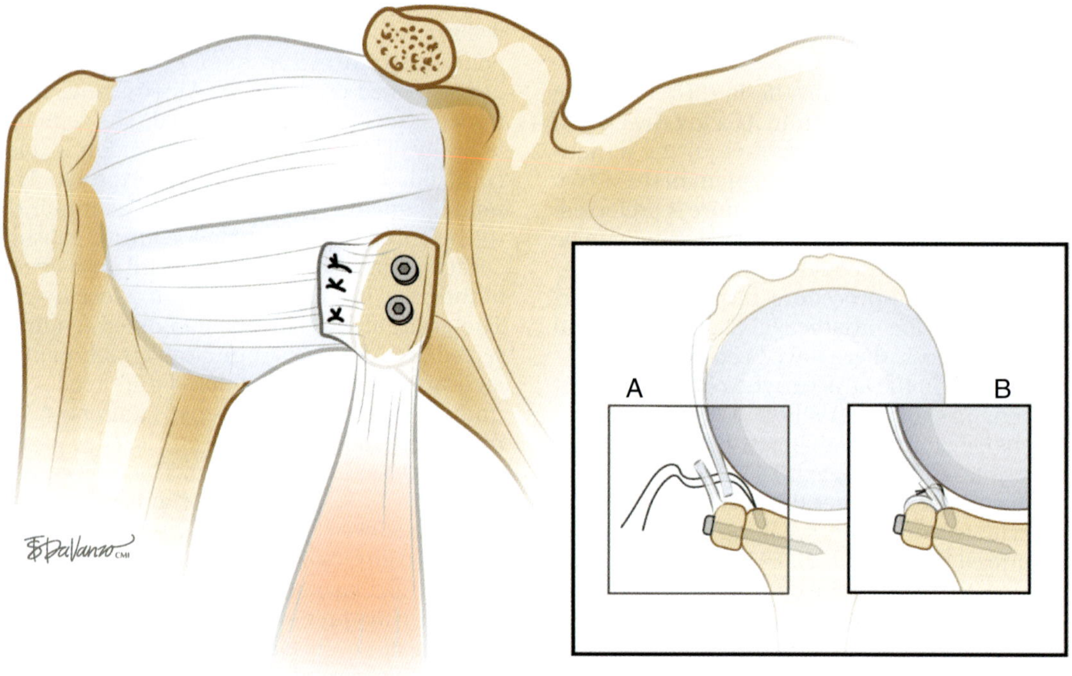

Fig. 1M.4 Illustration showing correct position of suture anchors for capsular repair producing an extraarticular coracoid transfer.

patient has 3+ anterior laxity with load and shift test (locks out anteriorly) and has a large Hill-Sachs lesion confirmed with imaging and arthroscopy, it is important to directly address the humeral head.

Humeral head bone grafting can be performed through a deltopectoral or posterior approach. With either approach, the humeral head defect is fully exposed and debrided. When using a deltopectoral approach, significant capsular releases are required so that the humeral head can be dislocated. A humeral head allograft is cut and shaped to fit the Hill-Sachs lesion and secured with counter-sunk screws. There has been recent interest in prosthetic resurfacing of focal humeral head defects as an alternative to autograft or allograft. Although use of these implants has been limited to case reports, this may be a good option in certain patients.

Conclusion

Shoulder instability results from a disruption in the delicate balance of static and dynamic factors. The bony architecture only contributes a portion to static glenohumeral joint stability. However, the bony anatomy plays an important role after disruption of the important capsuloligamentous restraints. The concept of the bipolar lesion is a relatively new one because the literature until recently focused on the contribution of glenoid and humeral head bone loss individually. There is a lack of high-level evidence to guide surgeons in the setting of bipolar bone loss. Future work must continue to investigate the interaction between glenoid and humeral head bone loss, as well as patient-specific factors that predispose to failure after surgical intervention, so that the surgeon can have well-defined parameters for success with arthroscopic, open soft tissue, or bone grafting techniques.

References

Arciero RA, Parrino A, Bernhardson AS, et al. The effect of a combined glenoid and Hill-Sachs defect on glenohumeral stability: a biomechanical cadaveric study using 3-dimensional modeling of 142 patients. *Am J Sports Med.* 2015;43(6):1422–1429.

Armitage MS, Faber KJ, Drosdowech DS, Litchfield RB, Athwal GS. Humeral head bone defects: remplissage, allograft, and arthroplasty. *Orthop Clin North Am.* 2010;41(3):417–425.

Balg F, Boileau P. The instability severity index score. A simple pre-operative score to select patients for arthroscopic or open shoulder stabilisation. *J Bone Joint Surg Br.* 2007;89(11):1470–1477.

Barcia AM, Rowles DJ, Bottoni CR, Dekker TJ, Tokish JM. Glenoid bare area: arthroscopic characterization and its implications on measurement of bone loss. *Arthroscopy.* 2013;29(10):1671–1675.

Baudi P, Campochiaro G, Rebuzzi M, Matino G, Catani F. Assessment of bone defects in anterior shoulder instability. *Joints.* 2013;1(1):40–48.

Bessière C, Trojani C, Carles M, Mehta SS, Boileau P. The open Latarjet procedure is more reliable in terms of shoulder stability than arthroscopic Bankart repair. *Clin Orthop Relat Res.* 2014;472(8):2345–2351.

Bollier MJ, Arciero R. Management of glenoid and humeral bone loss. *Sports Med Arthrosc.* 2010;18(3):140–148.

Boone JL, Arciero RA. Management of failed instability surgery: how to get it right the next time. *Orthop Clin North Am.* 2010;41(3):367–379.

Burkhart SS, De Beer JF. Traumatic glenohumeral bone defects and their relationship to failure of arthroscopic Bankart repairs: significance of the inverted-pear glenoid and the humeral engaging Hill-Sachs lesion. *Arthroscopy.* 2000;16(7):677–694.

Calandra JJ, Baker CL, Uribe J. The incidence of Hill-Sachs lesions in initial anterior shoulder dislocations. *Arthroscopy.* 1989;5(4):254–257.

Castagna A, Markopoulos N, Conti M, et al. Arthroscopic bankart suture-anchor repair: radiological and clinical outcome at minimum 10 years of follow-up. *Am J Sports Med.* 2010;38(10):2012–2016.

Charalambous CP, Eastwood S. The Bankart procedure: a long-term end-result study. *Classic Papers in Orthopaedics.* 2014;60:313–315.

Cho SH, Cho NS, Rhee YG. Preoperative analysis of the Hill-Sachs lesion in anterior shoulder instability: how to predict engagement of the lesion. *Am J Sports Med.* 2011;39(11):2389–2395.

Denard PJ, Dai X, Burkhart SS. Increasing preoperative dislocations and total time of dislocation affect surgical management of anterior shoulder instability. *Int J Shoulder Surg.* 2015;9(1):1–5.

Di Giacomo G, de Gasperis N, Scarso P. Bipolar bone defect in the shoulder anterior dislocation. *Knee Surgery Sport Traumatol Arthrosc.* 2016;24(2):479–488.

Di Giacomo G, Itoi E, Burkhart SS. Evolving concept of bipolar bone loss and the Hill-Sachs lesion: from "engaging/non-engaging" lesion to "on-track/off-track" lesion. *Arthroscopy.* 2014;30(1):90–98.

Friedman LGM, Ulloa SA, Braun DT, Saad HA, Jones MH, Miniaci AA. Glenoid bone loss measurement in recurrent shoulder dislocation: assessment of measurement agreement between CT and MRI. *Orthop J Sport Med.* 2014;2(9):1–7.

Garcia GH. Effect of bone loss in anterior shoulder instability. *World J Orthop.* 2015;6(5):421.

Griesser MJ, Harris JD, McCoy BW, et al. Complications and re-operations after Bristow-Latarjet shoulder stabilization: a systematic review. *J Shoulder Elbow Surg.* 2013;22(2):286–292.

Griffith JF, Antonio GE, Yung PSH, et al. Prevalence, pattern, and spectrum of glenoid bone loss in anterior shoulder dislocation: CT analysis of 218 patients. *AJR Am J Roentgenol.* 2008;190(5):1247–1254.

Hovelius L, Augustini BG, Fredin H, Johansson O, Norlin R, Thorling J. Primary anterior dislocation of the shoulder in young patients. *J Bone Joint Surg.* 1996;78(11):1677–1684.

Hovelius L, Sandström B, Sundgren K, Saebö M. One hundred eighteen Bristow-Latarjet repairs for recurrent anterior dislocation of the shoulder prospectively followed for fifteen years: study I—clinical results. *J Shoulder Elbow Surg.* 2004;13(5):509–516.

Itoi E, Lee S-B, Amrami KK, Wenger DE, An K-N. Quantitative assessment of classic anteroinferior bony Bankart lesions by radiography and computed tomography. *Am J Sports Med.* 2003;31(1):112–118.

Kaar SG, Fening SD, Jones MH, Colbrunn RW, Miniaci A. Effect of humeral head defect size on glenohumeral stability: a cadaveric study of simulated Hill-Sachs defects. *Am J Sports Med.* 2010;38(3):594–599.

Lippitt S, Matsen F. Mechanisms of glenohumeral joint stability. *Clin Orthop Relat Res.* 1993;291(291):20–28.

Lo IKY, Parten PM, Burkhart SS. The inverted pear glenoid: an indicator of significant glenoid bone loss. *Arthroscopy.* 2004;20(2):169–174.

Longo UG, Loppini M, Rizzello G, Romeo G, Huijsmans PE, Denaro V. Glenoid and humeral head bone loss in traumatic anterior glenohumeral instability: a systematic review. *Knee Surgery Sport Traumatol Arthrosc.* 2014;22(2):392–414.

Metzger PD, Barlow B, Leonardelli D, Peace W, Solomon DJ, Provencher MT. Clinical application of the "glenoid track" concept for defining humeral head engagement in anterior shoulder instability: a preliminary report. *Orthop J Sport Med.* 2013;1(2). 2325967113496213.

Milano G, Grasso A, Russo A, et al. Analysis of risk factors for glenoid bone defect in anterior shoulder instability. *Am J Sports Med.* 2011;39(9):1870–1876.

Miyatake K, Takeda Y, Fujii K, Takasago T, Iwame T. Validity of arthroscopic measurement of glenoid bone loss using the bare spot. *J Sport Med.* 2014;5:37–42.

Moroder P, Odorizzi M, Pizzinini S, Demetz E, Resch H, Moroder P. Open Bankart repair for the treatment of anterior shoulder instability without substantial osseous glenoid defects. *J Bone Joint Surg Am.* 2015;97(17):1398–1405.

Nakagawa S, Ozaki R, Take Y, Iuchi R, Mae T. Relationship between glenoid defects and Hill-Sachs lesions in shoulders with traumatic anterior instability. *Am J Sports Med.* 2015;43(11):2763–2773.

Nakagawa S, Ozaki R, Take Y, Mizuno N, Mae T. Enlargement of glenoid defects in traumatic anterior shoulder instability: influence of the number of recurrences and type of sport. *Orthop J Sport Med.* 2014;2(4):1–7.

Ozaki R, Nakagawa S, Mizuno N, Mae T, Yoneda M. Hill-Sachs lesions in shoulders with traumatic anterior instability: evaluation using computed tomography with 3-dimensional reconstruction. *Am J Sports Med.* 2014;42(11):2597–2605.

Ozturk BY, Maak TG, Fabricant P, et al. Return to sports after arthroscopic anterior stabilization in patients aged younger than 25 years. *Arthroscopy.* 2013;29(12):1922–1931.

Pagnani MJ. Open capsular repair without bone block for recurrent anterior shoulder instability in patients with and without bony defects of the glenoid and/or humeral head. *Am J Sports Med.* 2008;36(9):1805–1812.

Patel RM, Amin NH, Lynch TS, Miniaci A. Management of bone loss in glenohumeral instability. *Orthop Clin North Am.* 2014;45(4):523–539.

Patel RM, Walia P, Gottschalk L, et al. The effects of Latarjet reconstruction on glenohumeral kinematics in the presence of combined bony defects: a cadaveric model. *Am J Sports Med.* 2016.

Plewa MC, Delinger M. The false-positive rate of thoracic outlet syndrome shoulder maneuvers in healthy subjects. *Acad Emerg Med.* 1998;5(11):337–342.

Provencher MT, Frank RM, Leclere LE, et al. The Hill-Sachs lesion: diagnosis, classification, and management. *J Am Acad Orthop Surg.* 2012;20(4):242–252.

Provencher MT, Ghodadra N, LeClere L, Solomon DJ, Romeo AA. Anatomic osteochondral glenoid reconstruction for recurrent glenohumeral instability with glenoid deficiency using a distal tibia allograft. *Arthroscopy.* 2009;25(4):446–452.

Ranne JO, Sarimo JJ, Heinonen OJ, Orava SY. A combination of Latarjet and remplissage for treatment of severe glenohumeral instability and bone loss. A case report. *J Orthop.* 2013;10(1):46–48.

Rowe CR, Zarins B, Ciullo JV. Recurrent anterior dislocation of the shoulder after surgical repair. Apparent causes of failure and treatment. *J Bone Joint Surg Am.* 1984;66(2):159–168.

Sekiya JK, Wickwire A, Stehle J, Debski R. Biomechanical analysis of Hill-Sachs lesions: injuries and repair using osteoarticular allograft transplantation (SS-02). *Arthroscopy.* 2006;22(suppl 6):e1–e2.

Shaha JS, Cook JB, Song DJ, et al. Redefining "critical" bone loss in shoulder instability: functional outcomes worsen with "subcritical" bone loss. *Am J Sports Med.* 2015;43(7):1719–1725.

Streubel PN, Krych AJ, Simone JP, et al. Anterior glenohumeral instability: a pathology-based surgical treatment strategy. *J Am Acad Orthop Surg.* 2014;22(5):283–294.

Sugaya H, Moriishi J, Dohi M, Kon Y, Tsuchiya A. Glenoid rim morphology in recurrent anterior glenohumeral instability. *J Bone Joint Surg Am.* 2003;85-A(5):878–884.
Tauber M, Resch H, Forstner R, Raffl M, Schauer J. Reasons for failure after surgical repair of anterior shoulder instability. *J Shoulder Elbow Surg.* 2004;13(3):279–285.
Taylor DC, Arciero RA. Pathologic changes associated with shoulder dislocations. Arthroscopic and physical examination findings in first-time, traumatic anterior dislocations. *Am J Sports Med.* 1997;25(3):306–311.
Trivedi S, Pomerantz ML, Gross D, Golijanan P, Provencher MT. Shoulder instability in the setting of bipolar (glenoid and humeral head) bone loss: the glenoid track concept. In: *Clinical Orthopaedics and Related Research.* vol. 472. Springer: Philadelphia, Pennsylvania 2014:2352–2362.
van der Linde JA, van Kampen DA, Terwee CB, Dijksman LM, KleinJan G, Willems WJ. Long-term results after arthroscopic shoulder stabilization using suture anchors: an 8- to 10-year follow-up. *Am J Sports Med.* 2011;39(11):2396–2403.
Van Oostveen DPH, Temmerman OPP, Burger BJ, Van Noort A, Robinson M. Glenoid fractures: a review of pathology, classification, treatment and results. *Acta Orthop Belg.* 2014;80(1):88–98.
Voos JE, Livermore RW, Feeley BT, et al. Prospective evaluation of arthroscopic Bankart repairs for anterior instability. *Am J Sports Med.* 2010;38(2):302–307.
Wang RY, Arciero RA. Treating the athlete with anterior shoulder instability. *Clin Sports Med.* 2008;27(4):631–648.
Weber SC. The Instability Severity Index Score in Arthroscopic Instability Surgery (ISIS): failure to validate its predictive value in the selection of arthroscopic instability surgery. *J Shoulder Elbow Surg.* 2014;23(9):e231.
Widjaja AB, Tran A, Bailey M, Proper S. Correlation between Bankart and Hill-Sachs lesions in anterior shoulder dislocation. *ANZ J Surg.* 2006;76(6):436–438.
Yamamoto N, Itoi E, Abe H, et al. Contact between the glenoid and the humeral head in abduction, external rotation, and horizontal extension: a new concept of glenoid track. *J Shoulder Elbow Surg.* 2007;16(5): 649–656.
Yang JS, Mazzocca AD, Cote MP, Edgar CM, Arciero RA. Recurrent anterior shoulder instability with combined bone loss: treatment and results with the modified Latarjet procedure. *Am J Sports Med.* 2016;44(4):922–932.

1-1N OUTCOMES

MOLLY C. MEADOWS, MD, BONNIE P. GREGORY, MD, ROBERT J. THORSNESS, MD, and ANTHONY A. ROMEO, MD

Introduction

- Management of athletes after an anterior instability event is controversial, especially for in-season contact athletes.
- Nonoperative management with focus on guided physical therapy and rapid return to sport remains a reasonable option; surgical stabilization is the alternative.
- Many factors are considered to determine appropriate treatment, including the athlete's age, the timing of the injury (in or out of season), and the presence of glenoid or humeral bony lesions such as a bony Bankart lesion or Hill-Sachs defect.
- Joint decision making involving the patient, family, and surgeon is imperative to manage expectations and optimize the chances of a good outcome.

Nonoperative Management of Anterior Shoulder Instability

There is very little guidance provided in the literature for return to sport after an anterior instability event. Controversy exists with regard to optimal treatment, including acute surgical management versus nonoperative management with an emphasis on physical therapy and quick return to sport. This decision is guided by multiple variables, including whether the injury occurred early or late season, whether there is a bony injury including a bony Bankart or large Hill-Sachs defect, and whether the athlete is involved in contact sports (Buss et al, 2004; Dickens et al, 2014; Wheeler et al, 1989)

In a large multicenter study, Dickens et al (2014) evaluated 45 collegiate athletes involved in contact sports to assess return to play after an anterior glenohumeral instability event that occurred in season. All athletes underwent a guided rehabilitation program without shoulder immobilization and were followed during their season to evaluate for recurrence of instability and ability to return to play. Among these athletes, 73% returned to sport for either all or part of the season after a median 5 days lost from competition. Although 27% of the athletes completed the season without recurrence of instability, 64% had a recurrent instability event, and only 67% of these patients were able to successfully complete the season. Recurrent instability events were common regardless of whether the initial injury was a subluxation or dislocation.

Buss et al (2004) evaluated 30 athletes who experienced an anterior instability event. All patients were managed nonoperatively with guided physical therapy and were allowed to return to play with an anterior stabilization brace. The authors found that 87% of the athletes were able to return to play for the complete season, with the athletes missing an average of 10.2 days as a result of the injury. Ten athletes (37%) sustained a recurrent instability event. Sixteen athletes (53%) underwent anterior stabilization during the subsequent off-season.

Despite a lack of evidence of significant benefit, many clinicians elect for an anterior stabilization brace when patients return to sport after a nonoperatively managed anterior instability event. These braces are designed to limit motion of the shoulder, specifically abduction and external rotation. Buss et al (2004) reported that the athletes subjectively reported an improved sense of stability compared with playing without a brace but unfortunately provided no evidence to demonstrate the efficacy of the brace. The Dickens et al (2014) cohort demonstrated no significant protective effect of the brace, with no difference in recurrent instability in those who wore a brace compared with those who did not.

Table 1N.1 Bankart Repair with Suture Anchor

Authors	Journal	Year Published	Type of Study	Shoulders (*n*)	Mean Follow-up (yr)	Recurrence of Instability (%)	Complications (%)	Return to Play (at all) (%)	Return to Play (at previous level or higher)
Ide et al	*Am J Sports Med*	2004	Prospective cohort	55	3.5	7.3 (9.6 contact, 5.9 noncontact)	0	98.2	80.0
Rhee et al	*Am J Sports Med*	2006	Retrospective	48 (16 arthroscopic)	6	25.0	0	93.8	62.5
Castagna et al	*Am J Sports Med*	2010	Retrospective	31	10.9	23 (7 traumatic)	NR	NR	71.0
Franceschi et al	*Am J Sports Med*	2011	Retrospective	60	8	16.60	NR	100 (short term), 88 (at 8 yr)	NR
Castagna et al	*Arthroscopy*	2012	Retrospective	67	5.25	21 (10.7 traumatic)	0	100	81
Milchteim et al	*Arthroscopy*	2016	Retrospective	94	5	6.4	2.20	NR	82.50

NR, Not reported.

There is general consensus that athletes should be allowed to return to play when they can demonstrate symmetric range of motion and strength and when they can perform sport-specific exercises without pain. In our practice, we elect for acute surgical management in patients with a large bony Bankart lesion or a significant humeral head defect (>25%). If a patient lacks these features and this is his or her first instability event, we elect for nonoperative treatment if it is early in the patient's sports season. This includes a brief period of ice and immobilization in a simple sling followed by a guided rehabilitation program with the first goal of symmetric range of motion. The athlete then proceeds to strengthening of the rotator cuff and scapular stabilizing muscles and finally progresses to sport-specific drills. When the patient can complete these, she or he is allowed to return to sport, typically by 2 weeks postinjury.

Arthroscopic Stabilization for Anterior Shoulder Instability

Arthroscopic stabilization for anterior shoulder instability offers numerous advantages over traditional open procedures. Arthroscopic intervention has been shown to decrease surgical time, blood loss, and postoperative narcotic requirements and also allows the surgeon the opportunity to address concomitant intraarticular pathology. Perhaps most relevant to the athletic population, some evidence suggests that arthroscopic stabilization improves recovery time and allows for quicker return to sport (Green & Christensen, 1995). Whereas early arthroscopic techniques were associated with higher failure rates, modern techniques have demonstrated improved outcomes overall. Furthermore, with longer term data available, predictors of failure of arthroscopic stabilization have been readily identified to assist in identification of patients who will benefit from an arthroscopic procedure (Boileau et al, 2006; Burkhart & De Beer, 2000).

The earliest technique of arthroscopic shoulder stabilization, described by Johnson in 1980, included an arthroscopic Bankart repair and capsulorrhaphy using a staple to engage the Bankart lesion and capsule (Johnson, 1980). Later in the 1980s, techniques evolved to include arthroscopic transosseous suture fixation, which offered the advantage of providing multiple points of fixation. This technique was ultimately replaced by the use of suture anchors, which facilitated repair to the articular edge of the glenoid, rather than the glenoid neck (Abrams et al, 2002; Wolf, 1993). Fixation with suture anchors remains the most widely performed arthroscopic technique for management of Bankart lesions today. Additionally, other arthroscopic techniques such as capsular plication, arthroscopic coracoid transfer, and remplissage for management of Hill-Sachs lesions have been developed to address pathology contributing to anterior instability (Levy et al, 2016; Longo et al, 2014).

Outcomes of arthroscopic management of anterior instability in athletes have been largely favorable, with modern techniques demonstrating outcomes that rival their open counterparts. Although the reported recurrence rates after arthroscopic stabilization range from 0% to 49%, these numbers include studies that used historical fixation methods that have been proven to be less effective than modern techniques (Sperber et al, 2001). Even with earlier techniques, arthroscopic management of acute, traumatic anterior shoulder dislocations in athletic patients has been shown to significantly decrease recurrence rates as compared with nonoperative management. Arciero and colleagues (1994) at the United States Military Academy at West Point described a prospective study including 36 patients who underwent either arthroscopic transglenoid suture repair or immobilization and rehabilitation after an acute initial dislocation, and they demonstrated an 80% recurrence rate in the nonoperative cohort compared with only a 14% recurrence rate in those managed with arthroscopic stabilization.

Multiple subsequent studies have reported outcomes after stabilization with suture anchors in athletes with varying results (Table 1N.1). Rhee et al (2006) included 48 shoulders in collision athletes and reported a 25% recurrence rate postoperatively. Of their arthroscopic cohort, 25% of patients were able to return to sport at prior level of competition, 37.5% returned to near full (>90%) sports activities, 18.8% returned to sports with moderate limitations, and 6.2% were unable to return. Castagna et al (2010) described 10-year follow-up results after arthroscopic Bankart repair with suture anchors and noted a 36% recurrence rate in high-level athletes compared with only a 15% recurrence in all other athletes. The authors also reported a limitation in external rotation in abduction in 16.1% of patients, which they found to be correlated with risk of recurrence. In their study, 71% of patients were able to return to sport. In another series of 60 patients, including 55 athletes, Franceschi et al (2011) reported a recurrence rate of 16.1% at a minimum 5-year follow-up. Although all 55 athletes initially returned to sport, only 88% were actively participating in sports at 5 years. In a prospective study comparing outcomes in collision versus noncontact athletes, Ide and colleagues (2004) found a recurrence rate of 9.5% in collision athletes versus 5.9% in noncontact athletes; however, this difference was not statistically significant (Ide et al, 2004).

In a systematic review, Harris et al (2013) reported the outcomes of arthroscopic stabilization subdivided by fixation methods. The authors compared multiple outcome measures among studies using suture anchors, suture tacks, or transglenoid suture fixation. The authors reported a recurrent dislocation rate of 8.5% in the suture anchor group, 17% in the suture tack group, and 8% in the Caspari group. The recurrence rate was significantly greater in the overall arthroscopic group compared with the open group; however, there was no significant difference between the arthroscopic suture anchor and open groups. In the suture anchor group, 87% returned to sport at preinjury levels compared with 53% in the suture tack group and 88% in the Caspari group. Final follow-up Rowe and Constant scores showed no significant differences among groups.

In a recent study, Milchteim et al (2016) performed a retrospective review of arthroscopic Bankart repairs performed with bioabsorbable suture anchors in both contact and noncontact athletes. They included 94 patients undergoing either primary or revision stabilization with a mean follow-up of 5 years and reported significant improvement in shoulder outcome scores, with an 82.5% rate of return to sport and a low recurrence rate of 6.4%. The authors noted that all episodes of recurrent instability after stabilization occurred in the high school athlete population, with no episodes of recurrence in the collegiate and professional athletes. However, in their series of adolescent athletes undergoing arthroscopic stabilization, Castagna and colleagues (2012) noted a trend toward lower recurrence rates in younger patients.

In addition to soft tissue Bankart lesions, bony defects on both the glenoid and humeral side contribute to anterior shoulder instability. Significant glenoid bone loss was traditionally managed with open bone block procedures such as the Bristow-Latarjet procedure; however, arthroscopic techniques for coracoid transfer have recently been described (Boileau et al, 2010; Dumont et al, 2014; Lafosse et al, 2007). Boileau and colleagues (2010) reported outcomes after an all-arthroscopic Bankart-Bristow-Latarjet procedure in 47 shoulders, 6 of which were converted to an open procedure. Of their patient population, 92% were athletes, and 73% participated in contact or throwing sports. The authors reported no episodes of recurrence at a mean 16-month follow-up. A recent study of this procedure by the same authors reported a loss of 9 degrees of external rotation at the side, with 83% of patients returning to sport at a preinjury level (Boileau et al, 2014). Although the arthroscopic Latarjet procedure can be technically challenging, early outcomes have been favorable in an athletic population.

To address humeral osseous defects resulting from anterior shoulder instability, arthroscopic remplissage, or advancement of the infraspinatus and posterior capsule to the osseous surface of the Hill-Sachs lesion is a reasonable treatment strategy for smaller lesions (Garcia et al, 2016). In a systematic review of the literature describing arthroscopic remplissage combined with Bankart repair, Buza et al (2014) reported on 6 studies including 167 patients and noted "excellent" results, according to Rowe score, in 87.6% of patients. Looking specifically at the outcomes of arthroscopic remplissage in the athlete population, Garcia et al (2006b) examined the outcomes of remplissage for Hill-Sachs lesions in athletes at a minimum 2-year follow-up. They reported that 90% of patients were satisfied to very satisfied with their surgery, and 70% stated that the procedure improved their quality of life. The mean time to return to sports was 7 months, with 95.5% of patients returning to sport postoperatively, 80% of whom played at their preoperative levels. Of note, they did describe a significantly lower rate of return to sports in throwing athletes (51.7%) compared with nonthrowing athletes (95%). At final follow-up, 11.8% of patients suffered a recurrent dislocation event, all of whom ultimately underwent a revision procedure.

Careful patient selection is important to determine those who will benefit from an arthroscopic procedure. Boileau and colleagues (2006) identified multiple factors that place patients at risk of recurrence after arthroscopic stabilization, including significant bone loss on either the glenoid or humeral side (>25% of glenoid surface or >30% of humeral surface), anterior or inferior shoulder hyperlaxity, and those repaired with three suture anchors or fewer. Of note, the authors did not find patient age or type of sport (contact versus noncontact) to be correlated with risk of failure. The same group later developed the Instability Severity Index Score (ISIS), which uses age younger than 20 years at the time of surgery, type and degree of sport participation, shoulder hyperlaxity, presence of a Hill-Sachs lesion, and loss of glenoid contour as independent risk factors for failure of arthroscopic treatment (Balg & Boileau, 2007). Furthermore, in a systematic review comparing outcomes of arthroscopic stabilization in first-time versus recurrent instability patients, Grumet and colleagues (2010) found no difference in outcomes or complication rates between the two groups.

Whereas older publications report higher recurrence rates after arthroscopic stabilization compared with open procedures, the literature comparing modern arthroscopic techniques with their open counterparts describes similar recurrence rates. Indeed, in their comprehensive review of overlapping meta-analyses, Chalmers and colleagues (2015) concluded that the literature supports no significant difference in failure rates between open and arthroscopic shoulder stabilization. Furthermore, concomitant arthroscopic procedures to address glenoid and humeral bone loss may broaden the indications for arthroscopic intervention. With proper technique and patient selection, outcomes of arthroscopic management of anterior shoulder instability approach those of open procedures, with decreased perioperative morbidity to the affected shoulder.

Open Stabilization for Anterior Shoulder Instability

Although arthroscopic Bankart repair has recently become the gold standard for stabilization of primary anterior shoulder instability based on technologic improvements, open stabilization continues to be the preferred method for addressing instability in the revision setting. Many techniques for open stabilization have been described including largely historical procedures (Putti-Platt, Magnuson-Stack), anterior bone grafting procedures (iliac crest allograft or autograft, Latarjet, Bristow), anatomic reconstruction (open Bankart repair, capsular shift), and those that address humeral-sided lesions (humeral head bone grafting, remplissage).

Open stabilization has also been advocated by some surgeons in the primary setting for management of significant glenoid bone loss, engaging Hill-Sachs lesions, humeral avulsion of the glenohumeral ligament (HAGL) lesions, associated subscapularis tears, and patients with an ISIS greater than 7 (Balg & Boileau, 2007). The factors comprising ISIS and indicating increased risk of recurrence after arthroscopic Bankart include patients younger than 20 years of age, participation in contact sports or competitive sports, hyperlaxity, Hill-Sachs lesion visible on anteroposterior (AP) external rotation radiographs, and loss of glenoid contour on AP radiographs. In 2000, Burkhart and De Beer echoed these findings, reporting a recurrence rate of 4% after arthroscopic Bankart repair for anterior instability in patients without significant bone deficiency; the rate of recurrence was 67% in the presence of bony deficiency. They described significant glenoid bone loss as an "inverted pear glenoid," signifying greater than 25% loss of the inferior glenoid diameter.

In 1954, Latarjet first described a coracoid bone block technique to treat anterior instability. He described a technique in which the horizontal limb of the coracoid process was fixed to the anteroinferior margin of the glenoid with a screw to increase stability. Patte first described the "triple effect" in 1980 to explain the success of the procedure composed of the sling effect of the conjoined tendon on the subscapularis and anteroinferior capsule with abduction and external rotation, the "bony effect" of restoring anteroposterior diameter of the glenoid, and the capsular repair to the stump of the coracoacromial ligament (Young et al, 2011).

At an average 14-year follow-up, Allain et al (1998) reported long-term outcomes of 51 patients who underwent a primary Latarjet procedure for anterior instability. They reported no recurrent instability; however, 1 patient (2%) reported subjective instability, and 6 patients (10%) reported apprehension on examination. Fifty-one (88%) of patients reported having a stable shoulder at final follow-up. Rowe scores were excellent in 37 (64%), good in 14 (24%), fair in 5 (9%), and poor in 2 (3%). Of the 51 patients in the study who participated in sports, 41 (81%) returned to the same sport at the prior level, 6 (12%) at a lower level, 1 (2%) was unable to return to sport, and 3 (6%) changed sports.

Cerciello et al (2012) reported good results of the Latarjet procedure performed in 48 soccer players (51 shoulders). They noted one recurrence in a goalkeeper 74 months after surgery. All but 1 player (3.6%) returned to soccer at an average of 8 months (2–24 months), 71.4% of which were at the same level and 25% at a lower level. In a series of 34 rugby players (37 shoulders) at a mean 12-year follow-up, Neyton et al (2012) reported good results of the Latarjet procedure and demonstrated no recurrent instability events. Persistent apprehension was observed in 5 patients (14%) with 65% of patients returning to rugby.

Schmid et al (2012) reported on a series of 49 patients who underwent Latarjet procedure for recurrent anterior instability after prior anterior stabilization (19 capsulolabral repair, 30 arthroscopic Bankart repair). At an average follow-up period of 38 months, they reported no dislocations, 2 patients with subluxations not requiring treatment (4%), and 5 patients (10%) with apprehension but no subluxation. They showed significant improvement in activity level and subjective shoulder values but no difference in subjective scores, range of motion, or power.

In a series of 102 patients who underwent modified Latarjet procedures for significant (>25%) glenoid bone loss or engaging Hill-Sachs lesions, Burkhart et al (2007) reported a 4.9% instability recurrence rate at average 18.5 months of follow-up. Hovelius et al. (2014) reported a recurrent dislocation rate of 5%, subluxation rate of 13%, and revision rate of 1% after Latarjet procedures over a 24-year time period.

The Bristow procedure, which is still quite popular in Europe, consists of transferring just the tip of the coracoid (with the attached conjoined tendon, short head of the biceps, and coracobrachialis) to the inferomedial glenoid rim (Hovelius et al, 2004). Schroder et al (2006) reported 26-year outcomes of the modified Bristow procedure performed between 1975 and 1979 at the U.S. Naval Academy. They showed a recurrent instability rate of 14%, but those without recurrent instability had significantly higher Single Assessment Numeric Evaluation (SANE), Western Ontario Shoulder Instability Index (WOSI), and estimated Rowe scores. In the most recent series presented, Hovelius et al (2004) demonstrated a recurrence rate of 13.4% in 113 patients at 15 years, as well as a mean loss of external rotation in abduction of 12.4 degrees. The ability to throw normally was only preserved in 44% of patients.

In 2014, Bessiere et al (2014) compared patients treated with open Latarjet or arthroscopic Bankart repair for recurrent anterior instability. The Latarjet group had significantly less recurrent instability (10%) than the arthroscopic Bankart group (22%; $P = 0.026$), but reoperation rate was not significantly different. In both groups patients younger than 20 years had a higher recurrence risk ($P = 0.019$), and in the Bankart group, competitive sports and hyperlaxity were independent risk factors for recurrence.

In a recent systematic review, An et al (2016) compared open and arthroscopic Bankart repair with Latarjet in a total of 705 patients. In similar cohorts with no significant heterogeneity noted, they found significantly lower rates of recurrent instability in the Latarjet group (11.6%)

compared with the Bankart group (21.1%; $P = 0.0009$), as well as to open and arthroscopic Bankart repairs individually ($P = 0.01$ and $P = 0.03$, respectively). Furthermore, Rowe score was significantly higher in the Latarjet group (85.4 vs 79.0; $P < 0.001$). Mean loss in external rotation was also significantly less in the Latarjet group. There was no significant difference in complication rates, revision surgeries, or return to function. Alternatively, in a 2015 systematic review, Chalmers et al (2015) reported no significant difference in failure rates between open and arthroscopic stabilization for anterior instability.

In settings of significant glenoid bone loss, bone grafting of the glenoid with iliac crest auto- or allograft can be used. Warner et al (2006) reported on a group of 11 patients with significant glenoid bone loss (18–35 mm) and recurrent instability who underwent an anatomic glenoid reconstruction with autogenous tricortical iliac crest bone graft. They reported no recurrent instability or apprehension and noted all patients returned to their prior level of sports. Steffen and Hertel (2013) also reported on a group of 48 consecutive patients who underwent autogenous iliac crest bone graft for glenoid bone loss. At 9.2 years, they reported 1 patient with dislocation, 1 with subluxation, and 3 with subjective instability. They also reported a positive apprehension sign in 24 (60%) as well as an average external rotation loss of 4.1 degrees.

Alternatively, Weng et al (2009) described a technique using femoral head allograft to address significant glenoid bone loss. In 9 patients, they used a "quarter-graft" femoral head allograft slightly larger than the anatomic glenoid along with suture anchors to attach the capsule to the graft. They reported a change in average Rowe score from 24 preoperatively to 84 postoperatively ($P < 0.001$). Two patients sustained instability events (1 dislocation, 1 subluxation) after surgery secondary to having seizures but reported negative apprehension and relocation tests in all at final follow-up. They also reported a mean loss of 7 degrees of external rotation compared with the nonoperative side.

In the classic description of the open Bankart procedure by Rowe et al (1978), a dislocation rate of 3.9% was reported in 142 of 164 patients with a mean follow-up period of 6 years. At 20-year follow-up, Moroder et al (2015) reported on 47 patients who underwent primary open Bankart repair for recurrent instability without associated significant glenoid defects. They described significant decreases in abduction (4 degrees; $P = 0.009$), internal rotation (two vertebral levels; $P = 0.003$), and external rotation in neutral (7 degrees; $P < 0.001$) and 90 degrees of abduction (7 degrees; $P = 0.04$). They described good postoperative subjective outcomes scores but reported a 17.5 % rate of recurrent instability.

Yoneda et al (1999) reported on a group of 83 contact athletes (85 shoulders) who underwent open Bankart repair with coracoid transfer at a mean follow-up period of 5.8 years. Sports represented included rugby, football, judo, and handball. Rowe score was excellent or good in 93%, and return to sport was reported in 92% of patients, with 88% competing at preinjury levels. There was 1 redislocation (1.2%) in a traumatic rugby injury. Furthermore, in a systematic review of return to play after open Bankart repair, Stone and Pearsall (2014) reported a redislocation rate of 5.3%, with an average return to play at 23.2 weeks, with contact and throwing athletes requiring more time. Hatch and Hennrikus (2016) reported on a series of 21 teenage athletes with recurrent anterior instability and at minimum 2-year follow-up with no recurrence events and 100% excellent results based on Rowe score and 100% good or excellent results based on UCLA shoulder score, with all patients returning to preoperative high school sports. In 2015, Owens et al (2015) conducted a prospective randomized controlled trial comparing arthroscopic versus open Bankart repair in 40 patients with anterior shoulder instability. At final follow-up, they found no difference in recurrence, instability, American Shoulder and Elbow Surgeons (ASES) score, WOSII score, or complications (Table 1N.2).

When a lesion represents more than 20% of the diameter of the humeral head, the arc of motion available before the lesion engages the anterior glenoid rim in abduction and external rotation is reduced, facilitating an anterior dislocation (Itoi et al, 2013; Provencher et al, 2012). There are several treatment options to address large engaging Hill-Sachs lesions, including humeral head bone augmentation, remplissage, and Latarjet procedures. Degen et al (2014) performed a biomechanical evaluation of remplissage versus Latarjet procedure in the setting of a 25% Hill-Sachs lesion without associated glenoid bone loss. Recurrent instability was present in 16% of the remplissage model and 6% of the Latarjet model, but this difference was not statistically significant.

Complications of open stabilization in more of 25% of cases have been described, including neurovascular injury, infection, wound complications, hematoma formation, stiffness, hardware related failures, bony rim fractures, and humeral fractures (Allain et al, 1998; An et al, 2006; Kang et al, 2009). Anatomic studies have demonstrated that the axillary nerve is located just 1 to 1.5 cm below the inferior glenohumeral capsule, and the sensory branch lies close to the glenoid rim. Furthermore, the musculocutaneous nerve may penetrate the coracobrachialis muscle belly just 5 cm distal to the coracoid process (Eglseder & Goldman, 1997; Loomer & Graham, 1989). Neurologic complications have been reported in 0% to 10% of open stabilization procedures (Shah et al, 2012). Clearly, the surgeon must be cautious with respect to the neurovascular anatomy when performing open stabilization surgery.

Conclusion

Anterior shoulder instability is a common problem, and risk of recurrence after nonoperative management and anterior stabilization surgery is a concern. Although open bone-block procedures such as the Latarjet procedure have demonstrated significant advantages with regard to recurrence risk, open stabilization is not without risk of complications, including neurovascular injury. With regard to optimal initial treatment, age, timing of the injury, the presence of a bony lesion, and athlete involvement in contact sports all influence treatment decision making. Outcomes after both arthroscopic and open stabilization procedures can be excellent, but managing patient expectations with regard to recurrence risk and return to sport is paramount. We suggest early surgical intervention in overhead throwing athletes with dominant arm dislocations, as well as in athletes with large bone defects.

Table 1N.2 Open Stabilization Outcomes

Authors	Journal	Year Published	Type of Study	Patients (*n*)	Surgical Intervention	Mean Follow-up (yr)	Recurrence of Instability	Complications	Return to Play (at all) (%)	Return to Play (at Level Previous or Level Higher) (T)
Allain et al	*J Bone Joint Surg Am*	1998	Retrospective case series	58	Open Latarjet	14.3	0 dislocations; 1 patients/2% subjective instability; 6 patients/10% apprehension = 12% total	7%	93	81
Yoneda et al	*Am J Sports Med*	1999	Retrospective case series	83	Open Bankart + coracoid transfer	5.8	1.2% redislocation	4 patients/4.8%	92	88
Warner et al	*Am J Sports Med*	2006	Retrospective case series	11	Anatomic glenoid reconstruction with autogenous ICBG	2.8	0	NR	100	NR
Weng et al	*Am J Sports Med*	2009	Retrospective case series	9	Anatomic glenoid reconstruction with allogenic femoral head	4.5	1 patient/ (11%) dislocation, 1 patient (11%) subluxation = 22% total	NR	NR	NR
Schmid et al	*J Bone Joint Surg Am*	2012	Retrospective case series	49	Open Latarjet	3.2	0 dislocation; 2 patients/4% subluxation; 5 patients/14% apprehension = 14% total	12%	NR	NR
Ceriello et al	*J Orthopaed Traumatol*	2012	Retrospective case series	51	Open Latarjet	7.1	1 dislocation (3.6%)	NR	96.40	71.40
Shah et al	JBJS	2012	Retrospective case series	48	Open Latarjet	3.3	8%	25%	NR	NR
Hovelius et al	*J Shoulder Elbow Surg*	2012	Retrospective case series	319	Open Latarjet	15/17/6 for 3 series of patients reported	16/5% redislocation; 41 patients/13% subluxations	5/1.6%	NR	NR
Neyton et al	*J Shoulder Elbow Surg*	2012	Retrospective case series	34	Open Latarjet	12	0 dislocations/ subluxations; 5 patients (14%) apprehension on exam	5/14.7%	65	56
Steffen & Hertel	*J Shoulder Elbow Surg*	2013	Retrospective case series	48	Glenoid rim reconstruction with autogenous ICBG	9.2	1 patient/2% redislocation; 1 patient/2% subluxation; 3 patients/6% subjective instability; 24 patients/50% apprehension on exam	NR	NR	NR
Moroder et al	*J Bone Join Surg Am*	2015	Retrospective case series	47	Open Bankart	20	7 patients/17.5%	NR	NR	NR
Owens et al	*Orthop J Sports Med*	2015	Prospective RCT	10	Open Latarjet	1.4	Subluxations 3 patients (31%)	NR	NR	NR
Hatch & Hennrikus	*J Pediatr Orthop*	2016	Retrospective case series	21	Open Bankart	2	0	NR	100	100

ICBG, Iliac Crest Bone Graft; *NR,* not reported; *RCT,* randomized controlled trial.

References

Abrams JS, Savoie FH 3rd, Tauro JC, Bradley JP. Recent advances in the evaluation and treatment of shoulder instability: anterior, posterior, and multidirectional. *Arthroscopy*. 2002;18(9 suppl 2):1–13.

Allain J, Goutallier D, Glorion C. Long-term results of the Latarjet procedure for the treatment of anterior instability of the shoulder. *J Bone Joint Surg Am*. 1998;80(6):841–852.

An VV, Sivakumar BS, Phan K, Trantalis J. A systematic review and meta-analysis of clinical and patient-reported outcomes following two procedures for recurrent traumatic anterior instability of the shoulder: latarjet procedure vs. Bankart repair. *J Shoulder Elbow Surg*. 2016;25(5):853–863.

Arciero RA, Wheeler JH, Ryan JB, McBride JT. Arthroscopic Bankart repair versus nonoperative treatment for acute, initial anterior shoulder dislocations. *Am J Sports Med*. 1994;22(5):589–594.

Balg F, Boileau P. The instability severity index score. A simple pre-operative score to select patients for arthroscopic or open shoulder stabilisation. *J Bone Joint Surg Br*. 2007;89(11):1470–1477.

Bessière C, Trojani C, Carles M, Mehta SS, Boileau P. The open Latarjet procedure is more reliable in terms of shoulder stability than arthroscopic Bankart repair. *Clin Orthop Relat Res*. 2014;472(8):2345–2351.

Boileau P, Mercier N, Roussanne Y, Thélu CÉ, Old J. Arthroscopic Bankart-Bristow-Latarjet procedure: the development and early results of a safe and reproducible technique. *Arthroscopy*. 2010;26(11):1434–1450.

Boileau P, Thélu CÉ, Mercier N, et al. Arthroscopic Bristow-Latarjet combined with Bankart repair restores shoulder stability in patients with glenoid bone loss. *Clin Orthop Relat Res*. 2014;472(8):2413–2424.

Boileau P, Villalba M, Héry JY, Balg F, Ahrens P, Neyton L. Risk factors for recurrence of shoulder instability after arthroscopic Bankart repair. *J Bone Joint Surg Am*. 2006;88(8):1755–1763.

Burkhart SS, De Beer JF. Traumatic glenohumeral bone defects and their relationship to failure of arthroscopic Bankart repairs: significance of the inverted-pear glenoid and the humeral engaging Hill-Sachs lesion. *Arthroscopy*. 2000;16(7):677–694.

Burkhart SS, De Beer JF, Barth JR, Cresswell T, Roberts C, Richards DP. Results of modified Latarjet reconstruction in patients with anteroinferior instability and significant bone loss. *Arthroscopy*. 2007;23(10):1033–1041.

Buss DD, Lynch GP, Meyer CP, Huber SM, Freehill MQ. Nonoperative management for in-season athletes with anterior shoulder instability. *Am J Sports Med*. 2004;32(6):1430–1433.

Buza JA 3rd, Iyengar JJ, Anakwenze OA, Ahmad CS, Levine WN. Arthroscopic Hill-Sachs remplissage: a systematic review. *J Bone Joint Surg Am*. 2014;96(7):549–555.

Castagna A, Delle Rose G, Borroni M, et al. Arthroscopic stabilization of the shoulder in adolescent athletes participating in overhead or contact sports. *Arthroscopy*. 2012;28(3):309–315.

Castagna A, Markopoulos N, Conti M, Delle Rose G, Papadakou E, Garofalo R. Arthroscopic Bankart suture-anchor repair: radiological and clinical outcome at minimum 10 years of follow-up. *Am J Sports Med*. 2010;38(10):2012–2016.

Cerciello S, Edwards TB, Walch G. Chronic anterior glenohumeral instability in soccer players: results for a series of 28 shoulders treated with the Latarjet procedure. *J Orthop Traumatol*. 2012;13(4):197–202.

Chalmers PN, Mascarenhas R, Leroux T, et al. Do arthroscopic and open stabilization techniques restore equivalent stability to the shoulder in the setting of anterior glenohumeral instability? a systematic review of overlapping meta-analyses. *Arthroscopy*. 2015;31(2):355–363.

Degen RM, Giles JW, Johnson JA, Athwal GS. Remplissage versus Latarjet for engaging Hill-Sachs defects without substantial glenoid bone loss: a biomechanical comparison. *Clin Orthop Relat Res*. 2014;472(8):2363–2371.

Dickens JF, Owens BD, Cameron KL, et al. Return to play and recurrent instability after in-season anterior shoulder instability: a prospective multicenter study. *Am J Sports Med*. 2014;42(12):2842–2850.

Dumont GD, Fogerty S, Rosso C, Lafosse L. The arthroscopic Latarjet procedure for anterior shoulder instability: 5-year minimum follow-up. *Am J Sports Med*. 2014;42(11):2560–2566.

Eglseder WA Jr, Goldman M. Anatomic variations of the musculocutaneous nerve in the arm. *Am J Orthop (Belle Mead NJ)*. 1997;26(11):777–780.

Franceschi F, Papalia R, Del Buono A, Vasta S, Maffulli N, Denaro V. Glenohumeral osteoarthritis after arthroscopic Bankart repair for anterior instability. *Am J Sports Med*. 2011;39(8):1653–1659.

Garcia GH, Taylor SA, Fabricant PD, Dines JS. Shoulder instability management: a survey of the American Shoulder and Elbow Surgeons. *Am J Orthop (Belle Mead NJ)*. 2016a;45(3):E91–E97.

Garcia GH, Wu HH, Liu JN, Huffman GR, Kelly JD 4th. Outcomes of the remplissage procedure and its effects on return to sports: average 5-year follow-up. *Am J Sports Med*. 2016b;44(5):1124–1130.

Green MR, Christensen KP. Arthroscopic Bankart procedure: two- to five-year followup with clinical correlation to severity of glenoid labral lesion. *Am J Sports Med*. 1995;23(3):276–281.

Grumet RC, Bach BR Jr, Provencher MT. Arthroscopic stabilization for first-time versus recurrent shoulder instability. *Arthroscopy*. 2010;26(2):239–248.

Harris JD, Gupta AK, Mall NA, et al. Long-term outcomes after Bankart shoulder stabilization. *Arthroscopy*. 2013;29(5):920–933.

Hatch MD, Hennrikus WL. The open Bankart repair for traumatic anterior shoulder instability in teenage athletes. *J Pediatr Orthop*. 2016. Mar 3. [Epub ahead of print].

Hovelius L, Sandström B, Sundgren K, Saebö M. One hundred eighteen Bristow-Latarjet repairs for recurrent anterior dislocation of the shoulder prospectively followed for fifteen years: study I—clinical results. *J Shoulder Elbow Surg*. 2004;13(5):509–516.

Ide J, Maeda S, Takagi K. Arthroscopic Bankart repair using suture anchors in athletes: patient selection and postoperative sports activity. *Am J Sports Med*. 2004;32(8):1899–1905.

Itoi E, Yamamoto N, Kurokawa D, Sano H. Bone loss in anterior instability. *Curr Rev Musculoskelet Med*. 2013;6(1):88–94.

Johnson LL. Arthroscopy of the shoulder. *Orthop Clin North Am*. 1980;11(2):197–204.

Kang RW, Frank RM, Nho SJ, et al. Complications associated with anterior shoulder instability repair. *Arthroscopy*. 2009;25(8):909–920.

Lafosse L, Lejeune E, Bouchard A, Kakuda C, Gobezie R, Kochhar T. The arthroscopic Latarjet procedure for the treatment of anterior shoulder instability. *Arthroscopy*. 2007;23(11):1242.e1–1242.e5.

Levy DM, Cole BJ, Bach BR Jr. History of surgical intervention of anterior shoulder instability. *J Shoulder Elbow Surg*. 2016;25(6):e139–e150.

Longo UG, Loppini M, Rizzello G, et al. Remplissage, humeral osteochondral grafts, weber osteotomy, and shoulder arthroplasty for the management of humeral bone defects in shoulder instability: systematic review and quantitative synthesis of the literature. *Arthroscopy*. 2014;30(12):1650–1666.

Loomer R, Graham B. Anatomy of the axillary nerve and its relation to inferior capsular shift. *Clin Orthop Relat Res*. 1989;(243):100–105.

Milchteim C, Tucker SA, Nye DD, et al. Outcomes of Bankart repairs using modern arthroscopic technique in an athletic population. *Arthroscopy*. 2016;32(7):1263–1270.

Moroder P, Odorizzi M, Pizzinini S, Demetz E, Resch H, Moroder P. Open Bankart repair for the treatment of anterior shoulder instability without substantial osseous glenoid defects: results after a minimum follow-up of twenty years. *J Bone Joint Surg Am*. 2015;97(17):1398–1405.

Neyton L, Young A, Dawidziak B, et al. Surgical treatment of anterior instability in rugby union players: clinical and radiographic results of the Latarjet-Patte procedure with minimum 5-year follow-up. *J Shoulder Elbow Surg*. 2012;21(12):1721–1727.

Owens BD, Cameron KL, Peck KY, et al. Arthroscopic versus open stabilization for anterior shoulder subluxations. *Orthop J Sports Med*. 2015;3(1). 2325967115571084.

Provencher MT, Frank RM, Leclere LE, et al. The Hill-Sachs lesion: diagnosis, classification, and management. *J Am Acad Orthop Surg*. 2012;20(4):242–252.

Rhee YG, Ha JH, Cho NS. Anterior shoulder stabilization in collision athletes: arthroscopic versus open Bankart repair. *Am J Sports Med*. 2006;34(6):979–985.

Rowe CR, Patel D, Southmayd WW. The Bankart procedure: a long-term end-result study. *J Bone Joint Surg Am*. 1978;60(1):1–16.

Schmid SL, Farshad M, Catanzaro S, Gerber C. The Latarjet procedure for the treatment of recurrence of anterior instability of the shoulder after operative repair: a retrospective case series of forty-nine consecutive patients. *J Bone Joint Surg Am*. 2012;94(11):e75.

Schroder DT, Provencher MT, Mologne TS, Muldoon MP, Cox JS. The modified Bristow procedure for anterior shoulder instability: 26-year outcomes in Naval Academy midshipmen. *Am J Sports Med*. 2006;34(5):778–786.

Shah AA, Butler RB, Romanowski J, Goel D, Karadagli D, Warner JJ. Short-term complications of the Latarjet procedure. *J Bone Joint Surg Am*. 2012;94(6):495–501.

Sperber A, Hamberg P, Karlsson J, Swärd L, Wredmark T. Comparison of an arthroscopic and an open procedure for posttraumatic instability of the shoulder: a prospective, randomized multicenter study. *J Shoulder Elbow Surg*. 2001;10(2):105–108.
Steffen V, Hertel R. Rim reconstruction with autogenous iliac crest for anterior glenoid deficiency: forty-three instability cases followed for 5-19 years. *J Shoulder Elbow Surg*. 2013;22(4):550–559.
Stone GP, Pearsall 4th AW. Return to play after open Bankart repair: a systematic review. *Orthop J Sports Med*. 2014;2(2). 2325967114522960.
Warner JJ, Gill TJ, O'hollerhan JD, Pathare N, Millett PJ. Anatomical glenoid reconstruction for recurrent anterior glenohumeral instability with glenoid deficiency using an autogenous tricortical iliac crest bone graft. *Am J Sports Med*. 2006;34(2):205–212.
Weng PW, Shen HC, Lee HH, Wu SS, Lee CH. Open reconstruction of large bony glenoid erosion with allogeneic bone graft for recurrent anterior shoulder dislocation. *Am J Sports Med*. 2009;37(9):1792–1797.
Wheeler JH, Ryan JB, Arciero RA, Molinari RN. Arthroscopic versus nonoperative treatment of acute shoulder dislocations in young athletes. *Arthroscopy*. 1989;5(3):213–217.
Wolf EM. Arthroscopic capsulolabral repair using suture anchors. *Orthop Clin North Am*. 1993;24(1):59–69.
Yoneda M, Hayashida K, Wakitani S, Nakagawa S, Fukushima S. Bankart procedure augmented by coracoid transfer for contact athletes with traumatic anterior shoulder instability. *Am J Sports Med*. 1999;27(1):21–26.
Young AA, Maia R, Berhouet J, Walch G. Open Latarjet procedure for management of bone loss in anterior instability of the glenohumeral joint. *J Shoulder Elbow Surg*. 2011;20(suppl 2):S61–S69.

1-10 INTERNATIONAL PERSPECTIVE: FRANCE

PATRICK GENDRE, MD, CHARLES BESSIERE, MD, and PASCAL BOILEAU, MD

Introduction

- "Shoulder instability" constitutes a spectrum of disorders including dislocation, subluxation, and pain.
- The diagnosis of anterior instability is based on a thorough history, physical examination, and imaging.
- Early surgical intervention may be a consideration, especially in younger athlete patients.
- The key to more successful results is the ability to select patients for the adequate "a la carte" arthroscopic procedure.

Anterior shoulder dislocation is a common injury that represents 11% of shoulder injuries at all ages. The incidence of shoulder dislocation is estimated at 27 in 100,000 in men and at 22 in 100,000 in women (Nordqvist & Petersson, 1995). Ninety-five percent of shoulder dislocations are anteroinferior, 3% posterior, and 2% other types. Dislocations affect men three times more often than women. Men younger than 30 years of age are especially involved (mean age, 27 years). Family history of shoulder instability is found in one quarter of cases.

First, it is important to differentiate among laxity, hyperlaxity, and instability, which are three different concepts.

1. *Laxity* defines the physiological and asymptomatic translation of the humeral head on the glenoid, necessary for the normal function of the joint; this is the normal articular play.
2. *Hyperlaxity* is not a pathology but only a risk factor for the development of possible instability or a risk factor for recurrence of instability after arthroscopic Bankart stabilization. Hyperlaxity is difficult to analyze because its definition varies. Excessive external rotation with the arm at the side, that is, rotation of more than 90 degrees, has been reported to be an indicator of shoulder hyperlaxity (Coudane & Walch, 2000). This sign is almost always bilateral. In addition, we found that a stretched inferior glenohumeral ligament, defined as an asymmetric hyperabduction test of more than 20 degrees compared with the contralateral side (Coste et al, 1999; Gagey & Gagey, 2001), was associated with failure of arthroscopic Bankart stabilization (Boileau et al, 2006). It has been our experience that such inferior laxity is, most of the time, acquired and related to the amount of plastic deformation of the inferior axillary pouch after recurrent dislocations or subluxations.
3. *Instability* defines an excessive translation (nonphysiologic) of the humeral head on the glenoid cavity causing symptoms perceived by the patient as dislocations, subluxations, or pain (Boileau et al, 2011).
   - *Dislocation:* complete loss of contact between the joint surfaces, requiring a reduction maneuver
   - *Subluxation:* transient loss of contact of the articular surfaces that reduces spontaneously or without help

We describe the physiopathology of instability, the diagnostic elements, and finally our therapeutic practices based on current findings.

Physiopathology

Instability is more often traumatic. The mechanism can be direct (e.g., drop on the top of the shoulder) or indirect (e.g., forced abduction-external rotation). Traumatic dislocations commonly occur during sports (75% of cases). Instability may also be secondary to a single trauma, such as falling in external rotation-abduction, or can occur gradually because of overuse trauma. More rarely, it may be atraumatic, congenital, or secondary to neuromuscular lesions.

In patients older than 40 years of age, in one quarter of the cases, the shoulder dislocation is associated with other injuries (e.g., rotator cuff tears), which should be looked for systematically.

The glenohumeral joint is the most mobile one in the body. Various elements affect stability: the labrum, the inferior glenohumeral ligament (IGHL), the bony parts, and the muscles. These various elements can be injured when an anterior shoulder dislocation occurs.

BANKART LESION

The Bankart lesion (Bankart, 1938) is the essential lesion responsible for chronic anterior instability. It corresponds to an avulsion of the labrum to the anteroinferior part (Fig. 10.1). It is almost constantly present in traumatic anterior instability and tends to extend around the glenoid with repeated episodes of instability. Sometimes the labrum heals too medially (ALPSA [anterior labroligamentous periosteal sleeve avulsion]). This injury removes the wedge effect of the glenoid rim, decreasing the depth of the glenoid by half because of the detachment of the labrum and the removal of the *concavity–compression* in the joint.

CAPSULAR LESION

Capsuloligamentous damage is always associated with the Bankart lesion. Recurrent dislocations or subluxations are associated with earlier stretching or plastic deformation of the capsule, capsular rupture, or avulsion of the capsule of the humeral side (HAGL [humeral avulsion of the glenohumeral ligament] lesions).

This plastic deformation of the capsule should be treated during the arthroscopic treatment of instability, not just the Bankart lesion.

GLENOID BONE LESIONS

Lesions of the anteroinferior glenoid rim are very common quite variable and are roughly of two types:

- *Glenoid fracture* with a detached bone fragment (shear or avulsion fracture), called bony Bankart (Sugaya et al, 2005)
- *Glenoid bone defect* without any detached bone fragment (compression fracture), which usually reflects the chronic nature of the instability (Fig. 10.2)

The term "glenoid bone defect" applies if 25% or more of the anterior glenoid rim is missing (Boileau et al, 2006). This glenoid bone defect is associated with a higher rate of recurrent glenohumeral instability after arthroscopic Bankart repair (Balg & Boileau, 2007).

HILL-SACHS LESION

Posterosuperior humeral head bone defects, commonly known as Hill-Sachs lesions, have been reported to occur in 47% of individuals with a first-time glenohumeral dislocation and in up to 90% of those with recurrent anteroinferior glenohumeral instability (Calandra et al, 1989; Purchase et al, 2008; Spatschil et al, 2006). With recurrent episodes of glenohumeral instability, the lesions become larger and deeper, increasing the risk of further instability (Kralinger et al, 2002; Cetik et al, 2007). The term *engaging Hill-Sachs lesion* has been used by Burkhart and De Beer (2000) to describe a compression fracture of the humeral head that is large enough for the edge of the humeral head to drop over the glenoid rim as the arm is abducted and externally rotated. These large and engaging defects of the posterosuperior aspect of the humeral head are associated with a higher rate of recurrent glenohumeral instability after

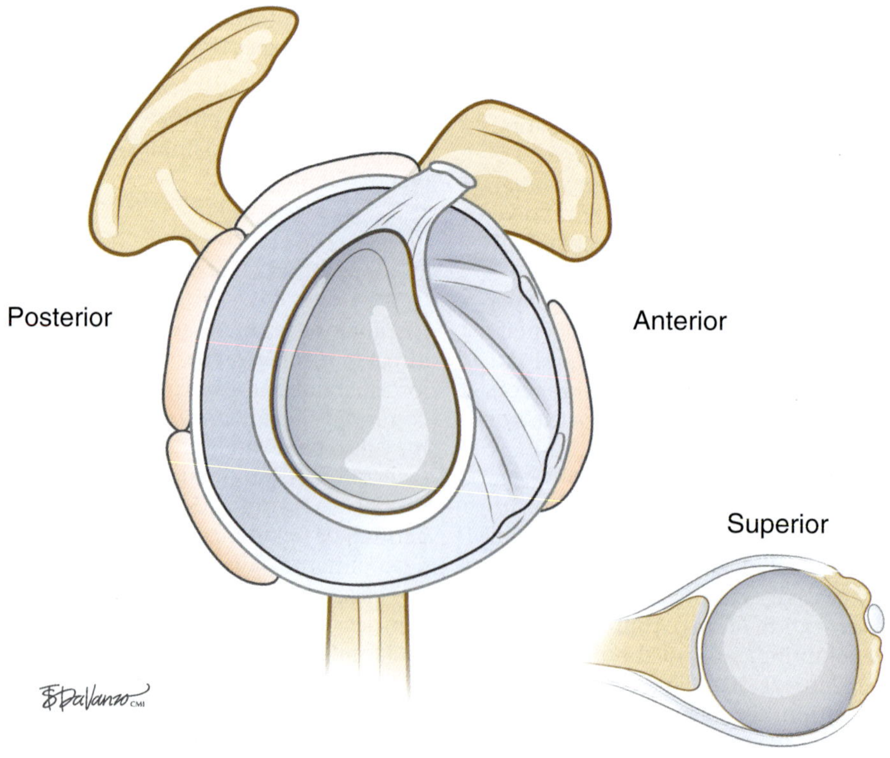

Fig. 10.1 Usual location of the Bankart lesion.

arthroscopic Bankart repair (Boileau et al, 2006; Voos et al, 2010).

ROTATOR CUFF TEARS

Partial tears of the deep surface of the supraspinatus tendon are relatively frequent after acute dislocation even in young patients (12%–23%). They are rare in chronic instabilities.

Full-thickness rotator cuff tears are rare, around 5% of cases. It is recommended to repair these injuries as soon as possible. The rotator cuff tears must be detected in patients older than 40 years, in whom they are more frequent: Any shoulder dislocation after 40 years of age is a traumatic rotator cuff tear until there is evidence of the contrary. Often the lack of active anterior elevation of the shoulder or loss of strength after the acute phase is attributed wrongly to axillary nerve palsy. Magnetic resonance imaging or computed tomography arthroscopy (CTA) imaging provides information on the size and length of lesions, which will determine repair options.

AXILLARY NERVE PALSY

Neurologic damage is caused by nerves stretching during trauma or during reduction maneuvers, and their reported incidence varies, according to studies, ranging from 19% to 55%. The frequency and severity increase with age, but they are almost always reversible. The testing of the sensitivity of the shoulder is indicative but not sufficient to affirm the absence of axillary nerve palsy because the existence of a disorder of the sensitivity reflects a severe attack. Deltoid muscle activity must be tested after reduction.

GREATER TUBEROSITY FRACTURE

The occurrence of a fracture of the greater tuberosity is caused by an extension of the Hill-Sachs lesion or a tear of the insertion of the rotator cuff tendons. Again, its frequency increases with age. Usually, the reduction of the dislocation reduces the greater tuberosity anatomically, but a displacement of more than 10 mm after reduction must be operated on. We recommend the use of a neutral rotation sling and slight abduction, which provides a more anatomic position of the bone fragment than an internal rotation sling. Strict immobilization for a maximum of 3 weeks is recommended followed by gentle mobilization with pendulum exercise and then passive motion. The sling should be removed at 4 weeks after the dislocation.

OSTEOARTHRITIS

There is preoperative arthropathy caused by instability in 15% of patients experiencing anterior instability. The risk of postoperative osteoarthritis is increased by the age at the first episode and at the time of the operation, the number of dislocations, and the length of time since the first dislocation (Buscayret et al, 2004).

Diagnosis

PHYSICAL EXAMINATION

Acute Dislocation

Most often, the initial pain is important. The patient maintains the injured limb with the healthy limb in the "traumatized upper limb attitude." The posterior and lateral aspect of the shoulder shows a hollow beneath the acromion. On palpation, there is a void under the acromion, and the humeral head can be palpated anteriorly. Because of the possible association of nerves and vascular injuries, an essential part of the physical examination of an anteriorly dislocated shoulder is the assessment of the neurovascular status of the upper extremity and charting of the findings before reduction.

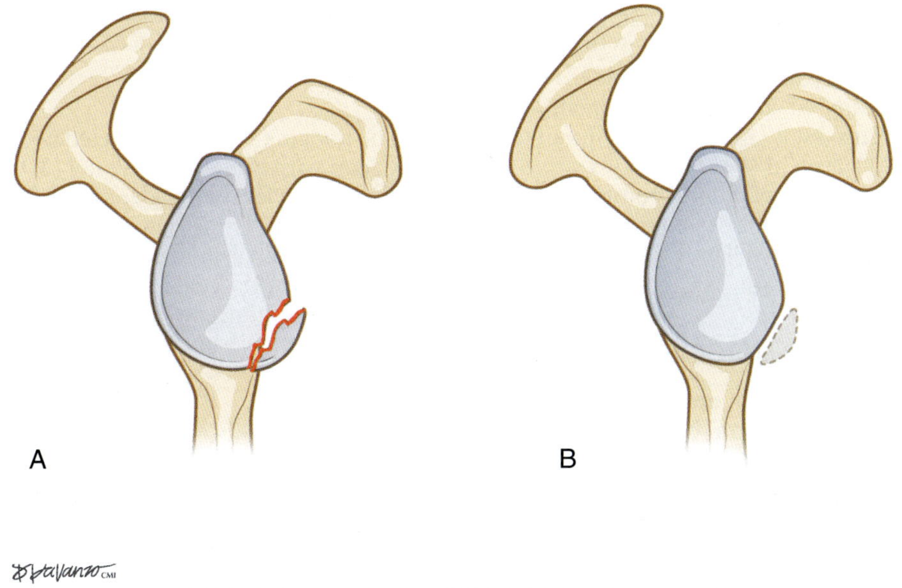

Fig. 10.2 A, Acute glenoid fracture. **B,** Glenoid bone defect.

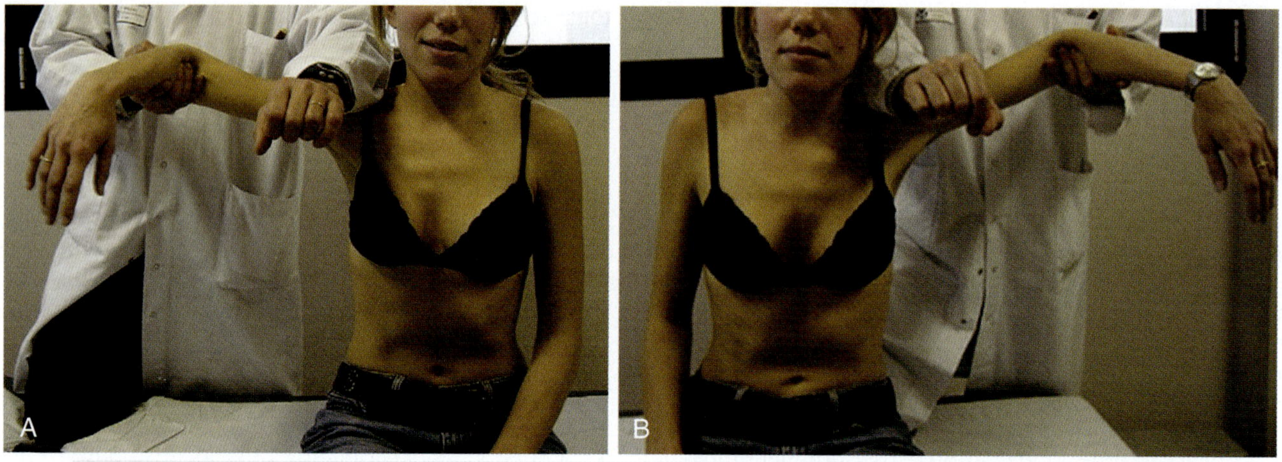

Fig. 10.3 A and B, Inferior hyperlaxity with asymmetry of greater than 20 degrees when performing the hyperabduction test.

Recurrent Anteroinferior Shoulder Instability

The occurrence of one or more episodes or persistence of subluxation or pain testifies to the chronicity.

- *The apprehension test.* The patient sits with his or her back to the examiner. The patient's arm is held in 90 degrees of abduction and external rotation. The examiner pulls the patient's wrist to the back with one hand while stabilizing the back of the shoulder with the other. A patient with anterior instability usually shows apprehension during this maneuver more or less associated with pain.
- *The relocation test* confirms the diagnosis: The patient lies supine at the edge of the examination table with the arm in 90 degrees of abduction and external rotation. The movement by the examiner causes apprehension or pain in cases of anterior instability. The test is repeated by pushing the humeral head from forward to backward to reduce the anterior subluxation and to obtain extreme amplitudes in abduction and external rotation while relieving the patient's apprehension and pain.
- *The comparative hyperabduction test* (Fig. 10.3) The result of this test is considered positive when (1) it reproduces the patient's pain (deep anterior pain recognized by the patient), (2) it is asymmetric compared with the contralateral side (>20 degrees of difference), and (3) there is a soft endpoint compared with the firm endpoint of the contralateral side. This test is called the "'Lachman test of the shoulder" (Boileau et al, 2011).

Inspection, palpation, search of painful points, and rotator cuff and deltoid testing must be systematic. These tests should be executed routinely, as well as the shoulder hyperlaxity test.

RADIOGRAPHS AND OTHER IMAGING

Standard radiographs, including an anteroposterior and a lateral view (Lamy view), can confirm the diagnosis of dislocation and are necessary to detect associated fractures (Fig. 10.4).

In the context of recurrent anteroinferior shoulder instability, four views are needed: anteroposterior view in neutral, internal and external rotation, and a glenoid profile (or Bernageau view).

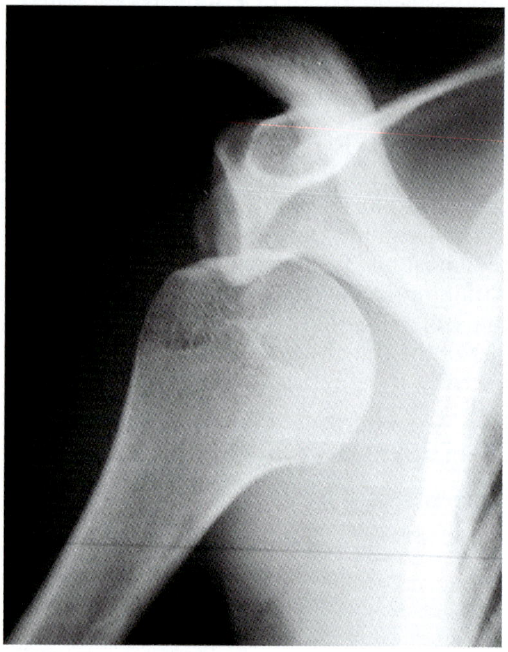

Fig. 10.4 Anteroposterior radiographic view shows an anteroinferior shoulder dislocation.

The imaging is to be completed with a computed tomography scan with three-dimensional (3D) reconstructions, especially with a view of the glenoid surface (after removal of the humeral head). These views are useful to detect humeral bone lesions or small glenoid bone loss. In the context of shoulder instability, we do not request injected imaging (CTA and magnetic resonance arthrography), except when an associated rotator cuff lesion is suspected clinically (Fig. 10.5).

Treatment

ACUTE TRAUMATIC ANTERIOR DISLOCATIONS

Reduction and Analgesia

Acute dislocations should be reduced as gently and expeditiously as possible, after a complete set of radiographs

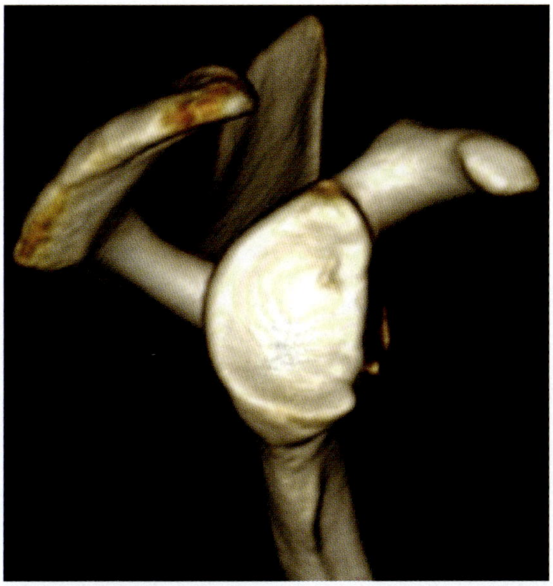

Fig. 10.5 Computed tomography scan with three-dimensional reconstruction after removal of the humeral head shows glenoid erosion.

is obtained to rule out associated bone injuries. After the diagnosis is made, the reduction must be done as soon as possible. A reduction without radiographs or anesthesia can pose legal problems and should be attempted only in extreme cases. Numerous techniques exist. The reduction must be done on a relaxed and reassured patient. A short general anaesthesia is preferable if the reduction is not achieved after two attempts.

There are two main types of reduction maneuvers:

- The first and oldest is the traction–countertraction technique with an axillary support. The support is obtained with a sheet placed around the thorax. This should always be done with an aide, never alone, and never using the foot for the countertraction.
- The second type is to mobilize the shoulder in a position that leads to a spontaneous reduction. In Kocher's method, the affected arm is bent at 90 degrees at the elbow, adducted against the body; the wrist and the elbow can be grasped by the examiner, who will slowly rotate the arm externally between 70 and 85 degrees until resistance is felt. In a conscious patient, the examiner should take plenty of time while distracting the patient with conversation. The externally rotated upper arm in the sagittal plane is lifted as far as possible forward and then the shoulder is rotated internally, bringing the patient's hand toward the opposite shoulder. The humeral head should now slip back into the glenoid fossa with the pain eliminated during this process.

Clinical examination must be systematic after reduction to check the absence of neurovascular complications. Any abnormalities should be documented in the medical record.

Similarly, a radiography control must be carried out systematically after reduction. It provides assessment of the effectiveness of the maneuver and detecting associated bone lesions.

Most authors propose an immobilization after reduction in internal rotation, but there is no consensus on the type of sling and the length of immobilization. Several studies have shown that a period of 3 weeks of immobilization is recommended. Immobilization in neutral or external rotation has not proven its usefulness. However, the duration of immobilization can be reduced, and it is less strict in patients older than 30 years of age because of the risk of a frozen shoulder.

NONOPERATIVE TREATMENT

The initiation of a specific rehabilitation program is an important element to prevent recurrence. It is based on the recovery of range of motion, strengthening the internal rotator muscles of the shoulder, and proprioceptive work. Furthermore, premature return to sport activities can promote recurrence in patients younger than 30 years of age.

WHEN TO OPERATE

There is a consensus on the indication of surgical stabilization for recurrent anteroinferior shoulder instability. But the decision to operate an isolated anterior shoulder dislocation cannot be made without knowledge of the spontaneous evolution of nonoperated anterior instability.

The risk of recurrence decreases with age. There is a maximum risk (60%–80%) before 20 years of age, and then it gradually decreases to 18% from 40 to 50 years, to 4% between 50 and 60 years, and to 1.9% after 60 years.

The studies of Hovelius et al (1996, 2008), following patients with unoperated anterior instability over 25 years, are fundamental. The two main findings of these studies are:

1. In a general population, the natural history of a first dislocation shows that 52% of patients have no recurrence at 15 years and 43% at 25 years of follow-up.
2. Only a quarter of patients (23%) will need an operative technique to stabilize the shoulder after 10 years of evolution and 27% after 25 years.

For Hovelius (1987), these data do not justify the indication of an arthroscopic Bankart stabilization after a first dislocation, even in young adults. However, extrapolation to a young and athletic population should be made with caution. Hovelius himself showed that the recurrence rate at 5 years was 50% before the age of 22 years, and the operation rate to stabilize the shoulder rose to 38% when looking at the population of 12- to 25-year-old patients after the first episode of dislocation (Hovelius, 1987).

The prospective randomized study by Kirkley et al (2005) and reported at two different time points is particularly interesting: The rate of recurrence after arthroscopic Bankart stabilization increases slightly over time (16% with 2 years to 27% with 5 years of follow-up) as well as after nonoperative treatment (45%–60%). In the group of initially nonoperated patients, 35% were due to be operated at 75 months of follow-up.

The randomized level I study by Robinson et al (2008) is instructive: Two groups of 42 patients younger than 35 years with an anterior shoulder dislocation were compared. One group had a single arthroscopic washing and the other an arthroscopic Bankart technique with anchors. At last follow-up, the Bankart group had significantly better results in terms of recurrence, satisfaction, and return to the same level of sport. The overall medical cost was also lower in the Bankart group.

Based on published studies, the recurrence rate of instability in a young athlete is approximately 70% after nonoperative treatment compared with 15% after an arthroscopic Bankart procedure after an isolated anterior shoulder dislocation. Thus, although the natural evolution after nonoperative treatment is favorable in most cases after an isolated anterior shoulder dislocation, there is a place for arthroscopic stabilization in a specific population of young athletes practicing high-risk sports.

SURGICAL TREATMENT: WHAT TECHNIQUE? WHAT RESULTS?

The gold standard of operative stabilization techniques remains the open coracoid bone block procedure (Latarjet, 1954) yielding the best results reported in the long term for unselected populations, with 5% to 10% of recurrence (subluxation or dislocation) (Bessiere et al, 2013; Lévigne, 2000). All other techniques do not have sufficient follow-up to judge the long-term results or have higher rates of recurrence. Other open techniques are also performed, including the Bankart technique with capsuloplasty (Cheung et al, 2008), Eden Hybbinette procedure (Hedman 1952), and Trillat procedure (Trillat, 1954), but are not widespread.

Arthroscopic Bankart techniques (with anchors and sutures) showed equivalent reliability on the short and medium term to historical open Bankart techniques (Harris, 2013) and now represent the alternative to the open coracoid bone block procedure.

New techniques and approaches have been developed in the past decades to improve the initial results of arthroscopic Bankart techniques: Bankart associated with the "Hill-Sachs remplissage" (Wolf and Arianjam, 2014), associated with the reinsertion of glenoid bone fragment fracture ("bony Bankart") (Sugaya et al, 2005), or associated with the Trillat procedure (Boileau et al, 2007) More recently, arthroscopic bone-block procedures have been developed using screws or double buttons to fix the coracoid (Boileau et al, 2010, 2016; Lafosse et al, 2007). (Video 10.1).

What are the indications of the different techniques, including the recent innovative techniques? Efforts have been made in recent years by the scientific community to improve patient selection; in fact, the study of the failures of arthroscopic Bankart repair helped highlight different risk factors of recurrence (Randelli et al, 2012). Most of them were included in the Instability Severity Index Score (ISIS) developed by Balg and Boileau (2007) and validated since (Table 10.1). Progress was also made in the diagnosis of bone lesions, including the use of regular 3D CT imaging.

Patients who are younger, hyperlax, practicing competitive at risk sports (with contact or with cocking of the arm), or with significant bone lesions are not good candidates for an isolated arthroscopic Bankart repair. These patients should instead undergo a coracoid bone block procedure or a previously described new technique combined with a Bankart repair (Fig. 10.6).

Today it seems that the key to more successful results is the ability to select patients for the adequate procedure to avoid recurrence. But today, the lack of high-level (I–II) comparative studies of the various techniques and the lack of long-term outcomes of the "new" techniques do not allow us to propose a consented and internationally recognized treatment course. The study conducted for the French symposium on anterior instability of the shoulder has also clearly shown that in 2010, the indications still depended more on the geographical origin, commercial arguments, and the type of training received by the surgeon than on science. There is a clear predominance in France of the open and arthroscopic coracoid bone block procedure compared with the domination of arthroscopic Bankart techniques in other countries in the management of recurrent anteroinferior shoulder instability (Thomazeau et al, 2010).

Table 10.1 Instability Severity Index Score Based on a Preoperative Questionnaire, Clinical Examination, and Radiographs

	Prognostic Factors		**Points**
Questionnaire	Age at surgery (yr)	≤20	2
		>20	0
	Degree of sport participation (preoperative)	Competitive	2
		Recreational or none	0
	Type of sport (preoperative)	Contact or forced overhead	1
		Other	0
Exam	Shoulder hyper-laxity	Anterior or inferior	1
		Normal laxity	0
AP radiography	Hill-Sachs lesion	Visible in external rotation	2
		Not visible in external rotation	0
	Glenoid loss of contour	Loss of contour	2
		No lesion	0
Total			**10**

AP, Anteroposterior.

Conclusions

Anterior shoulder instability is a common pathology in sports medicine and can be responsible for a true impairment in daily life. The treatment, as for all functional disorders of the shoulder, must be conservative at first and associated with a short immobilization followed by a specific rehabilitation program.

Surgical stabilization can be considered immediately after a single episode of dislocation in a young high-level athlete practicing a sport at risk. But for the vast majority of patients, the indication of surgical stabilization is for recurrent anteroinferior shoulder instability. For us, the gold standard technique is the coracoid bone block procedure, with the best results reported in the long term for unselected populations. Modern arthroscopic techniques should be reserved for selected patients and should be performed by surgeons well trained in shoulder arthroscopy surgery.

Although we are convinced of the future of the "all arthroscopic" surgical treatment of anterior shoulder instability, there is currently a lack of studies showing the long-term results of modern arthroscopic techniques (Hill Sachs remplissage, arthroscopic bone block technique). However, the last study for the French symposium showed the good

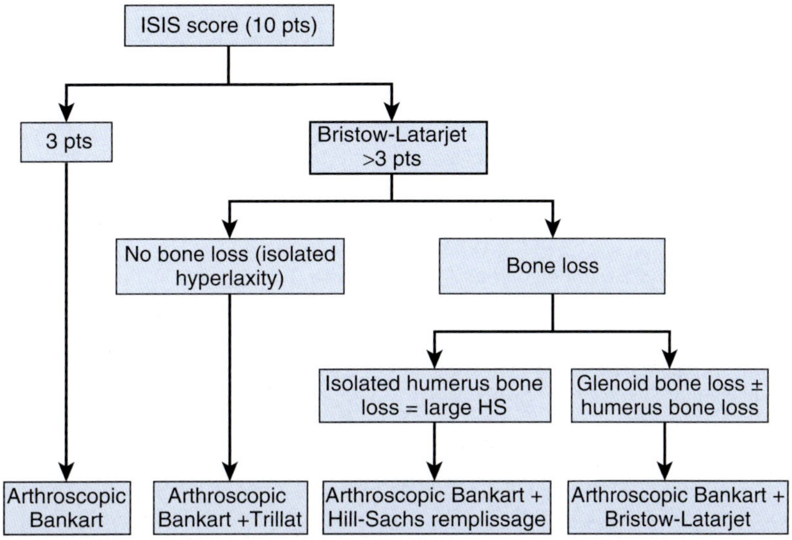

Fig. 10.6 "A la carte" arthroscopic management of recurrent anterior instability. Our treatment algorithm is based on (1) determination of risk factors for failures after isolated Bankart repair with the help of the Instability Severity Index Score (ISIS) and (2) selection of the additional procedure to perform according to the predominant (soft tissue or bony) lesion encountered. *pts,* Points.

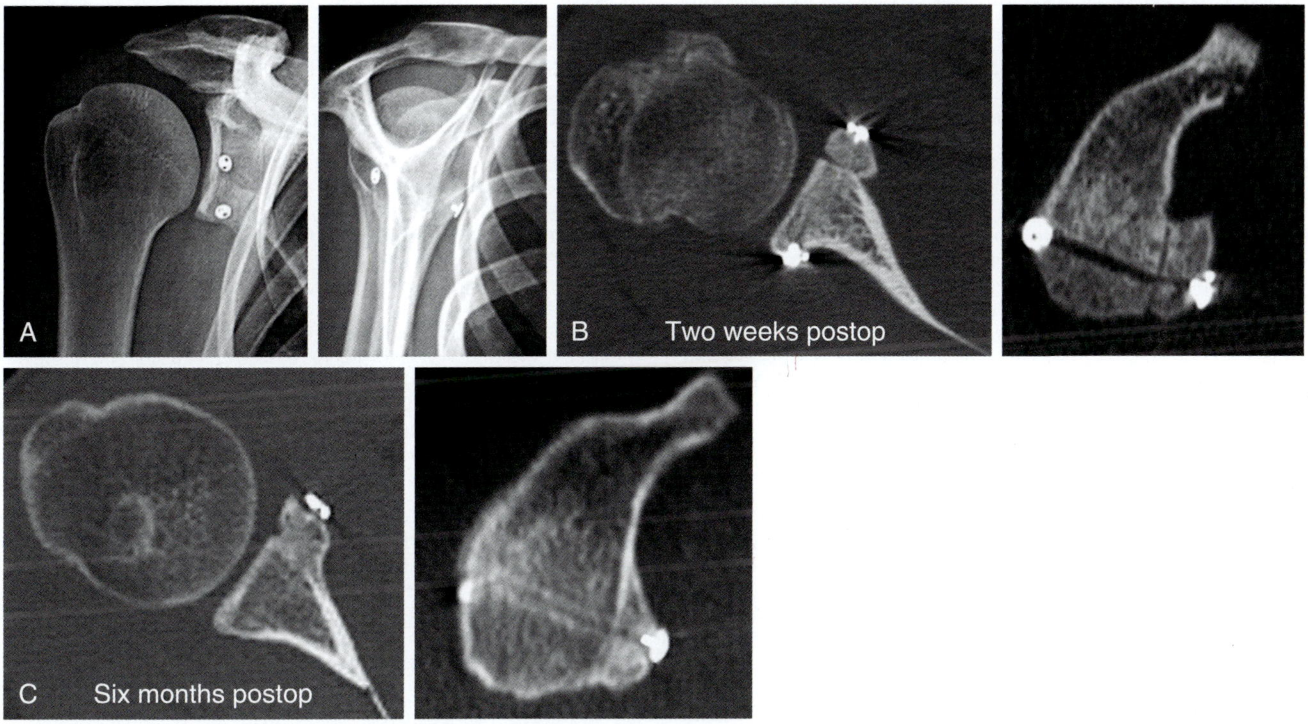

Fig. 10.7 Example of coracoid bone block positioning and healing after guided arthroscopic Latarjet procedure and fixation with suture and cortical buttons. **A,** Anteroposterior and lateral radiographs at 2 weeks. **B,** Two-dimensional computed tomography (CT) images at 2 weeks demonstrate perfect coracoid positioning (below the equator and flush to the glenoid surface). **C,** Two-dimensional CT images at 6 months demonstrate coracoid bone-block healing and remodeling.

reproducibility of bone-block positioning (under the equator and flush to the glenoid surface) of the arthroscopic bone block technique, which is a guarantee of future good long-term outcomes (Boileau et al, 2016; Walch & Lafosse, 2015) (Fig. 10.7).

References

Balg F, Boileau P. The instability severity index score. A simple pre-operative score to select patients for arthroscopic or open shoulder stabilisation. *J Bone Joint Surg Br*. 2007;89(11):1470–1477.

Bankart A. The pathology and treatment of recurrent dislocation of the shoulder joint. *Br J Surg*. 1938;26:23–29.

Bessiere C, Trojani C, Pelegri C, Carles M, Boileau P. Coracoid bone block versus arthroscopic Bankart repair: a comparative paired study with 5-year follow-up. *Orthop Traumatol Surg Res*. 2013;99(2):123–130.

Boileau P, Bicknell RT, Benchikh El, Fegoun A, Chuinard C. Arthroscopic Bristow procedure for anterior instability in shoulders with a stretched or deficient capsule: the "Belt-and-suspenders". Operative technique and preliminary results. *Arthroscopy*. 2007;23(6):593–601.

Boileau P, Gendre P, Baba M, Thélu CÉ, Baring T, Gonzalez JF, Trojani C. A guided surgical approach and novel fixation method for arthroscopic Latarjet. *J Shoulder Elbow Surg*. 2016;25(1):78–89.

Boileau P, Mercier N, Old J. Arthroscopic Bankart-Bristow-Latarjet (2B3) procedure: how to do it and tricks to make it easier and safe. *Orthop Clin North Am*. 2010;41:281–292.
Boileau P, Villalba M, Héry J, et al. Risk factors for recurrence of shoulder instability after arthroscopic Bankart repair. *J Bone Joint Surg Am*. 2006;88-A:1755–1763.
Boileau P, Zumstein M, Balg F, Penington S, Bicknell RT. The unstable painful shoulder (UPS) as a cause of pain from unrecognized anteroinferior instability in the young athlete. *J Shoulder Elbow Surg*. 2011;20(1):98–106.
Burkhart SS, De Beer JF. Traumatic glenohumeral bone defects and their relationship to failure of arthroscopic Bankart repairs: significance of the inverted-pear glenoid and the humeral engaging Hill-Sachs lesion. *Arthroscopy*. 2000;16:677–694.
Buscayret F, Edwards TB, Szabo I, Adeleine P, Coudane H, Walch G. Glenohumeral arthrosis in anterior instability before and after surgical treatment: incidence and contributing factors. *Am J Sports Med*. 2004;32(5):1165–1172.
Calandra JJ, Baker CL, Uribe J. The incidence of Hill-Sachs lesions in initial anterior shoulder dislocations. *Arthroscopy*. 1989;5:254–257.
Cetik O, Uslu M, Ozsar BK. The relationship between Hill-Sachs lesion and recurrent anterior shoulder dislocation. *Acta Orthop Belg*. 2007;73:175–178.
Cheung EV, Sperling JW, Hattrup SJ, Cofield RH. Long-term outcome of anterior stabilization of the shoulder. *J Shoulder Elbow Surg*. 2008;17(2):265–270.
Coste JS, Jund S, Lemaire M, Staccini P, Boileau P, Argenson C. Évaluation arthroscopique du test de laxité du ligament glénohuméral inférieur. *Rev Chir Orthop*. 1999;85:61.
Coudane H, Walch G. L'instabilité antérieure chronique de l'épaule chez l'adulte. Symposium de la Sofcot, Paris, 1999. *Rev Chir Orthop*. 2000;86(suppl 1):91–150.
Gagey OJ, Gagey N. The hyperabduction test. *J Bone Joint Surg Br*. 2001;83:69–74.
Harris JD, Gupta AK, Mall NA, et al. Long-term outcomes after Bankart shoulder stabilization. *Arthroscopy*. 2013;29(5):920–933.
Hovelius L. Anterior dislocation of the shoulder in teen-agers and young adults. Five-year prognosis. *J Bone Joint Surg Am*. 1987;69(3):393–399.
Hovelius L, Augustini BG, Fredin H, Johansson O, Norlin R, Thorling J. Primary anterior dislocation of the shoulder in young patients. A ten-year prospective study. *J Bone Joint Surg Am*. 1996;78(11):1677–1684.
Hovelius L, Olofsson A, Sandstrom B, et al. Nonoperative treatment of primary anterior shoulder dislocation in patients forty years of age and younger. a prospective twenty-five-year follow-up. *J Bone Joint Surg Am*. 2008;90(5):945–952.
Hedman D. The Edem-Hybbinette operation for recurrent dislocation of the shoulder; a clinical follow-up study. *Acta Chir Scand*. 1952;104(1):65–73.
Kirkley A, Werstine R, Ratjek A, Griffin S. Prospective randomized clinical trial comparing the effectiveness of immediate arthroscopic stabilization versus immobilization and rehabilitation in first traumatic anterior dislocations of the shoulder: long-term evaluation. *Arthroscopy*. 2005;21(1):55–63.
Kralinger FS, Golser K, Wischatta R, Wambacher M, Sperner G. Predicting recurrence after primary anterior shoulder dislocation. *Am J Sports Med*. 2002;30(1):116–120.
Lafosse L, Lejeune E, Bouchard A, Kakuda C, Gobezie R, Kochhar T. The arthroscopic Latarjet procedure for the treatment of anterior shoulder instability. *Arthroscopy*. 2007;23(11):1242. e1241–e1245.
Lafosse L, Walch G et al. Butée de Latarjet sous arthroscopie versus ciel ouvert. Symposium SFA. (grenoble, SFA 2015). *Orthop Traumatol Surg Res*, in press.
Latarjet M. Traitement des luxations récidivantes de l'épaule. *Lyon Chir*. 1954;49(8):994–997.
Lévigne C. Résultats à long terme des butées antérieures coracoïdiennes. *Rev Chir Orthop Reparatrice Appar Mot*. 2000;86(suppl 1):114–121.
Nordqvist A, Petersson CJ. Incidence and causes of shoulder girdle injuries in an urban population. *J Shoulder Elbow Surg*. 1995;4(2):107–112.
Purchase RJ, Wolf EM, Hobgood ER, Pollock ME, Smalley CC. Hill-Sachs "remplissage": an arthroscopic solution for the engaging Hill-Sachs lesion. *Arthroscopy*. 2008;24(6):723–726.
Randelli P, Ragone V, Carminati S, Cabitza P. Risk factors for recurrence after Bankart repair a systematic review. *Knee Surg Sports Traumatol Arthrosc*. 2012;20(11):2129–2138.
Robinson CM, Jenkins PJ, White TO, Ker A, Will E. Primary arthroscopic stabilization for a first-time anterior dislocation of the shoulder. A randomized, double-blind trial. *J Bone Joint Surg Am*. 2008;90(4):708–721.
Spatschil A, Landsiedl F, Anderl W, et al. Posttraumatic anterior-inferior instability of the shoulder: arthroscopic findings and clinical correlations. *Arch Orthop Trauma Surg*. 2006;126:217–222.
Sugaya H, Moriishi J, Kanisawa I, Tsuchiya A. Arthroscopic osseous Bankart repair for chronic recurrent traumatic anterior glenohumeral instability. *J Bone Joint Surg Am*. 2005;87(8):1752–1760.
Thomazeau HCO, Barth J, Pelegri C, Charousset C, Lespagnol F, et al. Can we improve the indication for Bankart arthroscopic repair? A preliminary clinical study using the ISIS score. *Orthop Traumatol Surg Res*. 2010;96(suppl 8):S77–S83.
Trillat A. Traitement des luxations récidivantes de l'épaule. *Lyon Chir*. 1954;49(8):986–993.
Voos JE, Livermore RW, Feeley BT, et al. HSS Sports Medicine Service. Prospective evaluation of arthroscopic bankart repairs for anterior instability. *Am J Sports Med*. 2010;38:302–307.
Wolf EM, Arianjam A. Hill-Sachs remplissage, an arthroscopic solution for the engaging Hill-Sachs lesion: 2- to 10-year follow-up and incidence of recurrence. *J Shoulder Elbow Surg*. 2014;23(6):814–820.

1-1P INTERNATIONAL PERSPECTIVE: ITALY

ANDREA PELLIGRINI, MD PAOLO PALADINI, MD GIOVANNI MEROLLA, MD GIUSEPPE PORCELLINI, MD

Introduction

- For patients with shoulder instability, it is important to conduct a clinical evaluation supported by appropriate imaging.
- Conservative treatment is reserved for patients in whom this approach has good chances of success.
- The arthroscopic approach includes complete joint evaluation and treatment.
- The open approach is reserved for complex cases that need accurate preparation.

Shoulder instability is characterized by symptomatic loosening of the contact area in the glenohumeral joint (Matsen et al, 1991). In Italy, trauma is the most common cause of shoulder instability; the estimated incidence is 24 new cases per 100,000 population per year. Notably, increased sports participation has resulted in greater exposure of the general population to overload injuries and microtraumas that may lead to shoulder instability (Merolla et al, 2016).

The clinical manifestations of shoulder instability include a wide spectrum of conditions that range from painful hyperlaxity to chronic locked shoulder dislocation. Glenoid or humeral bone loss or soft tissue lesions induced by shoulder dislocation can predispose to chronic unidirectional or multidirectional instability (MDI) (te Slaa et al, 2004). Sport type, the intensity of sport practice, joint laxity, and weakness of the humeral and scapular stabilizers are further causes of chronic instability (Matsen et al, 1991).

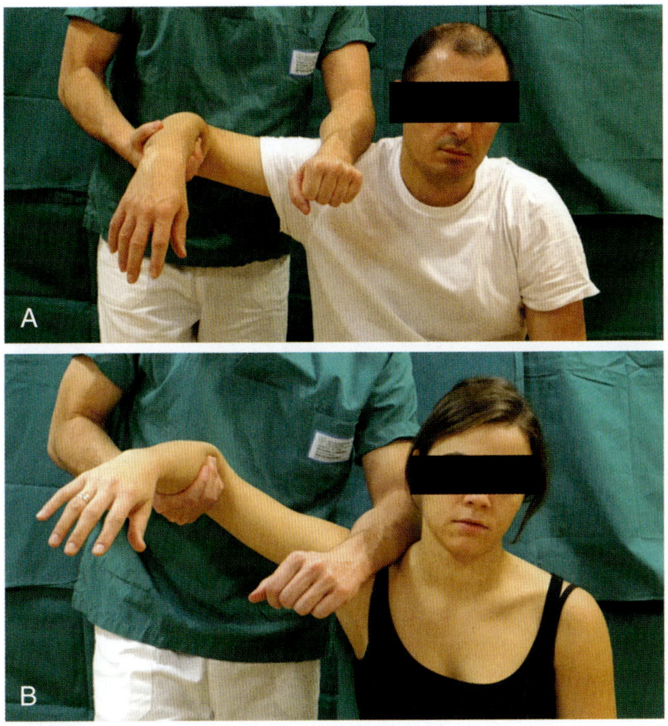

Fig. 1P.1 Gagey test during shoulder examination. The forearm of the physician holds the shoulder girdle firmly in the lower position, and the other hand lifts the patient's arm up in the frontal plane. The hyperabduction test result is negative (**A**) or positive (**B**).

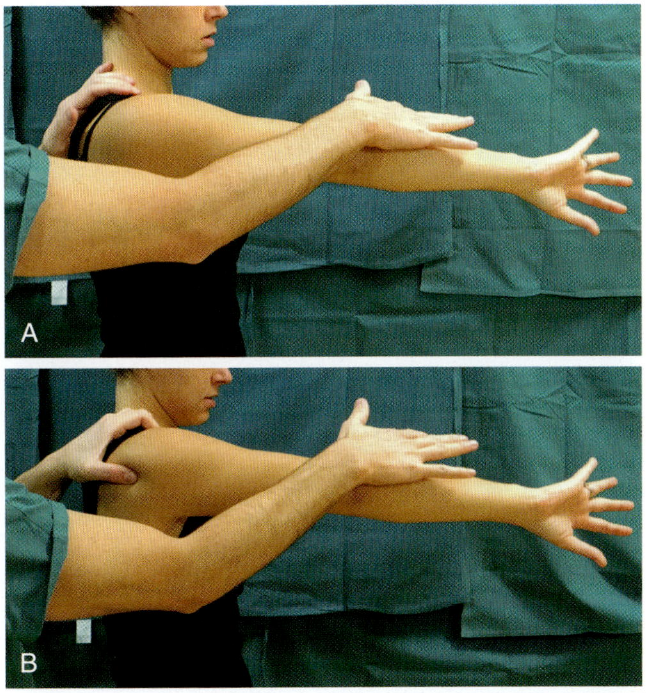

Fig. 1P.2 Porcellini test during shoulder examination. With the examiner standing behind the patient, the patient's arm is forward flexed to 90 degrees, adducted 10 to 15 degrees, and maximally internally rotated. After stabilizing the scapula with one hand, the patient is asked to elevate the arm against the resistance, and the pain and strength are noted (**A**). The thumb of the examiner's hand is placed just lateral to the posterior joint line, maintaining a moderate anterior force to prevent the humeral head from subluxating posteriorly, and then the maneuver is repeated. The test result is considered positive if the pain with or without weakness noticed during the first maneuver is reduced or eliminated during the second maneuver (**B**).

Clinical and Radiographic Evaluation of Shoulder Instability

The patient's clinical history should be carefully considered. Whereas the source of traumatic instability is easy to understand, the cause of MDI is often more difficult to establish and may depend on a variety of factors that include repetitive microtrauma, especially in individuals who practice overhead activities or sports; general laxity; and family history.

Symptoms are usually masked, especially in activities that patients have learned to avoid through compensatory movements.

The most common test for unidirectional traumatic glenohumeral instability is the "apprehension-relocation test" (Gerber & Ganz, 1984); those applied more often to evaluate MDI are the "sulcus test" (Matsen et al, 1991), the "load and shift test" (Gerber & Ganz, 1984), and the "Gagey test" (Gagey & Gagey, 2001) (Fig. 1P.1).

Patients with MDI often have a greater range of motion (ROM) in external rotation (ER) than internal rotation (IR) caused by posterior soft tissue retraction; the condition may lead to glenohumeral internal rotation deficit (GIRD), which is commonly seen in overhead athletes (Oyama et al, 2008). Walch (1996) has described ER exceeding 45 to 50 degrees with the arm adducted and the elbow flexed in patients with joint hyperlaxity. The authors have recently proposed the "Porcellini test" (Fig. 1P.2) for the preoperative diagnosis of posterior labral tears in patients with MDI and have demonstrated its excellent sensitivity and specificity (Morey et al, 2016). It has been suggested that in patients with shoulder instability, the examination should be extended to other joints, such as the knees, elbows, and spine, using Beighton's hypermobility score (Gaskill et al, 2011).

Radiologic evaluation of shoulder instability is primarily done by radiography in two standard views (anteroposterior and axillary), which depict the relationship between humeral head and glenoid surface and any bone loss and abnormalities, such as glenoid dysplasia. However, computed tomography (CT) allows quantification of humeral head (Hill-Sachs lesion) and glenoid bone loss (Fig. 1P.3). Over the past decade, three-dimensional (3D) CT scanning has acquired a key role in measuring the extent of humeral and glenoid bone defects. In particular, in the "PICO" method, the glenoid surface of the affected and contralateral shoulder is compared with software that calculates percent erosion (Provencher et al, 2010a); the result then guides the surgeon in selecting the most appropriate treatment. When the glenoid defect exceeds 15% to 20%, bone augmentation surgery may be required (Provencher et al, 2010b). The authors have recently demonstrated that the glenoid surface can be restored using the coracoid in patients with bone loss ranging from 20% to 34% (Paladini et al, 2016).

Magnetic resonance imaging (MRI) is the gold standard approach to assess shoulder instability because it affords optimal soft tissue, capsule, and ligament visualization. In MR arthrography, injection of contrast material into the intraarticular space accurately depicts labral lesions; the

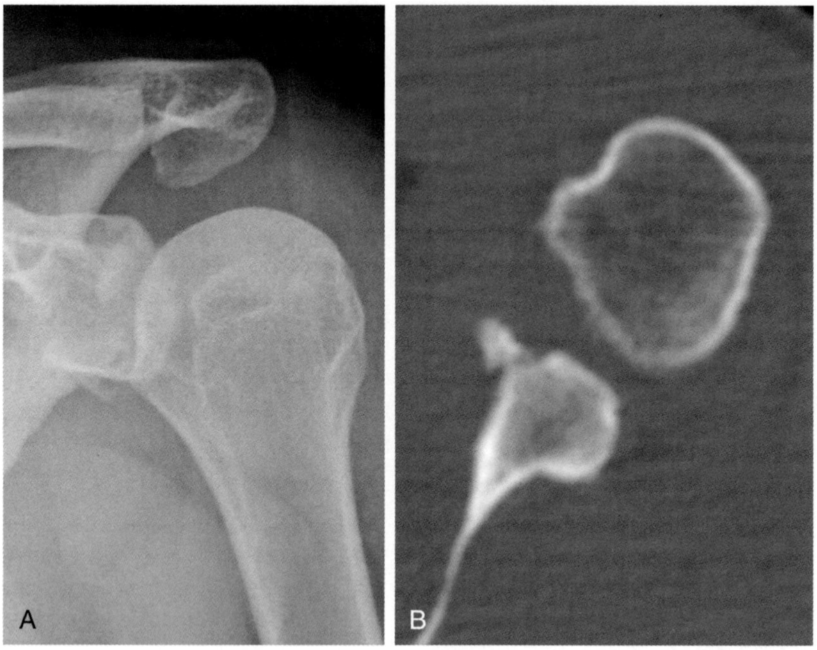

Fig. 1P.3 A bony Bankart lesion on radiography (**A**) and a computed tomography scan (**B**).

joint interval; the glenohumeral ligaments; and a number of conditions such as humeral avulsion of the glenohumeral ligament (HAGL), glenohumeral labrum articular disruption (GLAD), and superior labral pathology (SLAP) lesions (Dewing et al, 2008; Kim et al, 2007).

Whereas MRI examination of patients with traumatic shoulder instability often documents a Bankart lesion, patients with MDI typically exhibit increased joint space with capsule distention. Recent research has demonstrated that MRI in the "ABER" position provides excellent visualization of the capsule distention typical of MDI (Schaeffeler et al, 2014). Dynamic 3D MRI is expected to acquire an important role both in diagnosis and in the selection of treatment options (Tempelaere et al, 2016).

Conservative Treatment

In the authors' view, the first episode of anterior instability should be managed conservatively, beginning with 21 days of shoulder immobilization in a brace. Some researchers have found no differences in the recurrence of instability in patients immobilized for different periods of time, but others have reported better outcomes with an ER brace (Dodson & Cordasco, 2008); more recently, a review has found no improvement in recurrence with immobilization in ER (Whelan et al, 2016). Patients should then begin a rehabilitation protocol directed at ROM recovery and strengthening of scapular and humeral muscles, especially the scapular stabilizers (Dodson & Cordasco, 2008). The authors believe that immediate surgical management should be reserved for young elite athletes, who would otherwise experience a high rate of recurrence. In a study by Crall and colleagues (2012), recurrence was related to patient age (30 years or younger) and treatment (conservative or surgical). An earlier investigation had found a 92% rate of recurrence in cadets treated conservatively after the first dislocation (Wheeler et al, 1989).

Treatment for MDI is predominantly conservative and follows a specific protocol (Burkhead & Rockwood, 1992). The program includes proprioceptive neuromuscular exercises that improve dynamic shoulder stability and strengthen the scapular stabilizers, the glenohumeral protector muscles such as the subscapularis, and the scapulohumeral rhythm. This protocol was also able to restore passive stability and improve active control of the shoulder (Magarey & Jones, 2003). The authors have recently described the favorable effect of neuromuscular taping and a scapula-stabilizing T-shirt in helping scapular stabilization (Pellegrini et al, 2016).

Several researchers have described good outcomes of conservative treatment in patients with MDI. Rowe (1956) reported on results with a short-term follow-up, and Burkhead and Rockwood (1992) have obtained good to excellent outcomes in 80% of their MDI patients who underwent rehabilitation. In contrast, Misamore and colleagues (2005) have described poor outcomes of conservative management in young active athletes, suggesting that this population should be treated by surgery. Of course, shoulders in which conservative treatment has failed to restore stability can be managed by surgery, with high success rates.

Surgical Treatment

Surgical treatment is reserved for patients with capsulolabral tears, either isolated or associated with glenoid bone fracture or loss. Surgery provides anatomic restoration, reattachment of the capsulolabral complex to the glenoid, and capsular tensioning, which is usually required after the first dislocation episode (Provencher et al, 2010b). Surgeons should always take into consideration the rate of recurrence after the first dislocation, patient age; his or her life activities; and, in older patients, any associated lesions (Boone & Arciero, 2010; Porcellini et al, 2007, 2011).

Arthroscopic Approach

The authors usually evaluate the shoulder in the operating room. Here, with the patient under general anesthesia, the unstable joint is compared with the contralateral joint, and the severity and direction of instability are assessed for the last time before surgery.

The arthroscopic procedure is performed under general anesthesia combined with an interscalene brachial plexus block. The patient is placed in lateral decubitus position (other surgeons prefer the beach-chair position) with the arm in 30 degrees of abduction and 15 degrees of forward flexion and 5 kg of traction.

The camera is inserted through the posterior portal, 2 cm inferior to the posterior angle of the acromion (Snyder, 2003). An anterior portal is developed by the inside-out technique using a Wissinger rod to find the correct position (Matthews et al, 1985); a 6-mm cannula is inserted under the long head of the biceps; with the help of a needle, a third 8.5-mm cannula is passed over the subscapularis tendon, lateral to the coracoid process, by the outside-in technique (Wolf, 1989).

A general intraarticular examination is performed to confirm the diagnosis and identify all lesions. The camera is subsequently moved to the anterior portal, enabling easier visualization and treatment of anterior labral tears, beginning with labrum and capsule mobilization. The anchors should be implanted into the glenoid on the border between cartilage and bone, not into the glenoid neck (Snyder & Strafford, 1993), at a 45-degree angle and more proximal in relation to the capsule portion that needs tensioning. A suture shuttle relay (Linvatec, Key Largo, FL) is a useful tool to help pass the wires through the capsule and the glenoid labrum. The same procedure is applied for all anchor wires. Anchor number as well as degree of capsule and labrum tensioning are based on surgeon experience, lesion type, and injured tissue. Free wires for anterior or posterior capsule plication (simple suture) or absorbable anchors can be used in patients with MDI. Reasons for poor outcomes include missed glenoid bone loss and joint hyperlaxity (Boileau et al, 2006). Labrum and capsule repair may also be performed by an open deltopectoral approach and a subscapularis muscle split (Rhee et al, 2006). Because open and arthroscopic repair approaches share a similar failure rate (8% and 8.5%, respectively) (Harris et al, 2013), the authors prefer the less invasive approach.

In a 2009 study reporting the outcomes of arthroscopic capsulolabral repair in patients with instability but no bone defects (Porcellini et al, 2009), the authors found that young male patients had a higher rate of recurrence in relation to the time elapsed since the first episode of dislocation. The outcome of arthroscopic repair of bony Bankart lesions was also poorer in patients with chronic instability than in those with an acute condition (Fig. 1P.4) (Porcellini et al, 2002, 2007).

There is no consensus regarding the percent humeral bone loss that gives rise to instability and that can be managed by arthroscopy. According to Sekiya and colleagues (2009), defects exceeding 12.5% should be treated by open surgery. Wolf and coworkers (2004) have described an arthroscopic procedure involving infraspinatus tenodesis and posterior capsulodesis, called *remplissage*, to treat medium to large humeral head defects exhibiting the "engaging" mechanism in patients with limited glenoid bone loss. During the arthroscopic procedure, the engagement can be evaluated dynamically with the arm in the "ABER" position (Burkhart & De Beer, 2000). Recently, Di Giacomo et al (2016) have demonstrated the important role of the orientation and position of the humeral bone defect and its possible relationship to glenoid erosion, identifying off-track–on-track lesions and proposing a new treatment algorithm. The present authors have begun to use the new approach, besides the well-established "PICO" method, carefully assessing the position of the humeral bone defect shown on the MRI or CT scans and identifying the engaging lesions that are more amenable to treatment with a Bristow-Latarjet procedure.

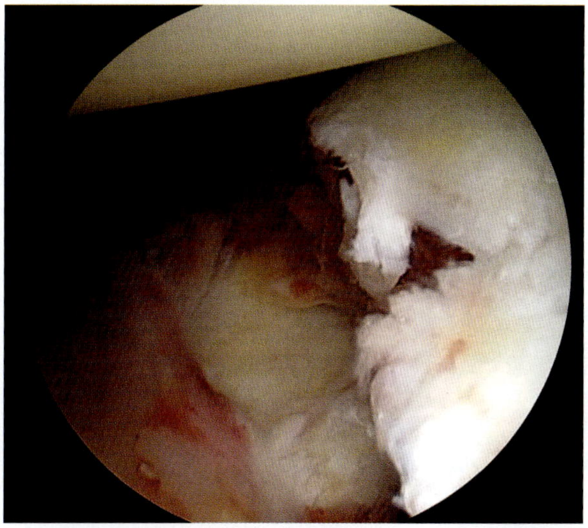

Fig. 1P.4 Arthroscopic view of a bony Bankart lesion.

In the *remplissage* technique (Video 1P.1), a bone bur passed through the posterior portal is used for debridement and identification of the bone defect; then a suture anchor is implanted in the middle of the defect using grasper wires passed through the capsule and the inferior portion of the infraspinatus tendon (Purchase et al, 2008). Optimal anchor positioning and soft tissue tensioning are crucial to avoid joint stiffness (Elkinson et al, 2013). Implantation of resorbable devices in the glenoid bone has been reported to cause glenoid rim fracture and hence recurrence of dislocation, even in patients exposed to low-impact traumas caused by formation of osteolysis around the devices (Augusti et al, 2015; Fritsch et al, 2010). The authors have recently reported excellent outcomes of humeral bone defects treated with *remplissage* (Merolla et al, 2015); the findings of this study show that fixation of the infraspinatus tendon to the humeral head defect induced a loss of ER with the arm at the side; conversely, ER with the shoulder abducted was satisfactory and not significantly different compared with the contralateral shoulder. Although these results are not explained by the available data, it is reasonable to hypothesize that a stiff, tight posterior capsule may affect humeral head rotation when the arm is adducted,

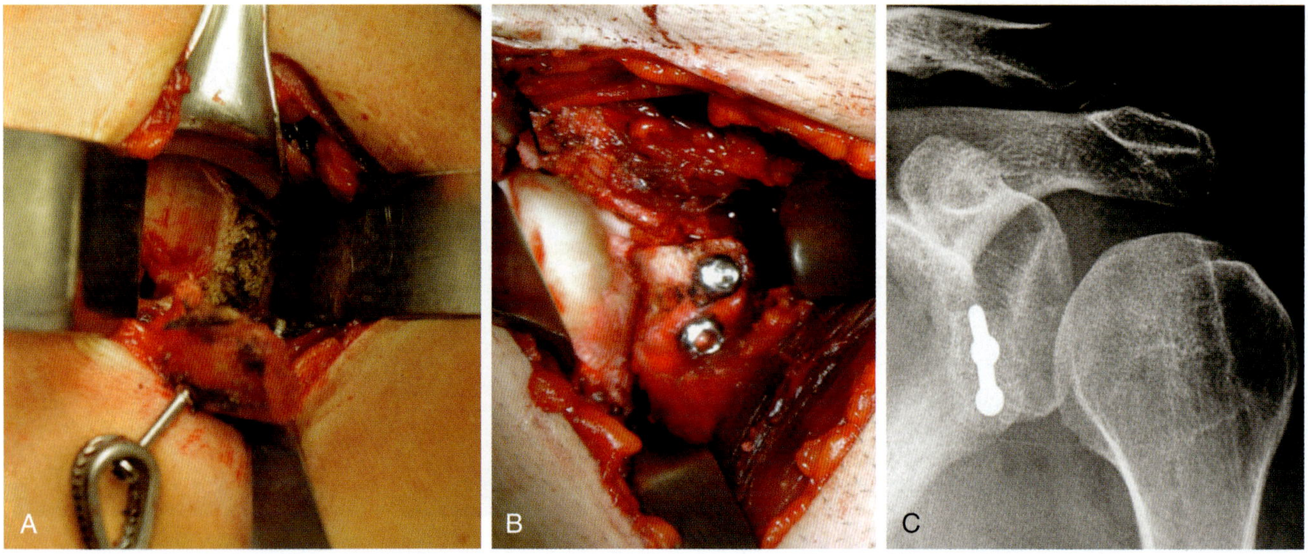

Fig. 1P.5 Bristow-Latarjet procedure. **A,** Glenoid preparation for grafting. **B,** Positioning of the coracoid graft. **C,** Postoperative radiographs.

inducing an anterosuperior shift of the humeral head that enhances ER. The surgical technique may also play a role because anchor fixation in the valley of the humeral head defect with sutures passed 1 cm more medial through the posterior soft tissues involves significantly reduced ER and IR and greater joint stiffness than anchor placement in the defect valley or the humeral head rim. These biomechanical considerations prompted us to place the anchor in the defect valley and to pass the sutures close to the anchor, not medially, to reduce the risk of severe joint stiffness. As noted earlier, none of our patients reported ER limitation because the ROM loss in this plane affected neither daily activities nor sport participation. Of course, the technique should be applied with caution in overhead athletes, whose delicate biomechanical equilibrium is easily affected.

The surgical approach to symptomatic MDI can be arthroscopic or open, even though most surgeons prefer the former technique. A recent systematic review (Elkinson et al, 2013) has shown that the two approaches are associated with similar rates of failure, return to sports, ER loss, and complications. The arthroscopic procedure involves multiple capsular plications, retensioning of the anterior and posterior band of the inferior glenohumeral ligament, and augmentation of labrum thickness. In the standard arthroscopic approach described earlier, passing the camera through the posterior portal affords accurate visualization of the joint space and allows the surgeon to choose the number of anchors required, decide the amount of plication looking for a positive "drive-through sign" and establish the degree of joint laxity. Capsular plication should be performed 1 cm lateral to the labrum insertion. An absorbable wire is passed through the anterior capsule using a 45-degree tool, from 5 to 4 o'clock, pushing the capsule in superomedial direction (Lubiatowski et al, 2012). The same step is performed posteriorly with capsule plication in the 6 o'clock position. The technique has achieved good to excellent results in 80% to 94% of patients with MDI (Cicak et al, 2005). Fleega and Shewy (2012) have reported complete ROM restoration after surgery with a failure rate of 4%. Some of the poorest results have been described in patients practicing intense sports activity (Cicak et al, 2005; Lubiatowski et al, 2012) and in MDI compared with unidirectional instability (Lubiatowski et al, 2012).

Open Approach

The failure rate of arthroscopy begins to increase when the anteroinferior glenoid defect approaches 20% to 25%. These patients can be managed by an open approach using a bone-block technique such as the Eden Hybinette procedure (Longo et al, 2014); the Bristow-Latarjet technique, in which the coracoid is grafted onto the glenoid defect, is the most reliable of such procedures. The deltopectoral approach is used most frequently. The coracoid process is easily identified after incision of the clavipectoral fascia; the coracoid osteotomy is made with a 90-degree saw at the level of the knee, carefully preserving the conjoined tendon; the fragment is mobilized carefully avoiding injury to the musculocutaneous nerve. The coracoid graft is prepared with debridement followed by drilling of two holes for 4-mm half-threaded screws. Splitting of the subscapularis muscle allows reaching the joint capsule and provides better results than the "L" technique in terms of postoperative strength recovery (Paladini et al, 2012). Then a vertical incision is performed to access the joint space. The glenoid neck is easily identified and prepared with debridement and two holes for the bicortical screws to fix the coracoid graft in the appropriate position on the glenoid surface (Mizuno et al, 2014). The Bristow-Latarjet procedure has a "triple effect" that is based on (1) the bone support provided by the coracoid graft, which enlarges the platform of the inverted-pear glenoid; (2) a sling effect because the conjoined tendon and the inferior portion of the subscapularis stabilize the anteroinferior glenohumeral joint in the ABER position; and (3) repair of the capsule with the coracoacromial ligament attached to the graft, if required (Latarjet, 1954). Graft positioning in the anterior glenoid neck is critical to avoid impingement with the humeral head laterally and a failure of the procedure medially (Fig. 1P.5) (Gupta et al, 2015).

Excellent outcomes, with a failure rate of 3.5%, have recently been described in professional athletes with

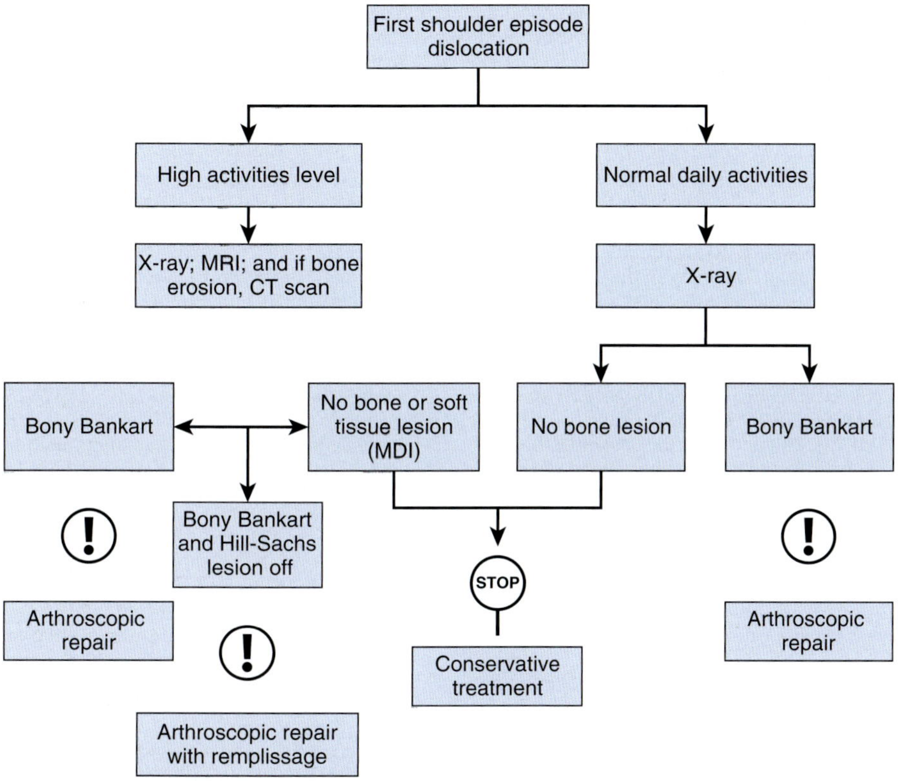

Fig. 1P.6 Treatment algorithm proposed by the authors facing a patient's first episode of dislocation. *CT,* Computed tomography; *MDI,* multidirectional instability; *MRI,* magnetic resonance imaging.

anterior glenoid bone loss treated with the Bristow-Latarjet procedure (Cerciello et al, 2012). Lafosse et al (2007, 2010) have proposed an arthroscopic Latarjet procedure. The arthroscopic Bristow-Latarjet approach is still in the hands of a small number of surgeons because of its high (10%) rate of complications involving nerves, vessels, and the bone graft (Athwal, 2016; Taverna et al, 2013). The authors believe that despite its technically highly demanding nature, the arthroscopic Bristow-Latarjet approach is useful because it combines the advantages of arthroscopy with the low failure rate of the Bristow-Latarjet technique.

Conclusion

Shoulder instability is still a challenge for orthopedic surgeons both in terms of diagnostic approach and of treatment selection. Accurate clinical examination is crucial to diagnose the type of instability and to select the imaging approach that will support and confirm the diagnosis. Advances in radiologic and surgical techniques have already improved the operative approach to first-time traumatic shoulder dislocation.

The authors prefer open surgery to treat medium to large bone defects in patients who are involved in contact sports, in whom the recurrence rate is very high. Patients with small defects can be treated with an arthroscopic approach such as the Bankart repair, an open procedure that can be performed by arthroscopy with clear benefit. The treatment algorithm proposed by the authors is reported in Fig. 1P.6.

In the authors' view, MDI requires careful management, which in the majority of patients should be primarily conservative; a surgical arthroscopic approach should be adopted only in case of its failure.

References

Athwal GS, Meislin R, Getz C, Weinstein D, Favorito P. Short-term complications of the arthroscopic Latarjet procedure: a North American experience. *Arthroscopy.* 2016;(16):S0749–S8063:00239-5.

Augusti CA, Paladini P, Campi F, Merolla G, Bigoni M, Porcellini G. Anterior glenoid rim fracture following use of resorbable devices for glenohumeral stabilization. *Orthop J Sports Med.* 2015;3(6).

Boileau P, Villalba M, Héry JY, et al. Risk factors for recurrence of shoulder instability after arthroscopic Bankart repair. *J Bone Joint Surg Am.* 2006;88:1755–1763.

Boone JL, Arciero RA. First-time anterior shoulder dislocations: has the standard changed? *Br J Sports Med.* 2010;44(5):355–360.

Burkhart SS, De Beer JF. Traumatic glenohumeral bone defects and their relationship to failure of arthroscopic Bankart repairs: significance of the inverted-pear glenoid and the humeral engaging Hill-Sachs lesion. *Arthroscopy.* 2000;16:677–694.

Burkhead WZ, Rockwood CA Jr. Treatment of instability of the shoulder with an exercise program. *J Bone Joint Surg Am.* 1992;74:890–896.

Cerciello S, Edwards TB, Walch G. Chronic anterior glenohumeral instability in soccer players: results for a series of 28 shoulders treated with the Latarjet procedure. *J Orthop Traumatol.* 2012;13:197–202.

Cicak N, Klobucar H, Bicanic G, Trsek D. Arthroscopic extracapsular plication to treat multidirectional instability of the shoulder. *Arthroscopy.* 2005;21:1278.

Crall TS, Bishop JA, Guttman D, Kocher M, Bozic K, Lubowitz JH. Cost-effectiveness analysis of primary arthroscopic stabilization versus non-operative treatment for first-time anterior glenohumeral dislocations. *Arthroscopy.* 2012;28:1755–1765.

Dewing CB, McCormick F, Bell SJ, et al. An analysis of capsular area in patients with anterior, posterior, and multidirectional shoulder instability. *Am J Sports Med.* 2008;36:515–522.

Di Giacomo G, Golijanin P, Sanchez G, Provencher MT. Radiographic Analysis of the Hill-Sachs Lesion in Anteroinferior Shoulder Instability After First-Time Dislocations. *Arthroscopy.* 2016;32(8):1509–1514.

Dodson CC, Cordasco FA. Anterior glenohumeral joint dislocations. *Orthop Clin North Am.* 2008;39:507–518.

Elkinson I, Giles JW, Boons HW, et al. The shoulder remplissage procedure for Hill-Sachs defects: does technique matter? *J Shoulder Elbow Surg.* 2013;22:835–841.

Fleega BA, El Shewy MT. Arthroscopic inferior capsular shift: long-term follow-up. *Am J Sports Med.* 2012;40:1126–1132.

Fritsch BA, Arciero RA, Taylor DC. Glenoid rim fracture after anchor repair: a report of 4 cases. *Am J Sports Med.* 2010;38(8):1682–1686.

Gagey OJ, Gagey N. The hyperabduction test. *J Bone Joint Surg Br.* 2001;83:69–74.

Gaskill TR, Taylor DC, Millett PJ. Management of multidirectional instability of the shoulder. *J Am Acad Orthop Surg.* 2011;19:758–767.

Gerber C, Ganz R. Clinical assessment of instability of the shoulder: with special reference to anterior and posterior drawer tests. *J Bone Joint Surg Br.* 1984;66:551–556.

Gupta A, Delaney R, Petkin K, Lafosse L. Complications of the Latarjet procedure. *Curr Rev Musculoskelet Med.* 2015;8:59–66.

Harris JD, Gupta AK, Mall NA, et al. Long term outcomes after Bankart shoulder stabilization. *Arthroscopy.* 2013;29:920–933.

Kim KC, Rhee KJ, Shin HD, Kim YM. Estimating the dimensions of the rotator interval with use of magnetic resonance arthrography. *J Bone Joint Surg Am.* 2007;89(11):2450–2455.

Lafosse L, Boyle S, Gutierrez-Aramberri M, Shah A, Meller R. Arthroscopic latarjet procedure. *Orthop Clin North Am.* 2010;41:393–405.

Lafosse L, Lejeune E, Bouchard A, Kakuda C, Gobezie R, Kochhar T. The arthroscopic Latarjet procedure for the treatment of anterior shoulder instability. *Arthroscopy.* 2007;23:1242.e1–1242.e5.

Latarjet M. Treatment of recurrent dislocation of the shoulder. *Lyon Chir.* 1954;49:994–997.

Longo UG, Rizzello G, Loppini M, et al. Multidirectional instability of the shoulder: a systematic review. *Arthroscopy.* 2015;31(12):2431–2443.

Lubiatowski P, Ogrodowicz P, Wojtaszek M, Breborowicz M, Długosz J, Romanowski L. Arthroscopic capsular shift technique and volume reduction. *Eur J Orthop Surg Traumatol.* 2012;22:437–441.

Magarey ME, Jones MA. Dynamic evaluation and early management of altered motor control around the shoulder complex. *Man Ther.* 2003;8:195–206.

Matsen FA, Harryman DT, Sidles JA. Mechanics of glenohumeral instability. *Clin Sports Med.* 1991;10:783–788.

Matthews LS, Zarins B, Michael RH, Helfet DL. Anterior portal selection for shoulder. *Arthroscopy.* 1985;1:33–39.

Merolla G, Paladini P, Di Napoli G, Campi F, Porcellini G. Outcomes of arthroscopic Hill-Sachs remplissage and anterior Bankart repair: a retrospective controlled study including ultrasound evaluation of posterior capsulotenodesis and infraspinatus strength assessment. *Am J Sports Med.* 2015;43(2):407–414.

Merolla G, De Falco M, Porcellini G. Traumatic and multidirectional glenohumeral instability: clinical biomechanics, treatment and results. *GIOT.* 2016;42:1–14.

Misamore GW, Sallay PI, Didelot W. A longitudinal study of patients with multidirectional instability of the shoulder with seven- to ten-year follow-up. *J Shoulder Elbow Surg.* 2005;14:466–470.

Mizuno N, Denard PJ, Raiss P, Melis B, Walch G. Long-term results of the Latarjet procedure for anterior instability of the shoulder. *J Shoulder Elbow Surg.* 2014;23:1691–1699.

Morey VM, Singh H, Paladini P, Merolla G, Phadke V, Porcellini G. The Porcellini test: a novel test for accurate diagnosis of posterior labral tears of the shoulder: comparative analysis with the established tests. *Musculoskelet Surg.* 2016;100:199–205.

Oyama S, Myers JB, Wassinger CA, Daniel Ricci R, Lephart SM. Asymmetric resting scapular posture in healthy overhead athletes. *J Athl Train.* 2008;43:565–570.

Paladini P, Singla R, Merolla G, Porcellini G. Latarjet procedure: is the coracoid enough to restore the glenoid surface? *Int Orthop.* 2016;40(8):1675–1681.

Paladini P, Merolla G, De Santis E, Campi F, Porcellini G. Long-term subscapularis strength assessment after Bristow-Latarjet procedure: isometric study. *J Shoulder Elbow Surg.* 2012;21(1):42–47.

Pellegrini A, Pogliacomi F, Costantino C, et al. Does scapula stabilizing t-shirt help over-head athletes in shoulder discomfort? A randomized control study. *Acta Biomed.* 2016;87(suppl 1):84–89.

Porcellini G, Campi F, Paladini P. Arthroscopic approach to acute bony Bankart lesion. *Arthroscopy.* 2002;18(7):764–769.

Porcellini G, Paladini P, Campi F, Paganelli M. Long-term outcome of acute versus chronic bony Bankart lesions managed arthroscopically. *Am J Sports Med.* 2007;35(12):2067–2072.

Porcellini G, Caranzano F, Campi F, Pellegrini A, Paladini P. Glenohumeral instability and rotator cuff tear. *Sports Med Arthrosc.* 2011;19(4): 348–353.

Porcellini G, Campi F, Pegreffi F, Castagna A, Paladini P. Predisposing factors for recurrent shoulder dislocation after arthroscopic treatment. *J Bone Joint Surg Am.* 2009;91(11):2537–2542.

Provencher MT, Bhatia S, Ghodadra NS, et al. Recurrent shoulder instability: current concepts for evaluation and management of glenoid bone loss. *J Bone Joint Surg Am.* 2010a;92:133–151.

Provencher MT, Ghodadra N, Romeo AA. Arthroscopic management of anterior instability: pearls, pitfalls, and lessons learned. *Orthop Clin North Am.* 2010b;41:325–337.

Purchase RJ, Wolf EM, Hobgood ER, Pollock ME, Smalley CC. Hill-Sachs "remplissage": an arthroscopic solution for the engaging Hill-Sachs lesion. *Arthroscopy.* 2008;24:723–726.

Rhee YG, Ha JH, Cho NS. Anterior shoulder stabilization in collision athletes: arthroscopic versus open Bankart repair. *Am J Sports Med.* 2006;34:979–985.

Rowe CR. Prognosis in dislocations of the shoulder. *J Bone Joint Surg Am.* 1956;38:957–977.

Schaeffeler C, Waldt S, Bauer JS, et al. MR arthrography including abduction and external rotation images in the assessment of traumatic multidirectional instability of the shoulder. *Eur Radiol.* 2014;24:1376–1385.

Sekiya JK, Wickwire AC, Stehle JH, Debski RE. Hill-Sachs defects and repair using osteoarticular allograft transplantation: biomechanical analysis using a joint compression model. *Am J Sports Med.* 2009;37: 2459–2466.

Snyder SJ, Strafford BB. Arthroscopic management of instability of the shoulder. *Orthopedics.* 1993;16:993–1002.

Snyder SJ. *Shoulder Arthroscopy.* New York: Lippincott Williams and Wilkins; 2003:22–28.

Taverna E, Ufenast H, Broffoni L, Garavaglia G. Arthroscopically assisted Latarjet procedure: a new surgical approach for accurate coracoid graft placement and compression. *Int J Shoulder Surg.* 2013;7(3):120–123.

Tempelaere C, Pierrart J, Lefèvre-Colau MM, et al. Dynamic three-dimensional shoulder MRI during active motion for investigation of rotator cuff diseases. *PLoS One.* 2016;11(7):e0158563.

te Slaa RL, Wijffels MP, Brand R, Marti RK. The prognosis following acute primary glenohumeral dislocation. *J Bone Joint Surg Br.* 2004;86:58–64.

Walch G. Chronic anterior glenohumeral instability. *J Boné Joint Surg Br.* 1996;78(4):670–677.

Wheeler JH, Ryan JB, Arciero RA, Molinari RN. Arthroscopic versus non-operative treatment of acute shoulder dislocations in young athletes. *Arthroscopy.* 1989;5(3):213–217.

Whelan DB, Kletke SN, Schemitsch G, Chahal J. Immobilization in external rotation versus internal rotation after primary anterior shoulder dislocation: a meta-analysis of randomized controlled trials. *Am J Sports Med.* 2016;44(2):521–532.

Wolf EM, Pollack ME. Hill-Sachs "remplissage": an arthroscopic solution for the engaging Hill-Sachs lesion. *Arthroscopy.* 2004;20:e14–e15.

Wolf EM. Anterior portals in shoulder arthroscopy. *Arthroscopy.* 1989;5:201–208.

1-1Q INTERNATIONAL PERSPECTIVE: JAPAN

NOBUYUKI YAMAMOTO, MD, PhD and EIJI ITOI, MD, PhD

Introduction

The Bristow procedure was used most in the 1980s and 1990s (Fig. 1Q.1). A review of the Japanese database (*Igaku Chuo Zasshi* [ICHUSHI]) indicated 189 articles related to the Bristow procedure. Since the 2000s, arthroscopic Bankart repair has become the most common procedure. The open Bankart and Bristow procedures were widely performed in Japan, but the clinical outcome of these procedures was not satisfactory in contact or collision athletes compared with noncontact athletes (Morioka, 1994). Some surgeons started to use a combined Bankart-Bristow procedure for contact and collision athletes. This chapter discusses how the surgical approach has been changed over the past 40 years in Japan, including surgical techniques and their clinical outcomes.

A Combined Bankart and Modified Bristow Procedure

Minoru Yoneda, one of the pioneers of shoulder arthroscopic surgery in Japan, reported good clinical outcomes with the Bankart procedure augmented by coracoid transfer (open Bankart and modified Bristow procedure) in contact athletes with recurrent anterior instability (Yoneda et al, 1999). The distal 1 to 1.5 cm of the coracoid tip was osteotomized with the conjoined tendon. The subscapularis tendon was divided from the anterior capsule. The Bankart lesion was repaired with the use of metal suture anchors. The capsular flap was shifted superiorly and was attached to the glenoid rim. The superior margin of the capsular flap was also sutured to the capsular portion of the supraspinatus tendon.

After the Bankart repair, the coracoid tip was transferred to the glenoid neck. According to the Rowe score,

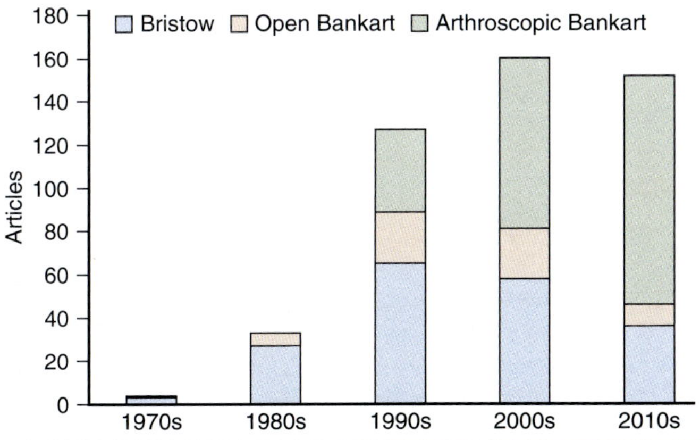

Fig. 1Q.1 The number of articles published in Japanese. The Bristow procedure was the most common procedure in the 1980s and 1990s. Since the 2000s, arthroscopic Bankart repair has become the most common procedure.

79 shoulders (93%) were graded as excellent or good. The recurrence rate was 1.2% at a mean follow-up period of 5.8 years. The mean losses of range of motion (ROM) compared with the uninvolved side were 3 degrees for forward elevation, 15 degrees for external rotation with the arm in adduction, and 7 degrees for external rotation at 90 degrees of abduction. After open Bankart and modified Bristow procedure, weakness of the muscle strength of the subscapularis was a concern because the subscapularis was separated at its insertion on the lesser tuberosity. The influence of rotational muscle strength on shoulder function after this procedure was investigated (Amako et al, 2008). Forty patients were measured with use of an isometric dynamometer at 12 months postoperatively. Their results indicated that sports activities should be delayed until 9 to 12 months after this procedure because the peak torque continued to increase until 12 months postoperatively.

Although the rate of recurrence after the open Bankart and modified Bristow procedures was very low as described, loss of ROM was observed postoperatively. Recently, an all-arthroscopic technique of a combined Bankart and modified Bristow procedure was reported by Suzuki et al (2013). They performed a combination of open Bankart repair and modified Bristow procedure in contact and collision athletes between 2007 and 2010. Since 2011, this procedure was arthroscopically performed. Suzuki et al's surgical technique was different from Boileau et al's (2010), in which seven portals were used and a specific guide, which was not commercially available in Japan, was used to insert a guide pin. In Suzuki et al's technique, five portals were used, and one of them was the Posteromedial (PM) portal, which was created by an outside-in technique through the pectoralis major muscle and was located 7 cm medial and 7 cm inferior to the tip of the coracoid process.

The subscapularis muscle was arthroscopically divided at the middle portion of the subscapularis. The coracoid fragment was arthroscopically osteotomized and fixed in the standing position with one cannulated screw on the glenoid neck. After the coracoid process was fixed, the capsulolabral complex was reattached on the glenoid rim using suture anchors. They reported excellent clinical results of this arthroscopic technique without any recurrence at a mean follow-up period of 25 months. The patients returned to contact or collision sports at mean 4.1 months. The mean ROMs were 170 degrees in forward elevation, 63 degrees in external rotation with the arm in adduction, and 90 degrees in external rotation at 90 degrees of abduction. These ROM results were better that those of open Bankart and modified Bristow procedures. Although the authors reported that there were no complications related to nerve injuries (musculocutaneous or axillary nerve), we need to be careful about the complications when performing this procedure. In addition, this arthroscopic procedure is technically demanding.

More recently, Tasaki et al (2015) introduced a new hybrid procedure performed in rugby players: a combination of an arthroscopic Bankart repair and an open Bristow procedure (Video 1Q.1). It seems easier to perform compared with that of Suzuki et al. In their technique, open Bristow procedure was performed first followed by arthroscopic Bankart repair. The subscapularis was separated in the direction of its fibers. After the coracoacromial ligament and the tendon of the pectoralis minor were severed from the coracoid process, the coracoid process was dissected. A 4.0-mm cannulated cancellous screw was used to fix the coracoid process to the anterior glenoid. Next, arthroscopic Bankart repair was performed. There were no recurrent dislocations at a mean follow-up period of 30 months. They concluded that this procedure was effective in preventing recurrent dislocation in rugby players; however, some players were not happy with their performance such as tackling probably because of the limited ROM, muscle weakness, or both.

Thus, a Bristow or combined Bankart and Bristow procedure has been widely performed in Japan. However, the Latarjet procedure, which is also one of coracoid transfer procedures, has gained popularity in Japan as in Europe. This is because complications such as nonunion of the coracoid process or screw breakage or migration are less common in the Latarjet procedure than in the Bristow procedure (Bouju et al, 2014). Although there have been some reports describing a high rate of postoperative osteoarthritis after Latarjet procedure, recent reports have shown that postoperative arthritis can be avoided by appropriate positioning of the coracoid bone graft (Walch, 1996; Walch & Boileau, 2000). Also, it has been demonstrated that the Latarjet procedure was effective even in patients with a large glenoid defect or in contact or collision athletes (Walch & Boileau, 2000). Searching the Japanese database ICHUSHI, which is a free full-text archive of biomedical and life sciences journal literature at the Japan Medical Abstracts Society, 15 articles were found since 2010 with the Latarjet procedure. It is more and more commonly performed in Japan.

Other Surgical Techniques

Katsuya Nobuhara, one of the founding members of the Japan Shoulder Society, modified the original Putti-Platt procedure and called it the N-H method (Nobuhara, 2013). There are several differences between the N-H method and the original Putti-Platt procedure: smaller incision, no resection of the conjoined tendon, the way to cut the subscapularis tendon and joint capsule, and the way to reattach the subscapularis tendon to the glenoid rim. A 5-cm-long longitudinal incision is made lateral to the coracoid process. The coracoacromial ligament is resected. With the arm in external rotation, three nonabsorbable stay sutures are placed at 2.5 cm medial to the bicipital groove. Then the subscapularis tendon is cut at 2.5 cm from its insertion to the lessor tuberosity. The medial stump of the subscapularis tendon is pulled laterally and sutured to the medial side of the bicipital groove with nonabsorbable sutures.

From 1970 to 1999, 340 patients were treated using the N-H method. Recurrent dislocation occurred in only 3 patients (0.9%). Nobuhara (2013) reported a long-term follow-up of 52 shoulders with a mean of 14 years. All patients had a limitation of external rotation to various degrees: more than 60 degrees of external rotation at the side was achieved in 44 patients (85%); 10 to 60 degrees in 6 patients (12%), and severe limitation of less than 10 degrees in 2 patients (4%). The recurrence rate was 2%. There were no clinical scores reported in this study. He emphasized that suturing of the subscapularis tendon should be done with the arm in neutral rotation to prevent the limitation of external rotation.

Some performed the conventional open Bankart procedure with modifications without using any suture anchor. Ogawa et al (2010) reported an excellent clinical outcome with a 4.8% recurrence rate after open Bankart procedure at a mean follow-up of 8.7 years. In their technique, the bone groove was created on the scapular neck 3 to 4 mm medial to the glenoid edge, and bone tunnels were created using a curved awl for the sutures to pass through and reattach the capsulolabral complex. The superior remnant of the joint capsule was sutured in layers with the overlaid superior glenohumeral ligament and coracohumeral ligament, with the arm in external rotation. They investigated the extent of the progression of postoperative osteoarthritis after open Bankart repair (Ogawa et al, 2010). A total of 167 shoulders were reviewed at a mean follow-up of 8.7 years. Preoperative computed tomography showed osteoarthritis in 44 shoulders (26%), among which 12 shoulders (7%) showed osteoarthritis on the preoperative radiographs. Radiographs taken at follow-up revealed osteoarthritis in 30 shoulders (18%), of which 24 (80%) had had osteoarthritis proven by preoperative imaging. They concluded that most osteoarthritis observed postoperatively had developed even before surgery. The preoperative factors seemed to be deeply involved in the development of osteoarthritis They reported that the preoperative factors associated with the development of osteoarthritis were the number of preoperative subluxation episodes, the total number of dislocation episodes, male gender, and greater glenoid bone defect.

In 2007, Mizuno and Yoneda developed a new technique of arthroscopic Bankart repair (the double-anchor footprint fixation [DAFF] technique) simulating a conventional open transosseous Bankart repair with good clinical results (Fig. 1Q.2). The DAFF technique consisted of a trough preparation and double-anchor footprint fixation to obtain a greater contact area of the repair site similar to dual-row repair of a rotator cuff tear. They reported that there was no recurrence at a mean follow-up of 12 months, and 80% of the patients fully returned to their sports. This is very good

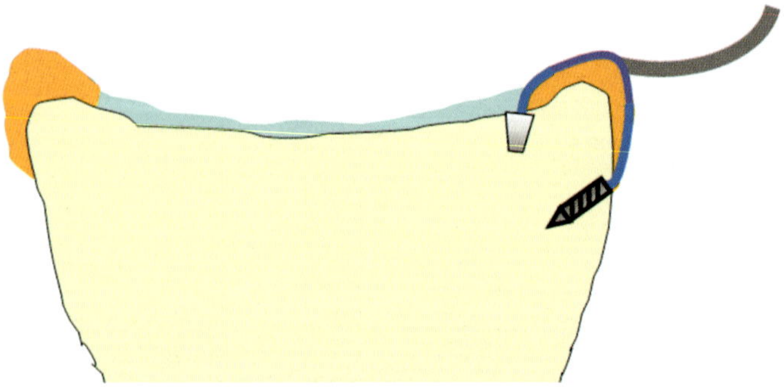

Fig. 1Q.2 Double-anchor footprint fixation technique. One suture anchor is placed on the articular surface of the glenoid, and another anchor is placed at the glenoid neck.

information because the construct resembles an open technique done with drill holes.

For patients with a large glenoid defect, iliac bone grafting was arthroscopically performed by Sugaya et al (2012). They described the short-term outcome after arthroscopic iliac bone grafting with capsulolabral reconstruction for 20 shoulders with a significant glenoid bone loss. The iliac crest was harvested with the patients in the supine position under general anesthesia. Arthroscopic iliac bone grafting was then performed in the beach-chair position followed by Bankart repair using suture anchors. Postoperative three-dimensional computed tomography performed more than 1 year after surgery showed optimal remodeling of the graft in 3, moderate remodeling and absorption in 4, and fair remodeling and distinct absorption in 3 patients. Although no patients experienced recurrence after the surgery, the position of the graft was strongly associated with postoperative bone remodeling and absorption. Although technically demanding, they concluded that arthroscopic iliac bone grafting in shoulders with a significant glenoid bone loss yielded successful outcomes with minimum morbidity.

References

Amako M, Imai T, Okamura K. Recovery of shoulder rotational muscle strength after a combined Bankart and modified Bristow procedure. *J Shoulder Elbow Surg*. 2008 Sep-Oct;17(5):738–743.

Boileau P, Mercier N, Roussanne Y, Thélu CÉ, Old J. Arthroscopic Bankart-Bristow-Latarjet procedure: the development and early results of a safe and reproducible technique. *Arthroscopy*. 2010;26(11):1434–1450.

Bouju Y, Gadéa F, Stanovici J, Moubarak H, Favard L. Shoulder stabilization by modified Latarjet-Patte procedure: results at a minimum 10 years' follow-up, and role in the prevention of osteoarthritis. *Orthop Traumatol Surg Res*. 2014;100(suppl 4):S213–S218.

Mizuno N, Yoneda M. Arthroscopic Bankart repair with a double anchor footprint fixation (DAFF) technique: a preliminary report. *Katakansetsu*. 2007;31(3):497–501.

Morioka K. Modified Bristow procedure (in Japanese). *Orthop Surg Traumatol*. 1994;37:1021–1027.

Nobuhara K. *The Shoulder. Its Function and Clinical Aspects*. Singapore: World Scientific Publishing; 2013:318–349.

Ogawa K, Yoshida A, Matsumoto H, Takeda T. Outcome of the open Bankart procedure for shoulder instability and development of osteoarthritis: a 5- to 20-year follow-up study. *Am J Sports Med*. 2010;38(8):1549–1557.

Sugaya H, Takahashi N, Kawai N, et al. Arthroscopic iliac bone grafting for unstable shoulders with significant glenoid bone loss. *Katakansetsu*. 2012;36(2):383–387.

Suzuki K, Nagai S, Uehara T, Tsutsui H. Arthroscopic Bankart-Bristow procedure for collision and contact athletes with traumatic anterior shoulder instability (in Japanese). *Katakansetsu*. 2013;37(2):527–530.

Tasaki A, Morita W, Yamakawa A, et al. Combined arthroscopic Bankart repair and coracoid process transfer to anterior glenoid for shoulder dislocation in rugby players: evaluation based on ability to perform sport-specific movements effectively. *Arthroscopy*. 2015;31(9):1693–1701.

Yoneda M, Hayashida K, Wakitani S, Nakagawa S, Fukushima S. Bankart procedure augmented by coracoid transfer for contact athletes with traumatic anterior shoulder instability. *Am J Sports Med*. 1999;27(1):21–26.

Walch G. Chronic anterior glenohumeral instability. *J Bone Joint Surg Br*. 1996;78(4):670–677.

Walch G, Boileau P. Latarjet-Bristow procedure for recurrent anterior instability. *Tech Shoulder Elbow Surg*. 2000;1(4):256–261.

1-1R REVISION ANTERIOR STABILIZATION: WORKUP, INDICATIONS, AND OUTCOMES

DAVID M. DARE, MD and RUSSELL F. WARREN, MD

Introduction

Acute anterior or anteroinferior instability is the most common injury pattern in shoulder instability. Numerous studies have demonstrated a high rate of recurrent dislocation in young, active patients. Recurrent instability rates can be as high as 94%. Given this exceedingly high rate, surgical repair is frequently advocated. Recent randomized controlled trials and a systematic review of level I and II studies have shown decreased rates of recurrence and improved outcomes after surgery (Chahal et al, 2012; Kirkley et al, 2005; Robinson et al, 2008). The goal of operative management is to restore stability by repairing the injured labrum or glenohumeral ligaments, and in some cases, retension a redundant capsule. Multiple studies in the previous decade have shown open and arthroscopic surgery to produce comparable results (Hobby et al, 2007).

Despite improved outcomes after primary stabilization surgery, persistent shoulder instability after surgery presents a challenging problem. The recurrence rate after surgery is reported to be between 3% and 25% (Bessiere et al, 2013; Owens et al, 2011; Uhorchak et al, 2000). Outcomes after revision surgery are inferior to primary surgery; therefore, the chief focus of the index surgery should be to prevent failure. It is critical that the surgeon identify all factors that predispose to failure (Table 1R.1). The most common reasons for recurrent instability can be identified in a careful preoperative history, physical examination, and certain imaging studies. In this chapter, we examine the most frequent causes of failure, evaluation in the setting of failure, and outcomes after revision shoulder stabilization.

Causes of Failure

Management of recurrent instability after a stabilization procedure requires identification of the specific causes of failure before developing a treatment course. Thorough investigation is imperative to avoid repeating potential errors and to appropriately counsel the patient on the risk of future instability.

Table 1R.1 Risk Factors for Recurrence After Bankart Repair

Patient factors	Young age
	Male sex
	Increased number of dislocations
	Number of prior procedures
Missed diagnoses	Significant anterior glenoid defect
	Large Hill-Sachs lesion
	HAGL lesion
	Capsular laxity
Technical errors	Medially placed glenoid anchors
	"High" placement of glenoid anchors
	Insufficient number of anchors
	Knot failure

HAGL, Humeral avulsion of the glenohumeral ligament.

Age and Gender

Age and gender are strongly correlated with recurrent instability after both primary open and arthroscopic stabilization. In a review of nearly 6000 patients, Wasserstein et al (2013) showed that patients younger than 20 years of age had a 12.6% risk of postoperative dislocation and a 7.7% revision rate after stabilization. In patients 29 years or older, in contrast, the risk of postoperative dislocation was 5.5%, and the revision rate was 2.8%. The increased risk of recurrence in young patients is attributed to increased soft tissue laxity, higher activity levels, decreased muscle bulk, and potentially poorer compliance with postoperative restrictions (Gwathmey & Warner, 2013; Randelli et al, 2012). Patients older than 40 years of age with persistent instability should be closely evaluated for a rotator cuff tear (Berbig et al, 1999).

Gender also seems to contribute to the recurrence rate because male patients have demonstrated an increased risk of instability after surgery (Porcellini et al, 2009). In a prospective, randomized clinical trial comparing open and arthroscopic stabilization, Mohtadi et al (2014) showed that recurrent instability was more likely in patients with a preoperative Hill-Sachs lesion and in male patients who were 25 years old and younger. The authors also showed a significantly higher recurrence rate in the arthroscopic group and suggested that open repair should be considered for this high-risk subgroup of young male patients. It should be noted, though, that the rate of participation in collision sports, although not significantly different between groups, was higher in the arthroscopic group (56% vs 44%). Participation in contact sports is a known risk factor for recurrent instability.

Activity

A large majority of patients who undergo shoulder stabilization are young, and their initial injuries are sustained during sporting activities. Consequently, failure secondary to a return to sport disproportionately affects this population. Tauber et al (2004) demonstrated that 85% of primary shoulder dislocations and 59% of recurrent dislocations after surgical stabilization were secondary to trauma. As expected, then, participation in collision or contact sports, particularly at higher levels of competition, has been shown to predict redislocation after both open and arthroscopic stabilization (Arce et al, 2012; Balg & Boileau, 2007; Porcellini et al, 2009; Randelli et al, 2012; Voos et al, 2010). Additionally, positional demands, such as those required by football linebackers and defensive backs, place them at increased risk of redislocation (Kaplan et al, 2005).

Previous Shoulder Stabilization

In a large retrospective analysis, Wasserstein et al (2013) demonstrated that patients with three or more dislocations have 10 times the risk of recurrent dislocation after stabilization and twice the risk of revision surgery. Both Randelli et al (2012) and Arce et al (2012) showed that the number of prior dislocations and the number of previous stabilization procedures negatively correlated with postsurgical outcomes. Marquardt et al (2007) also reported that patients with more than one stabilization surgery trended toward lower functional outcomes and patient satisfaction. Redislocation and revision surgery is progressively traumatizing to the bone and soft tissue. Bone loss, capsular attenuation, and distortion of native anatomy may lead to increased laxity.

Unaddressed Glenoid Defect

Glenoid bone loss is a well-recognized cause of failure in arthroscopic stabilization procedures. Burkhart & De Beer (2000) reported a 4% recurrence rate in those with minimal bone loss. This is compared with a 67% recurrence rate in those with significant bony deficiency. "Significant bone loss" was not quantified but rather was defined as a glenoid that assumed an "inverted pear" appearance on arthroscopic view. The authors concluded that these patients cannot be treated with a soft tissue procedure alone. Similarly, Tauber et al (2004) revealed that 51% of patients undergoing revision surgery had a bony Bankart lesion larger than 2 mm. An additional 5% possessed an attritional "eroded" anterior glenoid rim. Roughly 6 mm or less of bone anterior to the bare spot may confer significant bone loss (Burkhart & De Beer, 2000; Itoi et al, 2003; Mologne et al, 2007). In these patients, a soft tissue repair alone is likely insufficient.

Mologne et al (2007), though, proposed that arthroscopic Bankart repair was a good option in patients with 20% to 30% bone loss as long as the bony glenoid fragment could be incorporated into the repair. Arthroscopic repairs in the setting of attritional loss, however, were less predictable. These findings were corroborated in a systematic review (Randelli et al, 2012). The pooled data analysis demonstrated that the presence of a detached bony fragment did not increase the risk of failure compared to those patients without any glenoid bone defect. Kitayama et al (2015) proposed that arthroscopic osseous Bankart repair is an effective treatment for shoulders with more than 15% glenoid bone loss. In this series, there was a low rate of recurrence and a reconstitution of the glenoid morphology in the long term.

Compared with patients with a detached bony fragment, the risk of failure increases in patients with glenoid erosion. The "glenoid track" concept was developed to biomechanically quantify the effects of combined glenoid and humeral head bony defects on instability (Yamamoto et al, 2007). Clearly, anteroinferior bone loss contributes to a decrease in the functional length of the track. Moreover, progressive labral and bone loss increases the articular contact area and pressure across the glenohumeral joint under compressive loads (Greis et al, 2002). Thirty percent bone loss in the glenoid's anteroinferior quadrant resulted in a decreased contact area by 41% and increased the mean contact pressures in this quadrant by 300% to 400%. A soft tissue repair alone would be unlikely to withstand this overload at the soft tissue–glenoid interface.

Humeral Head Defect

A Hill-Sachs lesion decreases the "rotational arc length" of the humeral head on the glenoid. As first described by Burkhart & De Beer (2000), with progressive shoulder abduction and external rotation, large humeral head defects can engage the anterior glenoid rim and cause subluxation or dislocation. An engaging Hill-Sachs lesion was confirmed to be a risk factor for instability in further studies (Boileau et al, 2006; Randelli et al, 2012).

The size of a clinically relevant Hill-Sachs lesion has not been well established. Anecdotal evidence suggests that defects that occupy more than 20% of the humeral head predispose to instability and require surgical management. Elkinson et al (2012) showed that a 30% defect caused significant instability in abduction and external rotation, but a 15% head defect did not engage the glenoid rim in any position. The humeral head defect must be considered in conjunction with anterior glenoid bone loss because both contribute to a shortened glenoid track. Di Giacomo (2014) emphasized that the location and orientation of the humeral head lesion strongly correlates with instability. A more medially based defect oriented parallel to the anterior glenoid, for example, is more likely to engage the glenoid rim and cause subluxation or dislocation.

Capsular Laxity

Repeat dislocation results in progressively lax and redundant anterior capsular tissue. Failure to address capsular laxity is a common cause of stabilization failure (Meehan & Petersen, 2005; Rowe et al, 1984; Tauber et al, 2004; Zabinski et al, 1999). A biomechanical study showed that anterior capsular stretching occurs with or without labral disruption (Bigliani et al, 1992). Therefore incompetent anterior capsular tissue may be present even in the setting of Bankart repair. Rowe et al (1984) and Meehan et al (2005) demonstrated that 83% and 73%, respectively, of patients with a failed stabilization procedure had substantial capsular laxity. Capsular laxity has been confirmed by others to be an important cause of failure (Marquardt et al, 2007; Zabinski et al, 1999). Although capsular redundancy can be subtle, frank tears in the capsule or rotator interval are more conspicuous and should be repaired (Rhee & Cho, 2007). Last, it must be noted that humeral avulsion of the glenohumeral ligament (HAGL) is an infrequent but important cause of recurrent instability. A HAGL lesion occurs in roughly 10% of cases, and its diagnosis requires a high index of suspicion (Bui-Mansfield et al, 2007). Failure to treat a HAGL lesion may result in recurrent subluxation or dislocation (Rhee & Cho, 2007).

Technical Error

The goal of surgery is to restore the normal anatomy of the dynamic and active stabilizers of the glenohumeral joint, thereby preventing recurrent anterior instability without causing limitations in range of motion. The anterior band of the inferior glenohumeral ligament is the primary restraint to anterior translation with the arm in abduction and external rotation (O'Brien et al, 1989). The labrum and attached capsule and glenohumeral ligaments must be adequately mobilized and anatomically reduced to the glenoid to restore proper tension within the inferior glenohumeral complex (Bedi & Ryu, 2010; Boileau et al, 2006; Cole & Romeo, 2001). Suture anchors should be placed on the glenoid articular rim or 1 to 2 mm onto the face of the articular rim. Misplacement of the anchor medially on the glenoid neck fails to restore tension to the capsulolabral complex and functionally creates an anterior labroligamentous periosteal sleeve avulsion (ALPSA) and predisposes the repair to failure (Burkhart & De Beer, 2000; Kim et al, 2002).

Equally critical is the position of the anchors in the vertical plane. Although anchors must be placed in a position that addresses the injury, care must also be taken to ensure that suture anchors are placed sufficiently inferior on the glenoid. Superiorly positioned anchors fail to recruit and incorporate the lax inferior capsule and inferior glenohumeral ligament (Bartl et al, 2011; Shin et al, 2015). Given the correlation of residual capsular laxity and recurrent instability, reduction of capsular volume is critical to restoring stability. This pertains largely to the anterior capsule but also to the rotator interval and posterior capsule (Kim et al, 2002.; Neri et al, 2007; Rowe et al, 1984). It has been suggested that a reduction of capsular volume is better achieved by open compared with arthroscopic surgery (Cohen et al, 2005).

Despite adequate mobilization and anchor positioning, instability will persist if tension is not restored in the anterior capsule and inferior glenohumeral ligament. To this end, the tissue must be shifted from inferior to superior with each pass of suture through the avulsed capsulolabral complex and secured with a suture anchor superior to where the suture passes through the tissue. Yoo et al (2008) highlighted the importance of recreating this "bumper" or anterior buttress. As determined by magnetic resonance imaging (MRI), the "bumper," or anterior buttress, was more prominent in stable and normal shoulders compared with those with recurrent instability. In addition to surgical technique, the number of suture anchors is also important. Fixation strength may be inadequate if 3 or fewer suture anchors are used (Bartl et al, 2011; Boileau et al, 2006; Randelli et al, 2012). Recurrent instability has also been linked to suture failure in the form of soft tissue pull-out or knot breakage or loosening (Blackman et al, 2014).

The soft tissue quality may be affected by previous surgery. Thermal capsulorrhaphy, a technique that has been largely abandoned, is linked to significant capsular tissue damage and chondrolysis (Park et al, 2005). Capsular and ligamentous necrosis can cause initial failure and may also compromise the efficacy of a revision procedure. This may require an open capsular reconstruction with allograft. Poor technique in open stabilization, though, may increase the incidence of subscapularis insufficiency or scarring, leading to motion loss, recurrent instability, or the need for a more complex revision surgery (Boileau et al, 2009; Rowe et al, 1984; Vezeridis et al, 2010).

Failure to address pathology in the posterior shoulder may cause posterior instability and may also place stress on an anterior Bankart repair. Speer et al (1994) concluded that a Bankart lesion alone does not produce the amount of pathologic anterior translation necessary for anterior dislocation to occur. The tension-sharing relationships in the shoulder's capsuloligamentous system during motion of the shoulder have been demonstrated by strain-gauge analysis (Terry et al, 1991). Previous investigators have underscored the relationship between the anterior capsule and posterior instability, and likewise, the posterior stabilizers and anterior instability (Ovesen & Nielsen, 1986; Ovesen & Sojbjerg, 1986; Terry et al, 1991; Turkel et al, 1981). In a cadaveric study, these authors suggested that a posterior lesion is often involved in cases of anterior dislocation. These posterior lesions should be addressed to minimize the risk of recurrence.

Table 1R.2 Instability Severity Index Score Based on a Preoperative Questionnaire, Clinical Examination, and Radiographs

Prognostic Factors	Points
Age at Surgery (yr)	
≤ 20	2
≥ 20	0
DEGREE OF SPORT PARTICIPATION (PREOPERATIVE)	
Competitive	2
Recreational or none	0
TYPE OF SPORT (PREOPERATIVE)	
Contact or overhead	1
Other	0
SHOULDER HYPERLAXITY	
Shoulder hyperlaxity (anterior or inferior)	1
Normal laxity	0
HILL-SACHS ON AP RADIOGRAPH	
Visible on external rotation	2
Not visible on external rotation	0
GLENOID LOSS OF CONTOUR ON AP RADIOGRAPH	
Loss of contour	2
No lesion	0
Total (points)	10

AP, Anteroposterior.
(Balg & Boileau, 2007)

Postoperative Considerations

Postoperative rehabilitation and compliance are critical to the success of shoulder stabilization surgery. Shoulder immobilization for less than 3 weeks is associated with a higher risk of failure (Boileau et al, 2006). In contrast, prolonged immobilization can lead to unacceptable stiffness. A return to weight training should be delayed. Bench press, in particular, should be avoided for 12 to 14 weeks. Physicians should also be aware that return to contact sports or certain occupations may predispose to failure compared with less active, more sedentary patients (Mazzocca et al, 2005; Uhorchak et al, 2000).

Evaluation

When evaluating a patient with recurrent shoulder instability after a stabilization procedure, a comprehensive clinical workup is imperative in determining the cause of failure. Accurate diagnosis is critical to identifying the appropriate surgical treatment. Careful review of the history, physical examination, and appropriate imaging will enable the surgeon to avoid common mistakes and maximize the opportunity for successful revision.

History

A careful history can often reveal the cause of failure. Patient-specific risk factors associated with recurrence, such as younger age, hyperlaxity, male sex, and participation in collision sports should be noted (Arce et al, 2012; Balg & Boileau, 2007; Cho et al, 2006; Porcellini et al, 2009; Randelli et al, 2012; Voos, 2010). Balg and Boileau (2007) developed the instability severity index score (Table 1R.2) to identify patients at high risk of recurrent instability and to help guide treatment decisions. Patients older than age 40 years have a higher rate of rotator cuff tear with dislocation, but a concomitant rotator cuff tear should be ruled out in younger patients as well (Berbig et al, 1999; Porcellini et al, 2006). If this is not addressed at the index procedure, recurrent instability is more likely. A history of multidirectional instability or voluntary dislocation should be elucidated because results after revision in this population are less predictable (Levine et al, 2000; Zabinski et al, 1999). In a retrospective review of 50 patients who underwent revision anterior stabilization surgery, Levine et al (2000) reported that 7 of 11 patients with an unsatisfactory result had a history of voluntary dislocation. In Zabinski et al's (1999) report of 21 patients with multidirectional instability, 13 of 21 patients had a poor result after revision surgery. This is important to recognize because multidirectional and pathologic ligamentous laxity may have a lower risk of recurrence with open capsular shift procedures (Cohen, 2005).

The mechanism(s) of reinjury must be scrutinized because it implies important clues about possible reasons for failure. Reinjury caused by a high-energy mechanism may indicate rupture of a previously well-fixed labrum. In contrast, recurrent dislocation or subluxation with minimal trauma or motion suggests capsular laxity or large bony defects of the glenoid or humeral head (Burkhart & De Beer, 2000; Chen et al, 2007; Itoi et al, 2000; Mologne et al, 2007; Provencher et al, 2010; Tauber et al, 2004). The mechanism of injury might also help predict the efficacy of revision surgery. Excellent outcomes have been reported after revision stabilization following major trauma, but poor results are more common in patients who had redislocation in the setting of minimal trauma (Levine et al, 2000).

It is critical that the surgeon review all previous operative reports to assess for potential causes of failure and to facilitate preoperative planning. Operative reports that include anchor position, the number of anchors used, and an assessment of tissue quality are particularly helpful. These reports may also remark on concomitant intraarticular pathology, including capsular injury, superior labral tears, and rotator cuff tears. Knowledge of the type and location of previously used implants will aid in planning revision surgery.

Table 1R.3 Beighton scale Used in the Diagnosis of Congenital Joint Hyperlaxity

Characteristic	Scoring*
Passive dorsiflexion of the little finger beyond 90 degrees	1 point for each hand
Passive apposition of the thumb to the ipsilateral forearm	1 point for each hand
Active hyperextension of the elbow beyond 10 degrees	1 point for each elbow
Active hyperextension of the knee beyond 10 degrees	1 point for each knee
Forward flexion of the trunk, knees fully extended, hands flat on the floor	1 point

*A score of ≥4 points on a 9-point scale is diagnostic of hyperlaxity.
Beighton et al (1973)

Physical Examination

The physical examination should focus on range of motion, strength, stability, and laxity testing, with comparisons with the uninjured side. Range of motion should be tested to evaluate for stiffness; flexion, abduction, internal rotation, external rotation, and external rotation at 90 degrees of abduction should be measured. Increased passive external rotation with the arm at the side may indicate a subscapularis tear or incompetent anterior capsule. Loss of greater than 15 degrees of external rotation is seen in nearly half of patients that experienced postoperative recurrence (Castagna et al, 2010). Crepitus with abduction and external rotation may represent a Hill-Sachs lesion (Burkhart & De Beer, 2000; Chen et al, 2007; Itoi et al, 2000; Mologne et al, 2007). The patient should be evaluated for scapular dyskinesia because abnormal scapular mechanics may predispose to glenohumeral instability and cannot be corrected by surgery alone.

Shoulder instability is best detected with the apprehension and relocation tests. The degree of abduction at which point apprehension occurs should be noted. Apprehension at only 45 degrees of abduction may suggest substantial bone loss. Load and shift tests may be performed, but in-office findings are often unreliable because of patient guarding. A painful click on load and shift, however, should be noted and may represent a component of instability.

Ligamentous laxity is tested and may reveal laxity of an inherited (i.e., collagen disorders) or traumatic etiology. Generalized laxity is assessed using the Beighton score (Beighton et al, 1973) (Table 1R.3). A positive sulcus sign suggests inferior laxity. A positive sulcus sign that remains positive with external rotation suggests an incompetent rotator interval. The hyperabduction, or Gagey, test examines the competence of the inferior glenohumeral ligament complex, and a positive test may indicate capsular stretch or lengthening.

Imaging

Adequate and appropriate imaging is crucial because it allows for identification and quantification of causes of failure. Preoperative evaluation must include a complete series of shoulder radiographs. This should at least include a Grashey (true anteroposterior [AP]) view, internal and external AP views, Stryker notch view, and an axillary lateral view. The West Point and Stryker notch views are helpful in characterizing glenoid and humeral head defects. The West Point view has been shown to more accurately reflect true glenoid bone loss compared to standard axillary views (Itoi et al, 2007.). Radiographs, though, have a sensitivity of 50% in identifying bone loss and cannot be reliably used alone (Bushnell et al, 2008).

Computed tomography (CT) delivers a reliable and quantifiable assessment of glenoid bone loss and is critical in preoperative planning. Three-dimensional (3D) CT scans have recently been proven to be more useful than traditional two-dimensional (2D) scans. Several cadaveric studies have shown 3D CT scans to be more accurate and reliable than radiographs, 2D scans, and MRI in the evaluation of bone loss (Bishop et al, 2013; Rerko et al, 2013). This finding was corroborated in a saw bones study that compared 3D with 2D CT scans (Bois et al, 2012). Chuang et al (2008) reported a 96% correlation between 3D CT scan quantification of bone loss and intraoperative findings. These authors concluded that 3D CT scan was therefore an essential preoperative tool.

Evaluation of humeral head lesions has proven more elusive. A recent study detected only 90 of 118 Hill-Sachs lesions using CT imaging (Ozaki et al, 2014). Many of the 28 lesions missed were purely cartilaginous defects. Kodali et al (2011), though, showed that the depth, but not the width, of a humeral head defect could be reliably assessed on 2D CT. These authors concluded that the sagittal and axial plane measurements were more accurate for evaluation of these defects than the coronal plane.

Magnetic resonance imaging is essential for evaluation of capsulolabral pathology or other soft tissue injury, such as superior labrum anterior and posterior (SLAP), HAGL, or rotator cuff tears. Although MRI has not proven superior to CT for quantification of bony defects, it can still be used to accurately measure glenoid bone loss (e Souza et al, 2014; Gyftopoulos et al, 2014; Lee et al, 2013;).

Intraoperative Evaluation

Before the procedure, a comprehensive examination under anesthesia must be performed. This should include a range of motion assessment and load and shift testing,

Table 1R.4 Recurrence Rates After Revision Open Bankart Repairs

Study	Patients (*n*)	Mean Follow-up (months	Recurrence Rate (%)
Sisto et al (2007)	30	46	0
Genevra et al (2014)	73	44.2	5.5
Cho et al (2009)	26	42	11.5
Neviaser et al (2015)	30	122	0

which can be difficult to execute in the office. A thorough and systematic diagnostic arthroscopy is then performed. Particular attention should be paid to Bankart lesions, HAGL lesions, and capsular and labral tissue quality in addition to bony defects in both the glenoid and humeral head.

Although significant bone loss is often anticipated from the preoperative evaluation, intraoperative evaluation is equally critical. The glenoid should be scrutinized from a superior, rotator interval portal. "Inverted pear" glenoids should be identified. Approximately 6 mm or less of bone anterior to the glenoid bare spot, which corresponds to roughly 25% or more of bone loss, is associated with significant instability (Burkhart & De Beer, 2000; Chen et al, 2007; Itoi et al, 2000; Mologne et al, 2007). Hill-Sachs lesions can be quantified, and the potential for engagement in abduction and external rotation can be assessed. An engaging Hill-Sachs lesion may benefit from a remplissage procedure in addition to anterior stabilization.

Diagnostic arthroscopy should include evaluation for an ALPSA lesion. Despite adequate mobilization and repair of the ligamentous–labral complex, the mere presence of an ALPSA lesion has been associated with an increased failure rate after arthroscopic stabilization. ALPSA lesions are more common in patients who have sustained multiple dislocations, resulting in progressive capsular attenuation, and perhaps thereby explaining its association with failed stabilization (Ozbaydar et al, 2008). The presence of such a lesion may discourage arthroscopic revision.

Outcomes

Arthroscopic treatment of anterior shoulder instability as a primary procedure has proven to be a reliable and durable surgery (Garofalo et al, 2005; Hobby et al, 2007; Ide et al, 2004; Mazzocca et al, 2005). When compared with index procedures, however, revision surgery is associated with increased recurrence and poorer outcomes (Krueger et al, 2011; Marquardt et al, 2007). Open Bankart repair has shown recurrence rates ranging from 0% to -13% after revision (Cho et al, 2009; Genevra et al, 2014; Neviaser et al, 2015; Sisto, 2007) (Table 1R.4). Arthroscopic revision with modern implant designs and techniques has demonstrated recurrence rates from 6% to 27% (Alexander et al, 2013; Arce et al, 2012; Barnes et al, 2009; Bartl et al, 2011; Neri et al, 2007; Shin et al, 2015) (Table 1R.5). A recent meta-analysis showed comparable rates of recurrent instability after revision open and arthroscopic stabilization (Petrera et al, 2010).

Table 1R.5 Recurrence Rates After Revision Arthroscopic BANKART Repairs

Study	Patients (*n*)	Mean Follow-up (months	Recurrence Rate (%)
Arce et al (2012)	16	30.9	18.8
Bartl et al (2011)	56	37	11
Shin et al (2015)	63	46.9	19
Krueger et al (2011)	20	25	10
Neri et al (2007)	11	34.4	27
Barnes et al (2009)	17	38	5.9
Abouali et al (2013)	349	35.4	12.7

Revision surgery can be complicated by manipulated native anatomy and previously positioned hardware. Krueger et al (2011) showed that compared with initial arthroscopic stabilization, arthroscopic revision surgery is associated with lower subjective outcome scores and signs of radiographic instability arthropathy. Creighton et al (2007) retrospectively reviewed 18 patients who required revision stabilization who were treated with arthroscopic labral repair and capsular plication. Nine of the patients had previously undergone thermal capsulorrhaphy. Revision surgery used a mean of 4.6 suture anchors and 3 plication stitches. Fifteen of the 18 underwent rotator interval closure. At final follow-up at a mean of 30 months, 13 patients had satisfactory results. Five cases were considered clinical failures given continued pain or recurrent instability. In a retrospective review of 22 patients with recurrent instability after open stabilization, Boileau et al (2009) showed that failure was linked to trauma in 12 patients, a bone-block complication in 13 patients, and capsular laxity and Bankart lesions in all patients. The labrum and capsule was repaired and retensioned in all cases. Rotator interval closure was performed in 4 cases and inferior capsular plication in 12. Among 19 patients, a mean follow-up at 43 months showed a mean subjective shoulder value of 83%. One patient had recurrent subluxation, and 2 patients exhibited persistent apprehension.

Kim et al (2002) prospectively analyzed 23 patients with a failed Bankart repair treated with revision arthroscopic stabilization. Eight of these patients had previously undergone open Bankart repair, the remaining 15 an arthroscopic repair. Revision surgery included anterior labral repair with suture anchors, capsular plication, and proximal shift of the inferior capsule, with or without rotator interval closure. At final follow-up at a mean of 36 months, according to the UCLA scores, 15 patients had excellent results, 4 good, 3 fair, and 1 poor. The mean Rowe score improved from 87.3 to 91.2. Five patients experienced recurrence, and 18 of 23 patients achieved 90% of their preinjury activity level.

Franceschi et al (2008) performed a labral repair, capsular plication, and when indicated, rotator interval closure, in 10 patients after failed Bankart repair. At a minimum 4-year follow-up, UCLA scores significantly improved postoperatively (11.7–31.7). One of these 10 patients experienced recurrent dislocation, but the remaining patients returned to their previous activity levels. Barnes et al (2009) described similarly good results in a retrospective review of 18 shoulders that had revision arthroscopic stabilization after a failed primary open or arthroscopic repair. At a mean follow-up of 38 months, 94% of the shoulders were stable. One patient sustained a recurrent dislocation secondary to trauma 4 months after surgery. The mean Rowe score at final follow-up was 84. According to the Rowe scale, 9 shoulders were considered excellent, 4 good, and 3 fair.

Marquardt et al (2007) reported less favorable results. These authors followed 24 patients with a failed primary open or arthroscopic stabilization for a mean of 68 months. Eight of the 24 patients chose to be treated nonoperatively, and 16 underwent a revision stabilization procedure. A recurrent Bankart lesion was discovered in all 16 of these patients. Capsular redundancy was reported in 4 patients. Of the patients treated operatively, 8 reported persistent instability. Six of these 8 were stabilized for a third time. Although all shoulder scores improved after stabilization, only 7 patients (29%) reported good or excellent outcomes according to the Rowe score. The authors demonstrated that the number of stabilizing procedures adversely affected outcome scores, postoperative range of motion, and patient satisfaction.

Meehan and Petersen (2005) identified several factors that prognosticated a negative outcome. These factors included age older than 30 years, two or more previous instability procedures, a bony Bankart lesion, multidirectional instability, glenohumeral arthritis, and surgery involving the nondominant arm. These authors reported satisfactory results in 21 of 25 patients at a minimum of 24 months after revision surgery.

More recently, Shin et al (2015) reported clinical outcomes in 63 shoulders treated with revision arthroscopic surgery at a mean follow-up of 46.9 months. At final follow-up, the mean postoperative Western Ontario Shoulder Instability (WOSI) normalized score was 80.1. There were clinically significant improvements in American Shoulder and Elbow Surgeons (ASES) scores, Simple Shoulder Test scores, and the 10-point visual analog score for pain. Nonetheless, recurrent instability was present in 12 shoulders (19%). Similar to previous authors, they concluded that the number of prior surgeries and hyperlaxity were significant risk factors for failure. Several other studies that show that arthroscopic revision has high failure rates and should be used with caution (Blackman et al, 2014; McCabe et al, 2012).

Open stabilization has also been advocated after failed arthroscopic surgery. Sisto (2007) examined outcomes in 30 patients treated with open Bankart repair after failed arthroscopic stabilization. At final follow-up, the mean modified Rowe scores improved from 25 to 84.2. Excellent results were reported in 2 (6.7%), good in 24 (80%), and fair in 4 (13.3%). There were no poor results. These authors therefore concluded that open repair is a viable option in revision surgery. Cho et al (2009) demonstrated similar results. Open revision stabilization after arthroscopic failure rendered good or excellent results in 88.5% of patients. Recurrent instability was observed in three shoulders (11.5%), all of which had an engaging Hill-Sachs lesion and hyperlaxity. Neviaser et al (2015) used long-term outcomes to conclude that open repair is a reliable technique in revision stabilization. These authors analyzed outcomes of open Bankart repair for failed stabilization surgery at a mean follow-up of longer than 10 years. No patients had postoperative apprehension or instability. ASES and Rowe scores were 89.44 and 86.67, respectively and the WOSI index was 476.62. Radiography at final follow-up revealed 13 normal radiographs and 7 with mild, 2 with moderate, and 0 with severe arthritic changes.

Schmid et al (2012) showed that Latarjet coracoid transfer can be an effective revision procedure in the setting of previous shoulder stabilization. These authors reviewed 49 patients who underwent a Latarjet procedure subsequent to failure after at least one prior procedure. There were no subsequent dislocations, there were two subluxations, and five patients had unspecified shoulder symptoms. Forty-three shoulders (88%) were subjectively graded as excellent or good, 3 as fair, and 3 as poor. The mean subjective shoulder value increased from 53% preoperatively to 79% postoperatively.

Conclusion

The treatment of shoulders that have failed a stabilization surgery poses a challenging problem. Identification of risk factors that predispose to failure is crucial. These risk factors include young age, male gender, hyperlaxity, participation in collision sports, and a history of prior stabilization. Perhaps more important, investigation of the cause or causes of surgical failure is critical. Common pitfalls include failure to address bony defects and capsular laxity, along with technical errors, such as number of suture anchors used and their position on the glenoid. Surgical plans should be designed to address these deficiencies. Arthroscopic and open revision have proven equivalent in the treatment of simple, recurrent Bankart lesions and anterior capsular laxity. Significant glenoid bone loss requires either a Latarjet procedure or bone grafting. A large, engaging Hill-Sachs lesion may be most appropriately treated with coracoid transfer, remplissage, or bone grafting. Combined glenoid and humeral head bone loss may require simultaneous arthroscopic remplissage and an open anterior bone graft procedure.

References

Abouali JAK, Hatzantoni K, Holtby R, Veillette C, Theodoropoulos J. Revision arthroscopic Bankart repair. *Arthroscopy*. 2013;29:1572–1578.

Alexander J, Abouali K, Hatzantoni K, Holtby R, Veillette C, Theodoropoulos J. Revision Arthroscopic Bankart Repair. *Arthroscopy*. 2013;29:1572–1578.

Arce G, Arcuri F, Ferro D, Pereira E. Is selective arthroscopic revision beneficial for treating recurrent anterior shoulder instability? *Clin Orthop Relat Res*. 2012;470:965–971.

Balg F, Boileau P. The instability severity index score. A simple pre-operative score to select patients for arthroscopic or open shoulder stabilisation. *J Bone Joint Surg Br*. 2007;89:1470–1477.

Barnes CJ, Getelman MH, Snyder SJ. Results of arthroscopic revision anterior shoulder reconstruction. *Am J Sports Med*. 2009;37:715–719.

Bartl C, Schumann K, Paul J, Vogt S, Imhoff AB. Arthroscopic capsulolabral revision repair for recurrent anterior shoulder instability. *Am J Sports Med*. 2011;39:511–518.

Bedi A, Ryu RKN. Revision arthroscopic Bankart repair. *Sports Med Arthrosc*. 2010;18:130–139.

Beighton P, Solomon L, Soskolne CL. Articular mobility in an African population. *Ann Rheum Dis*. 1973;32:413–418.

Berbig R, Weishaupt D, Prim J, Shahin O. Primary anterior shoulder dislocation and rotator cuff tears. *J Shoulder Elbow Surg*. 1999;8:220–225.

Bessiere C, Trojani C, Pélégri C, Carles M, Boileau P. Coracoid bone block versus arthroscopic Bankart repair: a comparative paired study with 5-year follow-up. *Orthop Traumatol Surg Res*. 2013;99:123–130.

Bigliani LU, Pollock RG, Soslowsky LJ, Flatow EL, Pawluk RJ, Mow VC. Tensile properties of the inferior glenohumeral ligament. *J Orthop Res*. 1992;10:187–197.

Bishop JY, Jones GL, Rerko MA, Donaldson C. MOON Shoulder Group. 3-D CT is the most reliable imaging modality when quantifying glenoid bone loss. *Clin Orthop Relat Res.* 2013;471:1251–1256.

Blackman AJ, Krych AJ, Kuzma SA, Chow RM, Camp C, Dahm DL. Results of revision anterior shoulder stabilization surgery in adolescent athletes. *Arthroscopy.* 2014;30:1400–1405.

Boileau P, Richou J, Lisai A, Chuinard C, Bicknell RT. The role of arthroscopy. in revision of failed open anterior stabilization of the shoulder. *Arthroscopy.* 2009;25:1075–1084.

Boileau P, Villalba M, Héry JY, Balg F, Ahrens P, Neyton L. Risk factors for recurrence of shoulder instability after arthroscopic Bankart repair. *J Bone Joint Surg Am.* 2006;88:1755–1763.

Bois AJ, Fening SD, Polster J, Jones MH, Miniaci A. Quantifying glenoid bone loss in anterior shoulder instability: reliability and accuracy of 2-dimensional and 3-dimensional computed tomography measurement techniques. *Am J Sports Med.* 2012;40:2569–2577.

Bui-Mansfield LT, Banks KP, Taylor DC. Humeral avulsion of the glenohumeral ligaments: the HAGL lesion. *Am J Sports Med.* 2007;35:1960–1966.

Burkhart SS, De Beer JF. Traumatic glenohumeral bone defects and their relationship to failure of arthroscopic Bankart repairs: significance of the inverted-pear glenoid and the humeral engaging Hill-Sachs lesion. *Arthroscopy.* 2000;16:677–694.

Bushnell BD, Creighton RA, Herring MM. The Bony apprehension test for instability of the shoulder: a prospective pilot analysis. *Arthroscopy.* 2008;24:974–982.

Castagna A, Markopoulos N, Conti M. Delle Rose G, Papadakou E, Garofalo R Arthroscopic Bankart suture-anchor repair: radiological and clinical outcome at minimum 10 years of follow-up. *Am J Sports Med.* 2010;38:2012–2016.

Chahal J, Marks PH, MacDonald PB, et al. Anatomic Bankart repair compared with nonoperative treatment and/or arthroscopic lavage for first-time traumatic shoulder dislocation. *Arthroscopy.* 2012;28:565–575.

Chen AL, Hunt SA, Hawkins RJ, Zuckerman JD. Management of Bone loss associated with recurrent anterior glenohumeral instability. *Sports Med.* 2007:912–925.

Cho NS, Hwang JC, Rhee YG. Arthroscopic stabilization in anterior shoulder instability: collision athletes versus noncollision athletes. *Arthroscopy.* 2006;22:947–953.

Cho NS, Yi JW, Lee BG, Rhee YG. Revision open Bankart surgery after arthroscopic repair for traumatic anterior shoulder instability. *Am J Sports Med.* 2009;37:2158–2164.

Chuang TY, Adams CR, Burkhart SS. Use of preoperative three-dimensional computed tomography to quantify glenoid bone loss in shoulder instability. *Arthroscopy.* 2008;24:376–382.

Cohen SB, Wiley W, Goradia VK, Pearson S, Miller MD. Anterior capsulorrhaphy: an in vitro comparison of volume reduction—arthroscopic plication versus open capsular shift. *Arthroscopy.* 2005;21:659–664.

Cole BJ, Romeo AA. Arthroscopic shoulder stabilization with suture anchors: technique, technology, and pitfalls. *Clin Orthop Relat Res.* 2001;16:17–30.

Creighton RA, Romeo AA, Brown FM, Hayden JK, Verma NN. Revision arthroscopic shoulder instability repair. *Arthroscopy.* 2007;23:703–709.

Di Giacomo Di G, Itoi E, Burkhart SS. Evolving concept of bipolar bone loss and the Hill-Sachs lesion: from "engaging/non-engaging" lesion to "on-track/off-track" lesion. *Arthroscopy.* 2014;30:90–98.

e Souza PM, Brandão BL, Brown E, Motta G, Monteiro M, Marchiori E. Recurrent anterior glenohumeral instability: the quantification of glenoid bone loss using magnetic resonance imaging. *Skeletal Radiol.* 2014;43:1085–1092.

Elkinson I, Giles JW, Faber KJ, et al. The effect of the remplissage procedure on shoulder stability and range of motion an in vitro biomechanical assessment. *J Bone Joint Surg Am.* 2012;94(11):1003–1012.

Franceschi F, Longo UG, Ruzzini L, Rizzello G, Maffulli N, Denaro V. Arthroscopic salvage of failed arthroscopic Bankart repair: a prospective study with a minimum follow-up of 4 years. *Am J Sports Med.* 2008;36:1330–1336.

Garofalo R, Mocci A, Moretti B, et al. Arthroscopic treatment of anterior shoulder instability using knotless suture anchors. *Arthroscopy.* 2005;21:1283–1289.

Genevra L, Friedman M, Griesser MJ, Miniaci AA, Jones MH. Recurrent instability after revision anterior shoulder stabilization surgery. *Arthroscopy.* 2014;30:372–381.

Greis PE, Scuderi MG, Mohr A, Bachus KN, Burks RT. Glenohumeral articular contact areas and pressures following labral and osseous injury to the anteroinferior quadrant of the glenoid. *J Shoulder Elbow Surg.* 2002;11:442–451.

Gwathmey FW, Warner JJP. Management of the athlete with a failed shoulder instability procedure. *Clin Sports Med.* 2013;32:833–863.

Gyftopoulos S, Beltran LS, Yemin A, et al. Use of 3D MR reconstructions in the evaluation of glenoid bone loss: a clinical study. *Skeletal Radiol.* 2014;43:213–218.

Hobby J, Griffin D, Dunbar M, Boileau P. Is arthroscopic surgery for stabilisation of chronic shoulder instability as effective as open surgery? A systematic review and meta-analysis of 62 studies including 3044 arthroscopic operations. *J Bone Joint Surg Br.* 2007;89:1188–1196.

Ide J, Maeda S, Takagi K. Arthroscopic Bankart repair using suture anchors in athletes: patient selection and postoperative sports activity. *Am J Sports Med.* 2004;32:1899–1905.

Itoi E, Lee S-B, Amrami KK, Wenger DE, An K-N. Quantitative assessment of classic anteroinferior bony Bankart lesions by radiography and computed tomography. *Am J Sports Med.* 2003;31:112–118.

Itoi E, Lee SB, Berglund LJ, Berge LL, An KN. The effect of a glenoid defect on anteroinferior stability of the shoulder after Bankart repair: a cadaveric study. *J Bone Joint Surg Am.* 2000;82:35–46.

Kaplan LD, Flanigan DC, Norwig J, Jost P, Bradley J. Prevalence and variance of shoulder injuries in elite collegiate football players. *Am J Sports Med.* 2005;33:1142–1146.

Kim SH, Ha KI, Kim YM. Arthroscopic revision Bankart repair: a prospective outcome study. *Arthroscopy.* 2002;18:469–482.

Kirkley A, Werstine R, Ratjek A, Griffin S. Prospective randomized clinical trial comparing the effectiveness of immediate arthroscopic stabilization versus immobilization and rehabilitation in first traumatic anterior dislocations of the shoulder: long-term evaluation. *Arthroscopy.* 2005;21:55–63.

Kitayama S, Sugaya H, Takahashi N, et al. Clinical outcome and glenoid morphology after arthroscopic repair of chronic osseous Bankart lesions: a five to eight-year follow-up study. *J Bone Joint Surg Am.* 2015;97:1833–1843.

Kodali P, Jones MH, Polster J, Miniaci A, Fening SD. Accuracy of measurement of Hill-Sachs lesions with computed tomography. *J Shoulder Elbow Surg.* 2011;20:1328–1334.

Krueger D, Kraus N, Pauly S, Chen J, Scheibel M. Subjective and objective outcome after revision arthroscopic stabilization for recurrent anterior instability versus initial shoulder stabilization. *Am J Sports Med.* 2011;39:71–77.

Lee RKL, Griffith JF, Tong MMP, Sharma N, Yung P. Glenoid bone loss: assessment with MR imaging. *Radiology.* 2013;267:496–502.

Levine WN, Arroyo JS, Pollock RG, Flatow EL, Bigliani LU. Open revision stabilization surgery for recurrent anterior glenohumeral instability. *Am J Sports Med.* 2000;28:156–160.

Marquardt B, Garmann S, Schulte T, Witt K-A, Steinbeck J, Pötzl W. Outcome after failed traumatic anterior shoulder instability repair with and without surgical revision. *J Shoulder Elbow Surg.* 2007;16:742–747.

Mazzocca AD, Brown FM, Carreira DS, Hayden J, Romeo AA. Arthroscopic anterior shoulder stabilization of collision and contact athletes. *Am J Sports Med.* 2005;33:52–60.

McCabe MP, Savoie FH 3rd. Simple elbow dislocations: evaluation, management, and outcomes. *Phys Sportsmed.* 2012 Feb;40(1):62–71.

Meehan RE, Petersen SA. Results and factors affecting outcome of revision surgery for shoulder instability. *J Shoulder Elbow Surg.* 2005;14:31–37.

Mohtadi NG, Chan DS, Hollinshead RM, et al. A randomized clinical trial comparing open and arthroscopic stabilization for recurrent traumatic anterior shoulder instability: two-year follow-up with disease-specific quality-of-life outcomes. *J Bone Joint Surg Am.* 2014;96(5):353–360.

Mologne TS, Provencher MT, Menzel KA, Vachon TA, Dewing CB. Arthroscopic stabilization in patients with an inverted pear glenoid: results in patients with bone loss of the anterior glenoid. *Am J Sports Med.* 2007;35:1276–1283.

Neri BR, Tuckman DV, Bravman JT, Yim D, Sahajpal DT, Rokito AS. Arthroscopic revision of Bankart repair. *J Shoulder Elbow Surg.* 2007;16:419–424.

Neviaser AS, Benke MT, Neviaser RJ. Open Bankart repair for revision of failed prior stabilization: outcome analysis at a mean of more than 10 years. *J Shoulder Elbow Surg.* 2015;24:897–901.

O'Brien SJ, Neves MC, Arnoczky SP, et al. The anatomy and histology of the inferior glenohumeral ligament complex of the shoulder. *Am J Sports Med.* 1989;18:449–456.

Ovesen J, Nielsen S. Anterior and posterior shoulder instability. A cadaver study. *Acta Orthop Scand.* 1986;57:324–327.

Ovesen J, Sojbjerg JO. Lesions in different types of anterior glenohumeral joint dislocation. An experimental study. *Arch Orthop Trauma Surg.* 1986;105:216–218.

Owens BD, Harrast JJ, Hurwitz SR, Thompson TL. Wolf JM Surgical trends in Bankart repair: an analysis of data from the American Board of Orthopaedic Surgery Certification Examination. *Am J Sports Med.* 2011;39:1865–1869.

Ozaki R, Nakagawa S, Mizuno N, Mae T, Yoneda M. Hill-Sachs lesions in shoulders with traumatic anterior instability: evaluation using computed tomography with 3-dimensional reconstruction. *Am J Sports Med.* 2014;42:2597–2605.

Ozbaydar M, Elhassan B, Diller D, Massimini D, Higgins LD, Warner JJP. Results of arthroscopic capsulolabral repair: Bankart lesion versus anterior labroligamentous periosteal sleeve avulsion lesion. *Arthroscopy.* 2008;24:1277–1283.

Park HB, Yokota A, Gill HS, El Rassi G, McFarland EG. Revision surgery for failed thermal capsulorrhaphy. *Am J Sports Med.* 2005;33:1321–1326.

Petrera M, Patella V, Patella S, Theodoropoulos J. A meta-analysis of open versus arthroscopic Bankart repair using suture anchors. *Knee Surg Sports Traumatol Arthrosc.* 2010;18:1742–1747.

Porcellini G, Campi F, Pegreffi F, Castagna A, Paladini P. Predisposing factors for recurrent shoulder dislocation after arthroscopic treatment. *J Bone Joint Surg Am.* 2009;91:2537–2542.

Porcellini G, Paladini P, Campi F, Paganelli M. Shoulder instability and related rotator cuff tears: arthroscopic findings and treatment in patients aged 40 to 60 years. *Arthroscopy.* 2006;22(3):270–276.

Provencher MT, Bhatia S, Ghodadra NS, et al. Recurrent shoulder instability: current concepts for evaluation and management of glenoid bone loss. *J Bone Joint Surg Am.* 2010;92:133–151.

Randelli P, Ragone V, Carminati S, Cabitza P. Risk factors for recurrence after Bankart repair a systematic review. *Knee Surgery Sport Traumatol Arthrosc.* 2012;20:2129–2138.

Rerko MA, Pan X, Donaldson C, Jones GL, Bishop JY. Comparison of various imaging techniques to quantify glenoid bone loss in shoulder instability. *J Shoulder Elbow Surg.* 2013;22:528–534.

Rhee YG, Cho NS. Anterior shoulder instability with humeral avulsion of the glenohumeral ligament lesion. *J Shoulder Elbow Surg.* 2007;16:188–192.

Robinson CM, Jenkins PJ, White TO, Ker A, Will E. Primary arthroscopic stabilization for a first-time anterior dislocation of the shoulder. A randomized, double-blind trial. *J Bone Joint Surg Am.* 2008;90:708–721.

Rowe CR, Zarins B, Ciullo JV. Recurrent anterior dislocation of the shoulder after surgical repair. Apparent causes of failure and treatment. *J Bone Joint Surg Am.* 1984;66:159–168.

Schmid SL, Farshad M, Catanzaro S, Gerber C. The Latarjet procedure for the treatment of recurrence of anterior instability of the shoulder after operative repair: a retrospective case series of forty-nine consecutive patients. *J Bone Joint Surg Am.* 2012;94:e75.

Shin JJ, Mascarenhas R, Patel AV, et al. Clinical outcomes following revision anterior shoulder arthroscopic capsulolabral stabilization. *Arch Orthop Trauma Surg.* 2015;135:1553–1559.

Sisto DJ. Revision of failed arthroscopic Bankart repairs. *Am J Sports Med.* 2007;35:537–541.

Speer KP, Deng X, Borrero S, Torzilli PA, Altchek DA, Warren RF. Biomechanical evaluation of a simulated Bankart lesion. *J Bone Joint Surg.* 1994;76:1819–1826.

Tauber M, Resch H, Forstner R, Raffl M, Schauer J. Reasons for failure after surgical repair of anterior shoulder instability. *J Shoulder Elbow Surg.* 2004;13:279–285.

Terry G, Hammon D, France P, Norwood L. The stabilizing function of passive shoulder restraints. *Am J Sports Med.* 1991;19:26–34.

Turkel SJ, Panio MW, Marshall JL, Girgis FG. Stabilizing mechanisms preventing anterior dislocation of the glenohumeral joint. *J Bone Joint Surg Am.* 1981;63:1208–1217.

Uhorchak JM, Arciero RA, Huggard D, Taylor DC. Recurrent shoulder instability after open reconstruction in athletes involved in collision and contact sports. *Am J Sports Med.* 2000;28:794–799.

Vezeridis PS, Goel DP, Shah AA, Sung S-Y, Warner JJP. Postarthroscopic arthrofibrosis of the shoulder. *Sports Med Arthrosc.* 2010;18:198–206.

Voos JE, Livermore RW, Feeley BT, et al. Prospective evaluation of arthroscopic Bankart repairs for anterior instability. *Am J Sports Med.* 2010;38:302–307.

Wasserstein D, Dwyer T, Veillette C, et al. Predictors of dislocation and revision after shoulder stabilization in Ontario, Canada, from 2003 to 2008. *Am J Sports Med.* 2013;41:2034–2040.

Yamamoto N, Itoi E, Abe H, et al. Contact between the glenoid and the humeral head in abduction, external rotation, and horizontal extension: a new concept of glenoid track. *J Shoulder Elbow Surg.* 2007;16:649–656.

Yoo JC, Lee YS, Tae SK, Park JH, Park JW, Ha HC. Magnetic resonance imaging appearance of a repaired capsulolabral complex after arthroscopic Bankart repair. *Am J Sports Med.* 2008;36:2310–2316.

Zabinski SJ, Callaway GH, Cohen S, Warren RF. Revision shoulder stabilization: 2- to 10-year results. *J Shoulder Elbow Surg.* 1999;8:58–65.

2 Posterior Shoulder Instability

2-2A EPIDEMIOLOGY, MECHANISM OF INJURY, HISTORY, PHYSICAL EXAMINATION, AND IMAGING

JOSEPH A. GIL, MD and BRETT D. OWENS, MD

Introduction

- An injury to the shoulder may result in posterior shoulder instability, which ranges in severity from subluxation to dislocation.
- The incidence of unidirectional, posterior instability in young athletes is 10%.
- Posterior shoulder instability results from repetitive microtrauma, an acute traumatic event, or may be atraumatic.
- The most common presenting complaint is either generalized shoulder pain or deep pain in the posterior shoulder.
- Provocative examination maneuvers described for the assessment of posterior shoulder instability include the jerk test, Kim test, posterior stress test, and load and shift test.
- Diagnostic imaging required in the evaluation includes plain radiographs and magnetic resonance imaging.

The large range of motion allowed by the shoulder joint predisposes it to injury, particularly at the extremes of motion (Owens et al, 2007). An injury may result in posterior shoulder instability, which ranges in severity from subluxation to dislocation. A subluxation occurs when translation of the glenohumeral joint occurs beyond physiologic limits with some glenohumeral contact maintained (Owens et al, 2010a). In contrast, a dislocation occurs when translation of the glenohumeral joint occurs such that there is no residual contact between the humeral head and the glenoid fossa (Owens et al, 2010b, 2013). The diagnosis of shoulder dislocation requires radiographic evidence of complete disassociation of the humeral head and glenoid or the need for a manual reduction of the joint. Shoulder subluxation has been reported to account for 85% of traumatic, anterior shoulder instability events. However, shoulder subluxation events are often underreported because the diagnosis is not as straightforward as the diagnosis of a shoulder dislocation.

Epidemiology

Posterior shoulder instability most often presents in 15- to 40-year-old athletes (Lenart et al, 2012). The incidence of unidirectional, posterior instability in young athletes is 10% (Owens et al, 2007). The reported incidence of posterior shoulder instability has increased as the understanding of the pathoanatomy and awareness of this diagnosis increased over the past decade (Gerber & Ganz, 1984; Hawkins et al, 1984; Provencher et al, 2005). Although unidirectional posterior instability events can present as dislocation, more than 90% of these events are subluxations. More than 50% of patients present with recurrent, rather than first-time, subluxations.

Risk Factors

Patients with seizure disorders, a history of alcoholism, and those who sustain an electrical shock are at risk for a posterior shoulder dislocation (Gupta et al, 2013; Wooten et al, 2014). More commonly, the young, athletic population has been identified at risk for developing recurrent posterior shoulder instability that manifests as recurrent shoulder subluxation rather than dislocation (McIntyre et al, 1997; Owens et al, 2013; Provencher et al, 2011; Wooten et al, 2015). Athletes who have been identified to be at risk for developing posterior instability include weight lifters, football linemen, overhead throwers, rugby players, paddling sport athletes, swimmers, volleyball players, gymnasts, and climbers (Bradley et al, 2006; Chang et al, 2016; Lenart et al, 2012; McClincy et al, 2015; Provencher et al, 2011). More recently, batters have been identified to be at risk for developing episodic subluxation of the lead shoulder during the baseball swing (Wanich et al, 2012). Other activities that generate repetitive, posteriorly directed forces in the shoulder include archery and riflery, and wheelchair use also predisposes participants to developing posterior shoulder instability (Cho et al, 2012; DeLong et al, 2015).

Anatomic characteristics that predispose patients to recurrent posterior instability include increased glenoid retroversion (Fig. 2A.1) (Owens et al, 2013). A prospective evaluation of young athletes with posterior instability revealed that the most significant risk factor for posterior instability is increased glenoid retroversion. In their cohort, the median version in the noninjured participants was −7.7 degrees compared with −17.6 degrees in the participants with posterior instability (Owens et al, 2013).

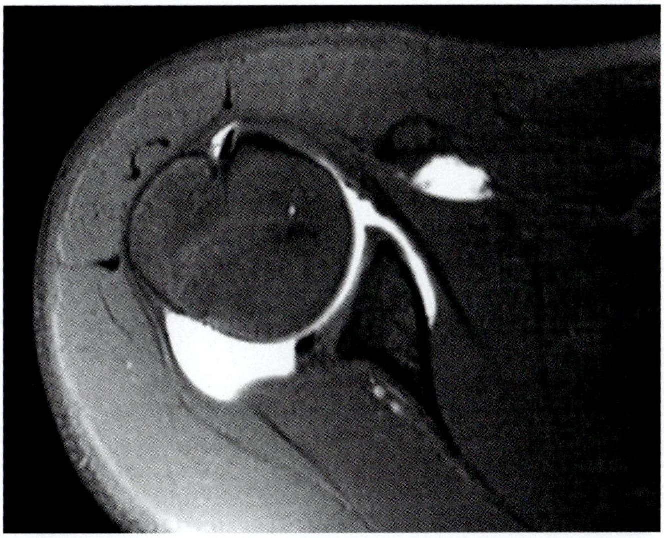

Fig. 2A.1 Axial T2-weighted magnetic resonance arthrogram image of the glenohumeral joint demonstrating excessive retroversion secondary to glenoid dysplasia.

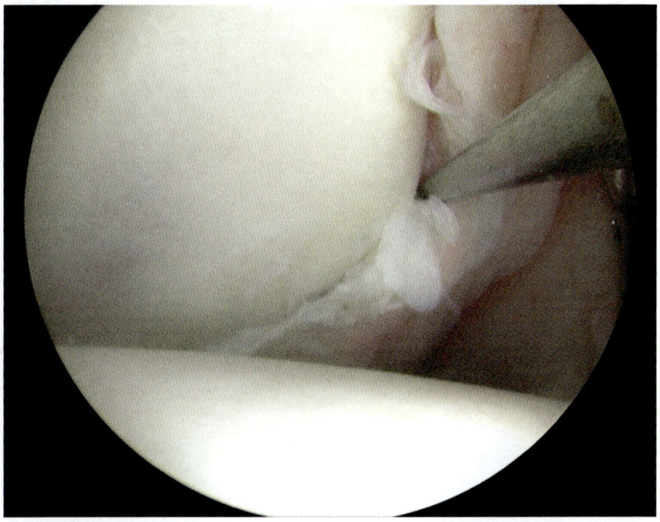

Fig. 2A.2 Arthroscopic image of a posterior labrum lesion.

Mechanism of Injury

Posterior shoulder instability results from repetitive microtrauma or an acute traumatic event, or it may be atraumatic (Lenart et al, 2012; Provencher et al, 2011). Patients who participate in activities in which the shoulder is repetitively posteriorly loaded in a flexed and internally rotated position are at risk for developing posterior shoulder instability. Over time, the cumulative microtrauma results in attenuation and tearing of the posterior capsulolabral complex and the posterior band of inferior glenohumeral ligament (PIGHL), which results in posterior instability (DeLong & Bradley, 2015).

An acute onset of posterior shoulder instability often results from a specific traumatic event. The classic traumatic event that results in acute, traumatic unidirectional posterior instability involves a posteriorly directed force that is applied to an adducted, internally rotated, and forward flexed upper extremity (Robinson et al, 2006). This results in shearing force of the humeral head along the glenoid that results in detachment of the capsulolabral complex. Acute, traumatic events generally predispose patients to recurrent instability (Mair et al, 1998; Pennington et al, 2010; Provencher et al, 2011). Similar to traumatic, anterior shoulder instability, the initial instability event in traumatic, posterior instability is most commonly a subluxation event rather than a dislocation (Hawkins & McCormack, 1988; Owens et al, 2007; Provencher et al, 2011).

Atraumatic posterior instability generally occurs in patients with generalized laxity (Provencher et al, 2011). Initially, instability symptoms are brought on by activities that posteriorly load the shoulder. As the tissues become more attenuated, these patients begin to have symptoms with activities of daily living.

Pathoanatomy

Posterior shoulder instability has been associated with injury to the osseous and soft tissue stabilizers. The congruity and stability of the shoulder joint depend on the soft tissue stabilizers because of the significant mismatch between the radius of curvature of the glenoid and humeral head (Lugo et al, 2008; Warner et al, 1993). The maximal area of the humeral head that articulates with the glenoid is 30%. Although the stability from the glenoid and humeral head alone is inadequate, the osseous anatomy of the shoulder plays a critical role in the overall stability of the shoulder. Increased glenoid retroversion has been demonstrated to predispose patients to loss of containment and resulting atraumatic posteroinferior instability (Kim et al, 2005a; Owens et al, 2013). Glenoid bone loss and glenoid dysplasia have also been associated with shoulder instability (Gerber & Ganz, 1984; Ghodadra et al, 2010; Gupta et al, 2013; Provencher et al, 2010, 2009; Schwartz et al, 2013). Operative intervention for posterior shoulder instability that does not address glenoid bone loss or dysplasia is at risk for an unsatisfactory result (Meuffels et al, 2010; Owens & Tucker, 2011; Schwartz et al, 2013).

The soft tissue stabilizers of the shoulder include static and dynamic soft tissue stabilizers (Lugo et al, 2008; Warner et al, 1993). The static stabilizers include the labrum, joint capsule, and glenohumeral ligaments. The glenoid labrum is a rim of fibrocartilaginous tissue that is attached to the periphery of the glenoid effectively increasing its depth by 50%, thereby increasing the contact area at the glenohumeral articulation. The labrum also allows for a negative-pressure suction phenomenon to occur that contributes to the overall stability of the shoulder joint. Nondisplaced posterior labral lesions, which are known as Kim lesions, are also associated with posterior instability (Fig. 2A.2) (Kim et al, 2003). These tend to occur in athletes who have repetitive microtrauma and who subject the shoulder to repetitive loads with the arm in adduction and internal rotation, such as swimmers. The labrum is attached to the posterior capsule, and the detached labrum is often found in continuity with the capsule (Leivadiotou & Ahrens, 2015). Additional pathology of the capsulolabral complex that is associated with posterior instability includes a redundant capsule, a tear in the posterior capsule, reverse humeral avulsion of the glenohumeral ligament (HAGL), and fraying of the posterior labrum (Leivadiotou & Ahrens, 2015).

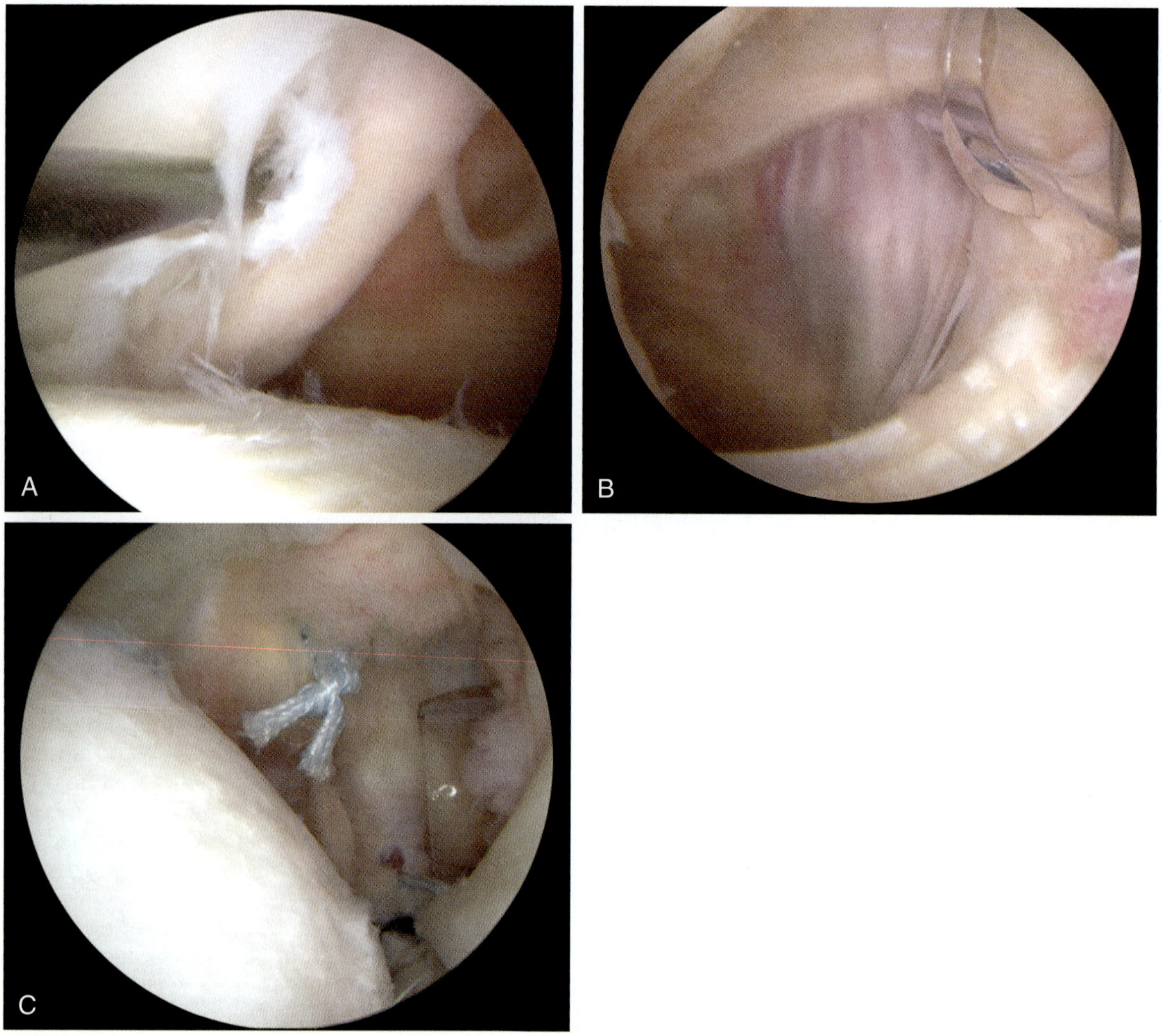

Fig. 2A.3 (A) Arthroscopic image of a reverse Bankart lesion in a 21-year-old wrestler with posterior shoulder instability. (B) Further arthroscopic evaluation of this patient's glenohumeral joint revealed a capsular rent. (C) Arthroscopic image after repair of the combined reverse Bankart lesion and the capsular rent.

The glenohumeral ligaments primarily function by limiting shoulder motion at the extremes of shoulder motion. In contrast to the anterior capsule and the anterior glenohumeral ligaments, the posterior capsule and the PIGHL are relatively thin (Provencher et al, 2011). The PIGHL primarily resists posterior translation when the shoulder is placed in the posterior loading position, which consists of internal rotation and forward flexion (Provencher et al, 2011). Although the PIGHL is the primary resistor to posterior translation, the middle glenohumeral ligament (MGHL) resists posterior translation of the shoulder in midrange shoulder abduction and the superior glenohumeral ligament (SGHL) resist posterior translation in midrange adduction (Provencher et al, 2011). Injury to or attenuation of the PIGHL results in posterior shoulder instability.

A reverse humeral avulsion of the glenohumeral ligament (RHAGL) lesion has also been identified as a source of posterior shoulder instability (Rebolledo et al, 2015). The majority (62%) of these lesions are associated with pathologic findings that may lead to missed RHAGL lesions, resulting in persistent instability. Therefore assessment of magnetic resonance imaging (MRI) for posterior shoulder instability must be carefully scrutinized with a high index of suspicion for this lesion. RHAGL lesions can be partial, complete, or floating, where the glenohumeral ligament is detached from the humerus and glenoid. It is important to note that the presence of a glenoid-based PIGHL lesion (reverse Bankart lesion) does not preclude the presence of a concomitant secondary disruption (RHAGL or capsular tear; Fig. 2A.3).

The dynamic soft tissue stabilizers include the rotator cuff and the scapulothoracic muscles (Lugo et al, 2008; Warner et al, 1993). The primary role of the rotator cuff on shoulder stability is to compress the humeral head against the glenoid and to maintain the humeral head in a relatively central position on the glenoid thereby limiting shear stress. The rotator cuff is the most important dynamic stabilizer in preventing posterior shoulder instability (Provencher et al, 2011). The subscapularis muscle is the primary muscle of the rotator cuff that dynamically resists posterior translation of the humeral head (Provencher et al, 2011). Injury to or attenuation of the rotator cuff, particularly the subscapularis, may result in posterior shoulder instability (Provencher et al, 2011).

Concomitant pathology associated with posterior instability events include reverse Hill-Sachs lesions and injury to any of the static and dynamic stabilizers (DeLong et al, 2015). Reverse Hill-Sachs lesions are humeral head compression fractures that result from impaction of the humeral head on the rim of the glenoid that occurs during a dislocation event. Hill-Sachs lesions that are larger than 1.5 cm^3 are associated with recurrent instability (Robinson et al, 2011).

History

Because of the high incidence of posterior shoulder instability in young athletes, especially collision athletes and weight lifters, this condition should be considered as part of the differential in athletes presenting with shoulder pain and any suspicion of instability. The history of posterior shoulder instability is often vague, and the onset may not be associated with a specific traumatic event (Gerber & Ganz, 1984; Lenart et al, 2012; Millett et al, 2006). The most common presenting complaint is either generalized shoulder pain or deep pain in the posterior shoulder (Hawkins et al, 1984; Provencher et al, 2005, 2011). The pain is often associated with decreased strength and endurance (Bradley et al, 2006; Kim et al, 2003; Robinson & Aderinto, 2005). The historical context will depend on the underlying etiology of the posterior instability. Commonly, a young athlete will report a gradual onset of pain and limitation in performance. In acute, traumatic posterior shoulder instability, the athlete will identify a specific event that resulted in a posteriorly directed force applied to an adducted, internally rotated, and forward flexed shoulder. It is often difficult to determine how much underlying repetitive microtrauma preceded this event. In cases of atraumatic posterior shoulder instability, the patient often may present with generalized laxity. Voluntary atraumatic posterior shoulder instability can be positional or voluntary (Millett et al, 2006). Voluntary instability that is positional is reproduced by placing the arm in a provocative position (flexion, adduction, and internal rotation). In contrast, voluntary instability that is muscular is more consistent with a muscular imbalance or generalized ligamentous laxity and is reproducible irrespective of the position of the shoulder. A patient who can demonstrate posterior subluxation with muscle contraction (posterior cuff) with the arm at the side may have an underlying psychiatric disorder. Extreme caution is advised in this scenario for any surgical treatment. Care should be taken to elicit history of contralateral instability or similar symptoms, as bilateral involvement can be common.

Physical Examination

The physical examination of a shoulder with suspected posterior shoulder instability should include a comprehensive and systematic evaluation of the shoulder given that the nonspecific symptoms of instability, including generalized pain and decreased strength and endurance, can be attributed to a wide range of etiologies (Millett et al, 2006; Provencher et al, 2011). Examination should begin with a general impression of the function of the patient's musculoskeletal; system, inspection, palpation, range of motion, neurovascular examination, rotator cuff evaluation, and assessment of stability (Silliman & Hawkins, 1993). Assessment for generalized laxity in the musculoskeletal system is determined by using the Beighton hypermobility scale (Remvig et al, 2007). It is critical to examine the contralateral shoulder for comparison, paying attention to obvious signs of muscle atrophy, instability, asymmetry, swelling, abnormal motion, and scapular dyskinesia (Provencher et al, 2011). In posterior shoulder instability, palpation can reveal tenderness at the posterior joint line (Millett et al, 2006; Provencher et al, 2011). Range of motion is often within normal limits with the exception of the overhead thrower population, which is predisposed to having increased external rotation while developing a glenohumeral internal rotation deficit (Mine et al, 2016).

Provocative examination maneuvers described for the assessment of posterior shoulder instability include the jerk test, Kim test, posterior stress test, and load and shift test (Blasier et al, 1997; Gerber & Ganz, 1984; Kim et al, 2005b; Pollock & Bigliani, 1993; Provencher et al, 2011). The jerk test is performed with the patient in a sitting position (Kim et al, 2005b). The examiner stabilizes the scapula with one hand and uses the other hand to abduct and internally rotate the shoulder by 90 degrees. In this position, the examiner applies an axial load to the abducted and internally rotated arm while simultaneously applying a horizontal adduction force. This test result is positive if it produces a sharp pain. The pain may be accompanied by a posterior clunk or click; however, a test result is positive if it produces a sharp pain irrespective of a clunk or click.

The Kim test was described for detecting posterior labral lesions of the shoulder (Kim et al, 2005b). This test is performed with the arm in 90 degrees of abduction. With the patient in a sitting position, the examiner holds the elbow and the lateral aspect of the proximal arm, applies an axial loading force, and elevates the distal arm to 45 degrees while applying an inferior and posterior force to the proximal arm. This test result is positive if this maneuver produces a sudden onset of pain, plus or minus a palpable clunk. It is important to perform this test in a chair with back support and with an assistant to provide counterpressure during axial loading.

The load and shift test can be performed with the patient supine or seated. The examiner holds the arm in 50 to 70 degrees of abduction in the scapular plane (Provencher et al, 2011). With the other hand, the examiner applies a compressive load to the humeral head within the glenoid and then applies posterior and anterior forces (Fig. 2A.4). The amount of translation that occurs can be graded using the McFarland grading system: grade I is translation limited to the glenoid fossa and grade II is translation that occurs to or beyond the glenoid rim (Owens et al, 2011).

The posterior apprehension sign can be elicited in the seated or supine position (Provencher et al, 2011). The examiner uses one hand to stabilize the scapula and the second hand to apply a force to the arm while it is held in 90 degrees of forward flexion, adduction, and internal rotation (Fig. 2A.5). The test result is positive if this maneuver produces pain or apprehension.

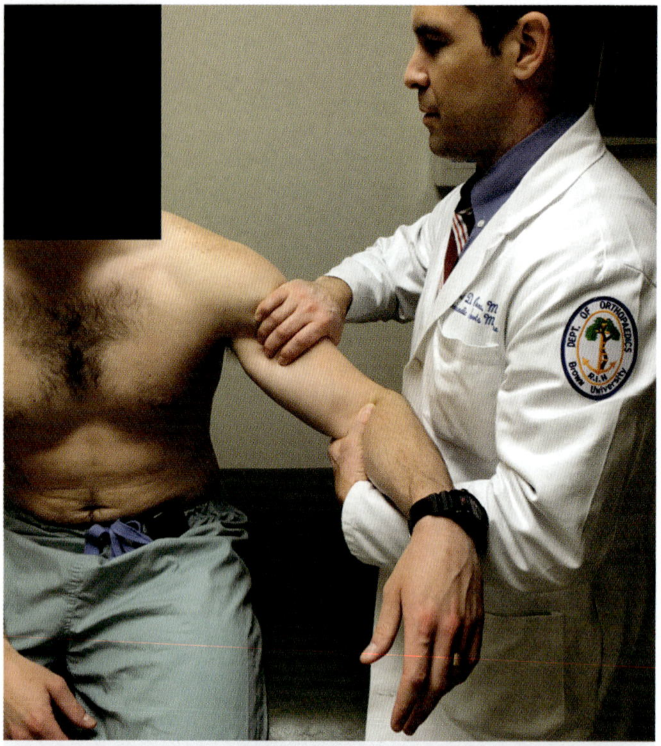

Fig. 2A.4 The load and shift test can be performed with the patient seated or supine. The examiner holds the arm in 20 degrees of forward flexion and abduction. With the other hand, the examiner applies a load to the humeral head while applying posterior and anterior forces.

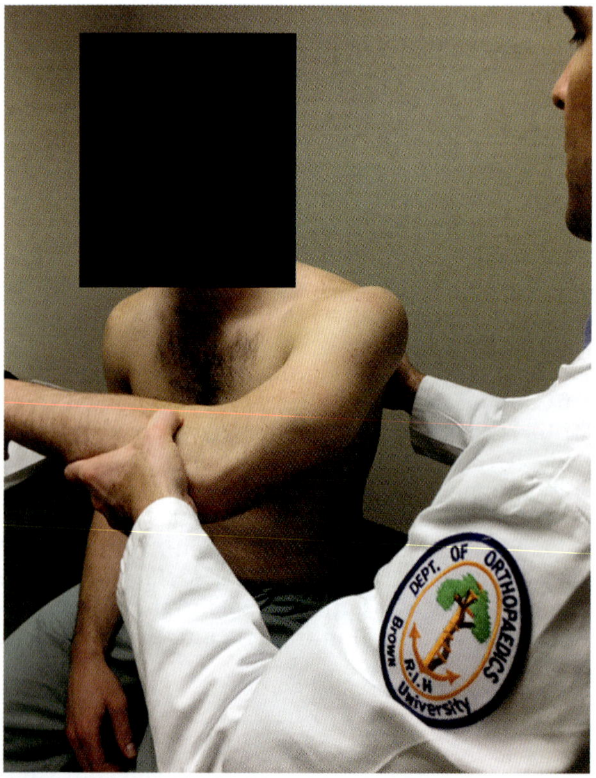

Fig. 2A.5 The posterior apprehension sign can be elicited in the seated or supine position. The examiner uses one hand to stabilize the scapula and the second hand to apply a force to the arm while it is held in 90 degrees of forward flexion, adduction, and internal rotation. The test result is positive if this maneuver produces pain or apprehension.

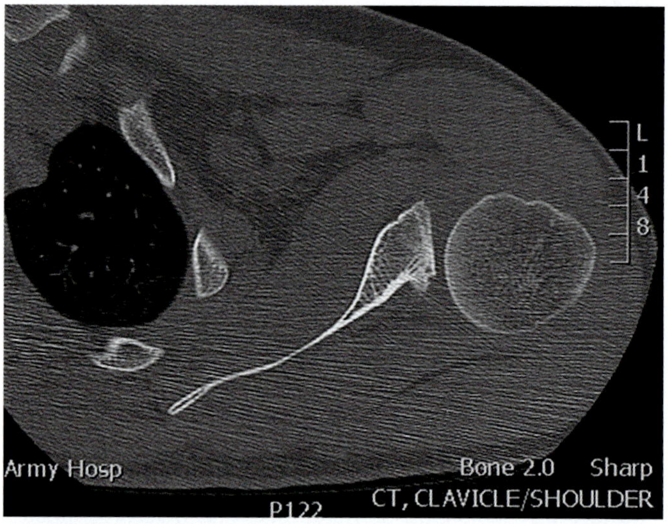

Fig. 2A.6 Axial computed tomography image of the left shoulder demonstrating excessive retroversion.

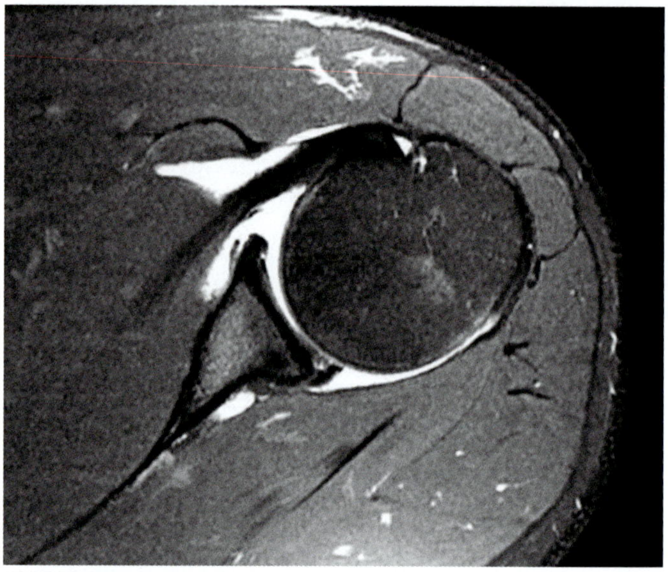

Fig. 2A.7 Axial T2-weighted magnetic resonance arthrogram image of the glenohumeral joint demonstrating a posterior labrum lesion.

Imaging

Routine plain radiographs should include anteroposterior, scapular Y, and axillary lateral views (Lenart et al, 2012). Although the plain radiographs are generally normal, the axillary lateral view provides the most relevant information for diagnosing posterior shoulder instability (Provencher et al, 2011). The axillary view can reveal reverse Hill-Sachs lesions, glenoid dysplasia, excessive glenoid retroversion, and sometimes even translation of the humeral head relative to the glenoid (Provencher et al, 2011). Computed tomography should be obtained to evaluate glenoid version and bone loss in suspicious cases (Fig. 2A.6) (Farrar et al, 2013). MR without contrast performed with an MRI scanner that has at least a 1.5-Telsa magnet should be obtained to evaluate the soft tissue static and dynamic stabilizers (Owens et al, 2010a). MR arthrograms have been demonstrated to have a higher sensitivity for detecting labral tears (Fig. 2A.7) and RHAGL lesions compared with MRI without contrast and can be helpful in chronic situations (Farrar et al, 2013). Obtaining an MRI or MRA is critical for identifying soft tissue pathology that is contributing to the instability and for surgical planning.

References

Blasier RB, Soslowsky LJ, Malicky DM, Palmer ML. Posterior glenohumeral subluxation: active and passive stabilization in a biomechanical model. *J Bone Joint Surg Am*. 1997;79:433–440.

Bradley JP, Baker CL, Kline AJ, Armfield DR, Chhabra A. Arthroscopic capsulolabral reconstruction for posterior instability of the shoulder: a prospective study of 100 shoulders. *Am J Sports Med*. 2006;34:1061–1071.

Chang ES, Greco NJ, McClincy MP, Bradley JP. Posterior shoulder instability in overhead athletes. *Orthop Clin North Am*. 2016;47(1):179–187.

Cho J-H, Chung N-S, Song H-K, Lee D-H. Recurrent posterior shoulder instability after rifle shooting. *Orthopedics*. 2012;35:e1677–e1679.

DeLong JM, Bradley JP. Posterior shoulder instability in the athletic population: variations in assessment, clinical outcomes, and return to sport. *World J Orthop*. 2015;6:927–934.

DeLong JM, Jiang K, Bradley JP. Posterior instability of the shoulder: a systematic review and meta-analysis of clinical outcomes. *Am J Sports Med*. 2015;43:1805–1817.

Farrar NG, Malal JJG, Fische J, Waseem M. An overview of shoulder instability and its management. *Open Orthop J*. 2013;7:338–346.

Gerber C, Ganz R. Clinical assessment of instability of the shoulder. With special reference to anterior and posterior drawer tests. *J Bone Joint Surg Br*. 1984;66:551–556.

Ghodadra N, Gupta A, Romeo AA, et al. Normalization of glenohumeral articular contact pressures after Latarjet or iliac crest bone-grafting. *J Bone Joint Surg Am*. 2010;92:1478–1489.

Gupta AK, Chalmers PN, Klosterman E, Harris JD, Provencher MT, Romeo AA. Arthroscopic distal tibial allograft augmentation for posterior shoulder instability with glenoid bone loss. *Arthrosc Tech*. 2013;2:e405–e411.

Hawkins RJ, Koppert G, Johnston G. Recurrent posterior instability (subluxation) of the shoulder. *J Bone Joint Surg Am*. 1984;66:169–174.

Hawkins RJ, McCormack RG. Posterior shoulder instability. *Orthopedics*. 1988;11:101–107.

Kim S-H, Ha K-I, Park J-H, et al. Arthroscopic posterior labral repair and capsular shift for traumatic unidirectional recurrent posterior subluxation of the shoulder. *J Bone Joint Surg Am*. 2003;85-A:1479–1487.

Kim S-H, Noh K-C, Park J-S, Ryu B-D, Oh I. Loss of chondrolabral containment of the glenohumeral joint in atraumatic posteroinferior multidirectional instability. *J Bone Joint Surg Am*. 2005a;87:92–98.

Kim S-H, Park J-S, Jeong W-K, Shin S-K. The Kim test: a novel test for posteroinferior labral lesion of the shoulder—a comparison to the jerk test. *Am J Sports Med*. 2005b;33:1188–1192.

Leivadiotou D, Ahrens P. Arthroscopic treatment of posterior shoulder instability: a systematic review. *Arthroscopy*. 2015;31:555–560.

Lenart BA, Sherman SL, Mall NA, Gochanour E, Twigg SL, Nicholson GP. Arthroscopic repair for posterior shoulder instability. *Arthroscopy*. 2012;28:1337–1343.

Mair SD, Zarzour RH, Speer KP. Posterior labral injury in contact athletes. *Am J Sports Med*. 1998;26:753–758.

McClincy MP, Arner JW, Bradley JP. Posterior shoulder instability in throwing athletes: a case-matched comparison of throwers and non-throwers. *Arthroscopy*. 2015;31:1041–1051.

McIntyre LF, Caspari RB, Savoie FH. The arthroscopic treatment of posterior shoulder instability: two-year results of a multiple suture technique. *Arthroscopy*. 1997;13:426–432.

Meuffels DE, Schuit H, van Biezen FC, Reijman M, Verhaar JAN. The posterior bone block procedure in posterior shoulder instability: a long-term follow-up study. *J Bone Joint Surg Br*. 2010;92:651–655.

Millett PJ, Clavert P, Hatch GFR, Warner JJP. Recurrent posterior shoulder instability. *J Am Acad Orthop Surg*. 2006;14:464–476.

Mine K, Nakayama T, Milanese S, Grimmer K. Effectiveness of stretching on posterior shoulder tightness and glenohumeral internal rotation deficit: a systematic review of randomised controlled trials. *J Sport Rehabil*. 2016 Aug; 24:1–28. [Epub ahead of print].

Owens BD, Campbell SE, Cameron KL. Risk factors for posterior shoulder instability in young athletes. *Am J Sports Med*. 2013;41:2645–2649.

Owens BD, Duffey ML, Deberardino TM, Cameron KL. Physical examination findings in young athletes correlate with history of shoulder instability. *Orthopedics*. 2011;34:460.

Owens BD, Duffey ML, Nelson BJ, DeBerardino TM, Taylor DC, Mountcastle SB. The incidence and characteristics of shoulder instability at the United States Military Academy. *Am J Sports Med*. 2007;35:1168–1173.

Owens BD, Nelson BJ, Duffey ML, et al. Pathoanatomy of first-time, traumatic, anterior glenohumeral subluxation events. *J Bone Joint Surg Am*. 2010a;92:1605–1611.

Owens BD, Nelson BJ, Duffey ML, et al. Pathoanatomy of first-time, traumatic, anterior glenohumeral subluxation events. *J Bone Joint Surg Am*. 2010b;92:1605–1611.

Owens BD, Tucker CJ. Surgical management of posterior shoulder instability. *Curr Orthop Pract*. 2011;22:474–482.

Pennington WT, Sytsma MA, Gibbons DJ, et al. Arthroscopic posterior labral repair in athletes: outcome analysis at 2-year follow-up. *Arthroscopy*. 2010;26:1162–1171.

Pollock RG, Bigliani LU. Recurrent posterior shoulder instability. Diagnosis and treatment. *Clin Orthop Relat Res*. 1993;85–96.

Provencher MT, Bell SJ, Menzel KA, Mologne TS. Arthroscopic treatment of posterior shoulder instability: results in 33 patients. *Am J Sports Med*. 2005;33:1463–1471.

Provencher MT, Bhatia S, Ghodadra NS, et al. Recurrent shoulder instability: current concepts for evaluation and management of glenoid bone loss. *J Bone Joint Surg Am*. 2010;92(suppl 2):133–151.

Provencher MT, Ghodadra N, LeClere L, Solomon DJ, Romeo AA. Anatomic osteochondral glenoid reconstruction for recurrent glenohumeral instability with glenoid deficiency using a distal tibia allograft. *Arthroscopy*. 2009;25:446–452.

Provencher MT, LeClere LE, King S, et al. Posterior instability of the shoulder: diagnosis and management. *Am J Sports Med*. 2011;39:874–886.

Rebolledo BJ, Nwachukwu BU, Konin GP, Coleman SH, Potter HG, Warren RF. Posterior humeral avulsion of the glenohumeral ligament and associated injuries: assessment using magnetic resonance imaging. *Am J Sports Med*. 2015;43:2913–2917.

Remvig L, Jensen DV, Ward RC. Epidemiology of general joint hypermobility and basis for the proposed criteria for benign joint hypermobility syndrome: review of the literature. *J Rheumatol*. 2007;34:804–809.

Robinson CM, Aderinto J. Recurrent posterior shoulder instability. *J Bone Joint Surg Am*. 2005;87:883–892.

Robinson CM, Howes J, Murdoch H, Will E, Graham C. Functional outcome and risk of recurrent instability after primary traumatic anterior shoulder dislocation in young patients. *J Bone Joint Surg Am*. 2006;88:2326–2336.

Robinson CM, Seah M, Akhtar MA. The epidemiology, risk of recurrence, and functional outcome after an acute traumatic posterior dislocation of the shoulder. *J Bone Joint Surg Am*. 2011;93:1605–1613.

Schwartz DG, Goebel S, Piper K, Kordasiewicz B, Boyle S, Lafosse L. Arthroscopic posterior bone block augmentation in posterior shoulder instability. *J Shoulder Elbow Surg*. 2013;22:1092–1101.

Silliman JF, Hawkins RJ. Classification and physical diagnosis of instability of the shoulder. *Clin Orthop Relat Res*. 1993;7–19.

Wanich T, Dines J, Dines D, Gambardella RA, Yocum LA. "Batter's shoulder": can athletes return to play at the same level after operative treatment? *Clin Orthop Relat Res*. 2012;470:1565–1570.

Warner JJ, Caborn DN, Berger R, Fu FH, Seel M. Dynamic capsuloligamentous anatomy of the glenohumeral joint. *J Shoulder Elbow Surg*. 1993;2:115–133.

Wooten C, Klika B, Schleck CD, Harmsen WS, Sperling JW, Cofield RH. Anatomic shoulder arthroplasty as treatment for locked posterior dislocation of the shoulder. *J Bone Joint Surg Am*. 2014;96:e19.

Wooten CJ, Krych AJ, Schleck CD, Hudgens JL, May JH, Dahm DL. Arthroscopic capsulolabral reconstruction for posterior shoulder instability in patients 18 years old or younger. *J Pediatr Orthop*. 2015;35:462–466.

2-2B ARTHROSCOPIC POSTERIOR CAPSULOLABRAL RECONSTRUCTION AND POSTERIOR HAGL LESION REPAIR AND OUTCOMES

KEVIN O'DONNELL, MD, FOTIOS P. TJOUMAKARIS, MD and JAMES P. BRADLEY, MD

Surgical Repair and Technique

INTRODUCTION

With the advent of advanced diagnostic imaging and the recognition of posterior labral and ligamentous pathology contributing to disability in the athlete, surgical techniques (including ours) have advanced considerably over the past several decades and years. The open techniques employed in the past met with high failure rates in an athletic population. This situation led to the advancement of arthroscopic techniques using transglenoid sutures, progressing to anchor fixation with traditional knot tying, and, more recently, knotless anchor fixation, which has reduced the incidence of knot impingement and postoperative clicking of the shoulder joint. Athletes and non-athletes alike who have undergone posterior shoulder instability repair have enjoyed high success rates and have seen a high return to athletic competition. There is no "classic" presentation for patients who present with posterior labral/capsular pathology; however, the majority of patients are younger, athletic patients involved in repetitive loading of the shoulder joint with activities. This joint loading can occur with axial compression (linemen in football or weight-lifters) or with repetitive high-demand activities such as overhead throwing (pitchers, quarterbacks, etc.) Patients rarely describe frank instability but more often complain of deep-seated shoulder pain, loss of velocity with throwing, difficulty warming up, or pain when the joint is loaded in flexion and adduction. Radiographs are routinely normal and magnetic resonance arthrography (MRA) is often diagnostic. The following section describes the technique that we currently employ in the treatment of patients requiring posterior capsulolabral reconstruction and posterior HAGL (humeral avulsion of the glenohumeral ligament) repair using an arthroscopic technique.

ARTHROSCOPIC POSTERIOR LABRAL REPAIR

See Video 2B.1.

Patient Positioning and Room Setup

We prefer to perform the procedure with the patient in the lateral decubitus position. This position allows the arm to be placed in gentle abduction (45 degrees) and slight forward flexion (20 degrees) with 10 to 15 lb of traction, giving excellent access to the posterior joint and capsule. After induction of general anesthesia and placement of an interscalene nerve block, the patient is transferred into the lateral decubitus position and held in place with an inflatable beanbag. Care is taken to ensure that all bony prominences are well padded, and an axillary gel roll is appropriately positioned under the dependent axilla to prevent an iatrogenic brachial plexopathy. Wide preparation and draping are performed to make sure that easy access to the shoulder both anteriorly and posteriorly is possible. We often angle the bed 45 degrees away from anesthesia machine/anesthesiologist work space and place the visualization tower across the surgical field and at eye level to the surgeon (Fig. 2B.1).

Portal Placement

All bony landmarks are marked with a marking pen (the acromion, coracoid process, and acromioclavicular joint). The anterior portal is typically placed in the rotator interval

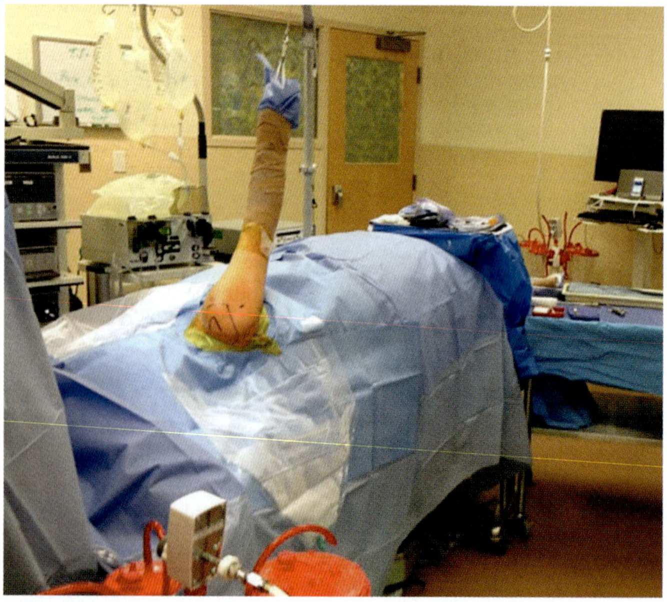

Fig. 2B.1 Patient is placed in the lateral decubitus position. The arm is abducted 45 degrees, is forward flexed 20 degrees, and is put under 15 to 20 lb of traction.

in a trajectory that is diagonal from the coracoid process to the anterolateral edge of the acromion. The posterior portal is created slightly lateral to a traditional posterior arthroscopy portal to allow tangential access to the posterior glenoid for anchor placement. The posterior portal is created first after insufflation of the joint with 30 mL of normal saline, and the anterior portal is created via an "inside-out" technique. Once portals are created a clear cannula is placed in the anterior portal with a traditional dilation technique. Either a 6-mm or 7-mm cannula can be used for the anterior portal.

Diagnostic Arthroscopy

A 30-degree arthroscope placed through a posterior viewing portal is used to perform an initial diagnostic arthroscopy. The joint is checked for concomitant pathology such as superior labral tears, rotator cuff tears, and osteochondral injury. Debridement of the joint can be carried out with a 4.5-mm shaver through the anterior portal as needed. Following an initial diagnostic arthroscopy, the camera is placed into the anterior cannula and the inflow cannula is placed on the side port on the cannula. A switching stick is placed in the posterior portal, which is dilated to 8 mm. An 8.25-mm cannula (Arthrex, Naples, FL) is then placed in the posterior portal. The 30-degree arthroscope can be switched for a 70-degree arthroscope, which allows slightly better visualization of the posterior and inferior capsule and posterior inferior band of the inferior glenohumeral ligament. Surgeons are encouraged to use both 30- and 70-degree arthroscopy cameras to obtain the best visualization possible during capsular and labral repair.

Glenoid and Labrum Preparation

A meticulous glenoid preparation is paramount to the success of the repair. An elevator is initially placed through the posterior portal and the labrum is sharply elevated off the glenoid. The labrum is mobilized as with anterior labral tears until the underside of the capsule edge of the glenoid rim is visualized. Care is taken during labral elevation and mobilization to not transect the labrum, and adequate trajectory through the posterior portal is critical in achieving this goal. If the angle is difficult, the elevator can be brought in through the anterior portal, and the labrum visualized posteriorly. Once adequate mobilization is achieved, a hooded bur is utilized to prepare the glenoid rim. Great care should be used to ensure that the labrum is protected during the bony debridement. A shaver is then utilized to remove any remaining soft tissue debris from the glenoid rim, followed by rasping to create a fresh, bleeding surface conducive to soft tissue healing (Fig. 2B.2).

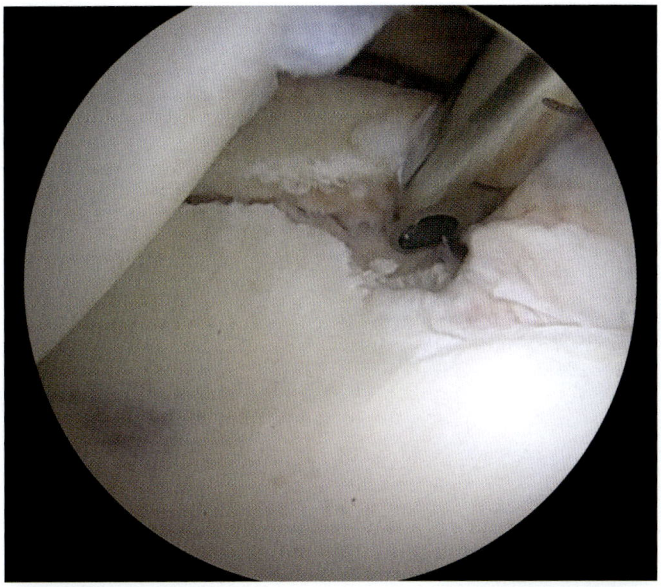

Fig. 2B.2 Complete mobilization of the labrum and glenoid preparation are achieved with a combination of an elevator, rasp, shaver, and bur.

Suture Passing and Labral Repair

We have evolved our technique to a knotless anchor system (2.4-mm biocomposite short PushLock anchors (Arthrex) with 1.3-mm flat braided SutureTape (Arthrex) as our primary fixation method. Knotless fixation superior to the equator of the glenoid may minimize the risk of humeral head chondral injury as well as articular-sided rotator cuff knot abrasion. Furthermore, SutureTape has fixation strength that is superior to FiberWire (Arthrex) and its low profile allows it to lie flat against the labrum, minimizing tear-through and providing excellent reduction without humeral abrasion. The first step in labral repair is predicated on the surgeon's understanding of the patient-specific pathology and how much strain the patient routinely puts on their shoulder as part of their lifestyle. Patients presenting with symptoms consistent with recurrent posterior subluxation (RPS) and insidious shoulder pain without gross macroinstability may benefit from a primary labral repair without significant capsular plication/advancement (e.g., throwing athletes). Patients with macroinstability or dislocation who participate in high-demand contact sports (e.g., offensive linemen) may require labral repair with plication of the posterior capsule.

For the standard posterior labral repair, we prefer to place anchors from approximately the 6 o'clock to the 11 o'clock position on the glenoid. To achieve positioning of the inferiormost anchor an accessory posterior portal may need to be created 45 degrees tangential to the glenoid. This portal is typically created slightly inferior and lateral to the posterior working portal. While viewing from the anterior portal, we use a spinal needle to localize the correct site of entry for the accessory posterior portal. Once the correct location and trajectory are identified for anchor placement, an accessory 5-mm cannula is introduced into the joint using a traditional Seldinger technique. Great care should be taken on cannula introduction to avoid damage to the axillary nerve, which lies at risk in this area. The anchors are all placed from inferior to superior after suture passage.

A curved suture hook (Spectrum, Linvatec, Edison, NJ) loaded with a No. 0 monofilament suture is placed through the posterior working cannula with the arthroscope placed in the anterior cannula. A bite of capsulolabral tissue is taken slightly inferior and lateral to the level of desired anchor location (to achieve capsular plication and advancement) (Fig. 2B.3), and the suture is delivered through the labrum against the glenoid articular margin. The monofilament suture is shuttled through the posterior working

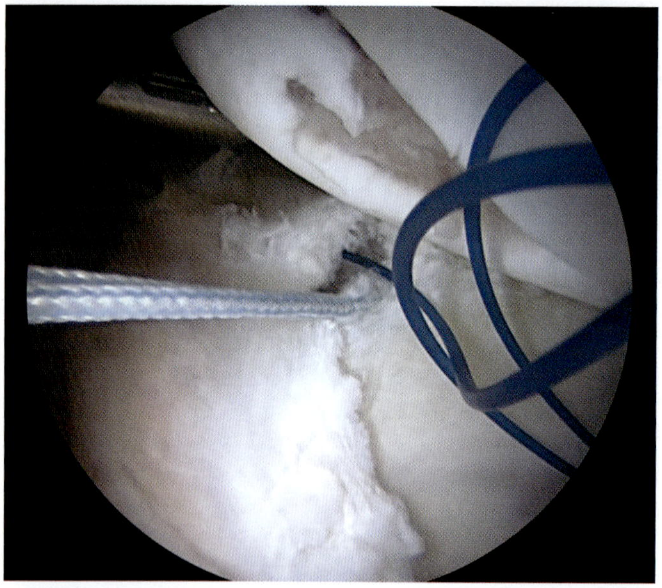

Fig. 2B.3 A curved suture hook is used to pass a monofilament shuttling suture next to the desired anchor location (note the osteochondral lesion on the posterior humeral head).

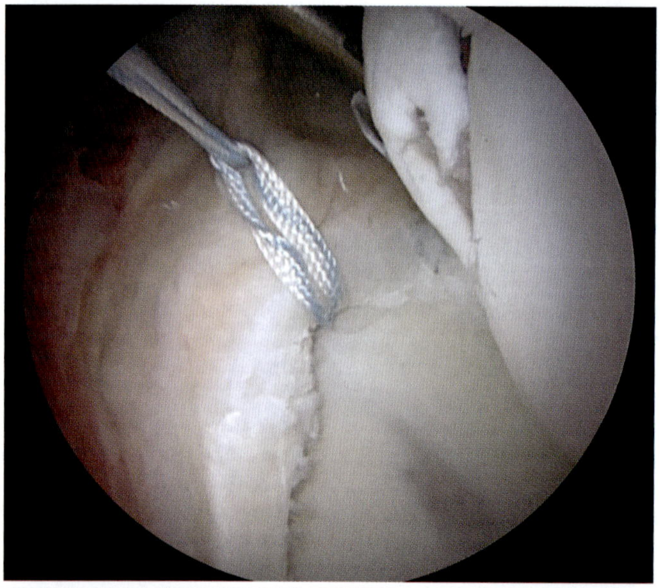

Fig. 2B.4 A luggage tag loop ("cinch stitch") made with SutureTape (Arthrex, Naples, FL) is secured down to the labrum. (This image provided courtesy of Arthrex, Inc.)

cannula, and a loop of SutureTape is placed in a knot of the monofilament suture. The goal is to create a "cinch" stitch akin to a luggage tag that will reduce the labrum and provide optimum suture security around the tissue. The loop of SutureTape is then shuttled back through the posterior working cannula, and the tail ends of the suture are delivered through the loop created in the tape. The two tails of the SutureTape are pulled and the cinch stitch is reduced to the labrum (Fig. 2B.4). A knot pusher can be used to help reduce the knot to the labral tissue if needed, when there is concern that the tissue is of poor quality. This creates 2.6 mm of SutureTape, because the tape is essentially doubled over to create a stable fixation construct around the labrum and capsular complex. The ends of the tape are

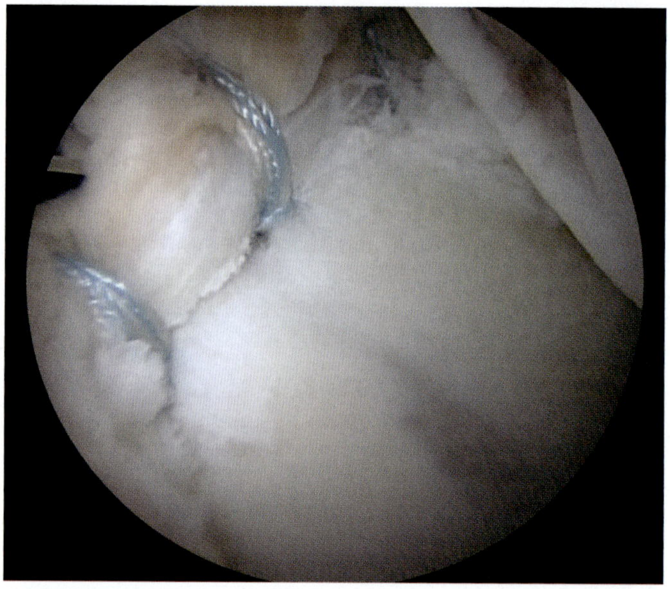

Fig. 2B.5 Anchors securing the labrum from the 8 o'clock to the 11 o'clock position (the osteochondral lesion has also been debrided and a microfracture can be performed if clinically indicated).

delivered through the accessory cannula for anchor placement. The drill guide is then placed through the accessory posterior cannula, and a pilot hole drilled in the desired location. The suture ends are shuttled through the eyelet of the knotless anchor, the anchor is slid to the level of the glenoid, and slight tension is applied to the limbs to reduce the labrum. The anchor is impacted into place within the pilot hole, and the labrum and capsule are reduced to the glenoid margin. Additional anchors can be placed in an identical fashion as needed. Anchors in the 8 o'clock to 11 o'clock position are generally placed through the standard posterior portal, which provides a better angle of approach in this zone (Fig. 2B.5).

Posterior Portal Closure

The posterior portal is closed using a No. 1 polydioxanone suture (PDS). The cannula is withdrawn to a level just external to the capsule. A suture passer is then used to pierce the capsule adjacent to the portal, and the PDS suture is introduced into the joint. A penetrating suture grasper is used to pierce the capsule on the opposite side of the portal, and the suture is retrieved. A sliding Weston knot is then used to close down the capsule. Additional sutures can be placed in a wider fashion if additional plication is required by the patient's needs as predetermined from the preoperative plan.

Rotator interval closure is not routinely performed as part of our technique for posterior instability repair. Indications for rotator interval closure are pathology specific to the rotator interval (capsular tear, injury to the superior glenohumeral/coracohumeral ligament complex) and excessive laxity in patients with multidirectional instability (sulcus sign, etc.). There is concern in the throwing athlete that excessive tightening of the rotator interval may serve to decrease glenohumeral external rotation and could compromise the ability to return to competitive throwing, despite its positive effects on restricting pathologic posterior glenohumeral translation.

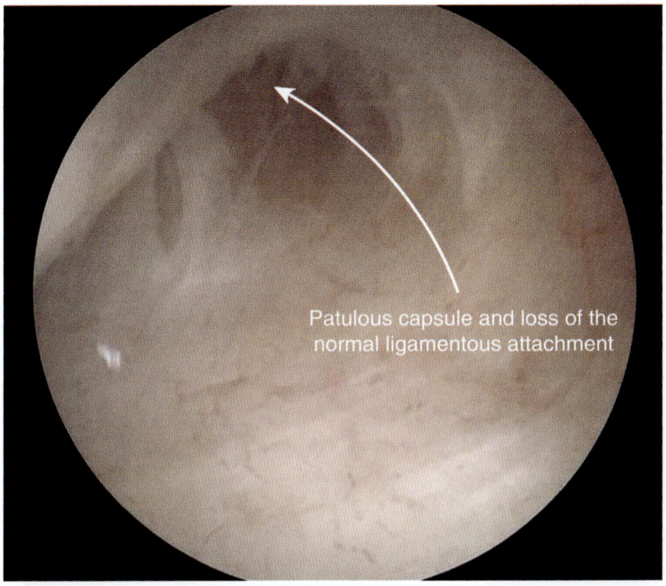

Fig. 2B.6 Arthroscopic view from the anterior portal viewing postero-inferiorly of an avulsed reverse HAGL lesion.

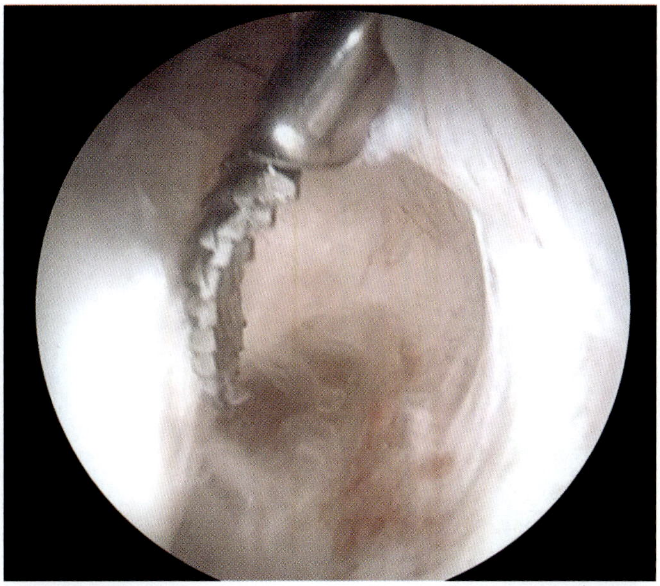

Fig. 2B.7 Preparation of the humeral attachment site for reverse HAGL lesion repair with a bony rasp.

ARTHROSCOPIC REVERSE HAGL LESION REPAIR

Patient Positioning, Setup, and Portal Placement

As with posterior labral repair, patients undergoing reverse HAGL lesion repair are optimally treated in the lateral decubitus position. The positioning, room setup, and portal placement are identical to those for primary posterior labral repair.

Diagnostic Arthroscopy

Diagnostic arthroscopy is carried out similarly to that for posterior labral repair. In evaluation of the HAGL lesion, viewing with a 70-degree arthroscope from the anterior portal greatly aids in visualization of both the lesion and the humeral attachment site of the ligament. The reverse HAGL lesion can be identified from the presence of a patulous posterior inferior capsule and the loss of the normal humeral attachment of the posterior inferior glenohumeral ligament (Fig. 2B.6). Either one working posterior portal or an accessory portal can be created in a fashion similar to that already described for labrum repair. Because the posterior capsule is fairly patulous, we have found that a single posterior portal typically gives us adequate access and excellent mobility. The humeral head can be rotated as needed by manipulation of the arm while it is in traction to expose the bare area of the humerus and the normal attachment site of the lesion.

Reverse HAGL Repair

After identification of the lesion the posterior humeral head is prepared to optimize the surface for bone to soft tissue healing (Fig. 2B.7). Working from the posterior portal, we use a rasp or bur to freshen the surface of the humeral head and soft tissues to create a bleeding surface amenable to healing.

Depending on the size of the lesion, either one or two anchors can be placed within the previously prepared humeral bed. Bone quality determines whether screw-in (rotator cuff style) anchors (4.5-mm double-loaded) or drill-in glenoid style anchors (ranging in size from 2.0 to 3.7 mm [SutureTak, Arthrex]) are placed percutaneously (through a 7 o'clock portal), through an accessory cannula, or through the posterior working portal. We prefer a double-loaded suture anchor to optimize reattachment of the ligament through a broad repair site. For smaller patients, one anchor may suffice; however, for the average size patient two anchors placed in a diagonal fashion adequately covers the defect. A double-loaded suture anchor is then placed into the humeral head at the level of the posteroinferior glenohumeral ligament attachment site (Fig. 2B.8A).

After placement of the anchor(s), the posterior cannula is withdrawn slightly just posterior to or "outside" and extraarticular to the posterior capsule, and the sutures are retrieved with a penetrating suture grasper in a mattress-stitch configuration. Each suture is passed individually to create two mattress stitches at the superior and inferior aspects of the ligament attachment site. While viewing intraarticularly from the anterior portal, we use a sliding locking knot to reduce the ligament and secure it to the humeral head (Fig. 2B.8B). The knots are then all tied in successive fashion to complete the repair.

POSTOPERATIVE CARE

Following surgery, the patient's arm is placed in a shoulder abduction sling to limit internal rotation. During the initial postoperative period, elbow and wrist active range-of-motion exercises are encouraged along with passive and active-assisted shoulder range-of-motion exercises. Most patients are progressed to complete passive and active range-of-motion exercises by postoperative week 8 to 12. Strengthening can begin at week 12, focusing on the periscapular musculature groups and the rotator cuff muscles. Throwing athletes may begin a light toss program by week 16. Final return to play and competitive

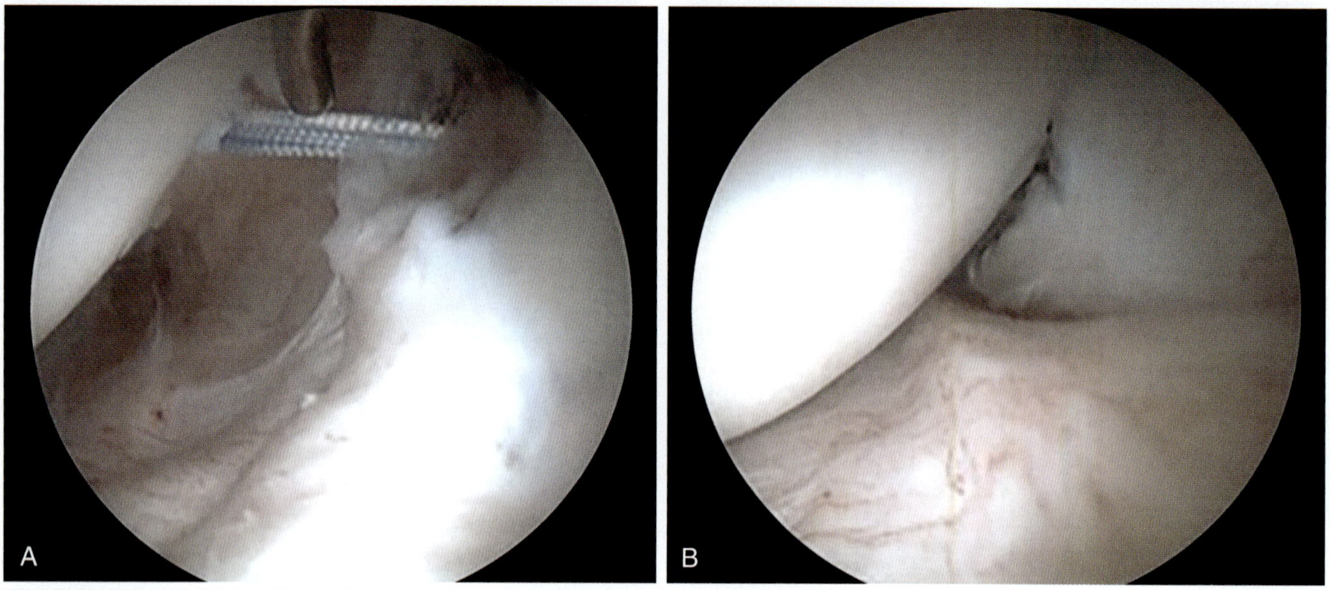

Fig. 2B.8 (A) Double-loaded anchor placed into the humeral insertion site; sutures are withdrawn out an 8.25-mm cannula docked superficial to the capsule. (B) Ligament is reduced and secured to the anatomic insertion site with a sliding locking knot.

sports is typically achieved at 6 months, but it may take up to a year for overhead throwing athletes to reach peak performance and throwing velocity. Patients are encouraged to wait until they have at least 80% of strength and near-normal range of motion prior to returning to full activities and athletics.

Operative Outcomes

POSTERIOR INSTABILITY REPAIR

A better understanding of the stress placed on an athlete's shoulder has led to increased recognition of posterior glenohumeral instability. Recognition and appropriate treatment of posterior instability are imperative to giving an athlete the best chance to return to the previous level of sports. Two types of athletes have been found to be at an increased risk for capsuloligamentous damage: overhead throwing athletes and athletes who bear significant loads with the arms forward flexed to 90 degrees. Despite the increased recognition of this pathology, there is still a lack of information with regard to the optimal fixation strategy and the outcomes of operative intervention. A summary of several studies analyzing the outcomes of posterior labral repair can be found in Table 2B.1.

The advent of advanced arthroscopic techniques has shifted the treatment of posterior instability from an open procedure to one done entirely arthroscopically. Bottoni et al (2005) compared the results of arthroscopic repair and open repair of posterior instability and found that although both techniques were associated with favorable outcomes, arthroscopic repair demonstrated superior results. Kim et al (2003) reported on 27 patients with traumatic unidirectional instability who were treated with arthroscopic labral repair and posterior capsular shift. All patients were able to return to their previous level of sport and 24 patients reported having more than 90% of their preinjury shoulder function level. Radkowski et al (2008) compared the results of arthroscopic posterior labral repair in throwing and nonthrowing athletes. They found similar outcomes with regard to range of motion, strength, and stability; however, only 55% of throwing athletes were able to return to the previous level of sport, versus 71% of nonthrowing athletes. Wooten et al (2015) showed a continuation of this trend in their study of athletes younger than 18 years. In direct contrast to the literature regarding anterior instability, they found that American Shoulder and Elbow Surgeons (ASES) scores improved most markedly in male patients participating in contact sports. Bradley et al (2006) compared the outcomes of arthroscopic stabilization for posterior unidirectional instability in athletes playing contact and noncontact sports. They found similar improvements in stability, pain, and function in the two cohorts, indicating that participation in a contact sport may not lead to a detrimental outcome following surgery. Of note, however, was that only 89% of patients were able to return to their sports and only 67% at the same level, rates that have been reproduced by multiple studies.

Reverse HAGL Lesion Repair

There is a relative paucity of literature reporting on the results of arthroscopic posterior glenohumeral ligament avulsion repair. The largest case series to date comes from Castagna et al (2007). In a retrospective review they reported on a series of nine patients who underwent posterior HAGL repair at a mean follow-up of 34.2 months. Of note, only three of the nine posterior HAGL lesions had occurred in isolation. Other concomitant injuries included posterior labral tears and superior labral anterior and posterior (SLAP) lesions. Following repair, there was a significant improvement in both University of California Los Angeles (UCLA) Shoulder Scale and Constant scores. All patients were able to return to their previous level of sport without any significant limitation.

Table 2B.1 Outcomes of Arthroscopic Posterior Labral Repair

Authors	Year	Journal	No. of Patients	Follow-Up (months)	Outcome Score(s)	Rate of Return to Sports	Failure Rate	Comments
Kim et al	2003	*JBJS Am*	27	39	ASES, Rowe, UCLA	100%	4%	>90% good to excellent results
Williams et al	2003	*AJSM*	27	61	L'Insalata, SF-36	92%	8%	Traumatic injury etiology
Goubier et al	2003	*JSES*	11	34	not recorded	100%	0%	72% at same level as prior to surgery in sport
Bottoni et al	2005	*AJSM*	19	34	SANE, WOSI, SST Rowe	NR	10%	Arthroscopic repair results better than open repairs
Bradley et al	2006	*AJSM*	91	27	ASES	89%	11%*	Athletes playing contact and noncontact sports show similar post-operative outcomes
Savoie et al	2008	*Arthroscopy*	131	28	Neer-Foster	NR	3%	
Radkowski et al	2008	*AJSM*	98	27	ASES	55% throwing athletes; 71% other	11% throwing; 10% other*	Nonthrowing athletes fared better than throwing athletes
Badge et al	2009	*International Journal of Shoulder Surgery*	29	32	Oxford, Constant, return to sport	100%		Return at 4.3 months
Pennington et al	2010	*Arthroscopy*	28	24	ASES, Rowe, UCLA, return to sport		7%	Athletes
Bahk et al	2010	*Arthroscopy*	29	66	ASES, Rowe, UCLA, SST	84%	3.4%	68% return to sport at same level
Lenart et al	2012	*Arthroscopy*	32	36	ASES, SST, VAS	100%	6%	
Bradley et al	2013	*AJSM*	183	36	ASES, return to sport	90%	7%*	Suture anchor repairs showed outcomes superior to those of anchorless repairs
Arner et al	2015	*Arthroscopy*	56	44.7	Return to sport, ASES	93%	3.5%*	Football players
Wooten et al	2015	*JPO*	22	63	ASES, Marx	67% return at same level	11%,† 20%*	Patients 18 years and younger

*Based on ASES instability rating greater or equal to 5.
†Failure rate—recurrent instability.
AJSM, *American Journal of Sports Medicine;* *ASES,* American Shoulder and Elbow Surgeons; *JBJS,* *Journal of Bone and Joint Surgery;* *JPO,* *Journal of Pediatric Orthopaedics;* *SANE,* Single Assessment Numeric Evaluation; *SST,* Simple Shoulder Test; *UCLA,* University of California Los Angeles Shoulder Scale; *VAS,* Visual Analog Scale; WOSI, Western Ontario Shoulder Instability index.

References

Arner JW, McClincy MP, Bradley JP. Arthroscopic stabilization of posterior shoulder instability is successful in American football players. *Arthroscopy*. 2015;31(8):1466–1471.

Badge R, Tambe A, Funk L. Arthroscopic isolated posterior labral repair in rugby players. *Int J Shoulder Surg*. 2009;3:4–7.

Bahk MS, Karzel RP, Snyder SJ. Arthroscopic posterior stabilization and anterior capsular plication for recurrent posterior glenohumeral instability. *Arthroscopy*. 2010;26:1172–1180.

Bottoni CR, Franks BR, Moore JH, DeBerardino TM, Taylor DC, Arciero RA. Operative stabilization of posterior shoulder instability. *Am J Sports Med*. 2005;33:996–1002.

Bradley JP, Baker CL III, Kline AJ, Armfield DR, Chhabra A. Arthroscopic capsulolabral reconstruction for posterior instability of the shoulder: a prospective study of 100 shoulders. *Am J Sports Med*. 2006;34:1061–1071.

Bradley JP, McClincy MP, Arner JW, Tejwani SG. Arthroscopic capsulolabral reconstruction for posterior instability of the shoulder: a prospective study of 200 shoulders. *Am J Sports Med*. 2013;41:2005–2014.

Castagna A, Snyder SJ, Conti M, Borroni M, Massazza G, Garofalo R. Posterior humeral avulsion of the glenohumeral ligament: a clinical review of 9 cases. *Arthroscopy*. 2007;23:809–815.

Goubier JN, Iserin A, Duranthon LD, Vandenbussche E, Augereau B. A 4-portal arthroscopic stabilization in posterior shoulder instability. *J Shoulder Elbow Surg*. 2003;12:337–341.

Kim SH, Ha KI, Park JH. Arthroscopic posterior labral repair and capsular shift for traumatic unidirectional recurrent posterior subluxation of the shoulder. *J Bone Joint Surg Am*. 2003;85:1479–1487.

Lenart BA, Sherman SL, Mall NA, Gochanour MA, Twigg SA, Nicholson GP. Arthroscopic repair for posterior shoulder instability. *Arthroscopy*. 2012;28:1337–1343.

Pennington WT, Sytsma MA, Gibbons DJ, et al. Arthroscopic posterior labral repair in athletes: outcome analysis at 2-year follow-up. *Arthroscopy*. 2010;26:1162–1171.

Radkowski CA, Chhabra A, Baker CL, Tejwani SG, Bradley JP. Arthroscopic capsulolabral repair for posterior shoulder instability in throwing athletes compared with nonthrowing athletes. *Am J Sports Med*. 2008;36:693–699.

Savoie FH III, Holt MS, Field LD, Ramsey JR. Arthroscopic management of posterior instability: evolution of technique and results. *Arthroscopy*. 2008;24:389–396.

Williams RJ, Strickland S, Cohen M, Altchek DW, Warren RF. Arthroscopic repair for traumatic posterior shoulder instability. *Am J Sports Med*. 2003;31:203–209.

Wooten CJ, Krych AJ, Schleck CD, Hudgens JL, May JH, Dahm DL. Arthroscopic capsulolabral reconstruction for posterior shoulder instability in patients 18 years old or younger. *J Pediatr Orthop*. 2015;35:462–466.

2-2C OPEN POSTERIOR CAPSULOLABRAL REPAIR AND RECONSTRUCTION

CRAIG R. BOTTONI, MD

Introduction

- Posterior glenohumeral instability is much less common than anterior instability.
- Injuries typically occur with an adducted, internally rotated shoulder.
- Physical therapy is the primary initial treatment in most cases.
- Operative intervention is indicated in recurrent posterior instability.
- Operative options include arthroscopic and open procedures.
- Open posterior stabilization may allow for a more extensive capsulorrhaphy.
- Posterior glenoid osteotomy may be required for posterior instability in the setting of excessive glenoid retroversion.
- Open posterior approach and osteochondral allograft transplantation may be necessary for a large, engaging reverse Hill-Sachs lesion.

Posterior glenohumeral instability occurs much less commonly than either anterior or multidirectional instability. Patients may have undefined and vague symptoms, such as posterior shoulder discomfort, pain, inability to participate in their sports, and repeated subluxation events. Further complexity exists because no single pathologic lesion occurs in all cases of posterior shoulder instability. Posterior shoulder subluxation is often accompanied by various lesions, which may result in instability in multiple directions rather than a single isolated direction. Historically, posterior instability has been reported to occur in approximately 2% to 5% of all cases of shoulder instability (Boyd & Sisk, 1972; Hawkins & McCormack, 1988; Hawkins et al, 1984; Rowe, 1956; Schwartz et al, 1987). However, the reported incidence of posterior instability in the competitive athletic population is increasing, most likely as a result of greater awareness of the associated pathophysiology and the ability to more reliably diagnose and treat patients with operative procedures (Chang et al, 2016; Leivadiotou & Ahrens, 2015; McClincy et al, 2015; Wootenet al, 2015). Traumatic posterior shoulder instability that develops after athletic or low-energy trauma represents a unique presentation within the spectrum of cases of posterior instability. Several later studies in specific athletic populations, including active duty military, have reported much higher rates of posterior and bidirectional instability than previously cited. Song et al (2015), in their series of 231 military patients who had operative stabilization for glenohumeral instability, reported more than 24% with isolated posterior instability and more than 18% with combined anterior and posterior instability.

One of the challenges of accurately diagnosing patients with posterior instability is that they typically do not complain of positional apprehension as those with anterior instability commonly do. The patient with posterior instability can frequently position the arm and demonstrate a subluxation pattern associated with the arm moving from abduction to forward elevation to adduction. Symptoms may be undefined and vague or patients may complain of an inability to participate or decreased performance in their respective sports. Activities that stress the posterior capsule and labrum, such as pushups, bench press, and blocking in football, can exacerbate the symptoms. Because of this common activity in football, isolated posterior shoulder instability has been increasingly recognized as a clinical problem in collision or contact athletes (Bradley et al, 2006, 2008, 2013; Mair et al, 1998; Williams et al, 2003). The initial mechanism of injury is typically a posteriorly directed force on a forward-flexed, adducted, and internally rotated arm. Although a frank dislocation can occur, posterior shoulder subluxation is more common with athletic injuries. Trauma is usually the precipitating factor in this group, but many patients may have a significant element of joint laxity in both shoulders and, possibly, in other joints as well, predisposing them to subluxation. It was once believed that patients with generalized laxity and complaints of shoulder instability were not candidates for operative management. In the more common current view, glenohumeral instability is a complex concept, with joint laxity a contributing factor, and often an initial traumatic event may result in symptomatic instability. A more thorough discussion of the presenting symptoms, diagnosis, and imaging is found in the previous section of this chapter.

The initial treatment for most patients with recurrent posterior instability is physical therapy. Rehabilitation and strengthening of the dynamic stabilizers of the shoulder joint are the primary focus. This treatment includes primarily strengthening of the external rotators and specifically the infraspinatus (Hawkins & Bell, 1989; Hawkins et al, 1984; Heinzelmann & Savoie, 2009). When nonoperative treatment is unsuccessful and recurrent symptoms preclude return to sports or affect daily activities, operative stabilization may be employed. Typically, operative stabilization for posterior glenohumeral instability is indicated for chronic recurrent posterior dislocation of the shoulder that is unresponsive to conservative measures. Bell and Noble (1991), more than two decades ago, described posterior shoulder instability as one of the most complex shoulder problems confronting surgeons. The advancement of shoulder arthroscopy over the past 30 years has allowed many procedures that were traditionally performed open to now be addressed arthroscopically, including the treatment of posterior glenohumeral instability. The use of arthroscopic techniques to address posterior labral pathology and capsular redundancy is described in detail in previous sections.

The focus of this section is on open operative stabilization of posterior instability.

When surgery is being considered, two factors must be evaluated: (1) the posterior labrum and posterior capsular redundancy and (2) anatomic or structural factors that may contribute to posterior instability, such as increased glenoid retroversion and reverse Hill-Sachs defect of the humeral head. If a posterior labral tear and/or posterior joint laxity is present without anatomic abnormalities, posterior labral repair and capsulorrhaphy may be all that are required. Historically, this was accomplished via an open posterior approach as described later. However, with greater understanding as well as advances in equipment and experience, the use of arthroscopic techniques has become the standard (Arner et al, 2015; Bottoni et al, 2005; Bradley et al, 2008; Chang et al, 2016; Leivadiotou & Ahrens, 2015; McClincy et al, 2015; Provencher et al, 2011;Wooten et al, 2015). The arthroscopic technique has several advantages over open stabilization. The joint can be more thoroughly evaluated arthroscopically. Concomitant pathology, including superior and anterior labral tears, rotator cuff tears, and biceps tendinopathy, can be addressed concomitantly via arthroscopic techniques. The incisions are more cosmetically acceptable, and postoperative pain is less severe with arthroscopic techniques in comparison with traditional open surgery. The arthroscopic techniques are described in detail in previous sections.

Open Posterior Capsulorrhaphy

PATIENT POSITION

The open posterior approach is utilized to access the posterior shoulder capsule and, if necessary, the posterior humerus or glenoid. The patient can be placed in the lateral decubitus or prone position with the operative arm draped free. This position allows full rotation and manipulation of the shoulder throughout the procedure. We do like to position the arm supported on a padded Mayo stand to place the arm into slight abduction, forward flexion, and neutral rotation. The arm is free, however, and can be manipulated into any position desired. The advantage of the lateral decubitus is the ability to first evaluate the shoulder arthroscopically prior to the posterior approach. The prone position on a radiolucent table allows for better intraoperative fluoroscopic assessment during a glenoid osteotomy but precludes concomitant arthroscopy.

An examination with the patient under anesthesia, prior to positioning for surgery, is very useful to confirm the direction and magnitude of glenohumeral instability. A comparison with the contralateral shoulder is mandatory to assess subtle differences in posterior glenohumeral laxity. The amount of humeral translation is quantified by the classification described by Altchek and Dines (1995). A shoulder with a grade 2 or higher posterior drawer test result is typically pathologic, except in the case of multidirectional instability. The other shoulder is then assessed to compare for asymmetry of glenohumeral laxity.

OPERATIVE APPROACH

See Video 2C.1.

For the posterior capsulorrhaphy, the posterior approach is made via a vertical incision starting at the posterior spine of the scapula and centered over the posterior glenohumeral articulation. Fasciocutaneous flaps are developed, and then the posterior deltoid is split in line with its fibers, ideally along the raphe between the middle and posterior components to expose the posterior rotator cuff (Fig. 2C.1). In a large patient it may be necessary to detach a portion of the deltoid from the scapular spine posteriorly to gain exposure; the detachment can be repaired during the closure. Care is taken to make sure the deltoid is not split more than 5 cm inferiorly to the spine of the acromion to prevent potential damage to the axillary nerve. The axillary nerve exits the quadrangular space, which is bound by the long and lateral heads of the triceps muscles and between the teres major and minor muscles. The axillary nerve must be protected when the deltoid is reflected off the scapular spine during the more extensive approach described later.

A continuous fascial sheet that spreads across the posterior rotator cuff muscles can make it difficult to expose the intervals between muscles (Fig. 2C.2). The spine of the scapula separates the supraspinatus from the infraspinatus,

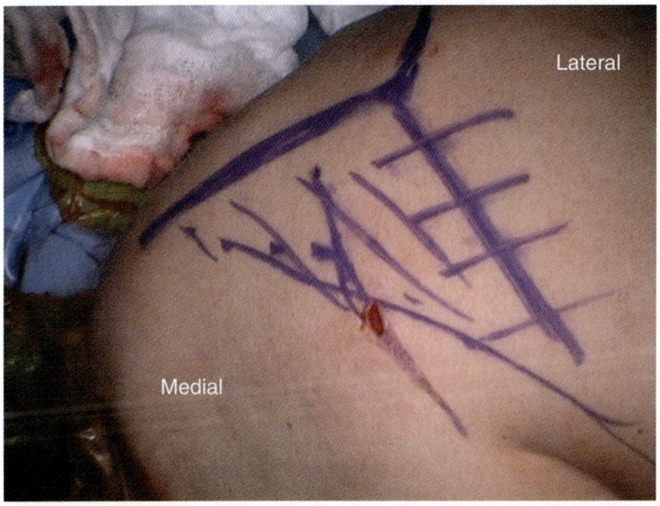

Fig. 2C.1 Operative view of posterior aspect of *right* shoulder demonstrating anatomic landmarks marked on the skin. The posterolateral acromion, scapular spine, posterior deltoid, and glenohumeral articulation are identified.

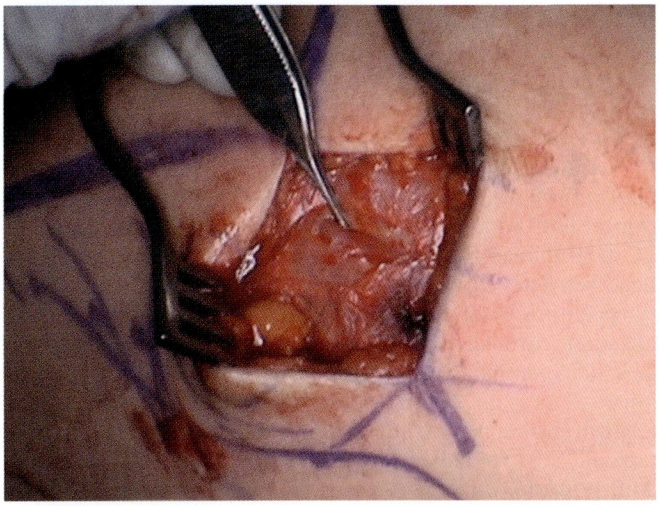

Fig. 2C.2 The skin is incised exposing the fascia over the posterior deltoid muscle.

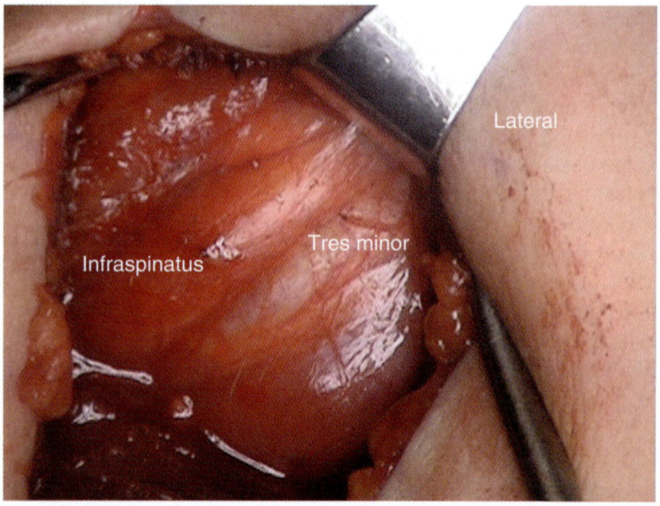

Fig. 2C.3 The deltoid is split between the middle and posterior segments and retracted to expose the posterior rotator cuff muscles, specifically the infraspinatus and teres minor.

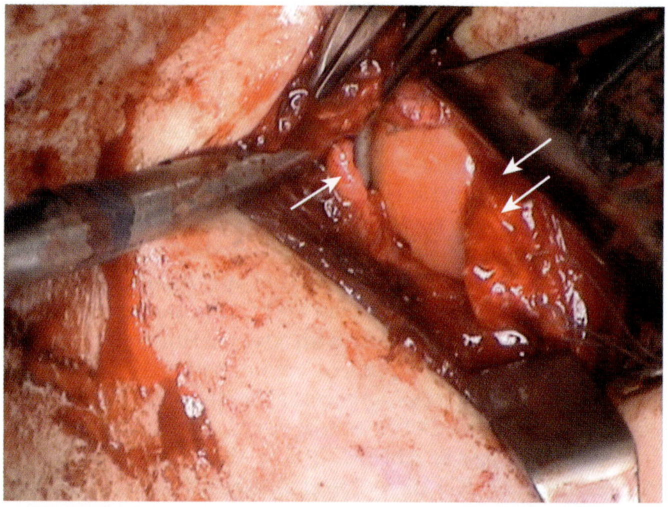

Fig. 2C.4 The interval between the infraspinatus and teres minor muscles is developed to expose the patulous posterior shoulder capsule. The capsule is split in a T shape with the vertical limb lateral and the horizontal limb at the lower portion of the posterior glenoid. The upper leaflet *(single arrow)* and the lower or inferior leaflet *(double arrows)* are demonstrated.

but their tendons converge as they pass laterally to insert on the greater tuberosity (Fig. 2C.3). The boundary between the tendons is nearly indistinguishable at their insertions. Therefore, separate the supraspinatus and infraspinatus, a line can be drawn from the scapular spine to the posterior aspect of the greater tuberosity, which splits the two muscles and their respective tendons. The innervation of both muscles is via the suprascapular nerve. The nerve courses from anterior to posterior after traversing the suprascapular notch underneath the suprascapular ligament. It then runs along the superior surface of the scapula in the supraspinatus fossa, after which it wraps around the spinoglenoid notch to innervate the infraspinatus. When the posterior glenoid is exposed during the osteotomy described later, the suprascapular nerve and vessels must be identified and protected as they exit the spinoglenoid notch.

The boundary between the infraspinatus and teres minor may be even more difficult to identify because the two muscle bellies blend together over the body of the scapula. However, at the point of insertion of the teres minor on the humerus, there is usually a distinct bony prominence. This may be traced more medially to split the two muscles. This interval can be developed medially without significant risk of damaging either the suprascapular or axillary nerve. To access the posterior capsule, the infraspinatus and teres minor are carefully reflected off the underlying capsule. A sharp self-retaining retractor then can be used to develop and maintain this interval.

The posterior capsule is then opened in a T-shaped configuration with the vertical limb based laterally and the horizontal limb in the middle of the palpable glenoid face (Fig. 2C.4). Unlike in the Bankart procedure, in which a humeral head retractor can be placed into the joint and hinged on the posterior lip of the glenoid to partially expose the glenoid articular surface, the posterior glenoid anatomy typically precludes similar exposure. However, if a posterior labral injury is present, the capsulotomy should allow adequate exposure to repair the labral injury. The posterior labrum is typically less robust than the anterior labrum. The redundant posterior capsule is separated inferiorly from the teres minor and pulled superiorly. The inferior leaflet is sewn to the lateral capsule, in a "pants over vest" pattern to eliminate the redundancy (Fig. 2C.5). The rotator cuff muscles and deltoid are allowed to resume their normal position when the retractors are removed. The skin is closed in standard fashion.

Glenoid Osteotomy

If excessive glenoid retroversion or a large reverse Hill-Sachs is present, a posterior capsulorrhaphy may be inadequate to address the posterior instability. Normal glenoid version in most studies has been reported close to 0 degrees, sometimes with slight anteversion but more often slight retroversion with values typically less than 10 degrees in either direction (Friedman et al, 1992; van de Bunt et al, 2015). The normal version can show great variability, and several studies have shown differences in measurements based on techniques utilized to determine version. Irrespective of the variation in glenoid version, it is clear that increased retroversion can lead to recurrent posterior instability owing to the posterior inclination of the glenoid articular surface. In cases of increased retroversion, a capsulorrhaphy alone may not be effective in maintaining joint stability.

The operative approach for a posterior glenoid osteotomy requires a more extensile exposure. Good visualization of the glenoid neck, including the suprascapular nerve and the glenoid articular surface, is paramount to being able to safely and effectively osteotomize the glenoid. Preoperative three-dimensional (3D) computed tomography (CT) is useful for assessing the true glenoid version and expected amount of posterior opening required to restore stability. Because of the tremendous variation in glenoid version for all shoulders, the procedure is typically considered only in patients who have posterior instability with glenoid retroversion greater than 20 degrees. The CT scan should also be carefully assessed for glenoid dysplasia. *Glenoid dysplasia, glenoid hypoplasia,* and *posterior glenoid rim deficiency* are all terms for a spectrum of abnormalities involving bone

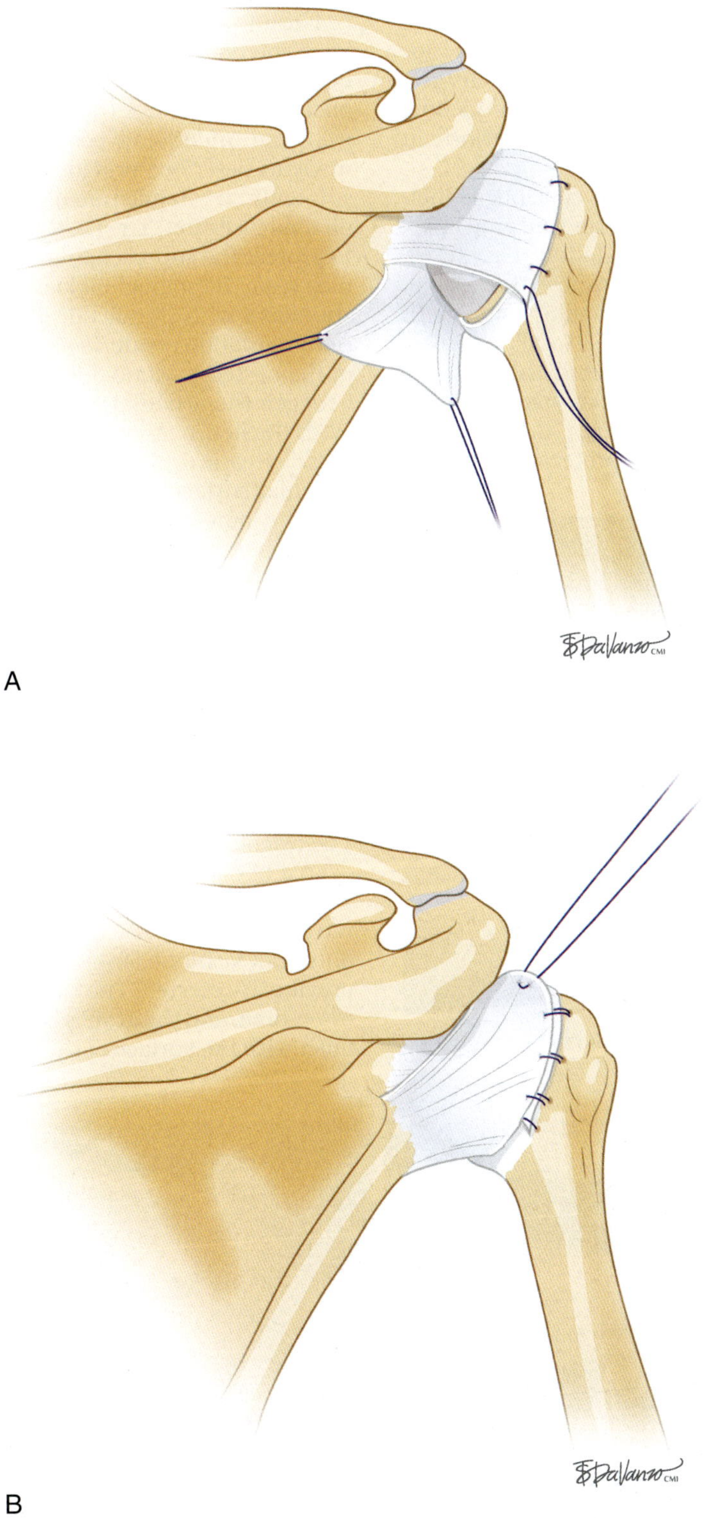

Fig. 2C.5 (A and B) Diagrammatic representation of the posterior capsulotomy and capsulorrhaphy. The lower leaflet is translated superiorly over the upper leaflet to eliminate the redundancy.

deficiency of the posteroinferior glenoid rim combined with hypertrophy of the adjacent cartilage. Harper et al (2005) at Duke University found a 14% incidence of glenoid dysplasia in 103 consecutive magnetic resonance imaging (MRI) sessions performed for shoulder pathology. They also noted a higher incidence of posterior labral tears in shoulders with moderate or severe glenoid dysplasia than in shoulders with no or mild dysplasia. Although associated with posterior instability, glenoid dysplasia appears to be an entity distinct from excessive glenoid retroversion, wherein the glenoid bone and the articular surface are angulated posteriorly in relation to the long axis of the scapular body.

The operative approach begins with a curvilinear incision stretching across the scapular spine and curving inferolaterally over the glenohumeral articulation (Fig. 2C.6). Fasciocutaneous flaps are developed to expose the deltoid. The deltoid is sharply released off the scapular spine, with care to ensure that a cuff of tendon is left to allow subsequent repair. The deltoid is released laterally all the way to the posterolateral corner of the scapular spine, and the muscle belly is reflected inferolaterally (Fig. 2C.7). The deltoid innervation, the axillary nerve, is protected as it exits inferior to the teres minor in the quadrangular space. The posterior rotator cuff is exposed in its entirety. However, to obtain better visualization superiorly, the posterior corner of the scapular spine is osteotomized. This bone is later utilized to provide bone graft and maintain the opening wedge glenoid osteotomy as described by Scott (1967).

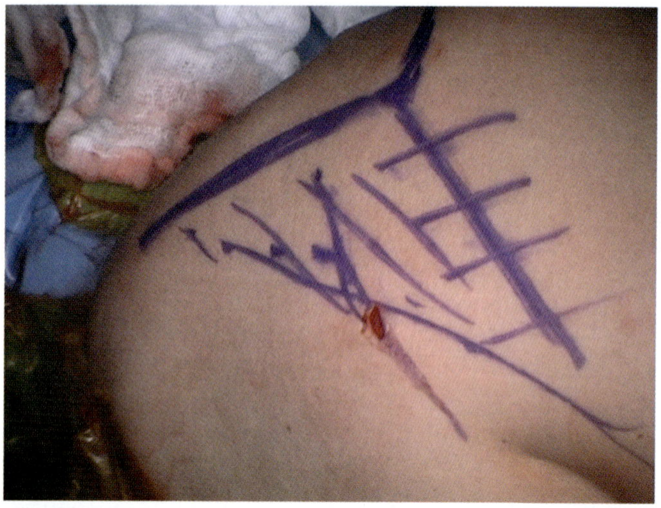

Fig. 2C.6 Operative view of *right* shoulder prior to extensile posterior shoulder. The anatomic landmarks are identified.

The infraspinatus tendon is now released from its humeral insertion on the greater tuberosity. Developing the interval between supraspinatus and infraspinatus is described previously. The tendon is then reflected medially and separated from the underlying posterior capsule. A capsulotomy is made as described previously. The medial limb of the capsulotomy is extended medially and then reflected from its glenoid insertion. The posterior glenoid is carefully exposed to protect the suprascapular nerve and artery, which emanate from the spinoglenoid notch. It should be noted that in shoulders with significant glenoid retroversion, the posterior angulation results in a shorter neck; therefore the width of the posterior glenoid is decreased, resulting in less bone between the articular surface and the spinoglenoid notch. With the neurovascular structures protected, two threaded guidewires are placed across the glenoid parallel to the articular surface. A humeral head retractor can be inserted into the joint to allow visualization of the articular surface. It is imperative that the guidewires and subsequent osteotomy do not breach the articular surface. Positioning the patient supine on a radiolucent table allows for fluoroscopic assessment and confirmation of guidewire placement.

The glenoid is cut with an oscillating saw along the guidewires 5 to 10 mm medial to the glenoid face and parallel to it while the suprascapular nerve is protected. It is helpful to measure the width of the glenoid on CT preoperatively to estimate the depth of the osteotomy. The surgeon must avoid cutting completely across the glenoid neck. The osteotomy is hinged anteriorly and slowly opened. The degree of correction can be measured on preoperative CT with a goal of restoring the version to neutral—that is, no retroversion. The osteotomy is kept open with a wedge of autograft fashioned from the bone of the posterior scapular previously resected. The osteotomy site is held open with an osteotome, and the graft is impacted into the osteotomy site, flush with the surface of the posterior glenoid. (Fig. 2C.8).

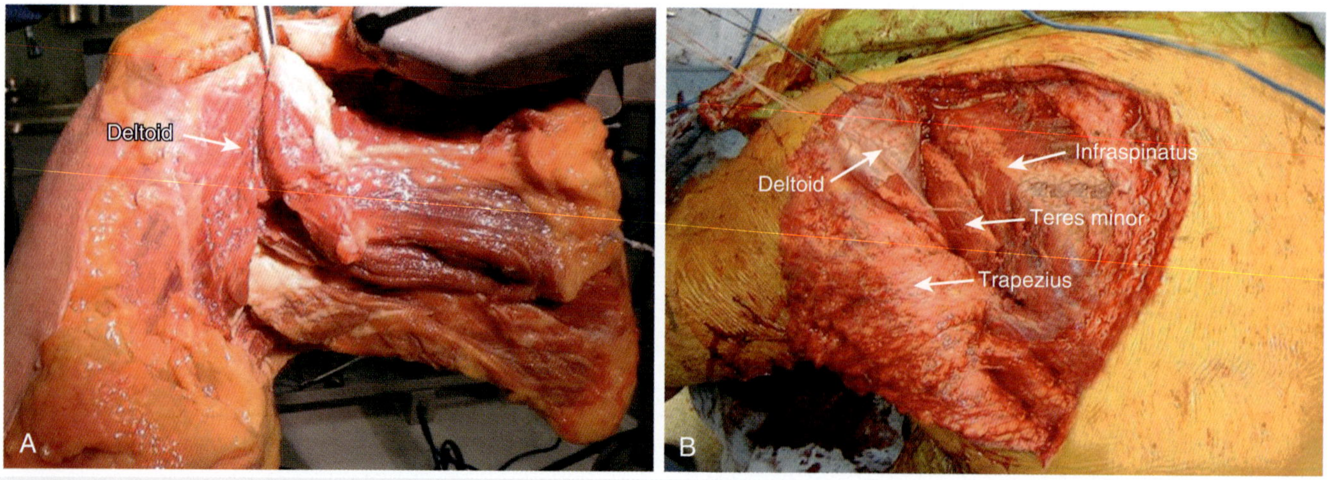

Fig. 2C.7 (A and B) Cadaveric dissection of left shoulder with the skin removed demonstrating extensile exposure. The deltoid's attachment to the scapular spine and posterolateral acromion is shown.

References

Altchek DW, Dines DM. Shoulder injuries in the throwing athlete. *J Am Acad Orthop Surg*. 1995;3(3):159–165.

Bell RH, Noble JS. An appreciation of posterior instability of the shoulder. *Clin Sports Med*. 1991;10(4):887–899.

Bottoni CR, Franks BR, Moore JH, et al. Operative stabilization of posterior shoulder instability. *Am J Sports Med*. 2005;33(7):996–1002.

Boyd HB, Sisk TD. Recurrent posterior dislocation of the shoulder. *J Bone Joint Surg Am*. 1972;54(4):779–786.

Bradley JP, Forsythe B, Mascarenhas R. Arthroscopic management of posterior shoulder instability: diagnosis, indications, and technique. *Clin Sports Med*. 2008;27(4):649–670.

Bradley JP, McClincy MP, Arner JW, Tejwani SG. Arthroscopic capsulolabral reconstruction for posterior instability of the shoulder: a prospective study of 200 shoulders. *Am J Sports Med*. 2013;41(9):2005–2014.

Bradley JP, Baker CL 3rd, Kline AJ, Armfield DR, Chhabra A. Arthroscopic capsulolabral reconstruction for posterior instability of the shoulder: a prospective study of 100 shoulders. *Am J Sports Med*. 2006;34(7):1061–1071.

Chang ES, Greco NJ, McClincy MP, Bradley JP. Posterior shoulder instability in overhead athletes. *Orthop Clin North Am*. 2016;47(1):179–187.

Friedman RJ, Hawthorne KB, Genez BM. The use of computerized tomography in the measurement of glenoid version. *J Bone Joint Surg Am*. 1992;74(7):1032–1037.

Harper KW, Helms CA, Haystead CM, Higgins LD. Glenoid dysplasia: incidence and association with posterior labral tears as evaluated on MRI. *AJR Am J Roentgenol*. 2005;184(3):984–988.

Hawkins RJ, McCormack RG. Posterior shoulder instability. *Orthopedics*. 1988;11(1):101–107.

Hawkins RJ, Belle RM. Posterior instability of the shoulder. *Instr Course Lect*. 1989;38:211–215.

Hawkins RJ, Koppert G, Johnston G. Recurrent posterior instability (subluxation) of the shoulder. *J Bone Joint Surg Am*. 1984;66(2):169–174.

Hawkins RJ, Neer CS 2nd, Pianta RM, Mendoza FX. Locked posterior dislocation of the shoulder. *J Bone Joint Surg Am*. 1987;69(1):9–18.

Heinzelmann AD, Savoie FH 3rd. Posterior and multidirectional instability of the shoulder. *Instr Course Lect*. 2009;58:315–321.

Hill HA, Sachs MD. The grooved defect of the humeral head: a frequently unrecognized complication of dislocations of the shoulder joint. *Radiology*. 1940;35:690–700.

Leivadiotou D, Ahrens P. Arthroscopic treatment of posterior shoulder instability: a systematic review. *Arthroscopy*. 2015;31(3):555–560.

Mair SD, Zarzour RH, Speer KP. Posterior labral injury in contact athletes. *Am J Sports Med*. 1998;26(6):753–758.

McClincy MP, Arner JW, Bradley JP. Posterior shoulder instability in throwing athletes: a case-matched comparison of throwers and non-throwers. *Arthroscopy*. 2015;31(6):1041–1051.

McLaughlin HL. Posterior dislocation of the shoulder. *J Bone Joint Surg Am*. 1952;24 A(3):584–590.

Provencher MT, LeClere LE, King S, et al. Posterior instability of the shoulder: diagnosis and management. *Am J Sports Med*. 2011;39(4):874–886.

Rowe CR. Prognosis in dislocations of the shoulder. *J Bone Joint Surg Am*. 1956;38-A(5):957–977.

Schwartz E, Warren RF, O'Brien SJ, Fronek J. Posterior shoulder instability. *Orthop Clin North Am*. 1987;18(3):409–419.

Scott DJ Jr. Treatment of recurrent posterior dislocations of the shoulder by glenoplasty. Report of three cases. *J Bone Joint Surg Am*. 1967;49(3):471–476.

Song DJ, Cook JB, Krul KP, et al. High frequency of posterior and combined shoulder instability in young active patients. *J Shoulder Elbow Surg*. 2015;24(2):186–190.

van de Bunt F, Pearl ML, Lee EK, Peng L, Didomenico P. Glenoid version by CT scan: an analysis of clinical measurement error and introduction of a protocol to reduce variability. *Skeletal Radiol*. 2015;44(11):1627–1635.

Williams RJ 3rd, Strickland S, Cohen M, Altchek DW, Warren RF. Arthroscopic repair for traumatic posterior shoulder instability. *Am J Sports Med*. 2003;31(2):203–209.

Wooten CJ, Krych AJ, Schleck CD, Hudgens JL, May JH, Dahm DL. Arthroscopic capsulolabral reconstruction for posterior shoulder instability in patients 18 years old or younger. *J Pediatr Orthop*. 2015;35(5):462–466.

2-2D ARTHROSCOPIC POSTERIOR GLENOID BONE GRAFT OPTIONS

EAMON BERNARDONI, MS, RACHEL M. FRANK, MD, JASON T. HAMAMOTO, BS, ANTHONY A. ROMEO, MD and NIKHIL N. VERMA, MD

Introduction

- Posterior glenohumeral instability is a rare condition that accounts for approximately 5% of all cases of shoulder instability.
- Posterior glenohumeral instability is typically seen in the setting of epilepsy, electrocution, alcoholism, and acute trauma, including competitive athletics.
- Classifications of posterior instability include acute posterior dislocation, chronic posterior dislocation, and recurrent posterior subluxation (most common).
- Athletic populations most at risk include overhead throwers, volleyball, footbll, and tennis players, swimmers, and weight lifters.
- Surgical candidates are those who have frank instability or those in whom an appropriate conservative treatment has failed and they continue to have symptoms of recurrent instability.
- Surgical options for posterior glenohumeral instability can be divided into soft tissue and osseous procedures.
  - Osseous procedures include posterior opening wedge osteotomy of the glenoid neck, posterior bone block, and posterior glenoid osteochondral allograft.
  - Osseous procedures aim to rebuild and extend the posterior glenoid surface to regain appropriate surface area and stability.

The focus of this section is to discuss posterior glenoid bone graft options for cases of posterior shoulder instability, including iliac crest bone autograft, distal clavicular autograft, iliac crest allograft, acromial autograft, and distal tibia allograft.

Anatomy and Biomechanics

The anatomy and biomechanics of the shoulder are complex, with several different static and dynamic stabilizers important in maintaining a stable joint throughout a large range of motion. The rotator cuff, deltoid, and long head of the biceps comprise the major dynamic stabilizers, while the labrum, capsular ligaments, cartilage surfaces, as well as intra-aticular pressure are responsible for static stabilization (Wang & Flatow, 2005). Disruption of any of these structures can lead to instability of the shoulder. Notably, the soft tissue capsulolabral structures of the posterior shoulder differ from those of the anterior shoulder. The posterior band of the inferior glenohumeral ligament (PIGHL) is relatively thin in comparison with the anteroinferior capsular tissue and thus, in addition to typical traumatic instability events, may be more subject to low-energy repetitive microtrauma. The contribution of the rotator interval tissue to overall shoulder stability, and specifically to posterior shoulder instability, remains controversial.

The overall osseous morphology of both the humeral head and glenoid are critical in providing static constraint to the glenohumeral joint. Anatomic variants, such as excessive glenoid retroversion and glenoid hypoplasia, are known risk factors for posterior subluxation and dislocation (Bradley et al, 2008; Brewer et al, 1986; Gottschalk et al, 2015). In addition, bony defects, including posterior glenoid erosion, glenoid dysplasia, posterior bony Bankart lesions, and reverse Hill-Sachs lesions, can lead to recurrent instability (Cerciello et al, 2016). Posterior glenoid bone loss resulting from acute traumatic injuries (i.e., posterior bony Bankart lesion) as well as from repetitive microtrauma resulting from recurrent instability (attrition-type bone loss), has become more commonly discussed in the literature in terms of its potential impact on surgical indications. Although indications for anterior glenoid bone reconstruction in the setting of clinically significant anterior glenoid bone loss are rather well defined, the amount of clinically relevant posterior glenoid bone loss that, if untreated, is likely to lead to recurrent posterior instability is poorly understood.

Indications for Osseous Augmentation

Currently, there are no clear guidelines for utilization of bone augmentation in patients with posterior instability. In the absence of an acute traumatic etiology with documented damage to the posterior glenoid, such as in the setting of an acute posterior bony Bankart lesion, most clinicians recommend that patients undergo nonoperative management before surgical treatment options are considered. Further, there is little evidence describing what percentage of bone loss correlates with increased risk of recurrent posterior instability (Longo et al, 2016), making it difficult to establish guidelines for when to treat with a bone-block procedure versus when to proceed with soft tissue–only stabilization procedures. In many cases, recurrence of posterior instability after soft tissue repair is thought to be due to stretching of the posterior capsule during the postoperative regain of range motion; the role of posterior glenoid osseous augmentation in these cases is unclear (Lafosse et al, 2012; Schwartz et al, 2013). Notably, patients with increased risk of posterior instability due to excessive glenoid retroversion or glenoid hypoplasia may be candidates for osseous augmentation at lesser degrees of glenoid bone loss (Tokish et al, 2014). Although there are no strict criteria, most clinicians agree that patients with posterior glenoid bone loss of 20% or more should be considered for osseous augmentation (Frank et al, 2014; Gupta et al, 2013; Provencher et al, 2010; Tokish et al, 2014). Patients with posterior glenoid bone loss in whom prior soft tissue repair has failed should also be considered for such augmentation (Arciero & Mazzocca, 2006). Surgical techniques for osseous augmentation of posterior glenoid bone loss include both open and arthroscopically assisted approaches, with bone-block options including iliac crest bone autograft, distal clavicular autograft, iliac crest allograft, and distal tibia allograft. Owing to anatomical constraints, coracoid transfer (Latarjet), and its associated stabilizing sling effect via the conjoined tendon, is not feasible for posterior glenoid reconstruction (Barbier et al, 2009).

Advantages of Arthroscopic versus Open Bone Augmentation

Traditionally, posterior glenoid osseous augmentation was performed with open surgical techniques. More recently, however, all-arthroscopic and arthroscopically assisted techniques have been performed, with encouraging results (Cerciello et al, 2016; Provencher et al, 2011). Open procedures may have greater associated morbidity than arthroscopic procedures, with described complications occurring as a result of aberrant retractor placement that causes neurovascular injury (Gupta et al, 2013), postoperative deltoid dysfunction, and unsatisfactory cosmesis (Barbier et al, 2009; Smith et al, 2012). Arthroscopic approaches allow for better visualization of the entire labrum and enable the surgeon to address concomitant pathologies that would otherwise be difficult to handle with an open approach (Smith et al, 2012). Arthroscopic technique also offers better visualization of the union and congruity of the articular surfaces, allowing for normalization of the joint contact pressures (Ghodadra et al, 2010; Gupta et al, 2013). A 2015 systematic review comparing open with arthroscopic posterior shoulder stabilization conducted by DeLong et al[18] found that patients treated arthroscopically had better outcomes with lower recurrence rates and higher return to play than those treated with open stabilization procedures. Despite the advantages of the arthroscopic technique, open procedures may need to be utilized in patients with significant glenoid bone loss (Provencher et al, 2011). Ultimately, the decision to use an open or arthroscopic technique is decided on a case-by-case basis, with patient-specific pathology and surgeon experience dictating the surgical approach. As described previously, bone-block options for posterior glenoid osseous reconstruction include iliac crest bone autograft, distal clavicular autograft, iliac crest allograft, and distal tibia allograft.

Iliac Crest Autograft

The iliac crest bone graft (ICBG) procedure has been described as a glenoid augmentation option for both anterior and posterior shoulder instability with clinically significant glenoid bone loss. For this procedure, patients can be placed in either the lateral decubitus or the beach-chair position, either of which allows for harvesting of the graft from the iliac crest and for placement of the graft along the glenoid (Schwartz et al, 2013). We typically prefer the lateral decubitus position for arthroscopically assisted posterior glenoid osseous augmentation procedures, including use of ICBG (see later discussion of our preferred approach for the technical steps of the procedure). An ICBG of at least 10 mm in width and 2 to 3 cm in length is taken for this procedure, typically from the anterior ipsilateral iliac wing (Barbier et al, 2009; Mulcahey et al, 2015). Graft harvesting can be done at the beginning of the operation or after exposure and preparation of the glenoid (Mulcahey et al, 2015). The ICBG procedure is advantageous for patients with large amounts of posterior bone loss, because a rather large bone graft can be harvested from the iliac wing. Another advantage of the iliac crest graft harvest site is the geometry of the donor site. The iliac wing is concave, matching the curvature of the native glenoid and allowing for excellent extension of the natural glenoid articular surface (Provencher et al, 2010). The graft is placed extraarticularly to act as a structural block to posterior humeral head translation.[12]

Despite several advantages to the ICBG procedure for posterior glenoid bone loss, several disadvantages do exist, including donor site morbidity as well as the risk of potential damage to the lateral femoral cutaneous nerve (Servien, 2007). Donor site morbidity associated with ICBG harvest includes postoperative hip pain, which may be undesirable for patients already undergoing a painful shoulder operation, and potential wound complications (Lynch et al, 2009). Outcomes of autograft ICBG procedures for posterior shoulder stabilization are generally acceptable, particularly with respect to maintaining stability postoperatively. Schwartz et al (2013) described their experience with arthroscopic posterior stabilization using an ICBG in 19 patients, which had excellent results at an average clinical follow-up of 20.5 months. Nine patients were able to return to their previous level of sport, three patients had persistent painful shoulders, one patient subsequently experienced instability, and one patient required hardware removal. Utilizing an all-arthroscopic technique using suture anchors, Boileau et al (2013) described their experience with the ICBG procedure in 15 consecutive patients, reporting overall good outcomes in 5 of the patients who reached an average follow-up of 17.6 months, with no postoperative recurrence of instability or apprehension. None of the patients in this group required revision surgery at short-term follow-up, although one patient described persistent donor site pain. By using suture anchors instead of conventional screw fixation, Boileau's group was able to limit some of the hardware complications described in other studies.

Distal Tibial Allograft

Glenoid reconstruction with distal tibial allograft (DTA) was first described by Provencher et al (2009) as an alternative solution to the Latarjet procedure for patients with anterior shoulder instability. This graft has since been described for use in posterior instability cases, with encouraging early outcomes (Gupta et al, 2013). For glenoid reconstruction with DTA, the lateral one third of a fresh distal tibia osteochondral allograft is cut and shaped to fit the geometry and size of the glenoid defect (Mulcahey et al, 2015). Because the DTA consists of the entire distal aspect of the tibia, the graft can be shaped and sized to match very large defects of the glenoid, an advantage not necessarily available with other autograft or allograft options. The distal tibia articular surface is substantial and allows for a graft that can accommodate large glenoid defects (Provencher et al, 2009). Further, the distal tibia is composed of dense weight-bearing corticocancellous bone, allowing for adequate screw fixation to the native glenoid. Use of the distal tibia is also advantageous as the articular surface of the distal tibia is a near-perfect congruent match to native glenoid concavity, resulting in an anatomic reconstruction of bone and cartilage (Gupta et al, 2013). The cartilage of the tibia is a weight-bearing cartilage with improved biomechanical performance in response to load and is thus able to withstand the forces of the glenohumeral joint (Provencher et al, 2009; Robinson & Aderinto, 2005).

Although use of an allograft eliminates the complication of donor site morbidity associated with the ICBG, risks associated with DTA (and any allograft, including iliac crest allograft) include infection, poor graft incorporation, and potential graft rejection, although the last has not been reported. Very few clinical studies have reported clinical outcomes of the use of a DTA for posterior glenoid stabilization. Millett et al (2013) described the outcome of posterior DTA placement in two patients at 2 years after surgery, noting that both patients had returned to noncontact recreational sports, had improvement in pain, reported good/stable shoulder function, and had resolution of mechanical symptoms. Additional research is necessary to develop an understanding of how the use of a DTA affects long-term clinical and functional outcomes.

Acromial Autograft

Several writers have described a novel use of an acromial bone block for posterior instability with an open approach (Arciero & Mazzocca, 2006; Kouvalchouk et al, 1993; Sirveaux et al, 2004). This graft is suitable for posterior glenoid bone grafting because the graft is in close proximity to the pathologic area, allowing for ease of harvest and placement through the same incision during an open approach (Robinson & Aderinto, 2005). For graft harvest, the patient can be placed in the lateral decubitus position with the arm in slight abduction and neutral rotation (Arciero & Mazzocca, 2006). After a posterior approach with the incision extending from the axilla to the scapular spine, the deltoid can be either split or detached from the acromial spine. The bone block is harvested from the midportion of the scapular spine, which has strong cortical bone allowing for durable screw fixation. The harvested bone graft is typically approximately 2.5 to 3 cm in length before it is shaped appropriately to match the glenoid bone defect. The surgeon then secures the bone block onto the posterior scapular neck with cannulated screws while preserving the labral attachments, extending the posterior articular surface, and supporting the posterior capsule and labral tissues. Use of this procedure has been reported in a small number of patients, in whom there were good outcomes at long-term follow-up with a low rate of osteoarthritis development (Kouvalchouk et al, 1993).

Distal Clavicular Autograft

Distal clavicular autograft has also been described as an option for the management of posterior instability with posterior glenoid bone loss. One of the advantages of the use of the distal clavicular autograft over other osseous augmentation options is that it is a readily available source of autologous osteochondral transplant material (Tokish et al, 2014). The thickness of the articular cartilage is often equivalent between the glenoid and distal clavicle, and further, the curvature of the articular surfaces is comparable, allowing for a congruent anatomic reconstruction of the glenoid surface. In addition, as with a DTA, the corticocancellous properties of the graft allow for strong fixation. A potential disadvantage of the distal clavicular graft is that it may not provide enough viable graft material to fix larger glenoid defects, because typically 6 to 8 mm of the distal clavicle is required (Tokish et al, 2014). Presence of any acromial clavicular arthritis may be a contraindication to the use of this graft type. To our knowledge, no clinical studies have been performed on this technique to date.

Selection of Bone Graft and Technique

To date, there is little evidence to draw upon to determine the superiority of one graft option over another for the treatment of posterior shoulder instability. Certainly this situation is due, at least in part, to the low incidence of posterior instability in general, and especially of posterior instability with clinically significant posterior glenoid bone loss (Schwartz et al, 2013). Most studies are case reports or involve small groups demonstrating encouraging short-term results; however, without longer-term follow-up, it remains unclear whether such short-term outcomes hold up over time (Cerciello et al, 2016). This uncertainty is particularly relevant when one considers the potential for allograft osteolysis over the long term. Currently, the choice of both graft and surgical approach is largely based on the surgeon's experience and comfort level (Gupta et al, 2013). One concern about grafts that lack an articular cartilage surface is the potential development of future joint arthrosis, as can be seen after Latarjet reconstruction for anterior shoulder instability, although it has been suggested that the occurrence of osteoarthritis is less prevalent with posterior than with anterior glenoid osseous augmentation (Sirveaux et al, 2004). Overall, each graft type has its advantages and disadvantages (Table 2D.1), and there is little evidence that any is superior.

Table 2D.1 A Comparison of Benefits (+) of Bone Graft Options for Posterior Glenoid Osseous Augmentation

	Iliac Crest Autograft	Distal Tibial Allograft	Distal Clavicular Autograft	Acromial Autograft
Cost	+	−	+	+
Availability	+	−	+	+
Arthroscopically feasible	+	+	+	−
Available graft size	+	+	−	+
Low risk of disease transmission	+	−	+	+
Viable cartilage surface	−	+	+	−

+, Benefit present for this option; −, benefit not present for this option.
Partially adapted from Tokish JM, Fitzpatrick K, Cook JB, Mallon WJ. Arthroscopic distal clavicular autograft for treating shoulder instability with glenoid bone loss. *Arthrosc Tech*. 2014;3:e475-481.

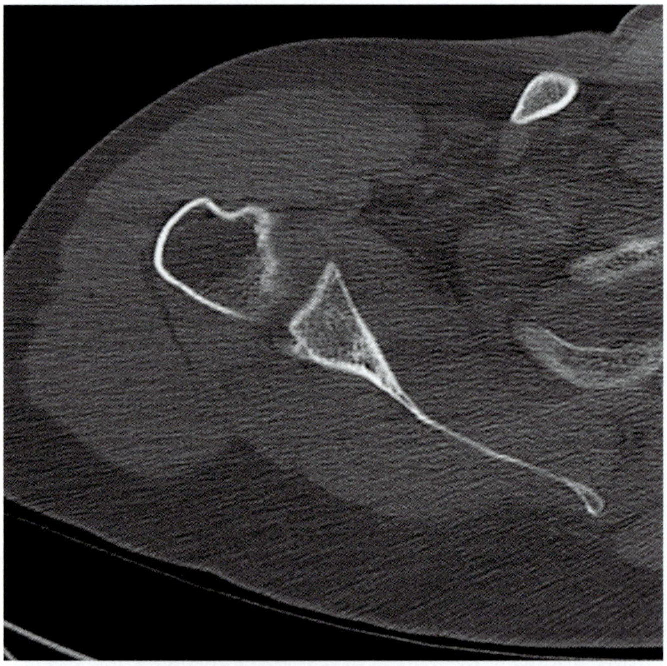

Fig. 2D.1 Preoperative computed tomography scan of a 33-year-old man with recurrent posterior instability with posterior glenoid bone loss of the right shoulder, after failure of a prior soft tissue stabilization.

Our Preferred Approach

For patients with clinically significant posterior glenoid bone loss in the setting of recurrent posterior instability (Fig. 2D.1), we perform posterior glenoid osseous reconstruction with the patient in the lateral decubitus position and under general and regional anesthesia (Video 2D.1). After an examination with the patient under anesthesia, a diagnostic arthroscopy via a standard posterior portal is performed to confirm the pathology and address any concomitant diagnoses. Typically, the diagnostic arthroscopy is notable for chronic posterior labral deficiency with capsular deficiency, with or without a reverse Hill-Sachs lesion on the humeral head (Fig. 2D.2). Next, two anterior portals—midglenoid and anterosuperior—are established, and the scope is switched to the anterosuperior portal. Working posteriorly through the posterior portal, we elevate the posterior labrum with an arthroscopic elevator (Fig. 2D.3). The posterior glenoid bony rim is then prepared using a

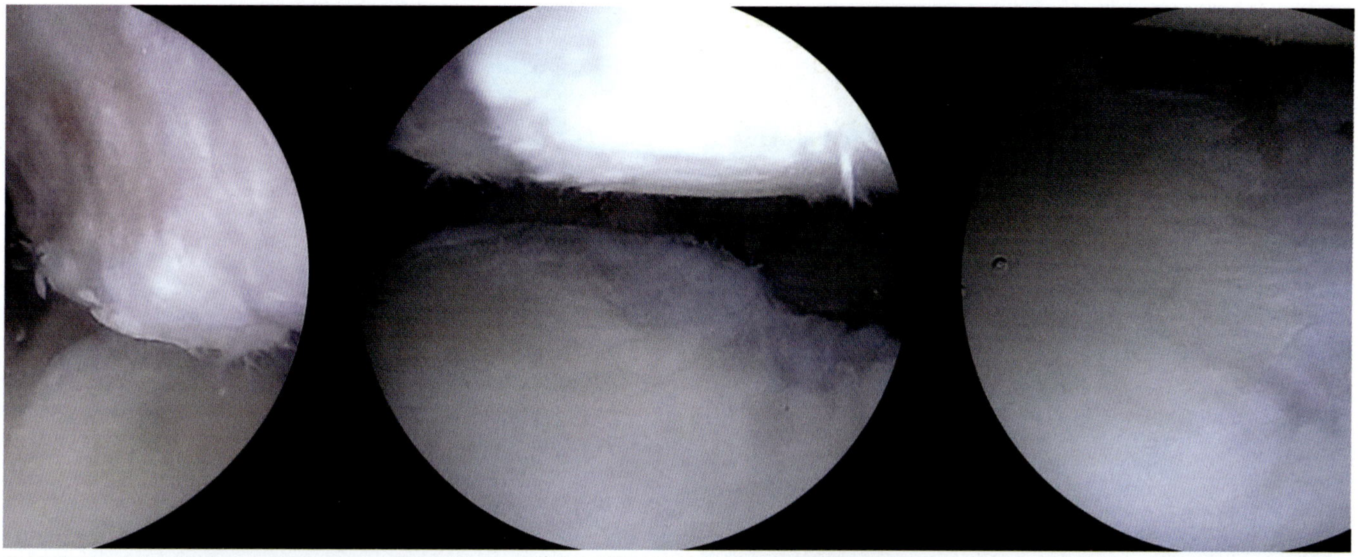

Fig. 2D.2 Arthroscopic images of a 33-year-old man undergoing right shoulder arthroscopically assisted distal tibia allograft reconstruction for recurrent posterior instability with posterior glenoid bone loss: Diagnostic arthroscopy photos demonstrated damage to the posterior labrum with posterior glenoid bone loss and a reverse Hill-Sachs lesion.

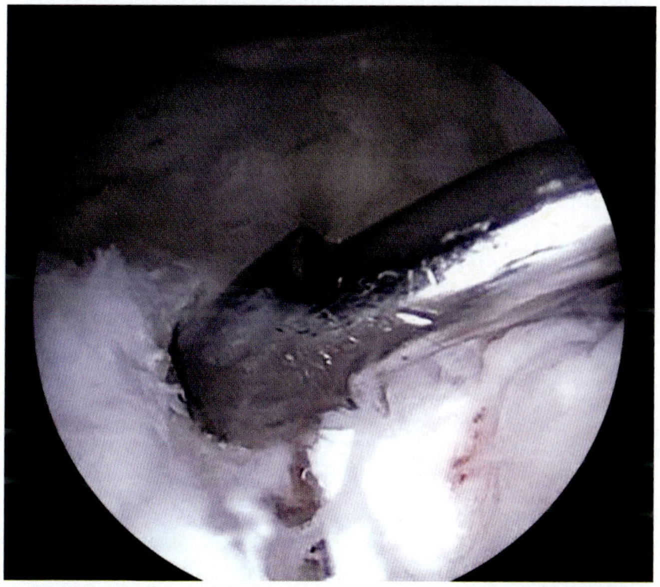

Fig. 2D.3 Arthroscopic image of a 33-year-old man undergoing right shoulder arthroscopically assisted distal tibia allograft reconstruction for recurrent posterior instability with posterior glenoid bone loss: Posterior labrum preparation with arthroscopic elevator.

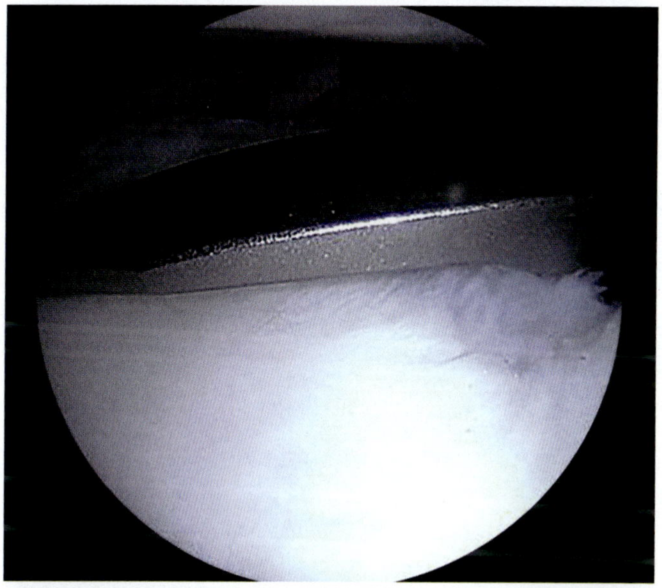

Fig. 2D.4 Arthroscopic image of a 33-year-old man undergoing right shoulder arthroscopically assisted distal tibia allograft reconstruction for recurrent posterior instability with posterior glenoid bone loss: Insertion of offset guide to drill first hole (inferior) in glenoid prior to graft insertion.

bone-cutting shaver with light decortication to create a flat surface for graft articulation.

Next, on the back table, the fresh DTA is prepared, with the dimensions of the graft matching the posterior glenoid defect. The typical graft size is approximately 15 to 20 mm in length, 8 to 12 mm in width, and 10 to 12 mm in depth. An offset guide is used to place drill holes through the graft in a parallel fashion, approximately 6 mm off the articular edge and separated by 10 mm. The graft is thoroughly washed with pulsatile lavage to remove any marrow elements.

At the level of the previously established posterior portal, an accessory 2- to 3-cm incision is made through the skin and subcutaneous tissues. A capsular incision is made in the same plane, and blunt finger dissection is used to dilate the tissue to allow for final glenoid preparation and passage of the allograft. The same offset guide is placed through the posterior incision (Fig. 2D.4), and an inferior drill hole in the glenoid is then made using the offset guide as a drill guide. Next, a small guidewire is placed through this inferior hole in the glenoid.

An articulating screwdriver is used to place a 4.0-mm cannulated screw through the allograft with a washer, and with use of the screwdriver, the graft is then inserted through the incision, with the screw providing provisional fixation to allow the graft to articulate with the native glenoid (Fig. 2D.5). The graft should be rotated so that the

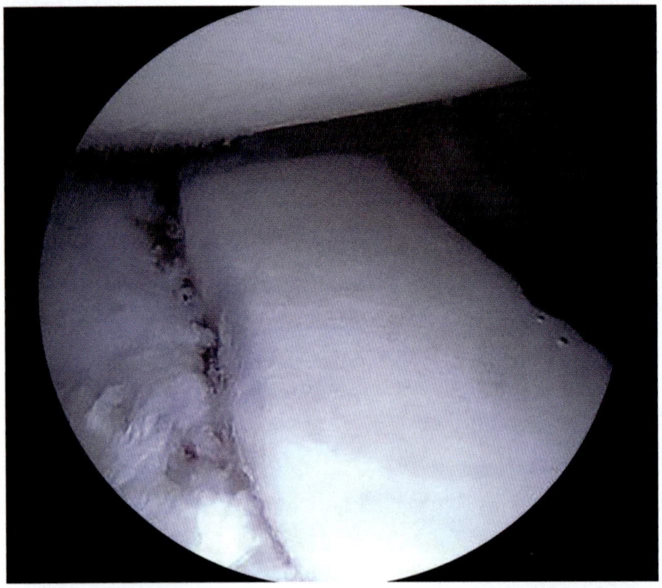

Fig. 2D.5 Arthroscopic image of a 33-year-old man undergoing right shoulder arthroscopically assisted distal tibia allograft reconstruction for recurrent posterior instability with posterior glenoid bone loss: Insertion and fixation of allograft to native glenoid.

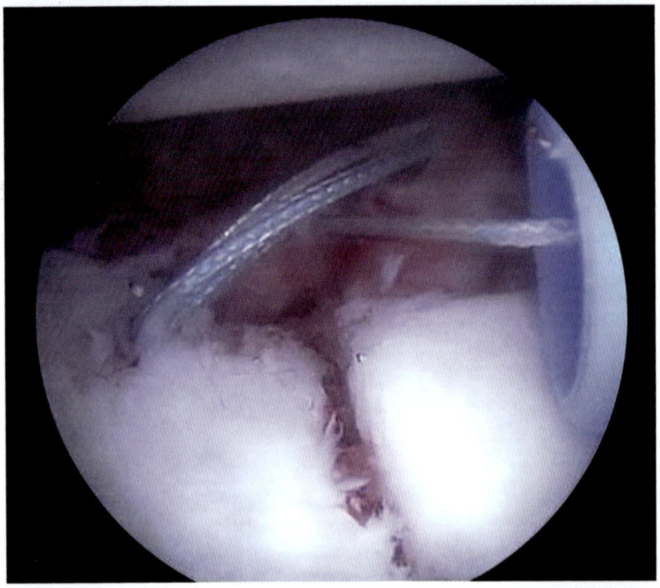

Fig. 2D.6 Arthroscopic image of a 33-year-old man undergoing right shoulder arthroscopically assisted distal tibia allograft reconstruction for recurrent posterior instability with posterior glenoid bone loss: Placement of suture anchor inferior to the graft, with sutures passing through the remaining capsulolabral complex, reestablishing the posterior inferior quadrant of the labrum and capsule tissues.

articular surface is parallel with the glenoid articular surface. A second guidewire is placed through the superior hole in the graft, followed by over-drilling and placement of a second 4.0-mm cannulated screw. The screws are typically 32 to 36 mm in length. Once the compression of the DTA against the native glenoid is satisfactory, a suture anchor can be placed inferior to the graft, with sutures passing through the remaining capsulolabral complex, thus reestablishing the posteroinferior quadrant of the labrum and capsule tissues (Fig. 2D.6). The wound is irrigated and

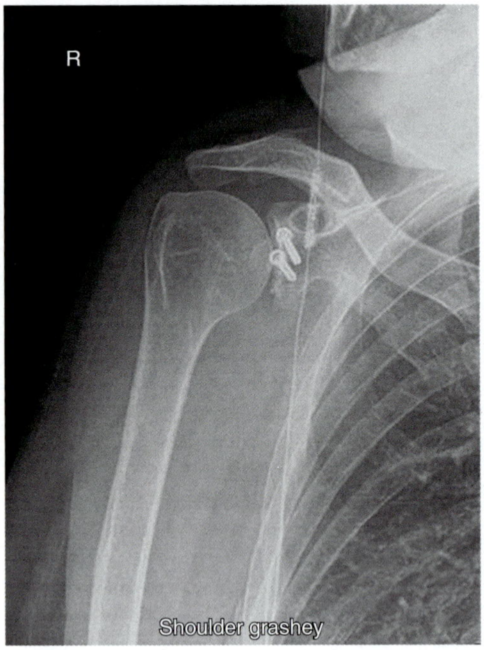

Fig. 2D.7 Initial postoperative Grashey radiograph of a 33-year-old man 10 days after right shoulder arthroscopically assisted distal tibia allograft reconstruction for recurrent posterior instability with posterior glenoid bone loss.

closed in layers in standard fashion. An abduction–external rotation brace is placed to maintain neutral rotation postoperatively, and its use is required for 4 to 6 weeks. Patients return for postoperative radiographs to ensure appropriate anatomic reconstruction of the glenohumeral joint structures (Fig. 2D.7). Return to sport-specific activity is expected at 6 months after surgery.

References

Arciero RA, Mazzocca AD. Posterior acromial bone block augmentation for the treatment of posterior glenoid bone loss associated with recurrent posterior shoulder instability. *Tech Shoulder Elbow Surg*. 2006;7:210–217.

Barbier O, Ollat D, Marchaland JP, Versier G. Iliac bone-block autograft for posterior shoulder instability. *Orthop Traumatol Surg Res OTSR*. 2009;95:100–107.

Boileau P, Hardy MB, McClelland WB Jr, Thelu CE, Schwartz DG. Arthroscopic posterior bone block procedure: a new technique using suture anchor fixation. *Arthrosc Tech*. 2013;2:e473–e477.

Bradley JP, Forsythe B, Mascarenhas R. Arthroscopic management of posterior shoulder instability: diagnosis, indications, and technique. *Clin Sports Med*. 2008;27:649–670.

Brewer BJ, Wubben RC, Carrera GF. Excessive retroversion of the glenoid cavity: a cause of non-traumatic posterior instability of the shoulder. *J Bone Joint Surg Am*. 1986;68:724–731.

Cerciello S, Visonà E, Morris BJ, Corona K. Bone block procedures in posterior shoulder instability. *Knee Surg Sports Traumatol Arthrosc*. 2016;24:604–611.

Frank RM, Shin J, Saccomanno MF, et al. Comparison of glenohumeral contact pressures and contact areas after posterior glenoid reconstruction with an iliac crest bone graft or distal tibial osteochondral allograft. *Am J Sports Med*. 2014;42:2574–2582.

Ghodadra N, Gupta A, Romeo AA, et al. Normalization of glenohumeral articular contact pressures after Latarjet or iliac crest bone-grafting. *J Bone Joint Surg Am*. 2010;92:1478–1489.

Gottschalk MB, Ghasem A, Todd D, Daruwalla J, Xerogeanes J, Karas S. Posterior shoulder instability: does glenoid retroversion predict recurrence and contralateral instability? *Arthroscopy*. 2015;31:488–493.

Gupta AK, Chalmers PN, Klosterman E, Harris JD, Provencher MT, Romeo AA. Arthroscopic distal tibial allograft augmentation for posterior shoulder instability with glenoid bone loss. *Arthrosc Tech*. 2013;2:e405–e411.

Kouvalchouk JF, Coudert X, Watin Augouard L, Da Silva Rosa R, Paszkowski A. Treatment of posterior instability of the shoulder joint using an acromial stop with a pediculated deltoid flap. *Rev Chirurg Orthop Reparatrice Appar Mot*. 1993;79:661–665.
Lafosse L, Franceschi G, Kordasiewicz B, Andrews WJ, Schwartz D. Arthroscopic posterior bone block: surgical technique. *Musculoskeletal Surg*. 2012;96:205–212.
Longo UG, Rizzello G, Locher J, et al. Bone loss in patients with posterior gleno-humeral instability: a systematic review. *Knee Surg Sports Traumatol Arthrosc*. 2016;24:612–617.
Lynch JR, Clinton JM, Dewing CB, Warme WJ, Matsen FA 3rd. Treatment of osseous defects associated with anterior shoulder instability. *J Shoulder Elbow Surg*. 2009;18:317–328.
Millett PJ, Schoenahl JY, Register B, Gaskill TR, van Deurzen DF, Martetschlager F. Reconstruction of posterior glenoid deficiency using distal tibial osteoarticular allograft. *Knee Surg Sports Traumatol Arthrosc*. 2013;21:445–449.
Mulcahey MK, Campbell KJ, Golijanan P, Gross D, Provencher MT. Posterior bone grafting for glenoid defects of the shoulder. *Oper Tech Sports Med*. 2015;23:32–42.
Provencher MT, Bhatia S, Ghodadra NS, et al. Recurrent shoulder instability: current concepts for evaluation and management of glenoid bone loss. *J Bone Joint Surg Am*. 2010;92(suppl 2):133–151.
Provencher MT, Ghodadra N, LeClere L, Solomon DJ, Romeo AA. Anatomic osteochondral glenoid reconstruction for recurrent glenohumeral instability with glenoid deficiency using a distal tibia allograft. *Arthroscopy*. 2009;25:446–452.
Provencher MT, LeClere LE, King S, et al. Posterior instability of the shoulder: diagnosis and management. *Am J Sports Med*. 2011;39:874–886.
Robinson CM, Aderinto J. Recurrent posterior shoulder instability. *J Bone Joint Surg Am*. 2005;87:883–892.
Schwartz DG, Goebel S, Piper K, Kordasiewicz B, Boyle S, Lafosse L. Arthroscopic posterior bone block augmentation in posterior shoulder instability. *J Shoulder Elbow Surg*. 2013;22:1092–1101.
Servien E, Walch G, Cortes ZE, Edwards TB, O'Connor DP. Posterior bone block procedure for posterior shoulder instability. *Knee Surg Sports Traumatol Arthrosc*. 2007;15:1130–1136.
Sirveaux F, Leroux J, Roche O, Gosselin O, De Gasperi M, Mole D. Surgical treatment of posterior instability of the shoulder joint using an iliac bone block or an acromial pediculated bone block: outcome in eighteen patients. *Rev Chirurgie Orthop Reparatrice Appar Mot*. 2004;90:411–419.
Smith T, Goede F, Struck M, Wellmann M. Arthroscopic posterior shoulder stabilization with an iliac bone graft and capsular repair: a novel technique. *Arthrosc Tech*. 2012;1:e181–e185.
Tokish JM, Fitzpatrick K, Cook JB, Mallon WJ. Arthroscopic distal clavicular autograft for treating shoulder instability with glenoid bone loss. *Arthrosc Tech*. 2014;3:e475–e481.
Wang VM, Flatow EL. Pathomechanics of acquired shoulder instability: a basic science perspective. *J Shoulder Elbow Surg*. 2005;14:2S–11S.

2-2E HUMERAL HEAD BONE LOSS: McLAUGHLIN AND NEER TRANSFERS

DAVID P. TROFA, MD, ANTHONY GUALTIERI, MD and WILLIAM N. LEVINE, MD

Introduction

- Posterior shoulder instability can result in an anterior humeral head defect known as a reverse Hill-Sachs lesion that can lead to recurrent instability or even a locked shoulder.
- Treatment options include the McLaughlin or Neer modification transfer.
- The McLaughlin transfer involves transferring the insertion of the subscapularis tendon into the anterior bony defect.
- The Neer modification involves transfer of the lesser tuberosity with the attached subscapularis into the bony defect.
- The Neer modification is the senior author's (DPT) preferred method for treating recurrent posterior instability associated with a reverse Hill-Sachs lesion involving less than 50% of the articular surface. The surgical technique is presented here.
- Further studies are necessary to better elucidate the outcomes of this procedure.

Epidemiology

Posterior shoulder dislocations represent 2% to 5% of all shoulder dislocation events (Detenbeck, 1972; Kowalsky & Levine, 2008; McLaughlin, 1952; Rowe, 1956). This number may not truly represent the full extent of all posterior shoulder dislocations, because the diagnosis is often missed.

In comparison with anterior shoulder dislocations, posterior dislocations tend to be more traumatic. A review of 475 posterior shoulder dislocation patients in 108 studies found the rate of fracture during posterior dislocations to be 34%, compared with 21% to 26% during anterior dislocations (Emond et al, 2004; Lee et al, 2005; Rouleau & Herbert-Davies, 2012). The same review cited the incidence of reverse hill-sachs lesion (RHSL) as 29%. Another retrospective study of 36 patients with posterior shoulder dislocations cited the incidence of RHSL at 86%, although of these lesions, roughly 68% accounted for less than 25% of the articular surface of the humeral head (Saupe et al, 2008). There is a higher incidence of RHSL with increasing patient age, likely owing to the presence of osteopenia (Emond et al, 2004).

Classification

Several classification methods have been proposed to describe posterior shoulder dislocations and RHSL. Prior classification systems focused only on the etiology of the posterior shoulder dislocation event or on the event's acuity and/or recurrence (Detenbeck, 1972; May, 1980). Hawkins and Bell improved upon these systems by distinguishing between dislocations associated with or without

RHSL as well as discriminating between chronically subluxating and locked dislocations (Detenbeck, 1972). Robinson and Aderinto (2005) further expanded upon this work by defining acute posterior shoulder dislocations as those occurring within 6 weeks of diagnosis and chronic dislocations as those that had been present for more than 6 months (Hawkins, 1985; Hawkins et al, 1987). Importantly, they also subdivided dislocations with RHSL on the basis of the defect's size relative to the articular surface: less than 20%, between 20% and 45%, and greater than 45% to 50% (Robinson & Aderinto, 2005). This distinction was made to assist in surgical decision-making.

Preoperative Planning

CLINICAL PRESENTATION

Because RHSLs occur at a high rate in posterior shoulder dislocations, maintaining a high index of suspicion for bony deficiency is necessary in the assessment of any patient with posterior instability (Rouleau & Herbert-Davies, 2012). When eliciting the history of a patient with a posterior glenohumeral dislocation, the interviewer must remember that the event can occur traumatically or atraumatically. A traumatic posterior dislocation typically occurs when an axial force is placed upon the upper extremity while in a state of adduction, internal rotation, and forward elevation (Bhatia et al, 2007). This type of dislocation can also occur from tetanic muscle contraction during convulsive seizures or electrocution when the internal rotators (i.e., subscapularis, teres minor, latissimus dorsi, and pectoralis major) overpower the static and dynamic posterior stabilizers of the shoulder (Ozer et al, 2005; Shaw, 1971; Tan, 2005).

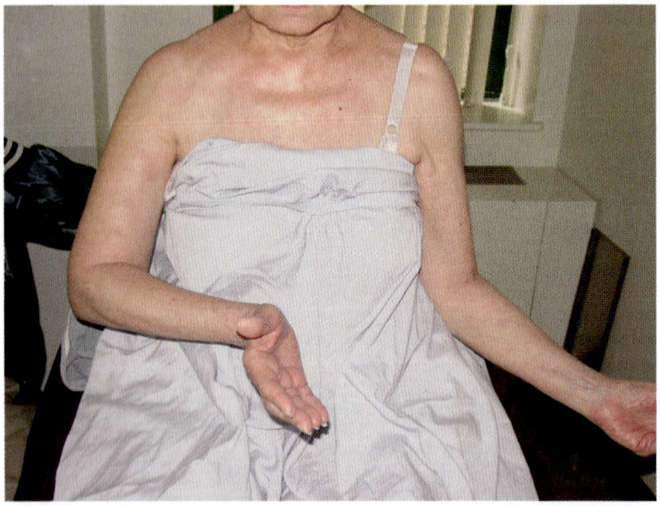

Fig. 2E.1 Clinical photograph of a 45-year-old right hand–dominant woman who had a seizure and suffered a posterior dislocation of the right glenohumeral joint. The shoulder is locked in internal rotation owing to the posterior dislocation. (Courtesy of Columbia University Center for Shoulder, Elbow and Sports Medicine.)

Physical examination is imperative to identification of posterior shoulder dislocations. Inspection may reveal a prominent coracoid, a glenohumeral void anteriorly from the posteriorly located humeral head, and/or a squared-off anterolateral acromion and overlying soft tissue (Hawkins, 1985; McLaughlin, 1952). The patient often holds the injured extremity in internal rotation and exhibits significant limitations in passive external rotation and abduction (Fig. 2E.1). It is important to not confuse limited passive range of motion from a posterior shoulder dislocation with a frozen shoulder. This confusion is a common cause of misdiagnosis and can cause a delay in treatment, adversely affecting outcomes (Hill & McLaughlin, 1963).

IMAGING

See Fig. 2E.2.

For a complete radiographic investigation of a shoulder for possible glenohumeral dislocation, anteroposterior, lateral (scapular-Y), and axillary views are required (Neer, 1970). More advanced radiographic methods are also useful for characterization of posterior shoulder dislocations and bone loss. A computed tomography (CT) scan more precisely defines the size of the RHSL and the proportion of the articular surface that remains (Wadlington et al, 1992). Magnetic resonance imaging (MRI) allows for investigation of contemporaneous injuries to the soft tissue, such as the

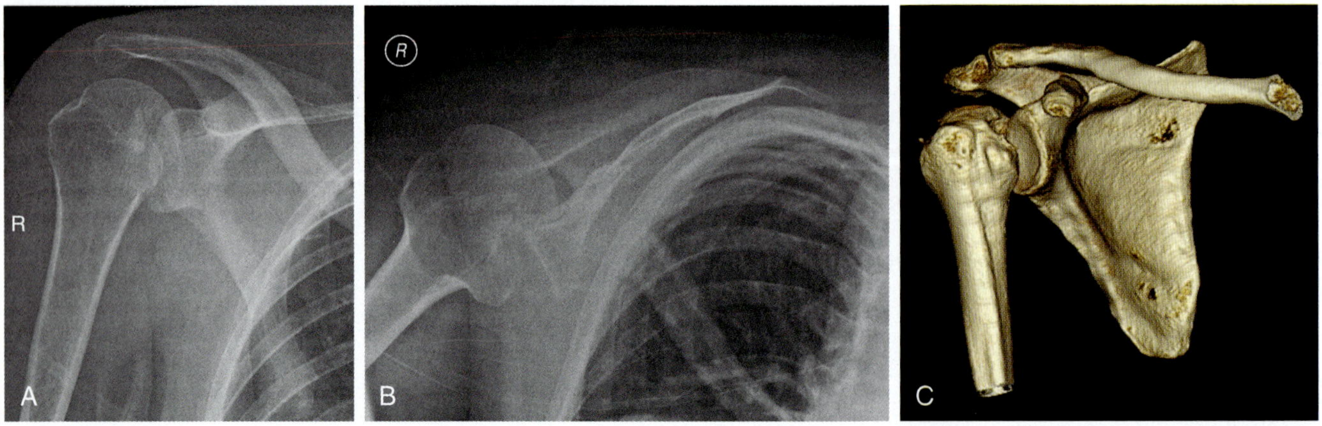

Fig. 2E.2 Imaging of a 52-year-old right hand–dominant man who suffered a seizure with resultant locked posterior dislocation of the right shoulder. (A) AP radiograph demonstrating no joint space and glenohumeral overlap; (B) axillary radiograph confirming the locked posterior dislocation; (C) three-dimensional CT scan demonstrating the locked posterior dislocation. (Courtesy of Columbia University Center for Shoulder, Elbow and Sports Medicine.)

posterior capsulolabral complex and rotator cuff (Schoenfeld & Lippitt, 2007; Simons et al, 1998).

Reviews of the literature have shown that estimation of the percentage of humeral head defect is the main determining criterion for choosing a treatment modality for RHSL (Cicak, 2004; Paul et al, 2011). However, this method is at risk for underestimation or over-estimation, even when performed by seasoned shoulder surgeons and musculoskeletal radiologists (Moroder et al, 2013). Moroder et al (2015) developed a method of assessing bony defects with high interobserver and intraobserver reliability. This method is based on centering a circle of best fit around the articular surface of the humeral head and measuring a variety of different angles and depths relative to landmarks such as the anterior defect margin, posterior defect margin, bicipital groove, anterior glenoid rim, and posterior glenoid rim. When interobserver and intraobserver reliability testing of this model was performed, high agreement was observed (Moroder et al, 2013). This system of lesion measurement is attractive because it allows for standardized comparisons among patients as well as the ability to generate treatment algorithms based on deficit size; however, whether it gains popularity in clinical practice remains to be seen.

TREATMENT OPTIONS

Owing to the paucity of high-level studies on RHSL, definitive treatment algorithms are lacking. Most of the existing literature is based on small case series and retrospective reviews. However, there is some consensus regarding the critical factors that determine proper treatment. These factors include duration of the dislocation event, size of the RHSL, presence or absence of concomitant fracture, and vascularity of the humeral head articular surface. Additionally, patient demographic information should be taken into account before the treatment strategy is chosen. A patient's health and functional status are critical factors in determining suitability for orthopedic intervention (Cicak, 2004; Kowalsky & Levine, 2008; Moroder et al, 2015; Paul et al, 2011). Surgery options should be approached with caution in patients who are elderly or debilitated or who have limited baseline functional status, who may instead benefit from "skillful neglect" (Loebenberg & Cuomo, 2000).

A comprehensive treatment approach to shoulder instability must be undertaken for every case (assessment of soft tissue destruction, glenoid bone loss, and humeral head bone loss), but when the humeral head defect is between 20% and 45% of the articular surface of the head, the procedures of choice include fracture disimpaction, restoration of the humeral head contour via grafting, and some form of transfer of the subscapularis tendon. This transfer can be done with the tendon alone (McLaughlin procedure) or via osteotomy of the lesser tuberosity (Neer modification), the latter of which is the senior author's (DPT) preferred method to address significant RHSL as described later (McLaughlin, 1952; Neer, 1970). The indication for this procedure is recurrent posterior shoulder instability or a chronic locked posterior dislocation associated with an RHSL involving less than 50% of the articular surface. We prefer the Neer modification (lesser tuberosity osteotomy) to better fill the defect and allow bone-to-bone healing. Larger lesions, comprising more than 50% of the articular surface, are contraindications to performing a McLaughlin or Neer procedure and require hemiarthroplasty, total shoulder arthroplasty, or reverse total shoulder arthroplasty to restore the normal humeral head contour.

Surgical Technique: Neer Modification of the McLaughlin Procedure

APPROACH

Either general or regional anesthesia may be used but we prefer regional anesthesia in most settings. The patient is placed in the beach-chair position with the head of the bed elevated appropriately. A pneumatic arm holder is used to provide adequate control of the operative extremity (Spyder Arm Holder, Tenet Medical, Calgary, Alberta). An examination with the patient under anesthesia is performed prior to the procedure so that the preoperative and postoperative ranges of motion can be compared. A standard deltopectoral approach is used to expose the shoulder joint, starting lateral to the coracoid process and extending laterally and distally (Fig. 2E.3). The skin is sharply divided, and the subcutaneous tissue dissected in the same plane with electrocautery. Medial and lateral flaps above the muscular layer are developed. Retractors are used at the superior and inferior aspects of the incision to aid in exposure. The cephalic vein is identified and retracted laterally with the deltoid, but the pectoralis major is retracted medially. If further exposure is necessary the superior 1 cm of the pectoralis major insertion can be released. A large self-retaining retractor is placed at the inferior aspect of the wound to retract the deltoid and pectoralis muscles, exposing the underlying subscapularis and the conjoined tendon medially. Medial retraction of the conjoined tendon may be performed with a right-angle retractor, but forceful retraction should be avoided to prevent injury to the musculocutaneous nerve. The subacromial space is bluntly released and a deltoid retractor can be placed for superior exposure. The biceps groove is identified and the long head of the biceps tendon

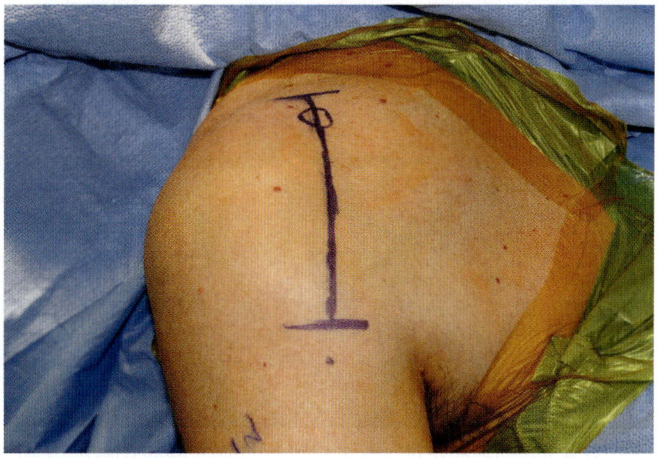

Fig. 2E.3 Intraoperative photo of a patient in the beach-chair position. The deltopectoral interval is marked in ink. (Courtesy of Columbia University Center for Shoulder, Elbow and Sports Medicine.)

Rouleau DM, Hebert-Davies J. Incidence of associated injury in posterior shoulder dislocation: systematic review of the literature. *J Orthop Trauma*. 2012;26(4):246–251.
Rowe CR. Prognosis in dislocations of the shoulder. *J Bone Joint Surg Am*. 1956;38-a(5):957–977.
Saupe N, White LM, Bleakney R, et al. Acute traumatic posterior shoulder dislocation: MR findings. *Radiology*. 2008;248(1):185–193.
Schliemann B, Muder D, Gessmann J, Schildhauer TA, Seybold D. Locked posterior shoulder dislocation: treatment options and clinical outcomes. *Arch Orthop Trauma Surg*. 2011;131(8):1127–1134.
Schoenfeld AJ, Lippitt SB. Rotator cuff tear associated with a posterior dislocation of the shoulder in a young adult: a case report and literature review. *J Orthop Trauma*. 2007;21(2):150–152.
Shaw JL. Bilateral posterior fracture-dislocation of the shoulder and other trauma caused by convulsive seizures. *J Bone Joint Surg Am*. 1971;53(7):1437–1440.
Simons P, Joekes E, Nelissen RG, Bloem JL. Posterior labrocapsular periosteal sleeve avulsion complicating locked posterior shoulder dislocation. *Skeletal Radiol*. 1998;27(10):588–590.
Spencer EE Jr, Brems JJ. A simple technique for management of locked posterior shoulder dislocations: report of two cases. *J Shoulder Elbow Surg*. 2005;14(6):650–652.
Tan AH. Missed posterior fracture-dislocation of the humeral head following an electrocution injury to the arm. *Singapore Med J*. 2005;46(4):189–192.
Wadlington VR, Hendrix RW, Rogers LF. Computed tomography of posterior fracture-dislocations of the shoulder: case reports. *J Trauma*. 1992;32(1):113–115.
Walch G, Boileau P, Martin B, Dejour H. Unreduced posterior luxations and fractures-luxations of the shoulder: apropos of 30 cases. *Rev Chir Orthop Reparatrice Appar Mot*. 1990;76(8):546–558.

2-2F REVISION POSTERIOR SHOULDER STABILIZATION: INDICATIONS, EVALUATIONS, AND OUTCOMES

MANDEEP S. VIRK, MD and ROBERT A. ARCIERO, MD

Introduction

- Failed posterior glenohumeral capsulolabral repair is relatively uncommon (≈8% of all posterior glenohumeral instability repairs).
- Failure to recognize and treat significant bone loss on the humerus side, the glenoid side, or both can result in early failure after primary posterior capsulolabral repair.
- The goal of a revision posterior glenohumeral instability procedure is to address soft tissue pathology (capsulolabral and rotator cuff), bony pathology (glenoid and/or humerus), or both.
- A reverse Hill-Sachs lesion that comprises more than 20% to 25% of the humeral head is an indication for reconstruction of the bone defect with subscapularis transfer, bone grafting (allograft, autograft), or arthroplasty, depending on the size of the lesion
- Posterior bone-block procedure is used to reconstruct the glenoid arc in a patient with a posterior glenoid bone defect.
- Proximal humeral derotation osteotomy and open wedge glenoid osteotomy are indicated for excessive retroversion of the humeral head and the glenoid, respectively, but are less commonly performed.

Failed posterior glenohumeral instability surgery is uncommon given the fact that primary posterior instability is not a common occurrence (accounting for <5%–10% of all instability events) (Antoniou et al, 2000; Blomquist et al, 2012; Owens et al, 2013; Robinson et al, 2011). It has been estimated that the average failure rate after primary posterior glenohumeral instability repair is approximately 8% (Bradley et al, 2006; DeLong et al, 2015; Kim et al, 2003; Leivadiotou & Ahrens, 2015; Lenart et al, 2012; Robinson et al, 2011; Savoie et al, 2007). However, failed posterior glenohumeral instability surgery is not very clearly defined in the literature. Adding to the complexity of managing patients with this problem is the diversity of presentation (Millett et al, 2006; Pollock & Bigliani, 1993; Provencher & Romeo, 2008). As with primary posterior glenohumeral instability, subluxation is a more commonly reported finding in failed repairs. The etiology of posterior glenohumeral instability is poorly understood and the diagnosis in a failed posterior instability repair is challenging and can be easily missed (DeLong et al, 2015; Leivadiotou & Ahrens, 2014; Pollock & Bigliani, 1993; Robinson et al, 2011). In this chapter, we have considered failed posterior glenohumeral instability repair as any situation that results in recurrence of symptoms or poor outcome after posterior instability repair but does not include missed diagnosis or wrong diagnosis.

Evaluation for Failed Posterior Glenohumeral Instability Repair

The first step in the management of a failed posterior glenohumeral instability repair is to understand why the primary or previous surgery failed. A systematic approach should be endorsed in order to answer this question. Although true failure of instability repair would strictly include recurrence of instability, it may not always be the case after posterior glenohumeral instability repair.

From a diagnostic standpoint, patients with failed posterior shoulder instability repair can present as one of three patterns, and each of these has implications with respect to the diagnosis:

1. The symptoms never improved after surgery (alternate etiology for symptoms [Table 2F.1], residual pathology, early postoperative complication-adhesive capsulitis)
2. Interval improvement in the symptoms but acute onset of pain in the index shoulder following a traumatic event (post traumatic recurrence, hardware complications)
3. Interval improvement in the symptoms followed by insidious recurrence of similar symptoms in the index shoulder (true recurrence)

If we assume that the primary posterior glenohumeral instability repair was performed for the correct diagnosis, there are multiple factors that can result in failure of repair (Table 2F.2) (Boileau et al, 2014; Chalmers et al, 2013; Fuchs et al, 2000; Longo et al, 2016; Provencher & Romeo, 2008; Rowe et al, 1973). Biologic failure is related to failure of capsulolabral tissues to heal to bone or failure of bone-to-bone healing. Infection in open repairs and less commonly in arthroscopic instability repair can negatively affect healing. Active smoking has been identified as a risk factor for poor bone and soft tissue healing in instability repairs (Boileau et al, 2014). Biomechanical failure can occur due to mechanical loss of fixation (excessive stress on the repair) during the healing phase of repair. Delayed bone healing and nonunion predisposes to eventual mechanical failure of fixation in bony procedures. If the primary surgery failed to address significant bone loss or excessive retroversion of humerus or glenoid or both, early failure of posterior capsulolabral repair will result (Longo et al, 2016; Owens et al, 2013; Wirth et al, 1994).

Table 2F.1 Causes of Persistent Shoulder Pain Following Posterior Glenohumeral Instability Repair

1. Cervical spine pathology: cervical radiculopathy
2. Suprascapular neuropathy
3. Acromioclavicular joint arthralgia
4. Intraarticular lesion (loose anchors, chondrolysis, postoperative stiffness)
5. Failed posterior glenohumeral instability repair

Table 2F.2 Factors Associated with Failure of Posterior Glenohumeral Instability Repair (Arthroscopic or Open)

BIOLOGIC FAILURE (FAILURE OF SOFT TISSUE OR BONY HEALING)

1. Poor quality tissue for healing: thin, stretched-out capsule, atrophic labrum
2. Non-union of posterior bone block or glenoid osteotomy or bone graft
3. Osteolysis of bone graft
4. Infection
5. Smoking

MECHANICAL FAILURE (STRUCTURAL FAILURE OF FIXATION)

1. Mechanical failure of fixation at the labrum-suture interface or bone-anchor interface
2. Implant breakage or loosening, graft fracture (posterior bone-block procedure, glenoid osteotomy, bone grafting for reverse Hill-Sachs defect)
3. Mechanical failure of soft tissues in presence of abnormal glenoid or humeral version
4. Early aggressive rehabilitation or noncompliance with postoperative rehabilitation plan
5. Voluntary instability (repeated stressing of the repair)

History

A detailed history is indispensable in the workup of a patient with a failed posterior instability repair. The patient's symptoms prior to the primary surgery as well as current symptoms should be explored in detail because doing so helps make the correct diagnosis and assists in decision-making for revision surgery. Unfortunately, symptoms of primary posterior glenohumeral instability and failed repair can be less well defined and often more vague than those of anterior shoulder instability.

Pain is one of the most frequently reported symptoms (Massoud et al, 2007; Provencher & Romeo, 2008). All aspects of pain, including its location, intensity, frequency, character, and aggravating and relieving factors as well as whether it occurs at night and with rest, should be inquired about. Pain associated with posterior shoulder instability is usually activity associated. Activities like pushups, bench presses, blocking tackles in football, boxing, and gymnastics involve a combination of axial loading of the arm in a posterior direction with the shoulder in either an adducted or internally rotated position or both and worsen the pain in a patient with failed posterior glenohumeral instability repair. Rest pain and night pain are unusual but can be present in association with paralabral cysts, persistent synovitis, chondrolysis, and instability arthropathy or in the presence of alternate diagnoses (cervical radiculopathy, acromioclavicular [AC] joint arthritis, suprascapular neuropathy).

Instability events in failed posterior glenohumeral instability repair are predominantly in the form of shoulder subluxation (Bradley et al, 2006; Kim et al, 2003; Wolf et al, 2005). Recurrent dislocation is commonly seen in the presence of traumatic dislocation with glenoid and humeral head bone loss (Barbier et al, 2009; Schwartz et al, 2012; Servien et al, 2007). The symptoms of posterior glenohumeral instability, especially in the absence of bone loss, are less well defined and may not always be associated with provocative positioning of the arm (flexion, adduction, and internal rotation in presence of a posteriorly directed load). However, the patient often perceives subluxation as a dislocation event even though in reality the shoulder may be subluxating posteroinferiorly or inferiorly. Patients often describe the sulcus sign as a dislocation event, however this actually demonstrate how they can dislocate and reduce the joint.

There can be a voluntary component to the posterior glenohumeral instability, and this element should be asked about during history taking (Fuchs et al, 2000; Huber & Gerber, 1994; Murachovsky et al, 2012; Pollock & Bigliani, 1993; Provencher & Romeo, 2008; Rowe et al, 1973). "Voluntary dislocators" have no history of trauma or may describe mild trauma before the onset of shoulder symptoms. The patient with a volitional pattern can demonstrate the ability to dislocate or subluxate and reduce the shoulder joint in a painless manner, although in certain cases a dramatic emotional overlay can be present. Psychiatric and emotional factors may play an important role in this condition and should be recognized (Rowe et al, 1973).

Positional posterior glenohumeral dislocation occurs when the arm is placed in a provocative position of flexion, adduction, and internal rotation. Such positioning can be a result of muscle patterning or could be secondary to structural lesions in the shoulder (posterior glenoid bone loss, excessive glenoid retroversion). Positional posterior shoulder instability due to muscle patterning results from neuromuscular imbalance of muscles around the shoulder girdle, with the internal rotators overpowering the external rotators (Takwale et al, 2000; Young, 1994). Muscle patterning is initially a voluntary event but transitions into involuntary phenomenon later on. Patients with voluntary dislocation and muscle patterning are poor surgical candidates but show good response to neuromuscular rehabilitation (proprioceptive and biofeedback program) and physical therapy (Beall et al, 1987; Merolla et al, 2015; Throckmorton et al, 2014).

Pertinent details related to primary shoulder symptoms and the first surgical procedure should be sought, including whether onset of symptoms was traumatic or atraumatic, duration of nonsurgical management prior to primary surgery and its result, and time interval between the onset of symptoms and surgery. The preoperative imaging, operative note, and intraoperative images (if the repair was performed arthroscopically) from the first procedure should be reviewed for more information about the pathology present during the primary repair. Use of thermal capsulorrhaphy predisposes to a higher failure rate and also makes revision surgery difficult (Massoud et al, 2007). Details related to compliance with postoperative immobilization and duration of shoulder rehabilitation should also be asked for. Occurrence of any wound complications, including drainage from the wound, and postoperative use of antibiotics, although uncommon, should be noted to detect a history of postoperative infection.

Physical Examination

A shoulder examination starts with a cervical spine examination to rule out cervical radiculopathy. Cervical range of motion, foraminal compression test or Spurling test, and shoulder abduction test are commonly used to differentiate shoulder and cervical spine pathology (Throckmorton et al, 2014). Cervical radiculopathy, especially C7 or C8 radiculopathy, can manifest as posterior shoulder or interscapular shoulder pain.

Important physical findings on inspection include atrophy of the rotator cuff muscles in the supraspinatus and infraspinatus fossae and the presence of scapular dyskinesis, including scapular winging (Provencher & Romeo, 2008). The patient should be asked to point to the site of maximum pain before the surgeon begins palpation. Location of the pain and site of maximum tenderness are valuable in the anatomic localization of the pain-generating structure. Range of motion (active and passive) is usually tested next and includes evaluation of glenohumeral as well as scapulothoracic motion. Shoulder stiffness patterns should be recognized during range of motion. Presence of glenohumeral internal rotation deficit (GIRD), posterior capsular tightness, and loss of external rotation in abduction or with the arm at the side are important capsular stiffness patterns.

Strength testing of the rotator cuff muscles against manual resistance and tests for external and internal shoulder impingement and for labral, biceps, and AC joint pathology should be performed (Millett et al, 2006; Provencher & Romeo, 2008). Tests to identify the direction of instability should be performed for anterior instability (anterior apprehension test, Jobe's relocation test) and posterior instability (posterior apprehension test, jerk test, Kim test) (Matsen et al, 2006; Millett et al, 2006; Provencher & Romeo, 2008). Physical signs of anterior laxity (anterior drawer or load and shift test, external rotation more than 85 degrees), inferior laxity (Gagey hyperabduction test), and posterior laxity (posterior load and shift test) should be sought bilaterally to estimate the degree of shoulder laxity in different directions (Boileau et al, 2006). The generalized joint laxity can be determined with the Beighton hypermobility scoring system (Remvig et al, 2007). Patients with a volitional component can demonstrate subluxation or dislocation maneuvers, and it is important to identify this subgroup preoperatively. A thorough neurovascular examination is important to identify focal neurological deficits preoperatively.

Imaging Studies

Abnormalities of the posterior labrum and capsule, posterior glenoid, humeral head, and rotator cuff can be identified on imaging studies. Three radiographic views of the shoulder, true anteroposterior view (Grashey view), axillary view, and scapular Y view, are routinely ordered (Walz et al, 2015). The glenoid profile view (Bernageau view), which can detect anterior glenoid bone loss, can also be used to identify posterior glenoid bone loss (Murachovsky et al, 2012; Schwartz et al, 2013; Servien et al, 2007). Plain radiographs are helpful in identifying posterior glenoid bone loss and glenoid rim insufficiency, shoulder dysplasia, and secondary degenerative changes but cannot demonstrate pathologic findings related to posterior labrum, capsule, and articular cartilage (Fig. 2F.1).

Magnetic resonance imaging (MRI), especially MR arthrography (MRA), is the advanced imaging of choice in patients with failed posterior glenohumeral instability repair. A recurrent tear of the posterior inferior labrum, paralabral cysts, loose bodies, rotator cuff tears (teres minor, infraspinatus), chondral wear, and arthritic changes can be well visualized on MRA (Saupe et al, 2008; Shah & Tung, 2009; Walz et al, 2015). In addition, this modality can demonstrate primary lesions like the Kim lesion, reverse Bankart lesion, and posterior labrocapsular sleeve avulsion (POLPSA) (Kim et al, 2004; Yu et al, 2002). POLPSA is one of the most common abnormalities seen in primary posterior glenohumeral instability. In POLPSA, the posteroinferior labrum along with the scapular periosteum is stripped off the posterior margin and neck of glenoid without a tear in the labrum (Fig. 2F.2) (Yu et al, 2002). Without sufficient scarring, the radiographic dye extends between the glenoid neck and periosteal sleeve avulsion. A reverse Bankart lesion, less common than a POLPSA lesion, is an avulsion tear of the posteroinferior labrum and scapular periosteum from the glenoid. The Kim lesion is a superficial tear at the junction of the posteroinferior labrum and the glenoid articular cartilage without complete

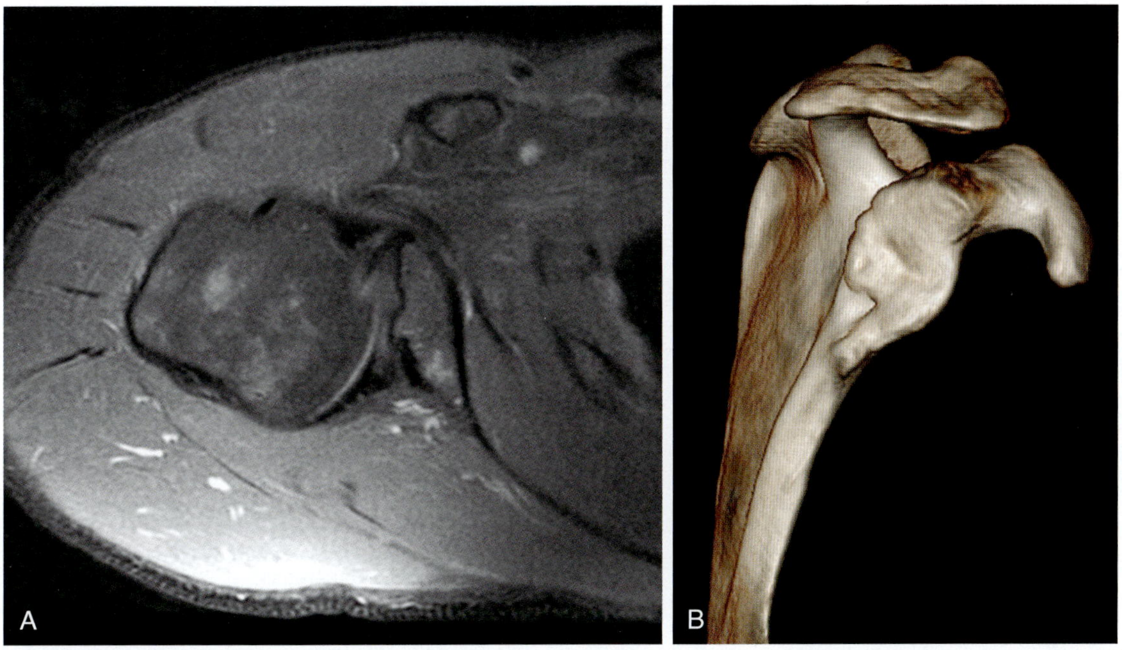

Fig. 2F.1 Glenoid dysplasia. Hypoplastic glenoid with increased glenoid version. (A) Axial T2-weighted MR image. (B) Three-dimensional (3D) CT scan.

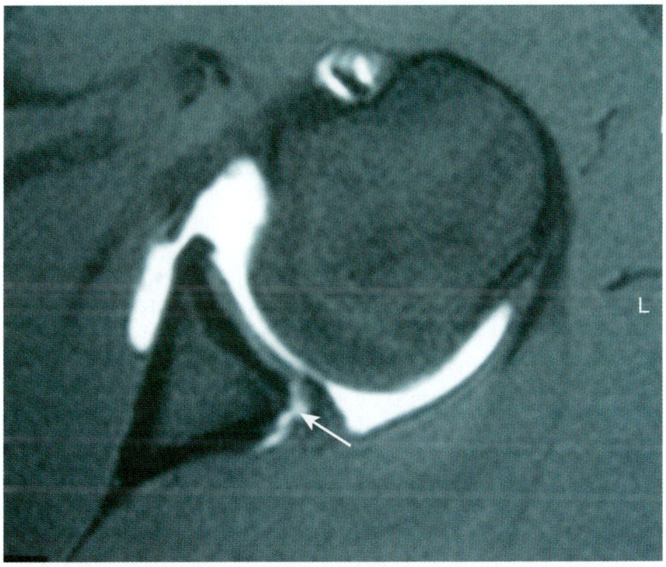

Fig. 2F.2 MR arthrogram demonstrating posterior labrocapsular sleeve avulsion (POLPSA). The posteroinferior labrum along with the scapular periosteum is stripped off the posterior margin and neck of glenoid without a tear in the labrum.

detachment of the glenoid labrum (Kim et al, 2004). It is associated with flattening of the posterior inferior labrum.

Computed tomography (CT) is the imaging modality of choice for determining the location and quantifying the amount of bone loss and can be performed in patients with contraindications to MRI (pacemaker, intraocular foreign body) (Chuang et al, 2007). Glenoid hypoplasia, increased glenoid retroversion, and humeral retrotorsion can be detected on MRI but CT is more sensitive for bony changes. Glenoid version angle, humeral retroversion, and humeral subluxation can be calculated on CT and MR images (Moroder et al, 2013). There are multiple methods for measuring anterior glenoid bone loss, but techniques for posterior glenoid bone loss and a reverse Hill-Sachs lesion are less well described (Saliken et al, 2015; Weishaupt et al, 2000). We prefer the best-fit circle method to diagnose percentage loss of bone on the posterior glenoid (Saliken et al, 2015). The size of the reverse Hill-Sachs lesion is commonly calculated as a percentage of the chondral arc involved by the defect as seen on axial CT scans or MR images (small [<25%], medium [25–50%], and large [>50%]) (Saliken et al, 2015).

Management

The management of failed posterior glenohumeral instability repair relies on identifying the cause of persistent, missed, recurring, or residual shoulder symptoms and determining a strategy for addressing this pathology (Fig. 2F.3). It is also important to identify risk factors for failure of revision surgery (failure to recognize bone loss in the glenoid and humeral head, presence of voluntary instability, capsular tear) (Longo et al, 2016; Weishaupt et al, 2000).

Both surgical and nonsurgical treatment options exist for failed posterior shoulder instability (Beall et al, 1987; Hurley et al, 1992; Millett et al, 2006; Provencher & Romeo, 2008). It is a reasonable option to start with nonsurgical management especially when there is no identifiable structural lesion in the shoulder. Oral antiinflammatory medications, intraarticular steroid injection, physical therapy, and therapeutic modalities are frequently used nonsurgical treatment options. Capsular stretching, rotator cuff strengthening, especially of the posterior and superior cuff, and achievement of scapular control, balance, and strength are important to the success of nonoperative rehabilitation for failed posterior shoulder instability repair.

Failure of nonsurgical management in the presence of structural pathology is an indication for revision posterior glenohumeral instability surgery. The type of revision

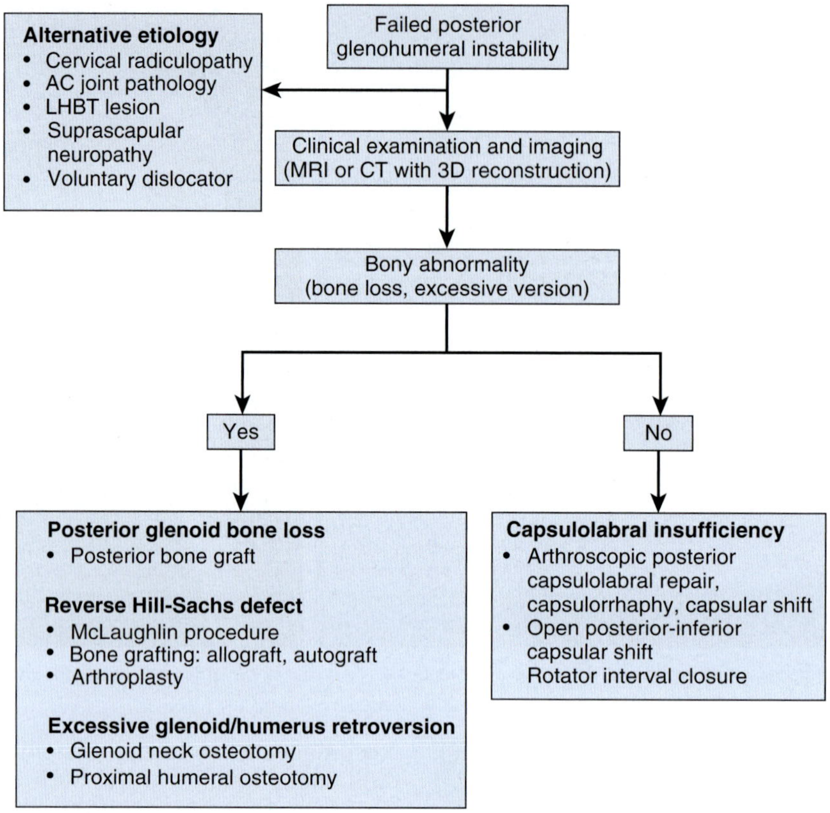

Fig. 2F.3 Treatment algorithm for the management of failed posterior glenohumeral instability repair. *AC,* acromioclavicular; *CT,* computed tomography; *LHBT,* long head of the biceps tendon; *MRI,* magnetic resonance imaging.

surgery is determined by the structural pathology identified on preoperative evaluation. The goal of revision posterior glenohumeral instability procedures is to address soft tissue pathology (capsulolabral and rotator cuff), bony pathology (glenoid and/or humerus), or both. There are no high-quality evidence-based guidelines available for this relatively uncommon pattern of glenohumeral instability. The treatment algorithms are based on case reports, small case series, or small cohorts as part of large case series of posterior shoulder instability.* Once recurrence of posterior shoulder instability has been determined to be the cause of the patient's symptoms, it is critical to identify bone loss (glenoid or humeral side) and voluntary dislocation , which are otherwise two important determinants of failure of revision surgery.

Posterior capsulolabral repair can be performed by open or arthroscopic techniques (DeLong et al, 2015; Kakar et al, 2007). Over the last two decades, advances in arthroscopy techniques, instrumentation, and fixation devices have made the arthroscopic approach popular, and the majority of the posterior glenohumeral instability repairs are performed arthroscopically (Blomquist et al, 2012; Bradley et al, 2006; Kakar et al, 2007; Kim et al, 2003; Savoie et al, 2007). Some investigators have proposed bony augmentation for failed arthroscopic posterior capsulolabral repair, especially if there is evidence of bone loss on the glenoid or humeral head side (Schwartz et al, 2013). However, if preoperative imaging demonstrates a recurrent posterior labral tear in the presence of good quality tissue, arthroscopic labral repair with capsulorrhaphy is successful (Chalmers et al, 2013). Capsular redundancy can be managed with arthroscopic capsular plication (with or without suture anchors) or via the open posterior capsular shift procedure (Kakar et al, 2007). Some researchers have recommended rotator interval closure to address inferior laxity. However, this procedure continues to be a topic of ongoing debate (Arciero & Mazzocca, 2006; Chalmers et al, 2013; Provencher & Romeo, 2008).

The presence of glenoid bone loss, humeral head defect, or both as well as the presence of abnormalities in glenohumeral alignment dictates the type of revision bony procedure. Glenoid realignment procedures are indicated for abnormal humeral head or glenoid version. Proximal humeral derotation osteotomy is indicated in severe humeral head retroversion or medium-sized reverse Hill-Sachs defect (Keppler et al, 1994; Kronberg & Brostrom, 1991; Ziran & Nourbakhsh, 2015). Loss of external rotation can be a limiting factor when this technique is used for treating large reverse Hill-Sachs lesions. Opening wedge glenoid neck osteotomy is indicated for correction of glenoid retroversion greater than 20 degrees (Bessems & Vegter, 1995; Brewer et al, 1986; Graichen et al, 1999; Hawkins, 1996). This procedure is performed via an open posterior approach, and the graft can be obtained locally from the scapula or from the iliac crest. However, higher rates of failure and of complications, including intraarticular glenoid

---

*Barbier et al, 2009; Boileau et al, 2013; Bradley et al, 2006; Chalmers et al, 2013; Gerber et al, 2014; Gupta et al, 2013; Hawkins, 1996; Kronberg & Brostrom, 1991; Leivadiotou & Ahrens, 2015; Lenart et al, 2012; Longo et al, 2016; Merolla et al, 2015; Owens et al, 2013; Provencher & Romeo, 2008; Schwartz et al, 2013; Servien et al, 2007; Weishaupt et al, 2000.

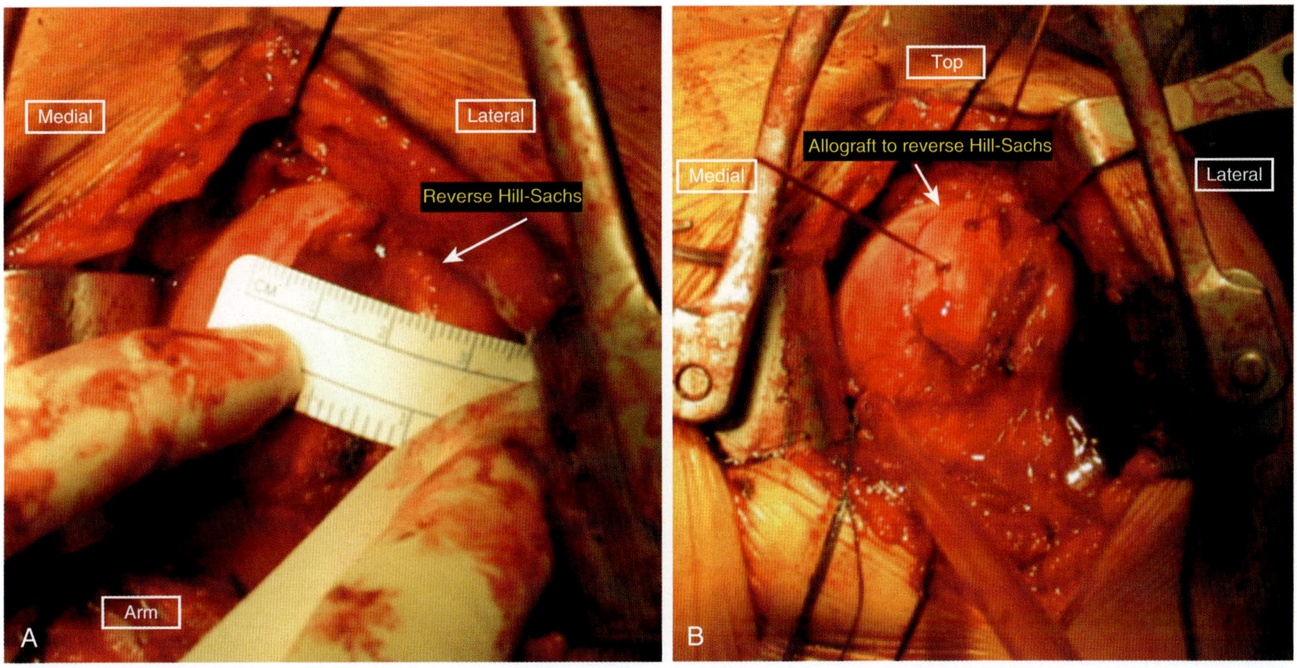

Fig. 2F.4 Allograft bone grafting for reverse Hill-Sachs lesion. A deltopectoral approach and subscapularis tenotomy are used to expose the lesion. After intraoperative measurement of the defect size (A), osteochondral allograft was provisionally fixed with K-wires prior to final fixation with headless screws (B).

fracture, injury to the axillary or suprascapular nerve, graft slippage and loss of reduction, and increased incidence of arthritis, have been reported (Bessems & Vegter, 1995; Graichen et al, 1999; Hawkins, 1996).

The presence of posterior glenoid bone loss and reverse Hill-Sachs defects in the humeral head have been identified as risk factors for recurrence of posterior glenohumeral instability (Longo et al, 2016; Weishaupt et al, 2000). The quantification method for measurement of reverse Hill-Sachs defect varies and the interobserver reliability is moderate at best. The percentage of the arc of the humeral head involved by the reverse Hill-Sachs defect in axial imaging slices is the most commonly used method for grading the size of the defect (Graichen et al, 1999). It is agreed that smaller lesions (<20% of the humeral head) can be observed. A reverse Hill-Sachs defect larger than 20% to 25% but smaller than 40% to 50% is managed by bone grafting (autograft, allograft, subscapularis tendon transfer [McLaughlin procedure], subscapularis tendon with osteotomized lesser tuberosity transfer [modified McLaughlin procedure]) (Charalambous et al, 2009; Diklic et al, 2010; Martetschlager et al, 2013; McLaughlin, 1952; Shams et al, 2016). Reverse Hill-Sachs defects larger than 40% to 50% or the presence of significant humeral head comminution is an indication for arthroplasty of the humeral head or osteochondral allograft reconstruction (Fig. 2F.4) (Gerber et al, 2014; Kappe et al, 2011).

The posterior bone-block procedure is used to reconstruct the glenoid arc in the presence of posterior glenoid bone defects (Arciero & Mazzocca, 2006; Barbier et al, 2009; Boileau et al, 2013; Chalmers et al, 2013; Gupta et al, 2013; Servien et al, 2007). However, there is no consensus on the amount of posterior bone loss that would be an indication for a posterior bone-block procedure. Posterior glenoid bone loss greater than 20%, or the loss of 12 mm of posterior glenoid (cranial-caudal direction) have been postulated as indications for posterior glenoid bone-block procedures (Arciero & Mazzocca, 2006; Weishaupt et al, 2000). Some investigators advocate a low threshold for posterior bone-block augmentation in failed posterior capsulolabral repair and recommend posterior glenoid augmentation for all cases of failed posterior soft tissue repair with any amount of posterior glenoid erosion (Arciero & Mazzocca, 2006; Schwartz et al, 2013). Both arthroscopic and open techniques have been described, and the graft can be placed extraarticularly or intraarticularly. Allograft bone (distal tibia osteochondral allograft) or autograft bone (iliac crest, acromion) can be used for reconstructing the glenoid arc. A proud graft and prominent hardware predisposes to degenerative arthritis and is a serious complication but can be avoided. Graft resorption, hardware irritation, recurrent instability, and nerve injury are other reported complications with this technique (Barbier et al, 2009; Schwartz et al, 2013; Servien et al, 2007).

Senior Author's Preferred Method for Failed Posterior Shoulder Stabilization and Glenoid Bone Loss: Posterior Open Acromial Bone-Block Repair and Capsulorrhaphy (Arciero & Mazzocca 2006)

The primary surgical indication for posterior glenoid bone grafting is posterior glenoid bone loss greater than 20% or glenoid bone erosion in the patient with failed arthroscopic or open capsulolabral repair and capsulorrhaphy (Fig. 2F.5) (Arciero & Mozzocca, 2006). In this technique bone

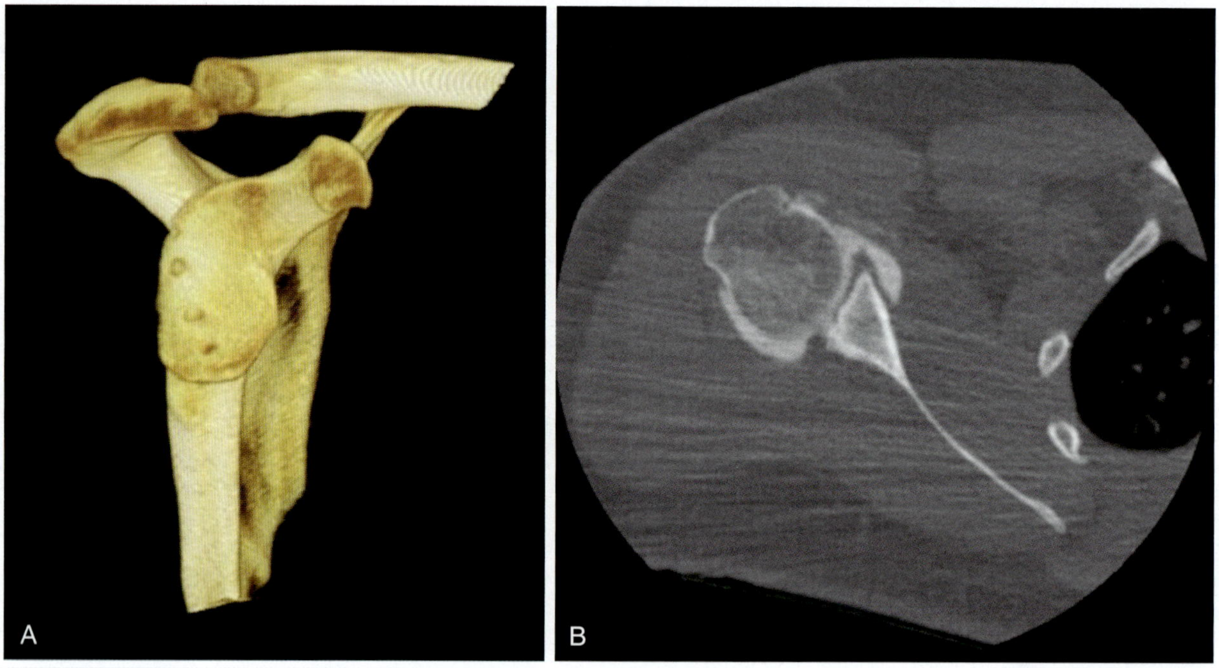

Fig. 2F.5 Posterior glenoid bone loss in a patient with failed prior posterior capsulolabral repair. (A) 3D CT scan; (B) axial section of a CT arthrogram.

graft is harvested from the spine of the acromion; this area is readily accessible in the posterior approach to the shoulder and the quality of the cortical bone allows stable and strong compression with screw fixation. The advantage of this reconstruction technique is that it avoids the morbidity of iliac crest bone graft harvest and the unpredictability of incorporation of allograft bone.

Patient Positioning

The patient is placed in a lateral decubitus position with overhead traction on the operated arm.

Glenohumeral Arthroscopy

Glenohumeral arthroscopy can be performed prior to open bone grafting because it allows treatment of pathology in the anterior part of the joint, closure of rotator interval, and retensioning of inferior glenohumeral ligaments.

Open Acromial Bone-Block Technique Using Scapular Spine

See Video 2F.1.

The arm is brought out of overhead traction and placed on a padded Mayo stand. A posterior approach to the shoulder is utilized with the incision placed somewhat medial to the standard posterior shoulder incision (Wirth et al, 1993). Full-thickness subcutaneous flaps are elevated and fascia overlying the deltoid is exposed. The raphe between the posterior and middle thirds of the deltoid muscle is dissected and elevated off its origin posteriorly to expose the spine of the scapula medial to the spinoglenoid notch (Fig. 2F.6).

A bone block measuring 2.5 to 3 cm in length and 1.5 cm in width is marked out on the spine of the scapula (see Fig. 2F.6). The midportion of the spine has good cortical bone, and an osteotome can be used to score the medial and the lateral extents of the bone block (see Fig. 2F.6). An osteotome or fine sagittal saw can then be used to cut in the coronal plane of the scapula. Once harvested, the free bone graft can be shaped with a bur to match the curvature of the articular surface and the posterior part of glenoid neck where the graft has to sit. For the posterior glenohumeral joint exposure, the interval between the infraspinatus and teres minor muscles is developed, with protection of the axillary nerve and the posterior circumflex vessels (Fig. 2F.7). The infraspinatus can be lifted off the posterior capsule with the use of a blunt Cobb elevator, not requiring an incision to reflect it. A laterally based T-shaped capsulotomy is then performed and the glenohumeral joint is exposed. At this stage, posterior labral avulsion can be treated with appropriate suture anchors, and anatomic repair of any disrupted posterior labral and capsular complex performed.

After the appropriate labral repair has been performed, the posterior scapular neck is debrided of all soft tissue right up to the labral reattachment to provide a flat, vascularized bed for healing of the autograft. The bone graft is then positioned in a lengthwise fashion along the posterior scapular neck, with care taken not to allow the graft to overhang. The graft is provisionally held with 2-mm K-wires out of the direction of final screw placement. Once it is confirmed that there is no overhang, the graft can be fixed with either fully threaded or partially threaded screws (see Fig. 2F.7). On completion of the bone-block fixation, a posterior and inferior capsular shift is performed (see Fig. 2F.7). The posterior deltoid is then reattached through transosseous holes and secured with high-strength nonabsorbable sutures. The surgical incision is closed in layers.

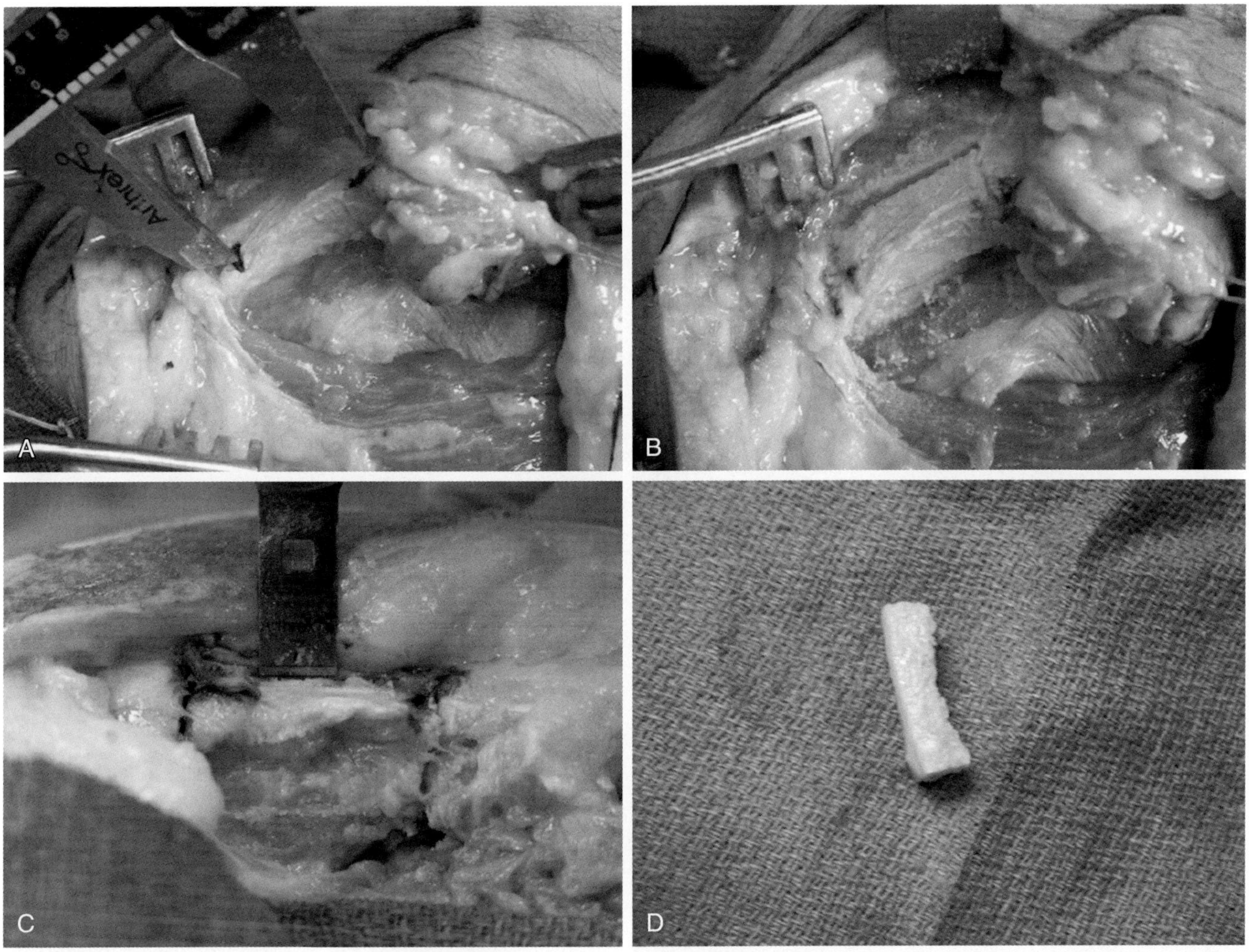

Fig. 2F.6 Acromial bone-block graft harvest in a cadaveric shoulder. (A) Exposure of the spine medial to the spinoglenoid notch. (B) Desired segment of scapular spine scored. (C) Bone block cut with saw or osteotome. (D) Harvested acromial bone graft.

Postoperative Rehabilitation

The arm is placed in an orthosis, an immobilizer, to keep it in external rotation and slight humeral extension, for 6 weeks. During the next 12 weeks a rehabilitation program to restore range of motion and rotator cuff strengthening is continued. Collision and contact sports are allowed after 6 months.

Outcomes

There are no large patient series or long-term clinical studies reporting the results of revision procedures for failed posterior glenohumeral instability repair. Scientific evidence is limited to case series and to systematic reviews that have reported on revision posterior glenohumeral stabilization as small fractions of their cohorts of posterior glenohumeral instability.*

There is considerable heterogeneity in available literature with regard to instability type (dislocation versus subluxation), procedure performed (soft tissue versus bony procedure), and reported outcomes in unidirectional primary posterior glenohumeral instability. Furthermore, the indications for different procedure types are not truly objective or well defined in the literature, instead being based on surgeon's experience or preference. However, these limitations are realistic because posterior glenohumeral instability and revision surgery is relatively uncommon and it is not practical or possible to have large series or randomized trials.

On the basis of data collected from systematic reviews and meta-analyses, the mean failure rate of posterior shoulder instability repair is reported to be approximately 8%. However, the majority of these series of primary posterior glenohumeral instability procedures do not report outcomes on revision cases as a separate subgroup (Bigliani & Pollock, 1995; Bradley et al, 2006; Kim et al, 2003; Lenart et al, 2012; Savoie et al, 2008). Chalmers et al (2013) reported their results on three patients with failed arthroscopic posterior instability repair who were treated with revision arthroscopic posterior capsulolabral stabilization. The investigators reported success in all

*Arciero & Mazzocca, 2006; Barbier et al, 2009; Bessems et al, 1995; Blomquist et al, 2012; Boileau et al, 2013; Bradley et al, 2006; Chalmers et al, 2013; Charalambous et al, 2009; Fuchs et al, 2000; Gerber et al, 2014; Graichen et al, 1999; Hawkins, 1996; Kakar et al, 2011; Kim et al, 2003; Kronberg et al, 1991; Leivadiotou & Ahrens, 2015; Lenart et al, 2012; Schwartz et al, 2013; Servien et al, 2007; Wolf et al, 2005; Ziran & Nourbakhsh, 2015.

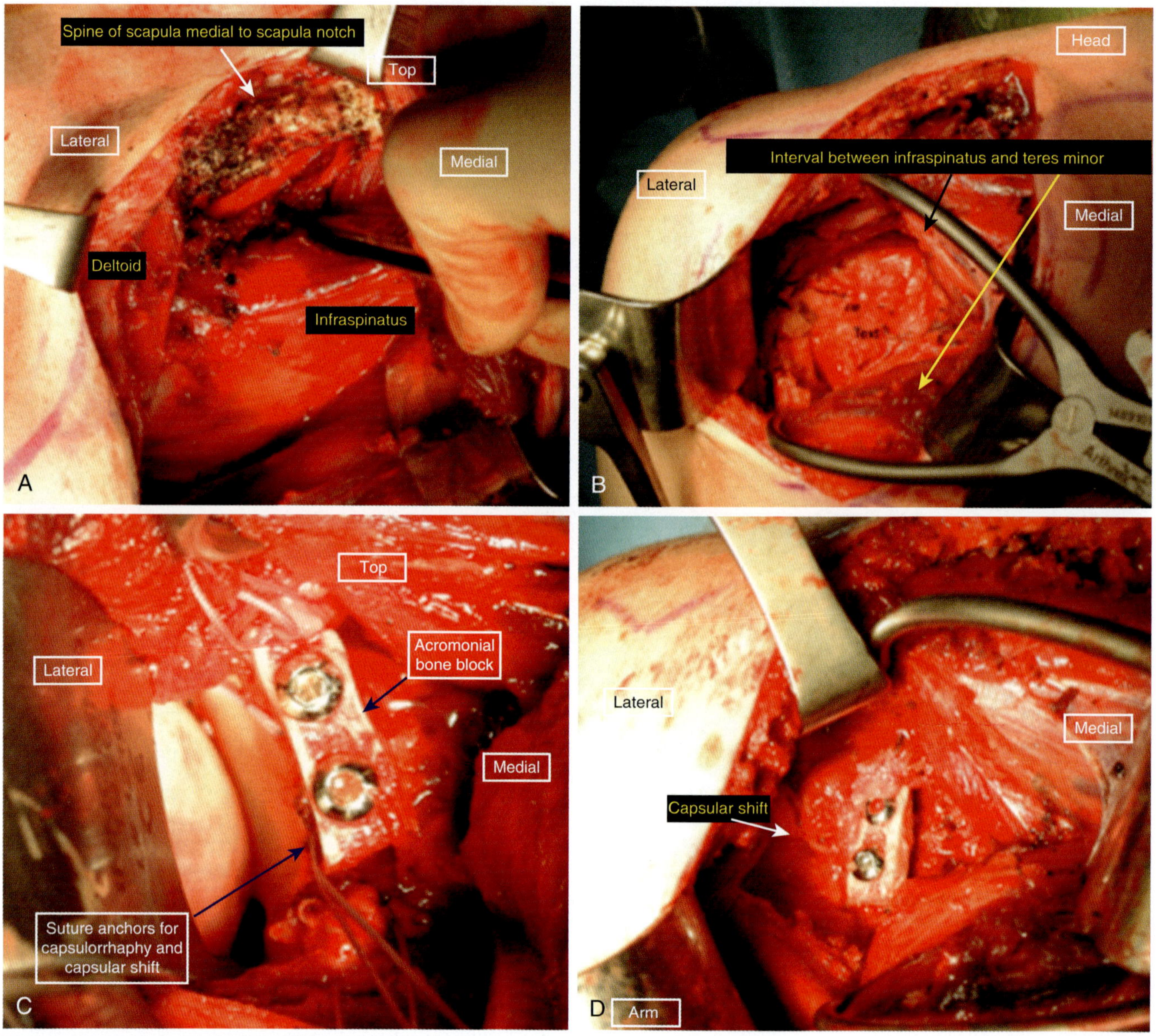

Fig. 2F.7 Acromial bone graft fixation. (A) Exposure of spine of the acromion for harvesting acromial bone block. (B) Exposure of the posterior capsule after dissection of the interval between the infraspinatus and teres minor muscles. (C) Fixation of the acromial bone graft flush with the glenoid articular surface. (D) Capsular shift and capsulorrhaphy.

three patients with their arthroscopic technique, in which they recommended using at least four suture anchors and addressing capsular abnormalities with capsular shift, reefing, and plication. Schwartz et al (2013) reported on the arthroscopic technique for posterior bone block augmentation in 18 patients, in 5 of whom prior arthroscopic or open labral repairs and capsular shift procedures had failed. Although radiographic healing was achieved in all cases, six patients required screw removal and one patient required revision because of graft resorption. Nine patients felt they had excellent results, six patients were satisfied with the results, and three had painful shoulders after the procedures. Barbier et al (2009) used iliac crest autografts for an open posterior bone-block technique in eight patients with posterior glenohumeral instability, in three of whom prior shoulder surgery, including arthroscopic repairs, had failed. Removal of screws was required in three patients and intermittent pain occurred in five patients, but no patient reported recurrence of instability.

Conclusion

Failed posterior glenohumeral instability repair is an infrequent presentation of posterior glenohumeral instability. A systematic approach should be followed preoperatively to identify pathology related to soft tissue and bony restraints for posterior glenohumeral stability. The goal of revision posterior glenohumeral instability procedures is to address soft tissue pathology (capsulolabral and rotator cuff), bony pathology (alignment or bone loss in glenoid and/or humerus), or both. Failure to identify and treat bone loss, capsular redundancy, and other preoperative risk factors (voluntary dislocation) can result in higher risk of recurrence after revision surgery.

References

Antoniou J, Duckworth DT, Harryman DT 2nd. Capsulolabral augmentation for the management of posteroinferior instability of the shoulder. *J Bone Joint Surg Am*. 2000;82:1220–1230.

Arciero RM, Mazzocca AD. Posterior acromial bone block augmentation for the treatment of posterior glenoid bone loss associated with recurrent posterior shoulder instability. *Tech Shoulder Elbow Surg*. 2006;7: 210–217.

Barbier O, Ollat D, Marchaland JP, Versier G. Iliac bone-block autograft for posterior shoulder instability. *Orthop Traumatol Surg Res*. 2009;95:100–107. http://dx.doi.org/10.1016/j.otsr.2008.09.008.

Beall MS Jr, Diefenbach G, Allen A. Electromyographic biofeedback in the treatment of voluntary posterior instability of the shoulder. *Am J Sports Med*. 1987;15:175–178.

Bessems JH, Vegter J. Glenoplasty for recurrent posterior shoulder instability: good results in 13 cases followed for 1-16 years. *Acta Orthop Scand*. 1995;66:535–537.

Bigliani LU, Pollock RG, McIlveen SJ, Endrizzi DP, Flatow EL. Shift of the posteroinferior aspect of the capsule for recurrent posterior glenohumeral instability. *J Bone Joint Surg Am*. 1995;77:1011–1020.

Blomquist J, Solheim E, Liavaag S, Schroder CP, Espehaug B, Havelin LI. Shoulder instability surgery in Norway: the first report from a multicenter register, with 1-year follow-up. *Acta Orthop*. 2012;83:165–170. http://dx.doi.org/10.3109/17453674.2011.641102.

Boileau P, Hardy MB, McClelland WB Jr, Thelu CE, Schwartz DG. Arthroscopic posterior bone block procedure: a new technique using suture anchor fixation. *Arthrosc Tech*. 2013;2:e473–e477. http://dx.doi.org/10.1016/j.eats.2013.07.004.

Boileau P, Thelu CE, Mercier N, et al. Arthroscopic Bristow-Latarjet combined with Bankart repair restores shoulder stability in patients with glenoid bone loss. *Clin Orthop Relat Res*. 2014;472:2413–2424. http://dx.doi.org/10.1007/s11999-014-3691-x.

Boileau P, Villalba M, Hery JY, Balg F, Ahrens P, Neyton L. Risk factors for recurrence of shoulder instability after arthroscopic Bankart repair. *J Bone Joint Surg Am*. 2006;88:1755–1763. http://dx.doi.org/10.2106/JBJS.E.00817.

Bradley JP, Baker CL 3rd, Kline AJ, Armfield DR, Chhabra A. Arthroscopic capsulolabral reconstruction for posterior instability of the shoulder: a prospective study of 100 shoulders. *Am J Sports Med*. 2006;34:1061–1071. http://dx.doi.org/10.1177/0363546505285585.

Brewer BJ, Wubben RC, Carrera GF. Excessive retroversion of the glenoid cavity: a cause of non-traumatic posterior instability of the shoulder. *J Bone Joint Surg Am*. 1986;68:724–731.

Chalmers PN, Hammond J, Juhan T, Romeo AA. Revision posterior shoulder stabilization. *J Shoulder Elbow Surg*. 2013;22:1209–1220. http://dx.doi.org/10.1016/j.jse.2012.11.019.

Charalambous CP, Gullett TK, Ravenscroft MJ. A modification of the McLaughlin procedure for persistent posterior shoulder instability: technical note. *Arch Orthop Trauma Surg*. 2009;129:753–755. http://dx.doi.org/10.1007/s00402-008-0721-8.

DeLong JM, Jiang K, Bradley JP. Posterior instability of the shoulder: a systematic review and meta-analysis of clinical outcomes. *Am J Sports Med*. 2015;43:1805–1817. http://dx.doi.org/10.1177/0363546515577622.

Diklic ID, Ganic ZD, Blagojevic ZD, Nho SJ, Romeo AA. Treatment of locked chronic posterior dislocation of the shoulder by reconstruction of the defect in the humeral head with an allograft. *J Bone Joint Surg Br*. 2010;92:71–76. http://dx.doi.org/10.1302/0301-620X.92B1.22142.

Fuchs B, Jost B, Gerber C. Posterior-inferior capsular shift for the treatment of recurrent, voluntary posterior subluxation of the shoulder. *J Bone Joint Surg Am*. 2000;82:16–25.

Gerber C, Catanzaro S, Jundt-Ecker M, Farshad M. Long-term outcome of segmental reconstruction of the humeral head for the treatment of locked posterior dislocation of the shoulder. *J Shoulder Elbow Surg*. 2014;23:1682–1690. http://dx.doi.org/10.1016/j.jse.2014.03.017.

Graichen H, Koydl P, Zichner L. Effectiveness of glenoid osteotomy in atraumatic posterior instability of the shoulder associated with excessive retroversion and flatness of the glenoid. *Int Orthop*. 1999;23:95–99.

Gupta AK, Chalmers PN, Klosterman E, Harris JD, Provencher MT, Romeo AA. Arthroscopic distal tibial allograft augmentation for posterior shoulder instability with glenoid bone loss. *Arthrosc Tech*. 2013;2:e405–e411. http://dx.doi.org/10.1016/j.eats.2013.06.009.

Hawkins RH. Glenoid osteotomy for recurrent posterior subluxation of the shoulder: assessment by computed axial tomography. *J Shoulder Elbow Surg*. 1996;5:393–400.

Huber H, Gerber C. Voluntary subluxation of the shoulder in children: a long-term follow-up study of 36 shoulders. *J Bone Joint Surg Br*. 1994;76:118–122.

Hurley JA, Anderson TE, Dear W, Andrish JT, Bergfeld JA, Weiker GG. Posterior shoulder instability: surgical versus conservative results with evaluation of glenoid version. *Am J Sports Med*. 1992;20:396–400.

Kakar S, Voloshin I, Kaye EK, et al. Posterior shoulder instability: comprehensive analysis of open and arthroscopic approaches. *Am J Orthop (Belle Mead NJ)*. 2007;36:655–659.

Kappe T, Elsharkawi M, Reichel H, Floren M. Cemented humeral surface replacement for a locked posterior fracture-dislocation: a case report. *J Orthop Trauma*. 2011;25:e90–e93. http://dx.doi.org/10.1097/BOT.0b013e3181fadb9f.

Keppler P, Holz U, Thielemann FW, Meinig R. Locked posterior dislocation of the shoulder: treatment using rotational osteotomy of the humerus. *J Orthop Trauma*. 1994;8:286–292.

Kim SH, Ha KI, Park JH, et al. Arthroscopic posterior labral repair and capsular shift for traumatic unidirectional recurrent posterior subluxation of the shoulder. *J Bone Joint Surg Am*. 2003;85A:1479–1487.

Kim SH, Ha KI, Yoo JC, Noh KC. Kim's lesion: an incomplete and concealed avulsion of the posteroinferior labrum in posterior or multidirectional posteroinferior instability of the shoulder. *Arthroscopy*. 2004;20:712–720. http://dx.doi.org/10.1016/j.arthro.2004.06.012.

Kronberg M, Brostrom LA. Proximal humeral osteotomy to correct the anatomy in patients with recurrent shoulder dislocations. *J Orthop Trauma*. 1991;5:129–133.

Leivadiotou D, Ahrens P. Arthroscopic treatment of posterior shoulder instability: a systematic review. *Arthroscopy*. 2015;31:555–560. http://dx.doi.org/10.1016/j.arthro.2014.11.009.

Lenart BA, Sherman SL, Mall NA, Gochanour E, Twigg SL, Nicholson GP. Arthroscopic repair for posterior shoulder instability. *Arthroscopy*. 2012;28:1337–1343. http://dx.doi.org/10.1016/j.arthro.2012.03.011.

Longo UG, Rizzello G, Locher J, et al. Bone loss in patients with posterior gleno-humeral instability: a systematic review. *Knee Surg Sports Traumatol Arthrosc*. 2016;24:612–617. http://dx.doi.org/10.1007/s00167-014-3161-8.

Martetschlager F, Padalecki JR, Millett PJ. Modified arthroscopic McLaughlin procedure for treatment of posterior instability of the shoulder with an associated reverse Hill-Sachs lesion. *Knee Surg Sports Traumatol Arthrosc*. 2013;21:1642–1646. http://dx.doi.org/10.1007/s00167-012-2237-6.

Massoud SN, Levy O, Copeland SA. Radiofrequency capsular shrinkage for voluntary shoulder instability. *J Shoulder Elbow Surg*. 2007;16:43–48. http://dx.doi.org/10.1016/j.jse.2005.11.011.

Matsen FA 3rd, Chebli C, Lippitt S, American Academy of Orthopaedic Surgeons. Principles for the evaluation and management of shoulder instability. *J Bone Joint Surg Am*. 2006;88:648–659.

McLaughlin LH. Posterior dislocation of the shoulder. *J Bone Joint Surg Am*. 1952;24A:584–590.

Merolla G, De Santis E, Cools AM, Porcellini G. Functional outcome and quality of life after rehabilitation for voluntary posterior shoulder dislocation: a prospective blinded cohort study. *Eur J Orthop Surg Traumatol*. 2015;25:263–272. http://dx.doi.org/10.1007/s00590-014-1486-0.

Millett PJ, Clavert P, Hatch GF 3rd, Warner JJ. Recurrent posterior shoulder instability. *J Am Acad Orthop Surg*. 2006;14:464–466.

Moroder P, Tauber M, Hoffelner T, et al. Reliability of a new standardized measurement technique for reverse Hill-Sachs lesions in posterior shoulder dislocations. *Arthroscopy*. 2013;29:478–484. http://dx.doi.org/10.1016/j.arthro.2012.10.016.

Murachovsky J, Bueno RS, Nascimento LG, et al. Calculating anterior glenoid bone loss using the Bernageau profile view. *Skeletal Radiol*. 2012;41:1231–1237. http://dx.doi.org/10.1007/s00256-012-1439-9.

Owens BD, Campbell SE, Cameron KL. Risk factors for posterior shoulder instability in young athletes. *Am J Sports Med*. 2013;41:2645–2649. http://dx.doi.org/10.1177/0363546513501508.

Pollock RG, Bigliani LU. Recurrent posterior shoulder instability: diagnosis and treatment. *Clin Orthop Relat Res*. 1993;(291):85–96.

Provencher MT, Romeo AA. Posterior and multidirectional instability of the shoulder: challenges associated with diagnosis and management. *Instr Course Lect*. 2008;57:133–152.

Remvig L, Jensen DV, Ward RC. Are diagnostic criteria for general joint hypermobility and benign joint hypermobility syndrome based on reproducible and valid tests? A review of the literature. *J Rheumatol*. 2007;34:798–803.

Robinson CM, Seah M, Akhtar MA. The epidemiology, risk of recurrence, and functional outcome after an acute traumatic posterior dislocation of the shoulder. *J Bone Joint Surg Am*. 2011;93:1605–1613. http://dx.doi.org/10.2106/JBJS.J.00973.

Rowe CR, Pierce DS, Clark JG. Voluntary dislocation of the shoulder: a preliminary report on a clinical, electromyographic, and psychiatric study of twenty-six patients. *J Bone Joint Surg Am*. 1973;55:445–460.

Saliken DJ, Bornes TD, Bouliane MJ, Sheps DM, Beaupre LA. Imaging methods for quantifying glenoid and Hill-Sachs bone loss in traumatic instability of the shoulder: a scoping review. *BMC Musculoskelet Disord*. 2015;16:164. http://dx.doi.org/10.1186/s12891-015-0607-1.

Saupe N, White LM, Bleakney R, et al. Acute traumatic posterior shoulder dislocation: MR findings. *Radiology*. 2008;248:185–193. http://dx.doi.org/10.1148/radiol.2481071003.

Savoie FH 3rd, Holt MS, Field LD, Ramsey JR. Arthroscopic management of posterior instability: evolution of technique and results. *Arthroscopy*. 2008;24:389–396. http://dx.doi.org/10.1016/j.arthro.2007.11.004.

Schwartz DG, Goebel S, Piper K, Kordasiewicz B, Boyle S, Lafosse L. Arthroscopic posterior bone block augmentation in posterior shoulder instability. *J Shoulder Elbow Surg*. 2013;22:1092–1101. http://dx.doi.org/10.1016/j.jse.2012.09.011.

Servien E, Walch G, Cortes ZE, Edwards TB, O'Connor DP. Posterior bone block procedure for posterior shoulder instability. *Knee Surg Sports Traumatol Arthrosc*. 2007;15:1130–1136. http://dx.doi.org/10.1007/s00167-007-0316-x.

Shah N, Tung GA. Imaging signs of posterior glenohumeral instability. *AJR Am J Roentgenol*. 2009;192:730–735. http://dx.doi.org/10.2214/AJR.07.3849.

Shams A, El-Sayed M, Gamal O, ElSawy M, Azzam W. Modified technique for reconstructing reverse Hill-Sachs lesion in locked chronic posterior shoulder dislocation. *Eur J Orthop Surg Traumatol*. 2016;26:843–849. http://dx.doi.org/10.1007/s00590-016-1825-4.

Takwale VJ, Calvert P, Rattue H. Involuntary positional instability of the shoulder in adolescents and young adults: is there any benefit from treatment? *J Bone Joint Surg Br*. 2000;82:719–723.

Throckmorton TQ, Kraemer P, Kuhn JE, Sasso RC. Differentiating cervical spine and shoulder pathology: common disorders and key points of evaluation and treatment. *Instr Course Lect*. 2014;63:401–408.

Walz DM, Burge AJ, Steinbach L. Imaging of shoulder instability. *Semin Musculoskelet Radiol*. 2015;19:254–268. http://dx.doi.org/10.1055/s-0035-1549319.

Weishaupt D, Zanetti M, Nyffeler RW, Gerber C, Hodler J. Posterior glenoid rim deficiency in recurrent (atraumatic) posterior shoulder instability. *Skeletal Radiol*. 2000;29:204–210.

Wirth MA, Butters KP, Rockwood CA Jr. The posterior deltoid-splitting approach to the shoulder. *Clin Orthop Relat Res*. 1993;(296):92–98.

Wirth MA, Seltzer DG, Rockwood CA Jr. Recurrent posterior glenohumeral dislocation associated with increased retroversion of the glenoid: a case report. *Clin Orthop Relat Res*. 1994;(308):98–101.

Wolf BR, Strickland S, Williams RJ, Allen AA, Altchek DW, Warren RF. Open posterior stabilization for recurrent posterior glenohumeral instability. *J Shoulder Elbow Surg*. 2005;14:157–164. http://dx.doi.org/10.1016/j.jse.2004.06.008.

Young MS. Electromyographic biofeedback use in the treatment of voluntary posterior dislocation of the shoulder: a case study. *J Orthop Sports Phys Ther*. 1994;20:171–175. http://dx.doi.org/10.2519/jospt.1994.20.3.171.

Yu JS, Ashman CJ, Jones G. The POLPSA lesion: MR imaging findings with arthroscopic correlation in patients with posterior instability. *Skeletal Radiol*. 2002;31:396–399. http://dx.doi.org/10.1007/s00256-002-0513-0.

Ziran B, Nourbakhsh A. Proximal humerus derotational osteotomy for internal rotation instability after locked posterior shoulder dislocation: early experience in four patients. *Patient Saf Surg*. 2015;9:15. http://dx.doi.org/10.1186/s13037-015-0062-9.

3 Multidirectional Shoulder Instability

3-3A EPIDEMIOLOGY, MECHANISM OF INJURY, HISTORY, IMAGING, AND PHYSICAL EXAMINATION

TRACEY DIDINGER, MD, JOSEPH D. COOPER, MD, and SETH C. GAMRADT, MD

Multidirectional Instability

- Epidemiology
  - Multidirectional instability (MDI) is characterized by symptomatic glenohumeral translation, subluxation, or dislocation in more than one direction that leads to functional impairment.
  - The relative incidence and prevalence of the disease are unknown, but it is most commonly seen in young female athletes who regularly perform overhead activities.
- Mechanism of Injury
  - Repetitive microtrauma and selective stretching to the shoulder capsule over time distend the joint and can lead to instability.
  - Muscular imbalance is a contributing factor in MDI with poor rotator cuff control or periscapular weakness leading to subjective shoulder instability.
- History and Physical Examination
  - Patients report insidious onset of shoulder pain and often subluxation without an emergency department (ED) visit.
  - A complete physical examination of the upper extremities should include inspection, palpation, range of motion of the bilateral shoulders, a neurologic examination, rotator cuff evaluation, and a stability assessment.
  - Diagnosis is largely based on clinical examination.
- Imaging
  - MDI is largely a clinical diagnosis; however, radiography and magnetic resonance imaging (MRI) and magnetic resonance arthrography (MRA) can be helpful to identify bony dysplasia, labral abnormalities, and possibly capsular redundancy, particularly involving the inferior pouch.

Epidemiology

The term *multidirectional instability* was first coined by Neer and Foster in 1980 (Neer & Foster, 1980) in their description of the inferior capsular shift operation. At the time, these patients were differentiated from patients with standard anterior instability because it was emphasized that the inferior component of the instability was the major pathoanatomic feature, and any success with surgical treatment required elimination of the inferior capsular redundancy. Similarly, Thomas and Matsen (1989) divided patients with recurrent glenohumeral instability into one of two categories. The first group tends to have a traumatic, unidirectional dislocation resulting in a Bankart lesion that would require surgical repair (TUBS). The second group has atraumatic MDI that is often bilateral and can be managed with rehabilitation but requires an inferior capsular shift for surgical treatment (AMBRI). Schenk and Brems (1998) characterized MDI as symptomatic global laxity of the shoulder with increased capsular volume and a rotator interval capsular deficiency. It is important to recognize patients with MDI and capsular hyperlaxity because the standard surgical procedures used to treat traumatic anterior instability are often not adequate to address the pathology involved in MDI (Neer & Foster, 1980). However, it is difficult to determine which patients have MDI and which do not because there is certainly overlapping pathology. Furthermore, there is no accepted universal criteria for diagnosing MDI.

When discussing MDI, it is important to differentiate between laxity and instability of the shoulder. Laxity describes the amount of humeral head translation with respect to the glenoid, which is intrinsic to an individual's normal anatomy and is asymptomatic. Put another way, certain patients have lax shoulders that have demonstrable physical examination findings (e.g., sulcus sign) without symptoms. Instability, on the other hand, is symptomatic glenohumeral translation, subluxation, or dislocation that leads to functional impairment (Savoie, 2010; Schenk & Brems, 1998). Kuhn (2010) reviewed 18 different shoulder instability classification schemes and proposed a new FEDS classification based on the *f*requency, *e*tiology, *d*irection, and *s*everity of instability. In this classification system, Kuhn proposed eliminating the term MDI because of a lack of an agreed-upon definition. However, the term is firmly entrenched in orthopaedic teaching worldwide and continues to imply certain patient characteristics summarized in Box 3A.1.

Box 3A.1 Features of Multidirectional Instability of the Shoulder

- Instability is in more than one direction, including inferior
- Often affects younger patients and females
- Often bilateral
- Atraumatic or attritional in origin
- Capsular laxity is a key component of the pathophysiology
- Subluxations are more common than true dislocations requiring reduction
- Can sometimes be associated with global ligamentous laxity or Ehlers-Danlos syndrome
- Certain patients can voluntarily demonstrate their shoulder instability

Box 3A.2 Pathophysiology of Multidirectional Instability

- Capsular redundancy or hyperlaxity
- Collagen disorders (e.g., Ehlers-Danlos syndrome)
- Attritional capsular laxity caused by overuse or overhead athletics
- Scapular position or scapular weakness
- Rotator cuff weakness
- Diminished glenolabral concavity

There is a paucity of literature evaluating the epidemiology of MDI. Three recent meta-analyses evaluating the surgical and nonsurgical management of MDI highlight the dearth of high-quality prospective literature evaluating the condition (Chen et al, 2016; Longo et al, 2015; Warby et al, 2014). In these studies, the average age of the pooled group of patients was the mid 20s, and the unifying physical examination findings were a positive sulcus sign and load and shift test. In addition, nearly all of the literature on MDI consisted of retrospective case series (level 4) evaluating the results of a specific treatment. Therefore the relative incidence and prevalence of MDI as a condition or group of conditions is unknown; thus long-term prospective data re needed.

Mechanism of Injury

The most common reason for MDI is thought to be a congenital redundancy or laxity of the shoulder capsule (Mallon & Speer, 1995; Neer & Foster, 1980; Schenck & Brems, 1998; Shafer et al, 2008). Asymptomatic shoulders can also have this capsuloligamentous laxity, which is why multiple factors can contribute to the pathophysiology of MDI. Box 3A.2 summarizes some prevailing theories as to the pathophysiology of MDI. Generalized joint laxity can be caused by a multitude of factors and is present in 40% to 70% of patients with MDI (Saccomanno et al, 2013). Most patients with hyperlaxity do not have an identifiable syndrome or condition, but patients with collagen abnormalities such as Ehlers-Danlos and Marfan syndromes are important to identify because these patients are known to have poorer surgical outcomes after stabilization procedures (Jerosch & Castro, 1990).

Box 3A.3 History Taking in Multidirectional Instability

- Duration of symptoms
- Age at onset
- Unilateral or bilateral symptoms
- Arm positions that incite symptoms
- Presence of neurovascular symptoms
- Family history of shoulder instability or collagen disorder (e.g., Marfan syndrome, Ehlers-Danlos syndrome)
- Recent activity or lifestyle changes
- Recent or distant shoulder trauma
- Level of athletic activity or sports participation (especially overhead sports)
- Whether the patient can reproduce the instability (voluntary)
- Previous treatment (nonoperative or operative)

The scapular stabilizers and rotator cuff provide dynamic stability to the shoulder. Recent studies have identified muscular imbalance as a contributing factor in MDI with poor rotator cuff control or periscapular weakness leading to subjective shoulder instability (Fleming, 2005; Morris et al, 2004; Ogsten, 2007). For this reason, sedentary individuals and women with poor muscular development present with MDI (Longo et al, 2015). Last, labral hypoplasia or abnormalities in glenoid size may diminish the congruency and static stability of the glenohumeral joint, contributing to instability (Doukas & Speer, 2000).

Overhead athletes in sports such as swimming, volleyball, and gymnastics are susceptible to MDI (Gaskill et al, 2011; Levine et al, 2001). MDI is thought to develop in response to repetitive microtrauma and selective stretching of the shoulder capsule, resulting in increased glenohumeral joint volume and capsular redundancy (Levine et al, 2001; Werner, 2009). These patients may not present with generalized laxity and may not have laxity of the opposite shoulder.

History and Physical Examination

In contradistinction to a traumatic anterior dislocation, the clinical presentation of MDI is often insidious, or a trivial mechanism may be identified leading to the onset of shoulder pain and subluxation without an ED visit (Hawkins et al, 1987). Patient age is typically the teens or 20s. In those with generalized hyperlaxity, there may be no identifiable inciting event. Trauma, athletic overuse, or inactivity can contribute to the onset of symptoms with MDI. It is important to remember that a history of a significant traumatic event does not exclude a patient from having MDI (Neer, 1985). A single traumatic event can result in labrum injury, rendering athletes with lax shoulders to begin with more unstable (Altchek et al, 1991; Bigliani et al, 1994). Overhead athletes can present with pain, subluxation, or neurologic symptoms such as numbness and paresthesias (Gaskill et al, 2011; Levine et al, 2001). Last, intentional or volitional instability of the shoulder should be identified because it certainly affects the potential for treatment success. Box 3A.3 summarizes our approach to taking a history on a patient with suspected MDI. In addition, although there is frequently global capsular laxity, in the clinical

Box 3A.4 Physical Examination in Multidirectional Instability

Inspection

- Posture
- Muscle atrophy
- Beighton Score for Hyperlaxity

Palpation

- Acromioclavicular
- Long head biceps
- Glenohumeral joint

Range of motion (with particular attention to hyperexternal rotation and hyperabduction)
Strength (rotator cuff and periscapular)
Provocative tests or stability examination

- Sulcus (in neutral and external rotation)
- Load and shift
- Apprehension/relocation
- Obrien's test
- Jerk test

Neurovascular examination

Box 3A.5 Beighton Scale*

- Passive hyperextension of the small finger >90 degrees (1 point for each extremity; 2 total)
- Passive thumb apposition to the ipsilateral forearm (1 point for each extremity; 2 total)
- Elbow and knee hyperextension >10 degrees (1 point for elbow 1 point for knee at each extremity; 4 total)
- Trunk flexion with knees straight and palms flat on the floor (1 point)

*A score of greater than 3 on a scale of 9 points is thought to be diagnostic of generalized joint laxity.

setting most patients complain of pain or instability with primarily an anteroinferior or posteroinferior presentation. In other words, for a patient with primarily an anteroinferior instability pattern, the patient will often complain that putting the arm in a position of abduction and external rotation provokes the greatest degree of symptoms. Conversely, those with primarily a posteroinferior problem will complain that placing the arm into forward flexion and adduction precipitates symptoms.

Box 3A.4 summarizes the physical examination checklist in MDI. First, the entire shoulder girdles of both shoulders need to be visible both anteriorly and posteriorly to compare the symptomatic and asymptomatic sides. Throughout the patient's physical examination, reproduction of the patient's symptoms is critical to note. The overall physical examination of the upper extremities should include inspection, palpation, range of motion of the bilateral shoulders, a neurologic examination, rotator cuff evaluation, and a stability assessment.

Begin by inspecting the shoulders for posture, scapular position, muscle atrophy, and symmetry. Next, the patient's degree of generalized ligamentous laxity should be determined using the Beighton scale (Box 3A.5) (Beighton & Horan, 1969). Generalized ligament laxity can be associated with connective tissue disorders such as Ehlers-Danlos syndrome or Marfan syndrome. It is important to recognize these connective tissue disorders because patients with them have poorer results after surgical stabilization (Jerosch & Castro, 1990; Vavken et al, 2016).

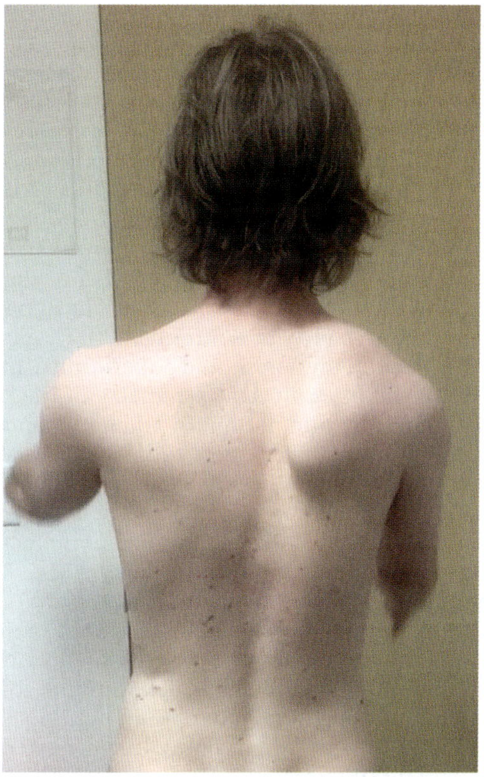

Fig. 3A.1 Scapular dyskinesis where the inferior angle is prominent and the scapular position is protracted and internally rotated. (Courtesy of George F. Rick Hatch, III, MD.)

Next, palpation of the anterior and posterior glenohumeral joint lines should be evaluated, noting any pain or fullness. Tenderness with palpation of either the anterior or posterior joint line is a common finding that can sometimes help differentiate anterior or posterior instability when present in isolation (Provencher et al, 2011). It is a nonspecific finding that can represent capsular stretching, labral pathology, or cuff pathology. Routine palpation to assess for concomitant pathology of the AC joint and biceps tendon is performed as well. Patients with MDI can also have tenderness to palpation at the medial angle of the scapula (Silliman & Hawkins, 1993).

Range of motion is then tested. A standard evaluation includes forward elevation in the frontal and scapular planes. External rotation at the side is measured; greater than 90 degrees of external rotation with the elbows at the side is common in MDI and hyperlaxity. Internal rotation behind the back is documented as the highest spinal level that the patient can reach. Internal and external rotation should also be measured at 90 degrees of abduction in the supine position. The hyperabduction test described by Gagey and Gagey (2001) can be used as well. The glenohumeral abduction is compared between the asymptomatic and symptomatic shoulders, and a difference of greater than 20 degrees is a positive finding. Hyperabduction past 180 degrees is representative of MDI.

Scapular motion and dyskinesis should be observed from behind the patient during arm elevation. Asymmetry in scapular motion should be noted (Fig. 3A.1). Scapular winging can also be observed by having the patient do a standing pushup against the wall. Scapulothoracic motion asymmetry is associated with MDI.

Strength testing is performed, beginning with the evaluation of deltoid strength in abduction. The empty can test evaluates the supraspinatus. External rotation strength evaluates the posterior rotator cuff. Liftoff, bear hug, and the belly press tests evaluate the internal rotation strength of the subscapularis. Although there is a low association of rotator cuff tears along with MDI, strength of the rotator cuff should be evaluated as well because of its dynamic stabilizing effect in MDI (Taylor & Arciero, 1997). A complete neurovascular examination should be performed, including evaluation of the integrity and symmetry of the patient's motor and sensory examination. In addition, concomitant pathology such as thoracic outlet syndrome should be ruled out in patients with paresthesias or numbness by using the Adson test. A positive test result is indicated by a diminished radial pulse provoked by head rotation while abducting and externally rotating the shoulder.

The final portion of the physical examination is the stability assessment. This portion includes both laxity tests, which examine the degree of humeral head translation, and provocative maneuvers, which attempt to reproduce the patient's instability symptoms. Inferior laxity is assessed first with the sulcus sign (Neer & Foster, 1980) (Fig. 3A.2). The sulcus sign is performed with the patient sitting upright with the shoulder in neutral rotation and the arm at the side. Axial traction is then applied to the upper arm and the amount of inferior subluxation of the humeral head in relation to the acromion is measured (Silliman & Hawkins, 1993). Grade 1 is a distance of less than 1 cm, grade 2 is 1 to 2 cm, and grade 3 is more than 2 cm. The sulcus sign is pathognomonic for inferior instability if it reproduces the patient's symptoms of apprehension and pain, but a sulcus sign can also be present in asymptomatic individuals (Johnson & Robinson, 2010). The sulcus sign is repeated with the arm in external rotation; persistent sulcus sign in external rotation can indicate a deficient rotator interval capsule (Ramsay & Klimkiewicz, 1999)

The load and shift test can be performed in both the anterior and posterior directions to measure the amount of humeral head translation in relation to the glenoid. This test is difficult to perform in a symptomatic, nonrelaxed patient. With the patient in a supine position, the patient's arm should be in approximately 20 degrees of abduction, 20 degrees of forward flexion, and neutral rotation. The humeral head is then axially loaded, and the examiner pushes the humeral head either anteriorly or posteriorly. The amount of translation of the humerus is graded 1 with 0 to 1 cm translation up the glenoid face, graded 2 with translation to the glenoid rim, and graded 3 with translation over the glenoid rim (Hawkins et al, 1996).

Anterior instability can be assessed with the apprehension test. This test is performed with the patient supine. The patient's shoulder is placed at 90 degrees of abduction while the arm is brought into maximum external rotation (Tzannes et al, 2004). Reproduction of the patient's symptoms of apprehension in this position is an indicator of anterior instability. In patients with a positive apprehension test result, the relocation test can be performed as an adjunct in the diagnosis of instability. With the patient in the same position, a posteriorly directed force is applied to the humeral head, relieving the symptoms and allowing the patient to tolerate more external rotation with the shoulder in abduction (Tzannes et al, 2004).

Posterior instability is best evaluated using the jerk test. The jerk test can be performed with the patient standing, supine, or in the lateral decubitus position. The examiner stabilizes the scapula by grasping the distal clavicle and the scapular spine with one hand and holds the patient's elbow with the other while placing the arm in 90 degrees of forward flexion and internal rotation. The flexed elbow is pushed posteriorly while the shoulder girdle is pushed anteriorly. A positive test result reproduces symptoms or provokes a sudden jerk as the humeral head slides over

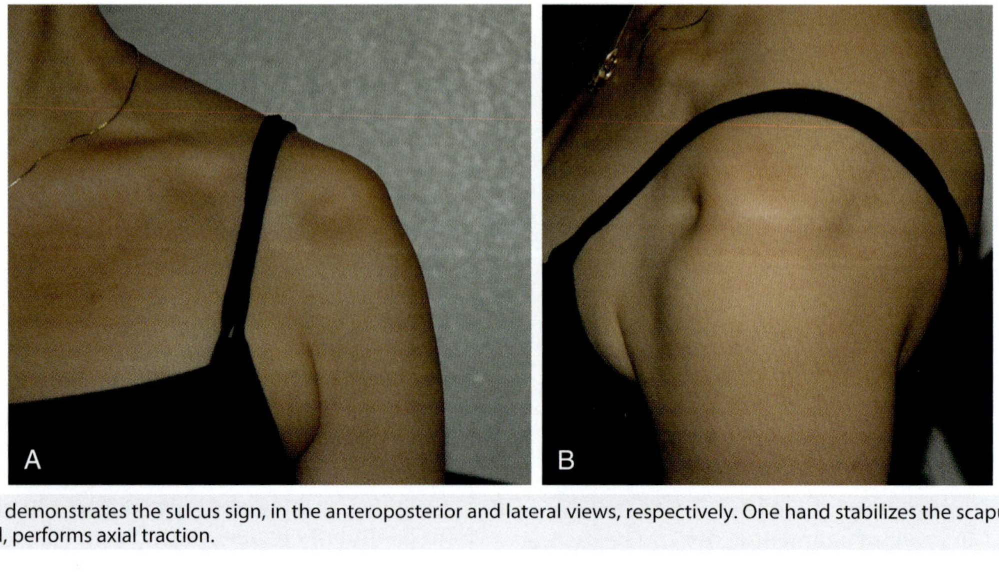

Fig. 3A.2 A and B demonstrates the sulcus sign, in the anteroposterior and lateral views, respectively. One hand stabilizes the scapula while the other hand, not pictured, performs axial traction.

the glenoid rim (Provencher et al, 2011). Posterior instability can also be reproduced by having the patient place her or his arm in a position of instability in adduction and forward flexion, creating discomfort, and transition to abduction and extension, leading to relief and reduction of the shoulder. The Kim test (Fig. 3A.3) is another useful test for evaluating posterior instability. With the patient seated, the arm is brought into 90 degrees of abduction. The examiner holds the patient's elbow and lateral aspect of the proximal arm while simultaneously applying an axial loading force and a 45-degree upward diagonal elevation to the distal arm and an inferior and posterior force to the proximal arm. The arm is then brought into adduction. A sudden onset of posterior shoulder pain is a positive result (Kim et al, 2005). O'Brien's test, or the active compression test, is performed by adduction of the shoulder in the standing position with the forearm pronated (thumb down). The arm is then loaded inferiorly, and pain is reproduced. In a positive test result, the pain is then relieved by supination of the forearm. This test is sensitive but not specific for superior labral tears.

Imaging

Multidirectional instability is largely a clinical diagnosis; however, imaging is important for identifying possible anatomic variations or pathologic causes. Routine radiographs in three views are standard (anteroposterior, scapular Y, and axillary). In the setting of acute trauma, it may be difficult to obtain an axillary view, so a Valpeau view can be obtained. Radiographs are reviewed for bone defects about the glenoid rim or humeral head. Anatomic variations in glenoid version, or glenoid dysplasia, can also be evaluated. A shallow or hypoplastic glenoid can be seen on the axillary view. If a bony defect is identified or suspected, computed tomography (CT) can help further delineate the osseous injury. CT is the best modality for evaluating glenoid bone loss and dysplasia.

Magnetic resonance imaging and specifically MRA are the best modalities for evaluating the soft tissue structures of the shoulder, including the labrum and the capsuloligamentous complex. Patients with multidirectional instability typically do not have frank labral detachment, and many have no labral pathology at all. However, there may be subtle labral abnormalities visualized on MRI or at arthroscopy. These can include labral splits, cracks, chondrolabral retroversion, or a redundant joint capsule (Jana & Gamanagatti, 2011; Schaeffeler et al, 2014). Multiple studies have attempted to quantify increased space within the joint capsule by measuring the width of the rotator interval or widening of the capsular space; however, these measurements are often not reliable based on the position of the shoulder and the volume of intraarticular contrast given (Bell, 2010; Dewing et al, 2008; Lee et al, 2013; Provencher et al, 2008). According to Neer and Foster (1980), bulging of the rotator interval with contrast is pathognomonic for MDI.

If labral injuries are present, they can be identified on axial MRA or MRI views. Structural pathology leading to posterior instability can be seen at the posterior glenoid, including posterior labral tears, labrocapsular avulsions, or humeral avulsion of the glenohumeral ligament. This can lead to posterior translation of the humeral head within the glenoid, which is also seen on this view (Tung & Hou, 2003).

Specific positioning of the arm can facilitate viewing of more subtle injuries if suspected. Positioning the arm in abduction and external rotation facilitates viewing of the anterior labrum and anterior capsuloligamentous structures, and flexion, adduction, and internal rotation allows visualization of the posterior shoulder (Chiavaras et al, 2010; Schaeffeler et al, 2014). Evaluation for other injuries, including rotator cuff tear, Bankart lesions, Hill-Sachs lesions, impaction fractures, and articular cartilage abnormalities, is also important to identify and although not associated with MDI can lead to shoulder pain and be a separate cause of instability.

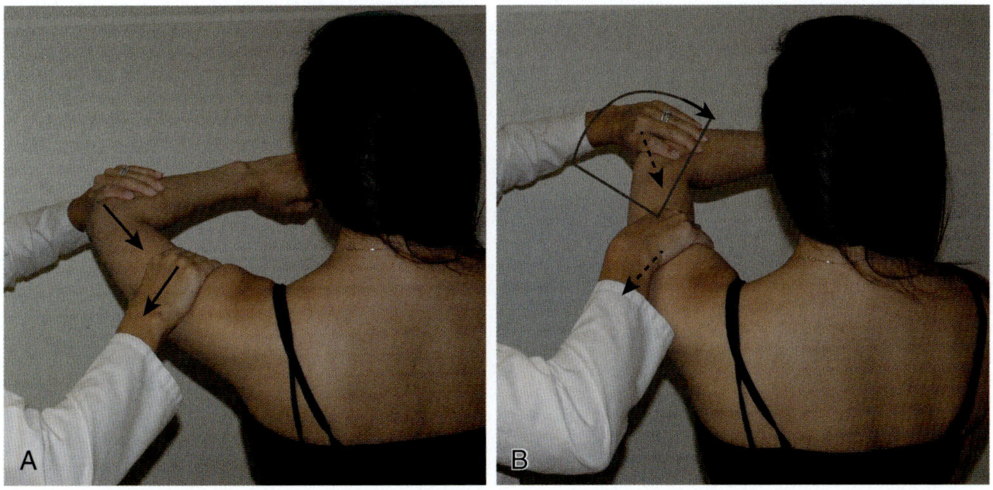

Fig. 3A.3 Demonstration of the Kim test. Position A is the patient's arm in abduction with the examiner applying an axial load and inferior posterior force on the proximal arm. As the patient's arm is brought into adduction, as seen in position B, the patient feels the onset of posterior shoulder pain.

Conclusion

The diagnosis of MDI is suspected in patients who develop atraumatic shoulder instability in their teens or 20s. A variety of causes lead to capsular laxity or redundancy. The key physical examination findings in MDI that identify this laxity, in our opinion, are the sulcus sign, glenohumeral hypermobility, generalized hyperlaxity, and the load and shift test. The presence or absence of the aforementioned physical examination findings can then be interpreted with the history and imaging to establish the degree, direction, and severity of the instability. Patients with MDI present with variable pathology and varying degrees of symptoms. Understanding the epidemiology, pathophysiology, and physical examination of these patients will result in an accurate diagnosis and lead to clinical success in nonoperative and surgical treatments to be discussed in the next section.

References

Altchek DW, Warren RF, Skyhar JM, Ortiz G. T-plasty modification of the Bankart procedure for multidirectional instability of the anterior and inferior types. *J Bone Joint Surg Am*. 1991;73:105–112.

Beighton P, Horan F. Orthopaedic aspects of the Ehlers-Danlos syndrome. *J Bone Joint Surg Br*. 1969;51(3):444–453.

Bell J. Arthroscopic management of multidirectional instability. *Orthop Clin North Am*. 2010;41:357–365.

Bigliani LU, Kurzweil PR, Schwartzbach CC, Wolfe IN, Flatow EL. Inferior capsular shift procedure for anterior-inferior shoulder instability in athletes. *Am J Sports Med*. 1994;22:578–584.

Fleming BC, Hulstyn MJ, Oksendahl HL, Fadale PD. Ligament Injury, Reconstruction and Osteoarthritis. *Curr Opin Orthop*. 2005;16(5): 354–362.

Chen D, Goldberg J, Herald J, Critchley I, Barmare A. Effects of surgical management on multidirectional instability of the shoulder: a meta-analysis. *Knee Surg Sports Traumatol Arthrosc*. 2016;24(2):630–639.

Chiavaras MM, Harish S, Burr J. MR arthrographic assessment of suspected posteroinferior labral lesions using flexion, adduction, and internal rotation positioning of the arm: preliminary experience. *Skeletal Radiol*. 2010;39(5):481–488.

Dewing CB, McCormick F, Bell SJ, et al. An analysis of capsular area in patients with anterior, posterior, and multidirectional shoulder instability. *Am J Sports Med*. 2008;36:515–522.

Doukas WC, Speer KP. Anatomy, pathophysiology, and biomechanics of shoulder instability. *Oper Tech Sports Med*. 2000;8:179–187.

Gagey OJ, Gagey N. The hyperabduction test. *J Bone Joint Surg Br*. 2001;83(1):69–74.

Gaskill TR, Taylor DC, Millett PJ. Management of multidirectional instability of the shoulder. *J Am Acad Orthop Surg*. 2011;19(12):758–767.

Hawkins RJ, Schutte JP, Janda DH, Huckell GH. Translation of the glenohumeral joint with the patient under anesthesia. *J Shoulder Elbow Surg*. 1996;5(4):286–292.

Hawkins RJ, Abrams JS, Schutte JP. Multidirectional instability of the shoulder: an approach to diagnosis. *Orthop Trans*. 1987;11:246.

Jana M, Gamanagatti S. Magnetic resonance imaging in the glenohumeral instability. *World J Radiol*. 2011;3(9):224–232.

Jerosch J, Castro WH. Shoulder instability in Ehlers-Danlos syndrome: an indication for surgical treatment? *Acta Orthop Belg*. 1990;56(2):451–453.

Johnson SM, Robinson CM. Shoulder instability in patients with joint hyperlaxity. *J Bone Joint Surg Am*. 2010;92(6):1545–1557.

Kim SH, Park JS, Jeong WK, Shin SK. The Kim test: a novel test for posteroinferior labral lesion of the shoulder—a comparison to the jerk test. *Am J Sports Med*. 2005;33(8):1188–1192.

Kuhn JE. A new classification system for shoulder instability. *Br J Sports Med*. 2010;44(5):341–346.

Lee HJ, Kim NR, Moon SG, Ko SM, Park J. Multidirectional instability of the shoulder: rotator interval dimension and capsular laxity evaluation using MR arthrography. *Skelet Radiol*. 2013;42:231–238.

Levine WN, Prickett WD, Prymka M, Yamaguchi K. Treatment of the athlete with multidirectional shoulder instability. *Orthop Clin North Am*. 2001;32(3):475–484.

Longo UG, Rizzello G, Loppini M, et al. Multidirectional instability of the shoulder: a systematic review. *Arthroscopy*. 2015;31(12):2431–2443.

Mallon WJ, Speer KP. Multidirectional instability: current concepts. *J Shoulder Elbow Surg*. 1995;4:54–64.

Morris AD, Kemp GJ, Frostick SP. Shoulder electromyography in multidirectional instability. *J Shoulder Elbow Surg*. 2004;13:24–29.

Neer CS II. Involuntary inferior and multidirectional instability of the shoulder: etiology, recognition, and treatment. *Instr Course Lect*. 1985;34:232–238.

Neer CS 2nd, Foster CR. Inferior capsular shift for involuntary inferior and multidirectional instability of the shoulder. A preliminary report. *J Bone Joint Surg Am*. 1980;62(6):897–908.

Ogston JB, Ludewig PM. Differences in 3-dimensional shoulder kinematics between persons with multidirectional instability and asymptomatic controls. *Am J Sports Med*. 2007;35:1361–1370.

Provencher MT, Dewing CB, Bell SJ, et al. An analysis of the rotator interval in patients with anterior, posterior, and multidirectional shoulder instability. *Arthroscopy*. 2008;24:921–929.

Provencher MT, LeClere LE, King S, et al. Posterior instability of the shoulder: diagnosis and management. *Am J Sports Med*. 2011;39(4):874–886.

Ramsay ML, Klimkiewicz JJ. Posterior instability: diagnosis and management. In: Iannotti JP, Williams GR, eds. *Disorders of the shoulder: diagnosis and management*. Philadelphia: Lippincott Williams and Wilkins; 1999:295–319.

Saccomanno MF, Fodale M, Capasso L, et al. Generalized joint laxity and multidirectional instability of the shoulder. *Joints*. 2013;1(4):171–179.

Savoie FH. Multidirectional instability of the glenohumeral joint. In: Ryu RK, ed. *The Shoulder*. Philadelphia: Saunders Elsevier; 2010:124–135.

Schaeffeler C, Waldt S, Bauer JS, et al. MR arthrography including abduction and external rotation images in the assessment of atraumatic multidirectional instability of the shoulder. *Eur Radiol*. 2014;24:1376–1385.

Schenk TJ, Brems JJ. Multidirectional instability of the shoulder: pathophysiology, diagnosis, and management. *J Am Acad Orthop Surg*. 1998;6:65–72.

Shafer BL, Mihata T, McGarry MH, Tibone JE, Lee TQ. Effects of capsular plication and rotator interval closure in simulated multidirectional shoulder instability. *J Bone Joint Surg Am*. 2008;90:136–144.

Silliman JF, Hawkins RJ. Classification and physical diagnosis of instability of the shoulder. *Clin Orthop Relat Res*. 1993;291:7–19.

Taylor DC, Arciero RA. Pathologic changes associated with shoulder dislocations. Arthroscopic and physical examination findings in first-time, traumatic anterior dislocations. *Am J Sports Med*. 1997;25(3):306–311.

Thomas SC, Matsen FA 3rd. An approach to the repair of avulsion of the glenohumeral ligaments in the management of traumatic anterior glenohumeral instability. *J Bone Joint Surg Am*. 1989;71(4):506–513.

Tung GA, Hou DD. MR arthrography of the posterior labrocapsular complex: relationship with glenohumeral joint alignment and clinical posterior instability. *AJR Am J Roentgenol*. 2003;180(2):369–375.

Tzannes A, Paxinos A, Callanan M, Murrell GA. An assessment of the interexaminer reliability of tests for shoulder instability. *J Shoulder Elbow Surg*. 2004;13(1):18–23.

Vavken P, Tepolt FA, Kocher MS. Open inferior capsular shift for multidirectional shoulder instability in adolescents with generalized ligamentous hyperlaxity or Ehlers-Danlos syndrome. *J Shoulder Elbow Surg*. 2016;25(6):907–912.

Warby SA, Pizzari T, Ford JJ, Hahne AJ, Watson L. The effect of exercise-based management for multidirectional instability of the glenohumeral joint: a systematic review. *J Shoulder Elbow Surg*. 2014;23(1):128–142.

Werner A. Multidirectional shoulder instability. Nonoperative and operative treatment strategies. *Orthopade*. 2009;38(1):64–69.

3-3B ARTHROSCOPIC CAPSULAR PLICATION AND SHIFT

JESSICA RYU, MD, JONATHAN-JAMES ENO, MD, and RICHARD RYU, MD

Introduction

- Since Neer and Foster's seminal work on multidirectional instability (MDI) (Neer, 1984), basic science and clinical research have helped to establish a better understanding of the basis for laxity, symptomatic laxity, and reestablishing glenohumeral stability in the management of this complex disorder (Gaskill et al, 2011; Rodeo et al, 1998).
- The diagnosis and treatment of patients with symptomatic MDI remains a challenging clinical entity for treating physicians (Field et al, 2016; Ryu, 2008). The multiple static and dynamic stabilizers, including glenoid shape and version, labral configuration, and glenohumeral ligament integrity, as well as the delicate balance of scapulothoracic musculature, rotator cuff strength, and proprioceptive control, all contribute to a perplexing clinical presentation. These factors can make it difficult to select the most appropriate and effective treatment.
- After this challenging diagnosis has been made, a conservative, nonoperative program to include lifestyle changes and therapeutic shoulder strengthening exercises should first be used in an effort to manage symptoms.
- Burkhead and Rockwood (1992) reported excellent and good outcomes in more than 80% of patients with atraumatic instability treated with a conservative strengthening program. Kuroda et al (2001) reported improvement in symptoms after rehabilitation exercises and permanent activity modifications were implemented.
- In contrast, a more recent study by Kiss and Damrel (2001) followed symptomatic MDI patients undergoing nonoperative management over an average of 4 years and found that one third of the patients still had moderate to total disability.
- Despite these revelations, a nonoperative rehabilitation program remains the gold standard for the initial treatment of MDI, with the targeting of scapulothoracic dyskinesis as one of the primary goals (Morris, 2004; Myers, 2004). It is noteworthy that in Misamore et al's (2005) longitudinal study, it was determined that if after 3 months of sound conservative care no significant progress was noted and symptoms persisted; further conservative measures were unlikely to be productive. In this setting, arthroscopic capsular plication becomes a reasonable alternative for patients with symptomatic MDI.
- Arthroscopic capsular plication is currently considered a reliable surgical alternative for patients with recalcitrant MDI disability (Gartsman et al, 2001; Jacobson et al, 2012; Treacy & Savoie, 1999; Wichman & Snyder, 1997), and its efficacy in the difficult athletic population has also been reported (Baker et al, 2009; Ma et al, 2012; Montgomery et al, 2010).
- An arthroscopic capsular plication can achieve the same goals of the time-honored open approach, and this has been elucidated in numerous studies focusing on volumetric measurements and surgical technique (Cohen et al, 2005; Luke et al, 2004; Ponce & Tokish, 2011; Provencher et al, 2008; Sekiya et al, 2007).
- The most difficult aspect of treating patients with symptomatic MDI is selecting the correct patients for more aggressive measures. The following section outlines the surgical technique in detail (Video 3B.1).

Surgical Technique: Arthroscopic Capsular Plication

STEP 1

The patient is examined under anesthesia (EUA), and the preoperative assessment is confirmed or modified. This should be performed in the supine position because comparison with the contralateral extremity can be critical to decision making. The cardinal feature of MDI is an obligate inferior component, and either the anterior or posterior component (or both) must be verified because it will impact the sequence of capsular volume reduction. A lateral decubitus position is implemented and is the preferred position because it permits unfettered access to the inferior capsule, which must be addressed in all cases.

STEP 2

A posterior portal (PP) is placed slightly lateral to avoid limitations imposed by the glenoid rim. Diagnostic arthroscopy is then undertaken to avoid missing any cogent associated pathology. In most cases, the labrum is intact or slightly frayed because MDI is a primary capsular pathology. In the late stages, labral tearing may be present. The rotator interval is commonly patulous, and the articulating surfaces and rotator cuff are typically intact. A markedly positive drive-through sign is often encountered (Fig. 3B.1). Dual anterior portals are established with the anterior-inferior portal (AIP) occupying the most inferior dimension of the rotator interval and the anterior-superior portal (ASP) at the most cephalad aspect of the interval.

STEP 3

Viewing from the ASP and using the AIP and PP as working portals, the capsule is carefully rasped to generate a healing response (Fig. 3B.2). Aggressive shavers and suction are to be avoided for fear of damaging the often thin capsular tissue, especially posteriorly. After the capsule has been roughened, a 60-degree angled suture hook is passed from the posterior portal, targeting the most inferior aspect of the

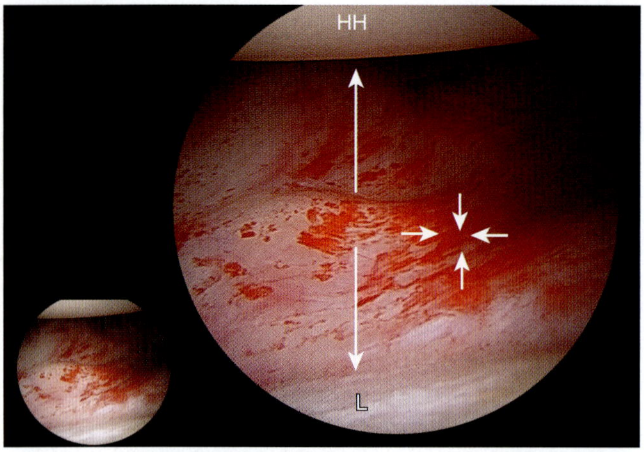

Fig. 3B.1 Viewing from a posterior portal in a right shoulder in the lateral decubitus position, capsulitis *(small arrows)* is readily evident with a significant drive-through sign present *(large arrows)*. (All subsequent images are in the same lateral position.) *HH,* Humeral head; *L,* labrum.

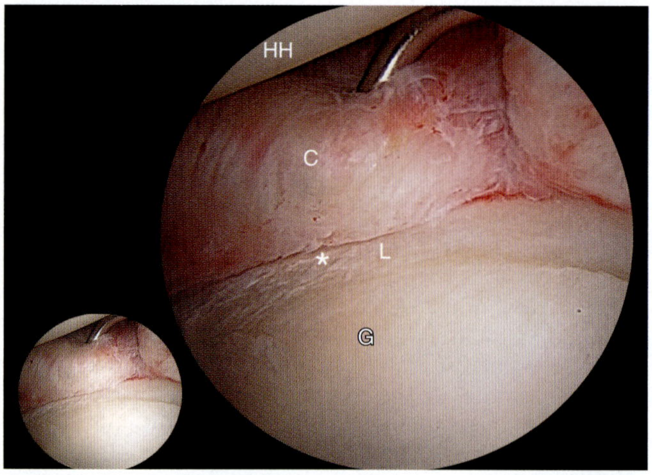

Fig. 3B.3 The pinch-tuck technique begins with an angled suture hook penetrating the capsule (C) at the 6 o'clock position *(asterisk)* from the posterior portal approximately 10 mm from the glenoid (G) rim. *HH,* Humeral head; *L,* labrum.

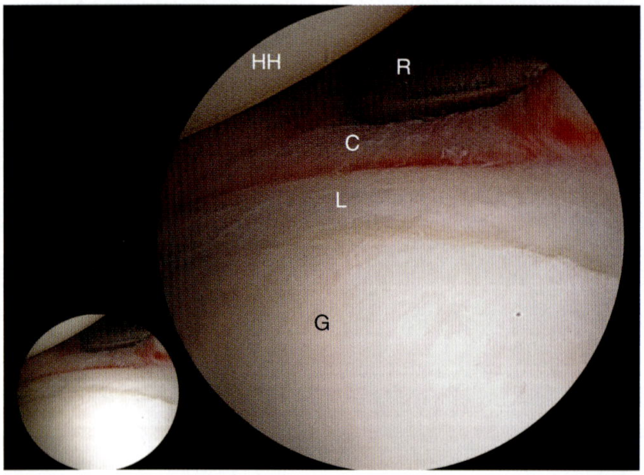

Fig. 3B.2 Viewing from an anterior superior portal, rasping of the capsule (C) is performed. *HH,* Humeral head; *L,* labrum; *R,* rasp; *G,* glenoid.

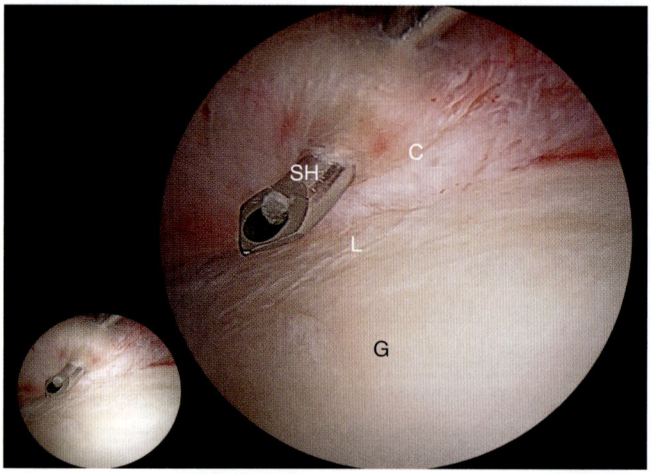

Fig. 3B.4 The suture hook (SH) captures a segment of the capsule (C), exiting the capsular tissue before engaging the labrum (L). *G,* Glenoid.

capsule at the 6 o'clock position (Fig. 3B.3). Using the Snyder pinch-tuck technique, the inferior capsule is penetrated 1 cm from the labral edge, and the tip is brought through the capsule tissue only (Fig. 3B.4). The hook is then advanced onto the glenoid labrum, which is pierced (Fig. 3B.5), shifting tissue superiorly and allowing the absorbable shuttling suture to be wheeled into the joint. If the labrum is of potentially poor quality, a suture anchor is placed in lieu of the labrum to ensure proper fixation of the shifted capsule. The shuttling suture is collected and then retrograded with a high strength, nonabsorbable suture in tow (Fig. 3B.6). A second pass is then made to complete a horizontal mattress suture configuration (Fig. 3B.7). The suture tails are passed such that the suture knots can be tied farthest from the articulating surfaces. Although the suture can theoretically be tied as a sliding knot, alternating half hitches and posts are used to complete the plication stitch in an effort to avoid traumatizing the compromised tissue with the potential abrasion associated with sliding knots (Fig. 3B.8).

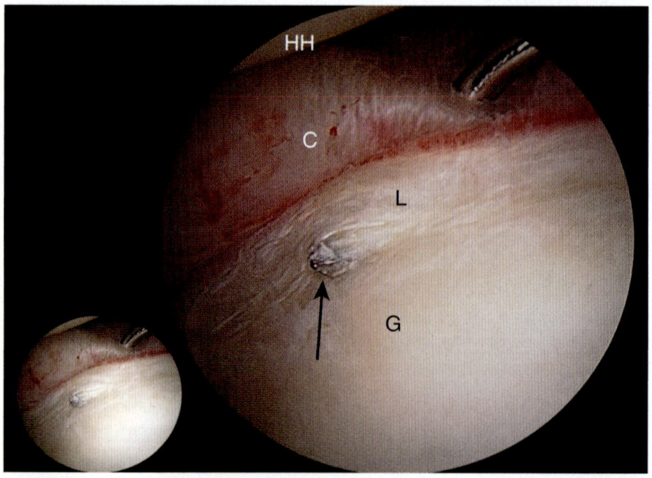

Fig. 3B.5 The pinch-tuck technique is completed as the "loaded" hook is passed through the intact labrum (L) *(small arrow)*. *C,* Capsule; *G,* glenoid; *HH,* humeral head.

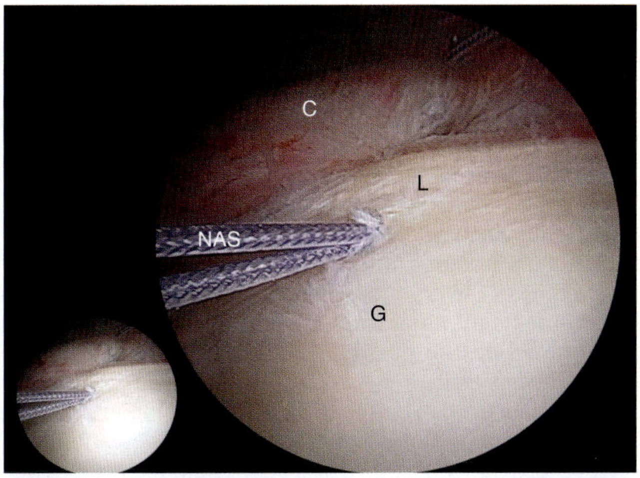

Fig. 3B.6 Using the absorbable suture as a shuttle, high-strength nonabsorbable suture (NAS) is retrograded through the labrum (L) and capsule (C). *G,* Glenoid.

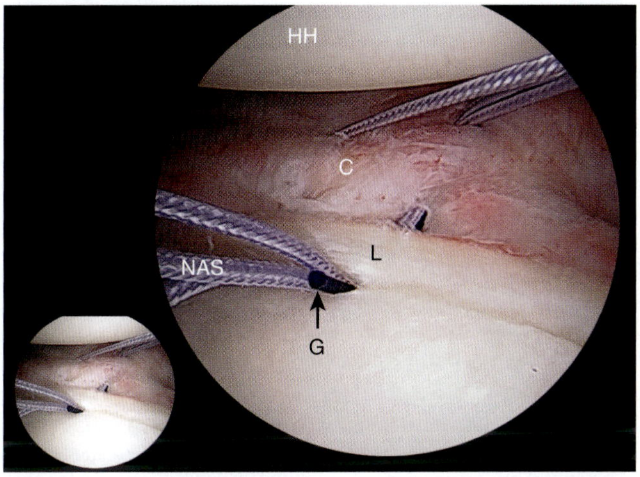

Fig. 3B.7 The second limb of the suture is passed through the labrum (L) and capsule (C), completing the horizontal mattress configuration. The *small arrow* points to the tail of nonabsorbable shuttling suture (NAS). *G,* Glenoid; *HH,* humeral head.

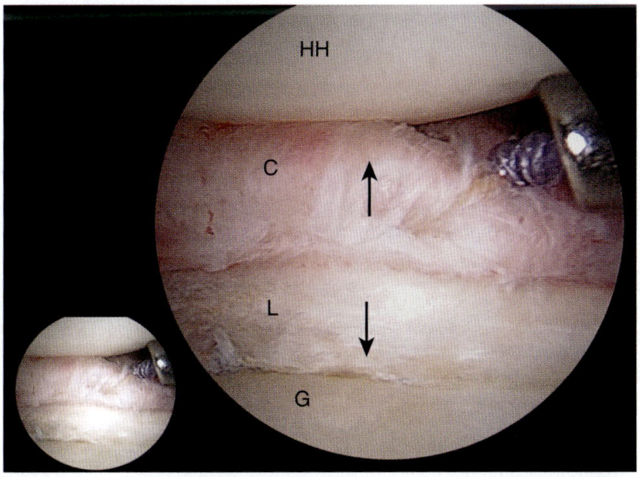

Fig. 3B.8 The suture is tied with alternating half hitches and posts rather than with a sliding knot to avoid abrading the atrophic capsule. A labral "bumper" *(arrows)* is created with the reinforced capsule. *HH,* humeral head; *C,* Capsule; *L,* labrum; *G,* Glenoid.

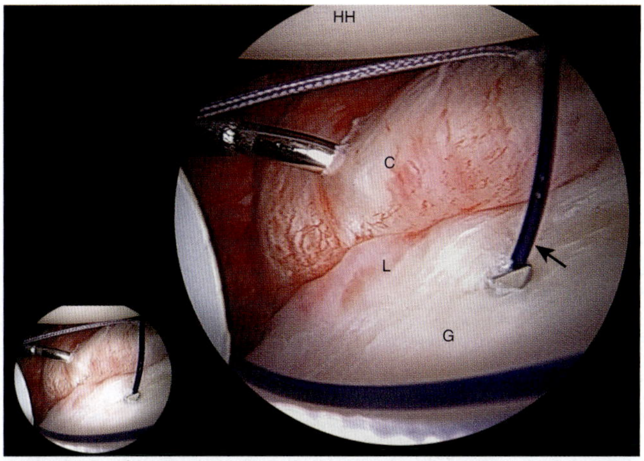

Fig. 3B.9 The second horizontal mattress suture is placed in identical fashion at the 5 o'clock position because anterior instability in this case is greater than posterior after the inferior capsule (C) has been addressed. The *arrow* points to the absorbable shuttling suture. *G,* Glenoid; *HH,* humeral head; *L,* labrum.

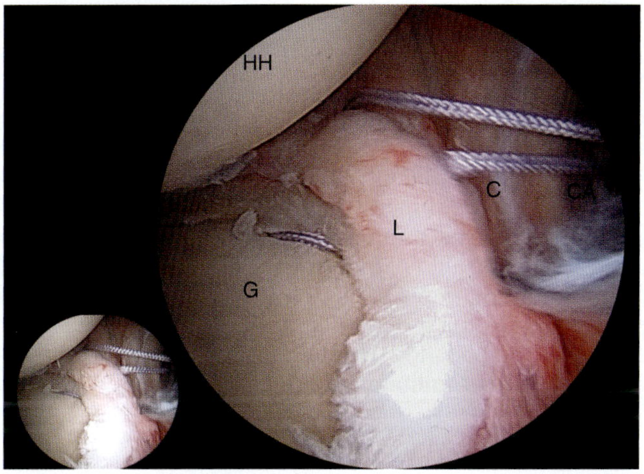

Fig. 3B.10 The third nonabsorbable horizontal mattress suture is placed posteriorly to balance the capsular plication. *C,* Capsule; *CA,* cannula; *G,* glenoid; *HH,* humeral head; *L,* labrum.

STEP 4

Based on the preoperative assessment and the EUA, the next most symptomatic direction of instability is addressed with the same horizontal mattress suture configuration and sequence (Fig. 3B.9). If anterior, the suture is placed at the 5 o'clock position. A subsequent mattress suture is then passed at the 7 o'clock position to balance the repair (Fig. 3B.10). If posterior instability is the focus, the sequence is reversed. After these three nonabsorbable sutures have been placed, the drive-through sign should be significantly reduced with the goal being at least 50% to 75% (Fig. 3B.11). Depending on the degree of instability, more sutures can be placed both anteriorly and posteriorly, working from inferior to superior. Concern for overcapturing the joint is always present, and the use of absorbable sutures at this time may be justified in the event that the shift is too tight. A simple stitch configuration can also diminish the risk of capturing the joint.

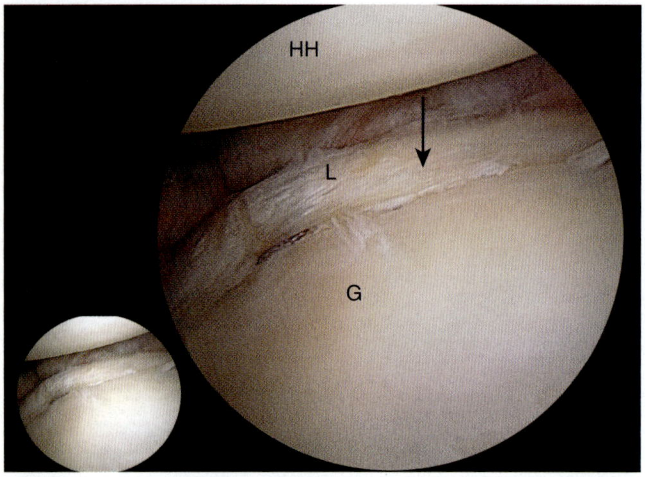

Fig. 3B.11 At the completion of the capsular plication, the drive-through sign is diminished by greater than 50% (*arrow*; compare with Fig. 3B.1). *G*, Glenoid; *HH*, humeral head; *L*, labrum.

STEP 5

Although much has been published about the rotator interval and whether it has an impact on posterior and inferior instability, passing the interval suture through the leading edge of the supraspinatus tendon ensures inclusion of the coracohumeral ligament. In conjunction with capturing the middle glenohumeral ligament, a more robust contribution from the rotator interval closure can be recognized. The possibility of overconstraining the shoulder and thereby limiting range of motion should be considered and externally rotating the shoulder before knot tying may help avoid this complication. Furthermore, the use of an absorbable suture may militate against the likelihood of motion loss as well.

STEP 6

In most cases, the posterior capsule is thinned and atrophic. The posterior portal should be closed at the conclusion of the capsular shift. An absorbable suture is passed with a straight suture hook inferior to the portal, and a grasping instrument is passed superior to the portal and the suture retrieved. This is performed through the posterior cannula, which has been withdrawn to an extracapsular position. The knot(s) is then tied blindly, closing the portal and further reducing volume.

After the procedure, the immobilization device is predicated on the treated directions of instability. For anterior-inferior instability, a standard shoulder immobilizer in internal rotation is applied while posterior-inferior or anterior-inferior and posterior instability is treated with an immobilization device in neutral rotation. Immediate scapular setting exercises are performed, but motion is delayed for at least 5 to 6 weeks. Patients should be counseled that a period of motion loss and stiffness will be encountered followed by a slow resumption of functional motion and strength. A major goal of plication surgery is to allow a degree of structural stability that achieves the previous balance of proprioception and dynamic and static stabilizing mechanisms.

Technical Pearls

1. The lateral decubitus position with the shoulder in 45 degrees of abduction facilitates plication of the inferior capsule while also decreasing the risk of overly constraining the shoulder because the inferior capsule is placed on some "traction." The axillary nerve must be carefully accounted for in this more abducted position.
2. Using a 45-degree angled hook from the posterior portal maximizes the ergonomic ease of addressing the inferior capsule as minimal torque is required to penetrate the tissue while the possibility of instrument breakage is lessened as well.
3. If the labrum is significantly frayed or incompetent, a suture anchor can be used without any deviation from the surgical technique described. The 6 o'clock anchor, if needed, can be placed with an accessory posterolateral portal.
4. Inclusion of the coracohumeral ligament in the rotator interval closure can be accomplished by placing the arthroscope in the subacromial space and verifying the location of the suture. (Follow the coracoacromial ligament to the base of the coracoid; the coracohumeral ligament originates from its medial border.)
5. When penetrating the capsule during the initial pinch-tuck maneuver, limit the excursion to 10 mm or less. Rather than incorporating more tissue, more sutures may be a more prudent approach to volumetric control.

References

Baker CL III, Mascarenhas R, Kline AJ, Chhabra A, Pombo MW, Bradley JP. Arthroscopic treatment of multidirectional shoulder instability in athletes: a retrospective analysis of 2-5 year clinical outcomes. *Am J Sports Med*. 2009;37:1712–1720.

Burkhead WZ, Rockwood CA. Treatment of instability of the shoulder with an exercise program. *J Bone Joint Surg Am*. 1992;74:890–896.

Cohen SB, Wiley W, Goradia VK, Pearson S, Miller MD. Anterior capsulorrhaphy: an in vitro comparison of volume reduction. Arthroscopic plication versus open capsular shift. *Arthroscopy*. 2005;21:659–664.

Field LD, Ryu RKN, Abrams JS, Provencher M. Arthroscopic management of anterior, posterior and multidirectional shoulder instabilities. *AAOS Instruct Course Lect*. 2016;65:411–435.

Gartsman GM, Roddey TS, Hammerman SM. Arthroscopic treatment of multidirectional glenohumeral instability: 2-5 year follow-up. *Arthroscopy*. 2001;17:236–243.

Gaskill TR, Taylor DC, Millett PJ. Management of multidirectional instability of the shoulder. *J Am Acad Orthop Surg*. 2011;19:758–767.

Jacobson M, Riggenbach M, Woolridge AN. Open capsular shift and arthroscopic capsular plication for treatment of multidirectional instability. *Arthroscopy*. 2012;28:1010–1017.

Kiss J, Damrel D. Non-operative treatment of multidirectional shoulder instability. *International Orthopaedics*. 2001;24:354–357.

Kuroda S, Sumiyoshi T, Moriishi J, Maruta K, Ishige N. The natural course of atraumatic shoulder instability. *J Shoulder Elbow Surg*. 2001;10:100–104.

Luke TA, Rovner AD, Karas SG, Hawkins RJ, Plancher KD. Volumetric change in the shoulder after open inferior capsular shift versus arthroscopic thermal capsular shrinkage: a cadaveric model. *J Shoulder Elbow Surg*. 2004;13:146–149.

Ma HL, Huang HK, Chiang ER, Wang ST, Hung SC, Liu CL. Arthroscopic pancapsular plication for multidirectional shoulder instability in the overhead athlete. *Orthopaedics*. 2012;35:e497–e502.

Misamore GW, Sallay PI, Didelot W. A longitudinal study of patients with multidirectional instability of the shoulder with seven- to ten-year follow-up. *J Shoulder Elbow Surg*. 2005;14:466–470.

Montgomery SR, Chen NC, Rodeo SA. Arthroscopic capsular plication in the treatment of shoulder pain in competitive swimmers. *HSS J*. 2010;6:145–149.

Morris AD, Kemp GJ, Frostick SP. Shoulder electromyography in multidirectional instability. *J Shoulder Elbow Surg*. 2004;13:24–29.

Myers JB, Ju Y, Hwang J, McMahon PY, Rodosky MW, Lephart SM. Reflexive muscle activation alterations in shoulders with anterior glenohumeral instability. *Am J Sports Med*. 2004;32:1013–1021.

Neer CS 2nd. Involuntary inferior and multidirectional instability of the shoulder: etiology, recognition and treatment. *Instr Course Lect*. 1984;34:232–238.

Ponce BA, Tokish JT. Sequential volume reduction with capsular plications: relationship between cumulative size of plications and volumetric reduction for multidirectional instability of the shoulder. *Am J Sports Med*. 2011;39:526–531.

Provencher MT, Verma N, Obopilwe E, et al. A biomechanical analysis of capsular plication versus anchor repair of the shoulder: can the labrum be used as a suture anchor? *Arthroscopy*. 2008;24:210–216.

Rodeo SA, Suzuki K, Yamauchi M, Bhargava M, Warren RF. Analysis of collagen and elastic fibers in shoulder capsule in patients with shoulder instability. *Am J Sports Med*. 1998;26:634–643.

Ryu RK. Multidirectional instability. In: Galatz LM, ed. *Orthopedic Knowledge Update. Shoulder and Elbow*. 3rd ed. Rosemont, IL: American Academy of Orthopedic Surgeons; 2008:303–311.

Sekiya JK, Willobee JA, Miller MD, Hickman AJ, Willobee A. Arthroscopic multi-pleated capsular plication compared with open inferior capsular shift for reduction of shoulder volume in a cadaveric model. *Arthroscopy*. 2007;23:1145–1151.

Treacy SH, Savoie FH. Arthroscopic treatment of multidirectional instability. *J Shoulder Elbow Surg*. 1999;8:345–350.

Wichman MT, Snyder SJ. Arthroscopic capsular plication for multidirectional instability of the shoulder. *Oper Tech Sports Med*. 1997;5: 238–243.

3-3C OPEN CAPSULAR SHIFT

CHARLES M. JOBIN, MD and JONATHAN B. TICKER, MD

Introduction

- Younger patients with multidirectional instability (MDI) are at higher risk for recurrence of instability (Hovelius, 1978), which significantly affects quality of life (Meller et al, 2007).
- Bankart (1938) described the essential lesion of the traumatic shoulder dislocation as an avulsion of the anterior-inferior glenoid labrum, but MDI is likely a result of redundant, stretched, and elastic capsule (Townley, 1950).
- A significantly higher rate of failure may be expected if both the labral and capsular pathology are not addressed at the time of surgery (Levine & Flatow, 2000; Rowe et al, 1984) .
- This chapter describes the rationale and technique for the open anterior-inferior capsular shift that was initially described by Neer and Foster (1980).
- An advantage of open anterior-inferior capsular shift includes exact titration of the capsular plication to match each patient's individual degree and direction of instability (Pollock et al, 2000).
- Open instability procedures have been shown to restore function and quality of life (Meller et al, 2007).

Indications

Surgical repair is recommended for patients with disability and pain caused by anteroinferior instability or MDI with a primary anterior component despite adequate nonoperative treatment. Primary posterior instability is not well suited to an anterior open approach. The choice of arthroscopic or open stabilization is largely a matter of surgeon preference. Previously, arthroscopic techniques were associated with higher recurrence rates than open repair (Lenters et al, 2007), and open repair remains the gold standard to compare the results of improving arthroscopic techniques. More recent reports demonstrate arthroscopic recurrence rates similar to those of open repair, particularly when there is no bony deficit (Longo et al, 2015). We favor open capsular shift and repair in revision cases, cases with multiple risk factors for arthroscopic failure such as patients younger than 20 years old who are contact athletes with some bipolar bone deficiency and some element of ligamentous laxity (Arciero et al, 2015; Ozturk et al, 2013). Even adolescent patients with Ehlers-Danlos syndrome have had successful outcomes with the open capsular shift procedure (Vavken et al, 2016). The open shift procedure also has very good success rates in patients with mild glenoid bone deficiency. The open anterior-inferior capsular shift is a reliable method for treating a wide variety of symptomatic shoulder instability patients. Voluntary instability with intentional muscular contraction and dislocation, active infection, and paralysis are contraindications to this procedure (Bigliani et al, 1994). Acute and semi-acute glenoid rim fractures as well as locked dislocations can be addressed with an open approach, but capsular shift is typically not required if the fracture is repaired.

Rationale for Surgical Capsular Shift

The inferior capsular shift was first designed to treat MDI of the shoulder described by Neer and Foster (1980). This procedure reduces capsular volume globally and restores tension on the glenohumeral ligaments by exposing the capsule laterally on the humerus and allows for a labral (Bankart) repair if torn. The posterior capsule can also be tensioned from an anterior approach by shifting the anterior and inferior capsule superiorly after releasing the capsule from the humerus. For unidirectional anterior instability, the capsular shift is modified with less extensive inferior capsular mobilization compared with Neer and Foster's original method.

An open anterior-inferior capsular shift allows titration of the capsular tensioning based on the differing

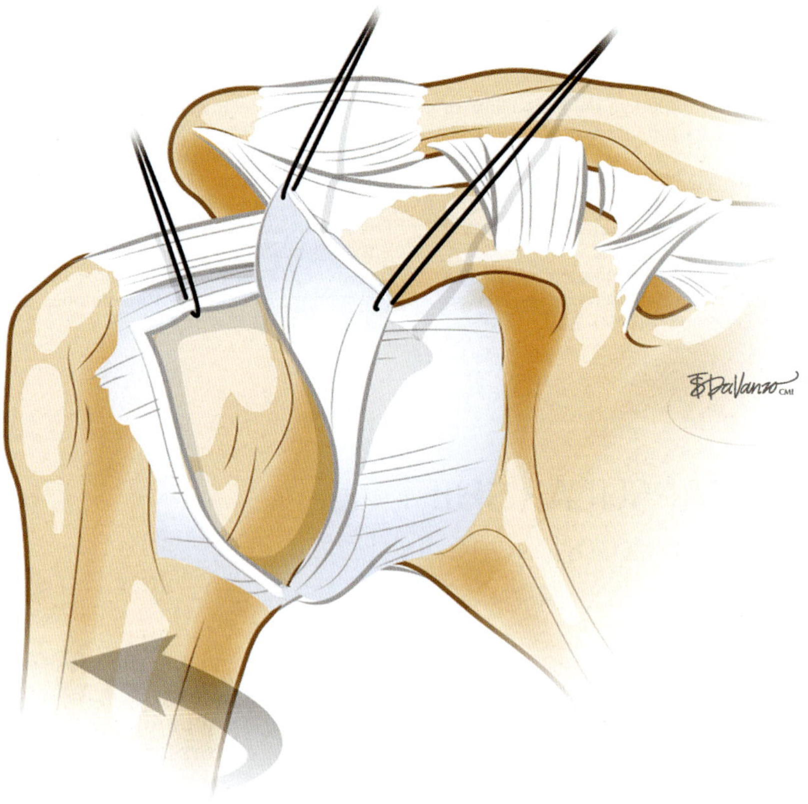

Fig. 3C.1 The humeral-based "L" capsulotomy shifts the entire anteroinferior capsule as one sleeve of tissue. Medial capsular redundancy near the glenoid labrum from recurrent stretch may be plicated using a "barrel" stitch that is passed vertically to plicate the medial capsule (Pollock et al, 2000). (Modified from Pollock RG, Owens JM, Flatow EL, Bigliani LU. Operative results of the inferior capsular shift procedure for multidirectional instability of the shoulder. *J Bone Joint Surg Am.* 2000;82-A(7):919-928.)

degrees of capsular redundancy in different patients. Experimental studies have demonstrated the importance of the inferior glenohumeral ligament as the primary static stabilizer against anterior inferior translation of the humeral head when the arm is abducted and externally rotated and the ligament is placed under significant tension (Mow et al, 1993; Ticker et al, 1996b; Turkel et al, 1981; Warner et al, 1993). Conversely, the superior and middle glenohumeral ligaments function to restrict anterior-inferior translation when the arm is adducted and externally rotated (Warner et al, 1993). The key maneuver to titration of the capsular tensioning is to adjust the degree of capsular takedown around the humeral neck as the redundancy of the inferior pouch is appreciated. The desired amount of capsule to shift is based on the size of the inferior pouch and the degree of laxity (Ticker & Warner, 2000). This ability to titrate the amount of capsule released and the degree of capsular shift is a large advantage because our experience has found that most patients do not fall into the classic two distinct categories of traumatic anterior or atraumatic MDI but represent a spectrum of pathology.

The choice of capsulotomy in a "T" or "L" configuration allows the surgeon to either independently tension the anterior and inferior capsule in a "T" capsulotomy versus a uniform sleeve of tissue with an "L" capsulotomy. An "L" capsulotomy releases the lateral capsule off the humerus and opens the rotator interval (Fig. 3C.1). A "T" capsulotomy separates the inferior and anterior capsule to independently tension these two sleeves of capsule (Fig. 3C.2). Either capsulotomy allows the surgeon to adjust capsular tension in the inferior to superior and medial to lateral directions (Levine & Flatow, 2000). If a Bankart labral tear is present, which is not common in MDI, it should be repaired. More commonly in MDI, there is a diminutive anterior labrum that is not torn, and there is medial capsular redundancy of the anterior capsule adjacent to the glenoid. This medial capsular redundancy is problematic with an "L"-type capsulotomy but can be plicated with a superior to inferior "barrel" stitch. The "T"-type capsulotomy allows repair of this medial capsule redundancy in a "pants over vest" plication. This is important because patients with medial capsular redundancy have been shown to have had a longer duration of symptoms and more repeat dislocations (Ahmad et al, 2003).

A humeral-based shift is preferred over the glenoid-based variation of this procedure. The capsule is funnel shaped with a larger circumference laterally on the humeral side. A laterally based capsulotomy therefore facilitates improved tensioning of the capsule and better reduction in capsular volume than a glenoid-based shift (Miller et al, 2003). An essential part of this procedure is the arm position during the capsular shift and repair. The

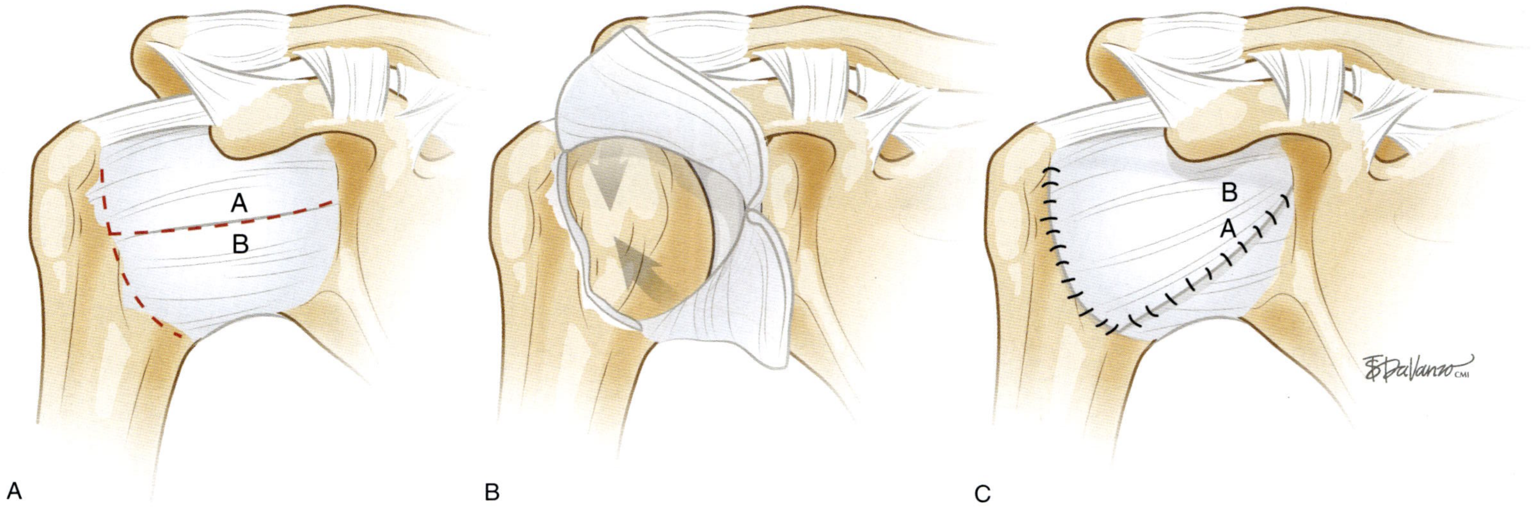

Fig. 3C.2 A. The capsule is sliced open in a "T" shape to separate the inferior and anterior capsule. B. The two separate sleeves are independently tensioned to adjust capsular tension in the inferior to superior and medial to lateral positions. C. The sleeves of the capsule are brought back together and repaired to restore anatomy. The humeral-based "T" capsulotomy and shift allows independent titration of the inferior and superior band to perform the capsular shift and reduce the capsular redundancy (Miller et al, 2003). (Modified from Miller MD, Larsen KM, Luke T, Leis HT, Plancher KD. Anterior capsular shift volume reduction: an in vitro comparison of 3 techniques. *J Shoulder Elbow Surg.* 2003;12(4):350-354.)

inferior flap is advanced superiorly and slightly laterally and secured to the humeral neck with the arm typically positioned in 30 degrees of abduction and 30 degrees of external rotation. The amount of abduction and external rotation is dependent upon the degree of capsular laxity. In overhead athletes, it is mandatory to allow for a sufficient amount of abduction and external rotation to perform overhead sports.

Surgical Technique

Interscalene regional anesthesia is preferred with supplemental local anesthesia in the T2 sensory dermatomal distribution at the inferior-medial aspect of the wound for pain control postoperatively. The modified beach-chair position is used and is amenable for arthroscopy of the glenohumeral joint if indicated before open capsular shift (Warner, 2001). Typically, an articulated arm holder helps facilitate arm position and exposure. Arm position and humeral rotation are critical during capsular repair of the inferior and then superior portions of the capsule to ensure appropriate plication and tightening. A self-retaining retractor may be used in the deltopectoral interval, and a humeral head retractor facilitates visualization of the anteroinferior glenoid rim and labrum. If a Bankart labral tear exists, then it should be repaired with suture anchors that are nonmetallic loaded with nonabsorbable suture size #2, #1, or #0.

When positioning and anesthesia are complete, an examination under anesthesia should be performed to confirm the degree and direction of instability. Drawer testing (Altchek et al, 1991) of the shoulder is performed in all directions and in varying degrees of abduction (0, 45, and 90 degrees) to yield maximum information about laxity in the inferior, anterior, posterior, and superior portions of the capsule. A large sulcus sign with the arm adducted and in external rotation may indicate a pathologic rotator interval lesion requiring closure.

An axillary incision is made 2 cm inferior to the coracoid, extending inferiorly toward the axillary crease (Video 3C.1). Skin flaps are developed, and the cephalic vein is identified and retracted laterally. A self-retaining retractor is placed in the deltopectoral interval after a combination of sharp and blunt dissection. The coracoid is identified, and the clavipectoral fascia is incised just lateral to the strap muscles. The position of the axillary nerve deep to the conjoint tendon and superficial to the subscapularis is identified by palpation. Using the arm holder, the arm is externally rotated in adduction to expose the subscapularis. At its inferior border, the anterior humeral circumflex vessels are identified and, if necessary, ligated for hemostasis. The upper border of the subscapularis is identified by visualizing and palpating the rotator interval. The subscapularis is incised 1 cm medial to its insertion onto the lesser tuberosity in its tendinous portion with care taken not to incise the underlying capsule (Fig. 3C.3). Next, the subscapularis is separated from the underlying glenohumeral capsule. This is the most important and demanding step of the procedure. The upper portion of the subscapularis is confluent with the capsule, but inferiorly, the capsule and subscapularis muscle are typically separate entities (Sugalski et al, 2005). Blunt dissection at the inferior aspect of the subscapularis allows identification of the plane between the capsule and subscapularis (Fig. 3C.4). After the plane is defined, an elevator and Mayo scissors are used to tease the confluent portion of the subscapularis off the anterior capsule. Tag sutures are placed to keep traction on the subscapularis tendon during separation. The axillary nerve should be protected during subscapularis release. The "tug test" (Flatow & Bigliani, 1992) may be helpful in identifying the axillary nerve. Adducting and externally rotating the humerus helps to move the axillary nerve farther from the operative dissection.

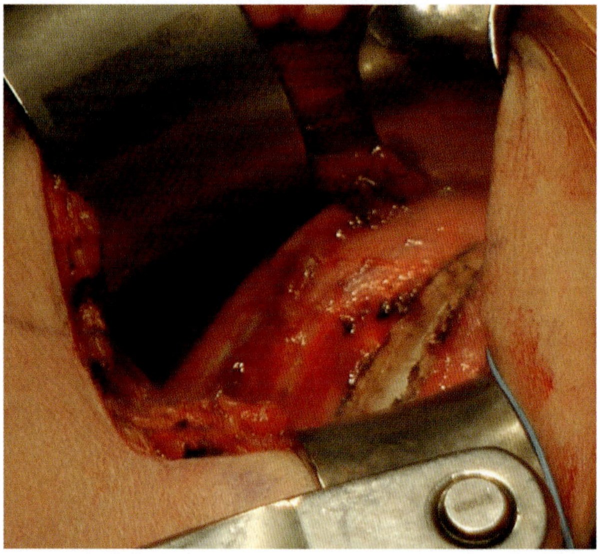

Fig. 3C.3 The location of the subscapularis tenotomy is marked 1 cm medial to the lesser tuberosity from the rotator interval stitch to the inferior border (right shoulder, deltopectoral approach).

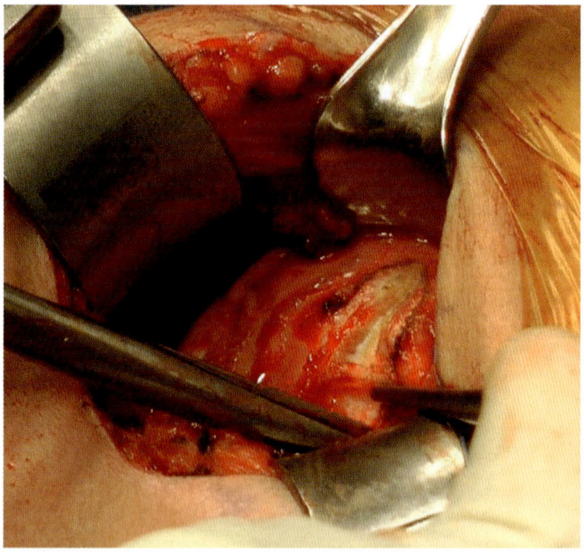

Fig. 3C.4 The subscapularis tendon is peeled off the anterior capsule beginning at the inferior subscapularis using scissors and blunt elevators (right shoulder, deltopectoral approach).

After the subscapularis is completely released from the capsule, the vertical capsulotomy is begun superiorly just medial to the stump of the subscapularis at the humeral attachment site. The capsular incision begins superiorly at the rotator interval and continues

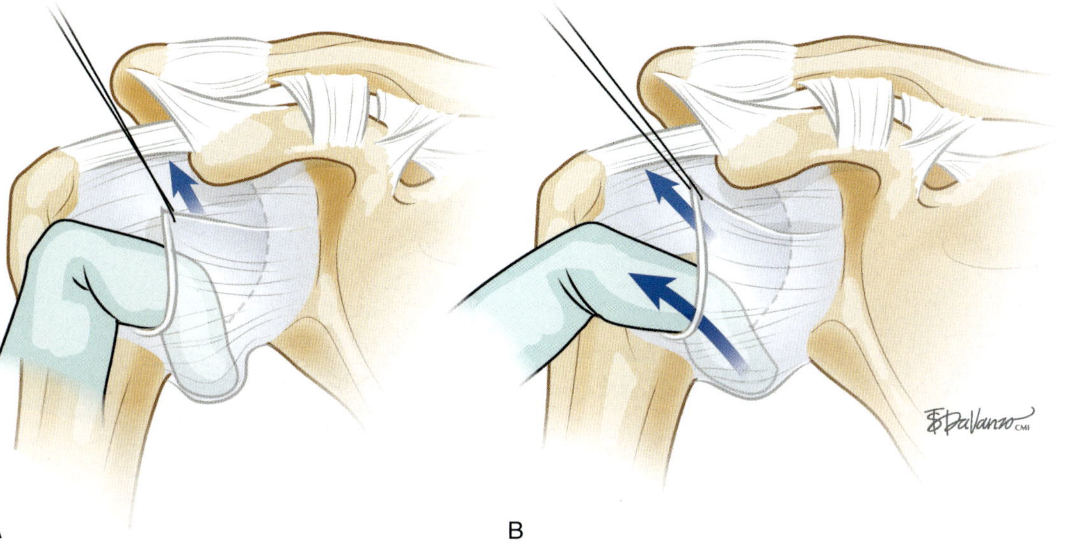

Fig. 3C.5 A. The surgeon's finger is placed in the inferior pouch to pull on the tag sutures to test the tension of the capsule. B. The surgeon's finger is pushed out of the pouch with tension on the tag sutures, demonstrating an adequate amount of capsule release. Digital assessment helps determine the amount of capsular release posteriorly by reduction of the inferior capsular space. Titration of the superior shift is also helped by digital palpation of capsular redundancy and the closure of space, forcing the finger out of the axillary pouch (Pollock et al, 2000). (Reproduced with permission from Pollock RG, Owens JM, Flatow EL, Bigliani LU. Operative results of the inferior capsular shift procedure for multidirectional instability of the shoulder. *J Bone Joint Surg Am.* 2000;82-A(7):919-928.)

inferiorly with traction sutures placed in the free edge. As the dissection is carried inferiorly, the arm is externally rotated for exposure while maintaining a safe distance from the axillary nerve. The amount of capsule released at the inferior humeral neck is determined by the degree of capsular redundancy. The surgeon places a finger in the inferior pouch and pulls on the tag sutures. If the pouch is obliterated and the finger is completely pushed out of the pouch with tension on the tag sutures, then an adequate amount of capsule has been released (Fig. 3C.5). The inferior extent of the capsular incision varies from 6 to 4 or 3 o'clock on the humeral neck for a right shoulder. In cases of traumatic instability, this is usually not carried farther than the 6 o'clock position. When excessive capsular laxity is anticipated, such as in patients with MDI, and a huge axillary pouch is encountered, dissection is carried farther posteriorly. The capsulotomy is complete when tension on the sutures in the capsular edge obliterates the pouch. A humeral head retractor, such as a Fukuda retractor, is inserted behind the posterior labrum to expose the glenoid surface and the anteroinferior labral attachment of the capsule. If a Bankart labral tear is encountered, it should be repaired, and it is elevated medially by stripping the capsulolabral attachments off the scapular neck. The anteroinferior portion of the glenoid rim is then decorticated with a small osteotome or rasp. Suture anchors are then placed for a single- or double-row repair with knots placed extracapsularly. Typically, at least three anchors are used with nonabsorbable suture. Both limbs of each suture are brought through the torn labrum and capsule from the inside to outside and tied down over the capsule after all sutures have been passed. No attempt is made to shift the capsule during Bankart repair. If there is excessive medial capsular redundancy or the anterior inferior labrum is intact but attenuated, an anterior crimping "barrel" stitch may be placed. The stitch is started on the external side of the capsule at the capsulolabral junction. It is passed through the capsule, inside the joint and then back out the capsule in a mattress fashion. Then the anterior medial redundancy is obliterated, and a bolster to the anterior labrum is created.

As mentioned, one of the advantages of a humeral-based shift is the ability to titrate the amount of capsular shift to the degree and direction of instability. For patients with isolated anterior instability, only the anterior capsule is mobilized in an "L" shape opening the rotator interval and lateral humeral attachment. However, for patients with multidirectional (primarily anterior and inferior) instability, the anterior capsule is split horizontally between the inferior and middle glenohumeral ligaments in a "T" configuration and overlapped in a pants-over-vest fashion to better reduce capsular volume and improve the superior shift of the inferior capsule (Fig. 3C.6). Before the capsular repair, the sulcus lateral to the humeral articular margin is decorticated with a curette and rongeur or a bur. Because the rim of capsular tissue inferiorly tends to be thin, a suture anchor can be placed into the humeral neck to insure a secure repair. During the inferior capsular shift and repair, the shoulder is typically placed in a position of 30 to 45 degrees of abduction and 30 degrees of external rotation. Less abduction and external rotation are used in patients with large Hill-Sachs lesions or anterior glenoid bone deficiency. The position of abduction and external rotation is determined individually based on the patient's functional requirements and arm dominance.

After the inferior capsule is repaired (Fig. 3C.7) the arm is repositioned in 0 degrees of abduction, approximately 45 degrees of external rotation, to repair the superior capsular flap. First, the rotator interval is closed; then the superior flap pulled inferiorly and laterally over

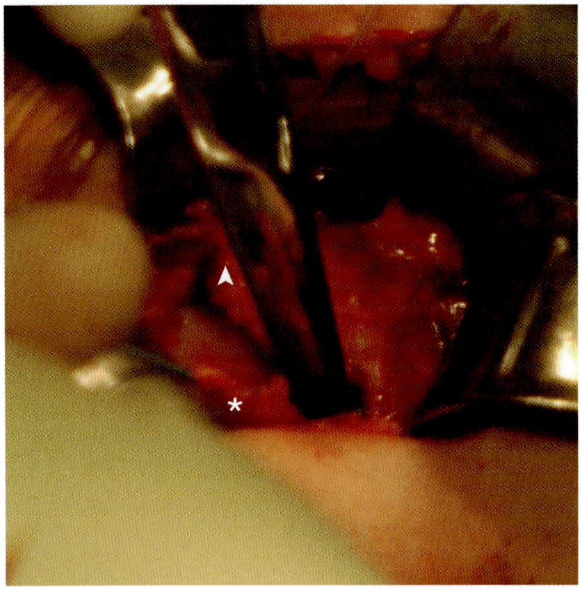

Fig. 3C.6 A "T"-shaped capsulotomy is performed with Mayo scissors from lateral to medial to separate the inferior *(*)* and anterior *(^)* capsule to allow independent tensioning and shifting of the capsular portions (right shoulder, deltopectoral approach).

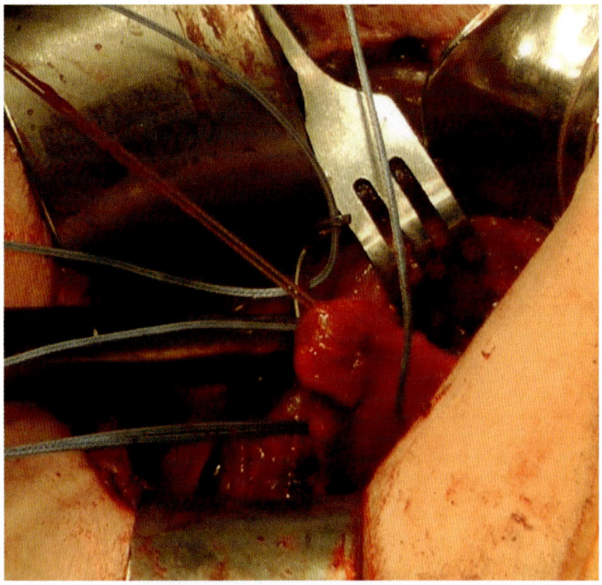

Fig. 3C.7 The inferior capsular flap is repaired to the superior anchor with the arm in a position of 30 degrees of abduction and 30 degrees of external rotation. The amount of capsule superior shift and lateralization depends on the amount of redundant capsule encountered in each patient (right shoulder, deltopectoral approach).

the inferior flap and sutured to the rim of capsular tissue in a "vest-over-pants" fashion, completing the capsular repair. The rotator interval is repaired if the preoperative sulcus sign remained positive in external rotation. The surgeon must be aware of overtightening the capsule. This will limit external rotation, particularly in overhead throwing athletes. The subscapularis is closed (Fig. 3C.8) anatomically with the modified Mason-Allen suture technique (Gerber et al, 1994) followed by a layered skin closure. Drains are not routinely used. A sling and swathe are applied in the operating room, and a device for cryotherapy with compression is applied over the shoulder if desired.

Postoperative Protocol

The patient is usually discharged on the day of surgery with the arm maintained in a sling for 4 weeks, except when the patient performs pendulum exercises, showers, or dresses. Skin sutures are typically removed at 10 to 14 days after surgery. Active assisted shoulder range of motion limitations are based on the repair but typically forward elevation up to 100 degrees by 2 weeks and 140 degrees by 4 weeks postoperatively. By 4 weeks, isometric strengthening is begun for external rotation, flexion, extension, and abduction of the arm, but internal rotation strengthening is delayed so as not to stress the subscapularis repair. At 6 weeks, isotonic strengthening is initiated using elastic bands, and range of motion is maximized. At 4 months postoperatively, the patient is permitted to swim and begin tossing a ball or hitting ground strokes in tennis. At 6 months, the patient is permitted to begin throwing with more force or swinging a racket overhead. A sport-specific reconditioning program is added as the patient progresses. Contact sports are avoided until 6 months postoperatively.

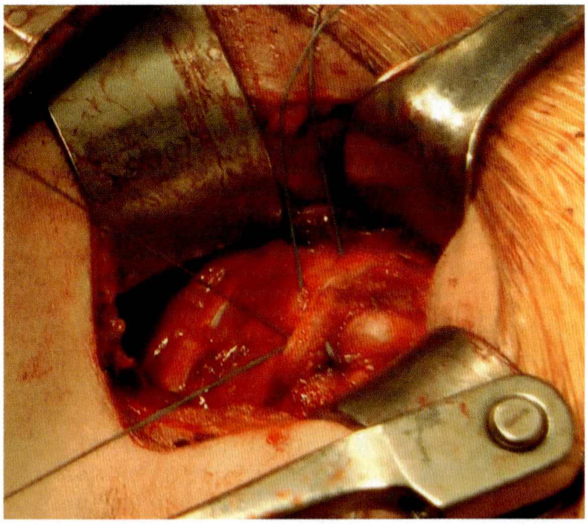

Fig. 3C.8 The subscapularis tenotomy is repaired with multiple Mason Allen suture technique (right shoulder, deltopectoral approach).

Complications

A number of potential problems must be recognized to avoid complications (Cooper et al, 1993; Norris, 1993; Warner, 1993). Errors in surgical technique or misjudgment on degree or direction of capsular shift can lead to recurrent instability or overtightening, leading to loss of motion, posterior instability, or early postcapsulorrhaphy arthropathy. Dissection along the inferior aspect of the subscapularis and along the inferior aspect of the humeral neck should be completed with the arm in adduction and progressive external rotation to avoid injury to the axillary nerve. The axillary nerve is palpable anteromedially to the inferior subscapularis muscle. When elevating the inferior portion of the capsule from the humeral neck, clear visualization should be maintained, and a blunt retractor or finger may be used to further protect the axillary nerve. Bleeding from the anterior humeral circumflex vessels at the inferior aspect of the subscapularis can be troublesome, and if possible, dissection should be kept superior to these vessels to preserve humeral head blood supply. Excessive or prolonged traction on the conjoined tendon may cause musculocutaneous nerve palsy. Postoperative infection is rare, but prolonged surgical time, incisions that encroach on the axilla, and patient factors contribute to increased infection risk (Ticker et al, 1996a).

Outcomes

An anterior-inferior capsular shift study performed at Columbia University in 68 shoulders in athletic patients found good or excellent results in 94% of patients, including 75% returning to their previous level of athletic competition. External rotation loss averaged 7 degrees, and only 2 patients had recurrence of dislocation (Bigliani et al, 1994). In a separate study of patients undergoing capsular shift, 38 patients with medial redundancy who received a crimping "barrel" suture were compared with 40 patients who did not have redundancy. Despite a higher number of dislocations and a longer duration of symptoms preoperatively, the incidence of good and excellent results and postoperative Rowe scores was similar for both groups (Ahmad e al, 2003). A landmark article on open Bankart repair on 162 shoulders found only a 2% recurrence of instability despite the high prevalence (73%) of glenoid rim bone lesions and Hill-Sachs lesions with good to excellent results in 98% of patients (Rowe et al, 1978).

Conclusion

Our understanding of the pathophysiology and treatment of shoulder instability has improved to better address the pathology of labral detachment, capsulolabral redundancy, and bony deficiency. When nonoperative intervention has failed, treatment should be directed at restoring the original anatomy. In the setting of adequate bony architecture, an anatomic reconstruction and early range of motion will yield successful results in patients with shoulder MDI. The anteroinferior capsular shift as described by Neer and Foster (1980) is preferred because the amount of capsule being shifted can easily be titrated to treat the amount and direction of pathology found at surgery. If Bankart repair is required, this technique allows for excellent exposure of the glenoid and the ability to individualize the procedure. If performed meticulously, the anteroinferior capsular shift provides excellent enduring results while allowing patients to return to full activity.

References

Ahmad CS, Freehill MQ, Blaine TA, Levine WN, Bigliani LU. Anteromedial capsular redundancy and labral deficiency in shoulder instability. *Am J Sports Med.* 2003;31(2):247–252.

Altchek DW, Warren RF, Skyhar MJ, Ortiz G. T-plasty modification of the Bankart procedure for multidirectional instability of the anterior and inferior types. *J Bone Joint Surg Am.* 1991;73(1):105–112.

Arciero RA, Parrino A, Bernhardson AS, et al. The effect of a combined glenoid and Hill-Sachs defect on glenohumeral stability: a biomechanical cadaveric study using 3-dimensional modeling of 142 patients. *Am J Sports Med.* 2015;43(6):1422–1429.

Bankart A. The pathology and treatment of recurrent dislocation of the shoulder joint. *Br Med J.* 1938;26:23–29.

Bigliani LU, Kurzweil PR, Schwartzbach CC, Wolfe IN, Flatow EL. Inferior capsular shift procedure for anterior-inferior shoulder instability in athletes. *Am J Sports Med.* 1994;22(5):578–584.

Cooper D, Warner J, Warren R. Complications of shoulder instability in the competitive athlete. In: Bigliani LU, ed. *Complications of Shoulder Surgery.* Philadelphia: Williams & Wilkins; 1993:240–257.

Flatow EL, Bigliani LU. Tips of the trade. Locating and protecting the axillary nerve in shoulder surgery: the tug test. *Orthop Rev.* 1992;21(4):503–505.

Gerber C, Schneeberger AG, Beck M, Schlegel U. Mechanical strength of repairs of the rotator cuff. *J Bone Joint Surg Br.* 1994;76(3):371–380.

Hovelius L. Shoulder dislocation in Swedish ice hockey players. *Am J Sports Med.* 1978;6(6):373–377.

Lenters TR, Franta AK, Wolf FM, et al. Arthroscopic compared with open repairs for recurrent anterior shoulder instability. A systematic review and meta-analysis of the literature. *J Bone Joint Surg Am.* 2007;89(2):244–254.

Levine WN, Flatow EL. The pathophysiology of shoulder instability. *Am J Sports Med.* 2000;28(6):910–917.

Longo UG, Rizzello G, Loppini M, et al. Multidirectional instability of the shoulder: a systematic review. *Arthroscopy.* 2015;31(12):2431–2443.

Meller R, Krettek C, Gosling T, et al. Recurrent shoulder instability among athletes: changes in quality of life, sports activity, and muscle function following open repair. *Knee Surg Sports Traumatol Arthrosc.* 2007;15(3):295–304.

Miller MD, Larsen KM, Luke T, Leis HT, Plancher KD. Anterior capsular shift volume reduction: an in vitro comparison of 3 techniques. *J Shoulder Elbow Surg.* 2003;12(4):350–354.

Mow V, Bigliani L, Flatow E, Ticker J, Ratcliffe A, Soslowsky L. Mechanical properties of the inferior glenohumeral ligament and the glenohumeral articular cartilage. In: Matsen FA, Fu FH, Hawkins RJ, eds. *The Shoulder: A Balance of Mobility and Stability.* Park Ridge, IL: AAOS Press; 1993:29–67.

Neer CS 2nd, Foster CR. Inferior capsular shift for involuntary inferior and multidirectional instability of the shoulder. A preliminary report. *J Bone Joint Surg Am.* 1980;62(6):897–908.

Norris T. Complications following anterior instability repairs. In: Bigliani LU, ed. *Complications of Shoulder Surgery.* Philadelphia: Williams & Wilkins; 1993:98–116.

Ozturk BY, Maak TG, Fabricant P, et al. Return to sports after arthroscopic anterior stabilization in patients aged younger than 25 years. *Arthroscopy.* 2013;29(12):1922–1931.

Pollock RG, Owens JM, Flatow EL, Bigliani LU. Operative results of the inferior capsular shift procedure for multidirectional instability of the shoulder. *J Bone Joint Surg Am.* 2000;82-A(7):919–928.

Rowe CR, Patel D, Southmayd WW. The Bankart procedure: a long-term end-result study. *J Bone Joint Surg Am.* 1978;60(1):1–16.

Rowe CR, Zarins B, Ciullo JV. Recurrent anterior dislocation of the shoulder after surgical repair. Apparent causes of failure and treatment. *J Bone Joint Surg Am.* 1984;66(2):159–168.

Sugalski MT, Wiater JM, Levine WN, Bigliani LU. An anatomic study of the humeral insertion of the inferior glenohumeral capsule. *J Shoulder Elbow Surg.* 2005;14(1):91–95.

Ticker J, Lippe R, Barkin D, Carroll M. Infected suture anchors in the shoulder. *Arthroscopy.* 1996a;12(5):613–615.

Ticker JB, Bigliani LU, Soslowsky LJ, Pawluk RJ, Flatow EL, Mow VC. Inferior glenohumeral ligament: geometric and strain-rate dependent properties. *J Shoulder Elbow Surg.* 1996b;5(4):269–279.

Ticker JB, Warner JJ. Selective capsular shift technique for anterior and anterior-inferior glenohumeral instability. *Clin Sports Med.* 2000;19(1):1–17.

Townley CO. The capsular mechanism in recurrent dislocation of the shoulder. *J Bone Joint Surg Am.* 1950;32A(2):370–380.

Turkel SJ, Panio MW, Marshall JL, Girgis FG. Stabilizing mechanisms preventing anterior dislocation of the glenohumeral joint. *J Bone Joint Surg Am.* 1981;63(8):1208–1217.

Vavken P, Tepolt FA, Kocher MS. Open inferior capsular shift for multidirectional shoulder instability in adolescents with generalized ligamentous hyperlaxity or Ehlers-Danlos syndrome. *J Shoulder Elbow Surg.* 2016;25(6):907–912.

Warner JJ. Management of massive irreparable rotator cuff tears: the role of tendon transfer. *Instr Course Lect.* 2001;50:63–71.

Warner JJ, Caborn DN, Berger R, Fu FH, Seel M. Dynamic capsuloligamentous anatomy of the glenohumeral joint. *J Shoulder Elbow Surg.* 1993;2(3):115–133.

4 Shoulder Instability Rehabilitation and Return to Sport

4-4A POSTOPERATIVE REHABILITATION: ANTERIOR STABILIZATION

TERRANCE A. SGROI, PT, DPT, SCS, MTC

The glenohumeral joint is an inherently unstable ball and socket joint that places high demands on both the static and dynamic stabilizers. The glenoid labrum approximately doubles the depth of the glenoid fossa and provides multidirectional stability to the shoulder joint (Howell, 1989). Laxity or disruption of the capsulolabral complex may require surgical fixation. Arthroscopic surgical anterior stabilization has been demonstrated as an effective procedure to help athletes to return to the highest level of athletics (Frank et al, 1987; Kim et al, 2002; Stein et al, 2011). Careful attention is given to progression of both range of motion (ROM) and strength during the rehabilitation process. This progression is criteria based and allows patients to be advanced in an individualized, safe, and protective manner.

As patients progress through postoperative rehabilitation, it is important to follow a few guiding principles:

- Ongoing effective communication with the surgical team about the details of the procedure and patient progression is essential.
- This progression should be individualized as healing and procedures may vary.
- Clinicians should progress active ROM (AROM) carefully to ensure high-quality capsulolabral healing.
- Reestablish scapular stability and rotator cuff activation before global strengthening.
- Restore dynamic stability and neuromuscular control with safe, pain-free progression of therapeutic exercises.

Throughout the rehabilitation process, it is important to manage patients' expectations. After anterior shoulder stabilization, it can be expected that shoulder strength will be restored by about 6 months (Rhee et al, 2007). Understanding of the passive and dynamic shoulder stabilizers is just as important. The three glenohumeral ligaments provide stability to the glenohumeral joint at different angles of shoulder abduction. The superior and middle glenohumeral ligaments develop most strain at 0 degrees of shoulder abduction. At 45 degrees of shoulder abduction, the inferior and middle glenohumeral ligaments develop most strain, and at 90 degrees of shoulder abduction, the inferior glenohumeral ligament (IGHL) develops the most strain (Ferrari, 1990; O'Connell et al, 1989; Turkel et al, 1981). The labrum also helps provide stability by deepening the socket from 2.5 to approximately 5 mm (Howell, 1989). The rotator cuff plays an important role in providing dynamic stability to the shoulder joint. The balanced function of the rotator cuff helps prevent superior displacement of the humeral head on the glenoid fossa and provides stability in the scapular plane (Sharkey & Marder, 1995). Wilk and Arrigo (1993) have also shown the important contribution to stability of the scapulothoracic musculature.

Phase 1: Protective Phase, 0 to 2 Weeks

(Video 4A.1) During the rotective phase, the primary goals are to reduce and minimize pain and swelling, prevent inhibition of dynamic stabilizers of the shoulder joint, and gradually control passive ROM (PROM) so as not to cause undue stress to the surgical repair. As Hurley et al (1994) demonstrated, pain can lead to joint instability, muscle inhibition, and weakness. More recently, pain has been shown to inhibit rotator cuff activation during specific exercises for shoulder strengthening (Stackhouse et al, 2013). Pain has also been shown to affect muscle coordination in the shoulder, which is why it is essential to minimize it as quickly as possible (Diederichsen et al, 2009).

After an anterior stabilization procedure, it is critical to respect ROM precautions and guidelines especially in the early phases. The purpose of the surgery is to provide stability to the joint, which can be compromised with PROM that is too early or too aggressive. Even subfailure strains can produce enough force to elongate and produce laxity in shoulder ligaments. This laxity, especially in the IGHL, can contribute to acquired shoulder instability (Pollock et al, 2000). Controlled motion in this phase must be respected in order to maintain capsular and ligamentous constraint. The position of abduction and external rotation (ER) produces the most stress in the anterior shoulder in both a native shoulder as well as shoulders with anterior labral repair (Penna et al, 2008). PROM is initiated in the scapular plane, which minimizes stress on passive and active shoulder stabilizers. Itoi et al (1999) showed that the edges of simulated Bankart lesions were kept approximated from full internal rotation (IR) to 30 degrees of ER.

Exercises in this phase are focused on scapular activation and postural correction as well as distal elbow, hand, and wrist movement. Submaximal isometric contractions of the scapular muscles are allowed, but we recommend against rotator cuff activation during this phase. Even though the rotator cuff is not affected during surgery, it is the experience of the author that early rotator cuff exercises can irritate the joint during the initial postoperative period. Distal muscle activation can help improve circulation and help minimize any swelling that has migrated beyond the elbow.

Immobilization

- A sling is to be worn at all times during the first 2 weeks.
- The sling can be taken off at home for exercise after week 2 and can be discharged at home starting week 4.
- The sling is to be worn outside the home for 6 weeks in all uncontrolled environments.

Range of Motion Progression

- Forward elevation: 0→ 90 degrees
- External rotation: 0→30 degrees (shoulder positioned in scapular plane)
- ER at 90 degrees shoulder abduction: contraindicated

Exercises

- Scapular isometrics
- Pendulums
- PROM shoulder to 90 degrees
- AROM elbow, wrist, hand

Modalities

- Cryotherapy and compression five times a day. (The author prefers the Game Ready system shoulder attachment.)

Phase 2: 3 to 6 Weeks

Progression to phase 2 is possible when pain is minimized, PROM shoulder flexion to 90 degrees has been achieved, and patients demonstrate good understanding of posture and precautions. During this phase, activation of the rotator cuff and other dynamic stabilizers is important to support the glenohumeral joint. It is important that the local stabilizers are initiated before global musculature, which will help maintain proper centralization of the humeral head in the glenoid. The rotator cuff muscles help stabilize the glenohumeral joint in all planes of movement. In flexion, the stabilizers are the infraspinatus, supraspinatus, and latissimus dorsi. In extension, the subscapularis and supraspinatus stabilize. In ER, the subscapularis is the stabilizer, and in abduction, the stabilizers are the infraspinatus and subscapularis (Kronberg et al, 1990). Without proper activation of these muscles, compromised GH stability would be imminent. Scapular protraction is not recommended until week 6 because of the excessive strain that it places on the anterior band of the IGHL (Weiser et al, 1999).

During this phase, scapulohumeral rhythm should also be emphasized. With the patient in a sidelying position, the therapist can palpate scapular musculature and provide manual resistance while cuing the patient to activate appropriate muscles. This manual resistance can be progressed to scapular proprioceptive neuromuscular facilitation (PNF) in the sidelying position. Closed kinetic chain activation can also be initiated in this phase. This type of exercise allows for distal fixation with proximal muscle activation while promoting centralization of the humeral head into the glenoid through compression.

IMMOBILIZATION

- Wean off sling at 4 to 6 weeks and discharge at 6 weeks

RANGE OF MOTION PROGRESSION

- Forward elevation 90→130 degrees
- ER 30→60 degrees
- ER at 90 degrees shoulder abduction: 0→45 degrees

EXERCISES

- Scapular and rotator cuff isometrics
- Isotonic band rows and low rows emphasizing scapular retraction
- Assisted active ROM (AAROM) flexion within ROM guidelines
  - Cane progression
    - AAROM supine with hands on cane in scapular plane
    - Incline table 15 to 20 degrees/week until patient is seated upright on table
- Prone row, prone extension emphasizing scapular retraction
- Closed-chain progression
  - Quadruped double-arm forward rock
  - Quadruped double-arm side-to-side rock
  - Quadruped double-arm rock on BOSU (Fig. 4A.1)

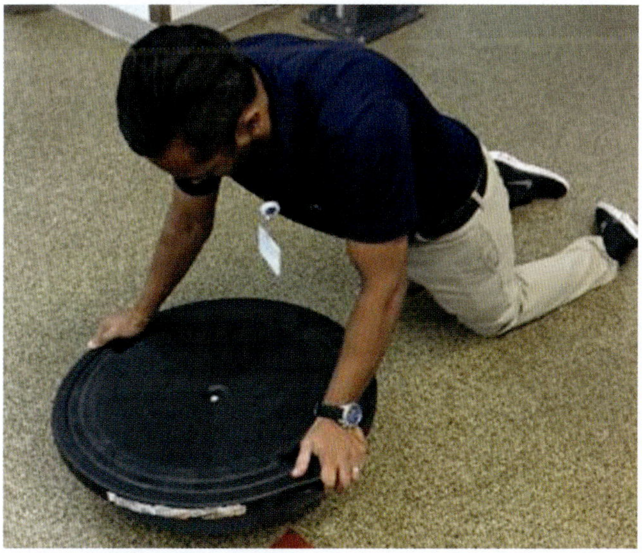

Fig. 4A.1 Quadruped double arm rock on BOSU. The patient rocks in multiple directions on an unstable surface while maintaining good core control with the scapula in a slightly protracted position.

MODALITY

- Cryotherapy as needed

Phase 3: 6 to 12 Weeks

The goals of this phase are to restore full shoulder ROM and normal scapulohumeral rhythm. Upper extremity strength should continue to be progressed, and by 12 weeks, patients are expected to have full pain-free AROM. If this is not achieved, consultation with the referring physician may be necessary to address limiting factors. AROM should be progressed from 0 degrees of abduction to the 90-degree/90-degree position by the end of this phase. Gentle glenohumeral joint mobilizations (grades II and III) can help restore mobility but should be used with caution because we do not want to stretch the joint capsule beyond its physiologic limit, on the other hand we do want to protect the integrity of the anterior capsule.

As strengthening progresses throughout this phase, caution is taken to avoid rotator cuff irritation, which can impede progress. Using current evidence and electromyographic (EMG) studies, careful exercise progression is used to advance strength with focus on rotator cuff and scapular muscles. Sidelying ER with a towel roll under the arm has been shown to elicit high levels of infraspinatus activation and is helpful in enhancing lower and mid trapezius activity ratios (Alizadehkhaiyat et al, 2015; De Mey et al, 2013). Using a towel roll has anatomic, neurologic, and biomechanical benefits. By using a towel roll under the arm for rotation exercises, a reduction is seen in the amount of compensatory abduction force through reciprocal inhibition, which will assist in improved rotator cuff isolation. Also, by raising the arm to about 30 degrees of abduction with a towel roll, there is decreased tension on the rotator cuff muscles (Kolber et al, 2008). During forward elevation, attention should be paid to the quality of movement, in particular shoulder shrug. If this is noticed, patients should stay within the "shrug-free" zone of movement until adequate dynamic GH centralization is achieved.

Scapulothoracic muscle strengthening is emphasized in this phase. Shoulder elevation in the scapular plane is introduced (30 degrees anteriorly from the frontal plane) as scaption maintains the humeral head into the glenoid and promotes shoulder stability (Moseley et al, 1992). Between 120 and 150 degrees of elevation, scaption elicits high lower trapezius and serratus anterior muscle activity. Rowing is an optimal exercise for middle trapezius and rhomboid activation, and prone extension is also optimal for middle trapezius activity (Moseley et al, 1992).

Serratus anterior activation can also commence in this phase, which will help to restore normal scapulohumeral rhythm. The push-up plus and dynamic hug both elicit high EMG activity (Decker et al, 1999). Two-arm press-ups in a quadruped position are a safe way to start closed-chain serratus activation. This can be progressed to tripod press-ups and then addition of an unstable surface. Finally, the patient can progress into a full plank tripod, double-arm and then single-arm press-up, which has been shown to have the highest EMG activity (Herrington et al, 2016).

As full ROM is achieved, overhead movement patterns can be initiated, including PNF. These exercises can be started in the supine position and gradually progressed to standing and then against resistance. PNF can be used to help increase ROM, increase muscular strength and power, and increase athletic performance (Hindle et al, 2012).

RANGE OF MOTION PROGRESSION

- Forward elevation 130→Within normal limits (WNL)
- ER 60→WNL
- ER at 90 degrees shoulder abduction: 45→WNL

EXERCISES

- Isotonic ER, IR with towel roll
- Sidelying ER with towel roll
- Isotonic rows
- Isotonic shoulder extension (prone)
- PNF (Fig. 4A.2)
- Thrower's ten exercises
- Closed-chain progression (correct for any winging of scapula)
  - Continue above
  - Quadruped opposite arm shoulder tap
  - Quadruped protraction
  - Quadruped band around wrists 3-point tap (Fig. 4A.3)
  - Quadruped perturbations on BOSU
- Endurance:
  - Initiate interval cardiovascular training (lower extremity)
- Core:
  - Sagittal, frontal, and transverse plane core strengthening
- Linking:
  - Modified side plank with shoulder ER
  - 3-month position with PNF shoulder patterns
  - Pallof press (Fig. 4A.4)

MODALITY

- Cryotherapy as needed

Phase 4: 12 to 18 Weeks

During phase 4, emphasis is on building the foundation for the athlete to return to her or his respective sport. Overhead strengthening and end range stability are focuses while maintaining previously established scapular rhythm and rotator cuff activation. This phase concentrates on whole-body strength and progresses to whole-body linking activities.

RANGE OF MOTION

- Full and pain-free in all motions
- Begin to stretch 90-degree/90-degree position for throwing athletes if appropriate

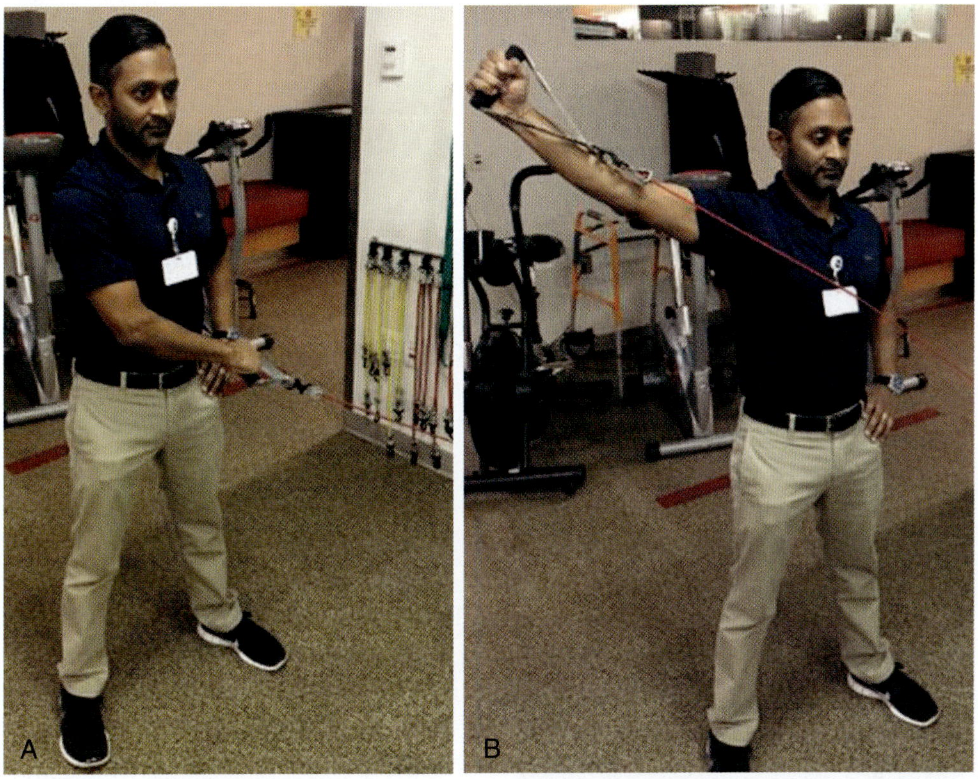

Fig. 4A.2 A, Proprioceptive neuromuscular facilitation diagonals. **B,** The patient brings the arm into shoulder flexion, abduction, and external rotation and forearm supination.

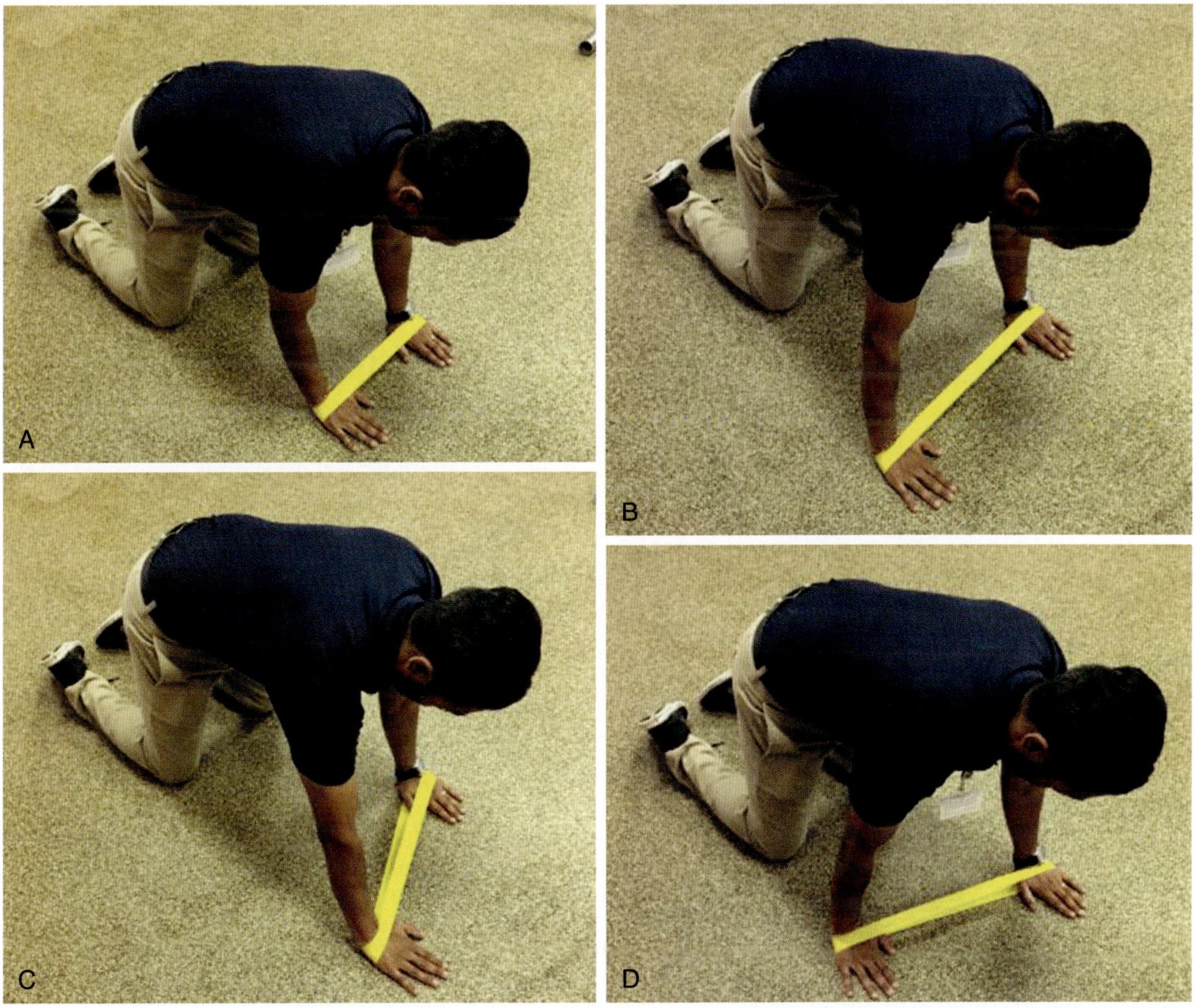

Fig. 4A.3 Quadruped band 3-point tap. **A,** The patient begins in a quadruped position with the band around the wrists, maintaining good core control and the scapula in a slightly protracted position. With one arm remaining stable, the opposite arm moves into an anterior (**B**), side (**C**), and posterior (**D**) position.

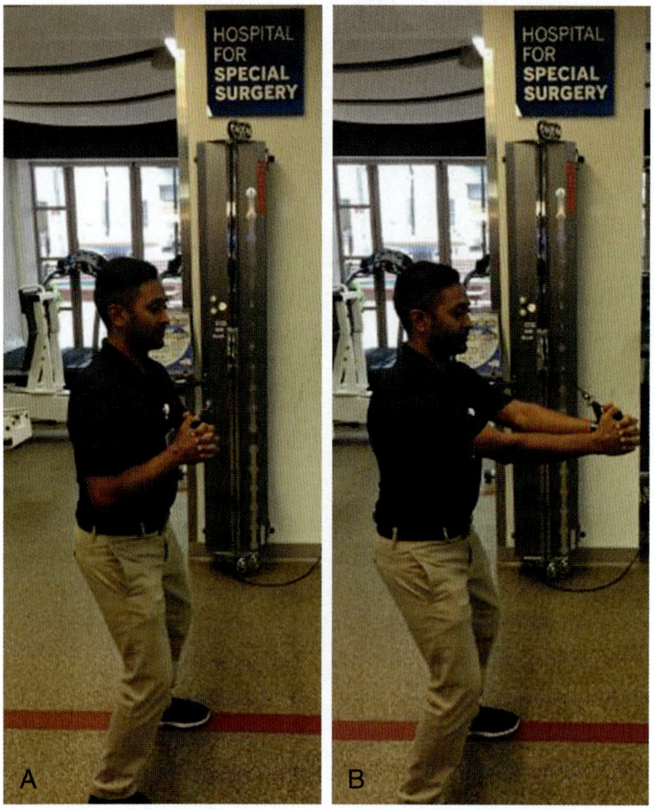

Fig. 4A.4 Pallof press. **A,** The patient stands with a cable column at chest level and then presses out until the elbows are fully extended, resisting trunk rotation. **B,** The cable is then brought back into the chest for a period of rest.

EXERCISES

- 90-degree/90-degree strengthening if applicable to patient's activities
- Prone row into ER→ seated on ball row into ER against band resistance
- Prone horizontal abduction with ER
- PNF
- Advanced thrower's ten exercises
- Closed-chain progression
  - Push-up progression: wall→ floor
  - Tripod: protraction →protraction on unstable surface
  - Plank wrist clocks
  - Plank position lateral step-up → step-up with unstable surface (Fig. 4A.5)
  - Plank position perturbations on BOSU→ stability ball
- Plyometrics (if applicable to patient's activities)
  - Double-hand chest ball toss plyoback
  - Single-arm ball toss with arm at side plyoback
  - Single-arm ball toss 90/90 against wall
  - Single arm ball toss 90/90 plyoback
  - Med ball forward slams
  - Rotational medical ball wall slams
  - TheraBand plyometrics

Phase 6: Weeks 18+

This phase focuses on sports-specific training and depends on the sport to which the athlete is returning. Baseball players will progress to a return to throwing program, tennis players to an interval tennis program, and so forth. These programs are structured to gradually apply increased load to the shoulder joint while building flexibility and endurance at the same time. The patient should consult his or her physical therapist with any onset of pain during this progression.

CRITERIA TO RETURN TO SPORT

- 0/10 pain Numerical Rating Pain score (NRPS)
- No shrug with any active movement
- 60-second plank on hands without scapular winging
- Isokinetic ER/IR <10% deficit
- Upper extremity Y balance test 80% limb length for all three reaches

THROWING ATHLETES

In addition to above:

- 90-degree/90-degree wall taps (2-lb ball) 60s without elbow dropping below shoulder height
- Overhead wall taps (4-lb ball) 60s without shrug
- 12, 1, 3 o'clock wall taps (2-lb ball) 45s without shrug
- 20 reverse catches with smooth follow-through and 0/10 pain on NRPS

EXERCISES

- Continued RC Progressive Resistance Exercises (PREs)
- Continued scapular PREs
- Continued 90-degree/90-degree strengthening with increasing speed and resistance
- Continued plyometric progression
- Continued closed-chain strengthening
- End-range perturbations
- Leg, hip, and core strengthening
- Cardiovascular training

Open Anterior Stabilization Considerations

If an open shoulder stabilization is performed, early rehabilitation restrictions must be followed because of surgical management of the subscapularis muscle or tendon. It is of primary importance to communicate with the surgeon to determine how much of the subscapularis and which portion was taken down during surgery, because ROM will affect upper and lower fibers differently. ROM should be progressively increased with both subscapularis split and subscapularis takedown. A recent study (Knesek et al, 2016) demonstrates that ER and ER plus 30 degrees of abduction places increased strain on both the upper and lower portions of the repaired subscapularis tendon. To protect the repair of the subscapularis, ER beyond neutral should be limited in the early postsurgical phase. Flexion in the scapular plane places less than 3% strain on the upper fibers of the subscapularis but places increased strain on the lower fibers. Active IR will also be contraindicated until 6 weeks after surgery due to the subscapularis contribution to this motion.

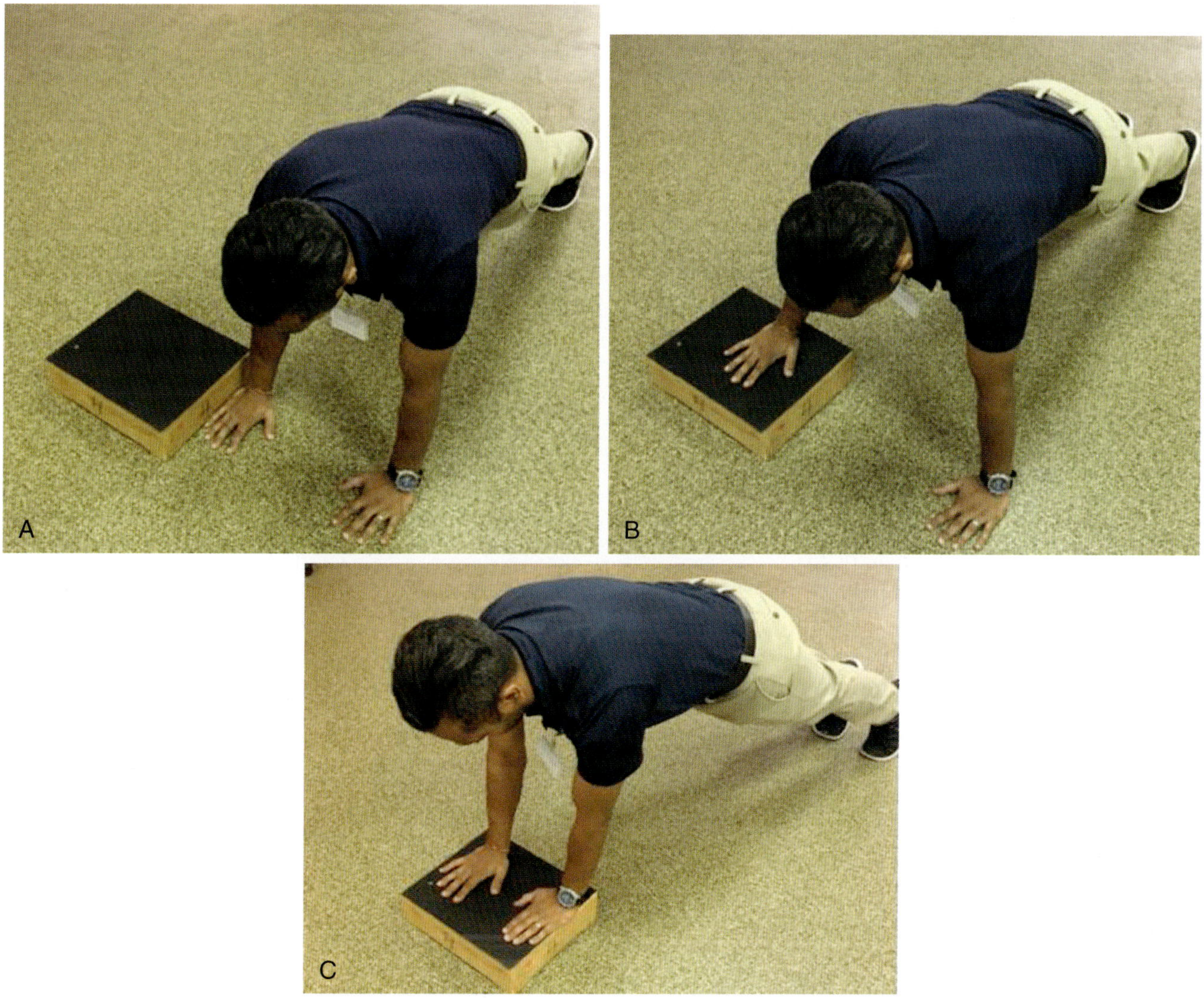

Fig. 4A.5 Plank lateral step-up. Starting in a plank position (**A**), the patient laterally walks onto a box of a set height (**B**). The trail arm is then brought up so that both hands are on top of box (**C**).

Weeks 0 to 6

Immobilization

- Sling discharged at 6 weeks

Range of Motion Progression

- Forward elevation 0→100 degrees until week 6; then progress per patient tolerance
- ER 0 degrees until week 6
- Shoulder abduction 90 degrees until week 6

Exercises

- Elbow, wrist, and hand AROM
- Scapular isometrics

Precautions

- No IR exercise until week 6; then progress slowly in weeks 6 to 12 to minimize strain to the healing subscapularis muscle. Isometric→ isotonic

WEEKS 6+

- Progress with arthroscopic stabilization guidelines with exception to ER ROM and IR strengthening.
- The patient's symptoms will dictate progression; keep in mind that patient should never be pushed through painful ROM or exercises.

References

Alizadehkhaiyat O, Hawkes DH, Kemp GJ, Frostick SP. Electromyographic analysis of the shoulder girdle musculature during external rotation exercises. *Orthop J Sports Med.* 2015;3(11). 2325967115613988.

Decker MJ, Hintermeister RA, Faber KJ, Hawkins RJ. Serratus anterior muscle activity during selected rehabilitation exercises. *Am J Sports Med.* 1999;27(6):784–791.

De Mey K, Danneels LA, Cagnie B, Huyghe L, Seyns E, Cools AM. Conscious correction of scapular orientation in overhead athletes performing selected shoulder rehabilitation exercises: the effect on trapezius muscle activation measured by surface electromyography. *J Orthop Sports Phys Ther.* 2013;43(1):3–10.

Diederichsen LP, Winther A, Dyhre-Poulsen P, Krogsgaard MR, Nørregaard J. The influence of experimentally induced pain on shoulder muscle activity. *Exp Brain Res.* 2009;194(3):329–337.

Ferrari DA. Capsular ligaments of the shoulder: Anatomical and functional study of the anterior superior capsule. *Am J Sports Med.* 1990;18(1):20–24.
Jobe FW, Giangarra CE, Kvitne RS, Glousman RE. Anterior capsulolabral reconstruction of the shoulder in athletes in overhand sports. *Am J Sports Med.* 1991;19(5):428–434.
Rhee YG, Lim CT, Cho NS. Muscle strength after anterior shoulder stabilization. *Am J Sports Med.* 2007;35(11):1859–1864.
Herrington L, Waterman R, Smith L. Electromyographic analysis of shoulder muscles during press-up variations and progressions. *J Electromyogr Kinesiol.* 2016;25(2015):100–106.
Hindle KB, Whitcomb TJ, Briggs WO. Hong J. Proprioceptive neuromuscular facilitation (PNF): its mechanisms and effects on range of motion and muscular function. *J Hum Kinet.* 2012;31:105–113.
Howell SM, Galinat BJ. The glenoid-labral socket. *Clin Orthop.* 1989;243: 122–125.
Hurley MV, Jones DW, Newham DJ. Arthrogenic quadriceps inhibition and rehabilitation of patients with extensive traumatic knee injuries. *Clin Sci (Lond).* 1994;310:305–310.
Itoi E, Hatakeyama Y, Urayama M, Pradhan RL, Kido T, Sato K. Position of immobilization after dislocation of the shoulder. A cadaveric study. *J Bone Joint Surg Am.* 1999;81(3):385–390.
Kim SH, Ha KI, Kim SH. Open versus arthroscopic technique. *Arthroscopy.* 2002;18(7):755–763.
Knesek M, Brunfeldt A, Korenczuk C, et al. Patterns of strain and the determination of the safe arc of motion after subscapularis repair—a biomechanical study. *J Orthop Res.* 2016;34(3):518–524.
Kolber MJ, Beekhuizen KS, Santore T, Fiers H. Implications for specific shoulder positioning during external rotator strengthening. *Strength Condition J.* 2008;30(4):12–16.
Kronberg M, Németh G, Broström LA. Muscle activity and coordination in the normal shoulder. *Clin Orthop Rel Res.* 1990:Aug;(257):76–85.
Moseley JB, Frank W, Perry J. EMG analysis of the scapular muscles during a shoulder rehabilitation program. *Am J Sports Med.* 1992;20(2):128–134.
O'Connell PW, Nuber GW, Mileski RA, Lautenschlager E. The contribution of the glenohumeral ligaments to anterior stability of the shoulder joint. *Am J Sports Med.* 1989;18(6):579–584.
Penna J, Deramo D, Nelson CO, et al. Determination of anterior labral repair stress during passive arm motion in a cadaveric model. *Arthroscopy.* 2008;24(8):930–935.
Pollock RG, Wang VM, Bucchieri JS, et al. Effects of repetitive subfailure strains on the mechanical behavior of the inferior glenohumeral ligament. *J Shoulder Elbow Surg.* 2000;9(5):427–435.
Sharkey NA, Marder RA. The rotator cuff opposes superior translation of the humeral head. *Am J Sports Med.* 1995;23(3):270–275.
Stackhouse SK, Eisennagel A, Eisennagel J, Lenker H, Sweitzer BA, McClure PW. Experimental pain inhibits infraspinatus activation during isometric external rotation. *J Shoulder Elbow Surg.* 2013;22(4):478–484.
Stein T, Linke RD, Buckup J, et al. Shoulder sport-specific impairments after arthroscopic Bankart repair: a prospective longitudinal assessment. *Am J Sports Med.* 2011;39(11):2404–2414.
Turkel SJ, Panio MW, Marshall JL, Girgis FG. Stabilizing mechanisms preventing anterior joint dislocation of the glenohumeral. *J Bone Joint Surg Am.* 1981;63-A(8):1208–1217.
Weiser WM, Lee TQ, McMaster WC, McMahon PJ. Effects of simulated scapular protraction on anterior glenohumeral stability. *Am J Sports Med.* 1999;27(6):801–805.
Wilk KE, Arrigo C. Current concepts in the rehabilitation of the athletic shoulder. *J Orthop Sports Phys Ther.* 1993;18:365–378.

4-4B POSTOPERATIVE REHABILITATION: POSTERIOR STABILIZATION AND MULTIDIRECTIONAL INSTABILITY

EMILIE SCHMIDT, DPT, SCS, ATC, CSCS, and AMY RESLER, DPT, CMP, CSCS

Introduction

- Postoperative course of rehabilitation for posterior and multidirectional instability (MDI) should be guided by a thorough appreciation of the structures involved or pathoanatomy, rates of tissue healing, and positions of stress and strain on the affected structures.
- Neuromuscular reeducation is a key component of rehabilitation to restore proper scapulohumeral rhythm to facilitate proper joint mechanics and resolve scapular dyskinesis, especially in the throwing population.
- Range of motion (ROM) should be gradually restored within pain-free ranges without undue stress on the ligamentous capsule.
- Postoperative ROM precautions depend on structures involved and their rates of physiologic healing.
- Thorough communication between surgeon and physical therapist or rehabilitation team is paramount when deciding on the appropriate postoperative rehabilitation protocol.
- Key differences between posterior stabilization and MDI rehabilitation postoperative protocols involve protection from arm movement in directions that will load the surgical repair and the timeframe for initiation of capsular stretching (Table 4B.1).
- Key similarities between posterior and MDI rehabilitation postoperative protocols include emphasis on neuromuscular reeducation to facilitate proper scapulohumeral and scapulothoracic mechanics, a gradual progression from passive ROM to active assisted ROM (AAROM) to active ROM (AROM) over a course of 4 to 12 weeks, and thorough strengthening of the periscapular muscle groups, including the rotator cuff complex and scapular stabilizers

Rehabilitation Overview

Although conservative management through rehabilitation is initially encouraged for patients with complaints and clinical signs of instability, many ultimately require surgical intervention for glenohumeral joint stabilization in cases of both posterior instability (PI), and MDI, especially athletes whose instability is limiting their participation in sport. Overall treatment success or failure is largely determined by a well-designed and appropriately implemented postoperative course of rehabilitation. Guiding principles for the postoperative course should be an understanding of the type and direction of instability and surgical stabilization technique performed, an understanding of the anatomic structures involved and their rates of healing, an understanding of positions and activities that stress the healing structures, the proper selection of manual therapy intervention applied at the appropriate

Table 4B.1 Postoperative Range of Motion Guidelines

	RANGE OF MOTION LIMITS (POSTERIOR INSTABILITY*/MULTIDIRECTIONAL INSTABILITY)					
Timeframe	**Scaption**	**Flexion**	**Adduction**	**Abduction**	**ER**	**IR**
0–14 days*	90/Codman	30/Codman	0/Codman	90/Codman	30/Codman	0/Codman
2–4 weeks†	120/90	90/90	0/0	100/90	30/30	0/20
5–8 weeks‡	140/120	120/120	0/20	120/120	45/45	0/30
9–12 weeks§	160/160	160/160	20/full	160/160	90/90	70/70
Weeks 13+§	Full/full	Full/full	Full/full	Full/full	Full/full	Full/full

*It may be the surgeon's preference in less stable repairs or revisions that flexion is avoided for 6 to 8 weeks instead performing rehabilitation only in the plane of the scapula.
†Passive range of motion.
‡Active assisted range of motion and active range of motion.
§Active range of motion

phase of healing, and a respect for the rate of ROM progression (Gaunt et al, 2010; Schmidt et al, 2015; van der Meijden et al, 2012).

Because of the paucity of research related to revascularization and rates of healing of the glenoid labrum and capsule after surgical repair, healing timelines have been modeled historically on the known physiology of the knee meniscus (Mulcahey et al, 2015). Thus, rehabilitation protocols for labral repairs have been extrapolated from the abundant literature related to the knee, as well as based on clinical experience. There has been, however, recent literature investigating the immunohistochemical changes within the labrum after injury, as well as the fibrous histologic makeup of the labrum (Mulcahey et al, 2015). Improved knowledge of these factors will allow for a better understanding of the healing timelines with respect to collagen formation, revascularization, and scar formation to optimize rehabilitation protocols and therefore calls for an updated approach to otherwise conventional treatment strategies (Hill et al, 2008).

The importance of proprioceptive joint position sense and an understanding of preinjury movement pattern faults have also garnered increased attention in this population, especially in athletes with chronic instability (De Mey et al, 2013; Halder et al, 2001; Lephart et al, 1994; Merolla et al, 2015; Myers & Lephart, 2000; Schiffern et al, 2002). One such rehabilitation advancement involves postoperative joint approximation. Patients with a history of MDI as well as chronic PI are known to lack proper neuromuscular control of the scapula, resulting in scapular dyskinesis thought to be partly caused by a lack of joint compression and congruency, thereby affecting known components of joint stability (Halder et al, 2001; Merolla et al, 2015; Provencher et al, 2011). Clinically, it has been observed that progressive manual joint approximation and compression help facilitate proprioception and kinesthesia of the shoulder. Therefore manually loading the glenohumeral joint during the early phases of rehabilitation when the upper extremity is maintained in a dependent position within the sling may be an important technique to incorporate into postoperative care until the onset of progressive closed-chain upper extremity exercises when weightbearing is permitted. This allows for a combination of humeral head centering as well as improved stability through concavity–compression, both key components of glenohumeral joint stability. In addition, manual compression may provide a sensation of stability for the patient because it optimizes joint congruency as well as maximizes proprioception and kinesthesia through the loading of mechanoreceptors of the joint and capsuloligamentous tissue (Halder et al, 2001).

Neuromuscular reeducation is essential for both PI and MDI. It is known that scapular position is a contributing factor to MDI both in its resting position and with activity (De May et al, 2013; Voight & Thomson, 2000). This impairment not only interferes with the ideal length–tension relationship of the stabilizing musculature but also prevents the humeral head from centering itself on the glenoid, reducing the above-noted concavity–compression mechanism, as well as affecting kinesthesia, resulting in muscle inhibition. In cases of glenoid insufficiency either caused by acute trauma glenoid dysplasia, manually (or physically) blocking abnormal translation of the humeral head during manual therapy or ROM may be beneficial in proprioceptive training while initiating rehabilitation (Video 4B.1).

Unfortunately, there is a high failure rate with PI and MDI preoperative rehabilitation because of an inherent or acquired pathoanatomy (Provencher et al, 2011; Tannenbam & Seklya, 2011). However, with the inclusion of proprioceptive neuromuscular training, success rates have been noted clinically to greatly improve (Cools et al, 2016; Lephart et al, 1994). Clinically, it has been observed that the application of these techniques also greatly improves postoperative outcomes. Therefore these techniques should be the foundation and emphasis throughout the course of postoperative rehabilitation for both PI and MDI, beginning with the conscientious correction of posture and scapulohumeral position and using tactile, compressive, and visual feedback and progressing to closed-chain weight-bearing activities before full resumption of sport-specific activity. (Please refer to Video 4B.1 to see an example of the implementation of joint position sense early on in the course of rehabilitation as demonstrated by incorporating blinded contralateral upper extremity movements to mirror passive ROM (PROM) of the involved extremity.) It cannot be emphasized enough that although there are specific anatomic differences between PI and MDI or explicit differences in the surgical stabilization techniques performed, the common underlying etiology is impaired neuromuscular control. Therefore the incorporation of proprioceptive and neuromuscular education

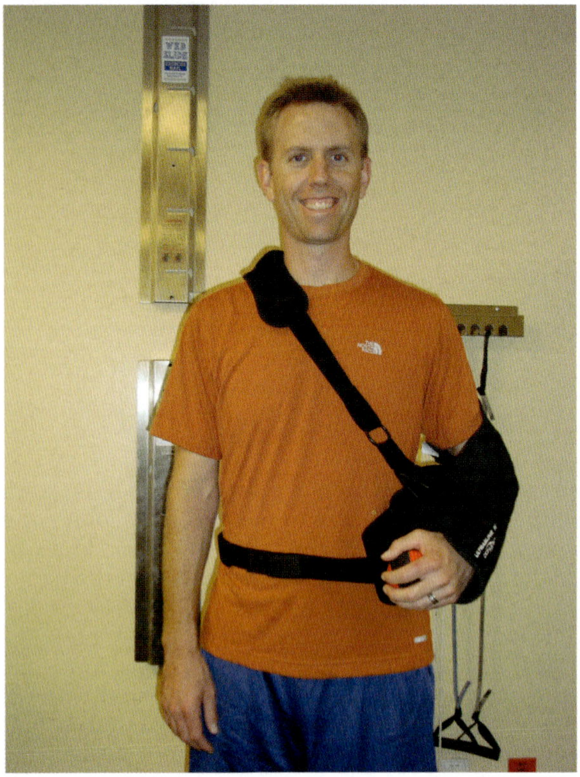

Fig. 4B.1 Abduction pillow sling.

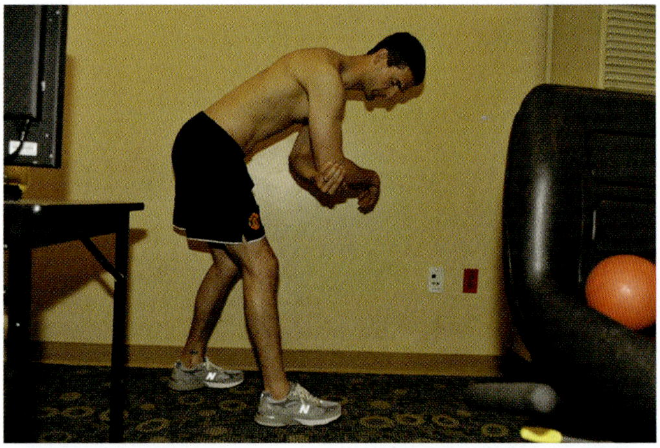

Fig. 4B.2 Supported Codman passive range of motion. Patients are instructed to fully relax the muscles surrounding the glenohumeral joint and use gravity to allow the arm to "hang" freely while moving the trunk to generate passive oscillations of the upper extremity.

components is a key element in all phases of both PI and MDI rehabilitation guidelines.

Phase 1: Weeks 0 to 2

Goals of rehabilitation for athletes undergoing glenohumeral joint stabilization procedures are to restore normal ROM, facilitate optimum motor control and scapulohumeral rhythm, and prevent future episodes of instability with the end goal of return to sport activity. During the initial phases of postoperative rehabilitation, protection of the surgical repair is paramount. This timeframe corresponds with the inflammatory period of healing, usually lasting approximately 10 to 14 days. Patients are placed in a protective sling using an abduction pillow with the arm in neutral rotation (MDI) or slight external rotation (ER) for posterior repairs (Fig. 4B.1). Patients should be thoroughly educated on the postoperative precautions and instructed how to properly don and doff their sling. Early PROM may be initiated within precautions via manual PROM for PI repairs; however, because of the likelihood of congenital laxity and a redundant capsule in patients diagnosed with MDI, PROM is initially recommended to be limited to a more protective supported Codman position (Fig. 4B.2), and extra care is taken to avoid active contraction of the biceps tendon so to reduce any strain throughout the capsule to allow it to tighten postoperatively as much as possible. Manual joint approximation is performed throughout PROM and during active postural correction. The capsular ligaments should not be put under any strain during this timeframe. Pain control is performed via modalities such as high-volt electrical stimulation, cryotherapy, and oral medications.

Phase 2: Weeks 3 to 5

Over the next several weeks, progressive PROM is initiated. This timeframe corresponds to the transition to the proliferative phase of healing as the body is beginning to lay the foundation for scar formation within the affected tissues. Protection of the repair continues via the use of a sling and PROM only. Pain mediation is also a continued focus. Submaximal isometrics are performed to the unaffected muscles, and scapular neuromuscular reeducation commences. Early application of rhythmic stabilization of the rotator cuff within precaution ranges may also be implemented. To facilitate scapular motor control, seated scapular retraction and depression as well as scapular clock exercises are begun, as are activities that emphasize trunk rotation. Patients are also cleared to begin cardiovascular training via stationary cycling or walking on level ground.

Phase 3: Weeks 6 to 8

In the early remodeling phase, from weeks 6 to 8, there is a transition from surgical structure protection to the application of gentle forces through the joint because the newly formed repair tissue, "scar," requires a certain degree of stress to develop appropriately (Mueller & Maluf, 2002). Sling use is discontinued, and ROM progresses to include AAROM and AROM while still respecting precaution ranges to avoid undue stress to the capsule. This can be achieved via cane/wand exercises within the pain-free precaution ranges and wall walks (Figs. 4B.3 and 4B.4). Scapular stabilization exercises progress to against gravity, and rotator cuff strengthening also progresses to light resistance unless concomitant repair has occurred (Figs. 4B.5 to 4B.7). Neuromuscular reeducation is the emphasis of this timeframe because it is imperative to restore proper motor control to prevent scapular dyskinesis or to perpetuate an

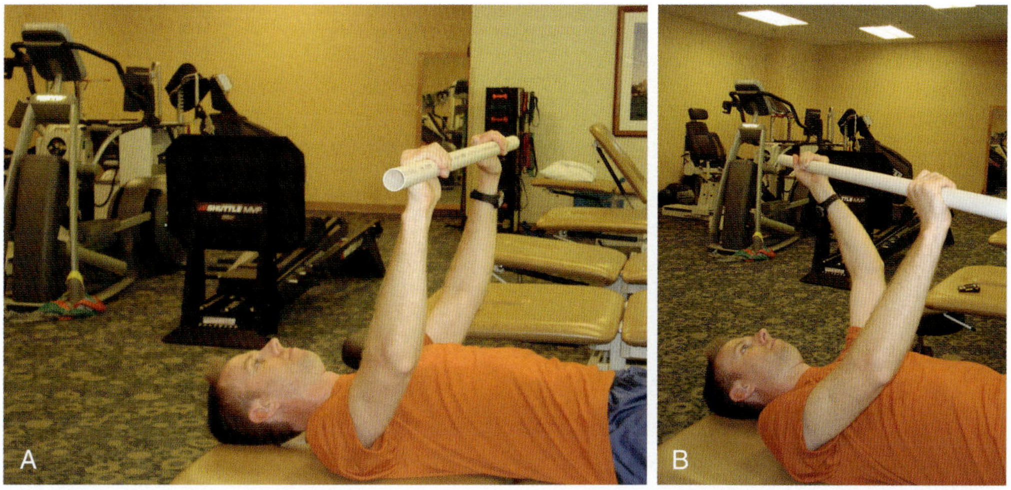

Fig. 4B.3 Cane-assisted active assisted range of motion for abduction (**A**) and scaption (**B**). Patients should be cued to avoid painful ranges and apply gentle stretch only within postoperative range of motion precautions. The unaffected upper extremity acts as the primary moving force, allowing the surgical arm gentle movement through available ranges of motion.

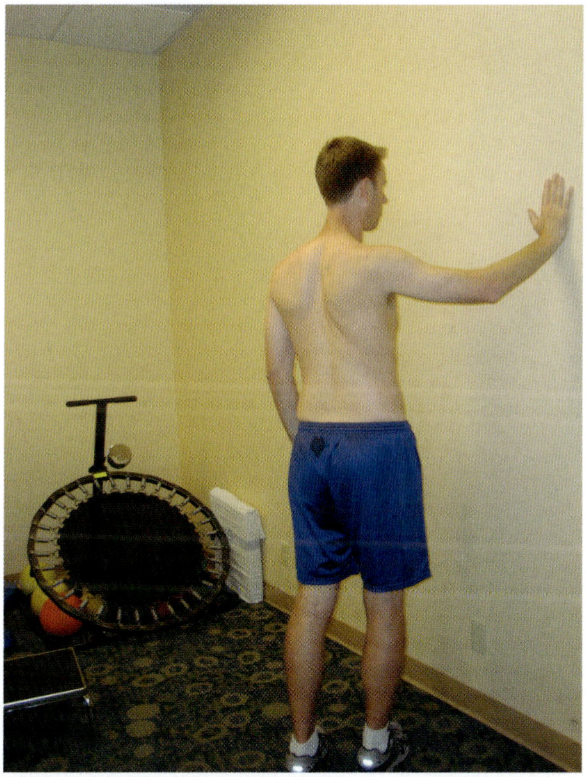

Fig. 4B.4 Wall walks. Patients are instructed to slowly advance the affected arm up the wall within pain-free ranges. They should be positioned so that the arm is in the scapular plane.

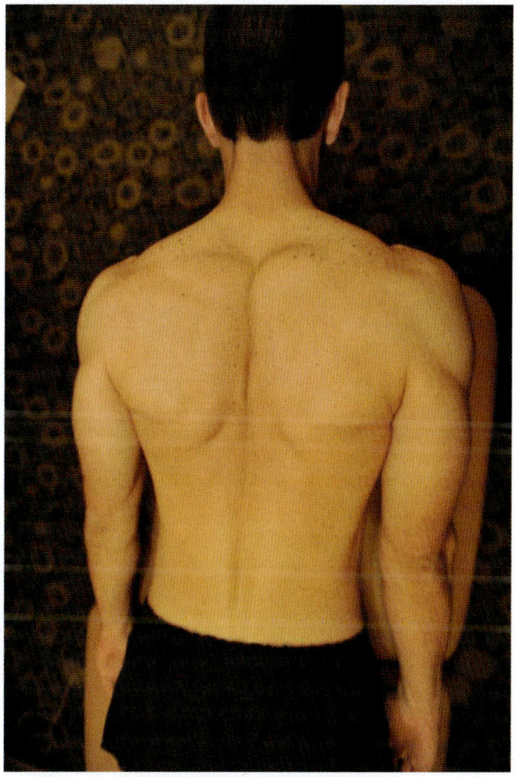

Fig. 4B.5 Prone scapular adduction "I." In prone, with arms in neutral at patient's side, the patient is instructed to sequentially depress the scapulae, retract the scapulae, and then extend the arm while maintaining the scapular position

already disadvantaged scapula (Figs. 4B.8 and 4B.9). (See Video 4B.1 for additional content demonstrating manual neuromuscular reeducation techniques.)

Phase 4: Weeks 8 to 12

As the healing process graduates to more mature collagen formation and progressively stronger repair tissue, more aggressive manual techniques are introduced as well as higher level strengthening and motor control activities. Over the next 4 weeks, the remodeling and maturation phase places emphasis on regaining both full PROM and AROM, and resisted strengthening exercises become the focus of rehabilitation. Active proprioceptive neuromuscular facilitation patterns are performed with resistance using bands, and other strengthening exercises begin the use of weights for resistance. Emphasis remains on the rotator cuff and periscapular muscles to ensure continued development of proper scapulohumeral rhythm patterns

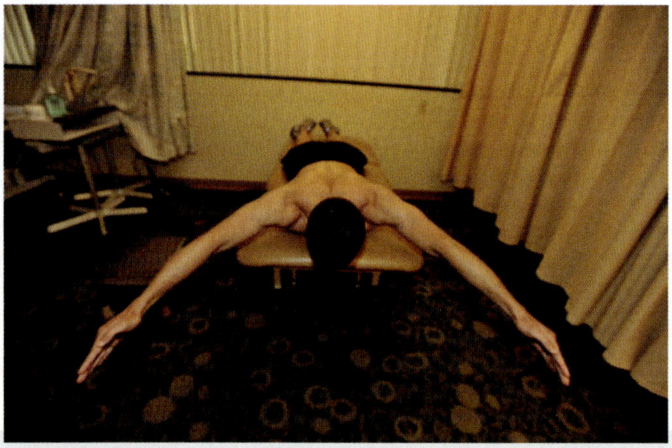

Fig. 4B.6 Prone lower trapezius "Y." In prone, the patient is instructed to elevate the arm in the scapular plane, making a "Y" by emphasizing scapular downward rotation and retraction.

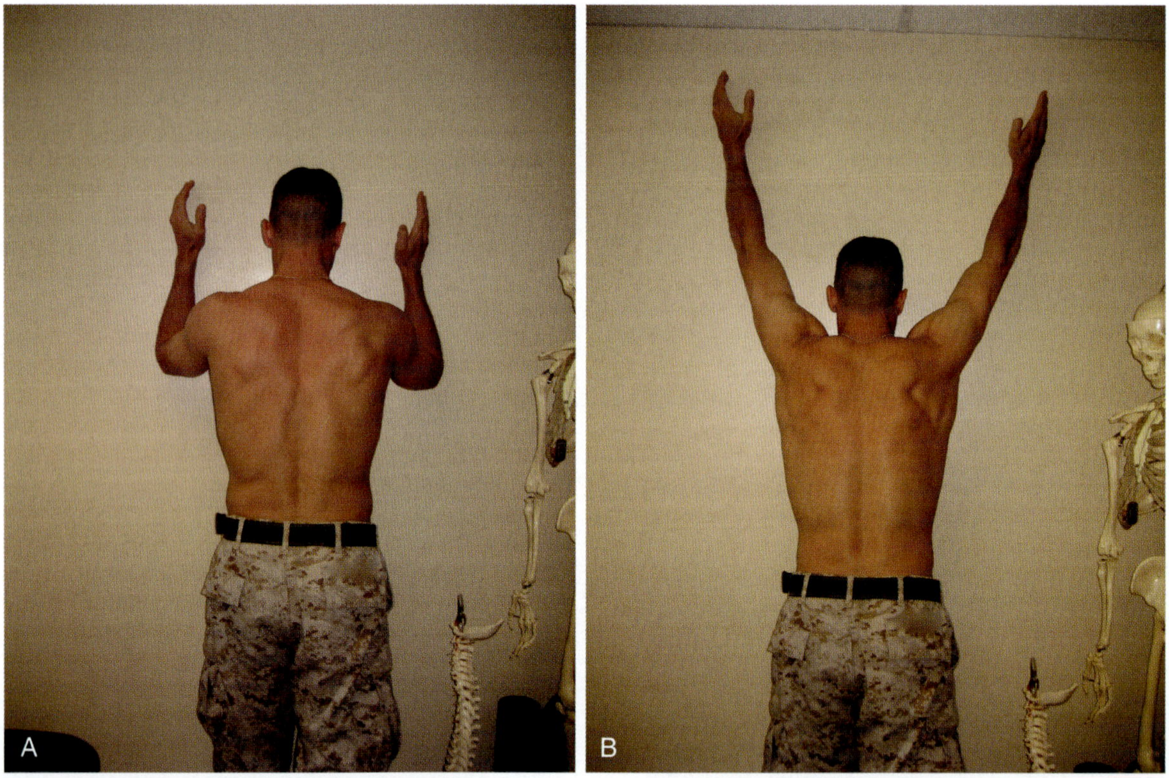

Fig. 4B.7 Wall slides for shoulder flexion/lower trapezius. The patient begins with the arms at a resting position with the palms lightly pressing into the wall while co-contracting the scapular adductors (**A**). The patient is instructed to slide the hands up the wall, continuing to press lightly against the wall (**B**) until the arms are overhead. At end range, the patient should perform active scapular depression with end-range glenohumeral flexion to facilitate the lower trapezius muscle.

(Figs. 4B.10 to 4B.13). For posterior stabilization cases, the emphasis is placed on subscapularis strength and motor control because of its role as a primary stabilizer for posterior translation. In patients with MDI, extra attention should be placed on scapular positioning with corrective exercises addressing any downward rotation faults that are commonly associated with the diagnosis. Throughout this timeframe and going forward, exercises should incorporate the entire functional kinetic chain. Muscular imbalances and asymmetries of the upper and lower extremities or core stability weaknesses should be addressed, as should any limitations in flexibility of the lower extremity, especially the hamstring musculature. This phase will set the foundation for the higher level sport-specific training that will ensue over the next 2 to 4 months. Athletes should be educated on the importance for full pain-free ROM and proper scapular mechanics as a requirement for progression toward return-to-sport activities.

Phase 5: Weeks 13 to 16

As the capsular repair continues to remodel and mature and as the patient's motor control regains appropriate

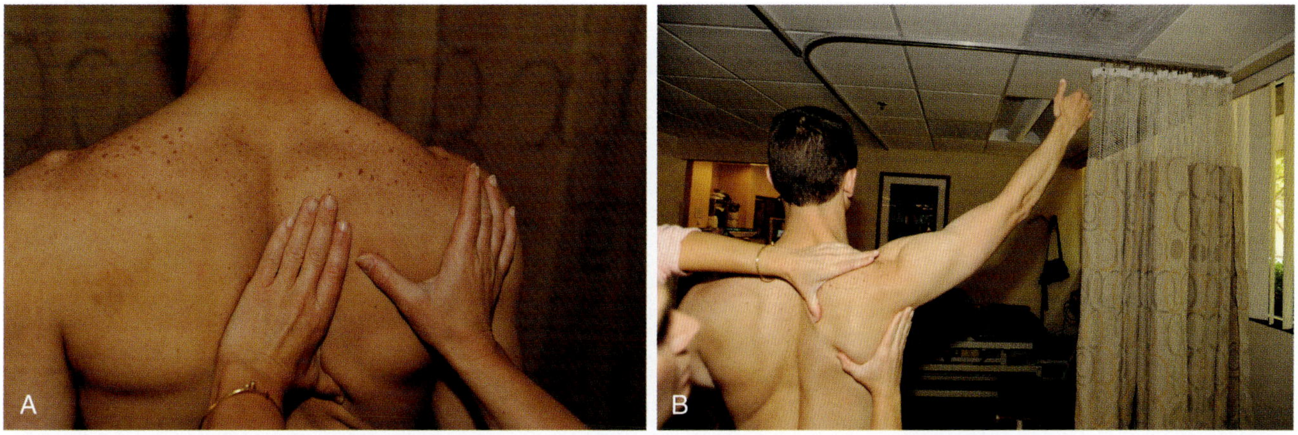

Fig. 4B.8 Scapular proprioceptive neuromuscular facilitation in standing. Manual resistance is applied to the medial border and inferior angle with the arm in neutral while the patient moves the scapula through diagonal patterns for upward and downward rotation as well as elevation and depression (**A**). Manual resistance is applied to the inferior angle and medial/superior border of the scapula while the patient performs scapular upward rotation in conjunction with arm scaption, as well as scapular downward rotation in conjunction with arm return to neutral (**B**).

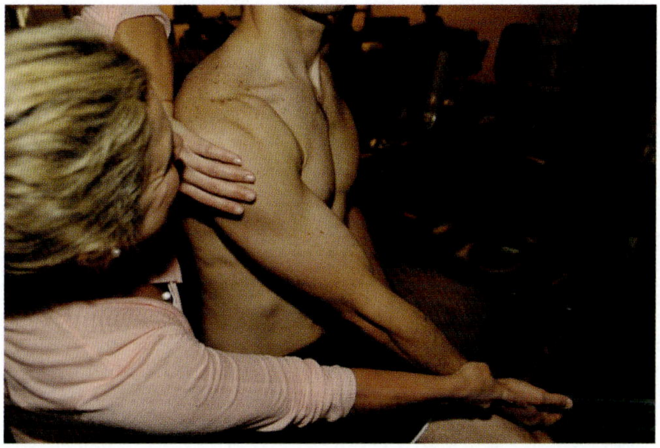

Fig. 4B.9 Scapular proprioceptive neuromuscular facilitation in sitting. This may be initiated while the patient is immobilized in a sling to stimulate periscapular muscle recruitment. Manual resistance is applied to the medial border and inferior angle with the arm in a sling or in neutral if no longer using a sling. The patient is cued to move the scapula through diagonal patterns for upward and downward rotation as well as elevation and depression. This may be enhanced with trunk rotation and cervical rotation.

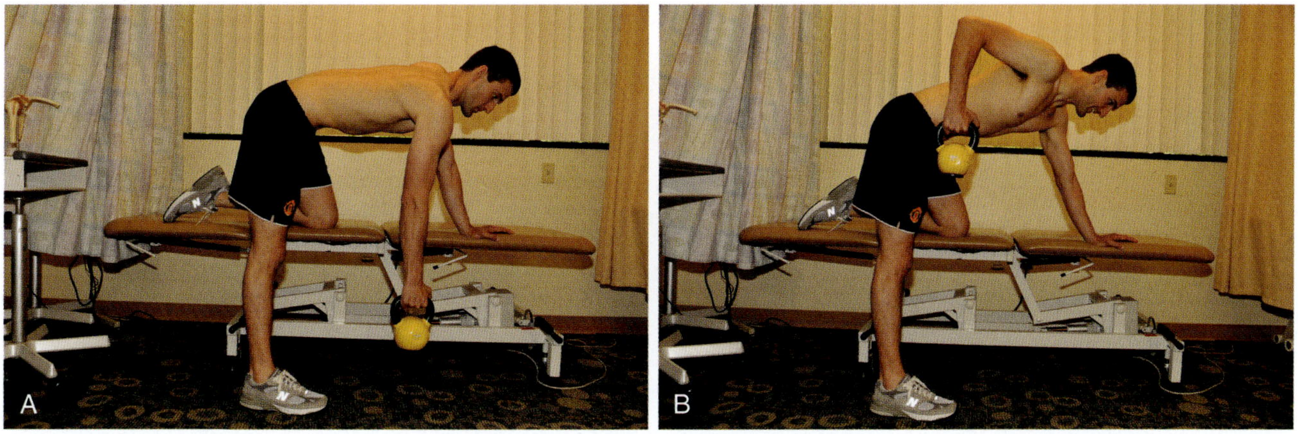

Fig. 4B.10 Bent-over row. **A,** Starting position. The patient is standing with the unaffected side upper and lower extremities supported on a flat surface with the hips flexed to 90 degrees and neutral spinal alignment with the affected upper extremity reaching to the floor while holding a weight. **B,** Ending position. The patient performs shoulder extension and elbow flexion until the shoulder is in approximately 30 degrees of extension.

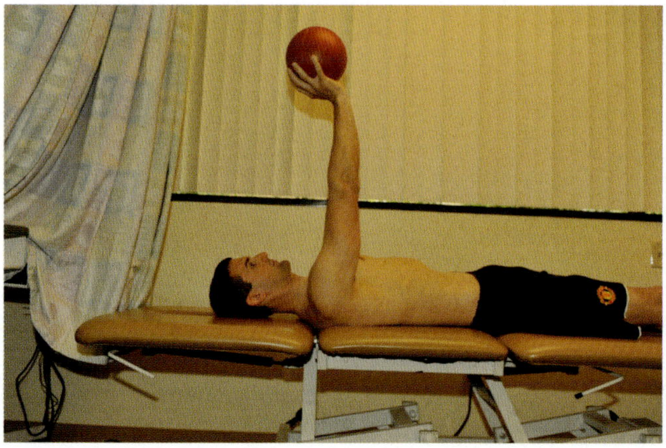

Fig. 4B.11 Supine serratus punch. Lying supine, the patient holds a weight in the hand with the arm outstretched to 90 degrees of flexion. The patient is instructed to keep the wrist and elbow locked straight while she or he punches the weight toward the ceiling by performing scapular protraction.

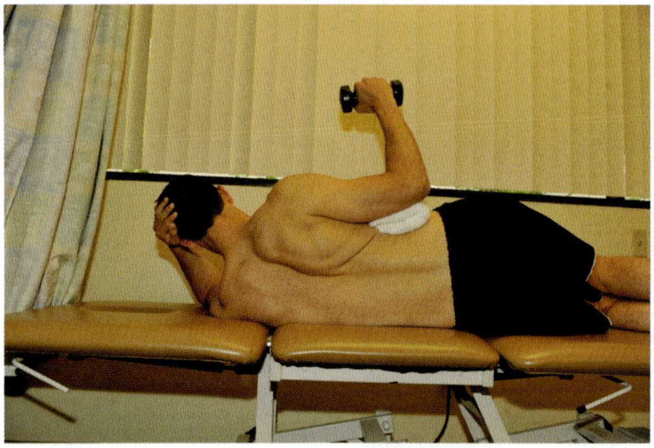

Fig. 4B.12 Sidelying external rotation with resistance. The patient is sidelying with the affected elbow supported on a towel roll to facilitate neutral glenohumeral abduction. The arm should rest on the abdomen while holding a weight. The patient is instructed to maintain scapular position while rotating the arm into approximately 45 degrees of external rotation.

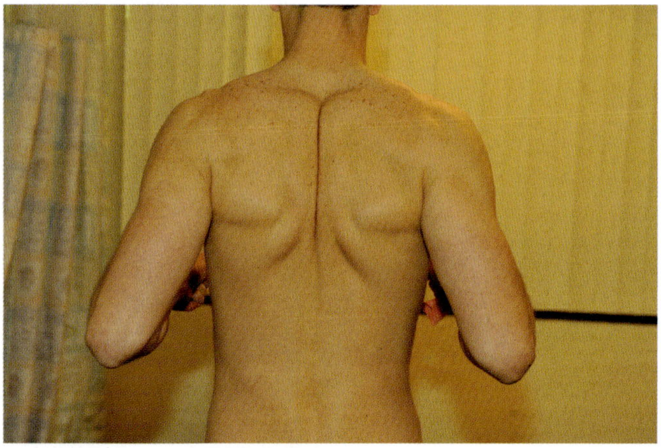

Fig. 4B.13 Scapular squeeze with resistance. The patient is instructed to hold a resistance band with the wrists in neutral pronation/supination (thumbs up) and perform light external rotation with both upper extremities while performing bilateral scapular adduction at the same time. The end position should be held for 10 to 15 seconds for each repetition to maximize the isometric contraction of the external rotator muscles.

scapulohumeral and scapulothoracic mechanics, exercises can progress to the early stages of plyometric and proprioceptive training over the next 4 weeks throughout phase 5. Total body strengthening continues combined with cardiovascular fitness activities, which can progress to an elliptical machine, upper body ergometer (UBE), VersaClimber, rowing machine, and jogging in a controlled setting. ROM should be full by this time; however, manual therapy techniques are continued to ensure adequate capsular mobility and continued stretching of the pectoralis muscles as well as latissimus dorsi and subscapularis. Gentle posterior capsule stretching may also be implemented after clearance by the surgeon via cross chest stretching or sidelying "sleeper stretch" because there is a delicate balance between flexibility and capsular stiffness to allow for optimal glenohumeral centering. This maneuver must be used with caution especially in postoperative rehabilitation of posterior instability patients.

Phase 6: Weeks 17 to 24

The final phase of postoperative rehabilitation encompasses the continued remodeling, maturation, and hypertrophic phases of tissue healing and usually begins approximately 4 months postoperatively and may continue into the first year after surgery. The athlete may begin the onset of sport-specific activities while still guarding against end range stresses in direction of the repair because it may take 12 months or longer for full scar formation and remodeling to occur. Continued progression of proprioceptive exercises and weight-bearing activities are encouraged to further ensure motor control and joint kinesthesia. Because of the chronicity of most shoulder instability complaints and the likelihood of preoperative faulty scapular movement patterns, continued neuromuscular reeducation is a key component in the prevention of future episodes of capsular instability (Figs. 4B.14 to 4B.16) (Schmidt et al, 2015). Thorough

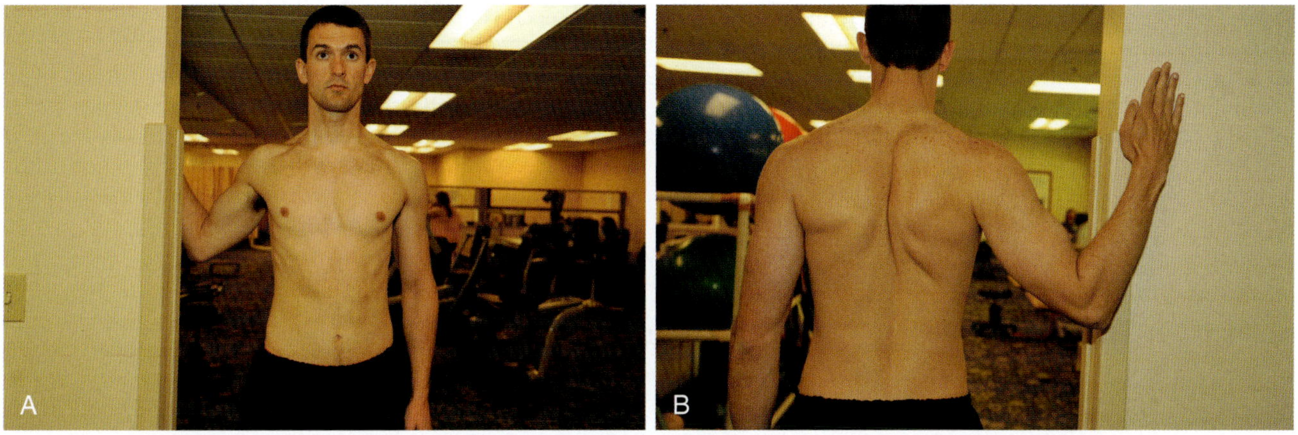

Fig. 4B.14 **A** and **B,** Pectoralis minor doorway stretch. The patient places the affected arm between 60 and 90 degrees of scaption against a doorframe or corner of the wall with palm flat. The patient is instructed to gently turn the trunk away from the arm until he or she feels a gentle stretch across the axilla. This stretch is progressed with the arm placed higher on the wall to a maximum of 120 degrees as pain ranges allow.

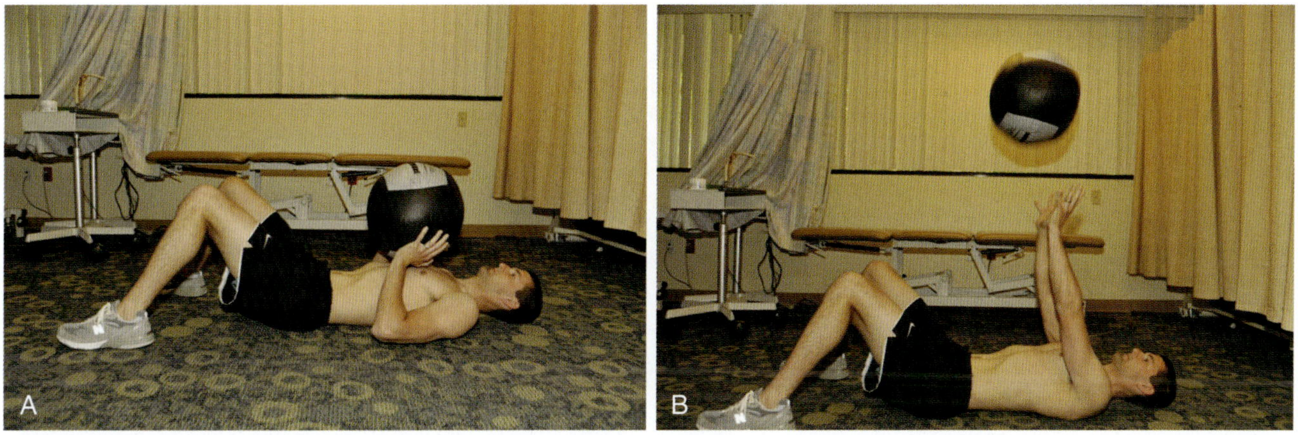

Fig. 4B.15 **A** and **B,** Dynamic medicine ball toss supine. The patient is supine holding a weighted medicine ball and instructed to perform a chest pass with active scapular protraction followed by catching the medicine ball and returning to the start position.

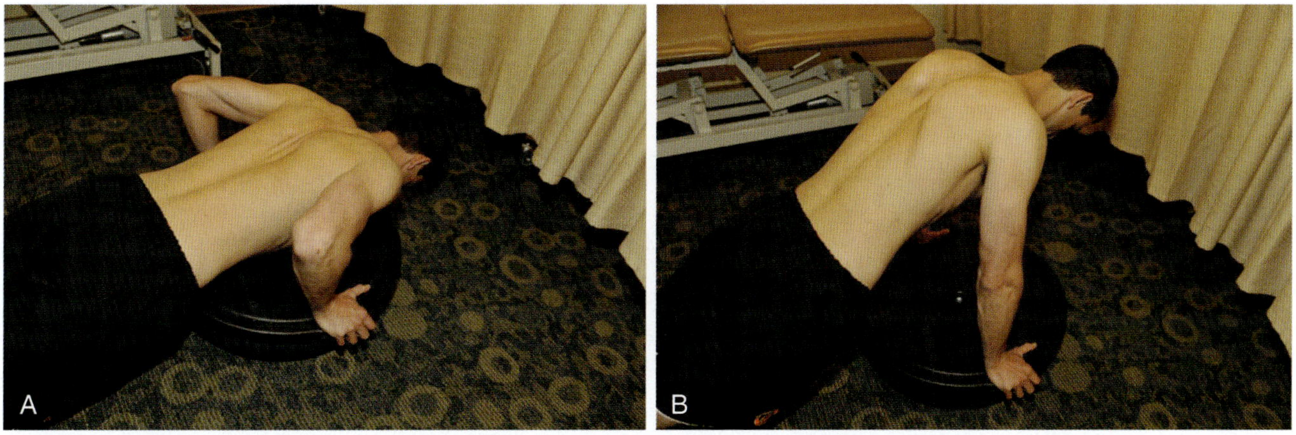

Fig. 4B.16 Closed-chain dynamic stability. Using an unstable surface, the patient is instructed to perform various activities, including the starting position of a push-up (**A**) and the end position of a push-up (**B**). The patient can also perform dynamic proprioceptive activities with rocking, circumduction, and plank activities.

communication with the sports medicine team is another key component during the transition from supervised rehabilitation to return to sport so that the strength training and athletic training providers are fully aware of the full scope of surgery performed to best design an appropriate periodized strength progression as the athlete transitions back to full team activities while minimizing the risk of repair failure.

Rehabilitation Guidelines

Tables 4B.1 and 4B.2 outline the suggested ROM precautions and postoperative rehabilitation guidelines for both posterior stabilization and MDI. These protocols are general in nature, and the clinician should alter them according to the patient's surgical procedure, affected structures, and any other complicating factors.

Table 4B.2 Postoperative Guidelines for Posterior Shoulder Instability and Multidirectional Shoulder Instability

	Posterior Instability	Multidirectional Instability
PHASE 1: WEEKS 0–2 (INFLAMMATORY PHASE)		
Precautions	▪ PROM only ▪ Flexion 30 degrees ▪ Abduction 90 degrees ▪ Scaption 90 degrees ▪ ER 30 degrees ▪ IR 0 degrees ▪ Adduction 0 degrees ▪ Abduction pillow sling at all times (including sleep) with arm in slight abduction and neutral rotation	▪ PROM via Codman exercises only ▪ Abduction pillow sling at all times (including sleep) ▪ No active biceps contraction (shoulder or elbow flexion)
Manual therapy	▪ PROM shoulder within precautions ▪ PROM scapula ▪ PROM elbow, wrist, and hand ▪ STM periscapular and cervical muscles ▪ Compression (Halder et al, 2001)	▪ PROM scapula ▪ PROM elbow, wrist, and hand ▪ STM periscapular and cervical muscles ▪ Compression
Therapeutic exercises	▪ Hand gripping exercises, active elbow and wrist flexion/extension ROM ▪ Codman/pendulums PASSIVE only ▪ Postural correction education ▪ Scapular joint position sense (use mirror)	▪ Hand gripping exercises, active wrist flexion/extension ROM ▪ Codman/pendulums PASSIVE only ▪ Postural correction education ▪ Scapular joint position sense (use mirror)
Modalities	▪ IFC estim for pain PRN ▪ Ice 10 minutes every hour as necessary ▪ High-volt estim for edema control ▪ Vasocompression/cryotherapy unit	▪ IFC estim for pain PRN ▪ Ice 10 minutes every hour as necessary ▪ High-volt estim for edema control ▪ Vasocompression/cryotherapy unit
PHASE 2: WEEKS 3–4 (INFLAMMATORY AND PROLIFERATIVE PHASE)		
Precautions	▪ Flexion 90 degrees ▪ Abduction 100 degrees ▪ Scaption 120 degrees ▪ ER 30 degrees ▪ IR 0 degrees ▪ Adduction 0 degrees ▪ Abduction pillow sling at all times (including sleep) with arm in slight abduction and neutral rotation	▪ Flexion 90 degrees ▪ Abduction 90 degrees ▪ Scaption 90 degrees ▪ ER 30 degrees in neutral abduction ▪ IR 20 degrees at 30 degrees abduction ▪ No active biceps contraction (active shoulder or elbow flexion) ▪ Abduction pillow sling at all times (including sleep)
Manual therapy	▪ PROM shoulder within precautions ▪ PROM scapula ▪ STM periscapular and cervical muscles ▪ Scapular PNF patterns ▪ GHJ centering and compression ▪ Glenohumeral joint position sense (Dover et al, 2003, Ulkar et al, 2004)	▪ PROM shoulder within precautions ▪ PROM scapula ▪ PROM elbow flexion, extension, supination, and pronation ▪ STM periscapular and cervical muscles ▪ Scapular PNF patterns ▪ Glenohumeral joint centering and compression ▪ Glenohumeral joint position sense
Therapeutic exercises	▪ Hand gripping exercises, active elbow and wrist flexion/extension ROM ▪ Codman/pendulums ▪ Postural correction education ▪ Cardiovascular activity 30 min/day stationary bike or walking on level ground ▪ Table slides abduction/flexion ▪ Gentle isometrics for ER/IR modified scapular plane ▪ AROM elbow flexion, extension, supination, and pronation ▪ Active trunk rotation ▪ Ipsilateral levator and upper trapezius stretching ▪ Seated scapular retraction/depression (scapular clocks) and scapular dumps ▪ Passive joint position sense	▪ Hand gripping exercises, active wrist flexion/extension ROM ▪ Codman/pendulums ▪ Postural correction education ▪ Cardiovascular activity 30 min/day stationary bike or walking on level ground ▪ Table slides abduction/flexion ▪ Gentle isometrics for ER/abduction/extension ▪ Active trunk rotation ▪ Ipsilateral levator and upper trapezius stretching ▪ Seated scapular retraction/depression ▪ Passive joint position sense

Table 4B.2 Postoperative Guidelines for Posterior Shoulder Instability and Multidirectional Shoulder Instability—cont'd

	Posterior Instability	Multidirectional Instability
Modalities	▪ IFC estim for pain PRN ▪ Ice 10 minutes every hour as necessary ▪ High-volt estim for edema control ▪ Vasocompression/cryotherapy unit	▪ IFC estim for pain PRN ▪ Ice 10 minutes every hour as necessary ▪ High-volt estim for edema control ▪ Vasocompression/cryotherapy unit
PHASE 3: WEEKS 5–8 (EARLY REMODELING PHASE)		
Precautions	▪ Flexion 120 degrees ▪ Abduction 120 degrees ▪ Scaption 140 degrees ▪ ER 45 degrees ▪ IR 0 degrees ▪ Progress to full PROM week 7 ▪ May discontinue sling at 6 weeks (if labral repair was performed without involvement of the rotator cuff or biceps tendon may discontinue at 4–5 weeks)	▪ Flexion 120 degrees ▪ Abduction 120 degrees ▪ Scaption 120 degrees ▪ ER 45 degrees ▪ IR 30 degrees ▪ Progress to full PROM week 7 ▪ No biceps strengthening until week 7 ▪ May discontinue sling at 6 weeks

Manual therapy	▪ Glenohumeral PROM all planes
	▪ Scapular PROM/mobilizations
	▪ Scapular PNF patterns
	▪ STM to pectoralis, latissimus, cervical, and periscapular muscles
	▪ ***Progress at 7 weeks to include:***
	  ▫ Manual PROM to full flexion/abduction and ER/IR at 45 degrees abduction
	  ▫ Glenohumeral mobs inferior and anterior capsule
	  ▫ Stretching of pectoralis and latissimus
		▪ Glenohumeral PROM all planes
		▪ Scapular PROM/mobilizations
		▪ Scapular PNF patterns
		▪ STM to pectoralis, latissimus, cervical, and periscapular muscles
		▪ ***Progress at 7 weeks to include:***
		  ▫ Manual PROM to full flexion/abduction and ER/IR at 45 degrees abduction
		  ▫ Glenohumeral mobs inferior and posterior capsule
		  ▫ Stretching of pectoralis and latissimus

Therapeutic exercises	▪ Pulleys ▪ Table slides abduction/flexion/scaption ▪ AAROM flex/abduction/ER via cane and progress to AROM, wall walks and standing two way ▪ Prone and standing scapular squeezes ▪ Prone row and prone abduction ▪ Wall slides for lower trapezius ▪ Submaximal isometrics at neutral rotation and 30 degrees abduction for flexion, abduction, ER, and extension ▪ Sidelying ER with scapular positioning and no resistance	▪ Pulleys ▪ Table slides abduction/flexion/scaption ▪ AAROM flex/abduction/ER via cane and progress to AROM, wall walks and standing two way ▪ Prone and standing scapular squeezes ▪ Prone row and prone abduction ▪ AROM elbow flexion, extension, supination, and pronation ▪ Submaximal isometrics at neutral rotation for abduction, ER, IR, and extension
Modalities	▪ Moist heat with pulleys for warm-up ▪ IFC PRN for pain ▪ Ice after PT session and HEP	▪ Moist heat for warm-up ▪ IFC PRN for pain ▪ Ice after PT session and HEP
PHASE 4: WEEKS 8–12 (REMODELING AND MATURATION PHASE)		
Precautions	▪ Avoid end-range resistance ▪ Horizontal adduction 20 degrees	▪ Avoid end-range resistance
Manual therapy	▪ As per phase 2 until full PROM achieved ▪ Rhythmic stabilization/in quadruped/PNF patterns	▪ As per phase 2 until full PROM achieved ▪ Rhythmic stabilization/in quadruped/PNF patterns
Therapeutic exercises	▪ UBE ▪ Ball on wall ▪ Prone two way (middle and lower trapezius) ▪ Standing two way (flexion and scaption) ▪ Prone row with resistance ▪ Sidelying ER with resistance as tolerated ▪ Scapular squeeze with resistance ▪ B ER with TB ▪ Seated low row ▪ IR/ER at neutral and progress to 45 degrees abduction with light resistance (may progress to 90 degrees of abduction at 10 weeks) ▪ Supine punch or standing punch (serratus anterior) ▪ Begin throwers 10 program at week 10: PNF patterns D1/D2, ER/IR at 45 degrees of abduction, scaption with IR limited to 30 degrees of abduction, seated press-ups, elbow and biceps flex, triceps extension ▪ Latissimus pull-downs in front of body ▪ Active joint position sense	▪ UBE ▪ Ball on wall ▪ Prone two way (middle and lower trapezius) ▪ Standing two way (flexion and scaption) ▪ Prone row with resistance ▪ Sidelying ER with resistance as tolerated ▪ Scapular squeeze with resistance ▪ B ER with TB ▪ Seated low row ▪ Wall slides for lower trapezius ▪ IR/ER at neutral and progress to 45 degrees of abduction with light resistance ▪ Supine punch or standing punch (serratus anterior) ▪ Begin throwers 10 program at week 10: PNF patterns D1/D2, ER/IR at 45 degrees of abduction, scaption with IR limited to 30 degrees of abduction, seated press-ups, elbow and biceps flex, triceps extension ▪ Latissimus pull-downs in front of body ▪ Sleeper stretch and cross-chest stretch ▪ Active joint position sense
Modalities	▪ Heat with UBE for warm-up ▪ Ice after PT session	▪ Heat with UBE for warm-up ▪ Ice after PT session

Continued

Table 4B.2 Postoperative Guidelines for Posterior Shoulder Instability and Multidirectional Shoulder Instability—cont'd

	Posterior Instability	Multidirectional Instability
PHASE 5: WEEKS 13–16 (MATURATION PHASE)		
Precautions	▪ None	▪ None
Manual therapy	▪ Manual capsular mobilization for full mobility ▪ Rhythmic stabilization in end ranges	▪ Manual capsular mobilization for full mobility ▪ Rhythmic stabilization in end ranges
Therapeutic exercises	▪ Throwers 10: progress resistance as tolerated ▪ May begin push-up progression ▪ Sleeper stretch and cross-chest stretch ▪ May progress ER/IR resistance to 90 degrees of abduction ▪ Begin plyometrics: shot toss and progress to shot throw and overhead toss ▪ Dynamic wall push-ups ▪ Progress push-ups to floor as tolerated	▪ Throwers 10: progress resistance as tolerated ▪ May begin push-up progression ▪ May progress ER/IR resistance to 90 degrees of abduction ▪ Begin plyometrics: shot toss and progress to shot throw and overhead toss ▪ Dynamic wall push-ups ▪ Progress push-ups to floor as tolerated
Modality	▪ Ice PRN	▪ Ice PRN
PHASE 6: WEEKS 17–24 (REMODELING, MATURATION AND HYPERTROPHIC PHASE)		
Precautions	▪ None	▪ None
Manual therapy	▪ Manual stretching/PNF/rhythmic stabilization PRN	▪ Manual stretching/PNF/rhythmic stabilization PRN
Therapeutic exercises	▪ Begin plyometrics: shot toss and progress to shot throw and overhead toss ▪ Sport-specific training ▪ Maximize cardiovascular fitness ▪ Gentle overhead motions and may progress to full overhead serve, swing, or throw at 20 weeks and full sports at 6 months	▪ Begin plyometrics: shot toss and progress to shot throw and overhead toss ▪ Dynamic wall pushups ▪ Sport-specific training exercises ▪ Throwing progression ▪ Maximize cardiovascular fitness ▪ Gentle overhead motions and may progress to full overhead serve, swing, or throw at 20 weeks and full sports at 6 months
Modality	▪ Ice PRN	▪ Ice PRN

AAROM, Active assisted range of motion; *AROM,* active range of motion; *B,* Bilateral; *ER,* external rotation; *estim,* electrical stimulation; *HEP,* Home Exercise Program; *IFC,* Interferential Current; *IR,* internal rotation; *PNF,* proprioceptive neuromuscular facilitation; *PRN,* as needed; *PROM,* passive range of motion; *PT,* physical therapy; *ROM,* range of motion; *STM,* Soft Tissue Mobilization; *UBE,* Upper Body Ergometer.

References

Cools AM, Borms D, Castelein F, Vanderstukken F, Johansson FR. Evidence-based rehabilitation of athletes with glenohumeral instability. *Knee Surg Sports Traumatol Arthrosc.* 2016;24:382–389.

De Mey K, Danneels L, Cagnie B, et al. Correction of scapular orientation in overhead athletes performing selected shoulder rehabilitation exercises: the effect on trapezius muscle activation measured by surface electromyography. *J Orthop Sports Phys Ther.* 2013;43(1):3–10.

Dover G, Kaminski T, Meister K, et al. Assessment of shoulder proprioception in the female softball athlete. *Am J Sports Med.* 2003;31(3):431–437.

Halder AM, Kuhl SG, Zobitz ME, et al. Effects of the glenoid labrum and glenohumeral abduction on stability of the shoulder joint through concavity-compression: an in vitro study. *J Bone Joint Surg Am.* 2001;83A(7):1062–1069.

Hill AM, Hoerning EJ, Brook K, et al. Collagenous microstructure of the glenoid labrum and biceps anchor. *J Anat.* 2008;212:853–862.

Gaunt BW, Shaffer MA, Sauers EL, et al. The American Society of Shoulder and Elbow Therapists' consensus rehabilitation guideline for arthroscopic anterior capsulolabral repair of the shoulder. *J Orthop Sports Phys Ther.* 2010;40(3):155–168.

Lephart S, Warner J, Borsa P, Fu F. Proprioception of the shoulder joint in healthy, unstable, and surgically repaired shoulders. *J Shoulder Elbow Surg.* 1994;3:371–380.

Merolla G, Cerciello S, Chillemi C, et al. Multidirectional instability of the shoulder: biomechanics, clinical presentation, and treatment strategies. *Eur J Orthop Surg Traumatol.* 2015;25:975–985.

Mueller MJ, Maluf KS. Tissue adaptation to physical stress: a proposed "physical stress theory" to guide physical therapist practice, education, and research. *Phy Ther.* 2002;82(4):383–403.

Mulcahey MK, Marshall M, Gallacher SE, et al. Factors expressed in an animal model of anteroinferior glenohumeral instability. *Orthop J Sports Med.* 2015;20(8). 2325967115599733.

Myers JB, Lephart SM. The role of the sensorimotor system in the athletic shoulder. *J Athl Train.* 2000;35(3):351–363.

Provencher MT, LeClere LE, King K, Frank R, et al. Current concepts: posterior instability of the shoulder diagnosis and management. *Am J Sports Med.* 2011;39(4):874–886.

Schiffern S, Rozencwaig R, Antoniou J, Richardson M, Matsen F. Anteroposterior centering of the humeral head on the glenoid in vivo. *Am J Sports Med.* 2002;30(3):382–387.

Schmidt E, Resler A, Rosenthal M, Provencher M. Postoperative rehabilitation after open or arthroscopic posterior shoulder stabilization. In: Reider B, Davies G, Provencher M, eds. *Orthopedic Rehabilitation of the Athlete.* Philadelphia: Saunders Elsevier; 2015:71–85.

Tannenbam E, Seklya J. Evaluation and management of posterior shoulder instability. *Sports Health.* 2011;3(3):253–263.

Ulkar B, Kunduracioglu B, Çetin C, Güner RS. Effect of positioning and bracing on passive position sense of shoulder joint. *Br J Sports Med.* 2004;38:549–552.

van der Meijden AO, Westgard P, Chandler Z, et al. Rehabilitation after arthroscopic rotator cuff repair: current concepts review and evidence-based guidelines. *Int J Sports Phys Ther.* 2012;7(2):197–218.

Voight ML, Thomson BC. The role of the scapula in the rehabilitation of shoulder injuries. *J Athl Train.* 2000;35(3):364–372.

4-4C RETURN TO SPORT

KEVIN E. WILK, PT, DPT, FAPTA, CHRISTOPHER A. ARRIGO, MS, PT, ATC, and
MICHAEL S. BAGWELL, PT, DPT

Introduction

- The shoulder complex has the greatest range of motion (ROM) of any joint in the human body. Because of the large quantity of motion available at the joint, it is also the most commonly dislocated joint, both in the general population and in contact sports.
- The inherent mobility of the shoulder makes returning to sport participation after a shoulder instability episode, whether it is an anterior or posterior incident, non-operative, or postoperative treatment, a challenging task for both the clinician and the athlete.
- "When can I play again?" is possibly the most frequently asked question of an athlete after any type of limiting shoulder injury. The simple answer is the patient can resume athletic activity again when he or she is ready and not before. Although this answer may sound flippant, it is in fact very true.
- Nothing is more demoralizing to an athlete and produces a more problematic setback in the rehabilitation process than developing reactive symptoms when trying to resume athletic activity before an athlete is functionally ready and capable. Additionally, the use of time as the sole determination of when an athlete may resume practice or play after a shoulder instability episode is a critical error.
- The time from the injury itself is not the primary element that will determine readiness to return to practice or competition. This has been well documented at the knee joint after anterior cruciate ligament (ACL) injury in athletes. Myer et al (2012) documented no association between time from surgery to return to play after ACL reconstruction. In addition, Hartigan et al (2013) reported no specific time frame returning to sport in ACL-deficient knee patients; rather, it was based on neuromuscular performance.
- We advocate for the use of objective criteria, patient-reported confidence, and the successful performance of specific tests to determine when an athlete is ready to begin practice and return to participation. Using specific criteria to progress an athlete through the rehabilitation course assists in guiding the process and in progressing the athlete only when he or she is physically capable of advancement rather than based solely on an arbitrary timeframe.
- The purpose of this chapter is to review the current literature on the return-to-play criteria that is currently available. In addition, we will discuss the tests the authors prefer to use. Although in the current literature more than 500 articles have been written on return-to-play guidelines, criteria, and suggestions after knee injuries, few articles have addressed return to play after shoulder instability. Our goal is to provide some useful information for clinicians.

Review of Literature

Alentorn-Geli et al (2016) looked at return to sports after arthroscopic capsulolabral repair of anterior shoulder instability in soccer players with a minimum 5-year follow-up. Participants in their study had shoulder instability during soccer play and had not responded to conservative treatment. They underwent primary capsulolabral repair with knotless anchors with the absence of a glenoid or tuberosity fracture. Fifty-seven male soccer players participated;, 80% had Bankart lesions, 20% had labroligamentous periosteal sleeve avulsion, and 100% had a Hill-Sachs lesion. Five had a type 1 SLAP (superior labrum anterior and posterior) lesion, which were not surgically repaired. The participants underwent a standardized 12+ week rehabilitation program that discontinued when complete pain-free ROM and 80% or greater strength (strength of what muscles and how was it measured) compared with the contralateral side was achieved in which return to sport was allowed. The authors report that 49 players (86%) were able to return to soccer, and 36 players (73%) were able to return at the same preinjury level. Of those who did not return, the main reasons were knee injuries (2 players), changes in personal life (2 players), and job-related reasons (3 players). Nobody quit playing because of shoulder injury. The authors report that there was, however, a total of 6 (10.5%) redislocations, but all of these were of traumatic origin postoperatively (Alentom-Geli et al, 2016).

Witney-Lagen et al (2016) looked at 50 (32 males and 18 females) patients who underwent arthroscopic plication for multidirectional instability. All patients had symptomatic subluxations or dislocations that reduced spontaneously. All had not responded to 6 months to 5 years of physical therapy, shoulder laxity as defined by a positive sulcus sign, and external rotation of 90 or greater with the arm in neutral as well as positive drawer tests in two or more directions during examination under anesthesia. No radiographic abnormalities were identified. Patients were excluded if they had labral lesions, voluntary dislocators, or were younger than 16 years of age. A single surgeon performed anterior-inferior capsular placation. All patients underwent specialized physical therapy for 4 to 6 weeks. Patients regained appropriate ROM around 3 months postoperatively in which return to noncontact sport was allowed. Return to contact sport was allowed at the 6-month mark. The primary outcome measures used were the Oxford Instability scores compared pre- and postoperatively. Patients were monitored for a minimum of 2 years (average, 5.1 years). Of the 50 patients, 45 returned to the same level of sport, 2 returned to a reduced level of sport, and 3 were unable to return to any sport. Of the 2 who returned to a reduced level, 1 was a judo player, and the other was a patient who was unable to lift very heavy weight overhead. Two rugby players and 1 cricket player did not return to sport because of apprehension (Witney-Lagen et al, 2016).

Using specific tests and predetermined criteria takes the subjective element out of athlete progression and provides everyone involved in the process with known, preestablished, measurable markers and goals that must be achieved before progressing to practice and returning to competition. An objective format serves both to motivate the athlete and to eliminate as much of the guesswork as possible out of answering the question of, "When can I play again?" In addition, athlete-patient psychological feedback is necessary as well. The patient must return to sport without the fear of reinjury, fear that the shoulder is not ready, or apprehension. This has been well reported in the knee literature after ACL injury and surgery (Ardern et al, 2011, 2016).

Table 4C.1 3P Program: Performance, Practice, and Play

Component	Description
P1: Performance training	Restoration of function through sport-specific training for athletes returning to competition
P2: Practice participation	Gradual progression of participation via sequentially increasing the time, intensity, and repetitions performed by the athlete during practice.
P3: Play	After the successful advancement through a controlled practice progression, the athlete is evaluated for readiness to resume competition in game situations at 100% effort

RETURN TO PARTICIPATION CRITERIA

1. Appropriate time from injury or surgery for healing
2. Successful completion of a formal rehabilitation program
3. Full sport-specific nonpainful ROM
4. Excellent stability with no pain during special tests
5. Strength that meets specific participation criteria
6. Satisfactory functional scoring
7. Patient-reported subjective score.

ROM, Range of motion.

Return to Participation Process and Criteria

The transition from rehabilitation back into play after an episode of shoulder instability follows three sequential steps. The first is a return to high-level performance rehabilitation and training. The second step is the resumption of participation in practice that sequentially progresses from limited, controlled activity to unrestricted practice. Finally, the third step is a return to unrestricted participation and competitive play. We refer to this program as the 3 P program: performance, practice, and play (Table 4C.1). The first two steps must be successfully accomplished before the athlete attempts any level of unrestricted play.

P1: Performance training: The last step in the sequential progression of shoulder instability rehabilitation involves the restoration of function through sport-specific training for athletes returning to competition. This must include the ability to successfully and asymptomatically perform sport-specific drills including plyometrics, agility drills, end-range proprioceptive exercises, and perturbation drills. These drills differ by sport and activity but should mimic the activity demands and nature of the sport in a progressive and sequential manner. During this mode of training, the specific movement patterns required for asymptomatic shoulder function are learned and integrated. A progression of challenges is provided in a controlled setting that focuses on achieving and maintaining end-range stability during challenging athletic activities similar to those encountered during competition.

P2: Practice participation: Next an athlete advances from the performance training phase of rehabilitation into controlled participation in a practice setting. This process involves the gradual progression of participation via sequentially increasing the time, intensity, and repetitions performed by the athlete during practice. This progression begins at lower intensities and gradually increases from 50% to 60% up to a 75% level, advancing to 80% to 90% and finally 100% effort and exertion. When 100% intensity and effort is obtained in practice, the athlete should be advanced to a practice game or scrimmage activities. In addition, in this practice phase, exposure time is also controlled to gradually improve endurance, In baseball, the pitcher would be on a pitch count. In football, the player will be on a play count- or time-monitored program.

P3: Play: After the successful advancement through a controlled practice progression, the athlete is evaluated for readiness to resume competition in game situations at 100% effort.

Successfully advancing functional activity beyond performance training back into participation in practice and then competitive play requires more than just a decision based on how the athlete says her or his shoulder feels. The complex nature of progressing an athlete back into unrestricted participation after any shoulder instability episode requires assessing and measuring the key functional elements necessary for symptom-free athletic performance of the shoulder and upper extremity. The athlete must also demonstrate sufficient confidence in the affected extremity to successfully return to sport without any fears or limitations. The criteria we evaluate to assist in determining when an athlete can return to practice and then unrestricted competition include (1) appropriate time from injury or surgery for healing, (2) successful completion of a formal rehabilitation program, (3) full sport-specific nonpainful ROM, (4) excellent stability with no pain during special tests, (5) strength that meets specific participation criteria, (6) satisfactory functional scoring, and (7) patient-reported subjective score (see Table 4C.1).

We incorporate a battery of tests designed to determine activity readiness before the introduction of demanding functional athletic practice or competitive participation to reduce the risk of reinjury or contralateral injury as well as promote psychological confidence in the involved shoulder. This program rank orders the relative demand of functional activities required for athletic participation and guides advancement back to unlimited activity via defined criteria to determine readiness for resuming practice and then unrestricted participation after shoulder injury. The tests performed and criteria used to progress an athlete back to participation in practice and then competition are outlined in Table 4C.2.

Table 4C.2 Shoulder Instability Performance Progression Assessment Testing

Name: _______________ Date: ____________
____
____

Right left bilateral injury/procedure: ________________________________
____

Evaluation for clearance to begin: Practice participation Competition

1. WOSI shoulder evaluation form: Score_____ Pass_____ Fail_____
2. Full sport-specific ROM: Pass_____ Fail_____
3. Satisfactory clinical examination: Pass_____ Fail_____
4. Ball drop test: Score ____ Pass_____ Fail_____
5. Push-up test: Score ____ Pass_____ Fail_____
6. CKCUEST: Score ____ Pass_____ Fail_____
7. Bench press assessment: Score ____ Pass_____ Fail_____
8. Unilateral pulling assessment: Score ____ Pass_____ Fail_____
9. Unilateral pushing assessment: Score_____ Pass_____ Fail_____
10. Isokinetic testing (or handheld dynamometer): Pass_____ Fail_____

Test summary: Pass Fail

Rationale for failure:

CRITERIA TO BEGIN PARTICIPATION IN PRACTICE

- WOSI shoulder score of ≥ 90
- Full, nonpainful PROM
- Satisfactory clinical examination without positive findings or apprehension
- Ball drop test: 90% involved to uninvolved
- Push-up test: Ability to perform more repetitions in second testing bout
- CKCUEST ≥21 repetitions
- Bench press ≥ 75% of preinjury 1RM without substitution
- Unilateral pulling assessment
- Unilateral pushing assessment
- Isokinetic test that fulfills criteria

CLEARANCE CRITERIA FOR RETURN TO SPORT

- WOSI shoulder score of ≥95
- Full, nonpainful PROM
- Satisfactory clinical examination without positive findings or apprehension
- Ball drop test: 100% involved to uninvolved
- Push-up test: Ability to perform more repetitions in second testing bout
- CKCUEST ≥25 repetitions
- Bench press ≥95% of preinjury 1RM without substitution
- Unilateral pulling assessment
- Unilateral pushing assessment
- Isokinetic test that fulfills criteria

ISOKINETIC TEST CRITERIA

External rotator peak torque/BW ratio 180 degrees/sec: 18%–23%
Internal rotator peak torque/BW ratio 180 degrees /sec: 26%–32%
ER-to-IR ratios 180 degrees/sec: 72%–76%
Bilateral comparison: ER 95%–100%, IR 100%–1100%
No pain during test

CKCUEST, Closed Kinetic Chain Upper Extremity Stability Test; *ER,* external rotation; *1RM,* one repetition maximum; *IR,* internal rotation; *PROM,* passive range of motion; *ROM,* range of motion; *WOSI,* Western Ontario Shoulder Instability Index.

OUTCOMES TOOL

The American Shoulder and Elbow Surgeons (ASES) Shoulder Score assessment tool is administered to assist in determining the athlete's self-assessment of the functional status and confidence in his or her shoulder (Table 4C.3). The patient's self-reporting scoring can be performed with one of these two self-assessment forms. Kirkley et al (1998) developed the Western Ontario Shoulder Instability Index (WOSI). It includes 21 questions that evaluate the physical and psychological components of the patient's recovery (Table 4C.4). Alberta et al (2010) developed the self-assessment for overhead athletes. This evaluation form is beneficial for overhead athletes who have been treated for shoulder instability.

Table 4C.3 Patient's Subjective Scoring

How does your shoulder feel?

0__________25%______50%______________75%____________100%

Feels terrible	Feels OK	Feels perfect
▪ Does your shoulder feel like it is slipping out of joint?	Yes	No (20 points)
▪ Has your shoulder popped out since the injury or surgery?	Yes	No (20 points)
▪ Do you have shoulder pain?	Yes	No (20 points)
▪ Does your shoulder ache at night?	Yes	No (20 points)
▪ Does your shoulder feel weak?	Yes	No (20 points)
▪ Are you ready to play?	Yes	No

The design and testing of the Degree of Shoulder Involvement in Sports (DOSIS) scale is a scale described by Blonna et al (2015). This scale was developed to assess athletes affected by shoulder instability. It was based on three parameters: (1) type of sport, (2) frequency with which sport is played, and (3) level at which sport is played. It was developed with 85 patients who were affected by recurrent anterior shoulder instability who underwent either a Bristow-Latarjet procedure (41 of 85) or Bankart repair (44 of 85). The average age of follow-up was 33 years old (range, 19–63 years). The scale showed good criterion validity compared with the Tegner activity scale. The test–retest reliability was found to be 0.96. The authors reported that it represented acceptable psychometric features and was a valid instrument for shoulder assessment after instability (Blonna et al, 2015).

RANGE OF MOTION

Active and passive ROM of the shoulder are evaluated to ensure that the athlete exhibits full sport-specific, nonpainful, and nonapprehensive ROM of the shoulder joint. Elevation, internal and external rotation in the supine 90/90 position, and horizontal abduction and adduction are all assessed. Along with full nonpainful ROM, the athlete should present with a normal clinical examination. No pain, tenderness, apprehension, or other abnormal findings should be evident, particularly in the assessment of provocative instability signs. In patients who have experienced episodes of instability, it is important to evaluate apprehensiveness with passive ROM.

BALL DROP TEST

We have developed a specific test to evaluate endurance, willingness to move quickly, and dynamic stability. It is called the ball drop test. It is performed in the prone position using a 2-lb weighted ball with the arm being tested completely off the plinth as a measure of dynamic stability of the shoulder (Fig. 4C.1). The test is performed for a bout of 30 seconds counting the number of releases and catches, and then involved and uninvolved sides are compared for a performance percentage. We have determined a satisfactory score of 110% or greater on the dominant extremity.

PUSH-UP TEST

A push-up test is performed as a measure of muscular endurance of the upper body and shoulder complex. The test is performed in a standard push-up position measuring the number of correct form push-ups an athlete can perform down to one fist distance off the floor in 60 seconds. Two bouts of the test are performed with 1 minute of rest in between. There is an expectation that the athlete will be able to perform a greater number of push-ups during the second bout of the examination (Department of the Army, 2009).

CLOSED KINETIC CHAIN UPPER EXTREMITY STABILITY TEST

The Closed Kinetic Chain Upper Extremity Stability Test (CKCUEST) is administered as a measure of upper quarter stability, agility, and power (Fig. 4C.2) The test is performed in a push-up position with the hands placed 36

Table 4C.4 Western Ontario Shoulder Instability Index (WOSI)

Date: ____________

Clinician's name: ______________ Patient's name: ______________

The following questions concern the symptoms you have experienced because of your shoulder problem. In all cases, please record the amount of the symptom you have experienced in the past week on the scale provided. (Please place a mark at the appropriate part on the line.)

1. How much pain do you experience in your shoulder with overhead activities?

   0 25 50 75 100

   ----

2. How much aching or throbbing do you experience in your shoulder?

   0 25 50 75 100

   ----

3. How much weakness or lack of strength do you experience in your shoulder?

   0 25 50 75 100

   ----

4. How much fatigue or lack of stamina do you experience in your shoulder?

   0 25 50 75 100

   ----

5. How much clicking, cracking, or snapping do you experience in your shoulder?

   0 25 50 75 100

   ----

6. How much stiffness do you experience in your shoulder?

   0 25 50 75 100

   ----

7. How much discomfort do you experience in your neck muscles as a result of your shoulder?

   0 25 50 75 100

   ----

8. How much feeling of instability or looseness do you experience in your shoulder?

   0 25 50 75 100

   ----

9. How much do you compensate for your shoulder with other muscles?

   0 25 50 75 100

   ----

10. How much loss of range of motion do you have in your shoulder?

    0 25 50 75 100

    ----

11. How much has your shoulder limited the amount you can participate in sports or recreational activities?

    0 25 50 75 100

    ----

12. How much has your shoulder affected your ability to perform the specific skills required for your sport or work? (If your shoulder affects both sports and work, consider the area that is most affected.)

    0 25 50 75 100

    ----

13. How much do you feel the need to protect your arm during activities?

    0 25 50 75 100

    ----

14. How much difficulty do you experience lifting heavy objects below shoulder level?

    0 25 50 75 100

    ----

15. How much fear do you have of falling on your shoulder?

    0 25 50 75 100

    ----

16. How much difficulty do you experience maintaining your desired level of fitness?

    0 25 50 75 100

    ----

17. How much difficulty do you have rough-housing or horsing around with friends?

    0 25 50 75 100

    ----

18. How much difficulty do you have sleeping because of your shoulder?

    0 25 50 75 100

    ----

19. How conscious are you of your shoulder?

    0 25 50 75 100

    ----

20. How concerned are you about your shoulder becoming worse?

    0 25 50 75 100

    ----

21. How much frustration do you feel because of your shoulder?

    0 25 50 75 100

Physical symptoms score: ___ ___%
Sports/recreation/work score: ___ ___%
Lifestyle score: ___ ___%
Emotion score: ___ ___%

The WOSI score is: ___ ___%.

inches apart on strips of athletic tape. The person reaches with alternating hands across the body to touch the piece of tape under the opposing hand. The number of cross-body touches performed in 15 seconds is recorded (Goldbeck et al, 2000; Pontillo et al, 2014; Roush et al, 2007; Tucci et al, 2014).

ONE REPETITION MAXIMUM BENCH PRESS TEST

A one repetition maximum (1RM) bench press is used as an assessment of upper extremity strength. The test is evaluated for symmetrical performance without compensation, lag, or substitution. If available, preinjury 1RM maximum lift scores are used as a comparison to assist in determination of functional strength (Seo et al, 2012).

UNILATERAL MAXIMUM CHEST PRESS TEST

A unilateral maximum (1RM) chest press test can be used by the clinician using a chest press isotonic weight machine (Fig. 4C.3). The senior author of this chapter (KEW) has used this test on athletic patients with the goal being 80% or greater on the involved side compared with the uninvolved side. Although a clinically useful test, we have no data or research to validate this test method.

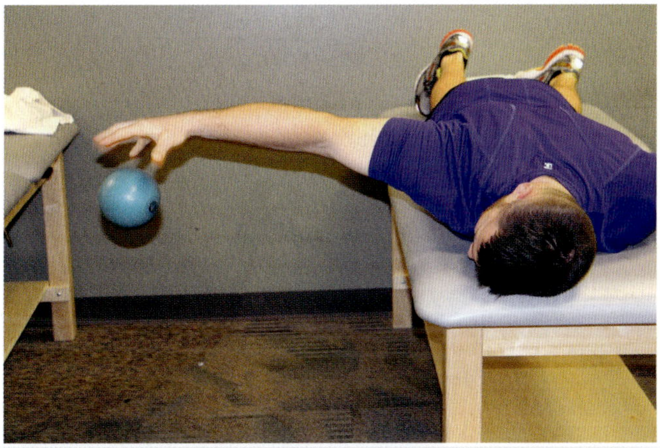

Fig. 4C.1 Ball drop test. The patient is in a prone position on the table with 2-lb plyoball in hand. The patient performs ball drops and catches for 30 seconds.

UNILATERAL PULLING ASSESSMENT

A unilateral pulling assessment using a cable machine to perform a standing pull-back is performed for 20 repetitions with each arm to assess efficiency and imbalances during pulling movements. In addition to a side-to-side strength comparison, the movement is evaluated for undesired compensations, such as arching the low back, shoulder elevation, and forward head positioning (Clark et al, 2014).

SINGLE-ARM PUSHING ASSESSMENT

Similar to the pulling assessment, a single-arm pushing assessment is performed to assess movement efficiency and imbalances during pushing activity. Again, the test is administered using a cable machine, and 20 repetitions are performed with each arm. This evaluates both the amount of weight that the athlete can use for the test and the presence of undesired movement compensations (Clark et al, 2014).

ISOKINETIC TEST AND HANDHELD DYNAMOMETER

Isokinetic testing or handheld dynamometer assessment of the shoulder internal and external rotators is also conducted to assess shoulder strength and power. It is important to evaluate specific parameters to ensure that the athlete exhibits appropriate strength and power relative to the ratio between the shoulder internal and external rotators, the ability to generate torque in relation to his or her body weight, and a pure bilateral comparison of strength. Expected values for these key parameters include ratios of external rotation (ER) to internal rotation (IR) of 72% to 76%, ER torque to body weight ratio of 18% to 23%, IR torque to body weight ratio of 26% to 32%, bilateral

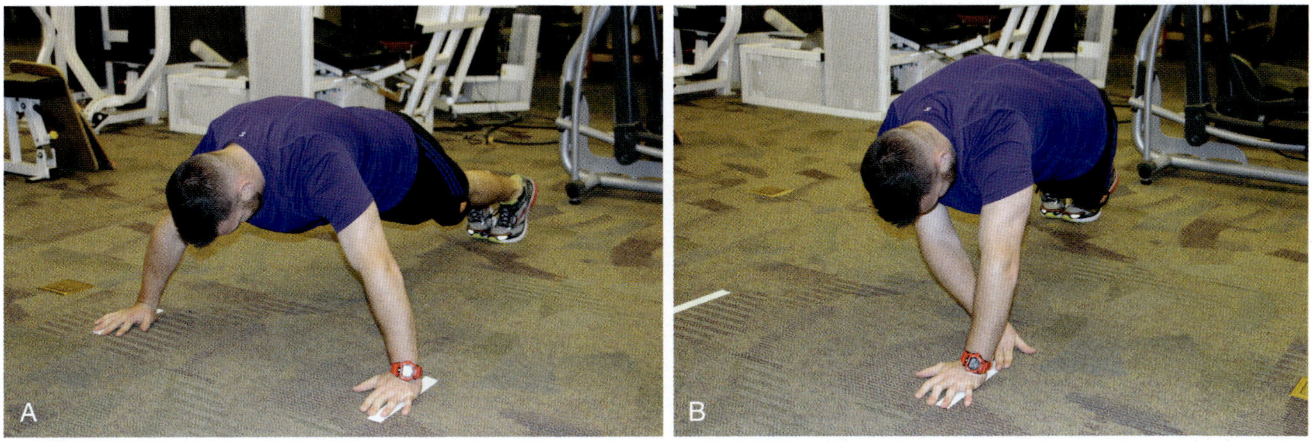

Fig. 4C.2 Closed Kinetic Chain Upper Extremity Stability Test (CKCUEST) **A,** The patient assumes the push-up position with the hands placed 36 inches apart on strips of athletic tape. **B,** The patient reaches with alternating hands across the body to touch the opposing piece of tape as many times as possible in 15 seconds.

comparison of ER of 95% to 100%, and bilateral comparison of IR of 100% to 115%.

UPPER QUADRANT Y-BALANCE TEST

The Upper Quadrant Y-Balance Test (YBT-UQ), a test similar to the Lower Quadrant Y-Balance Test (YBT-LQ) except for the upper quadrant, was first studied by Westrick et al (2012) an assessment of upper quarter closed kinetic chain performance in the rehabilitation setting. The test involves maintaining sustained unilateral stance with one upper extremity while the other reaches out in a smooth and controlled manner in the medial, superolateral, and inferolateral directions. The average distance reached based on three trials is then recorded. Westrick et al (2012) and Gorman et al (2012) have demonstrated good test–retest (Intraclass Correlation Coefficient (ICC) 0.91, 0.92, and 0.80–0.99, respectively) and interrater reliability (ICC, 1.00) as well as the establishment of normative data for active adults and young adults. Taylor et al (2016) have also documented normative data for male and female collegiate athletes.

SINGLE-ARM SEATED SHOT PUT TEST

The single-arm seated shot put test was first described in the literature as an assessment of upper body power in adolescent wrestlers in 1992 by Mayhew et al. The test uses a 6-lb ball, and the participant is seated with her or his back against the wall and the knees bent so the feet are flat on the floor. The participant is then required to push the ball from shoulder level, maintaining contact with the wall behind her or him, minimizing the use of the legs and trunk. After two practice trials, the distances of three maximal effort trials are then recorded for a successful test session, with an average distance being used as the final test value. Negrete et al (2010) have also recorded good test–retest reliability for the nondominant (ICC, 0.97) and dominant arm (ICC, 0.99) in young male and female participants within the literature. Negrete et al (2010) and Chmielewski et al (2014) document normative data in the literature for select populations, including young males and females (average age, 24.3 years) and the following collegiate sports: men's football, men's baseball, women's basketball, women's lacrosse, women's softball, and women's volleyball.

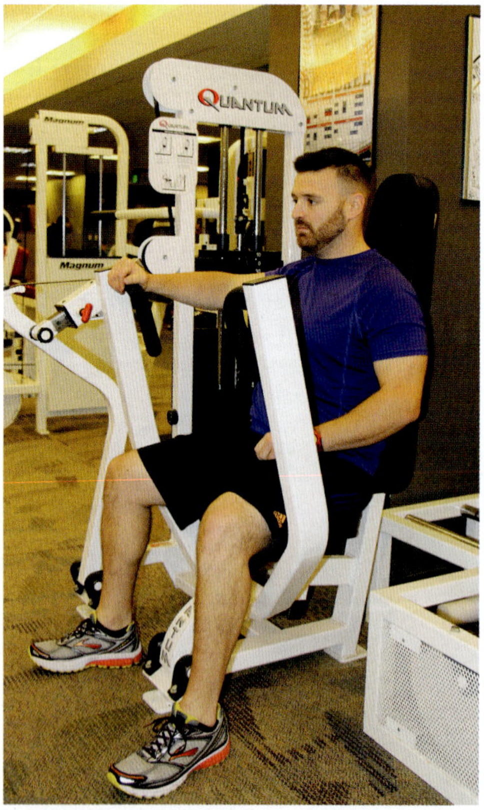

Fig. 4C.3 Unilateral seated isotonic chest press test (one repetition maximum [1 RM]. The patient is seated on an isotonic chest press machine. With one upper extremity at a time, the patient performs a unilateral press while the contralateral upper extremity is relaxed in a neutral position. The test is complete after a RM has been achieved for each upper extremity.

FUNCTIONAL THROWING PERFORMANCE INDEX

The Functional Throwing Performance Index (FTPI), a test described by Davies et al (1993), is a functional assessment of throwing athletes. The FTPI is a test that involves throwing a ball 21 inches in diameter at a target 1 square foot in size. The test requires a warm-up four submaximal throws and five maximal throws and then records three trials of the number of accurate throws within a 30-second timeframe. Davies et al (1993) also described FTPI normative data for both males (47%) and females (29%).

UPPER EXTREMITY HOP TEST

The upper extremity hop test is a test described by Falsone et al (2002). The test was designed by the University of North Carolina Sports Medicine staff. It is a test used to simulate the axial loading required in sports such as wrestling, gymnastics, and football. The test requires the patient to place one arm in weight bearing in a push-up position while the non–weight-bearing limb is placed on the lumbar spine. The patient then uses the weight-bearing extremity to hop onto the step (10.2 cm in height) and off the step five times as quickly as possible. Falsone et al documented test–retest reliability among male collegiate wrestlers (ICC, 0.81) and male collegiate football players (ICC, 0.78). Also documented within the study, Falsone et al (2002) found on average that the nondominant upper extremity performance times were 4.4% slower than the dominant. Although this was not found to be statistically significant, it may be of clinical significance.

TESTS WE USE

Numerous tests are available to clinicians to determine whether a patient is ready to return sports after a shoulder instability injury or surgery. Table 4C.2 outlines the tests we most commonly use. Each component of the testing is important, but we believe there certain components that are vital to the successful and nonrestricted return to sports. These include ROM, no apprehension, clinical stability on specific testing (drawer and fulcrum tests), appropriate strength and endurance (ball drop test), and patient's psychological response (level of confidence). The WOSI subjective scoring is an excellent and valid indicator of shoulder stability in general orthopedic patients or collision athletes.

Conclusion

This type of performance progression assessment testing provides the clinician with a useful set of tools to objectively assist and guide the determination regarding when an athlete can safely progress back to practice and then return to unrestricted athletic activities. In addition, it may provide incentive for patients who require additional strength and neuromuscular retraining. The testing battery purposely incorporates a subjective analysis, conducted by the clinician, regarding the athlete's function ability. A lack of confidence or any compensation strategies used during these tasks indicates an athlete who requires continued training and counseling before returning to unrestricted athletics.

References

Alberta FG, ElAttrache NS, Bissell S, et al. The development and validation of a functional assessment tool for the upper extremity in the overhead athlete. *Am J Sports Med.* 2010;38:903–911.

Alentorn-Geli E, Alverez-Diaz P, Doblas J, et al. Return to sports after arthroscopic capsulolabral repair using knotless suture anchors for anterior shoulder instability in soccer players: minimum 5 year follow up study. *Knee Surg Sports Traumatol.* 2016;24:440–446.

Ardern CL, Glasgow P, Schneiders A, et al. 2016 Consensus Statement on Return to Sport from the First World Congress in Sports Physical Therapy, Bern. *Br J Sports Med.* 2016;50(14):853–864.

Ardern CL, Webster KE, Taylor NF, Feller JA. Return to sport following anterior cruciate ligament reconstruction surgery: a systematic review and meta-analysis of the state of play. *Br J Sports Med.* 2011;45(7): 596–606.

Blonna D, Bellato E, Bonasia DE, et al. Design and testing of the degree of shoulder involvement in sports (DOSIS) scale. *Am J Sports Med.* 2015;43: 2423–2430.

Chmielewski TL, Martin C, Lentz TA, et al. Normalization considerations for using the unilateral seated shot put test in rehabilitation. *J Orthop Sports Phys Ther.* 2014;44(7):518–524.

Clark MA, Sutton BG, Lucett SC. *NASM Essentials of Personal Fitness Training.* 4th ed. Burlington, MA: Jones and Bartlett Learning; 2014. rev.

Davies GJ, Dickoff-Hoffman S. Neuromuscular testing and rehabilitation of the shoulder complex. *J Orthop Sports Phys Ther.* 1993;18(2): 449–458.

Department of the Army. Army Regulation 350-1, Army Training and Leader Development, Washington, DC: Headquarters, Section VI, Army Training Programs, 1-24. *Army Phys Fitness Train.* December 18, 2009:10–13.

Falsone SA, Gross MT, Guskiewicz KM, Schneider RA. One-arm hop test: reliability and effects of arm dominance. *J Orthop Sports Phys Ther.* 2002;32(3):98–103.

Goldbeck TG, Davies GJ. Test-Retest reliability of the closed kinetic chain upper extremity stability test: a clinical field test. *J Sport Rehabil.* 2000;9(1):35–46.

Gorman PP, Butler RJ, Plisky PJ, Kiesel KB. Upper quarter Y balance test: reliability and performance comparison between genders in active adults. *J Strength Cond Res.* 2012;26(11):3043–3048.

Hartigan EH, Lynch AD, Logerstedt DS, Chmielewski TL, Snyder-Mackler L. Kinesiophobia after anterior cruciate ligament rupture and reconstruction: noncopers versus potential copers. *J Orthop Sports Phys Ther.* 2013;43(11):821–832.

Kirkley A, Griffin S, McLintock H, Ng L. The development and evaluation of a disease-specific quality of life measurement tool for shoulder instability: the Western Ontario Shoulder Instability Index (WOSI). *Am J Sports Med.* 1998;26(6):764–772.

Mayhew JL, Bemben MG, Rohrs DM. Seated shot put as a measure of upper body power in adolescent wrestlers. *Pediatr Exerc Sci.* 1992;4:78–84.

Myer GD, Martin L Jr, Ford KR, et al. No association of time from surgery with functional deficits in athletes after anterior cruciate ligament reconstruction: evidence for objective return-to-sport criteria. *Am J Sports Med.* 2012;40(10):2256–2263.

Negrete RJ, Hanney WJ, Davies GJ. Reliability, minimal detectable change, and normative values for tests of upper extremity function and power. *J Strength Cond Res.* 2010;24(12):3318–3325.

Pontillo M, Spinelli BA, Sennet BJ. Prediction of in-season shoulder injury from preseason testing in Division I collegiate football players. *Sports Health.* 2014;6(6):497–503.

Roush JR, Kitamura J, Waits MC. Reference values for the closed kinetic chain upper extremity stability test (CKCUEST) for collegiate baseball players. *N Am J Sports Phys Ther.* 2007;2(3):159–163.

Seo D, Kim E, Fahs CA, Rossow L, et al. Reliability of the one-repetition maximum test based on muscle group and gender. *J Sports Sci Med.* 2012;11(2):221–225.

Taylor JB, Wright AA, Smoliga JM, DePew JT, Hegedus EJ. Upper extremity physical performance tests in collegiate athletes. *J Sport Rehabil.* 2016;25(2):146–154.

Tucci HT, Martins J, Sposito Gde C, Camarini PM, de Oliveira AS. Closed kinetic chain upper extremity stability test (CKCUES Test): a reliability study in persons with and without shoulder impingement syndrome. *BMC Musculoskel Disord.* 2014;15:1.

Westrick R, Miller JM, Carow SD, Gerber JP. Exploration of the Y-balance test for assessment of upper quarter closed kinetic chain performance. *Int J Sports Phys Ther.* 2012;7(2):139–147.

Witney-Lagen C, Hassan A, Doodson A, Venkateswaran B. Arthroscopic plication for multidirectional instability:50 patients with a minimum of 2 years of follow-up. *J Shoulder Elbow Surg.* 2016;(16):30242–30247.

SECTION **II**

Rotator Cuff Injury

SECTION OUTLINE

5 Overview

JARED THOMAS, MD; MOIN KHAN, MD, MSC, FRCSC; M. TYRRELL BURRUS, MD; and ASHEESH BEDI, MD

Introduction

- Rotator cuff tears are common in throwers and contact athletes.
- A thorough knowledge of shoulder anatomy is essential to translating patient history, physical examination, and imaging findings into a treatment plan.
- In the athletic population, the mechanism of injury and host factors are often quite different from the typical degenerative tears seen in older patients.
- Many rotator cuff tear classification systems exist, and although no one system alone can guide treatment or provide prognostic certainty, some have been shown to be useful guides when formulating a surgical plan and establishing patient expectations.

Anatomy, Epidemiology, and Pathomechanics

ANATOMY

A detailed understanding of the rotator cuff anatomy and its associated structures is required of the treating physician. Consisting of four muscle–tendon units, the rotator cuff originates from the scapula to insert on the proximal humerus. Extending from the anterior surface of the scapula, the subscapularis inserts onto the lesser tuberosity and humeral neck just medial to the long head of the biceps tendon. The subscapularis receives its innervation from both the upper and lower subscapular nerves, which arise from the posterior cord of the brachial plexus. Next, the teres minor takes its origin from the middle third of the lateral border of the scapula and inserts onto the inferior facet of the greater tuberosity of the humerus. The teres minor is innervated by a terminal branch of the brachial plexus, the posterior branch of the axillary nerve. Last, the supraspinatus and infraspinatus arise and travel along their respectively named fossae on the posterior aspect of the scapula and insert onto the greater tuberosity. The supraspinatus has been further described as having an anterior and posterior belly. The infraspinatus and supraspinatus take their nervous supply from the suprascapular nerve, which arises from the upper trunk of the brachial plexus.

The tendinous portions of these four muscles ultimately fuse with one another in addition to blending with the fibrous capsule before their final insertion onto the humerus. Intervals exist both anteriorly between the supraspinatus and subscapularis and posteriorly between the supraspinatus and infraspinatus. Referred to as the rotator interval, the more easily defined anterior interval between the supraspinatus and subscapularis contains the coracohumeral ligament, superior glenohumeral ligament, glenohumeral capsule, and biceps tendon.

The insertion of the rotator cuff and its so-called footprint have been extensively studied. Cadaveric studies have elucidated it both qualitatively and quantitatively and form the basis of anatomic repair. The insertional footprint of the supraspinatus is trapezoidal or triangular in shape with an average length between 6.9 and 23 mm and average width of 12.6 to 16 mm (Curtis et al, 2006; Minagawa et al, 1998). Normally, there is a 1.5-mm margin of exposed bone between the articular edge and the insertion of the supraspinatus. This normal or expected margin can be used to estimate the amount of detachment of articular-sided tears. The infraspinatus has a trapezoidal footprint with an average length of 10 to 29 mm and width of 19 to 32.7 mm (Fig. 5.1). Additionally, the thickness of the tendons is between 10 and 14 mm.

As mentioned previously, these two tendons are intimately intertwined by the footprint, making anatomic repair difficult without the use of an external landmark. The bare area of the humerus can be used to consistently identify the interval between the infraspinatus and supraspinatus tendons and is a useful arthroscopic landmark. Additionally, the supraspinatus and infraspinatus tendons form a crescent-shaped thickened area of tendon referred to as the rotator cable, which runs from the anterior border of the supraspinatus to the posterior border of the infraspinatus (Fig. 5.2). First described by Burkhart et al (1993), this cable protects the tendon–bone interface from the forces generated by the rotator cuff muscles. Some have hypothesized that this may also partially explain why some patients who have an intact cable are able to maintain functional strength despite the presence of a full-thickness tear (Burkhart et al, 1993; Halder et al, 2002; Mesiha et al, 2013; Oh et al, 2011); conversely, some have hypothesized that the presence of this load-sharing cable may be responsible for tear propagation (Keener et al, 2015; Kim et al, 2010).

Ultimately, understanding the anatomy of the rotator cuff and its relationship to the other structures within the shoulder girdle is paramount to successful diagnosis and treatment of rotator cuff injuries.

EPIDEMIOLOGY

Rotator cuff tear is the most common cause of presenting shoulder complaints, and its incidence increases with age. It is estimated that rotator cuff tears result in 4.5 million physician visits annually (Mather et al, 2013) with roughly 250,000 repairs performed each year (Oh et al, 2007).

Age-related degenerative rotator cuff tears are far more common than traumatic tears in the general population.

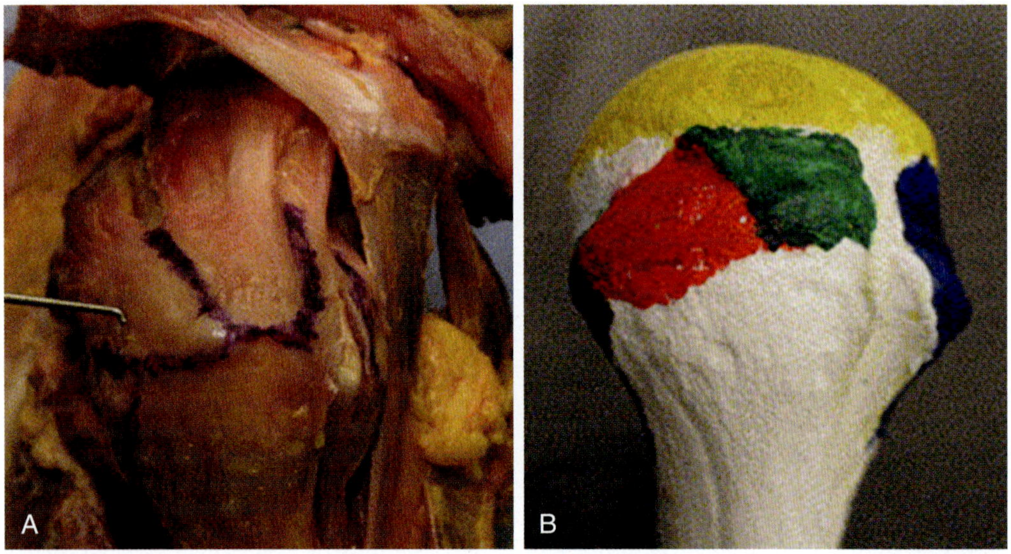

Fig. 5.1 Rotator cuff footprint. **A,** Lateral view of an intact rotator cuff with intervals marked before dissection. **B,** Model of the humeral head showing the articular surface *(yellow)* and insertional footprints of the supraspinatus *(green)* and infraspinatus *(red)*. The subscapularis footprint *(blue)* is anterior to the biceps groove and the teres minor *(black)* is posterior-inferior. (Reprinted from Curtis AS, Burbank KM, Tierney JJ, Scheller AD, Curran AR. The insertional footprint of the rotator cuff: an anatomic study. *Arthroscopy*. 2006;22(6):609e1.)

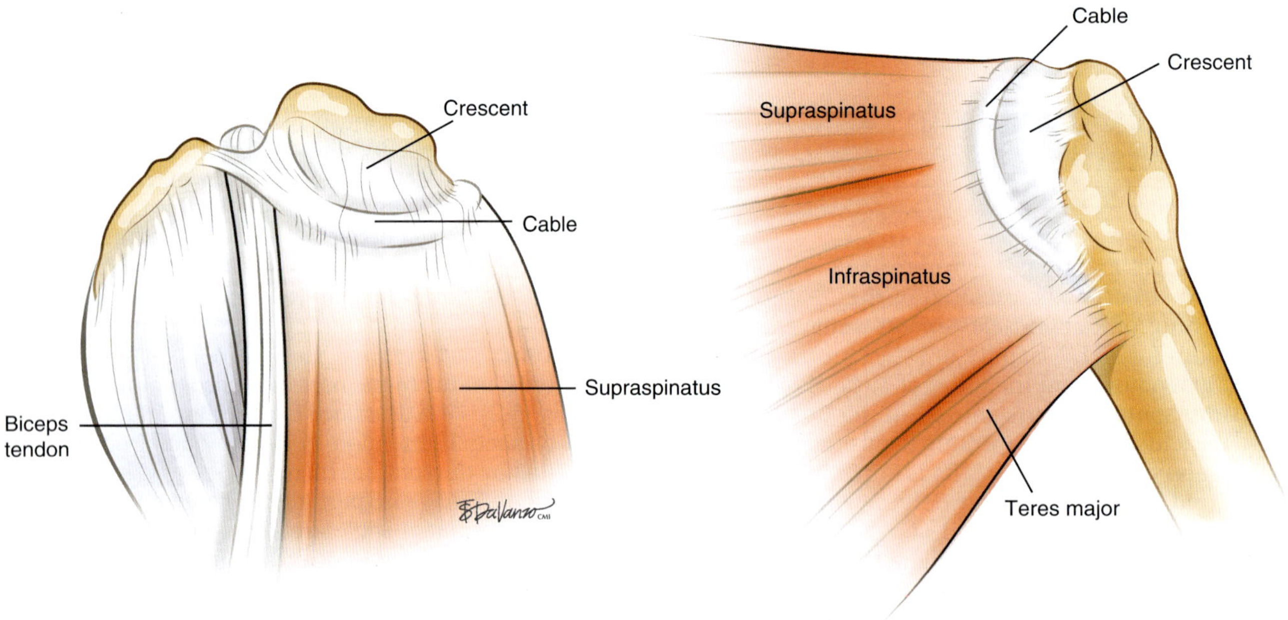

Fig. 5.2 Superior *(left)* and posterior *(right)* projections of the rotator cable and crescent. The rotator cable extends from the biceps to the inferior margin of the infraspinatus (I) tendon, spanning the supraspinatus and infraspinatus tendon insertions. Mediolateral diameter of rotator crescent; biceps tendon; width of rotator cable; teres minor. (Reprinted from Lo IK, Burkhart SS. Current concepts in arthroscopic rotator cuff repair. *Am J Sports Med.* 2003;31:308-324.)

Similarly, throwing athletes more commonly sustain degenerative tears related to overuse, but other athletes, especially contact athletes, are more likely to sustain traumatic tears during competition or training. A recent systematic review reinforced what has been previously believed, that throwers tend to develop partial-thickness articular-sided tears due to chronic overuse, but nonthrowers are more likely to suffer full-thickness tears during a single traumatic event. This same systematic review noted that studies evaluating rotator cuff tears in patients under the age of 40 years are lacking in both quality and quantity (Lazarides et al, 2015).

It is important to note that not all rotator cuff tears are symptomatic, and care should be taken to determine if the patient's symptoms correlate to imaging findings. This point is highlighted by ultrasonography, magnetic resonance imaging (MRI), and arthrography findings that have shown full-thickness tears in 4% to 13% of asymptomatic individuals 40 to 60 years old, 20% of subjects 60 to 70 years old, 31% to 50% of subjects 70 to 80 years of age, and 50% to 80% of subjects older than 80 years old. Perhaps more germane to the athlete population, it should also be noted that partial-thickness tears have been found in 4% of asymptomatic patients younger than 40 years (Minagawa et al, 2013; Moosmayer et al, 2009; Sher et al, 1995; Tempelhof et al, 1999).

PATHOMECHANICS

Although all athletes are subject to rotator cuff injury, the pathomechanics discussed in this section are most pertinent to throwing athletes. The other category of tears tends to be acute injuries caused by a single catastrophic event resulting in traumatic avulsion of the rotator cuff. The pathomechanics of rotator cuff injury in the athlete are thought to arise from three proposed mechanisms (Economopoulos & Brockmeier, 2012; Halbrecht et al, 1999; Walch et al, 1992): internal impingement, external or outlet impingement, or tensile overload.

Thought to be a common cause of partial articular-sided tears in throwers, the pathomechanics of internal impingement are described as abnormal contact of the rotator cuff, glenoid, and labrum during the throwing motion (Fig. 5.3). Because this repetitively occurs during the late cocking and acceleration phase of the overhead throwing motion, it can lead to a predictable pattern of injury involving partial articular-sided tears of the posterior portion of the supraspinatus and the superior portion of the infraspinatus in addition to posterosuperior labral injury. This initial description by Walch et al (1992) was expanded on by Burkhart et al (2003), who described a mechanism that placed posterior capsular tightness as the key pathologic change leading to the internal impingement pathway. The proposed pathomechanical cascade begins with the high and repetitive deceleration forces seen by the posterior rotator cuff and capsule. This repetitive stress leads to hypertrophy and capsular contracture that over time forces the humeral head into a less stable posterosuperior position when the arm is abducted and externally rotated. In this less stable position, the humerus is permitted to go into a position of supraphysiologic external rotation that creates increased shearing forces on the rotator cuff and labrum, thereby exacerbating the innate impingement of these structures during the normal overhead throwing motion.

Subacromial or outlet impingement is thought to be a less common cause of rotator cuff tear in throwing athletes. The pathomechanics of rotator cuff tear caused by subacromial impingement are well understood because of its suspected role in older patients with the vastly more common and well-studied degenerative rotator cuff tear. Under normal conditions, the contents of the subacromial space must pass under and through the coracoacromial arch during abduction. As the rotator cuff tendons and the subacromial bursa pass through this anatomic arch formed by the acromion, coracoacromial ligament, and coracoid process, they are subjected to impinging and shearing forces. These forces are further amplified when a thrower has rotator cuff or periscapular weakness caused by fatigue or poor training. Weakness of the rotator cuff can lead to altered throwing mechanics by allowing the deltoid to overpower the weakened or fatigued rotator cuff, disrupting normal force coupling and leading to dynamic superior migration of the humeral head. This superior migration of the humeral head further reduces the volume of the subacromial space and thereby causes further impingement on the rotator cuff tendons and bursa. Periscapular weakness can lead to scapular dyskinesia during the throwing motion, which ultimately leads to compensatory alterations in both scapular and humeral head position, further exacerbating the impinging forces on the rotator cuff. The bursa then becomes inflamed, which may alter the local environment and lead to pain and possible poor tendon tissue quality over time. The rotator cuff tendons have been shown to have altered vascular patterns in response to repetitive stress, thereby reducing the structural strength of the tendon and making it more susceptible to injury (Fukuda, 2003); this mechanism is also thought to play a prominent role in tears caused by tensile overload. Regardless of the cause of outlet impingement, during the acceleration phase of the overhead throwing motion, these forces are further amplified and thus can explain bursal-sided or rarely even full-thickness tears of the rotator cuff.

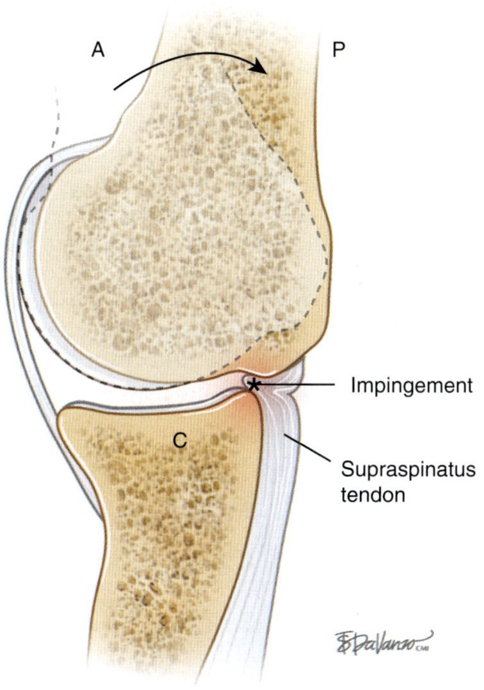

Fig. 5.3 Internal impingement. With the shoulder fully abducted and externally rotated, the posterior superior rotator cuff *(asterisk)* becomes entrapped between the greater tuberosity of the humerus and the glenoid, leading to damage to both the rotator cuff and the glenoid labrum. *A*, Anterior; *C*, glenohumeral center of rotation; *P*, posterior. (Reprinted from Burkhart SS, Morgan CD, Kibler WB. The disabled throwing shoulder: spectrum of pathology. Part I: pathoanatomy and biomechanics. *Arthroscopy*. 2003;19(4):404-420.)

Tensile overload refers to attritional degeneration and eventual tear of the rotator cuff in response to the cumulative and repetitive stresses caused by overhead throwing. Most of the injury and preceding stress placed on the rotator cuff in this setting occur during the deceleration phase of throwing, as eccentric contracture of the posterior rotator cuff attempts to slow the arm from its maximum angular velocity. As these posterior structures slow the arm, they experience considerable strain, leading to the aforementioned vascular changes, which creates the conditions for articular-sided wear and eventually partial-thickness tear.

These attritional injuries occur most commonly in the posterior portion of the supraspinatus and anterior half of the infraspinatus, as the rotator cuff maintains the humeral head within the glenoid while simultaneously slowing the arm against tremendous force. The deceleration phase is also implicated as the pathologic force in Burkhart's mechanism of internal impingement-driven rotator cuff injury in throwers previously discussed in this chapter.

Although each mechanism is described separately, it is important to recognize that significant overlap likely occurs in throwers presenting with suspected rotator cuff injury. An understanding of these mechanisms highlights the need for strength training, proper throwing mechanics, and rest for the throwing athlete so that intervention can be made proactively before significant injury occurs.

History, Physical Examination, Imaging, and Classification

HISTORY

As with any clinical encounter, a thorough history is paramount to guiding the clinician to a timely and accurate diagnosis. Questioning should be targeted at determining the acuity or chronicity of the chief complaint as well as aggravating and alleviating activities. Areas of special focus include the sport, position, level of participation, and expectations of the patient. Previous treatments as well as the patient's response should be recorded.

Throwers may present with a variety of complaints, from discomfort, decreased velocity or stamina, to a generalized ache and inability to throw. A detailed throwing history should be obtained, including any recent changes in mechanics, training program, or workload. High-level throwers can often identify the exact phase of their throwing motion where symptoms occur. Throwing or contact athletes may complain of persistent symptoms or acute onset that correlates to a traumatic event. Symptoms of rotator cuff injury are often localized to the subdeltoid region and exacerbated by activities of daily living that place the arm away from the body or overhead. Complaints of night pain are common.

Patients with acute traumatic tears often present with severe pain accompanied by profound loss of function after an identifiable inciting event. An inability to elevate the arm for days to weeks after the injury is not uncommon. A contact athlete with an acute rotator cuff tear may report a history of shoulder dislocation at the time of injury.

PHYSICAL EXAMINATION

Evaluating the rotator cuff via physical examination can be challenging because of its intimate relationship with other commonly injured structures in and about the shoulder. Common pathologies in this patient population that have significant examination findings that overlap with rotator cuff injury findings include proximal biceps tendon pathology, labral injury, acromioclavicular joint arthrosis, and symptomatic os acromiale. It should not be surprising then that many of the physical examination findings described have been reported to have modest sensitivity and even lower specificity for rotator cuff tear (Table 5.1).

Inspection

The physical examination should commence with careful inspection of the patient's undressed shoulder girdle from multiple perspectives, noting symmetry, muscular bulk and tone, swelling, bruising, scarring, and deformity. Asymmetry may be due to normal hand dominance or may be a pathologic sign of guarding or atrophy. Muscular atrophy should always be interpreted as abnormal and may be a sign of rotator cuff tear or central or peripheral nerve compression.

Palpation

The examiner should attempt to identify areas of tenderness about the shoulder girdle. Areas of interest include the acromioclavicular joint, long head of the biceps tendon–bicipital groove, deltoid, posterior capsule, and rotator cuff muscles and their insertions.

Range of Motion

Active and passive range of motion (ROM) should be assessed in all planes. Instability and apprehension can be tested as part of the passive ROM examination. Overhead athletes often exhibit increased external rotation and concomitantly decreased internal rotation as a result of adaptive changes caused by repetitive throwing; this is commonly referred to as *glenohumeral internal rotation deficit*. Normal laxity is often present in athletes such as swimmers and overhead throwers and should not be interpreted as pathologic. However, limited internal rotation may also reflect posterior capsule tightness secondary to early pathology in throwers. Deficits in active and passive ROM should be noted. Pain with active ROM within the so-called painful arc between 60 and 120 degrees of flexion in the scapular plane has been associated with

Table 5.1 Reported Sensitivities and Specificities of Physical Examination Maneuvers

Physical Examination Maneuver	Reported Sensitivity/ Specificity (%)	References
INFRASPINATUS		
External rotation lag	46–98/72–98	Miller et al, 2008 Hertel et al, 1996 Walch et al, 1998
SUPRASPINATUS		
Jobe or empty can	53–89/65–82	Park et al, 2005 Yuen et al, 2012
Drop arm	10–73/77–98	Miller et al, 2008 Park et al, 2005 Yuen et al, 2012
TERES MINOR		
Hornblower's sign	100/93	Walch et al, 1998
SUBSCAPULARIS		
Lift off/lag	17–100/60–98	Barth et al, 2006 Gerber & Krushell, 1991 Hertel et al, 1996 Miller et al, 2008 Scheibel et al, 2005
Belly press	40–43/93–98	Barth et al, 2006 Yuen et al, 2012
Bear hug	60/92	Barth et al, 2006

rotator cuff pathology. During ROM testing, it is important to observe both scapulae from behind the patient as the arm is brought through the full range of abduction and forward flexion. Care should be taken to examine for the presence of winging and abnormal or asymmetric motion concerning for scapula dyskinesia, which can be a common cause of shoulder pain in throwers and may accompany a rotator cuff injury.

Strength Testing and Special Maneuvers Specific to the Rotator Cuff

Infraspinatus. Strength of the infraspinatus is tested by resisted external shoulder rotation with the arm fully adducted and in a neutral to slightly internally rotated position. In addition to strength testing, pain may be elicited in the aforementioned position in patients with infraspinatus pathology.

External rotation lag at 0 and 90 degrees can be used to test for infraspinatus competence. To test at 0 degrees, the seated patient's back is to the physician with the elbow flexed to 90 degrees and the shoulder positioned 20 degrees in the scapular plane. While supporting the limb at the elbow, the examiner grasps the wrist and brings the shoulder to near maximal external rotation. Care should be taken not to place the patient in maximal external rotation because this will cause a false-positive result when the arm recoils; a false-positive result may also be appreciated in patients with an anterior capsular contracture, but a false-negative result may be caused by subscapularis insufficiency. The patient then attempts to maintain the position of external rotation as the examiner releases the wrist while support of the limb at the elbow is maintained. The test is considered positive when the arm falls into internal rotation. The test can be performed similarly with the arm held at 90 degrees of abduction and near maximal external rotation. Neither of these tests is thought to completely isolate the infraspinatus, and as such, sensitivity and specificity are 46% to 98% and 72% to 98%, respectively, in the literature.

Supraspinatus. Strength of the supraspinatus is tested with resisted elevation in the scapular plane with the arm held in 90 degrees of abduction and neutral rotation. As with infraspinatus testing, pain may be a sign of supraspinatus pathology even in the setting of full manual strength, and this is the basis of the Jobe or empty can maneuver.

Special maneuvers thought to be more specific for supraspinatus pathology are the Jobe (also known as "empty can") test and the drop sign. To perform the Jobe or empty can test, the arm is placed in 90 degrees of abduction and brought forward 30 degrees into the scapular plane. Internally rotating the arm rotates the thumb toward the ground, and the patient attempts to resist a downward force. Pain or weakness is interpreted as a positive test result; however, with a reported sensitivity and specificity of 53% to 89% and 65% to 82%, respectively, it should be noted that this test can also be a sign of impingement. The drop arm sign is elicited by having the patient abduct the arm past 90 degrees before slowly adducting the arm back to his or her side. The test result is considered positive if at any time the patient drops the arm to the side because of pain or weakness.

Teres minor. Strength of the teres minor is tested by having the patient externally rotate against resistance with the arm held in 90 degrees of abduction.

The hornblower sign has been shown to have high sensitivity and specificity for teres minor pathology. Originally described in the obstetrics literature in the context of birth-related brachial plexus injury and later adapted by Walch et al (1998) as a test for rotator cuff tears involving the teres minor, this special maneuver has been variously described. Ultimately, the test is used to demonstrate profound external rotation weakness with the arm held in the position of strength testing described earlier. The test result is considered positive when the patient's hand falls into internal rotation requiring abduction of the shoulder to bring hand to mouth, thereby assuming the characteristic "hornblower" position (Fig. 5.4).

Subscapularis. Subscapularis strength is tested with resisted internal rotation with the arm adducted at the side. In addition to strength testing, one physical examination finding that should raise suspicions for subscapularis tear is markedly increased external rotation compared with the contralateral side, which may be noted during ROM testing.

Several physical examination maneuvers may identify subscapularis pathology. The most commonly used special maneuvers for detecting subscapularis injury are the lift-off test, belly press test, internal rotation lag sign, and bear hug test. The lift-off test commences with the affected arm extended and internally rotated so that the dorsum of the hand comes to rest on the lumbosacral spine. The patient is then asked to lift her hand off her back; a positive test occurs when the patient is unable to lift the hand. The

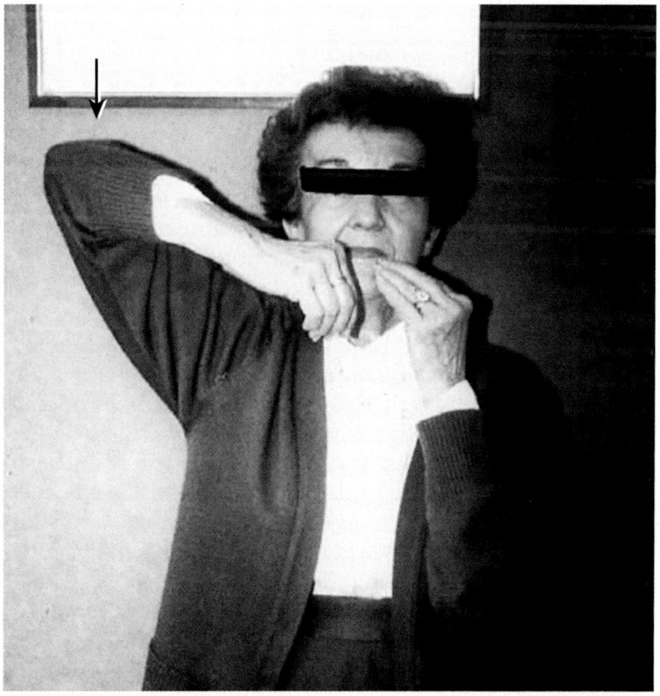

Fig. 5.4 Hornblower's sign. The patient assumes the characteristic hornblower position when asked to bring her hand to her mouth. (Reproduced with permission from Walch G, Boulahia A, Calderone S, Robinson AH. The 'dropping' and 'hornblower's' signs in evaluation of rotator-cuff tears. *J Bone Joint Surg Br*. 1998;80(4): 624-628.)

lift-off test is thought to be more specific for the inferior portion of the subscapularis. The lag sign, also referred to as the passive lift-off test, is started in an identical fashion to the lift-off test but is carried out by passively placing the patient's hand off the lumbar spine and asking the patient to maintain that position after the arm is released. The lag sign is positive when the hand falls to the back. The belly press test is performed by having the patient press the palm of the hand flat against the abdomen while maintaining internal rotation. The test result is considered positive for subscapularis pathology when the patient is unable to maintain internal rotation, causing the elbow to fall back behind the trunk. The bear hug test described by Barth et al (2006) has been shown to be a sensitive examination maneuver for detecting tear of the upper portion of the subscapularis. The patient places the palm of the affected arm flat against the contralateral shoulder and is then asked to resist the examiner as the hand is pulled off the shoulder. A positive bear hug test result is documented when the patient is either unable to keep the hand pressed against the shoulder or exhibits pain or weakness during testing.

IMAGING

Imaging of the painful shoulder in this population presents several challenges because it can be difficult to correlate imaging findings to the patient's symptoms. This is most obvious in overhead athletes because partial-thickness rotator cuff and labral tears have been reported in up to 45% of asymptomatic throwing athletes (Connor et al, 2003; Halbrecht et al, 1999; Jerosch et al, 1993; Jost et al, 2005; Miniaci et al, 2002). The clinician must keep this in mind when interpreting imaging findings and do so with the understanding that diagnostic imaging is only one component in making a diagnosis and formulating a subsequent treatment plan.

Plain Radiographs

Imaging of the painful shoulder should commence with plain radiographs, including anteroposterior (AP), true AP (Grashey), axillary lateral, and scapular Y views; an outlet view may be obtained to evaluate the shape of the acromion. Fracture or dislocation of the humerus, clavicle, and scapula should be ruled out; the presence of an os acromiale should be noted. In patients with rotator cuff tears, radiographs are typically normal, although there are a few characteristic findings that, if present, should not be missed. Although more typically associated with age-related degenerative tears of the rotator cuff, the presence of enthesophyte, cyst, or notching of the greater tuberosity has been reported in throwing athletes with articular-sided partial-thickness tears (Nakagawa et al, 2001). Additionally, cortical irregularity at the greater tuberosity has been shown in a separate study to have a sensitivity of 90% and negative predictive value of 96% for the presence of a rotator cuff tear when noted at the expected insertion site of the supraspinatus (Wohlwend et al, 1998). Other findings such as humeral head migration, calcification of the rotator cuff or bursa, or bony or soft tissue lesions concerning for malignancy are not expected in this population but should be noted.

Magnetic Resonance Imaging

Magnetic resonance imaging remains the gold standard for diagnosis of partial- and full-thickness rotator cuff tears. Noncontrast MRI is reported to have 69% sensitivity and 94% specificity with regards to the diagnosis of partial-thickness tears (de Jesus et al, 2009). MR arthrography has been reported to improve on detection of partial-thickness rotator cuff tears that involve more than 25% of the tendon by increasing sensitivity to 85% (Chun et al, 2010; de Jesus et al, 2009; Meister et al, 2004). MR arthrography with the patient's arm in abduction and extra rotation (ABER position) has been suggested and may be helpful to increase the diagnostic accuracy of articular-sided tears because it increases the distance between the rotator cuff tendons and the humeral head, enabling contrast to more effectively infiltrate the tear (Lee & Lee, 2002).

Full-thickness tears are seen as fluid extending through the tendon, and MRI can assist with assessing tear dimension, degree of tendon retraction, and associated muscular atrophy. When diagnosing full-thickness tears, MRI and MR arthrography have been demonstrated to have similar sensitivity (92%–95%) and specificity (93%–98%) (Ryu et al, 2002). In addition to being highly accurate, MRI is advantageous because it allows for imaging of the glenohumeral joint, labrum, and other surrounding structures in addition to the rotator cuff. Noted disadvantages of MRI include patient reluctance because of claustrophobia or anxiety, increased cost, decreased availability and portability, and more contraindications because of comorbidities or implanted medical devices when compared to ultrasound.

Ultrasonography

Once considered an emerging option for imaging of the rotator cuff, ultrasonography is quickly establishing itself as a fast, accurate, and cost-effective imaging modality. Ultrasonography has a reported sensitivity of 64% and specificity of 94% for detecting partial-thickness tears (de Jesus et al, 2009), although some maintain that these numbers may be lower when trying to detect articular-sided tears. The numbers are even more encouraging when using ultrasonography to detect full-thickness tears, with a reported sensitivity and specificity of 93% and 94%, respectively (de Jesus et al, 2009; Wiener & Seitz, 1993). Several studies have compared ultrasonography with MRI in diagnosing full-thickness rotator cuff tears, with more than one systematic review and accompanying meta-analysis concluding that, for the diagnosis of full-thickness rotator cuff tears, the use of ultrasonography is comparable and in many cases equivalent to MRI (de Jesus et al, 2009; Lenza et al, 2013). Ultrasonography has also been shown to reliably evaluate rotator cuff atrophy and fatty infiltration (Kavanagh et al, 2008; Khoury et al, 2008). Most experienced clinicians add the caveat that ultrasonography be performed by a skilled ultrasonographer and interpreted by a skilled physician; however, this distinction is not well defined because the reported intra- and interobserved reliabilities have varied widely in the literature, especially with regards to partial-thickness tears. Despite these promising results, in athletes, MRI is still preferred in most cases

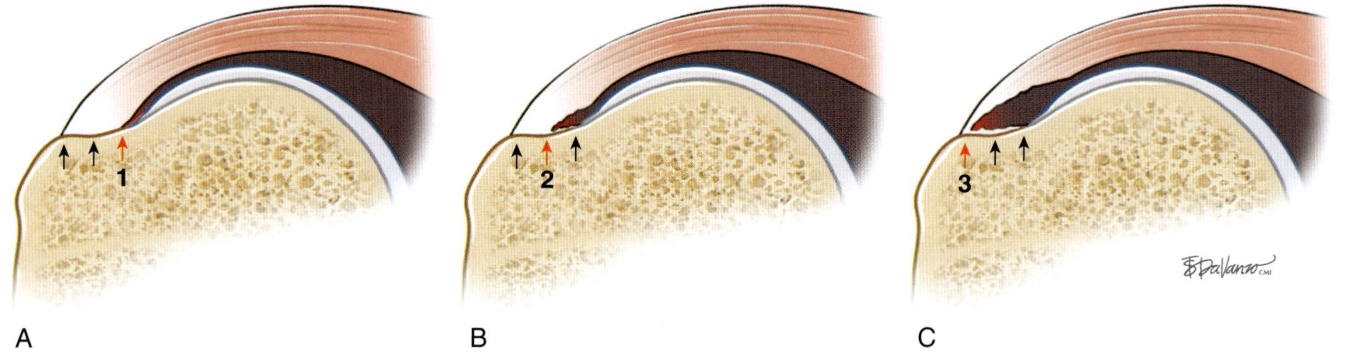

Fig. 5.5 Longitudinal extension of articular-sided supraspinatus tendon tears in coronal plane, as classified by Habermeyer et al (2008). **A,** Type 1 tear: small tear within transition zone from cartilage to bone. **B,** Type 2 tear: extension of tear to center of footprint. **C,** Type 3 tear: extension of tear to the greater tuberosity. (Reprinted from Habermeyer P, Krieter C, Tang KL, Lichtenberg S, Magosch P. A new arthroscopic classification of articular-sided supraspinatus footprint lesions: a prospective comparison with Snyder's and Ellman's classification. *J Shoulder Elbow Surg*. 2008;17(6):909-913.)

for its ability to evaluate more of the relevant structures about the shoulder girdle.

CLASSIFICATION

Although no single classification system of rotator cuff tear succeeds at accounting for all the factors thought to be important to both reliable diagnosis and subsequently prognosis, several systems do exist to aid the clinician with decision making, surgical planning, and setting of expectations for patients.

Partial-Thickness Tears

Ellman (1990), Snyder (2003), and Habermeyer et al (2008) have all described partial-thickness rotator cuff tear classification systems based on intraoperative findings. Ellman's system was the first to gain widespread popularity and classified partial-thickness tears as grade 1 for tears less than 3 mm deep, grade 2 for tears 3 to 6 mm deep but not exceeding half of the tendon's thickness, and grade 3 for tears greater than 6 mm deep (Ellman, 1990).

Snyder (2003) laid out a comprehensive classification that describes the extent of the tear in addition to its location and size. First, the location of the tear is described as articular, bursal, or full thickness. Partial-thickness tears are further subclassified as normal cuff with smooth synovial and bursal covering (0), minimal superficial bursal or synovial irritation or slight capsular fraying over a small area (1), fraying with failure of some rotator cuff fibers in addition to synovial bursal or capsular injury (2), more severe rotator cuff injury fraying and fragmentation of tendon fibers often involving the whole of a cuff tendon, usually greater than 3 cm (3) or very severe partial rotator cuff tear that contains a sizeable flap tear and often more than one tendon (4). A special lesion was described as a variation of articular-sided type 3 or 4; this partial articular supraspinatus tendon avulsion is the "PASTA" lesion often found in throwing athletes (Snyder, 2003). Although very descriptive, this classification has not been well validated and lacks adequate interobserver reliability.

Although limited to the classification of articular-sided tears, Habermeyer et al's (2008) system does address the three-dimensional nature of a tear. This classification is also based on arthroscopic findings, and although more thorough in its descriptive capabilities, the system does neglect to classify bursal-sided and interstitial tears and has not been validated. Habermeyer et al (2008) classifies partial-thickness articular-sided rotator cuff tears as type 1 if there is a small tear within the transition zone from cartilage to bone, type 2 when the tear is up to the center of the footprint, and finally type 3 when it extends to the greater tuberosity (Fig. 5.5). When describing the sagittal extension in the transverse plane, the authors describe a tear of the coracohumeral ligament that continues into the medial border of supraspinatus tendon (type A), an isolated tear within the crescent zone (type B), and a tear from the lateral border of pulley system extending to the crescent zone of the supraspinatus tendon (type C) (Fig. 5.6).

Full-Thickness Tears

Injury to the rotator cuff and more specifically full-thickness tears can be classified in a number of ways. Perhaps most simply, tears are described in terms of their anatomic location in the supraspinatus, infraspinatus, teres minor, subscapularis, or some combination of two or more of these rotator cuff tendons. Similarly, Harryman et al (1991) developed a classification system for posterosuperior tears based on the number of involved tendons identified at the time of surgery. Stages Ia and Ib describe partial- and full-thickness tears, respectively, isolated to the supraspinatus. Stage II tears involve both the supraspinatus and infraspinatus. Stage III tears involve the supraspinatus, infraspinatus, and subscapularis. The classification ends with stage IV, which describes patients who progressed to rotator cuff arthropathy.

Size

DeOrio and Cofield (1984) developed one of the most commonly used classification systems for rotator cuff tears. Using the AP length of the tendon noted to be detached from the humeral head intraoperatively, they defined a

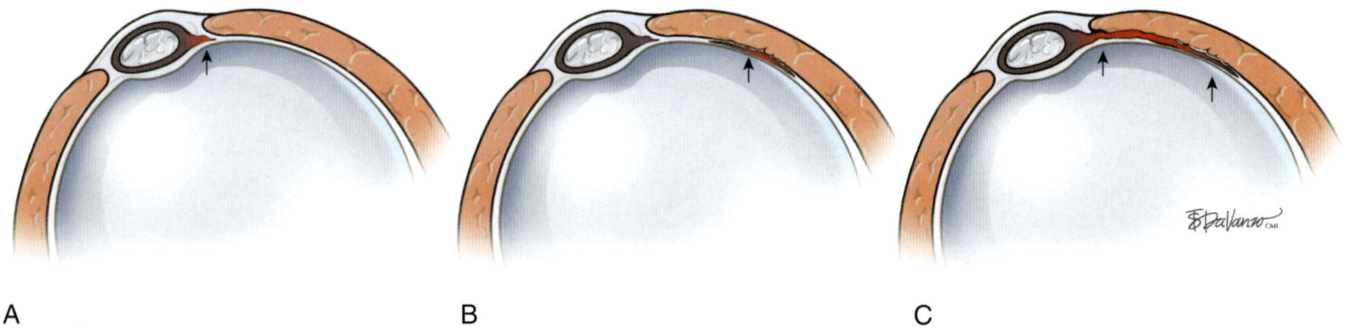

Fig. 5.6 Sagittal extension of articular-sided supraspinatus tendon tears in transverse plane, as classified by Habermeyer et al (2008). **A,** Type A tear: tear of coracohumeral ligament continuing into medial border of supraspinatus tendon. **B,** Type B tear: isolated tear within crescent zone. **C,** Type C tear: tear extending from lateral border of pulley system over medial border of supraspinatus tendon up to area of crescent zone. (Reprinted from Habermeyer P, Krieter C, Tang KL, Lichtenberg S, Magosch P. A new arthroscopic classification of articular-sided supraspinatus footprint lesions: a prospective comparison with Snyder's and Ellman's classification. *J Shoulder Elbow Surg*. 2008; 17(6): 909-913.)

classification system based on the size of a tear. This system classifies tears as small when less than 1 cm, medium if the tear is between 1 and 3 cm, large if between 3 and 5 cm, and massive when greater than 5 cm in length (DeOrio & Cofield, 1984). Several studies have combined the size of the tear with other factors to create a model for predicting outcomes; however, this classification system alone seems to provide limited prognostic information. Critics point out that this widely used classification system does not account for which tendon(s) are involved, tear shape, tissue quality, fatty infiltration, or differences in patient size. It should be mentioned that Bayne and Bateman (1984) came up with a similar classification based on the size of the tear after debridement ranging from grade 1 to 4 correlating to the same dimensions as DeOrio and Cofield's small, medium, large and massive tears.

Shape

Taking into account the three-dimensional shape of the rotator cuff tear morphology, Ellman (1993) developed a classification system based on the shape of the tear characterized at the time of surgery. This description has been further expanded and has evolved to include four commonly described shapes (Fig. 5.7). Crescent-shaped tears are described as being wider in the AP plane with minimally medial retraction making them amenable to a relatively low-tension repair back to their previous bony attachment. Tears that detach from the humeral insertion and extend medially into the tendons posteriorly or anteriorly are referred to as L-shaped and reverse L-shaped tears, respectively. A U-shaped tear can be characterized as a crescent tear with significant medial retraction past the rotator cable. Last, the more variably appearing massive tear can be U-shaped, trapezoidal, or longitudinal and can often be immobile because of profound retraction and scarring.

Atrophy

Goutallier et al's (1994) classification, initially described on the basis of axial computed tomography scans and later modified by Fuchs et al (1999) to be used with oblique sagittal T1-weighted MRI, has become a standard system for describing the chronicity and by proxy the reparability or healing potential of a rotator cuff tear. Progressing from stage 0, which is normal, this classification system describes the changes as stage I, muscle with some fatty streaks; stage II, fatty infiltration with more muscle than fat; stage III, equal fat and muscle content; and stage IV, more fat than muscle. Additionally, classifications systems by Thomazeau et al (1996) and Warner et al (2001) have used oblique sagittal T1-weighted MRI to classify rotator cuff tears according to the degree of atrophy. Thomazeau et al (1996) described the occupation ratio of the supraspinatus muscle belly within its fossa, with stage I being normal or slightly atrophied, stage II showing moderate atrophy, and stage III characterized by serious or severe atrophy. Warner et al's (2001) system described atrophy of either the infraspinatus or supraspinatus as none, mild, moderate, or severe. Although intra- and interobserver reliabilities of these classification systems have been moderate at best, preoperative knowledge of fatty changes and atrophy has been shown to be very useful in predicting likelihood of retear when coupled with tear size and patient age (Goutallier et al, 1994; Oh et al, 2009).

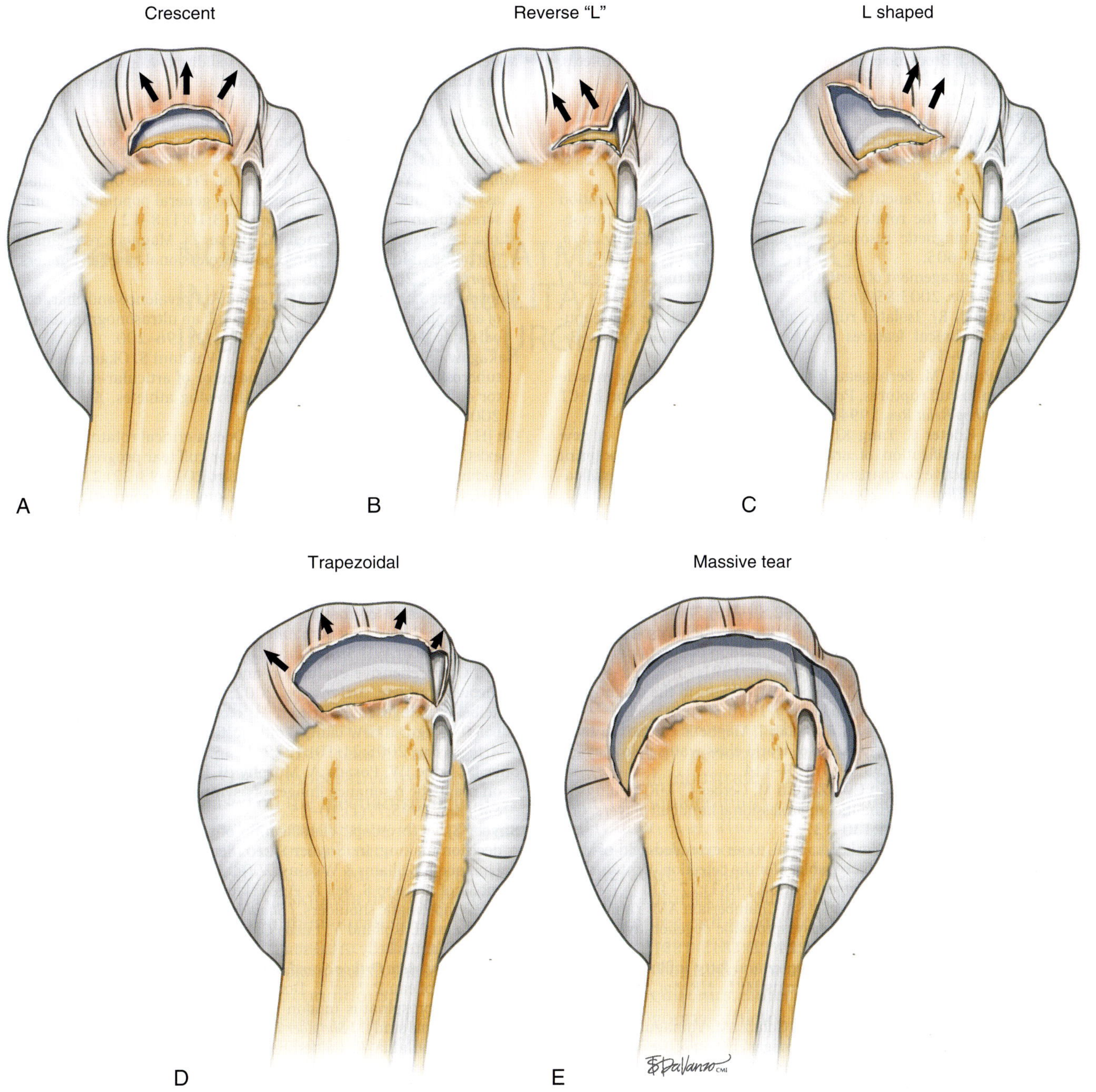

Fig. 5.7 Classification of full-thickness rotator cuff tears by shape: crescent (**A**), reverse "L" (**B**), "L" (**C**), trapezoidal (**D**), and massive (**E**). (Reprinted from Ellman H, Gartsman GM. Open repair of full-thickness rotator cuff tears. In: Ellman H, Gartsman GM, eds. *Arthroscopic Shoulder Surgery and Related Disorders.* Philadelphia: Lea & Febiger; 1993:181-202.)

References

Barth JR, Burkhart SS, De Beer JF. The bear-hug test: a new and sensitive test for diagnosing a subscapularis tear. *Arthroscopy*. 2006;22(10): 1076–1084.

Bayne O, Bateman JE. Long-term results of surgical repair of full-thickness rotator cuff tears. In: Bateman JE, Welsh R, eds. *Surgery of the Shoulder*. Philadelphia: CV Mosby; 1984:161–171.

Burkhart SS, Esch JC, Jolson RS. The rotator crescent and rotator cable: an anatomic description of the shoulder's "suspension bridge.". *Arthroscopy*. 1993;9(6):611–616.

Burkhart SS, Morgan CD, Kibler WB. The disabled throwing shoulder: spectrum of pathology Part I: pathoanatomy and biomechanics. *Arthroscopy*. 2003;19(4):404–420.

Chun KA, Kim MS, Kim YJ. Comparisons of the various partial-thickness rotator cuff tears on MR arthrography and arthroscopic correlation. *Korean J Radiol*. 2010;11(5):528–535.

Connor PM, Banks DM, Tyson AB, Coumas JS, D'Alessandro DF. Magnetic resonance imaging of the asymptomatic shoulder of overhead athletes: a 5-year follow-up study. *Am J Sports Med*. 2003;31(5): 724–727.

Curtis AS, Burbank KM, Tierney JJ, Scheller AD, Curran AR. The insertional footprint of the rotator cuff: an anatomic study. *Arthroscopy*. 2006;22(6):609e1.

de Jesus JO, Parker L, Frangos AJ, Nazarian LN. Accuracy of MRI, MR arthrography, and ultrasound in the diagnosis of rotator cuff tears: a meta-analysis. *AJR Am J Roentgenol*. 2009;192(6):1701–1707.

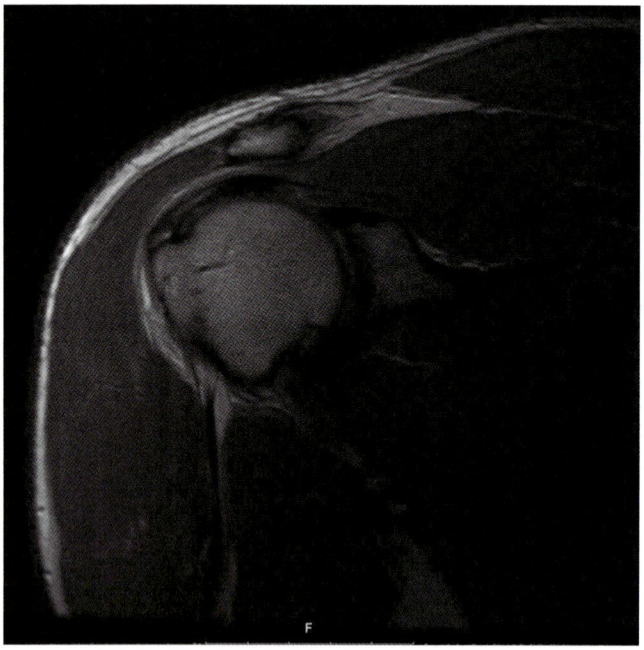

Fig. 6A.1 MR image of supraspinatus contusion. A contusion of the supraspinatus muscle, demonstrated on this coronal proton density weighted sequence, accounts for the hyperintensity at the bursal margin of the tendon without delamination of a bursal sideslip.

importance of the intratendinous extension of the tear has been recommended (Conway, 2001). The interstitial tendon tear has also been described to be an important factor determining the treatment of partial rotator cuff tears (Fukuda, 2003).

The mechanism of injury in overhead throwing athletes is due mostly to repetitive microtrauma. Extreme loads are placed on the shoulder in the such athletes. Forces at the shoulder of up to 108% of body weight (Werner et al, 2001) as well as peak humeral angular velocities up to 7000 degrees per second (Dillman et al, 1993) have been recorded in throwing athletes. Since most partial tears in athletes are on the articular side or intrinsic in nature (Payne et al, 1997), the two most likely mechanisms are tensile overload and internal impingement. (Andrews and Wilcox) found that most of the partial tears they have treated included the posterior portion of the supraspinatus and the anterior portion of the infraspinatus tendons several millimeters proximal to the tendon insertion. They concluded that the injury is created by compression with shearing of the tendons. The deceleration phase of throwing creates high eccentric loads on the rotator cuff that mostly involve the supraspinatus. If the timing and force of the contraction are not adequate, the tensile forces placed on the rotator cuff can lead to injury (Williams & Kelley, 2000). The fact the tendon has poor vascularity is believed to contribute to an increased risk of injury due to microtrauma (Rathburn & Macnab, 1970).

Internal impingement refers to compression of the articular side of the rotator cuff by the superior glenoid during the throwing motion (Walch et al, 1992). Most writers believe that this compression occurs in the late cocking and acceleration phases of the throwing motion. Several observations have provided insight into the cause of this "pinching" effect. Initially proposed as a contributing factor in internal impingement is subtle anterior shoulder instability related to attritional changes to the anterior band of the inferior glenohumeral ligament (Bigliani et al, 1997; Paley et al, 2000). The increased anterior translation of the humeral head in an abducted and externally rotated position results in entrapment of the rotator cuff between the greater tuberosity and the glenoid. Subsequently it has been proposed that athletes with contracted posterior capsules are predisposed to internal impingement. This results in a loss of internal rotation (glenohumeral internal rotation deficit [GIRD]) (Burkhart et al, 2003). Repetitive forces on the infraspinatus and the posterior shoulder capsule during the deceleration and follow-through phases of throwing create hypertrophy and stiffness in these structures. The result of these changes shifts the center of rotation of the shoulder to a more posterosuperior position. This abnormal position then creates the internal impingement. Poor scapula control may also lead to internal impingement. During the late cocking phase of throwing upward, scapula rotation helps maintain glenohumeral articular congruency (Myers et al, 2005). Scapular dyskinesia allows the scapula to move into a protracted and upwardly tilted position, directing the glenoid anteriorly and superiorly (Burkhart et al, 2003). The resulting greater external rotation during the throwing motion can produce internal impingement (Kibler & McMullen, 2003).

Adaptive changes occur in the throwing shoulder. Kibler et al (2013) observed that "the throwing athlete can be considered on the edge of a cliff in terms of the demands of the throwing motion on the anatomic structures." Signal abnormalities involving the rotator cuff on MRI are common in asymptomatic overhead throwing athletes. A study of asymptomatic minor league baseball players demonstrated that 40% had abnormal rotator cuff findings (Connor et al, 2003). Studies also show changes to the rotator cuff can take up to 6 days to normalize after a pitcher throws (Lesniak et al, 2013) Most writers agree that losses of internal rotation and of total arc of motion place the athlete's shoulder at risk (Tokish, 2014). Wilk et al (2011) demonstrated that a loss of more than 5 degrees in total arc of motion in pitchers put them at increased risk of injury and that associated loss of internal rotation increased risk of injury at least twofold.

Rotator cuff contusions and partial rotator cuff tears in the athletes have various mechanisms. This diagnosis has resulted from direct injury or trauma in contact sport athletes. The overhead throwing athlete is at increased risk for this injury owing to microtrauma related to the forces generated in a repetitive nature. It is also likely, on the basis of literature findings, that various factors, possibly in combination, create the observed pathology. Knowledge of all the possible contributing factors is key to direct treatment strategies. An understanding of the adaptive changes that are seen in the overhead throwing athlete is necessary for the clinician to assure an accurate diagnosis.

Treatment

There is currently a lack of guidelines based on randomized, prospective studies to aid the clinician treating partial rotator cuff tears and contusions. Also, most of the available studies lack adequate statistical power. The results of nonoperative management of partial-thickness tears are largely

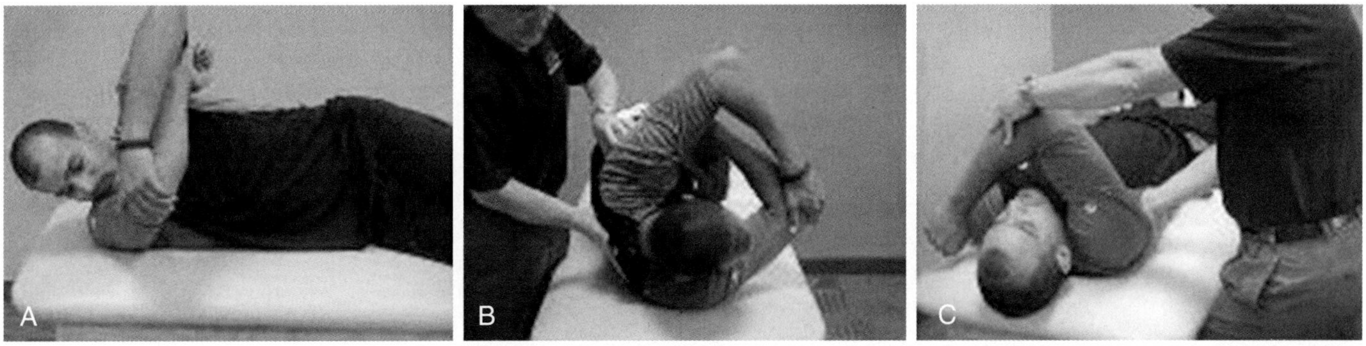

Fig. 6A.2 **(A)** Front view of a modified sleeper stretch with a lift to improve posterior soft tissue mobility. **(B)** Caudal view of the modified sleeper stretch. **(C)** Supine horizontal adduction with the scapula stabilized by the rehabilitation specialist. (From Wilk KE, Macrina LC. Nonoperative and postoperative rehabilitation for injuries of the throwing shoulder. *Sports Med Arthrosc Rev.* 2014;22[2]:137-50.)

unknown because there are no long-term follow-up studies using a standardized treatment protocol. Nonsurgical treatment is still regarded as the initial management step. The goal of treatment in athletes with a partial rotator cuff tear is to eliminate pain and restore function. Treatment of the athlete with a rotator cuff contusion has the same objective. The goals could evolve if biologic interventions are developed that lead to a true healing response (Ferhat et al, 2016).

Determining whether the injury is traumatic or is related to overuse is the first step to frame the treatment strategies. In the athlete with a trauma history, the initial goal is to control the pain and to restore full shoulder/scapula mobility and strength. The treatment for a partial rotator cuff tear in the overhead throwing athlete centers on the underlying deficiencies seen, such as loss of shoulder motion, scapula dyskinesia, and rotator cuff weakness. Mechanical flaws in the throwing or overhead motion may also need to be corrected.

The majority of patients in the study by Cohen et al (2007) examining rotator cuff contusions showed quick responses to treatment with modalities such as, pulse ultrasound and cuff/scapula strenthening. It was noted that the athletes who had significant subentheseal bone bruises and what the researchers called "chronic tendinopathy" had more prolonged recovery. In the patients who did not demonstrate significant improvement by the third day after injury (23%) a subacromial corticosteroid injection was utilized; this step was described to be of benefit, because only one of the six athletes who received a cortisone injection later needed surgery. Minimal morbidity was noted overall as a result of the contusions but 11% of the patients required later surgical intervention.

Separate Cochrane Systematic Reviews evaluating the benefits of electrotherapy modalities as well as assessing the value of manual therapy and exercise for rotator cuff disease have been performed (Page, Green, McBain, et al, 2016; Page, Green, Mrocki, et al, 2016). Modalities such as transcutaneous electric nerve stimulation, therapeutic ultrasound, low-level laser therapy (LLLT), and pulsed electromagnetic field therapy are examples of the modalities potentially utilized in the electrotherapy evaluation. On the basis of low-quality evidence, therapeutic ultrasound may have short-term benefits for patients with calcific tendinitis, and LLLT may have short-term benefits in patients with rotator cuff disease. The review of the literature identified only 1 of 60 trials to be of high quality regarding manual therapy and exercise, and no benefit was noted.

In the overhead throwing athlete, shoulder rehabilitation should be directed at the underlying deficits, most commonly loss of shoulder internal rotation and poor control of the scapula. A four-phase approach is described by Wilk & Macrina (2014) in the nonoperative treatment of throwing shoulder injuries. In phase 1, the "acute phase," the primary goals are to diminish pain/inflammation, improve motion, activate the appropriate muscles, create dynamic stability and muscle balance, and restore proprioception. The athlete's level of activity is adjusted according to symptoms, which usually require the athlete to abstain from activity. Internal rotation motion is addressed; the preferred stretches are the modified sleeper's stretch and supine horizontal adduction with internal rotation stretch (Fig. 6A.2). A horizontal adduction stretch with manual patient assistance into internal rotation is performed. Assessment of scapula positioning is also recommended, with strengthening of the scapula retractors and the lower trapezius and additional stretching of the pectoralis minor. The primary goals of phase 2, the "intermediate phase," are to progress the strengthening program, improve the range of motion, and facilitate neuromuscular control. Core strengthening is also initiated during this phase. Kibler et al (2013) have emphasized the need to evaluate and treat the entire system to restore the athlete's kinetic chain. Phase 3, the "advanced strengthening phase," involves aggressive strengthening drills to promote power and endurance as well as functional drills, and throwing is gradually introduced. "Return to throwing phase," phase 4, incorporates the progression of an interval-throwing program. This program controls for distance, intensity, and surface, in that for pitchers, throwing from the mound is the last advancement. It is important to be aware that when athletes are told to throw with 50% effort, they actually throw at 83% of their maximal speed, and when asked to throw at 75% they are actually throwing at 90% of their maximal effort (Fleisig et al, 1996).

Corticosteroid injections have been commonly utilized in treating rotator cuff disease. Koester et al (2007) performed a systematic review of the literature and analyzed nine randomized controlled studies comparing subacromial corticosteroid injection with placebo. One study demonstrated significant pain relief and two studies showed an increased range of motion in the injection group. No significant complications were identified. In a study comparing a corticosteroid injection with a platelet-rich plasma (PRP) injection for subacromial impingement syndrome, the investigators found the Constant score and VAS for pain to be significantly better at both 6 weeks and 6 months in the corticosteroid-treated group. Good patient candidates for a single subacromial corticosteroid injection to achieve pain control are those with significant night pain or patients who will not tolerate phase 1 rehabilitation because of pain.

PRP injections are being utilized for partial rotator cuff tears. There are mixed results in the literature. A randomized controlled trial (level I evidence) with a 1-year follow-up demonstrated no benefit from a single PRP injection in comparison with placebo (Kesikburun et al, 2013). Biologic type injections may have a role in the treatment of partial rotator cuff tears; however, the exact platelet count and leukocyte concentration in PRP for optimal growth factor activity has yet to be definitively proven in the literature.

Surgical Indications

Consensus has been reached on the correct management of patients with rotator cuff tears (Dunn et al, 2005). There are data showing that rotator cuff repairs in younger patients with a traumatic history are more successful than those in older patients with chronic tears (Braune et al, 2003). Rotator cuff repair has not been as successful however in young overhead throwing athletes. (Lazarides et al, 2015). Level I evidence is not available for surgical repair of partial rotator cuff tears in athletes. Reynolds et al (2008), in a level IV therapeutic study, reported that 55% of elite throwing athletes were able to return to their previous levels of competition or better, and 85% were determined to have good or excellent results following debridement of partial-thickness rotator cuff tears.

The other consideration is that the natural history of a partial-thickness tear is not fully known. Yamanaka & Matsumoto (1994) demonstrated that 80% of partial tears they studied did progress during a 2-year period, 10% decreased in size, and 10% resolved. Concern exists that potential tear progression and possible muscle atrophy may compromise future surgical results. A randomized controlled trial in patients diagnosed with impingement syndrome was performed comparing a structured exercise program with arthroscopic acromioplasty. An MRI study performed at baseline was then compared with a study performed 5 years later for each patient. The nonsurgically treated patients did not demonstrate increased frequency of complete tears, and the two groups were similar in terms of muscle volume (Ketola et al, 2016). The mean age in the study was 47 years so these data may not be fully applicable to the young athlete.

Surgical intervention should be considered in the athlete whose injury does not respond to nonoperative treatment in 8 to 12 weeks. In a group of contact sport athletes undergoing surgery for rotator cuff injury, the average time from the time of injury to surgery was 9 weeks (Blevins et al, 1996). In the overhead throwing athlete, all deficiencies should be identified and corrected before surgical intervention is considered. This approach would mandate improving shoulder flexibility and strength as discussed, requiring at least 8 to 12 weeks.

References

Andrews JR, Wilcox L. Decision making in the throwing athlete. *Sports Med Arthrosc Rev.* 2014;22(2):130–136.

Bigliani LU, Codd TP, Connor PM, et al. Shoulder motion and laxity in the professional baseball player. *Am J Sports Med.* 1997;25:609–613.

Blevins FT, Hayes WM, Warren RF. Rotator cuff injury in contact athletes. *Am J Sports Med.* 1996;24(3):263–267.

Braune C, von Eisenhart-Rothe R, Welsch F, et al. Midterm results and quantitative comparison of postoperative shoulder function in traumatic and non-traumatic rotator cuff tears. *Arch Orthop Trauma Surg.* 2003;123:419–424.

Burkhart SS, Morgan CD, Kibler WB. The disabled throwing shoulder: Spectrum of pathology part I: Pathoanatomy and biomechanics. *Arthroscopy.* 2003;19(4):404–420.

Burkhart SS, Morgan CD, Kibler WB. The disabled throwing shoulder: Spectrum of pathology part III: The SICK scapula, scapula dyskinesis, the kinetic chain and rehabilitation. *Arthroscopy.* 2003;9(6): 641–661.

Cohen SB, Towers JD, Bradley JP. Rotator cuff contusions of the shoulder in professional football players: epidemiology and magnetic resonance imaging findings. *Am J Sports Med.* 2007;35(3):442–447.

Connor PM, Banks DM, Tyson AB, et al. Magnetic resonance imaging of the asymptomatic shoulder of overhead athletes: a 5-year follow-up study. *Am J Sports Med.* 2003;31:724–727.

Conway JE. Arthroscopic repair of partial-thickness rotator cuff tears and SLAP lesions in professional baseball players. *Orthop Clin North Am.* 2001;32:443–456.

Dillman CJ, Fleisig GS, Andrews JR. Biomechanics of pitching with emphasis upon shoulder kinematics. *J Orthop Sports Phys Ther.* 1993;18:402–408.

Dunn WR, Schackman BR, Walsh C, et al. Variation in orthopaedic surgeons' perception about the indications for rotator cuff surgery. *J Bone Joint Surg Am.* 2005;87:1978–1984.

Ellman H. Diagnosis and treatment of incomplete rotator cuff tears. *Clin Orthop Relat Res.* 1990;254:64–74.

Ferhat S, Gurler D, Bulbul M. Platelet-rich plasma versus steroid injection for subacromial impingement syndrome. *J Orthop Surg (Hong Kong).* 2016;24(1):62–66.

Fleisig GS, Zheng N, Barrentine S. Kinematic and kinetic comparison of full effort and partial effort baseball pitching. In: American Society of Biomechanics, ed. *Biomechanics: Conference Proceedings of the 20th Annual Meeting.* Atlanta: American Society of Biomechanics; 1996:151–152.

Fukuda H. The management of partial-thickness tears of the rotator cuff. *J Bone Joint Surg Br.* 2003;85:3–11.

Kaplan LD, Flanigan DC, Norwig J, et al. Prevalence and variance of shoulder injuries in elite collegiate football players. *Am J Sports Med.* 2005;33(8):1142–1146.

Kesikburun S, Tan AK, Yilmaz B, et al. Platelet-rich plasma injections in the treatment of chronic rotator cuff tendinopathy: a randomized controlled trial with 1-year follow-up. *Am J Sports Med.* 2013;41(1): 2609–2616.

Ketola S, Lehtinen J, Elo P, et al. No difference in long-term development of rotator cuff rupture and muscle volumes in impingement patients with or without decompression. *Acta Orthop.* 2016;87(4):351–355.

Kibler WB, Kuhn JE, Wilk K, et al. The disabled throwing shoulder: spectrum of pathology:10 year update. *Arthroscopy.* 2013;29(1):141–161.

Kibler WB, McMullen J. Scapular dyskinesis and its relation to shoulder pain. *J Am Acad Orthop Surg.* 2003;11(2):142–151.

Koester MC, Dunn WR, Kuhn JE, Spindler KP. The efficacy of subacromial corticosteroid injection in the treatment of rotator cuff disease: a systematic review. *J Am Acad Orthop Surg.* 2007;15(1):3–11.

Lazarides AL, Alentorn-Geli E, Choi JHJ, et al. Rotator cuff tears in young patients: a different disease than rotator cuff tears in elderly patients. *J Shoulder Elbow Surg.* 2015;24:1834–1843.

Lesniak BP, Baraga MG, Jose J, et al. Glenohumeral findings on magnetic resonance imaging correlate with innings pitched in asymptomatic pitchers. *Am J Sports Med.* 2013;41:22–27.

Luo ZP, Hsu HC, Morrey BF, et al. Etiologic environment of rotator cuff tears: intrinsic or extrinsic? *Orthop Trans.* 1997;20:799–800.

Myers JB, Laudner KG, Pasquale MR, et al. Scapula position and orientation in the throwing athlete. *Am J Sports Med.* 2005;33(2):263–271.

Neer CS II. Impingement lesions. *Clin Orthop Relat Res.* 1983;173:70–77.

Page MJ, Green S, McBain B, et al. Manual therapy and exercise for rotator cuff disease. *Cochrane Database Syst Rev.* 2016;10(6). CD012224.

Page MJ, Green S, Mrocki MA, et al. Electrotherapy modalities for rotator cuff disease. *Cochrane Database Syst Rev*. 2016;10(6). CD012225.

Paley KJ, Jobe FW, Pink MM, Kvitne RS, El Attrache NS. Arthroscopic findings in the overhand throwing athlete: evidence for posterior internal impingement of the rotator cuff. *Arthroscopy*. 2000;16:35–40.

Payne LZ, Altchek DW, Craig EV, Warren RF. Arthroscopic treatment of partial rotator cuff tears in young athletes: a preliminary report. *Am J Sports Med*. 1997;25:299–305.

Rathburn JB, Macnab I. The microvascular pattern of the rotator cuff. *J Bone Joint Surg Br*. 1970;11:530–536.

Reynolds SB, Dugas JR, Cain EL, et al. Debridement of small partial-thickness rotator cuff tears in elite overhead throwers. *Clin Orthop Relat Res*. 2008;466:614–621.

Sakurai G, Ozaki J, Tomita Y, Kondo T, Tamai S. Incomplete tears of the subscapularis tendon associated with tears of the supraspinatus tendon: cadaveric and clinical studies. *J Shoulder Elbow Surg*. 1998;7:510–515.

Sher JS, Uribe JW, Posada A, Murphy BJ, Zlatkin MB. Abnormal findings on magnetic resonance images of asymptomatic shoulders. *J Bone Joint Surg Am*. 1995;77:10–15.

Snyder SJ, Pachelli AF, Del Pizzo W, Friedman MJ, Ferkel RD, Pattee G. Partial thickness rotator cuff tears: result of arthroscopic treatment. *Arthroscopy*. 1991;7:1–7.

Tokish JM. Acquired and adaptive changes in the throwing athlete: implications on the disabled throwing shoulder. *Sports Med Arthrosc Rev*. 2014;22(2):88–93.

Walch G, Boileau J, Noel E, et al. Impingement of the deep surface of the supraspinatus tendon on the posterosuperior glenoid rim: an arthroscopic study. *J Shoulder Elbow Surg*. 1992;1:238–243.

Werner SL, Gill TJ, Murray TA, et al. Relationship between throwing mechanics and shoulder distraction in professional baseball pitchers. *Am J Sports Med*. 2001;29:354–358.

Wilk KE, Macrina LC, Fleisig GS, et al. Correlation of glenohumeral internal rotation deficit and total rotational motion to shoulder injuries in professional baseball pitchers. *Am J Sports Med*. 2011;39:329–335.

Wilk KE, Macrina LC. Nonoperative and postoperative rehabilitation for injuries of the throwing shoulder. *Sports Med Arthrosc Rev*. 2014;22(2):137–150.

Williams GR, Kelley M. Management of rotator cuff and impingement injuries in the athlete. *J Athl Train*. 2000;35(3):300–315.

Yamanaka K, Matsumoto T. The joint side tear of the rotator cuff: a follow-up study by arthrography. *Clin Orthop Relat Res*. 1994;304:68–73.

6-6B ARTHROSCOPIC MANAGEMENT

CHRISTOPHER C. DODSON, MD and KIRSTEN L. POEHLING-MONAGHAN, MD

Introduction

Partial-thickness tears of the rotator cuff are certainly not an uncommon phenomenon, and they can encompass a broad range of pathology, etiologies, and demographics. The intricacies of each of these variables play a large role in determining the adequate arthroscopic treatment once nonoperative methods have failed.

Articular-Sided Injuries

OVERVIEW/PATIENT DEMOGRAPHICS

Articular-sided partial-thickness rotator cuff tears affect both younger and older patients, although mechanism of injury varies greatly. Those older than 40 years tend to have underlying degenerative tissue with fraying and partial detachment of the anterior cuff at the hypovascular critical zone of the supraspinatus insertion. This phenomenon occurs relatively frequently, with some studies reporting partial-thickness rotator cuff tears in 18% to 38% of asymptomatic patients older than 40 (Reilly et al, 2006).

In contrast, patients younger than 40 with even small articular-sided tears tend to have symptoms. Most often these injuries occur at the posterior footprint near the supraspinatus-infraspinatus interval and can involve a component of intratendinous delamination. These patients are often overhead throwing athletes with chronic internal impingement that occurs during the late cocking/early acceleration phases of throwing owing to irritation of the supraspinatus at its insertion on the tuberosity as it abuts the posterosuperior glenoid. These injuries are often associated with concomitant pathology, including posterior labral and superior labrum anterior and posterior (SLAP) tears, Bennett lesions (hypertrophy of posterior capsule), and posterior glenoid cartilage delamination.

ARTHROSCOPIC DEBRIDEMENT

In both young and old patients in whom less than 50% (or less than 6 mm) of tendon thickness is involved, arthroscopic debridement may be considered.

Our technique involves placing the patient in the beach-chair position, although an alternate positioning such as the lateral decubitus may be used depending on surgeon experience and comfort level. A standard diagnostic arthroscopy is performed through the posterior portal and must include evaluation of the biceps anchor at the glenoid, the anterior and posterior labrum, the capsuloligamentous structures, and the integrity of both the humeral and glenoid articular cartilage. Any concomitant pathology should be addressed after the arthroscopic debridement.

Once fraying or partial tearing of the underside of the cuff is identified, the arm is placed in 45 degrees of abduction and external rotation with slight traction to better visualize the cuff at its insertion. For younger patients, in whom extent of the tear into the posterior aspect of the footprint is more likely, it may be necessary to switch the camera to the anterior portal for adequate visualization. The cuff tear is probed, and depth as well as anteroposterior extension is estimated with use of a probe with a 3-mm tip. The arthroscope is then switched to a subacromial viewing portal, and the insertion of the cuff is once again probed to ensure that no full-thickness extension exists.

Once the cuff has been assessed, the arthroscope is switched back to a posterior viewing portal, and a 4.0-mm shaver is introduced from an anterior working portal. The cuff edges can be first lightly abraded with a high-oscillation setting without suction. This process abrades the edges without taking too much tissue until the boundaries of the tear are clearly established. Then, with suction on intermittently, the cuff is debrided until viable fibers are seen attaching to the tuberosity. If intratendinous delamination is seen, the articular flap may be debrided or abraded, with care taken not to resect too much tissue and thereby compromise the depth of the tear. In younger patients in whom the tear extends more posteriorly on the footprint, the same process may need to be repeated with the surgeon viewing from an anterior portal, or with a 70-degree arthroscope from the posterior portal to better visualize the supraspinatus-infraspinatus interval.

TRANSTENDINOUS REPAIR

In young, overhead throwing athletes with tears comprising any percentage of cuff thickness but with a significant component of intratendinous delamination, fixation of the cuff without formal completion of the tear may be considered (Brockmeier et al, 2008).

Setup and initial arthroscopic assessment are performed as previously described. The opposing delaminated surfaces of tendon are lightly abraded with the shaver to promote healing. Likewise, the footprint is debrided down to lightly bleeding bone. When viewing from the subacromial space, the surgeon should perform extensive bursectomy to facilitate suture management.

The surgeon begins the repair process with the arthroscope once again viewing from the posterior portal, while an assistant uses a tissue grasper to hold the articular-sided flap in a reduced position back to the tuberosity. The surgeon then places two percutaneous spinal needles across the cuff and into the joint. A polydioxanone (PDS) suture is then advanced through each spinal needle, and a grasper is used to shuttle these sutures out of the anterior working cannula. The sutures are then tied to each other and pulled into the joint, and the knot is shuttled externally by pulling on one of the sutures. This process results in the placement of a mattress suture that secures the articular-sided flap to the intact peripheral cuff, thereby reducing the articular defect while also closing any intrasubstance delamination. For the ultimate fixation the surgeon uses a nonabsorbable suture by shuttling it through the tear with the PDS. Multiple mattress sutures can be placed with this technique as dictated by tear size and morphology. The sutures are then individually retrieved and tied in the subacromial space with use of standard arthroscopic knot-tying techniques.

TEAR COMPLETION AND FORMAL CUFF REPAIR

In older patients in whom greater than 50% (or greater than 6 mm) of cuff depth is involved, the remaining tissue may be subjected to excessive stresses if not formally repaired, leading to inevitable progression of the tear or unacceptable strain on the remaining cuff tissue (Mazzocca et al, 2008). In such patients, formal debridement to complete the tear may be performed, and the cuff repaired with use of traditional arthroscopic techniques from the subacromial space. The surgeon may debride the cuff tear from the articular side, viewing from a posterior portal with a shaver introduced from the anterior portal. During debridement care should be taken not to damage the adjacent biceps or rotator interval if these structures are currently intact. Alternately, a percutaneous spinal needle can be introduced across the cuff into the area of maximal fraying, and a PDS suture passed through the needle and retrieved with a grasper out the anterior portal. This grasper is then clipped together to the drapes while the arthroscope is switched to the subacromial portal, and an anterolateral working portal is created through which the shaver may be introduced. After an extensive subacromial bursectomy the PDS suture is identified and the tear is completed with the shaver until tuberosity is exposed. The surgeon may then proceed with arthroscopic rotator cuff repair using a preferred technique.

Intrasubstance Injuries

OVERVIEW/PATIENT DEMOGRAPHICS

Partial-thickness tears of the rotator cuff often manifest as pain in a patient in whom intrasubstance signal and inflammation are seen on advanced imaging. Such patients may have a history of inflammatory or rheumatologic disorders. Less often, the tissue may simply be degenerative with preservation of the bursal and articular sides of the tendon. Additionally, patients with calcific tendinitis may present with radiographic and MRI findings of calcification embedded within the tendon and surrounding inflammation.

ARTHROSCOPIC TREATMENT

The debridement of degenerative or inflammatory intrasubstance partial-thickness rotator cuff tears largely involves ultimate completion of the tear because of the location. It can, however, involve preservation of the tendon in instances of calcific tendinitis.

After a thorough diagnostic arthroscopy using the previously mentioned technique, the arthroscope is inserted into the subacromial space through a posterior viewing portal. If visualization permits, a spinal needle may be used to percutaneously locate the foci of calcification and aid in the placement of an optimal working portal. A cannula should be utilized to prevent the deposition of debris in the soft tissues outside the subacromial space during introduction and removal of instruments (Fig. 6B.1A). An arthroscopic probe is used to gently open the area of calcification, allowing pieces to be expressed (Fig. 6B.1B). This is alternated with a 4.0-mm shaver and, if needed, the grasper, to debride and remove these calcifications (Fig. 6B.1C and D). Once all mobile debris has been removed, the area of calcific tendon

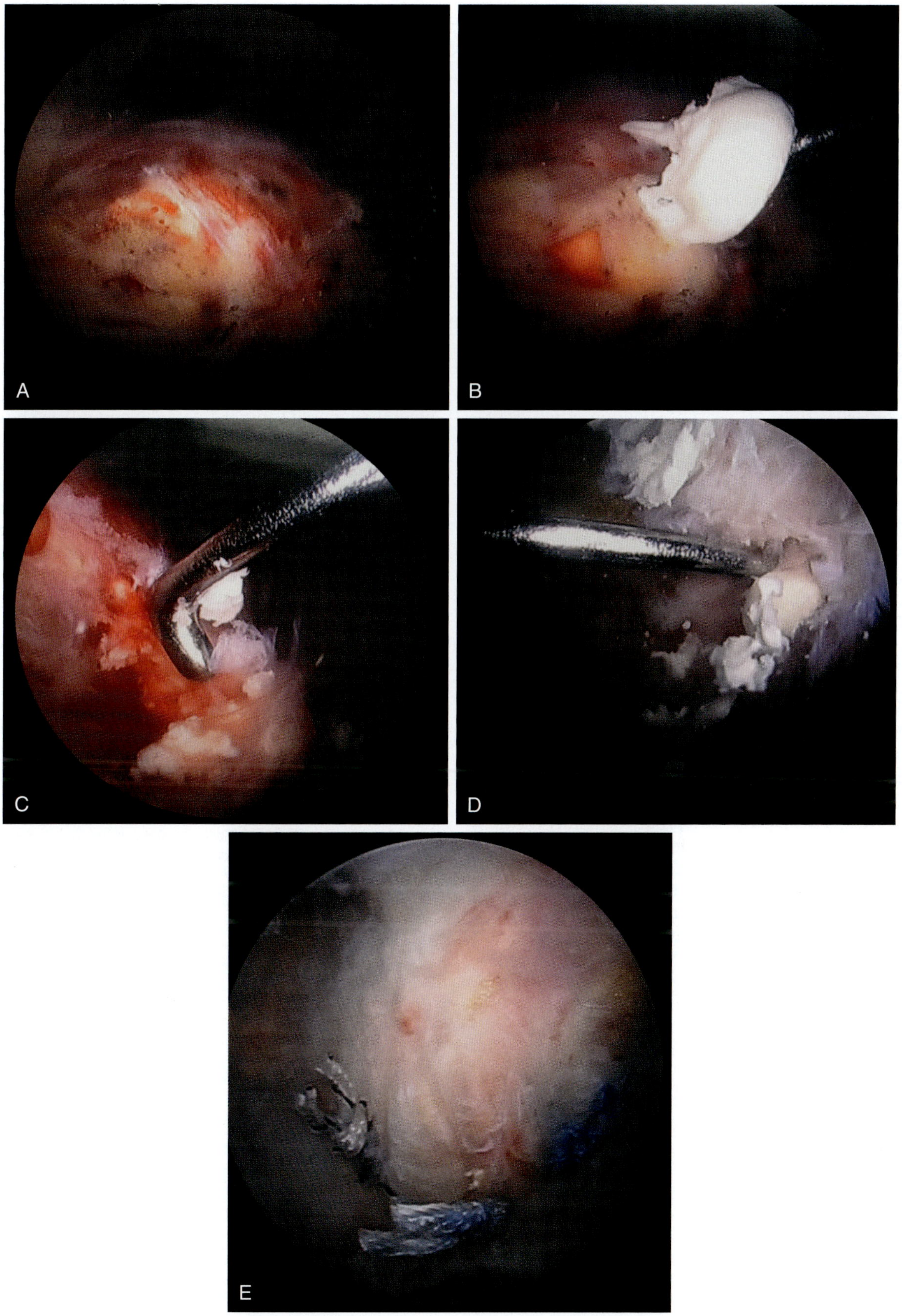

Fig. 6B.1 (**A**) The calcific tendinitis is identified over the tuberosity. (**B**) With a probe, the tissue overlying the lesion is gently removed, and the calcification can be expressed. (**C** and **D**) The calcifications are removed with a combination of a probe, a grasper, and a shaver. (**E**) Once the remaining defect is assessed, if it is more than 3 mm in depth, it can be formally repaired.

is lightly shaved, with care taken to ensure that the remaining tendon bed is left intact. The probe can be used to feel the thickness of the remaining tendon: if tuberosity can easily be felt, the debridement was too extensive and the tendon will likely need to be taken down and repaired per the techniques described in the previous and preceding sections (Fig. 6B.1E).

Bursal-Sided Injuries

ETIOLOGY AND DEMOGRAPHICS

Partial-thickness bursal-sided injuries of the rotator cuff are far more prevalent in older patients, representing the sequelae of a combination of subacromial impingement from a hypertrophic coracoacromial arch and degenerative cuff tissue. It is a common phenomenon, with some studies reporting bursal-sided partial-thickness tears in 48% of Senior Olympics athletes older than 60 years (McMahon et al, 2014). Arthroscopic treatment ranges from simple debridement to formal tear completion and arthroscopic rotator cuff repair.

ARTHROSCOPIC TREATMENT

Tears less than 3 mm in depth can often be successfully managed with arthroscopic debridement alone, and such treatment can have successful outcomes, with some studies reporting less than 10% of such tears progress to full thickness at 10 years (Maman et al, 2009).

After a thorough diagnostic arthroscopy documenting concomitant pathology and the absence or presence of any partial articular-sided tearing, the subacromial space is viewed through a posterior portal. A spinal needle is inserted percutaneously and an accessory working portal is created. An extensive subacromial bursectomy is performed with a 4.0-mm shaver until the rotator cuff is easily visualized. The shaver itself may be used as a probe to identify the area of partial tearing or softening of the cuff. The arthroscopic shaver is turned on its side initially to debride any residual bursa that may be masking a deeper defect. Once the true tear is identified, the shaver is brushed lightly over the edges of the cuff so that only degenerative or torn tissue is removed and intact cuff remains. The arthroscopic probe is used to verify that the residual defect remains an adequate depth. Any subacromial impingement is then addressed per the surgeon's usual technique. In general, fraying of the coracoacromial ligament suggests underlying impingement and the need for a subacromial bony decompression.

TEAR COMPLETION AND FORMAL CUFF REPAIR

Partial-thickness tears deeper than 3 mm are at higher risk for progression to full-thickness tears and respond less predictably to arthroscopic debridement. Such tears often require formal completion of the tear followed by repair.

After a thorough diagnostic arthroscopy, any concomitant articular-sided tears can be lightly debrided and tagged with a PDS suture per the previously mentioned techniques. Once the procedure has reached the subacromial space, the cuff tear can be identified either via the PDS suture tag or with previously mentioned methods after a thorough bursectomy. The tear is debrided with the shaver down to exposed tuberosity, which should also be debrided down to bleeding bone to promote healing. The surgeon should use light pressure with the shaver as a guide to distinguish between healthy and degenerative cuff and thus discern the extent of the debridement and resultant complete cuff tear. Thereafter the cuff may be repaired via the surgeon's usual preferred technique. As mentioned previously, fraying of the coracoacromial ligament suggests underlying impingement and the need for a subacromial bony decompression.

References

Brockmeier SF, Dodson CC, Gamradt SC, Coleman SH, Altchek DW. Arthroscopic intratendinous repair of the delaminated partial-thickness rotator cuff tear in overhead athletes. *Arthroscopy*. 2008;24(8):961–965.

Maman E, Harris C, White L, Tomlinson G, Shashank M, Boynton E. Outcome of nonoperative treatment of symptomatic rotator cuff tears monitored by magnetic resonance imaging. *J Bone Joint Surg Am*. 2009;91(8):1898–1906.

Mazzocca AD, Rincon LM, O'Connor RW, et al. Intra-articular partial-thickness rotator cuff tears: analysis of injured and repaired strain behavior. *Am J Sports Med*. 2008;36(1):110–116.

McMahon PJ, Prasad A, Francis KA. What is the prevalence of senior-athlete rotator cuff injuries and are they associated with pain and dysfunction? *Clin Orthop Relat Res*. 2014;472(8):2427–2432.

Reilly P, Macleod I, Macfarlane R, Windley J, Emery RJ. Dead men and radiologists don't lie: a review of cadaveric and radiological studies of rotator cuff tear prevalence. *Ann R Coll Surg Engl*. 2006;88(2):116–121.

7 Full Thickness Posterior Rotator Cuff Tear

7-7A ARTHROSCOPIC POSTEROSUPERIOR ROTATOR CUFF REPAIR FOR FULL-THICKNESS TEARS

MATTHEW P. NOYES, MD; PATRICK J. DENARD, MD; and STEPHEN S. BURKHART MA, MD

Introduction

- Advancements in shoulder arthroscopy have allowed for better tear pattern recognition of the posterosuperior rotator cuff, which allows for anatomic repair and restoration of external rotation strength.
- The subscapularis generates the largest amount of force of any rotator cuff muscle and is generally believed to be the most important single rotator cuff muscle.
- The choice of knotted or knotless repair techniques is based on tissue quality.
- Massive rotator cuff tears are a subset of rotator cuff tears that remain a problematic condition to treat because the force couples are no longer balanced, resulting in an unstable fulcrum of motion and painful dysfunction.
- The Diamondback repair is an enhanced suture bridging repair construct that provides twice as many linked diagonal compression sutures with three times the number of intersection points.
- The load-sharing rip-stop construct is the authors' preferred method for massive rotator cuff repair with poor tissue quality in which a double-row repair is not possible because of limited mobility.

TEAR PATTERN RECOGNITION

One of the major advancements of arthroscopy has been the ability to more thoroughly evaluate rotator cuff tears compared to a traditional open approach. This has led to recognition of four major types of rotator cuff tears: (1) crescent tears, (2) U-shaped tears, (3) L-shaped tears, and (4) massive contracted tears. Recognition of these distinct tear patterns is crucial because the tear pattern dictates the repair pattern. Anatomic reconstruction of the posterosuperior footprint is important to restore external rotation strength and balance force couples, and repairing tears according to their tear pattern can lead to excellent results (Burkhart et al, 2001).

Crescent-shaped tears are the simplest of all tears. These tears have good medial-to-lateral mobility and can be repaired directly to bone with minimal tension. Essentially, all crescent-shaped tears are repaired with a double-row construct.

In contrast, U-shaped rotator cuff tears extend much farther medially. The apex of the tear is usually adjacent to the glenoid rim medially. These tears demonstrate significant mobility in the anterior-to-posterior direction and should be initially repaired in a side-to-side fashion using margin convergence sutures. Failure in recognizing this tear pattern will result in overwhelming tensile stresses if an attempt is made to repair a lateral bone bed. However, sequential medial to lateral suturing of the anterior and posterior leaflets causes the free margin of the rotator cuff to converge toward the bone bed on the humerus. The free margin of the tear is then directly repaired to bone in a tension-free manner. This technique both allows repair of possible irreparable tears and minimizes strain on the repair site (Burkhart et al, 2004).

L-shaped and reverse L-shaped tears have a leaflet that is more mobile than the other leaflet. In these cases, side-to-side suturing along the longitudinal split is required followed by repair to the greater tuberosity bone bed. The use of traction stitches is useful in assisting reduction and repair of these more complex tear patterns.

Massive contracted tears have limited mobility in both the anteroposterior and medial-lateral planes. These tears typically require advanced mobilization techniques such as interval slides to achieve repair. Based on their limited mobility and frequent tendon loss, these are often best addressed with a single-row or load-sharing rip-stop (LSRS) repair.

IMPORTANCE OF THE SUBSCAPULARIS

Although this chapter focuses on posterosuperior tears, one must not neglect the subscapularis tendon. The subscapularis generates the largest amount of force of any rotator cuff muscle and is generally believed to be the most important single rotator cuff muscle because it is the only anterior muscle that can balance the posterior forces of the rotator cuff. In addition, the anterior attachment of the rotator cable extends to the upper subscapularis insertion. Therefore repair of the upper subscapularis decreases the stress on the adjacent repair of the supraspinatus, thereby protecting the supraspinatus repair. After the subscapularis has been repaired, the *comma sign* is very useful in locating the anterolateral corner of the supraspinatus tendon, to which it remains attached. For these reasons, we strongly recommend repairing all subscapularis tears before proceeding with arthroscopic repair of the supraspinatus and infraspinatus tendons.

Surgical Technique: Setup and Preparation

In shoulder arthroscopy, angles and soft tissue and bone preparation play integral parts in anatomic rotator cuff repair.

ANGLE

The angle of visualization is influenced by the position of the patient, the angle of the arthroscope, and the position of the portal the surgeon is viewing through. We perform rotator cuff repairs in the lateral decubitus position. The arm is held in 20 to 30 degrees of abduction combined with 20 degrees of forward flexion with 5 to 10 lb of lateral weight suspended from a standard arthroscopic boom. We palpate the "soft spot" created by the glenoid medially and humeral head laterally and insert the arthroscope below the equator of the glenohumeral joint at about 7 o'clock. We have found that the often-used posterior portal tends to move too superior as soft tissue swelling increases and provides a poor angle of approach to the subacromial space. Therefore we avoid this by placing our skin incision more inferiorly. We also use 30- and 70-degree scopes interchangeably during the case.

BONE-BED PREPARATION

A complete bursectomy is essential in all rotator cuff repair cases for two reasons. First, it is essential to see the entire rotator cuff margin to recognize the tear pattern. This includes removing all bursal leaders that attach to the internal deltoid fascia. We routinely release the internal deltoid fascia to achieve greater freedom for the instruments to move. Second, it removes the pain-generating cytokines that reside in the inflamed bursa in the subacromial space. With bone preparation, it is useful to remove all soft tissues from the greater tuberosity with an electrocautery device and then lightly use a high-speed bur to create a uniformly bleeding bone bed to facilitate healing.

Repair Techniques for Full-Thickness Tears

We strongly believe in restoration of anatomy. Therefore we perform a suture-bridging double-row repair whenever possible. However, the repair must respect the tear mobility and tendon length. A variety of suture-bridging techniques are available. As described further later, we base the choice of knotted and knotless techniques on tissue quality.

SUTURE-BRIDGING DOUBLE-ROW REPAIR

The original double-row repair was described as two independent rows of anchors. The technique has progressed to linking of the medial and lateral row anchors, which has improved biomechanical properties and decreased retear rates (Fig. 7A.1) (Denard et al, 2012a; Lo & Burkhart, 2003)

The tear is initially visualized through a posterior subacromial viewing portal with a 30-degree arthroscope. A 70-degree arthroscope is also often helpful, particularly for lateral row placement. Additionally, the scope may be placed in the lateral viewing portal as necessary to better visualize the posteromedial aspect of the footprint. The medial anchors are placed through separate percutaneous portals. This allows the proper angle of approach and aids in suture management. A threaded double-loaded anchor (5.5-mm BioComposite Corkscrew FT; Arthrex, Naples, FL) is placed anteromedially adjacent to the articular margin and approximately 5 mm posterior the bicipital groove. A second anchor is placed posteromedially.

Medial mattress sutures are then passed with a self-retrieving antegrade suture passer. The mattress sutures should be evenly spaced to prevent suture cut-out. We have a simple way of restoring the normal length–tendon relationship, even in tendon loss, to achieve anatomic repair with normal biomechanics. In the setting of a mobile tear, an anatomic and properly tensioned double-row repair can be obtained if the surgeon passes the medial-row sutures 2 to 3 mm lateral to musculotendinous junction. This always restores proper length–tendon relationship. In the case of tendon loss in which only a single-row repair is possible, anchors are placed slightly lateral to the articular margin. In such cases of single-row repair, the sutures are placed more lateral, 6 to 7 mm from the musculotendinous junction. This allows the musculotendinous junction to be within 2 mm of the articular margin, preventing overtensioning and reducing the probability of retear.

Traditionally, only one suture pair from each anchor is used for the SutureBridge, but the use of the second suture pair may add fixation in poor quality tendons. The mattress sutures are tied with a static six-throw surgeon's knot using a double-diameter knot pusher (Surgeon's Sixth Finger; Arthrex). After each pair is tied, the suture limbs are preserved by retrieving them out the same portal used for anchor insertion. The lateral row is then established by crisscrossing the medial row suture limbs. One limb from each medial row anchor is retrieved out the lateral cannula and the combined suture limbs are secured with two 4.75- or 5.5-mm BioComposite SwiveLock C anchors (Arthrex). The sutures are tensioned through the cannula before inserting the anchor to determine the appropriate location of the lateral anchors. The lateral anchors are placed on the metaphyseal cortex lateral to the "corner" of the greater tuberosity. One anchor is placed anteriorly and another posteriorly. The sutures are cut flush with the anchor for a low-profile knotless lateral repair.

KNOTLESS DOUBLE-ROW ROTATOR CUFF REPAIR

In the setting of good-quality tissue, we use a knotless technique (Video 7A.1). The steps in the repair are essentially the same as previously described. Medial threaded anchors (BioComposite SwiveLock C; Arthrex) preloaded with a 2-mm suture tape (FiberTape; Arthrex) are placed adjacent to the articular margin.

One of two techniques is then used for suture passage depending on the desired construct. The medial anchors have #2 safety sutures in the anchor eyelet that may be incorporated into the repair. We often use these to create a broad double-mattress suture between the two anchors using a double-pulley technique. The suture tape and safety sutures from one anchor are retrieved out the lateral working portal. The free end of a FiberLink suture (Arthrex) is loaded onto an antegrade suture passer and passed through the rotator cuff. The sutures from the anchor are then passed through the opposite end of the FiberLink, which is a closed loop. The free end of the FiberLink is then retrieved out the portal used for anchor placement and used to shuttle the sutures through the rotator cuff. These steps are repeated for the other anchor.

Next one #2 suture from each anchor is retrieved out the lateral portal. A six-throw surgeon's knot is tied over an instrument and limbs are cut. Pulling the opposite limbs of the #2 sutures delivers the knot into the subacromial space so that it rests over one of the anchors. The remaining two #2 suture limbs are then retrieved and tied with a

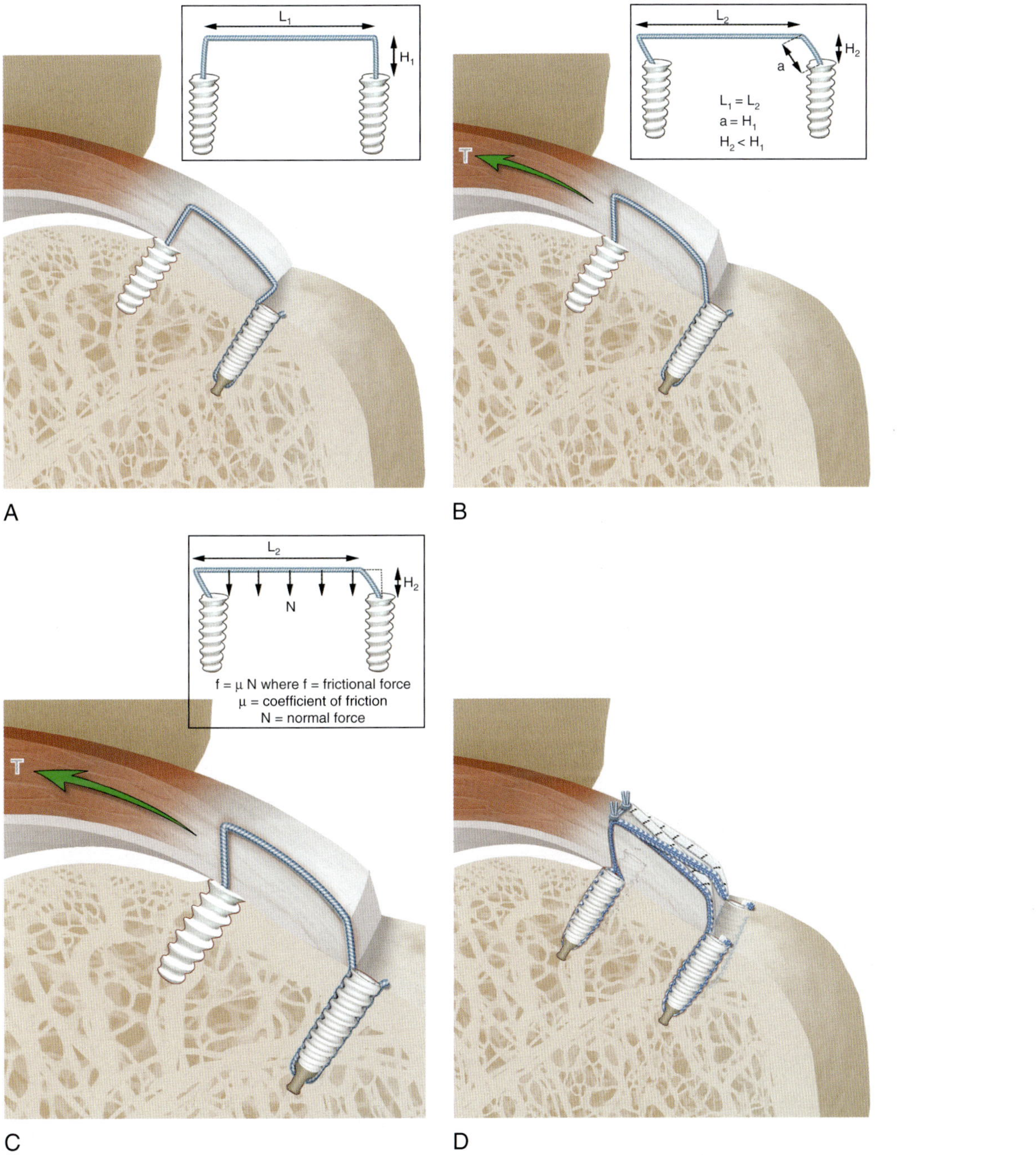

Fig. 7A.1 Schematic of the self-reinforcing suture bridge technique. **A,** Linked double-row construct before loading. *Inset,* Free body diagram of the construct. *H1,* Thickness of rotator cuff before loading; *L1,* length of tendon beneath suture. **B,** Loading of the linked double-row construct results in compression of rotator cuff footprint. *Inset,* Free body diagram of the construct. *a,* Length of suture between tendon edge and lateral anchor; *H2,* thickness of compressed rotator cuff under tensile load; *L2,* length of tendon beneath suture; *T,* tensile loading force. **C,** Up-close view of the linked double-row construct after loading. *Inset,* Free body diagram showing distributed normal force (N) resulting from elastic deformation of tendon beneath the suture. The frictional force (f) increases as the normal force (N) increases under load. **D,** Linked double-row construct with two medial anchors linked to two lateral anchors provides maximal footprint compression under loading. Additionally, a medial double-mattress stitch in this case provides a seal to joint fluid. (Reprinted with permission from Burkhart SS, Lo IK, Brady PC, Denard PJ. *The Cowboy's Companion.* Philadelphia: Lippincott Williams & Wilkins, 2012.)

static knot (a sliding knot cannot be used since the previous knot prevents sliding) over the opposite anchor. This medial double-mattress creates a medial seal between the rotator cuff and the glenohumeral joint.

Before lateral fixation, the tendon repair is assessed for dog ears. The same FiberLink used for shuttling can be used to create cinch loops at the anterior and posterior margins of the tear to reduce dog ears and reinforce the rotator cable attachments. Finally, the suture tape limbs (and dog-ear sutures if placed) are crisscrossed and secured laterally with two knotless anchors as previously described (Figs. 7A.2 and 7A.3).

If tissue quality is excellent, a completely knotless technique can be used. In this setting, the medial #2 safety sutures are removed and the suture tapes alone are passed through the rotator cuff in the standard fashion. Because the limbs of these tapes come prewedged into a single limb at the end of the suture, a shuttling technique is not required in this case.

Massive Tears

Massive rotator cuff tears are a subset of rotator cuff tears that remain a problematic condition to treat. With a significant tear, the force couples are no longer balanced, resulting in an unstable fulcrum of motion and painful dysfunction. However, not all tears will result in an unstable fulcrum. This is because many tears occur in the avascular crescent region of the posterior rotator cuff (e.g., supraspinatus tendon and anterior half of the infraspinatus tendon). Enclosed within the arc of the rotator cable is the classical crescent region of the rotator cuff, which is the area where the majority of tears begin. When a tear begins in this region, the muscle exerts its force on the humeral head through the rotator cable in much the same way that a suspension bridge exerts its force through a distributed load from its cable to its columns. Because of this preserved function, most tears that are contained within the rotator cable region still have a stable fulcrum, allowing for preserved motion and minimal strength

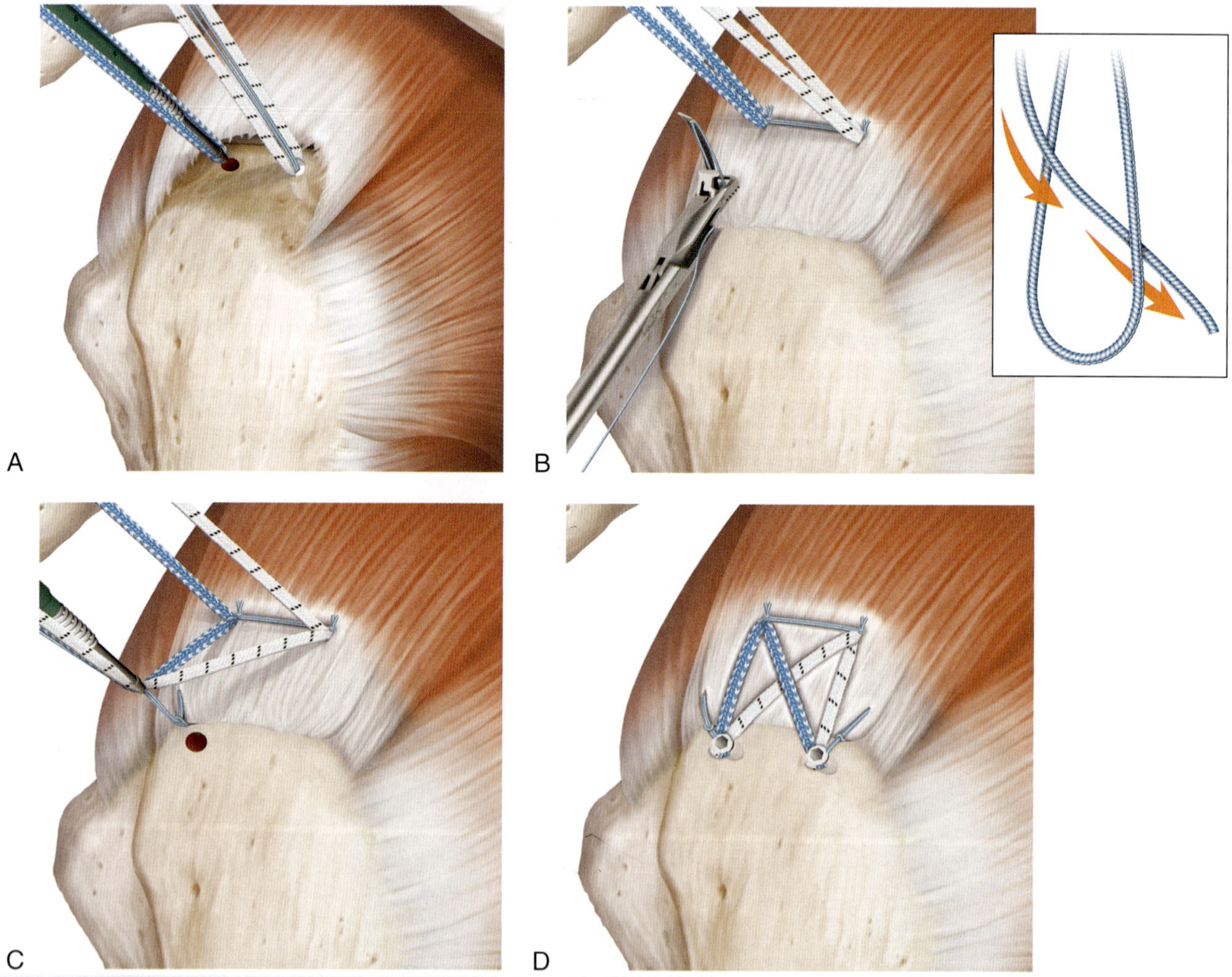

Fig. 7A.2 Schematic of a SpeedBridge (Arthrex, Naples, FL) rotator cuff repair with medial double-pulley and dog-ear reduction. **A,** Two medial anchors are placed for a SpeedBridge repair **B,** Medial sutures are passed through the rotator cuff in a single pass using a FiberLink (Arthrex). Then a mattress stitch is tied between the two anchors using the #2 FiberWire Eyelet safety stitches with a double-pulley technique. The FiberLink can then be used for dog-ear reduction. The closed end of the FiberLink is passed through the rotator cuff at the margin of the tear and is retrieved out the same portal as used for insertion. *Inset,* Extracorporeally, the closed end of the FiberLink is passed through the looped end to create a cinch loop. **C,** The cinch loop, a suture from the anteromedial anchor, and a suture from the posteromedial anchor are secured laterally with a BioComposite SwivelLock C anchor. **D,** Final appearance after placement of a posterior FiberLink and a posterolateral anchor. (This image provided courtesy of Arthrex, Inc.)

deficits. Conversely, tears that extended through the rotator cable attachments usually result in an unstable fulcrum, with loss of strength and the possible development of pseudoparalysis (Denard et al, 2012b).

INTERVAL SLIDES AND OTHER ADVANCED MOBILIZATION TECHNIQUES

Although partial rotator cuff repairs have been shown to work very well with regard to improving pain and function in the short term, a complete anatomic rotator cuff repair is desirable, particularly in younger patients. In two separate studies, Denard et al (2012c, 2015) showed that an anatomic repair of a massive rotator cuff tear is possible even in the setting of pseudoparalysis and results in restoration of the cable region with resultant improvement in function in 90% of cases or greater. It is critical to exhaust all efforts to mobilize the rotator cuff in the medial to lateral and anterior to posterior planes based on the tear pattern. Most massive rotator cuff tears may be reparable without releases after properly evaluating for the natural mobility. One of the keys in repairing massive tears is to first address and repair the subscapularis tendon, which is torn in the majority of massive rotator cuff tears. We also perform a limited subacromial decompression that preserves the coracoacromial arch. The other major key to success is to excavate the tendon and bursal leaders. This requires visualization of the scapular spine and clearing of the posterolateral gutter. While viewing through the lateral portal using a combination of motorized shaver and cautery placed through the posterior portal, the scapular spine is exposed. Bouncing the shaver off the scapular spine to enter the space ensures protection of the underlying rotator cuff. The scapular spine is a keel-shaped structure that delineates the interval between the supraspinatus and the infraspinatus tendons. Work can then be carried laterally to safely remove bursal leaders or false cuff that inserts on the deltoid.

The need for interval slides is based on the mobility of the rotator cuff tendon margins. When a tear has been determined to be irreparable despite standard releases, interval slides should be considered to improve mobility. The decision is based on a number of factors, including patient age, symptoms, tissue quality, and initial tear mobility. This is particularly relevant in patients with greater than 50% fatty atrophy on magnetic resonance imaging (Burkhart et al, 2012).

Two slides are relevant to repairs of the posterior rotator cuff: the anterior interval slide in continuity and the posterior interval slide. The anterior interval slide is a release of the anterior leading edge of the supraspinatus tendon from the rotator interval. Our preferred method (anterior interval slide in continuity) is to use an electrocautery to release the coracohumeral ligament from the base of the coracoid while preserving the comma tissue (Lo & Burkhart, 2004). This preserves the tissue adjacent to the anterior leading edge of the subscapularis. The anterior interval slide typically provides an additional 1 cm of excursion, and we use this in nearly all massive tears. The release is typically done while viewing with a 70-degree arthroscope through a posterior portal and working through an anterosuperolateral portal.

In contrast, the posterior slide is a release of the posterior edge of the supraspinatus from the infraspinatus. Our experience has been that the posterior interval slide provides more mobility than the anterior interval slide, with up to 4 cm of increased excursion noted after performing the slide. The posterior interval slide is performed while viewing through a lateral portal with a 30-degree arthroscope or from a posterior portal while viewing with a 70-degree arthroscope. Traction stitches are placed in the supraspinatus and infraspinatus tendons. A spinal needle is used to identify the correct angle approach in line with the posterior interval and toward the scapular spine. An arthroscopic scissor is then introduced and begins the posterior interval slide along the lateral margin of the rotator cuff directing the tendon incision toward the base of the scapular spine. The release is continued toward the scapular spine until the perineural fat pad lateral to the spine is encountered. This identifies the proximity of the suprascapular nerve. With an isolated posterior interval slide only, the mobility of the infraspinatus tendon is usually sufficiently improved to permit for repair

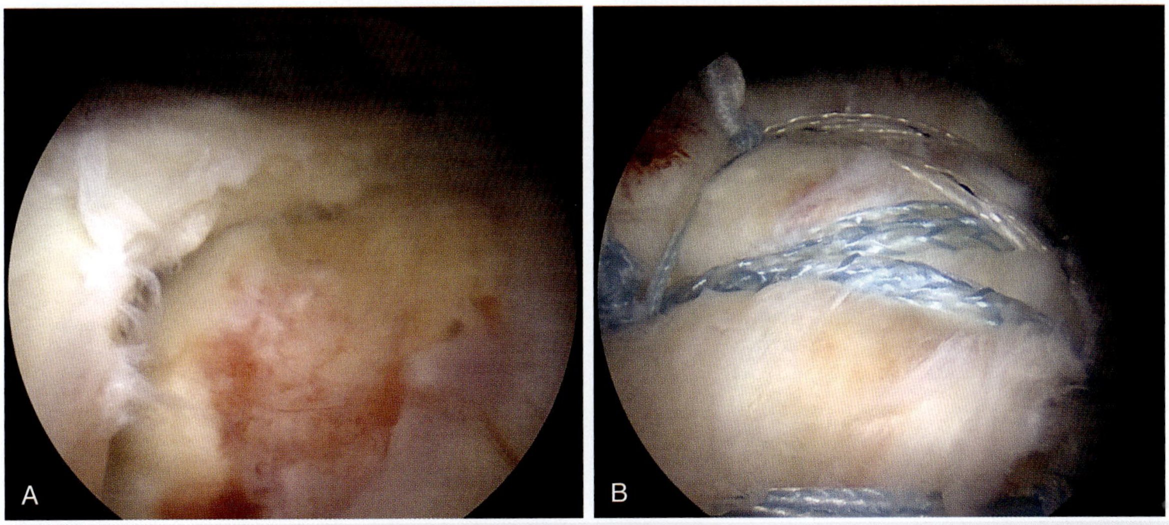

Fig. 7A.3 A, Right shoulder, posterior subacromial viewing portal demonstrating a crescent-type full-thickness posterosuperior rotator cuff tear. **B,** Right shoulder, posterior subacromial viewing portal demonstrating SpeedBridge (Arthrex, Naples, FL) rotator cuff repair with medial double-pulley and dog-ear reduction. (This image provided courtesy of Arthrex, Inc.)

to bone. After repair of the tendon to bone, the separation between the supraspinatus and infraspinatus is closed with margin convergence sutures, which reduces strain, thereby protecting the tendon–bone repair interface during critical phases of healing.

DIAMONDBACK REPAIR

The repair pattern must be adapted to the tear pattern. As such, in the setting of a large uncovered footprint from anterior to posterior, additional lateral or medial anchors may be placed as needed. One adaptation is the Diamondback repair. This repair was developed by the senior author (SSB) as an enhanced suture bridging repair construct that provides twice as many linked diagonal compression sutures with three times the number of intersection points.

Two medial double-loaded anchors (5.5-mm BioComposite Corkscrew FT; Arthrex) are placed just lateral to the articular margin in the fashion described previously for the knotted suture-bridging technique. All eight suture limbs are passed in a mattress fashion 2 to 3 mm lateral to the musculotendinous junction. The four central limbs are used in a double-pulley technique to create broad double-mattress sutures. The first two suture limbs are cut short, but the tails of the second pair are preserved. Mattress sutures are tied with the anterior-most two limbs and repeated posteriorly. A total of 3 BioComposite SwiveLock C anchors are placed laterally accepting two suture limbs for each SwiveLock in a crisscross fashion creating a diamondback pattern of repair. Biomechanical testing of the diamondback configuration demonstrated the highest initial footprint contact area and lowest decrease in contact pressure over time when compared with single- and double-row repairs (Burkhart et al, 2012)

LOAD-SHARING RIP-STOP TECHNIQUE FOR MASSIVE ROTATOR CUFF REPAIR

A Load-Sharing Rip-Stop technique (LSRS) technique was developed by the authors that combines the advantages of a wide rip-stop suture tape and load-sharing properties of a double-row repair (Denard et al, 2012a). Ma et al (2004) demonstrated that a rip-stop suture with a double-loaded anchor had load to failure equivalent to a modified Mason-Allen stitch. This construct is particularly useful for cases in which there is limited medial tendon that precludes a standard double-row repair.

While viewing through a posterior portal, a FiberTape suture is passed through the rotator cuff as an inverted mattress stitch placed 3 mm lateral to the musculotendinous junction. If the tear has a large anterior-to-posterior dimension, then a second FiberTape may be placed in similar fashion. The limbs are retrieved out of an accessory portal. These rip-stop suture tapes must not be tensioned and repaired to bone until after the sutures from the medial anchors have been passed circumferentially around them.

Next, two double-loaded 5.5-mm anchors are placed anteromedially and posteromedially along the articular margin. Beginning posteriorly, the sutures are passed from the medial anchors as simple stiches that penetrate the rotator cuff medial to the rip-stop suture. After the medial sutures are passed, the FiberTape rip-stop sutures are retrieved from an accessory portal and secured laterally with two knotless suture anchors, making sure they encircle the sutures from the medial anchors.

Finally, simple sutures from the medial anchors are retrieved, and static knots are tied. It is important to delay knot tying until after the rip-stop stitch is secured laterally. This is done for two reasons. First, it is important to have a firm, taut rip stop. Second, the FiberTape serves to unload the medial sutures because the rip-stop construct is secured laterally to an anchor.

Burkhart et al (2014) were the first to report a biomechanical study of an LSRS construct for repair of tissue-deficient rotator cuff tears. The mean load to failure for LSRS was nearly twice that for a single-row repair construct. The LSRS construct is the authors' preferred method for massive rotator cuff repair with poor tissue quality in which a double-row repair is not possible because of limited mobility.

References

Burkhart SS, Danaceau SM, Pearce CE. Arthroscopic rotator cuff repair: analysis of results by tear size and repair technique-margin convergence versus direct tendon to bone repair. *Arthroscopy*. 2001;17:905–912.

Burkhart SS, Denard PJ, Obopilwe E, Mazzoca AD. Optimizing pressurized contact area in rotator cuff repair: the diamondback repair. *Arthroscopy*. 2012;28(2):188–195.

Burkhart SS, Barth JR, Richards DP, Zlatkin B, Larsen M. Arthroscopic repair of massive rotator cuff tears with stage 3 and 4 fatty degeneration. *Arthroscopy*. 2007;23(4):347–354.

Burkhart SS, Denard PJ, Konicek J, Hanypsiak BT. Biomechanical validation of load sharing rip stop fixation for the repair of tissue deficit rotator cuff tears. *Am J Sports Med*. 2014;42(2):457–462.

Burkhart SS. The principle of margin convergence in rotator cuff repair as a means of strain reduction at the tear margin. *Ann Biomed Eng*. 2004;32(1):166–170.

Denard PJ, Burkhart SS. A load sharing rip stop fixation construct for arthroscopic rotator cuff repair. *Arthrosc Tech*. 2012;15(1):37–42.

Denard PJ, Jiwani AZ, Ladermann A, Burkhart SS. Long term outcome of arthroscopic massive rotator cuff repair: the importance of double row fixation. *Arthroscopy*. 2012a;28(7):909–915.

Denard PJ, Koo SS, Murena L, Burkhart SS. Pseudoparalysis: the importance of the rotator cable integrity. *Orthopaedics*. 2012b;35(9):1353–1357.

Denard PJ, Ladermann A, Brady PC, et al. Pseudoparalysis from a massive rotator cuff tear is reliably reversed with an arthroscopic rotator cuff repair in patients without preoperative glenohumeral arthritis. *Am J Sports Med*. 2015;43(10):2373–2378.

Denard PJ, Ladermann A, Jiwani AZ, Burkhart SS. Functional outcome after arthroscopic repair of massive rotator cuff tears in individual with pseudoparalysis. *Arthroscopy*. 2012c;28(9):1214–1219.

Lo IK, Burkhart SS. Arthroscopic repair of massive, contracted, immobile rotator cuff tears using single and double interval slides: technique and preliminary results. *Arthroscopy*. 2004;20(1).

Lo IK, Burkhart SS. Double row arthroscopic rotator cuff repair: re-establishing the footprint of the rotator cuff. *Arthroscopy*. 2003;19(9):1035–1042.

Ma CB, MacGillivray JD, Clabeaux J. Biomechanical of arthroscopic rotator cuff stitches. *J Bone Joint Surg Am*. 2004;86:1211–1216.

7-7B OUTCOMES

BRIAN C. LAU, MD; ALAN L. ZHANG, MD; and C. BENJAMIN MA, MD

Introduction

- The diagnosis and surgical management of posterior rotator cuff tears have evolved over the past several decades. Improved imaging protocols, in particular magnetic resonance imaging (MRI), have enhanced our characterization of size and tear pattern (Davidson & Burkhart, 2010; Lansdown & Feeley, 2012).
- Improved techniques have expanded surgical treatment to include open, mini-open, and all-arthroscopic techniques.
- Efforts to study and determine outcomes have also seen the development of new tools to assess repairs including ultrasonography, MRI, and patient-reported outcome measures (PROMs) (Makhni et al, 2015).
- To critically assess the literature and determine optimal treatments, a thorough understanding of outcomes measurements must first be achieved.

PATIENT-REPORTED OUTCOMES

A study by Makhni et al (2015) reviewed 156 studies that evaluated rotator repair outcomes and found significant variability exists in outcomes reporting. The type of validated PROMs usage ranged greatly between 16% and 61%. Constant-Murley (Constant) score was the most frequently used in 61% of studies, the American Shoulder and Elbow Surgeons (ASES) score was the second most used at 59%, the University of California Los Angeles (UCLA) shoulder rating scale was the third most used at 35%, and the Simple Shoulder Test (SST) was the fourth most used at 28%. The Constant score was developed in 1986 and is a summative scale that provides a global score based on weighted measures of physical impairments in range of motion (ROM) and strength along with patient reported pain and activity limitation (Constant & Murley, 1987). The distinguishing part of the Constant score from other PROMs is that 65% of the final score is based on an objective component scored by a health professional. The Constant score also allows for age- and sex-related changes in the musculoskeletal system by converting the absolute score to a relative score to adjust for age and sex (Constant & Murley, 1987). The UCLA shoulder rating scale was developed in 1981 and is also a combination of physical examination findings (active forward elevation and strength) and subjective patient-reported measures (pain, satisfaction, and function) with a higher score indicating better function (Amstutz et al, 1981). The distinguishing part of the UCLA score is that it preferentially weighs the subjective component (Amstutz et al, 1981). Similarly, the ASES contains a physician and patient-rated component; however, only the patient-reported subjective pain visual analog scale and 10 functional questions are typically used to tabulate the reported ASES score (Richards et al, 1994). The total score is evenly weighted between 50% pain and 50% function (Richards et al, 1994). The SST relies solely on patient-subjective data and is composed of 12 yes-or-no questions (Lippitt et al, 1993). Several studies appeared in fewer than 4% to 10% of all studies, including the Penn Shoulder Score, L'Insalata/Shoulder Rating Questionnaire, Shoulder Pain and Disability Index, Rotator Cuff-Quality of Life, EuroQol-5D, Shoulder Activity Scale, Marx Activity Scale, Korean Shoulder Score, and Rowe score, making it difficult to assess their utility (Makhni et al, 2015) (Table 7B.1).

IMAGING ASSESSMENT

Tendon integrity and retear rates were evaluated with MRI in 38% and ultrasonography in 31% of studies (Makhni et al, 2015). The accuracy of these measures has been assessed in preoperative characterization of rotator cuff tears. In preoperative preimaging, MRI and ultrasonography have been shown to have similar sensitivity in rotator cuff diagnosis (90.4% and 92%, respectively) (de Jesus et al, 2009). Postoperatively, however, the characterization of the rotator cuff and accuracy of detecting a tear become more difficult because of surgical changes and placement of hardware. Motamedi et al (2002) determined a 91% sensitivity but a 25% specificity of a musculoskeletal radiologist diagnosing a recurrent rotator cuff after repair with MRI and cautioned at the high false-positive rate. Recent literature evaluated the interobserver agreement among seven fellowship-trained orthopaedic shoulder surgeons on MRI and determined that recurrent full-thickness tears had moderate agreement of 80%, but characterization of partial tears, rotator cuff footprint coverage, biceps tendon tear, bone marrow edema, and cyst formation had poor reliability (Khazzam et al, 2012). Given the high costs of MRI, ultrasonography has been increasingly used for postoperative evaluation of rotator cuff repairs (Fig. 7B.1). A recent prospective, multicenter study identified that ultrasonography had an 85% concordance with MRI for detecting a recurrent rotator cuff tear (Codsi et al, 2014).

LENGTH OF FOLLOW-UP

Length of follow-up is another consideration when evaluating outcome studies in rotator cuff repairs. Short-term refers to follow-up of 2 years and long-term follow-up at 10 or more years. Short-term follow-up allows assessment of time to return to function and early pain relief. Long-term follow-up allows assessment of the durability of repairs.

Outcomes for Conservative versus Operative Treatment

Conservative treatment including physiotherapy is a mainstay of early care for rotator cuff tears. However,

Table 7B.1 Patient-Reported Outcome Measures

Patient-Reported Measure	Percentage Used in Literature*	Defining Characteristic
Constant-Murley (Constant)	61	Score combined patient subjective and physician objective with 65% based on Physician Objective component
American Shoulder and Elbow Surgeons (ASES)	59	Combination of patient subjective and physician objective but only patient-subjective data are used in generating the score with 50% based on pain and function
University of California Los Angeles (UCLA) Shoulder Rating	35	Score combines patient subjective and physician objective with 57% based on Patient Subjective component
Simple Shoulder Test	28	Patient-subjective component only with 12 yes/no questions

*Many studies used multiple outcome scores.
Based on Makhni EC, Steinhaus ME, Morrow ZS, et al. Outcomes assessment in rotator cuff pathology: what are we measuring? *J Shoulder Elbow Surg.* 2015;24(12):2008-2015.

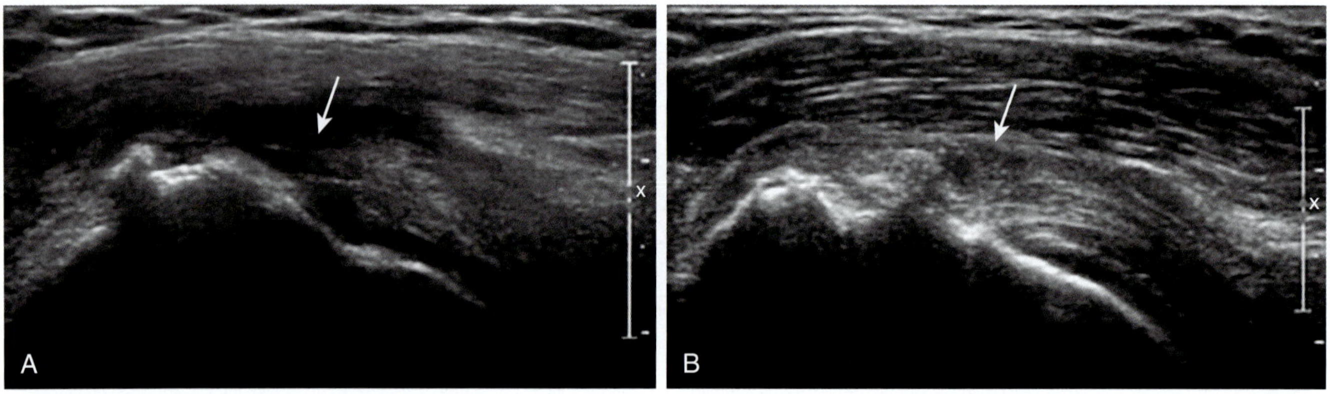

Fig. 7B.1 Ultrasound examination after rotator cuff repair. Images from a 63-year-old woman with a near full-thickness defect 5 weeks after surgery, mimicking a retear. **A,** Longitudinal sonogram 5 weeks after surgery shows a hypoechoic area within the repaired tendon *(arrow)*. **B,** This area *(arrow)* gradually improved on follow-up sonography 6 months after surgery. (From Yoo HJ, Choi JY, Hong SH, et al. Assessment of the postoperative appearance of the rotator cuff tendon using serial sonography after arthroscopic repair of a rotator cuff tear. *J Ultrasound Med* 2015;34 1183-1190.)

there has been a trend toward surgical rotator cuff repair with a rise of the incidence of rotator cuff repairs over the past decade by 238% (Ensor et al, 2013). Both treatments have possible side effects, including risks associated with surgery such as infection and postoperative stiffness for surgical repairs versus progression of tears with physiotherapy alone. There have been several recent cohort and randomized studies directly comparing the two treatment options that support an initial trial of physical therapy.

The MOON Shoulder Group evaluated 452 patients in a prospective cohort study and treated patients with atraumatic full-thickness rotator cuff tears with a directed physical therapy program. At follow-up visits, patients who were not satisfied with their responses to physical therapy were allowed to convert to surgical treatment. Patients elected to convert to surgical fixation less than 25% of the time, and most did so within the first 6 to 12 weeks of treatment (Kuhn et al, 2013).

Moosmayer et al (2014) randomized 103 patients with rotator cuffs smaller than 3 cm into primary repair (open or mini-open) or physiotherapy alone and found that patients who underwent primary repair had statistically significant improved results in ASES and Constant scores compared with physiotherapy alone. However, this was at or near the minimally clinically significant important difference. The study also found that in 37% of patients treated with physiotherapy alone, there was progression of tear size that was associated with inferior outcomes. In the physiotherapy treatment group, nearly a quarter of patients converted to the repair group with the majority choosing to convert within the first year. In the patients who underwent secondary repair, there were no significant differences in ASES or Constant scores at 5 years. The authors suggest that a primary trial of physiotherapy is supported in most patients with small to medium tears (Moonsmayer et al, 2014).

Lambers et al (2015) randomized 56 patients with degenerative tears to a physiotherapy-only group and a surgical repair with mini-open technique group and found no difference in Constant scores. There was; however, a difference in pain and disability in favor of surgical treatment. Of note, at 1 year postoperatively, 73.7% of surgically repaired patients demonstrated retear of the rotator cuff. In a subgroup analysis, patients who had a retear after surgical repair did not have any significant difference with the physiotherapy group only (Lambers et al, 2015).

BOTTOM LINE

- Conservative treatment is an effective initial option for rotator cuff tears.
- Patients who fail conservative treatment tend to convert to operative treatment early in physical therapy treatment.
- Delayed operative fixation after initial trial of conservative management has similar outcomes to initial operative fixation.
- Older patients with degenerative tears have improved pain and disability with surgical repair despite high retear rates.

Outcomes for Rotator Cuff Repair Based on Tear Thickness

FULL-THICKNESS TEARS

Full-thickness tears include involvement of all fibers in a superior-to-inferior direction, from the bursal side to the articular side. Repair techniques of full-thickness tears have been extensively studied and have demonstrated good to excellent PROMs, quality of life, and tendon integrity regardless of whether open, mini-open, or all arthroscopic techniques have been used.

Outcomes after open repair of full-thickness rotator cuffs identified that 88% of patients had good to excellent Constant scores and that all patients who were gainfully employed before surgery returned to employment after surgery (Iannotti et al, 1996). In a randomized study comparing open repairs with mini-open repairs, there was improved early quality of life in the mini-open group up to 3 months postoperatively; however, in subsequent follow-ups, there was no difference in ROM or PROMs (Mohtadi et al, 2008).

FIXATION CONFIGURATION

All arthroscopic repairs also have demonstrated good to excellent functional outcome whether using a suture-bridge or double-row technique (Kim et al, 2012a; Mihata et al, 2011). Kim et al (2012a) evaluated 52 consecutive rotator cuff tears; at 2 years, the study identified significant improvement in Constant, ASES, and UCLA scores. Mihata et al (2011) compared single-row, double-row, and combined double-row and suture-bridge repairs in full-thickness rotator cuff tears and found retear rates of 10.8%, 26.1%, and 4.7%, respectively. They suggested that the combination of double-row with suture-bridge techniques may be beneficial. A randomized study of 86 patients with full-thickness all-arthroscopic repair identified similar ASES and quality of life indices with or without acromioplasty; however, 9% (4 of 45) patients without acromioplasty required reoperation versus none in the acromioplasty group (MacDonald et al, 2011). Regarding the durability of an arthroscopic repair, a recent study of 59 patients with 1-year and 10-year follow-up after full-thickness arthroscopic repair demonstrated that improvements in ASES scores and ROM over that time period were retained (Mihata et al, 2011).

Bottom Line

- Full-thickness tears have good to excellent short- and long-term outcomes after surgical repair.
- A combination of double-row with suture-bridge techniques may be beneficial.
- Concurrent acromioplasty may help prevent reoperation but does not affect ROM or PROMs.

PARTIAL-THICKNESS TEARS

Partial-thickness tears can be divided into articular- or bursal-sided tears. There are two main approaches to repair of partial-thickness tears, including debridement and transtendon repair, to prevent progression or conversion to full-thickness tear followed by more traditional repair. Proponents of transtendon repair suggest that the maintenance of the intact rotator cuff tissues may strengthen the repair, but some authors suggest that transtendon repair may lead to stiffness (Huberty et al, 2009; Lo & Burkhart, 2004). It is common practice to use 50% thickness as an indicator of supporting one particular management approach over another (Bollier & Shea, 2012; Strauss et al, 2011).

A recent study by Ranalletta et al (2016) evaluated articular-sided partial tears at 2 years from arthroscopic debridement and transtendon repair and found average improvement of 31.7 on the ASES and 17.9 on the UCLA score with 92.5% of patients reporting satisfaction with results. Despite concerns for increased stiffness, only 5 patients developed postoperative adhesive capsulitis, and all responded well to physical therapy.

A number of studies that directly compared transtendon repair with completion of tears with repair have found no significant difference in functional outcomes. Franceschi et al (2013) prospectively compared arthroscopic transtendon repair with arthroscopic full-thickness conversion and repair and found no differences in functional outcome, return to sports, and retear rates. Castagna et al (2015) also prospectively randomized patients into one of the two repair groups and concluded satisfactory functional improvement and pain resolution with no significant difference between groups. These studies also found no significant difference in postoperative stiffness between treatment groups.

Several studies comparing partial-thickness tears based on the 50% thickness criteria also found no significant difference between treatment groups. A prospectively randomized study between transtendon repair and conversion to full-thickness and repair in partial rotator cuff tears greater than 50% thickness concluded there was no difference in functional improvements, PROMs, or pain relief (Shin, 2012) (Fig. 7B.2). In an evaluation between articular- and bursal-sided tears exceeding 50% thickness, there was no significant difference in PROMs. There was, however, an increase in retear rate in the conversion and repair group for bursal-sided tears but no difference in articular-sided tears (Kim et al, 2015). Other studies comparing articular- and bursal-sided tears identified similar improvement in PROMs and functional outcomes with greater trend toward retears in bursal-sided tears compared with articular-sided tears in the conversion of tear and repair (Kim et al, 2014; Koh et al, 2011).

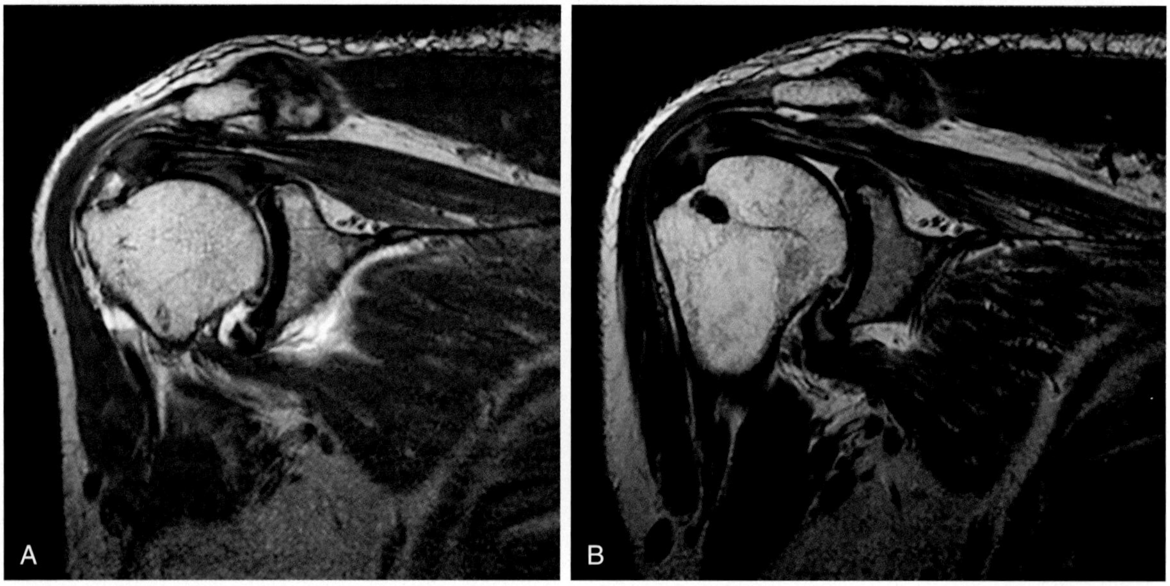

Fig. 7B.2 Articular-sided tears on magnetic resonance images before and after repair. **A,** Preoperative oblique coronal T2-weighted image shows that more than 50% of tendon thickness was torn on the articular surface of the supraspinatus tendon. **B,** Postoperative oblique coronal T2-weighted image shows normal tendon integrity with continuity and sufficient thickness of the tendon. Granulation tissue was observed filling the preoperative tendon defect area in the supraspinatus. (From Shin SJ. A comparison of 2 repair techniques for partial-thickness articular-sided rotator cuff tears. *Arthroscopy.* 2012;28(1):25-33.)

Bottom Line

- There are two techniques for partial cuff tears: (1) transtendon repair and (2) completion of tear and then repair.
- PROMs, rate of stiffness, and return to sport are similar between repair techniques.
- In partial bursal tears that exceed 50%, there may be an increase in retear rate with completion of the tear and then repair.

Outcomes Based on Tear Size

Tear size is measured in the anteroposterior dimension and has been evaluated as a possible predictor of outcome. Small is defined as smaller than 1 cm, medium as less than 3 cm, large as less than 5 cm, and massive as larger than 5 cm.

Outcomes for small to medium-sized tears repaired all-arthroscopically with and without acromioplasty demonstrated excellent ROM and average ASES and Constant scores (Shin et al, 2012). Although studies suggest that there may not be a difference between small and medium tears, several studies show that large and massive tears have lower healing rates and higher retear rates after rotator cuff repair. Failure rates after arthroscopic repair of large or massive rotator cuff tears have been reported to range from 34% to 94% depending on various series (Galatz et al, 2004). There is also a high retear rate as demonstrated in a recent systematic review of massive rotator cuff tears by Henry et al (2015) of 18 studies and pooled data that demonstrated a 79% retear rate. Gulotta et al (2011) through the rotator cuff registry of all-arthroscopic repairs found that predictors of rotator cuff defect at 5 years postoperatively were larger size of preoperative tear (odds ratio [OR], 1.72), and multiple tendon involvement (OR 5.56). Poor tendon healing is also associated with poorer outcomes (Namdari et al, 2014).

Interestingly, despite poor healing and high retear rates of large and massive tears, functional outcomes and return to daily activities have been generally good after repairs and not correlated to postoperative radiographic defects (Chung et al, 2013; Galatz et al, 2004; Gulotta et al, 2011). Burkhart et al (2001) followed 59 patients (3 small tears, 31 medium tears, 12 large tears, and 13 massive tears) who underwent mini-open or all-arthroscopic repair and found that good to excellent UCLA, visual analog scale pain score, and ROM in 95% of cases. A possible explanation is that despite residual rotator cuff tendon defect or recurrent defect, there is enhancement in overall tendon integrity, resulting in functional improvement but not to the degree of smaller tears that have complete healing and tendon integrity at follow-up.

BOTTOM LINE

- Small and medium tears have excellent functional outcomes and healing rates with low retear rates.
- Large and massive tears have poor healing and high retear rates.
- Large and massive tears may still have good functional and patient-reported outcomes and still benefit from repair.

Outcomes Based on Fatty Infiltration and Muscle Atrophy

As rotator cuff tears become larger than 5 cm (massive), there is an association with muscle fatty infiltration and atrophy. Two components that may lead to development of these changes appear to be unloading of the muscle–tendon unit and denervation of the muscle. Clinically, these changes have been found to be irreversible and correlated with poor functional outcomes following repair (Gladstone et al, 2007; Shen et al, 2008).

Fatty infiltration, as described by Goutallier et al. (1994), uses degree of fat (grade 0 to 4) as seen on CT within a muscle: grade 0 no fat; grade 1 thin streaks of fat; grade 2, less fat than muscle; grade 3, equal amounts fat and muscle; and grade 4, more fat than muscle and has been validated on T1-weighted MRI by several groups (Lippe et al, 2012; Schiefer et al, 2015; Slabaugh et al, 2012). Muscle atrophy is described based on a scale proposed by Warner et al (2001) and is described as none, mild, moderate, or severe based on the oblique sagittal MRI.

Outcomes after rotator cuff repair with preoperative fatty infiltration and muscle atrophy have a strong correlation with worse outcomes on ASES, Constant, and strength (Gladstone et al, 2007; Shen et al, 2008). Furthermore, atrophy and fatty infiltration progressed despite repair, and in cases with retear, the progression was found to be worse (Gladstone et al, 2007). Goutallier et al (2003) in a series of 220 shoulders determined that there was a greater likelihood for retear at 3 years if the degree of fatty infiltration was 2 or greater. The study also found that fatty infiltration of the infraspinatus and subscapularis muscle had an influence on the supraspinatus tendon outcome.

The role of fatty infiltration and atrophy of the teres minor without tear but with tears of the supraspinatus and infraspinatus has demonstrated similar outcomes with SST and ASES scores (Kim et al, 2016). Moreover, there was no significant change in fatty infiltration of the teres minor muscle after repair (Kim et al, 2016) (Fig. 7B.3).

Although patients with fatty infiltration and rotator cuff atrophy have lower rates of healing and greater retear rates, they may still benefit from rotator cuff repair. Outcomes in Goutallier grade 3 or 4 fatty degeneration reported improvement in ROM, UCLA, and Constant scores (Burkhart et al, 2007). Additionally, successful repair of the rotator cuff appears to prevent progression of fatty infiltration and muscle atrophy, but those with retears develop significant progression (Liem et al, 2007).

BOTTOM LINE

- Preoperative fatty infiltration and rotator cuff atrophy are associated with worse functional outcomes and are irreversible.
- Outcomes from repair of supraspinatus tears may be affected by fatty infiltration of infraspinatus and subscapularis.
- Fatty infiltration of the teres minor muscle may not appear to affect outcomes in supraspinatus and infraspinatus tears.
- Patients with significant fatty infiltration and atrophy may still benefit from repair.

Outcomes Based on Tear Pattern

Tears may also be classified by their pattern or shape; common descriptions are crescent, U shaped, or L shaped. Crescent-shaped tears are the most common and account for 40% of tears; they are characterized by direct avulsion from the greater tuberosity without extension into the rotator interval (Sallay et al, 2007). U-shaped tears account for 15% of all tears and are characterized by farther medial extension toward the glenoid than crescent-shaped tears (Sallay et al, 2007). L-shaped tears account for approximately 30% of all tears and are described as having both transverse and longitudinal components (Sallay et al, 2007). Various repair techniques may include tendon–bone repair, marginal convergence, or interval slides.

Burkhart et al (2001) evaluated crescent tear repaired with direct tendon-to-bone and U-shaped tears repaired by marginal convergence and found comparable results in UCLA outcome scores and ROM and concluded that tear pattern and repair technique did not influence outcome. A recent study by Park et al (2014) found similar findings in a cohort of L-shaped and U-shaped tears that underwent all-arthroscopic

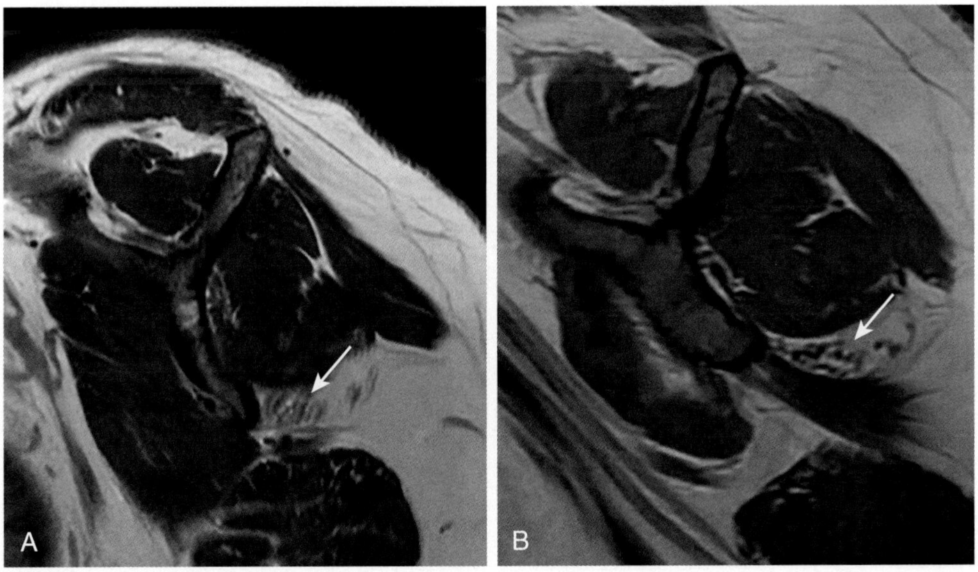

Fig. 7B.3 Teres minor fatty infiltration. Preoperative (**A**) and postoperative (**B**) T1-weighted oblique sagittal magnetic resonance images (right shoulder) of a 53-year-old female patient. The patient had a supraspinatus tear with minimal retraction (5 mm). Severe fatty infiltration (FI) could be observed preoperatively in the teres minor *(arrow)*. FI of the teres minor did not recover after successful rotator cuff repair. (From Kim JK, Yoo HJ, Jeong JH, Kim SH. Effect of teres minor fatty infiltration on rotator cuff repair outcomes. *Arthroscopy*. 2016; 32(4):552-558.)

repair and also demonstrated similar retear rates among tear shapes. The authors suggested that arthroscopic repair yielded substantial improvements in shoulder function regardless of tear pattern (Park et al, 2014).

BOTTOM LINE

- There are good to excellent patient-reported and functional outcomes regardless of tear pattern.
- There are similar retear rates between crescent- and U-shaped tears.

Outcomes for Open versus Mini-Open versus Arthroscopic Repair

Traditional repair of rotator cuffs involved open repair, but as arthroscopic techniques improved, rotator cuff repair evolved to include mini-open and subsequently all-arthroscopic repairs (Zhang et al, 2013a). Many studies have demonstrated that all repair types have good to excellent outcomes.

Outcomes between open and mini-open repair in a randomized clinical trial demonstrated no significant difference with PROMs, quality of life, and functional outcomes from 6 months to 1 and 2 years (Mohtadi et al, 2008). Similarly, in a randomized trial between mini-open and all-arthroscopic repairs, there was no difference in pain level, ROM, or complications after 5 days postoperatively (Cho et al, 2012). Interestingly, all-arthroscopic patients had lower pain visual analog scales at days 1 and 2 and less analgesic use throughout recovery compared with patients undergoing mini-open repair (Cho et al, 2012).

The durability of the different repairs has not been directly compared, but evidence supports good long-term results for each type of repair. At 10-year follow-up for 33 patients from open repair of full-thickness rotator cuff tears, Galatz et al (2001) found that there was no change in Constant scores from their 2 year follow-up. Forty-two percent of patients continued to work, with 36% at the same level as at 2-year follow-up; the remaining patients were retired (Galatz et al, 2001). Bell et al (2013) had 15-year follow-up after mini-open rotator cuff repair and demonstrated that 69% of patients had good or excellent UCLA outcome scores with 84% satisfied with their final outcomes. Marrero et al (2011) evaluated 24 patients with 33 rotator cuff repairs at 10 years after all-arthroscopic repair and found that 87.7% of patients had excellent results on UCLA outcome measure, with 97% of patients reporting that surgery was successful with excellent shoulder ROM and strength.

BOTTOM LINE

- Excellent to good outcomes have been seen for all repair types, including open, mini-open, and all-arthroscopic repairs.
- All-arthroscopic repairs may decrease pain in acute postoperative period (<5 days) and decrease overall analgesic use during recovery.
- All repair types demonstrate durability.

Outcomes for Single Row- versus Double-Row Repairs

The ideal rotator cuff repair construct would provide high fixation strength to minimize gap formation and allow healing. Biomechanical studies have shown increased load to failure, improved contact areas and pressures, and decreased gap formation with double-row compared with single-row repairs (Kim et al, 2006; Meier & Meier, 2006; Smith et al, 2006). These findings, however, have not translated to differences in clinical outcomes. See Fig. 7B.4 for postoperative MR images of double-row repair.

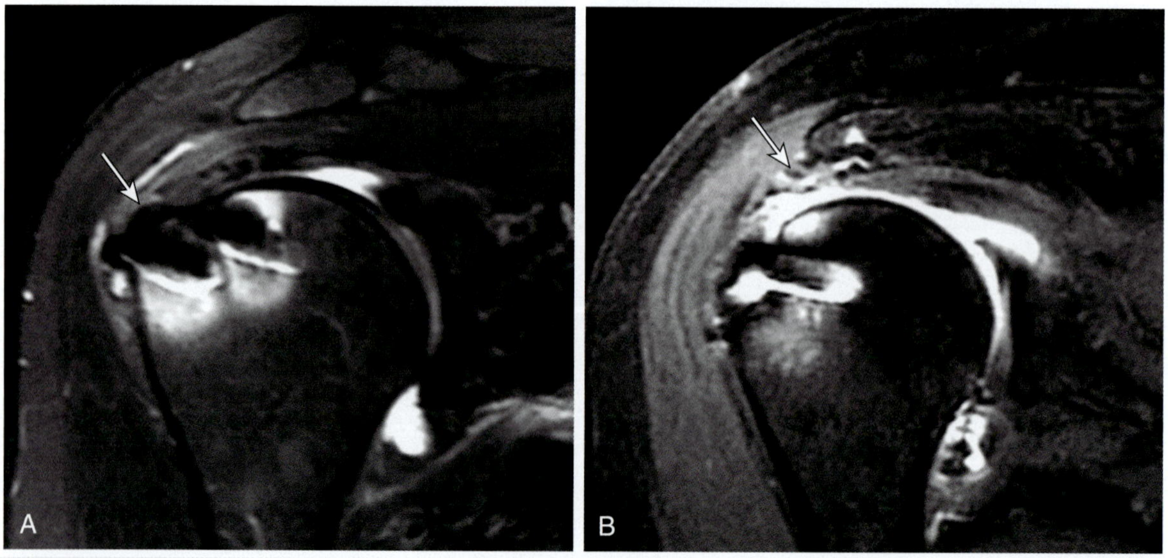

Fig. 7B.4 Postoperative images of a double-row repair. **A,** Coronal T1-weighted image showing intact tendon after double-row repair. The *arrow* shows complete footprint coverage by tendon. **B,** Coronal T1-weighted image showing full-thickness tear at insertion site after double-row repair. The *arrow* shows the tendon defect. (From Ma HL, Chiang ER, Wu HT, et al. Clinical outcome and imaging of arthroscopic single-row and double-row rotator cuff repair: a prospective randomized trial. *Arthroscopy*. 2012;28(1):16-24.)

Grasso et al (2009) and Ma et al (2012) performed prospective randomized studies that determined there were no significant differences in clinical PROMs, strength, or tendon integrity at 6 months and 2 years.

Several meta-analyses performed by Dehaan et al (2012) and Zhang et al (2013b) demonstrate similar findings with no significant difference in functional outcomes between single- or double-row repairs. However, a trend toward higher retear rates in single-row repairs was shown (Dehaan et al, 2012; Zhang et al, 2013b). Zhang et al (2013b) further determined that the increased retear rate for single-row repair was found in rotator cuff tears larger than 3 cm and that there was no difference in retear rates between single- or double-row repairs for tears smaller than 3 cm. Interestingly, in a systematic review of 8 meta-analyses with a Jadad algorithm to determine the studies with the highest level of evidence, the authors demonstrated superior structural healing and outcomes with double-row fixation over single-row fixation (Mascarenhas et al, 2014).

Mihata et al (2011) also demonstrated, however, that in the subcategory of large massive rotator cuff tears, the retear rate in double-row with suture-bridge group (7.5%) was significantly less than double-row (41.7%) or single-row group (62.5%). The study also noted postoperative functional outcome was inferior in the patients with retear compared with those without retear.

BOTTOM LINE

- Functional and patient-reported outcomes are similar between single- or double-row repairs.
- Large to massive tears may have decreased retear rates with double-row repair.
- In large to massive tears, double-row with suture-bridge repair may decrease the retear rate.

Outcomes Based on Rehabilitation Protocol

Recent studies have evaluated the effect of early mobilization (<6 weeks) and delayed mobilization (>6 weeks). The proposed benefit of early mobilization was to prevent stiffness but with the risk of early failure of a healing repair. Lee et al (2012) compared early and delayed rehabilitation protocols in a randomized study of all-arthroscopic single-row repair for a full-thickness tear. Early rehabilitation began at postoperative day 1 with passive ROM twice a day with a therapist and home exercises. The delayed group had minimal passive exercises starting at 3 weeks and then began work with a therapist at 6 weeks. Patients in the early mobilization group noted rapid improvement in forward flexion, external rotation, abduction, and abduction until 3 months postoperatively when differences normalized between groups. MRIs obtained at average 7.6 months after repair demonstrated a trend but no statistical significance in retear rates of early (23.3%) versus delayed (8.8%) rehabilitation protocols. The authors recommended a gentle early rehabilitation protocol within normal limits of shoulder motion (Lee et al, 2012). In contrast, a randomized study of 56 patients by Kim et al (2012b) found a trend toward less retear rates in early (12%) versus delayed (18%) ROM and found no significant difference between healing rates.

A recent systematic review and meta-analysis by Kluczynski et al (2016) determined that early active ROM was associated with increased risk of structural defect for small and large rotator cuff repairs. In a related meta-analysis, however, Kluczynski et al (2015) found that there was no significant difference in retear rates between early and delayed rehabilitation alone. The authors, however, concluded there was insufficient evidence to recommend the optimal timing of ROM following rotator cuff repair.

BOTTOM LINE

- Early and delayed mobilization had similar functional outcomes and retear rates.
- Early mobilization does not guarantee early gain of ROM, pain relief, or improved patient-reported outcomes.
- Delayed mobilization is not detrimental to outcomes.

Outcomes in Rotator Cuff Repair with or without Platelet-Rich Plasma

Platelet-rich plasma (PRP) has received increased attention for possible augmentation of rotator cuff repairs (Fig. 7B.5). The rationale is that the high concentrations of several growth factors within platelets may stimulate cell proliferation and provide a temporary matrix to fill defect sites, which may serve as a framework for cell migration and tissue remodeling (Alsousou et al, 2009).

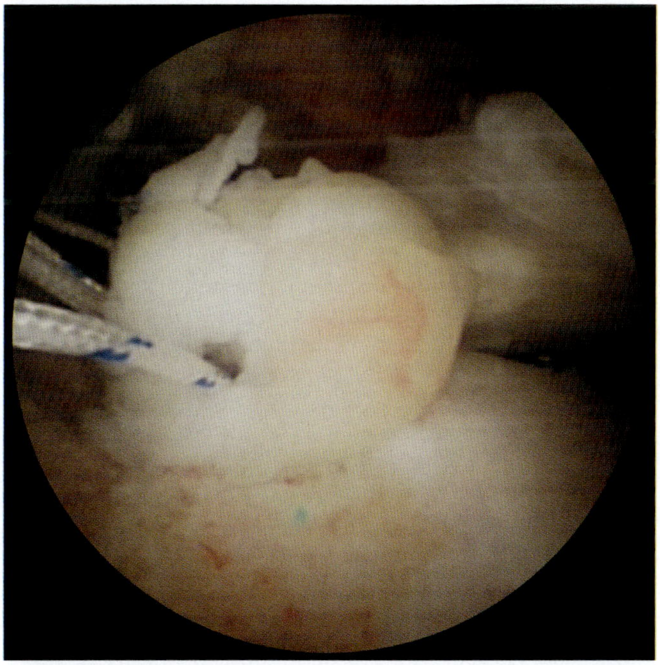

Fig. 7B.5 Platelet-rich plasma (PRP) construct. A PRP globule threaded onto the suture anchor suture was delivered to the repair site. (From Barber FA, Hrnack SA, Snyder SJ, Hapa O. Rotator cuff repair healing influenced by platelet-rich plasma construct augmentation. *Arthroscopy*. 2011;27(8):1029-1035.)

Zhao et al (2015) performed a meta-analysis of 8 randomized controlled trials of 464 patients that compared outcomes of arthroscopic full-thickness tears with and without PRP. The analysis found that there was no difference in retear rate in the PRP group (26%) with group without PRP (28%). The Constant and UCLA scores also demonstrated no significant difference between treatment groups. The authors concluded that they did not support use of PRP with full-thickness tears. A similar meta-analysis by Cai et al (2015) published in the same year, however, noted that patients with PRP demonstrated greater healing potential as determined by MRI at 12 months postoperatively. The authors concluded that platelet-rich therapy may improve tendon-to-bone healing in small or moderate rotator cuff tears. Although controversy remains regarding the clinical benefit of platelet-rich therapy, Samuelson et al (2016) performed a cost analysis and determined at this time that use of PRP currently was not cost effective.

BOTTOM LINE

- There is insufficient evidence to advocate routine use of PRP in rotator cuff repairs.

Conclusions and Future Research

Rotator cuff disease accounts for more than 4.5 million annual visits to physicians, and more than 75,000 surgical repairs are performed a year (Vitale et al, 2007). Despite the increase in surgical repairs, there is evidence that conservative treatment with physiotherapy alone may have comparable outcomes compared with open or mini-open repairs for rotator cuff tears smaller than 3 cm. All-arthroscopic repair has become the mainstay of treatment and has demonstrated comparable outcomes compared with mini-open and open repairs. It should be noted, however, that no studies have demonstrated superiority in functional or patient-reported outcomes or retear rates when comparing arthroscopic with mini-open or open repairs. Large and massive tears have greater failure rates and high retear rates, up to 94%. Fatty infiltration and muscle atrophy are predictors of poor outcomes and are irreversible. Preliminary studies demonstrate that repair techniques such as single-row and double-row repairs demonstrate comparable results. Early rehabilitation and delayed rehabilitation demonstrate similar functional outcomes and risk of retear. Currently, the use of PRPs has not been shown to be cost effective, and their clinical benefit is uncertain.

Future research is needed to evaluate outcomes between physiotherapy only and all-arthroscopic repair, as well as for large to massive rotator cuff tears. Further randomized comparison of individual surgical repair techniques is warranted to determine the ideal repair constructs for different types of tears. There also needs to be research into the best types of exercises and training in rehabilitation that will optimize ROM while limiting the risk of retear after rotator cuff repair. Overall, the review of current literature available demonstrates that rotator cuff surgery yields good outcomes for appropriately selected patients. The best treatment is one that is tailored for each individual patient as well as each individual surgeon based on experience and comfort level.

References

Alsousou J, Thompson M, Hulley P, Noble A, Willett K. The biology of platelet-rich plasma and its application in trauma and orthopaedic surgery: a review of the literature. *J Bone Joint Surg Br*. 2009;91:987–996.

Amstutz HC, Sew Hoy AL, Clarke IC. UCLA anatomic total shoulder arthroplasty. *Clin Orthop Relat Res*. 1981;155:7–20.

Bell S, Lim YI, Coghlan J. Long-term longitudinal follow up of mini-open rotator cuff repair. *J Bone Joint Surg Am*. 2013;95:151–157.

Bollier M, Shea K. Systematic review: what surgical technique provides the best outcome for symptomatic partial articular-sided rotator cuff tears? *Iowa Orthop J*. 2012;32:164–172.

Burkhart SS, Barth JR, Richards DP, Zlatkin MB, Larsen M. Arthroscopic repair of massive rotator cuff tears with stage 3 and 4 fatty degeneration. *Arthroscopy*. 2007;23:347–354.

Burkhart SS, Danaceau SM, Pearce CE Jr. Arthroscopic rotator cuff repair: analysis of results by tear size and by repair technique-margin convergence versus direct tendon-to-bone repair. *Arthroscopy*. 2001;17(9):905–912.

Cai YZ, Zhang C, Lin XJ. Efficacy of platelet-rich plasma in arthroscopic repair of full-thickness rotator cuff tears: a meta-analysis. *J Shoulder Elbow Surg*. 2015;24(12):1852–1859.

Castagna A, Borroni M, Garofalo R, et al. Deep partial rotator cuff tear: transtendon repair or tear completion and repair? A randomized clinical trial. *Knee Surg Sports Traumatol Arthrosc*. 2015;23:460–463.

Cho CH, Song KS, Jung GH, Lee YK, Shin HK. Early postoperative outcomes between arthroscopic and mini-open repair for rotator cuff tears. *Orthopedics*. 2012;35(9):e1347–e1352.

Chung SW, Kim JY, Kim MH, Kim SH, Oh JH. Arthroscopic repair of massive rotator cuff tears: outcome and analysis of factors associated with healing failure or poor postoperative function. *Am J Sports Med*. 2013;41:1674–1683.

Codsi MJ, Rodeo SA, Scalise JJ, Moorehead TM, Ma CB. Assessment of rotator cuff repair integrity using ultrasound and magnetic resonance imaging in a multicenter study. *J Shoulder Elbow Surg*. 2014;23(10):1448–1472.

Constant CR, Murley AH. A clinical method of functional assessment of the shoulder. *Clin Orthop Relat Res*. 1987;214:160–164.

DeHaan AM, Axelrad TW, Kaye E, Silvestri L, Puskas B, Foster TE. Does double-row rotator cuff repair improve functional outcome of patients compared with single-row technique? A systematic review. *Am J Sports Med*. 2012;40(5):1176–1185.

Davidson JF, Burkhart SS. The geometric classification of rotator cuff tears: a system linking tear pattern to treatment and prognosis. *Arthroscopy*. 2010;26(3):417–424.

de Jesus JO, Parker L, Frangos AJ, Nazarian LN. Accuracy of MRI, MR arthrography, and ultrasound in the diagnosis of rotator cuff tears: a meta analysis. *AJR Am J Roentgenol*. 2009;192(6):1701–1707.

Ensor KL, Kwon YW, Dibeneditto MR, Zuckerman JD, Rokito AS. The rising incidence of rotator cuff repairs. *J Shoulder Elbow Surg*. 2013;22(12):1628–1632.

Franceschi F, Papalia R, Del Buono A, et al. Articular sided rotator cuff tears: which is the best repair? A three year prospective randomised controlled trial. *Int Orthop*. 2013;37:1487–1493.

Galatz LM, Ball CM, Teefey SA, Middleton WD, Yamaguchi K. The outcome and repair integrity of completely arthroscopically repaired large and massive rotator cuff tears. *J Bone Joint Surg Am*. 2004;86-A:219–224.

Galatz LM, Griggs S, Cameron BD, Iannotti JP. Prospective longitudinal analysis of postoperative shoulder function: a ten-year follow up study of full-thickness rotator cuff tears. *J Bone Joint Surg Am*. 2001;83-A(7):1052–1056.

Gladstone JN, Bishop JY, Lo IK, Flatow EL. Fatty infiltration and atrophy of the rotator cuff do not improve after rotator cuff repair and correlate with poor functional outcome. *Am J Sports Med*. 2007;35(5):719–728.

Goutallier D, Postel J, Bernageau J, Lavau L, Voisin MC. Fatty muscle degeneration in cuff ruptures. Pre- and postoperative evaluation by CT scan. *Clin Orthop Relat Res*. 1994;304:78–83.

Goutallier D, Postel JM, Gleyze P, Leguilloux P, Van Driessche S. Influence of cuff muscle fatty degeneration on anatomic and functional outcomes after simple suture of full-thickness tears. *J Shoulder Elbow Surg*. 2003;12:550–554.

Grasso A, Milano G, Salvatore M, Falcone G, Deriu L, Fabbriciani C. Single-row versus double-row arthroscopic rotator cuff repair: a prospective randomized clinical study. *Arthroscopy*. 2009;25:4–12.

Gulotta LV, Nho SJ, Dodson CC, Adler RS, Altchek DW, MacGillivray JD. Prospective evaluation of arthroscopic rotator cuff repairs at 5 years: part II—prognostic factors for clinical and radiographic outcomes. *J Shoulder Elbow Surg*. 2011;20:941–946.

Henry P, Wasserstein D, Park S, et al. Arthroscopic repair for chronic massive rotator cuff tears: a systemic review. *Arthroscopy*. 2015;31(12):2472–2480.

Huberty DP, Schoolfield JD, Brady PC, Vadala AP, Arrigoni P, Burkhart SS. Incidence and treatment of postoperative stiffness following arthroscopic rotator cuff repair. *Arthroscopy*. 2009;25:880–890.

Iannotti JP, Bernot MP, Kuhlman JR, Kelley MJ, Williams GR. Postoperative assessment of shoulder function: a prospective study of full-thickness rotator cuff tears. *J Shoulder Elbow Surg*. 1996;5(6):449–457.

Khazzam M, Kuhn JE, Mulligan E, et al. Magnetic resonance imaging identification of rotator cuff retears after repair: interobserver and intraobserver agreement. *Am J Sports Med*. 2012;40(8):1722–1727.

Kim DH, Elattrache NS, Tibone JE, et al. Biomechanical comparison of a single-row versus double-row suture anchor technique for rotator cuff repair. *Am J Sports Med*. 2006;34:407.

Kim KC, Shin HD, Cha SM, Park JY. Repair integrity and functional outcome after arthroscopic conversion to a full-thickness rotator cuff tear: articular-versus bursal-side partial tears. *Am J Sports Med*. 2014;42(2):451–456.

Kim KC, Shin HD, Lee WY, Han SC. Repair integrity and functional outcome after arthroscopic rotator cuff repair: double-row versus suture-bridge technique. *Am J Sports Med*. 2012a;40(2):294–299.

Kim JK, Yoo HJ, Jeong JH, Kim SH. Effect of teres minor fatty infiltration on rotator cuff repair outcomes. *Arthroscopy*. 2016;32(4):552–558.

Kim YS, Chung SW, Kim JY, Ok JH, Park I, Oh JH. Is early passive motion exercise necessary after arthroscopic rotator cuff repair? *Am J Sports Med*. 2012b;40:815–821.

Kim YS, Lee HJ, Bae SH, Jin H, Song HS. Outcome comparison between in situ repair versus tear completion repair for partial thickness rotator cuff tears. *Arthroscopy*. 2015;31(11):2191–2198.

Kluczynski MA, Nayyar S, Marzo JM, Bisson LJ. Early versus delayed passive range of motion after rotator cuff repair: a systematic review and meta-analysis. *Am J Sports Med*. 2015;43(8):2057–2063.

Kluczynski MA, Isenburg MM, Marzo JM, Bisson LJ. Does early versus delayed active range of motion affect rotator cuff healing after surgical repair? A systematic review and meta-analysis. *Am J Sports Med*. 2016;44(3):785–791.

Koh KH, Shon MS, Lim TK, Yoo JC. Clinical and magnetic resonance imaging results of arthroscopic full-layer repair of bursal-side partial thickness rotator cuff tears. *Am J Sports Med*. 2011;39(8):1660–1667.

Kuhn JE, Dunn WR, Sanders R, et al. MOON Shoulder Group. Effectiveness of physical therapy in treating atraumatic full-thickness rotator cuff tears: a multicenter prospective cohort study. *J Shoulder Elbow Surg*. 2013;22(10):1371–1379.

Lansdown DA, Feeley BT. Evaluation and treatment of rotator cuff tears. *Phys Sportsmed*. 2012;40(2):73–86.

Lambers Heerspink FO, van Raay JJ, Koorevaar RC, et al. Comparing surgical repair with conservative treatment for degenerative rotator cuff tears: a randomized controlled trial. *J Shoulder Elbow Surg*. 2015;24(8):1274–1281.

Lee BG, Cho NS, Rhee YG. Effect of two rehabilitation protocols on range of motion and healing rates after arthroscopic rotator cuff repair: aggressive versus limited early passive exercises. *Arthroscopy*. 2012;28(1):34–42.

Liem D, Lichtenberg S, Magosch P, Habermeyer P. Magnetic resonance imaging of arthroscopic supraspinatus tendon repair. *J Bone Joint Surg Am*. 2007;89:1770–1776.

Lippe J, Spang JT, Leger RR, Arciero RA, Mazzocca AD, Shea KP. Inter-rater agreement of Goutallier, Patte, and Warner classification scores using preoperative magnetic resonance imaging in patients with rotator cuff tears. *Arthroscopy*. 2012;28(2):154–159.

Lippitt S, Harryman D, Matsen F. *A Practical Tool FOR Evaluating Function: The Simple Shoulder Test*. Rosemont, IL: American Academy of Orthopaedic Surgeons; 1993:501–518.

Lo IK, Burkhart SS. Transtendon arthroscopic repair of partial- thickness, articular surface tears of the rotator cuff. *Arthroscopy*. 2004;20:214–220.

Ma HL, Chiang ER, Wu HT, et al. Clinical outcome and imaging of arthroscopic single-row and double-row rotator cuff repair: a prospective randomized trial. *Arthroscopy*. 2012;28(1):16–24.

Macdonald P, McRae S, Leiter J, Mascarenhas R, Lapner P. Arthroscopic rotator cuff repair with and without acromioplasty in the treatment of full-thickness rotator cuff tears: a multicenter, randomized controlled trial. *J Bone Joint Surg Am*. 2011;93(21):1953–1960.

Makhni EC, Steinhaus ME, Morrow ZS, et al. Outcomes assessment in rotator cuff pathology: what are we measuring? *J Shoulder Elbow Surg*. 2015;24(12):2008–2015.

Marrero LG, Nelman KR, Nottage WM. Long-term follow-up of arthroscopic rotator cuff repair. *Arthroscopy*. 2011;27(7):885–888.

Mascarenhas R, Chalmers PN, Sayegh ET, et al. Is double-row rotator cuff repair clinically superior to single-row rotator cuff repair: a systematic review of overlapping meta-analysis. *Arthroscopy*. 2014;30(9):1156–1165.

Meier SW, Meier JD. The effect of double-row fixation on initial repair strength in rotator cuff repair: a biomechanical study. *Arthroscopy*. 2006;22:1168–1173.

Mihata T, Watanabe C, Fukunishi K, et al. Functional and structural outcomes of single-row versus double-row versus combined double-row and suture-bridge for rotator cuff tears. *Am J Sports Med*. 2011;39(10):2091–2098.

Mohtadi NG, Hollinshead RM, Sasyniuk TM, Fletcher JA, Chan DS, Li FX. A randomized clinical trial comparing open to arthroscopic acromioplasty with mini-open rotator cuff repair for full-thickness rotator cuff tears: disease-specific quality of life outcome at an average 2-year follow up. *Am J Sports Med*. 2008;36(6):1043–1051.

Moonsmayer S, Lund G, Seljom US, et al. Tendon repair compared with physiotherapy in the treatment of rotator cuff tears: a randomized controlled study in 103 cases with a five-year follow-up. *J Bone Joint Surg Am*. 2014 Sep 17;96(18):1504–1514.

Motamedi AR, Urrea LH, Hancock RE, Hawkins RJ, Ho C. Accuracy of magnetic resonance imaging in determining the presence and size of recurrent rotator cuff tears. *J Shoulder Elbow Surg*. 2002;11(1):6–10.

Namdari S, Donegan RP, Chamberlain AM, Galatz LM, Yamaguchi K, Keener JD. Factors affecting outcome after structural failure of repaired rotator cuff tears. *J Bone Joint Surg Am*. 2014;96:99–105.

Park JY, Jung SW, Jeon SH, Cho HW, Choi JH, Oh KS. Arthroscopic repair of large U-shaped rotator cuff tears without margin convergence versus repair of crescent- or L-shaped tears. *Am J Sports Med*. 2014;42(1):103–111.

Ranalletta M, Rossi LA, Bertona AB, et al. Arthroscopic transtendon repair of partial-thickness articular-side rotator cuff tears. *Arthroscopy*. 2016 Mar 31. [Epub available prior to print].

Richards RR, An KN, Bigliani LU, et al. A standardized method for the assessment of shoulder function. *J Shoulder Elbow Surg*. 1994;3:347–352.

Sallay PI, Hunker PJ, Lim JK. Frequency of various tear patterns in full-thickness tears of the rotator cuff. *Arthroscopy*. 2007;23(10):1052–1059.

Samuelson EM, Odum SM, Fleischli JE. The cost-effectiveness of using platelet-rich plasma during rotator cuff repair: a Markov model analysis. *Arthroscopy*. 2016;32(7):1237–1244.

Schiefer M, Mendonca R, Magnanini MM, et al. Intraobserver and interobserver agreement of Goutallier classification applied to magnetic resonance images. *J Shoulder Elbow Surg*. 2015;24(8):1314–1321.

Shen PH, Lien SB, Shen HC, Lee CH, Wu SS, Lin LC. Long-term functional outcomes after repair of rotator cuff tears correlated with atrophy of the supraspinatus muscles on magnetic resonance images. *J Shoulder Elbow Surg*. 2008;17(suppl 1):1S–7S.

Shin SJ. A comparison of 2 repair techniques for partial-thickness articular-sided rotator cuff tears. *Arthroscopy*. 2012;28(1):25–33.

Shin SJ, Oh JH, Chung SW, Song MH. The efficacy of acromioplasty in the arthroscopic repair of small-to medium-sized rotator cuff tears without acromial spur: prospective comparative study. *Arthroscopy*. 2012;28(5):628–635.

Slabaugh MA, Friel NA, Karas V, Romeo AA, Verma NN, Cole BJ. Interobserver and intraobserver reliability of the Goutallier classification using magnetic resonance imaging: proposal of a simplified classification system to increase reliability. *Am J Sports Med*. 2012;40(8):1728–1734.

Smith CD, Alexander S, Hill AM, et al. A biomechanical comparison of single and double-row fixation in arthroscopic rotator cuff repair. *J Bone Joint Surg Am*. 2006;88:2425–2431.

Strauss EJ, Salata MJ, Kercher J, et al. The arthroscopic management of partial-thickness rotator cuff tears: a systematic review of the literature. *Arthroscopy*. 2011;27:568–580.

Vitale MA, Vitale MG, Zivin JG, et al. Rotator cuff repair: an analysis of utility scores and cost-effectiveness. *J Shoulder Elbow Surg*. 2007;16:181–187.

Warner JJP, Higgins L, Parsons IM 4th, Dowdy P. Diagnosis and treatment of anterosuperior rotator cuff tears. *J Shoulder Elbow Surg*. 2001;10:37–46.

Zhang AL, Montgomery SR, Sgo SS, Hame SL, Wang JC, Gamradt SC. Analysis of rotator cuff repair trends in a large private insurance population. *Arthroscopy*. 2013a;29(4):623–629.

Zhang Q, Ge H, Zhou J, Yuan C, Chen K, Cheng B. Single-row or double-row fixation technique for full-thickness rotator cuff tears: a meta-analysis. *PLoS One*. 2013b;8(7):e68515.

Zhao JG, Zhao L, Jiang YX, Wang ZL, Wang J, Zhang P. Platelet-rich plasma in arthroscopic rotator cuff repair: a meta-analysis of randomized controlled trials. *Arthroscopy*. 2015;31(1):125–135.

7-7C SUPRASCAPULAR NERVE: WHEN TO DECOMPRESS?

HENRY M. FOX, BS, MA; CORY STEWART, MD; and JON J.P. WARNER, MD

Introduction

- Pain in the shoulder can arise from many causes.
- Suprascapular nerve (SSN) neuropathy has been shown to be a rare cause of shoulder pain, either in isolation or with other concomitant pathologies.
- Patients with SSN neuropathy often present with posterosuperior shoulder pain, muscular atrophy, and weakness of the supraspinatus and infraspinatus.
- Diagnosis of SSN and determination of optimum treatment is challenging.
- Magnetic resonance imaging (MRI) can be used to evaluate rotator cuff anatomy and nerve pathology.
- Electromyography (EMG) findings may be falsely negative, but if positive, they are likely accurate for the diagnosis.
- Nonoperative treatment options include activity modification, physical therapy, and guided injections.
- In patients who fail conservative measures, arthroscopic release can be performed; open release is largely a historical treatment.
- Reliable pain relief after SSN release has been confirmed in the literature, mainly in small level IV cohort studies.
- If there is significant associated fatty muscle degeneration, it does not reliably reverse after SSN release.

Suprascapular nerve pathology has been an area of increasing interest because both general orthopedic surgeons and shoulder specialists may miss this rare condition. This is not only the case as an isolated entity causing pain, but it may also occur in association with rotator cuff disease (Boykin et al, 2010; Murphy & Carr, 2010; Piasecki et al, 2009). Once considered primarily a diagnosis of exclusion, causes of SSN neuropathy can include excessive tension on the nerve as part of massive rotator cuff tears, traction and microtrauma from repetitive overhead activities, and compression from space-occupying lesions (Habermeyer et al, 1987; Lafosse et al, 2011).

Advanced modalities for evaluating SSN neuropathy include MRI as well as EMG and nerve conduction velocity (NCV) studies. MRI is valuable in evaluating muscle bulk and fatty infiltration in the setting of rotator cuff tears, as well as evaluating for compressive sources of SSN neuropathy related to cysts or tumors. However, most cases of SSN neuropathy do not have obvious muscle changes. EMG and NCV have been suggested as the gold standard for diagnosis of SSN neuropathy, although several studies have pointed to the limited intra- and interobserver reliability as well as limitations in the type of nerves evaluated and the manner in which evaluation occurs (Collin et al, 2014; Freehill et al, 2012; Hill et al, 2014). Early, nonoperative treatment of SSN neuropathy can include injections, activity modifications, and physical therapy. When weakness or pain is persistent, arthroscopic release of the nerve has been demonstrated to be very effective (Freehill et al, 2012; LaFosse et al, 2011,). We have found fluoroscopic-guided injection into the SSN notch to be diagnostic, although scientific study has not confirmed this to date (Bennett et al, 2014).

Anatomy

The SSN arises from the upper trunk of the brachial plexus and is derived from the fifth and sixth cervical nerve roots. The motor supply of the SSN is to the supraspinatus and infraspinatus muscles (Piasecki et al, 2009) with a small branch of the nerve supplying the skin overlying the posterior shoulder. After branching from the brachial plexus, the SSN passes through two principal areas of potential compression—the suprascapular and spinoglenoid notches. Whereas compression at the suprascapular notch affects both the supraspinatus and infraspinatus muscles, compression at the spinoglenoid notch results in denervation of the infraspinatus alone (J Salata et al, 2013) (Fig. 7C.1).

Prevalence

Significant variability exists in studies describing the prevalence of SSN neuropathy. Zehetgruber et al (2002) performed a systematic review of the literature, which found only 44 described instances of SSN neuropathy. In their study, SSN dysfunction was more common in male patients younger than 40 years of age. They found that compression caused by mass effect from ganglion cysts more commonly affected only the infraspinatus, but patients with combined infra- and supraspinatus pathology more commonly had nerve compression at the level of the transverse scapular ligament. More recently, in patients with chronic shoulder pain, Clavert and Thomazeau (2014) found a prevalence of SSN neuropathy of 2% of all patients presenting with shoulder pain, while Boykin et al (2011) found that SSN pathology accounted for 4% of new patient visits seen over the course of 1 year at a tertiary referral shoulder center.

In certain subsets of the population, the prevalence of SSN neuropathy would appear to be much higher. In athletes undergoing EMGs and NCVs for sports injuries, Krivickas and Wilbourn (1989) found that SSN pathology was present in 8.3% of patients. Multiple authors have found that male volleyball players similarly demonstrate clinical evidence of SSN neuropathy (Ferretti et al, 2016; Witvrouw et al, 2000) and postulated that it was caused by repetitive traction as part of overhead play. In many of these athletes, the presentation is of painless atrophy of the spinati with preserved function. In an older population of patients with full-thickness rotator cuff tears, the prevalence of SSN neuropathy has ranged from 8% to 100% (Brown et al, 2000; Mallon et al, 2003; Vad et al, 2003).

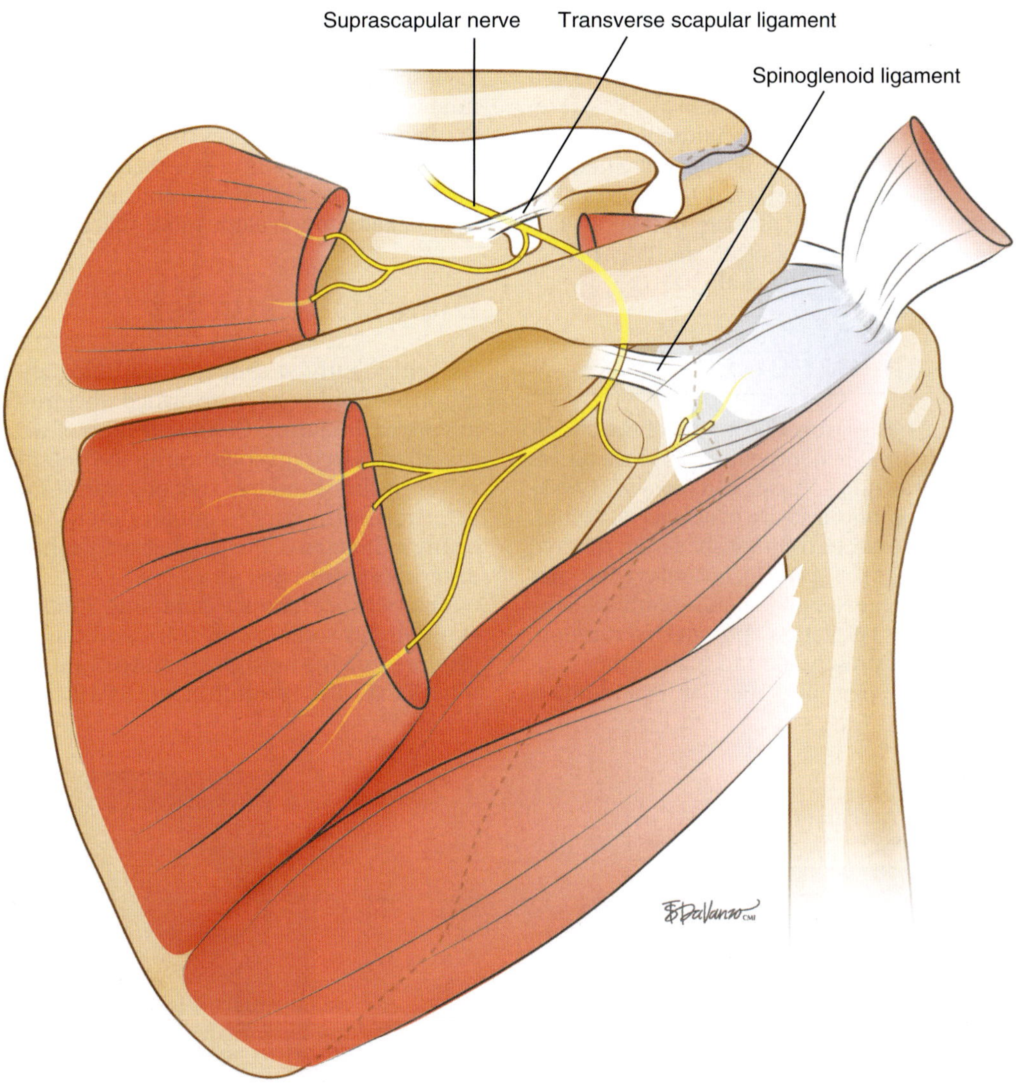

Fig. 7C.1 **Course of the suprascapular nerve. After branching from the superior trunk of the brachial plexus, the nerve passes underneath the transverse scapular ligament before wrapping around the spinoglenoid notch.** (From Boykin, RE, Friedman DJ, Higgins LD, Warner JJ. Suprascapular neuropathy. *J Bone Joint Surg Am*. 2010;92(13):2348-2364.)

Etiology

A variety of pathologies exist that can predispose one to SSN dysfunction. SSN neuropathy can be caused by traction or compression of the nerve at several different points along its path. In the majority of individuals, at the suprascapular notch, the nerve travels inferior to the transverse scapular ligament, and the suprascapular artery and vein run superior to the ligament. Although this is the most commonly found orientation of structures, multiple variations in normal anatomy have been described. Accessory ligaments about the suprascapular notch can cause impingement (Polguj et al, 2012a), and the transverse scapular ligament can be bifid or trifid, reducing the amount of space available for the nerve to pass (Joy et al, 2015).

Accessory musculature running from the first costal cartilage to the superior aspect of the scapula (subclavius posticus) can also result in SSN neuropathy (Cogar et al, 2015). In addition, multiple variations in the bony morphology of the suprascapular notch have been described, including complete ossification of the suprascapular notch, seen in Fig. 7C.2, *A* (Edelson 1995; Polguj et al, 2013; Kharay et al, 2016; Kumar et al, 2014; Yang et al, 2012).The spinoglenoid ligament has been noted to be variably present in several cadaver studies and has been thought to play a role in isolated infraspinatus dysfunction, especially in overhead athletes (Demirhan et al, 2003, 2016; Plancher et al, 2005). Regarding vascular abnormalities, the suprascapular artery has been demonstrated in some individuals to run underneath the transverse scapular ligament in immediate proximity to the nerve (Reineck et al, 2007), and multiple suprascapular veins can be present and can run either over or under the transverse scapular ligament (Yang et al, 2012).

Suprascapular nerve dysfunction has been noted in association with retracted rotator cuff tears (Brown et al, 2000; Vad et al, 2003) and caused by compression from suprascapular and spinoglenoid notch cysts (Fernandes & Fernandes, 2010; Lee et al, 2007), specifically in association with superior labrum from anterior to posterior (SLAP) tears (Hashiguchi et al, 2016; Lee et al, 2015; Tan & Lee 2012). SSN neuropathy can also arise secondary to neuropathic diseases such as Parsonage-Turner syndrome (Camargo et al, 2014).

Suprascapular nerve dysfunction has also been noted with ganglion cysts caused by posterior labral tears (Fig. 7.2, C) (Westrick et al, 2013) and in association with swimmer's shoulder (Arriaza et al, 2013). Iatrogenic causes of SSN dysfunction must also be considered (Tragord et al, 2015), and SSN neuropathy should also be considered as a possible cause of persistent pain after other shoulder procedures (Murphy & Carr, 2010; Strauss et al, 2010).

History and Examination Findings

Dull, deep pain over the posterosuperior aspect of the shoulder is often associated with SSN neuropathy, as is weakness and atrophy of the supra- and infraspinatus fossae. Weakness is generally most pronounced in overhead activities. This complaint must, of course, be distinguished from referred pain from cervical disk disease or acromioclavicular (AC) joint disease. A handheld dynamometer allows quantitative assessment of weakness in forward elevation and external rotation. Because of the similarity in presentation to many other conditions, complete cervical spine and thoracic examination should also be performed at the time of the initial evaluation to rule out confounding sources of pain. In some instances, a cervical spine MRI is indicated and an AC joint injection will distinguish pain arising from the AC joint from pain arising from the SSN. In chronic cases, the teres minor may hypertrophy to compensate for loss of external rotation strength secondary to infraspinatus dysfunction and may make diagnosis through motor examination alone more difficult (Ferretti et al, 2016).

Diagnostic Studies

As with many orthopedic pathologies, dedicated radiographs should be performed before obtaining more advanced imaging. Ossified lesions, fractures, and suprascapular notch dysplasia can be identified on standard views of the shoulder. Osseous variants can be best characterized by the suprascapular notch view. In this view, the beam is directed 15 to 30 degrees cephalad from the direct anteroposterior view.

Magnetic resonance imaging studies can be used to evaluate for rotator cuff tears and the amount of fat atrophy present in the supraspinatus and infraspinatus fossae (Fig. 7C.2, *B*) (Freehill et al, 2012; Leclere et al, 2014;

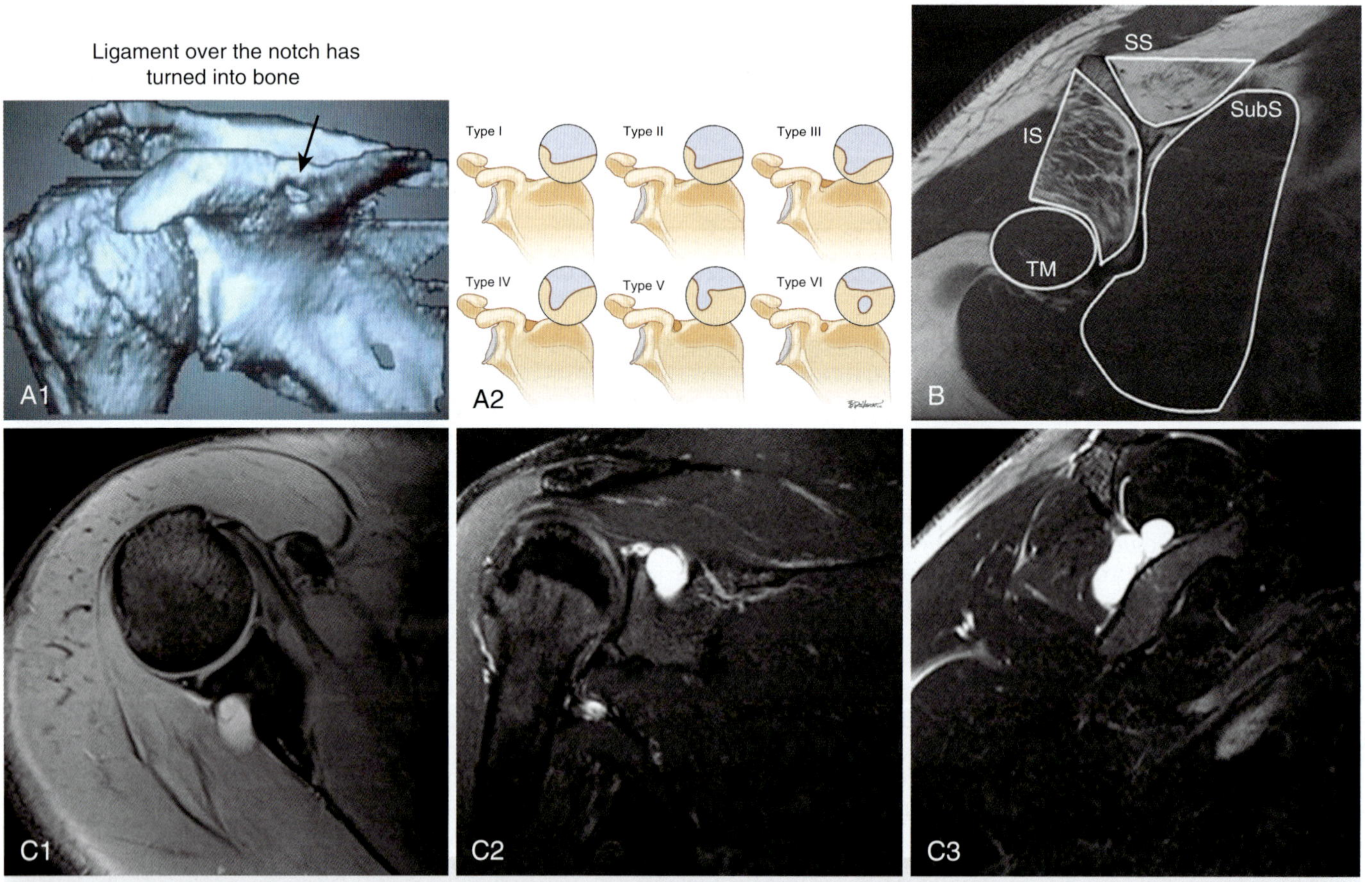

Fig. 7C.2 A1, Three-dimensional computed tomography scan demonstrating complete ossification of the suprascapular notch. **A2,** Anatomical variants in the suprascapular notch are detailed in the *center panel*. **B.** Sagittal T1-weighted magnetic resonance image (MRI) demonstrating fat atrophy of the supraspinatus and infraspinatus secondary to suprascapular neuropathy. Axial (C1), coronal (C2), and sagittal (C3) MR images of a patient with multiple paralabral cysts in the suprascapular notch and spinoglenoid notch. IS, infraspinatus; SubS, subscapularis; SS, supraspinatus; TM, teres minor. (A1, from Boykin RE, Friedman DJ, Higgins LD, Warner JJ. Suprascapular neuropathy. *J Bone Joint Surg Am.* 2010;92(13):2348-2364. A2, from Rengachary SS, Burr D, Lucas S, Brackett CE. Suprascapular entrapment neuropathy: a clinical, anatomical, and comparative study. Part 3: comparative Study. *Neurosurgery.* 1979;5:452-455. B,C, from Shi LL, Freehill MT, Yannopoulos P, Warner JJ. Suprascapular nerve: is it important in cuff pathology? *Adv Orthop.* 2012;2012:516985.)

Shimokobe et al, 2013). Computed tomography (CT) scans can be helpful in characterizing the suprascapular notch in the case of aberrant bony anatomy (Polguj et al, 2013). Ultrasonography in skilled hands can be used similarly to MRI to evaluate for rotator cuff tears, suprascapular notch morphology, and space-occupying lesions but is primarily used for image guidance during injections (Moriggl, 1997). Ultrasonography has also been used in conjunction with arthroscopic procedures (Hashiuchi et al, 2013).

Historically EMG and NCV have been suggested to be the gold standard in diagnosis of SSN pathology. Because EMG and NCV criteria for diagnosing SSN pathology differ among centers and EMG and NCV studies are unable to evaluate pain fibers, some have criticized the overreliance on nerve studies as the sole means for definitive diagnosis. Boykin et al (2011) noted that EMG is unreliable for determining SSN pathology. The most common abnormalities noted in their study were abnormal motor unit action potentials. They cautioned against using nerve denervation as a primary criteria for SSN neuropathy because only 33% of patients in their study had evidence of denervation (Boykin et al, 2011). Some authors have found EMG and NCV to be predictive of outcomes after surgery. Antoniou et al (2001) found that limited response to treatment was noted in patients with minimal EMG changes associated with denervation and that this was most pronounced in patients with nerve compression secondary to spinoglenoid notch cyst.

Nonoperative Treatment

In the absence of concomitant pathology such as a labral tear with associated ganglion cyst formation or a retracted rotator cuff tear, a short course of nonoperative treatment can be attempted. In cases of isolated SSN neuropathy, activity modification, physical therapy, and antiinflammatory medications can provide relief. Martin et al reviewed 15 patients with confirmed SSN neuropathy by EMG treated nonoperatively. These patients were treated primarily with physical therapy alone and had an average follow-up period of 3 years, 11 months. The final evaluation included EMG and NCV studies and dynamic strength testing of bilateral upper extremities. Five patients had excellent results, and three patients had good results. The remaining three patients underwent operative treatment because of persistence of symptoms. Of these, one patient had an excellent result, one had a good result, and one had a poor result. The authors suggested that patients without clear mechanical compression of the SSN can be treated effectively by nonoperative means (Martin et al, 1997). Guided injections to the suprascapular notch can also provide diagnostic and therapeutic data. Improvement in pain after injection was thought to be predictive of reliable pain relief after SSN decompression (Shi et al, 2012; Steiman, 1988).

Operative Interventions and Outcomes

In patients with SSN dysfunction with concomitant pathology such as compressive cysts or retracted rotator cuff tears, surgical intervention is generally indicated acutely without a trial of nonoperative management. In patients with isolated SSN neuropathy who have failed nonoperative treatment, surgical intervention is similarly indicated. Modern operative technique is usually arthroscopic (Fig. 7C.3) (Fernandes & Fernandes, 2010; Ghodadra et al, 2009; Gupta et al, 2015; Hashiguchi et al, 2016; Kim et al, 2009). Most commonly, the technique performed is based on that originally described by Lafosse et al (2011) (Video 7C.1).

In a study by Costouros et al (2007), 26 patients were identified with massive, retracted rotator cuff tears. Twenty-seven percent (7 of 26) of these patients were found to have EMG abnormalities consistent with SSN dysfunction. All six patients who underwent rotator cuff repair had notable improvement in pain relief and partial or complete recovery of the SSN function based on EMG and NCV testing (Costouros et al, 2007). Fernandez et al (2010) presented two cases of isolated infraspinatus atrophy secondary to spinoglenoid notch cysts treated with arthroscopic repair and cyst decompression. In both instances, there was significant improvement in pain and muscle strength.

Shah et al (2011) reported on 27 patients with isolated SSN neuropathy in the absence of concomitant pathology who were followed for an average of 22.5 months. Seventy-one percent (17 of 24) of patients reported pain relief based on visual analog scale testing at an average of 9 weeks after surgery. Seventy-five percent (18 of 24) of patients had improvements in ASES scores, and 71% (17 of 24) would have the surgery again (Shah et al, 2011). Kim et al (2005) retrospectively reviewed 42 patients with SSN entrapment. Improvements in supraspinatus muscle strength occurred more reliably than infraspinatus strength in their series and of 8 patients whose complaints were predominantly pain related; 7 had significant improvements in pain postoperatively. Regarding patients with preoperative paresthesias, Oizumi et al (2012) performed arthroscopic decompressions on 25 patients with sensory disturbances consistent with SSN neuropathy and found complete resolution of sensory abnormalities in all patients.

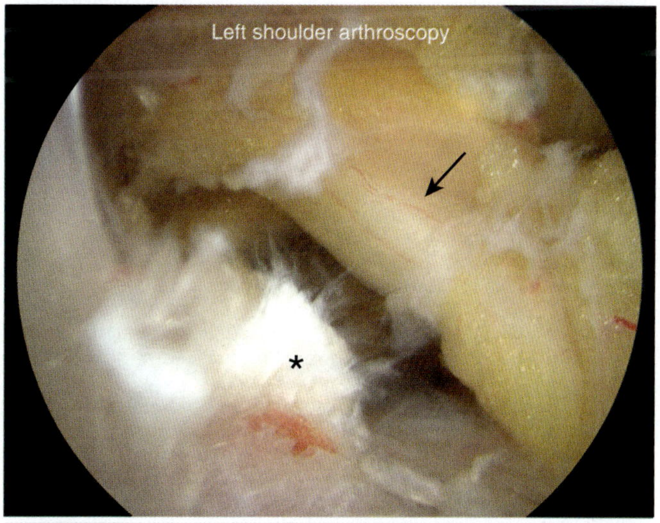

Fig. 7C.3 Arthroscopic images of a left shoulder viewed from the lateral position after suprascapular nerve *(arrow)* decompression by release of the transverse scapular ligament *(asterisk)*. Note the abundant fat tissue present. (From LeClere LE, Shi LL, Lin A, Yannopoulos P, Higgins L, Warner JP. Complete fatty infiltration of intact rotator cuffs caused by suprascapular neuropathy. *Arthroscopy*. 2014;30(5):639-644.)

Fabre et al (1999) identified 34 patients who underwent operative release for SSN neuropathy. In their study, pain relief after surgery was less reliable with 15 of 34 patients having complete resolution of pain, 1 patient having slight pain, and 8 patients having moderate pain postoperatively. Of the 25 patients who had atrophy of both the infraspinatus and supraspinatus, 13 had full recovery of muscle bulk in both supra- and infraspinatus musculature, 7 had improvement in atrophy in both, and in 5 there was no noticeable atrophy of the supraspinatus with interval improvement in infraspinatus muscle bulk. Isolated atrophy of infraspinatus persisted in 4 of 7 patients for whom it was identified preoperatively (Fabre et al, 1999). Hill et al (2014) found that patients with structural causes of SSN neuropathy did better than those without clear mechanical processes.

Discussion

Increasing interest has been directed at SSN pathology as a cause of significant pain and disability in patients, with and without concomitant pathology involving the shoulder. Diagnosis of SSN dysfunction is frequently complicated by vague presenting symptoms of pain over the superior and posterior aspect of the shoulder. EMG and NCV studies may be equivocal. Surgeons should consider SSN neuropathy in patients with unexplained posterosuperior shoulder pain with external rotation weakness and supra- and infraspinatus atrophy. SSN dysfunction in the absence of concomitant pathology can be managed with a trial of conservative management. In patients who fail conservative management and patients with SSN dysfunction in the setting of concomitant shoulder pathology, operative decompression is recommended. Pain relief is more assured than return of strength.

References

Antoniou J, Tae SK, Williams GR, Bird S, Ramsey ML, Iannotti JJ. Suprascapular neuropathy. Variability in the diagnosis, treatment, and outcome. *Clin Orthop Relat Res.* 2001;386:131–138.

Arriaza R, Ballesteros J, López-Vidriero E. Suprascapular neuropathy as a cause of swimmer's shoulder: results after arthroscopic treatment in 4 patients. *Am J Sports Med.* 2013;41(4):887–893.

Bennett DL, Cronin AM, Palmer WE, Kattapuram SV, Huang AJ. Optimization and standardization of technique for fluoroscopically guided suprascapular nerve blocks. *Am J Roentgenol.* 2014;202(3):576–584.

Boykin RE, Friedman DJ, Higgins LD, Warner JJ. Suprascapular neuropathy. *J Bone Joint Surg Am.* 2010;92(13):2348–2364.

Boykin RE, Friedman DJ, Zimmer ZR, Oaklander AL, Higgins LD, Warner JJ. Suprascapular neuropathy in a shoulder referral practice. *J Shoulder Elbow Surg.* 2011;20(6):983–988.

Brown TD, Newton PM, Steinmann SP, Levine WN, Bigliani LU. Rotator cuff tears and associated nerve injuries. *Orthopedics.* 2000;23(4):329–332.

Camargo PR, Zanca GG, Okino PS, et al. Scapular kinematics and muscle performance in a single case of Parsonage-Turner. *Man Ther.* 2014;19(1):77–81.

Clavert P, Thomazeau H. Peri-articular suprascapular neuropathy. *Orthop Traumatol Surg Res.* 2014;100(suppl 8):S409–S411.

Cogar AC, Johnsen PH, Potter HG, Wolfe SW. Subclavius posticus: an anomalous muscle in association with suprascapular nerve compression in an athlete. *Hand (N Y).* 2015;10(1):76–79.

Collin P, Treseder T, Lädermann A, et al. Neuropathy of the suprascapular nerve and massive rotator cuff tears: a prospective electromyographic study. *J Shoulder Elbow Surg.* 2014;23(1):28–34.

Costouros JG, Porramatikul M, Lie DT, Warner JJ. Reversal of suprascapular neuropathy following arthroscopic repair of massive supraspinatus and infraspinatus rotator cuff tears. *Arthroscopy.* 2007;23(11):1152–1161.

Demirhan M, Imhoff AB, Debski RE, Patel PR, Fu FH, Woo SL. The spinoglenoid ligament and its relationship to the suprascapular nerve. *J Shoulder Elbow Surg.* 2016;7(3):238–243.

Demirkan AF, Sargon MF, Erkula G, Kiter E. The spinoglenoid ligament: an anatomic study. *Clin Anat.* 2003;16(6):511–513.

Edelson JG. Bony bridges and other variations of the suprascapular notch. *J Bone Joint Surg Br.* 1995;77(3):505–506.

Fabre T, Piton C, Leclouerec G, Gervais-Delion F, Durandeau A. Entrapment of the suprascapular nerve. *J Bone Joint Surg Br.* 1999;81:414–419.

Fernandes MR, Fernandes RJ. Indirect arthroscopic decompression of spinoglenoid cyst with suprascapular neuropathy: report of two cases and literature review. *Rev Bras Ortop.* 2010;45(3):306–311.

Ferretti A, Carli AD, Fontana M. Injury of the suprascapular nerve at the spinoglenoid notch. the natural history of infraspinatus atrophy in volleyball players. *Am J Sports Med.* 2016;26(6):759–763.

Freehill MT, Shi LL, Tompson JD, Warner JJ. Suprascapular neuropathy: diagnosis and management. *Phys Sportsmed.* 2012;40(1):72–83.

Ghodadra N, Nho SJ, Verma NN, et al. Arthroscopic decompression of the suprascapular nerve at the spinoglenoid notch and suprascapular notch through the subacromial space. *Arthroscopy.* 2009;25(4):439–445.

Gupta R, Kapoor L, Shagotar S. Arthroscopic decompression of paralabral cyst around suprascapular notch causing suprascapular neuropathy. *J Clin Orthop Trauma.* 2015;6(3):184–186.

Habermeyer P, Brunner U, Wiedemann E, Wilhelm K. Compression syndromes of the shoulder and their differential diagnosis. *Orthopäde.* 1987;16(6):448–457.

Hashiguchi H, Iwashita S, Ohkubo A, Takai S. SLAP repair with arthroscopic decompression of spinoglenoid cyst. *SICOT J.* 2016;2:1.

Hashiuchi T, Sakurai G, Sawai K, et al. Ultrasound-guided arthroscope insertion and decompression of a supraspinous fossa. *J Med Ultrason (2001).* 2013;40(4):475–481.

Hill LJN, Jelsing EJ, Terry MJ, et al. Evaluation, treatment, and outcomes of suprascapular neuropathy: a 5-year review. *PM R.* 2014;6(9):774–780.

J Salata M, J Nho S, Chahal J, Van Thiel G, et al. Arthroscopic anatomy of the subdeltoid space. *Orthop Rev.* 2013;5(3):e25.

Joy P, Sinha MB, Satapathy BC. The ossified bifid superior transverse scapular ligament causing a double suprascapular foramen: a case report. *J Clin Diagn Res.* 2015;9(6). AD03-04.

Kharay SS, Sharma A, Singh P. Unusual morphology of scapulae: incidence and dimensions of ossified ligaments and supraspinous bony tunnels for clinical consideration. *Singapore Med J.* 2016;57(1):29–32.

Kim DH, Murovic JA, Tiel RL, Kline DG. Management and outcomes of 42 surgical suprascapular nerve injuries and entrapments. *Neurosurgery.* 2005;57(1):120–127.

Kim SH, Kim SJ, Sung CH, Koh YG, Kim YC, Park YS. Arthroscopic suprascapular nerve decompression at the suprascapular notch. *Knee Surg Sports Traumatol Arthrosc.* 2009;17(12):1504–1507.

Krivickas LS, Wilbourn AJ. Sports and peripheral nerve injuries: report of 190 injuries evaluated in a single electromyography laboratory. *Muscle Nerve.* 1998;21(8):1092–1094.

Kumar A, Sharma A, Singh P. Anatomical study of the suprascapular notch: quantitative analysis and clinical considerations for suprascapular nerve entrapment. *Singapore Med J.* 2014;55(1):41–44.

Lafosse L, Piper K, Lanz U, Costouros JG, et al. arthroscopic suprascapular nerve release: indications and technique. *J Shoulder Elbow Surg.* 2011;20(suppl 2):S9–S13.

Leclere LE, Shi LL, Lin A, Yannopoulos P, Higgins LD, Warner JJ. Complete fatty infiltration of intact rotator cuffs caused by suprascapular neuropathy. *Arthroscopy.* 2014;30(5):639–644.

Lee BCS, Yegappan M, Thiagarajan P. Suprascapular nerve neuropathy secondary to spinoglenoid notch ganglion cyst: case reports and review of literature. *Ann Acad Med.* 2007;36(12):1032–1035.

Lee YKi, Han EY, Choi SW, Kim BY, Suh MJ. Type 2 superior labral anterior to posterior lesion-related paralabral cyst causing isolated infraspinatus paralysis: two case reports. *Ann Rehabil Med.* 2015;39(5):848–852.

Mallon WJ, Wilson RJ, Albritton MJ, et al. The association of suprascapular neuropathy with massive rotator cuff tears: a preliminary report. *J Shoulder Elbow Surg.* 2003;15(4):395–398.

Martin SD, Warren RF, Martin TL, Kennedy K, O'Brien SJ, Wickiewicz TL. Suprascapular neuropathy. Results of non-operative treatment. *J Bone Joint Surg Am.* 1997;79(8):1159–1165.

Moriggl B. Fundamentals, possibilities and limitations of sonography of osteofibrous tunnels in the shoulder area. 1. *Ann Anat.* 1997;179(4):355–373.

Murphy RJ, Carr AJ. Shoulder pain. *BMJ Clin Evid*. 2010;07(1107):1–37.

Oizumi N, Suenaga N, Funakoshi T, et al. Recovery of sensory disturbance after arthroscopic decompression of the suprascapular nerve. *J Shoulder Elbow Surg*. 2012;21(6):759–764.

Piasecki DP, Anthony AR, Bach BR, Nicholson GP. Suprascapular neuropathy. *J Am Acad Orthop Surg*. 2009;17(11):665–676.

Plancher KD, Peterson RK, Johnston JC, et al. The spinoglenoid ligament. Anatomy, morphology, and histological findings. *J Shoulder Elbow Surg*. 2005;87(2):361–365.

Polguj M, Jędrzejewski K, Majos A, Topol M. The trifid superior transverse scapular ligament: a case report and review of the literature. *Folia Morphol (Warsz)*. 2012a;71(2):118–120.

Polguj M, Jędrzejewski K, Topol M. The bifid anterior coracoscapular ligament: a new morphological variation and its potential clinical implications. *Folia Morphol (Warsz)*. 2012b;71(4):282–284.

Polguj M, Sibiński M, Grzegorzewski A, Grzelak P, Majos A, Topol M. Variation in morphology of suprascapular notch as a factor of suprascapular nerve entrapment. *Int Orthop*. 2013;37(11):2185–2192.

Reineck JR, Krishnan SG, Barwood SA, et al. Subligamentous suprascapular artery encountered during arthroscopic suprascapular nerve release: a report of three cases. *J Shoulder Elbow Surg*. 2007;18(3):1–3.

Shah AA, Butler RB, Sung SY, Wells JH, Higgins LD, Warner JJ. Clinical outcomes of suprascapular nerve decompression. *J Shoulder Elbow Surg*. 2011;20(6):975–982.

Shi LL, Freehill MT, Yannopoulos P, Warner JJ. Suprascapular nerve: is it important in cuff pathology? *Adv Orthop*. 2012;2012:516985.

Shimokobe H, Gotoh M, Mitsui Y, et al. Ganglion cyst in the supraspinous fossa: arthroscopically undetectable cases. *Kurume Med J*. 2013;60(1):21–24.

Steiman I. Painless infraspinatus atrophy due to suprascapular nerve entrapment. *Arch Phys Med Rehabil*. 1988;69(8):641–643.

Strauss EJ, Barker JU, McGill K, Verma NN. The evaluation and management of failed distal clavicle excision. *Sports Med Arthrosc Rev*. 2010;18(3):213–219.

Tan BY, Lee KT. SLAP lesion with supraglenoid labral cyst causing suprascapular nerve compression: a case report. *Malays Orthop J*. 2012;6(suppl A):46–48.

Tragord BS, Bui-Mansfield LT, Croy T, Shaffer SW. Suprascapular neuropathy after distal clavicle resection and coracoclavicular ligament reconstruction: a resident's case problem. *J Orthop Sports Phys Ther*. 2015;45(4):299–305.

Vad VB, Southern D, Warren RF, et al. Prevalence of peripheral neurologic injuries in rotator cuff tears with atrophy. *J Shoulder Elbow Surg*. 2003;12(4):333–336.

Westrick RB, Fogarty BT, Johnson MP. Posterior labral tear with a paralabral cyst causing suprascapular nerve compression. *J Orthop Sports Phys Ther*. 2013;43(7):511.

Witvrouw E, Cools A, Lysens R, et al. Suprascapular neuropathy in volleyball players. *Br J Sports Med*. 2000;34(3):174–180.

Yang HJ, Gil YC, Jin JD, Ahn SV, Lee HY. Topographical anatomy of the suprascapular nerve and vessels at the suprascapular notch. *Clin Anat*. 2012;25(3):359–365.

Zehetgruber H, Noske H, Lang T, Wurnig C. Suprascapular nerve entrapment. a meta-analysis. *Int Orthop*. 2002;26(6):339–343.

8 Isolated Subscapularis Tendon Tear

8-8A PHYSICAL EXAMINATION AND IMAGING

DAVID BERNHOLT, MD and ROBERT H. BROPHY, MD

Introduction

- History:
  - Most common mechanisms are forced external rotation/hyperextension and anterior dislocation.
  - Common complaints are anterior shoulder pain and weakness.
- Examination:
  - Assessment should be made for increased passive external rotation.
  - Focused testing of subscapularis can be done through a variety of examination maneuvers, including lift-off test, internal rotation lag sign, belly press/Napoleon test, belly-off test, and bear hug test.
- Imaging:
  - Magnetic resonance imaging (MRI) is the modality of choice.
  - Ultrasonography is similar in sensitivity to MRI for full-thickness tears.
  - Arthroscopy remains the gold standard for diagnosis of subscapularis tears.

History

As with any injury, a thorough history should be obtained with emphasis on mechanism and symptoms. Traumatic injuries of the subscapularis may occur through forced external rotation or hyperextension of the shoulder (Gerber & Krushell, 1991; Kreuz et al, 2005) or in association with an anterior dislocation of the shoulder (Gerber & Krushell, 1991; Neviaser et al, 1988). One study reported a direct blow to the shoulder as the mechanism for 13 of their patients with either full or partial subscapularis tears (Kreuz et al, 2005). Alternatively, a subscapularis tear may manifest without any known traumatic event, as is often the case for other rotator cuff tears. Patients typically complain of anterior shoulder pain (Gerber & Krushell, 1991; Kreuz et al, 2005; Resch et al, 2000); however, anterior shoulder pain has neither high sensitivity nor high specificity for subscapularis tears. Patients with any rotator cuff pathology most often report anterior or lateral pain irrespective of which tendons are involved (Itoi et al, 2006). In addition to pain, patients may complain of weakness about the shoulder, especially with internal rotation. When associated with an anterior dislocation, subscapularis ruptures may also manifest as subjective or clinical instability; however, instability is not typically present in forced external rotation or hyperextension injuries (Gerber & Krushell, 1991).

Physical Examination

Physical examination for a subscapularis injury should begin with visual inspection of the shoulder, noting areas of swelling, ecchymosis, or atrophy. Careful palpation of the shoulder can identify area(s) of maximal tenderness; tenderness may be present over the anterior aspect of the glenohumeral joint or at the intertubercular groove (Deutsch et al, 1997; Kreuz et al, 2005). Active and passive ranges of motion of the shoulder should be assessed. An increase in passive external rotation greater than 10 degrees relative to the unaffected side is supportive of a complete subscapularis tendon rupture (Resch et al, 2000; Gerber et al, 1996). This finding was present during office examination in 10 of 16 patients in the series reported by Gerber et al and in 5 of 8 described by Resch et al, and was present in all of the Gerber group's patients under anesthesia. If the patient sustains only a partial tear of the subscapularis, a significant increase in passive external rotation is not expected to be present.

There are six examination maneuvers described in the English literature that attempt to diagnose injury to the subscapularis tendon by isolating its motor function (Video 8A.1):

LIFT-OFF TEST

The lift-off test, initially described by Gerber and Krushell (1991), is performed by having the patient place the hand on the affected side behind the back with the elbow flexed to approximately 90 degrees and the dorsum of the hand resting against the midlumbar region of the back or, if possible, the lower border of the scapula. The patient is then asked to lift the hand off of the back through additional internal rotation of the shoulder (Fig. 8A.1). The result is positive when the patient is unable to lift the hand away from the back. This test can be performed only in patients who have full passive internal rotation of the shoulder and who are not limited by pain when attempting active internal rotation of the shoulder.

The lift-off test places the shoulder near maximal internal rotation and extension, which Gerber and Krushell (1991) suggested would best isolate the motor function of the subscapularis. Electromyography (EMG) studies have shown that the subscapularis is the primary internal rotator of the shoulder in the lift-off position (Greis et al, 1996; Kadaba et al, 1992 Stefko et al, 1997; Tokish et al, 2003); however there are still contributions from other internal rotators of the shoulder as well as extensors of the shoulder and elbow (Stefko et al, 1997; Tokish et al, 2003). Increasing the amount of shoulder internal rotation at the start point of the lift-off test helps increase the activity of the subscapularis and further isolate its function (Greis et al, 1996; Stefko et al, 1997). In one study, patients with a visually confirmed subscapularis rupture, as well as patients given a targeted nerve block to prevent any subscapularis function, were able to perform the lift-off maneuver with the hand at the buttocks and midlumbar region but were unable to do so with the shoulder in maximal internal rotation with the hand at the lower border of the scapula (Stefko et al, 1997).

INTERNAL ROTATION LAG SIGN

The internal rotation lag sign was first described by Hertel et al in 1996. This test is carried out using the same positioning as in the lift-off test. The examiner then lifts the hand passively away from the back by internally rotating the patient's shoulder. The patient is instructed to maintain the position of the hand away from the back, and the examiner lets go of the hand while still supporting the patient's elbow (Fig. 8A.2). The result is positive if there is an internal rotation lag, meaning that the patient's hand falls toward the back. The amount of lag can also be measured quantitatively, and Hertel et al (1996) suggested recording this lag to the nearest 5 degrees . Like the lift-off test, the internal rotation lag test requires full passive internal rotation and painless active internal rotation to provide accurate results. Because this test uses the same positioning as the lift-off test, the afore mentioned EMG studies likely apply to it as well, although these studies did not assess the internal rotation lag sign specifically.

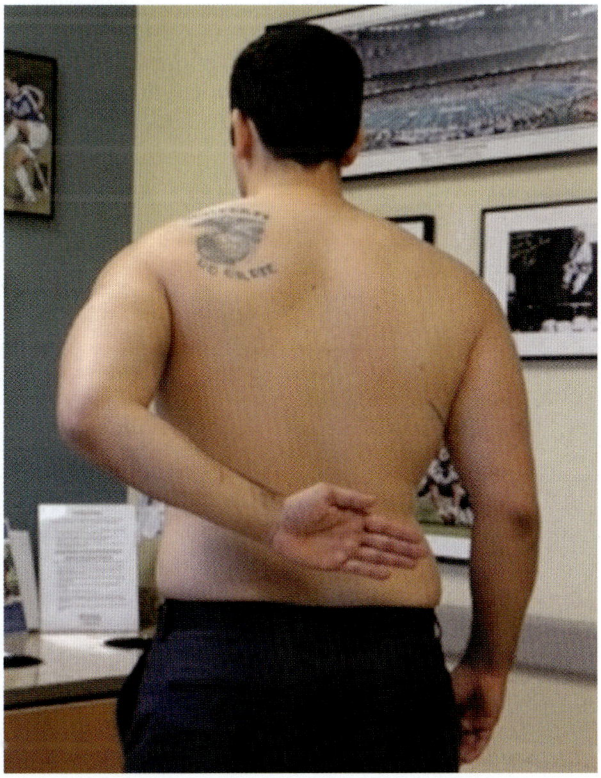

Fig. 8A.1 Photograph of lift-off test being performed.

BELLY PRESS TEST OR NAPOLEON TEST

The belly press test was first described by Gerber et al in their 1996 study. They developed it to test subscapularis function in patients in whom passive internal rotation is too short for positioning for the lift-off test. To perform the test, the patient places the palm of the hand against the abdomen and then pushes the hand against the abdomen with the wrist in neutral while internally rotating the shoulder to bring the elbow anterior to the trunk. A positive result occurs when the patient is unable to keep the elbow anterior to the trunk (Gerber et al, 1996) (Fig. 8A.3).

The modified belly press test and Napoleon test (Ballmer et al, 1997) have been presented as alternatives to the originally described belly press test. The tests are performed the same way by the patient, but the results are determined by the amount of wrist flexion required to keep the elbow anterior

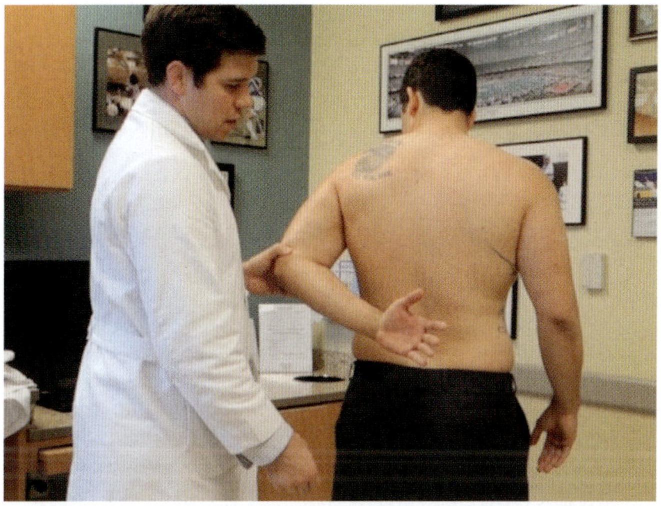

Fig. 8A.2 Photograph of internal rotation lag test being performed.

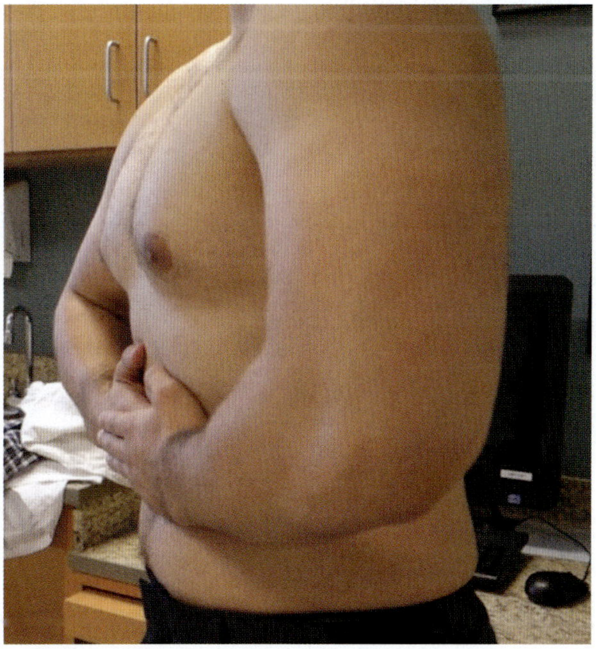

Fig. 8A.3 Photograph of belly press test being performed.

to the trunk (Fig. 8A.4). The modified belly press test is performed on both sides and a positive result occurs when there is 10 degrees or greater increased wrist flexion on the affected side (Barstch et al, 2010; Scheibel et al, 2006). For the Napoleon test (Ballmer et al, 1997), a positive result consists of wrist flexion from 60 to 90 degrees, an intermediate result of wrist flexion from 30 to 60 degrees, and a negative result with wrist remaining neutral (Burkhart & Tehrany, 2002). These three categorizations for the Napoleon test are meaningful because in the series reported by Burkhart and Tehrany (2002), all the patients with complete subscapularis tears had a positive result, patients with partial tears greater than 50% most often had an intermediate result, and patients with partial tears less than 50% tended to have a negative result.

BELLY-OFF TEST

The belly-off test is another test for the internal rotation lag sign but is performed with positioning similar to that for the belly press test. The examiner performs the test by flexing the patient's elbow to 90 degrees and passively flexing and maximally internally rotating the shoulder to bring the patient's palm against the abdomen. One of the examiner's hands should be used to stabilize the patient's elbow while the other holds the hand/wrist of the patient in position against the abdomen. The examiner then releases the patient's hand/wrist while instructing the patient to maintain the position of the hand against the abdomen (Fig. 8A.5). If the hand lifts off of the abdomen, the result is considered positive (Scheibel et al, 2005).

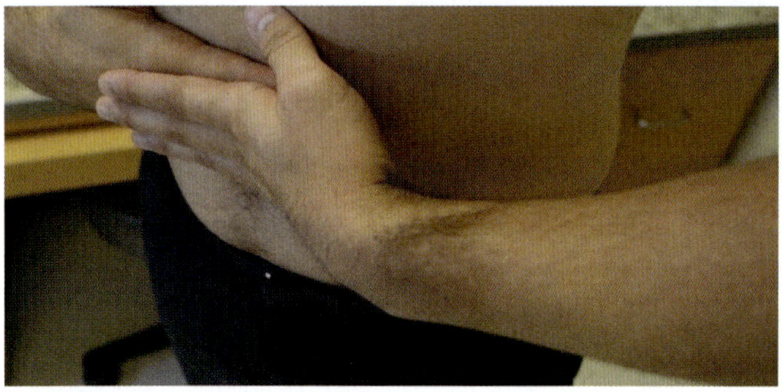

Fig. 8A.4 Photograph demonstrating wrist flexion during performance of the belly press test.

BEAR HUG TEST

To perform the bear hug test, the examiner places the palm of the patient's hand belonging to the injured extremity on the contralateral acromioclavicular (AC) joint with the shoulder flexed to either 45 or 90 degrees. With the palm in this position, the elbow should be positioned directly anterior to the shoulder and should be kept directly in line with the shoulder, maintaining the same craniocaudal level. The patient is then asked to keep this position while the examiner applies an external rotation force to the patient's wrist in an attempt to pull the wrist/palm away from the contralateral AC joint (Fig. 8A.6). A positive result occurs when the patient is unable to maintain the palm against the AC joint or the position of the arm/elbow or when there is detectable weakness relative to the contralateral extremity (Barth et al, 2006). EMG analysis of upper and lower subscapularis firing during this test has shown that the test better isolates the subscapularis muscle with 45 or 90 degrees of shoulder flexion than with 0 degrees of flexion; the analysis also found that when the test is performed at 45 degrees of flexion, it better isolates the upper subscapularis, whereas at 90 degrees of flexion it better isolates the lower subscapularis (Chao et al, 2008).

INTERNAL ROTATION RESISTANCE TEST

The internal rotation resistance test as presented by Lin et al (2015) is performed with the patient in two different positions: (1) 0 degrees of shoulder abduction and external rotation, and (2) 90 degrees of abduction and maximal external rotation. For the 0-degree test, the patient flexes the elbows to 90 degrees bilaterally with the arms adducted at the side

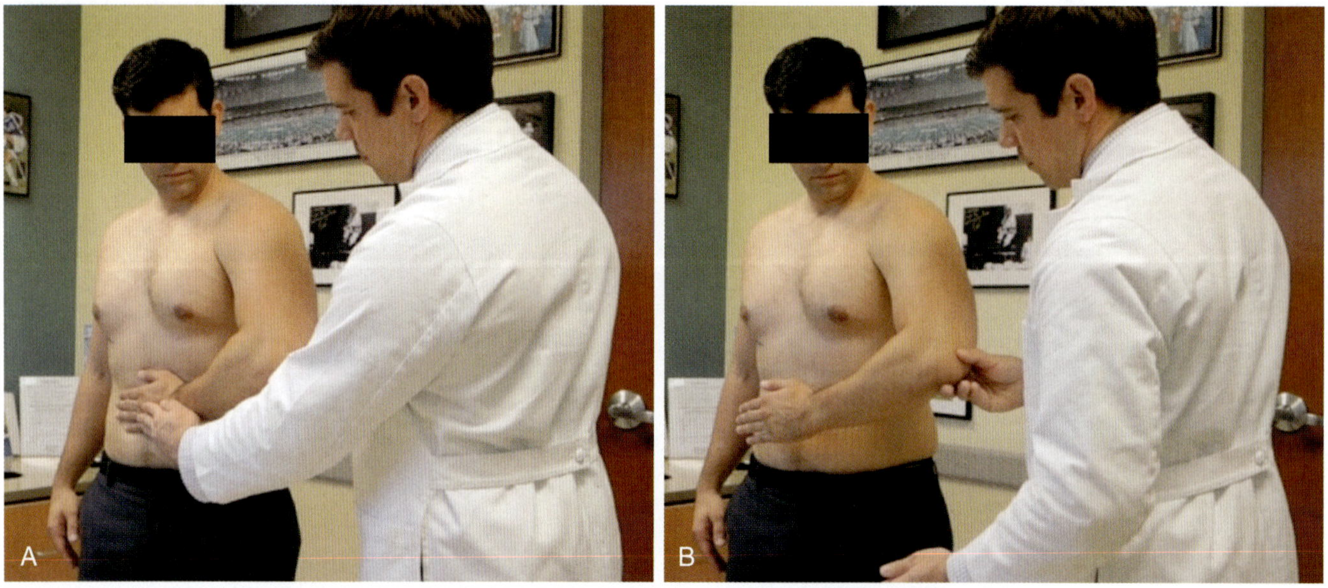

Fig. 8A.5 (A) Photograph of belly-off test being performed. (B) Positive result of this test.

and the fingertips facing forward to indicate 0 degrees of shoulder external rotation. The examiner then applies an internal rotation force perpendicular to the patient's forearm while asking the patient to maintain the position. For the 90-degree test, the patient flexes the elbow to 90 degrees, and then the shoulder is abducted to 90 degrees and externally rotated to a maximal degree by the examiner. The examiner then applies an internal rotation force perpendicular to the patient's forearm while asking the patient to maintain the position. A positive result occurs when the patient cannot maintain the position or when there is detectable weakness in comparison to the contralateral side (Lin et al, 2015).

UTILITY OF SUBSCAPULARIS CLINICAL TESTS

Owing to the low frequency of isolated complete subscapularis tendon ruptures, there are no well-established sensitivity and specificity values for clinical subscapularis tests. This situation is further complicated by the fact that many studies combine partial-thickness and full-thickness subscapularis tendon tears in assessing test sensitivity and specificity. The lift-off test has shown nearly perfect sensitivity for full-thickness tendon tears in many series (Gerber & Krushell, 1991; Kreuz et al, 2005; Resch et al, 2000); however, when partial subscapularis tendon tears are included, the sensitivity has been reported as low as 12% to 69% (Bartsch et al, 2010; Hegedus et al, 2012; Kim et al, 2003; Yoon et al, 2013). When initially presented by Hertel et al (1996), the internal rotation lag sign showed a much higher sensitivity than the lift-off test, but this figure has not been replicated in all studies, and the sensitivity now ranges from 20% to 71% (Bartsch et al, 2010; Lin et al, 2015; Yoon et al, 2013) The modified belly press and belly-off tests were reported as much more sensitive (88% and 87%, respectively) than the lift-off and internal rotation lag sign tests (71% and 40%, respectively) in one of the larger studies comparing the effectiveness of the various clinical examination maneuvers in diagnosing partial subscapularis tears (Bartsch et al, 2010). Similarly, the bear hug test has been reported to have a higher sensitivity for partial tears than the lift-off test (60% vs 17%) (Barth et al, 2006). The greater sensitivities of the belly press, belly-off, and bear hug tests for partial subscapularis tears have been suggested to result from more recruitment of the upper subscapularis than of the lower subscapularis with the test movements, because most partial tears occur at the upper portion of the tendon. Although one EMG study supported this explanation (Tokish et al, 2003), a later EMG study showed no difference in recruitment of the upper and lower subscapularis by the bear hug or belly press test and the lift-off test (Greis et al, 1996; Pennock et al, 2011). Despite the problematic lack of sensitivity with the various subscapularis examination maneuvers, these tests do show high specificity (Yoon et al, 2013).

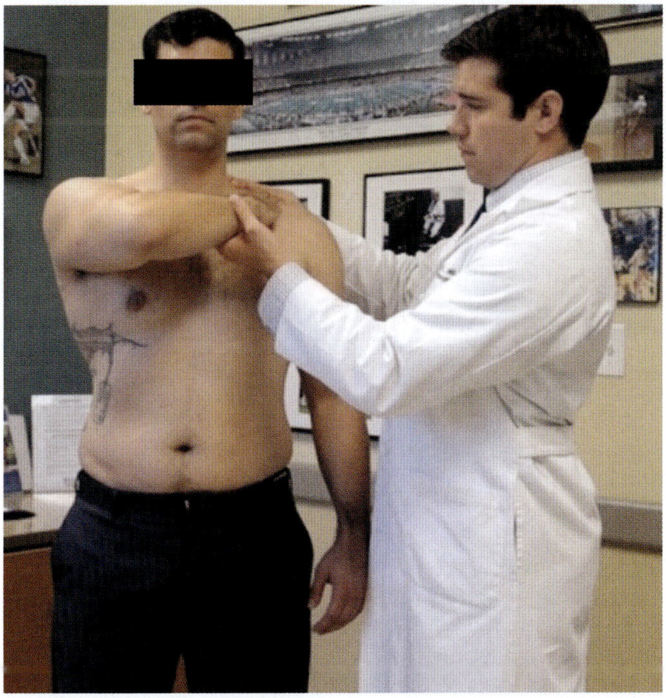

Fig. 8A.6 Photograph of bear hug test being performed.

Imaging

Because a subscapularis tear cannot often be diagnosed clinically, imaging is important to the diagnosis, although arthroscopy does remain the gold standard for diagnosis of subscapularis pathology. MRI is the primary imaging modality used to evaluate the integrity of the subscapularis. Unfortunately, just as with the clinical examination, MRI is very sensitive for identifying complete tears of the subscapularis tendon, but identifying partial tears comprising less than 50% of the tendon width with this imaging modality is difficult (Adams et al, 2010, 2012; Gryftopoulis et al, 2013; Smucny et al, 2016). To best view the subscapularis on MRI, a combination of the sagittal oblique and axial planes is used (Morag et al, 2011); using only one plane decreases the accuracy for diagnosis (Pfirmann et al, 1999). Furthermore, one study has suggested that the addition of radially sliced MR images can be used to increase sensitivity for subscapularis tears, particularly partial tears (Furukawa et al, 2014). Partial tears typically occur in the anterosuperior portion of the tendon, which is susceptible to the partial-volume effect, making them hard to visualize, and addition of radially sliced images helps mitigate this problem (Furukawa et al, 2014). Although use of intraarticular contrast for MR angiography (MRA) has been shown to enhance the diagnosis of supraspinatus and infraspinatus rotator cuff tears, one study showed MRA and MRI to be equivalent for diagnosis of subscapularis tears (Foad & Wijdicks, 2012). However, the ability to better assess for other shoulder pathology that may be responsible for the patient's symptoms makes MRA the preferred choice (de Jesus et al, 2009).

Overall, the reported accuracy for MRI is inconsistent across the literature. One of the biggest factors contributing to this may be the experience and training of the examiners reading the images. Multiple studies have reported very low sensitivity for detecting subscapularis tears on MRI, ranging between 31% and 39% (Adams et al, 2010; Foad & Wijdicks, 2012; Tung et al, 2001). In contrast, in two studies in which musculoskeletal radiologists read

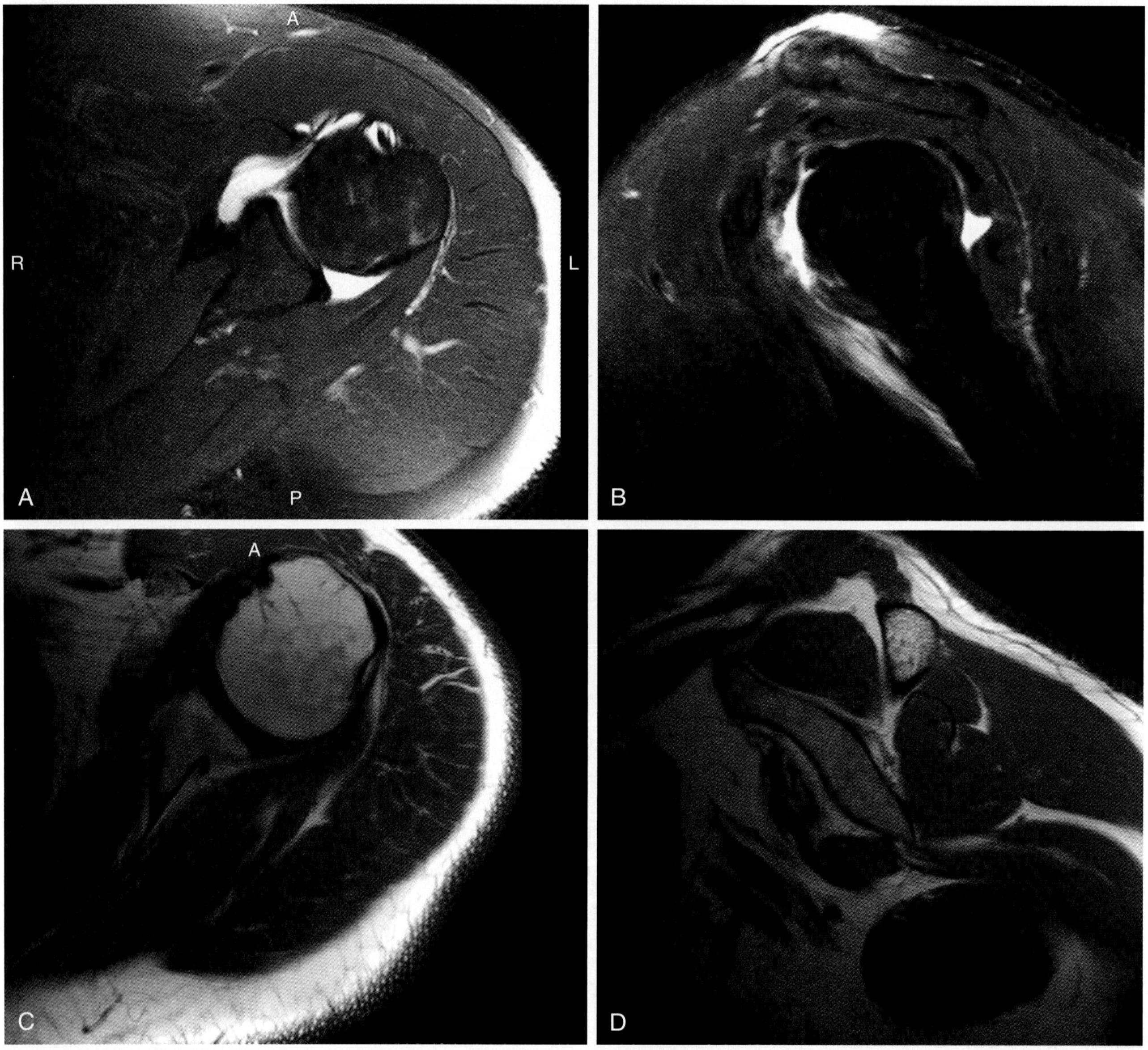

Fig. 8A.7 MR arthrography images demonstrating the four MRI diagnostic criteria proposed by Adams et al (2012) for subscapularis tears. (A) T2-weighted fat suppression axial slice demonstrating full-thickness tear of subscapularis tendon with retraction. (B) T2-weighted fat suppression sagittal slice demonstrating absence of subscapularis attachment to lesser tuberosity. (C) T1-weighted axial slice demonstrating medial subluxation of the long head of the biceps tendon. (D) T1-weighted sagittal slice demonstrating fatty atrophy of the subscapularis muscle belly.

the images, the sensitivity was reported at 80% and 91% and specificity at 91% and 86% for any tear, and sensitivity at 100% for full-thickness tears (Gryftopoulis et al, 2013; Pfirrman et al, 1999). In a follow-up study, whose initial study found a 39% sensitivity, Adams et al (2012) were able to markedly increase the sensitivity to 73% and specificity to 94% by employing strict diagnostic criteria to assess for subscapularis tears. These diagnostic criteria require that two of the following conditions be met: (1) the presence of tendon tear on the axial or (2) sagittal images, (3) presence of subluxation or dislocation of the biceps tendon on the axial images, and (4) presence of atrophy of the subscapularis muscle on the sagittal images (Adams et al, 2012) (Fig. 8A.7). Importantly, in this study all MR images were read by five orthopedic surgeons at different institutions, suggesting that use of these criteria may be generalizable and may allow for more accurate interpretation of MRI for subscapularis tears even in the absence of a trained musculoskeletal radiologist.

Although MRI is the imaging modality of choice for evaluating subscapularis injuries, ultrasonography also has been shown to have utility. It has been validated in the diagnosis of rotator cuff tears in general (de Jesus et al, 2009; Teefey et al, 2000, 2004). There are limited data pertaining to ultrasonography for the subscapularis tendon specifically, but ultrasound has been demonstrated to be able to accurately diagnosis full-thickness tears (Farin & Jaroma, 1996; Teefey et al, 2005). The largest study of ultrasonography for subscapularis ruptures demonstrated a sensitivity of 86% for full-thickness subscapularis tendon tears; however, ultrasound is less sensitive for evaluating small partial-thickness subscapularis tears (Farin & Jaroma, 1996; Teefey et al, 2005). It should be noted that accurate ultrasound evaluation of the subscapularis tendon requires that the patient have full external rotation of the shoulder, a potential limitation of this imaging modality.

Plain radiographs are of minimal utility in the diagnosis of a subscapularis tendon injury, but shoulder radiographs should be obtained in the patient presenting with a traumatic shoulder injury or chronic shoulder pain to rule out fracture, arthritic change, and any bony lesions. In the case of a complete subscapularis rupture, it is possible to see anterior subluxation of the humeral head on a radiograph. Subscapularis tendon injuries may occur after anterior dislocation, and in this case radiographs may demonstrate a bony Bankart or Hill-Sachs lesion. Computed tomography could be used to better evaluate any of these bony lesions, but it is not helpful for diagnosis of a subscapularis tendon rupture.

References

Adams CR, Brady PC, Koo SS, et al. A systematic approach for diagnosing subscapularis tendon tears with preoperative magnetic resonance imaging scans. *Arthroscopy*. 2012;28:1592–1600.

Adams CR, Schoolfield JD, Burkhart SS. Accuracy of preoperative magnetic resonance imaging in predicting a subscapularis tendon tear based on arthroscopy. *Arthroscopy*. 2010;26:1427–1433.

Barth JRH, Burkhart S, De Beer JF. The bear-hug test: A new and sensitive test for diagnosing a subscapularis tear. *Arthroscopy*. 2006;22:1076–1084.

Bartsch M, Greiner S, Haas NP, Scheibel M. Diagnostic values of clinical tests for subscapularis lesions. *Knee Surg Sports Traumatol Arthrosc*. 2010;18:1712–1717.

Ballmer FT, Lambert SM, Hertel R. Napoleon's sign: a test to assess subscapularis function. *J Shoulder Elbow Surg*. 1997;6:193.

Burkhart SS, Tehrany AM. Arthroscopic subscapularis tendon repair: technique and preliminary results. *Arthroscopy*. 2002;17:454–463.

Chao S, Thomas S, Yucha D, Kelly JD, Driban J, Swanik K. An electromyographic assessment of the "bear hug": an examination for the evaluation of the subscapularis muscle. *Arthroscopy*. 2008;24:1265–1270.

Deutsch A, Altchek DW, Veltri DM, Potter HG, Warren RF. Traumatic tears of the subscapularis tendon: clinical diagnosis, magnetic resonance imaging findings, and operative treatment. *Am J Sports Med*. 1997;25:13–22.

de Jesus JO, Parker L, Frangos AJ, Nazarian LN. Accuracy of MRI, MR arthrography, and ultrasound in the diagnosis of rotator cuff tears: a meta-analysis. *Am J Roentgenol*. 2009;192:1701–1707.

Farin P, Jaroma H. Sonographic detection of tears of the anterior portion of the rotator cuff (subscapularis tendon tears). *J Ultrasound Med*. 1996;15:221–225.

Foad A, Wijdicks CA. The accuracy of magnetic resonance imaging and magnetic resonance arthrogram versus arthroscopy in the diagnosis of subscapularis tendon injury. *Arthroscopy*. 2012;28:636–641.

Furukawa R, Morihara T, Arai Y, et al. Diagnostic accuracy of magnetic resonance imaging for subscapularis tendon tears using radial-slice magnetic resonance images. *J Shoulder Elbow Surg*. 2014;23: 283–290.

Gerber C, Krushell RJ. Isolated tears of the subscapularis muscle: clinical features in sixteen cases. *J Bone Joint Surg Br*. 1991;73B:389–394.

Gerber C, Hersche O, Farron A. Isolated rupture of the subscapularis tendon. *J Bone Joint Surg Am*. 1996;78:1015–1023.

Greis PE, Kuhn JE, Schultheis J, Hintermeister R, Hawkins R. Validation of the liftoff test and analysis of subscapularis activity during maximal internal rotation. *Am J Sports Med*. 1996;24:589–593.

Gyftopoulos S, O'Donnell J, Shah NP, Goss J, Babb J, Recht MP. Correlation of MRI with arthroscopy for the evaluation of the subscapularis tendon: a musculoskeletal division's experience. *Skelet Radiol*. 2013;42: 1269–1275.

Hegedus EJ, Goode A, Cook C, et al. Which physical examination tests provide clinicians with the most value when examining the shoulder? Update of a systematic review with meta-analysis of individual tests. *Br J Sports Med*. 2012;46:964–978.

Hertel R, Ballmer FT, Lambert SM, Gerber C. Lag signs in the diagnosis of rotator cuff rupture. *J Shoulder Elbow Surg*. 1996;5:307–313.

Itoi E, Minagawa H, Yamamoto N, Seki N, Abe H. Are pain location and physical examinations useful in locating a tear site of the rotator cuff? *Am J Sports Med*. 2006;34:256–264.

Kadaba MP, Cole A, Wootten ME, et al. Intramuscular wire electromyography of the subscapularis. *J Orthop Res*. 1992;10:394–397.

Kim TK, Rauh PB, McFarland EG. Partial tears of the subscapularis tendon found during arthroscopic procedures on the shoulder: a statistical analysis of sixty cases. *Am J Sports Med*. 2003;31:744–750.

Kreuz PC, Remiger A, Erggelet C, Hinterwimmer S, Niemeyer P, Gächter A. Isolated and combined tears of the subscapularis tendon. *Am J Sports Med*. 2005;33:1831–1837.

Lin L, Yan H, Xiao J, Ao Y, Cui G. Internal rotation resistance test at abduction and external rotation: a new clinical test for diagnosing subscapularis lesions. *Knee Surg Sports Traumatol Arthrosc*. 2015;23:1247–1252.

Morag Y, Jamadar DA, Miller B, Dong Q, Jacobson JA. The subscapularis: anatomy, injury, and imaging. *Skeletal Radiol*. 2011;40:255–269.

Neviaser RJ, Neviaser TJ, Neviaser JS. Concurrent rupture of the rotator cuff and anterior dislocation of the shoulder in the older patient. *J Bone Joint Surg*. 1988;70:1308–1311.

Pennock AT, Pennington WW, Torry MR, et al. The influence of arm and shoulder position on the bear-hug, belly-press, and lift-off tests: an electromyographic study. *Am J Sports Med*. 2011;39:2338–2346.

Pfirrmann CW, Zanetti M, Weishaupt D, Gerber C, Hodler J. Subscapularis tendon tears: detection and grading at MR arthrography. *Radiology*. 1999;213:709–714.

Resch H, Povacz P, Ritter E, Matschi W. Transfer of the pectoralis major muscle for the treatment of irreparable rupture of the subscapularis tendon. *J Bone Joint Surg Am*. 2000;82:372–382.

Scheibel M, Magosch P, Pritsch M, Lichtenberg S, Habermeyer P. The belly-off sign: a new clinical diagnostic sign for subscapularis lesions. *Arthroscopy*. 2005;21:1229–1235.

Scheibel M, Tsynman A, Magosch P, Schroeder RJ, Habermeyer P. Postoperative subscapularis muscle insufficiency after primary and revision open shoulder stabilization. *Am J Sports Med*. 2006;34:1586–1593.

Smucny M, Shin EC, Zhang AL, et al. Poor agreement on classification and treatment of subscapularis tendon tears. *Arthroscopy*. 2016;32: 246–251.

Stefko JM, Jobe FW, VanderWilde RS, Carden E, Pink M. Electromyographic and nerve block analysis of the subscapularis liftoff test. *J Shoulder Elbow Surg*. 1997;6:347–355.

Teefey SA, Hasan SA, Middleton WD, Patel M, Wright RW, Yamaguchi K. Ultrasonography of the rotator cuff: a comparison of ultrasonographic and arthroscopic findings in one hundred consecutive cases. *J Bone Joint Surg Am*. 2000;82:498–504.

Teefey SA, Rubin DA, Middleton WD, Hildebolt CF, Leibold RA, Yamaguchi K. Detection and quantification of rotator cuff tears: comparison of ultrasonographic, magnetic resonance imaging, and arthroscopic findings in seventy-one consecutive cases. *J Bone Joint Surg Am*. 2004;86:708–716.

Teefey SA, Middleton WD, Payne WT, Yamaguchi K. Detection and measurement of rotator cuff tears with sonography: analysis of diagnostic errors. *Am J Roentgenol*. 2005;184:1768–1773.

Tokish JM, Decker MJ, Ellis HB, Torry MR, Hawkins RJ. The belly-press test for the physical examination of the subscapularis muscle: electromyographic validation and comparison to the lift-off test. *J Shoulder Elbow Surg*. 2003;12:427–430.

Tung GA, Yoo DC, Levine SM, Brody JM, Green A. Subscapularis tendon tear: primary and associated signs on MRI. *J Comput Assist Tomogr*. 2001;25:417–424.

Yoon JP, Chung SW, Kim SH, Oh JH. Diagnostic value of four clinical tests for the evaluation of subscapularis integrity. *J Shoulder Elbow Surg*. 2013;22:1186–1192.

8-8B SURGICAL TREATMENT: ARTHROSCOPIC REPAIR

LAURENCE D. HIGGINS, MD, MBA; M. DANIEL HATCH, MD; and TYLER J. HUNT, BS

Introduction

- Arthroscopic repairs to the subscapularis tendon are unique because of the increased retraction, proximity to neurovascular structures, and limited visualization associated with this structure.
- The techniques for repair of these tears are varied, but for the surgeon it is most important to remember the principle of anatomic tension-free repair.
- The patient can be placed in the beach-chair or lateral position for this procedure.
- Repairs of isolated type I through III tears can be performed almost entirely intraarticularly, but type IV repairs require extraarticular work.
- The medial sling of the biceps tendon can be used to identify the superolateral portion of the retracted subscapularis tendon.
- Arthroscopic repair of isolated subscapularis tendon tears is as good as open repair.

Subscapularis tears were historically treated with an open technique and were the last rotator cuff tendon tears to be repaired arthroscopically owing to the unique challenges that arise from repair of that specific tendon (Burkhart & Brady, 2006). First, the subscapularis tendon, secondary to its relative excursion, retracts more than the rest of the rotator cuff when torn, making mobilization more difficult. Second, the difficulty in mobilization is compounded by the fact that this tendon tends to scar to the coracoid near important neurovascular structures, namely the axillary artery and both the axillary and musculocutaneous nerves. Finally, visualization to mobilize the retracted and scarred subscapularis is challenging in the restricted subcoracoid space, particularly because of the close proximity to the previously mentioned neurovascular structures. Although techniques have been described for every type and variety of tear, adhering to the well-established principles of repair is more important than following any specific technique.

On the basis of preoperative imaging and intraoperative evaluation, Lafosse et al (2007) classified subscapularis tears into five distinct types (Table 8B.1). Type I tears are partial tears that involve the deep fibers of the superior one-third of the tendon. Type II through V tears are complete tears that are broken into thirds, from superior to inferior. Type II is a full-thickness tear of the superior one-third of the tendon, Type III a full-thickness tear of the superior two-thirds of the tendon, and Type IV a full-thickness tear involving the entire tendon with a well-centered head and fatty degeneration less than or equal to Goutallier stage 3. Type V is similar to type IV in dimension, but with an eccentric head that causes coracoid impingement and fatty degeneration greater than Goutallier stage 3.

In the following section, we specifically detail our approach and technique for arthroscopically treating type I through type IV tears.

Surgical Options

POSITIONING

All patients receive an interscalene block prior to surgery. The patient is positioned in the beach-chair position (T-Max/Shoulder Positioner, Smith & Nephew, York, UK) at 70 degrees of inclination after having been intubated and receiving general anesthesia. The hips and knees should be flexed gently to relieve pressure on the sciatic nerve. The head and neck are positioned with a mask in a neutral position.

The entire operative extremity is prepared for surgery and draped free. The drapes should extend across the chest wall just above the nipple line, medially to about the sternoclavicular (SC) joint and across the lower neck, and posteriorly along the medial border of the scapula. The arm is then placed in a pneumatic arm holder (Spider Limb Positioner, Smith & Nephew) to allow free manipulation of the arm in space.

PORTALS

Three portals are typically used (Fig. 8B.1). First, a 30-degree arthroscope is introduced through the posterior soft spot portal approximately 2 cm inferior and medial to the posterolateral corner of the acromion (viewing portal). Next, the anterior portal is created, via an outside-in technique by placement of a spinal needle into the joint just lateral to the coracoid through the rotator interval, as a working portal to place the anchor and to pass sutures through the torn tendon. The third portal is an anterolateral accessory portal placed via the outside-in technique approximately 1 cm lateral and inferior to the anterolateral acromial edge. This last portal is parallel to the lesser tuberosity and is useful to assist in pulling traction to evaluate the tear pattern, release the tendon, debride the subcoracoid space and lesser tuberosity, and place suture anchors. A cannula is optionally placed in this portal.

Table 8B.1 Lafosse Classification of Subscapularis Tears

Type	Tear Description
I	Partial-thickness tear
II	Full-thickness tear of superior one-third
III	Full-thickness tear of superior two-thirds
IV	Complete subscapularis tear with well-centered head and ≤ Goutallier stage 3 fatty degeneration
V	Complete subscapularis tear with eccentric head and > Goutallier stage 3 fatty degeneration

Modified from Lafosse L, Jost B, Riland Y, et al. Structural integrity and clinical outcomes after arthroscopic repair of isolated subscapularis tears. *J Bone Joint Surg Am*. 2007;89(6):1184-1193.

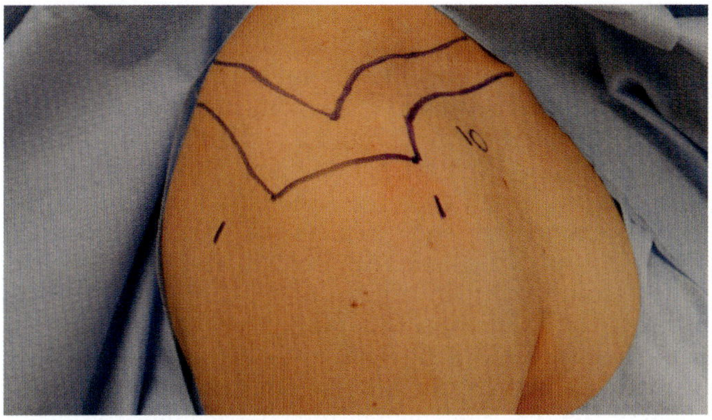

Fig. 8B.1 Outside view, right shoulder portal placement.

SURGICAL TECHNIQUE

The first step in any repair is to perform diagnostic arthroscopy to ensure that there is no other intraarticular pathology (i.e., biceps disease, labral tears, concomitant supraspinatus or infraspinatus tears, arthritis). If biceps pathology is discovered— biceps instability is a common concomitant problem in subscapularis tears—it may be addressed by tenotomy or tenodesis, and immediate management of a subluxated biceps tendon may facilitate both visualization and management of subscapularis tears. During the diagnostic portion of the arthroscopy, it is also useful to evaluate firsthand the tear pattern and reparability. A standard subacromial and subcoracoid decompression assists in providing space for repair as well as for evaluating the bursal-sided cuff tears.

Isolated type I through III subscapularis tears can be evaluated and treated almost entirely through intraarticular visualization from the posterior portal, but type IV tears typically require some extraarticular work. With electrocautery the rotator interval should be opened to delineate the borders of the subscapularis as well as specify the tear pattern. With the interval open, the anterior surface of the subscapularis can be visualized, although a 70-degree arthroscope is sometimes required. A probe inserted into the anterior portal is used to evaluate the tear and delineate any partial tearing or tears in continuity (when the subscapularis is torn off of the lesser tuberosity but held in a lateral position by a superficial band of tissue).

Appropriate releases of the tendon may be necessary to adequately mobilize the tendon (especially important in type IV tears). The placement of a traction suture, with a line of pull parallel to the subscapularis tendon, is often critical to the success of mobilization. Releases are performed with a combination of electrocautery and a shaver. A circumferential release requires the separating of the middle glenohumeral ligament (MGHL) from the posterior surface of the subscapularis in conjunction with release of subdeltoid and subcoracoid adhesions and the coracohumeral ligament. If the tendon tear is more chronic and the tendon retracted, it may have scarred to the anterior surface of the glenoid and/or the coracoid and need to be released. To safely perform releases anteriorly and inferiorly, one needs to identify and protect the axillary nerve with blunt dissection. After the tendon edge has been delineated and appropriately mobilized to allow tension-free mobilization to the lesser tuberosity footprint, the shaver and bur are used to decorticate and prepare the lesser tuberosity for repair.

Complete disruption of the subscapularis tendon is usually associated with tearing and medial retraction of the biceps tendon's medial sling. This tissue, commonly known as the "comma sign," assists the surgeon in identifying the superolateral portion of the retracted subscapularis tendon (Lo & Burkhart, 2003).

REPAIR OF SUBSCAPULARIS TEARS

Partial-Thickness Repair

(Video 8B.1)

Type I tears involve only the deep fibers of the subscapularis, making the repair markedly different from that used for full-thickness tears (types II–IV). Type I tears can be repaired fully intraarticularly and require minimal to no mobilization. The viewing portal is the standard posterior portal and the working portal is anterior through the rotator interval, cheating laterally. One double-loaded metal or biocomposite anchor (Arthrex, Naples, FL) is placed at the top portion of the subscapularis. We use a CleverHook (DePuysSynthes, Warsaw, IN) to shuttle sutures through the tendon and a lasso-loop technique with one end of the suture, and then pass the other end of the suture in a horizontal mattress fashion through the tissue, and then repeat this process with the other suture. This lasso-loop method allows the tendon to be advanced to the anchor in the footprint without creating undue tension on the repair. The knots are then tied with five reverse-post half-hitches.

Full-Thickness Repair

See Video 8B.2.

Type II through IV tears are repaired in similar fashion, but we focus here on type IV tears. A lateral portal is used as the viewing portal and an anterolateral portal as the working portal. The arm is placed in a forward-flexed and internally rotated position to open the subcoracoid space. If necessary for visualization and tendon mobilization a coracoplasty of the posterior coracoid is performed. The axillary nerve is visualized and isolated with blunt dissection, and then a traction suture is placed through the subscapularis tendon and pulled out through a small percutaneous hole in line with the direction of the native subscapularis. The traction suture is pulled by an assistant while the subscapularis is mobilized on the bursal and articular side (as noted previously). The lesser tuberosity is prepared by removal of soft tissue with a shaver and bur, but we avoid removing cortical bone. Our preferred technique for an isolated type IV subscapularis repair is to use two or three 4.5-mm metal corkscrew anchors double-loaded with FiberWire suture (Arthrex). We prefer metal anchors because the placement into the lesser tuberosity can be more difficult to visualize and there is no need to tap a metal anchor, thus decreasing the number of steps for repair. Additionally, the bone of the lesser tuberosity may be quite dense, and metal anchors will not suffer the fatigue fractures occasionally seen with biocomposite anchors. If the subscapularis tendon edges are frayed and weak, they are first debrided and then a horizontal mattress stitch with a lasso-loop technique (as described previously for partial tears) is employed. If the tissue edge is less frayed and strong the stitches are passed in a horizontal mattress pattern without a lasso loop.

The sutures are retrieved with a CleverHook or are shuttled with an ACCU-PASS Suture Shuttle (Smith & Nephew) through the anterior portal while traction (traction stitch or locking grasper) is pulled through the anterolateral portal and visualized from the lateral portal. It is most difficult to visualize the inferior aspect of the repair, so the inferior anchor is placed first, at the junction between the inferior one-third and superior two-thirds. Those sutures are then pulled out of another portal to keep them out of the way. Next, the superior anchor is placed between the inferior two-thirds and the superior one-third of the subscapularis tendon. The sutures are retrieved with CleverHooks, as described previously. Finally, the knots are tied with five reverse-post half-hitches, and the excess suture is cut.

POSTOPERATIVE CARE AND REHABILITATION

The arm and shoulder are placed in a shoulder immobilizer with an abduction pillow in neutral, which may be removed only for showers and changing clothes. The patient may remove dressings on postoperative day 3 for a shower. Passive range of motion starts at week 3 with formal physical therapy, and active motion starts at week 6. Strengthening is delayed until week 12. The patient is seen at 10 to 14 days for a wound check, and then at 6 weeks, 3 months, 6 months, and 1 year after surgery.

OUTCOMES

All studies on isolated subscapularis repairs are level IV retrospective studies, and there is one systematic review comparing open and arthroscopic results. The first report of an all-arthroscopic repair of the subscapularis was made by Burkhart and Tehrany (2002). The study consisted of 25 patients with an average follow-up of 10.7 months. At that early time-point, the patient's UCLA scores had improved from 10.7 (preoperatively) to 30.5 (postoperatively). The same patient cohort with the addition of 17 patients was reported on with a median follow-up of 5 years (Adams et al, 2008). The results showed that the improvement in functional scores was maintained, with the UCLA score improving from 15.7 to 31.6 and the American Shoulder and Elbow Surgeons (ASES) score rising from 40.5 to 91.2, with good or excellent results in 80% of patients. A third study with the same cohort at minimum 7-year follow-up found good to excellent results in 83.3% of patients, with 92.4% satisfied with their outcome, and showed that UCLA score improvement was still maintained (Denard et al, 2012).

Lafosse et al (2007), evaluating outcomes in 17 patients following arthroscopic repair of isolated subscapularis tendon tears at an average follow-up of 29 months, found results to those reported in the three Burkhart group studies. The UCLA score improved from 16 to 32, and the Constant score from 58 to 96. Postoperative computed tomographic arthrography found complete healing of the repair in 15 patients and partial retear in 2. Bartl et al (2011) reported on a cohort of 21 patients with isolated subscapularis tears who were treated with arthroscopic repair at an average follow-up of 27 months; they found the Constant score to have risen from 50 to 82. Even though postoperative magnetic resonance imaging (MRI) demonstrated that 20 of 21 patients (95.2%) had tendon-to-bone healing, the belly-press test result remained positive in 24%.

Mall et al (2012) compared the results of open and arthroscopic repairs in isolated subscapularis tears in a systematic review. They reviewed three arthroscopic and six open studies and found similar healing rates of 90% to 95% with no apparent difference in outcome measures.

Conclusion

Over the last 15 years, arthroscopic subscapularis tendon repair has become more commonplace with improved instrumentation and techniques. Understanding the principles of establishing good visualization and obtaining proper mobilization are key to accomplishing a tension-free, secure repair construct. The literature has found arthroscopic repair to be at least as good as open repair, and it allows concomitant visualization and repair of other intraarticular shoulder pathology.

References

Adams CR, Schoolfield JD, Burkhart SS. The Results of Arthroscopic Subscapularis Tendon Repairs. *Arthroscopy*. 2008;24(12):1381–1389. http://doi.org/10.1016/j.arthro.2008.08.004.

Bartl C, Salzmann GM, Seppel G, et al. Subscapularis function and structural integrity after arthroscopic repair of isolated subscapularis tears. *Am J Sports Med*. 2011;39(6):1255–1262. http://doi.org/10.1177/0363546510396317.

Burkhart SS, Brady PC. Arthroscopic subscapularis repair: Surgical Tips and Pearls A to Z. *Arthroscopy*. 2006;22(9):1014–1027. http://doi.org/10.1016/j.arthro.2006.07.020.

Burkhart SS, Tehrany AM. Arthroscopic subscapularis tendon repair: technique and preliminary results. *Arthroscopy*. 2002;18(5):454–463. http://doi.org/10.1053/jars.2002.30648.

Denard PJ, Jiwani AZ, Lädermann A, Burkhart SS. Long-term outcome of a consecutive series of subscapularis tendon tears repaired arthroscopically. *Arthroscopy*. 2012;28(11):1587–1591. http://doi.org/10.1016/j.arthro.2012.02.031.

LafosseL, Jost B, Reiland Y, Audebert S, Toussaint B, Gobezie R. Structural integrity and clinical outcomes after arthroscopic repair of isolated subscapularis tears. *J Bone Joint Surg Am*. 2007;89(6):1184–1193. http://doi.org/doi:10.2106/JBJS.F.00007.

Lo IKY, Burkhart SS. The comma sign: an arthroscopic guide to the torn subscapularis tendon. *Arthroscopy*. 2003;19(3):334–337. http://doi.org/10.1053/jars.2003.50080.

Mall NA, Chahal J, Heard WM, et al. Outcomes of arthroscopic and open surgical repair of isolated subscapularis tendon tears. *Arthroscopy*. 2012;28(9):1306–1314. http://doi.org/10.1016/j.arthro.2012.02.018.

8-8C SURGICAL TREATMENT: OPEN REPAIR

ANDREW GREEN, MD

Introduction

- The rotator cuff, comprising the subscapularis, supraspinatus, infraspinatus, and teres minor muscles and tendons, is critically important to athletic shoulder function.
- Most attention is focused on treatment of superior and posterior cuff tears, isolated subscapularis tears being much less common.
- Gerber and Krushell (1991) described the clinical features of 16 cases of isolated subscapularis tendon tear.
- Shoulder arthroscopy provides an additional opportunity to both identify and treat subscapularis tendon tears.
- Surgical treatment is predicated on correlation of the clinical presentation with the pathologic anatomy.
- Although arthroscopic treatment has received increasing focus there remains a role for open repair of isolated subscapularis tendon tears.

Relevant Anatomy

The subscapularis is the largest and most powerful of the rotator cuff muscles. The muscle originates from the anterior surface of the scapula and is innervated by the upper and lower subscapular nerves, which are branches of the posterior cord of the brachial plexus (Fig. 8C.1) (Kasper et al, 2008; Lyons & Green, 2005). The upper 60% inserts as a tendon onto the lesser tuberosity, and the upper border has a discrete rolled edge that firmly inserts on the upper facet of the lesser tuberosity (Yoo et al, 2015) (Fig. 8C.2). The lower 40% of the subscapularis muscle inserts directly onto the lower aspect of the lesser tuberosity and the surgical neck. The anterior capsule covers the posterior aspect of the tendon and muscle, and the rotator cuff interval capsule anterosuperiorly connects the superior edge of the subscapularis tendon to the supraspinatus. The subscapularis muscle and tendon have an intimate relationship with important neurovascular structures. The muscle and tendon pass inferior to the coracoid process and posterior to the conjoint tendon, and lie close to the musculocutaneous and axillary nerves. In addition, the anterior humeral circumflex artery courses along the anterior surface of the inferior aspect of the subscapularis muscle, whereas the posterior humeral circumflex artery passes inferior to the muscle and through the quadrangular space under the inferior capsule with the axillary nerve.

Pathophysiology

Isolated subscapularis tendon tears manifest as a spectrum, resulting from traumatic and atraumatic mechanisms and ranging from partial-thickness to complete full-thickness tears. The usual traumatic mechanism is forced extension or external rotation of the shoulder against resistance (Deutsch et al, 1997). Traumatic anterior dislocations in older patients can be associated with subscapularis tearing, although this is often combined with supraspinatus and infraspinatus tearing. The tendon is usually avulsed from the lesser tuberosity and retracted medially (Neviaser & Neviaser, 1995). It is not uncommon for the lower muscular portion to remain intact, with the tear extending longitudinally from lateral to medial. Associated pathology of the long head of the biceps, including partial tear, complete rupture, and instability, is common (Lyons & Green, 2005). In contrast, chronic atraumatic tears most commonly manifest as articular-side tears and have an intact connection to the transverse humeral ligament across the biceps groove that limits retraction. The tendon may be attenuated, depending on the extent of the degeneration. Disruption of the biceps sling results in long head tendon instability with the biceps typically dislocating under or posterior to the subscapularis. The biceps can also dislocate into the subscapularis if there is an intrasubstance or delaminated tear.

Indications and Contraindications

Indications for open repair are as follows:
- Early repair of acute traumatic partial-thickness or complete full-thickness subscapularis tears
- Failure of nonoperative treatment of chronic atraumatic subscapularis tear
- Inability of surgeon to technically perform an arthroscopic repair

Contraindications to open repair are as follows:
- Chronic retracted subscapularis tears with advanced fatty muscle degeneration
- Advanced glenohumeral joint arthritis
- Inability of patient to comply with postoperative rehabilitation

Open Repair Technique

In most cases of an isolated subscapularis tear the deltopectoral approach provides excellent exposure for the repair. When there is associated acromial spurring and impingement an arthroscopic acromioplasty can be performed before the open repair. Alternatively, the anterior deltoid can be retracted superiorly to allow access for an open anterior acromioplasty. A very cosmetic skin incision can be made, following the axillary skin crease and extending several centimeters superiorly in Langer's lines. Alternatively, an anterior incision that begins at the coracoid and extends distally over the deltopectoral interval can be used. Skin and subcutaneous tissue flaps are elevated to expose the deltopectoral interval, which is usually identified from the fat stripe that overlies the cephalic vein.

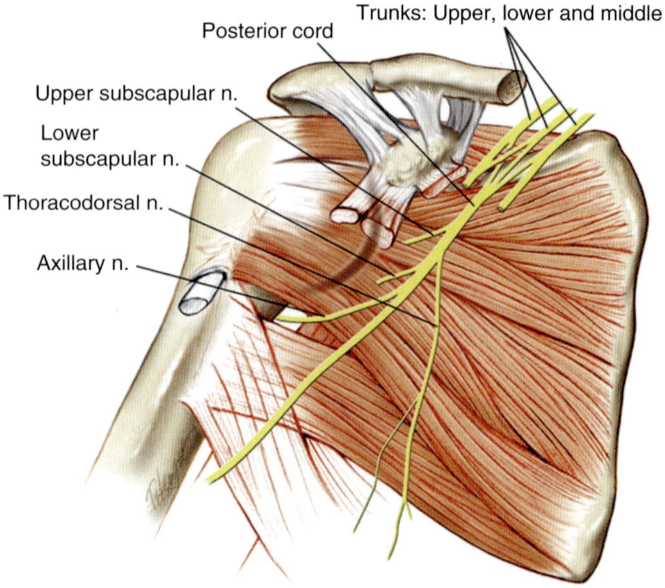

Fig. 8C.1 **Diagram of the subscapularis muscle demonstrating innervation from the upper and lower subscapular nerves (n.) on the anterior surface of the muscle. Note the axillary nerve passing inferior to the subscapularis muscle.** (From Kasper JC, Itamura JM, Tibone JE, Levin SL, Stevanovic MV. Human cadaveric study of subscapularis muscle innervation and guidelines to prevent denervation. *J Shoulder Elbow Surg.*2008;17:659-662.)

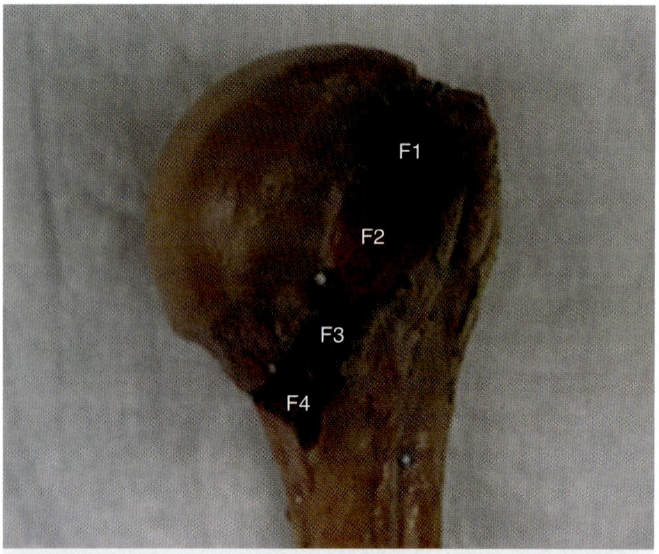

Fig. 8C.2 **Dissected left shoulder demonstrating the four facets of the lesser tuberosity insertion site (F1–F4) of the subscapularis tendon and muscle. The tendon inserts on F1 and F2.** (From Yoo JC, Rhee YG, Shin SJ, et al. Subscapularis tendon tear classification based on 3-dimensional anatomic footprint: A cadaveric and prospective clinical observational study. *Arthroscopy.* 2015;31:19-28.)

The cephalic vein is dissected so that it can be retracted laterally with the deltoid muscle. Lateral mobilization of the vein is preferred because there are fewer branches on the medial side. The coracoid is identified proximally in the wound, and the deltopectoral interval is opened to expose the clavipectoral fascia. The clavipectoral fascia is incised to expose the subscapularis muscle and tendon and the proximal humerus. Any subacromial and subdeltoid adhesions are released by an elevator slid under the acromion and upper deltoid. The shoulder is then internally rotated to expose the greater tuberosity and allow inspection of the supraspinatus insertion for any tearing.

At this point the anatomy of the subscapularis tear can be fully evaluated. The axillary nerve is palpated posterior to the conjoined tendon and inferior to the subscapularis muscle. The status of the long head of the biceps is assessed, and if there is any pathology or instability, a biceps tenodesis should be performed. The biceps can be released at the superior labrum and tagged until the tenodesis is performed. If the subscapularis tear is an articular-side tear the transverse humeral ligament is incised over the biceps groove. It is important to not be misled and incise the subscapularis tendon too medially. In some cases of full-thickness retracted subscapularis tears, there may be a thin layer of scar tissue overlying the anterior aspect of the glenohumeral joint.

The rotator interval is opened along the superior edge of the subscapularis tendon. Careful evaluation of the superior glenohumeral ligament (SGHL) and the coracohumeral ligament (CHL) portions of the biceps pulley complex are performed, and the biceps tendon is inspected for instability, fraying, and tearing.

Depending on the extent of retraction and chronicity of the tear, some degree of mobilization of the subscapularis muscle-tendon unit may be required. Traction sutures are placed in the tendon to pull the tendon and muscle laterally. A complete 360-degree release of the subscapularis requires freeing the superior margin from the coracoid, the posterior surface from the anterior capsule and scapular neck, the inferior border from the axillary nerve and circumflex vessels, and the anterior surface from the conjoined tendon (Yung et al, 1996) (Fig. 8C.3). Adhesions superficial to the subscapularis muscle are released with careful dissection under strap muscles. To avoid injuring the subscapular nerves, the superficial dissection should not be excessive. Any connections to the coracoid are released. The muscle and tendon are pulled laterally to determine whether a capsular release is needed. If the capsule is preventing reduction of the tendon, then the capsule is released lateral to the glenoid labrum.

Once the subscapularis tendon and muscle are adequately mobilized the subscapularis footprint on the lesser tuberosity is debrided and prepared with curettes, rongeur, or bur to remove soft tissue and create a vascular bed for healing. A variety of techniques can be used to repair the subscapularis tendon to the lesser tuberosity, including transosseous sutures and various suture anchor constructs (Bartl et al, 2011; Deutsch et al, 1997; Edwards et al, 2006). The anatomy of the lesser tuberosity and the adjacent biceps groove dictate the best technique. Proximally, where the biceps groove is relatively shallow, it is difficult to perform a transosseous repair ,but more distally, where the biceps groove is deeper, transosseous suture placement is relatively easy.

The author prefers a combined approach, using suture anchors proximally and transosseous sutures distally (Figs. 8C.4 and 8C.5). The goal of the repair is to reattach the tendon securely in an anatomic position that facilitates healing. If there is inadequate length such that the repair would substantially limit external rotation, additional techniques may be need to augment the repair. The long head biceps

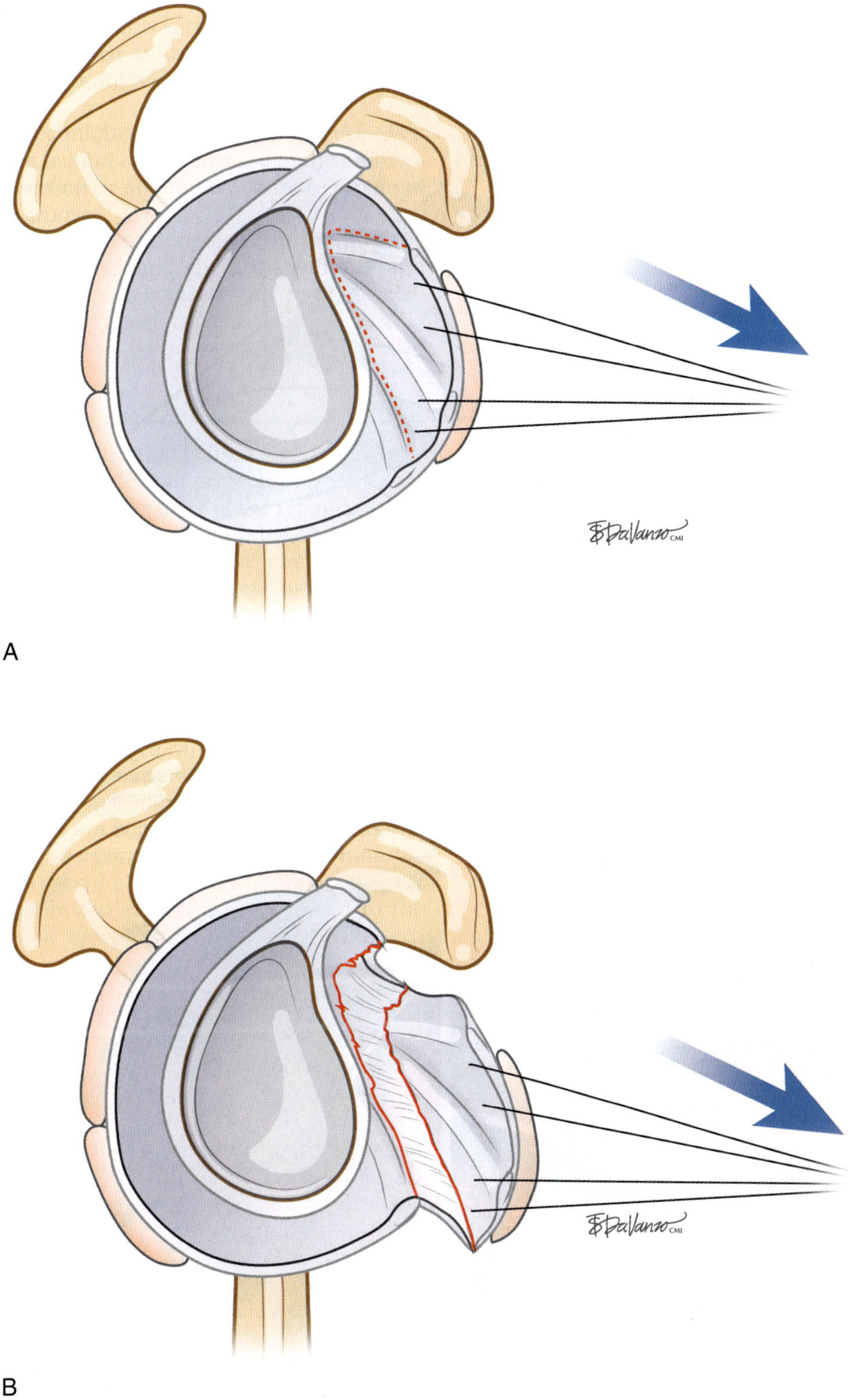

Fig. 8C.3 Subscapularis mobilization. **(A)** *Dashed line* indicates the cut along the rotator cuff superiorly, anterior capsule medially, and anterior inferior capsule. **(B)** Mobilization of the subscapularis muscle and tendon with traction sutures. The arrow indicates the direction of traction from the sutures. (From Boileau P, Kontakis GM, Trossarello P, Coste JS. Release of the subscapularis tendon and muscle: A limited gain in length. *Orthopedics.* 2007;30[8]:657-661.)

Table 8C.1 Published Outcomes of Open Repair of Isolated Subscapularis Tendon Tears

Study	Constant, Preop (mean range)	Constant, Postop (mean range)	Constant Pain Score, Preop	Constant Pain Score, Postop	Satisfaction (n [%])	Postop Imaging (% Intact)	Belly Press Result (% Positive, Preop/Postop)	Lift-Off Test Result (% Positive, Preop/Postop)	Constant Strength, Preop/Postop
Bartl et al (2011)	51.3 (39-62)	82.2 (65-98)	4.2	12.6	G/E, 27 (90)	MRI and US (93)	90/20	57/10	9.3/15.5
Fuchs et al (2006)	51.8	72.9	5	11.8		MRI (100)			9.25/11.8
Edwards et al (2005)	55 (14-84)	79.5 (25-101)	4.6	11.2	G/E, 74 (88)		90/18	71/20	10.3/15.2
Kreuz et al (2005)	44 (35-65)	89 (79-98)			G/E, 15 (94)			81/0	
Deutsch et al (1997)								100/0	93% grade 4/100% grade 5
Gerber et al (1996)		82		10.4	G/E, 13 (81)		100/31	81/19	

G/E, good to excellent; MRI, magnetic resonance imaging; *preop*, preoperative; *postop*, postoperative; US, ultrasound.

References

Bartl C, Scheibel M, Magosch P, Lichtenberg S, Habermeyer P. Open repair of isolated traumatic subscapularis tendon tears. *Am J Sports Med.* 2011;39:490–496.

Boileau P, Kontakis GM, Trossarello P, Coste JS. Release of the subscapularis tendon and muscle: a limited gain in length. *Orthopedics.* 2007;30(8):657–661.

Deutsch A, Altchek DW, Veltri DM, Potter HG, Warren RF. Traumatic tears of the subscapularis tendon: clinical diagnosis, magnetic resonance imaging findings, and operative treatment. *Am J Sports Med.* 1997;25:13–22. .

Edwards TB, Walch G, Sirveaux F, et al. Repair of tears of the subscapularis. *J Bone Joint Surg Am.* 2005;87:725–730. .

Edwards TB, Walch G, Sirveaux F, et al. Repair of tears of the subscapularis: Surgical Technique. *J Bone Joint Surg Am.* 2006;88(suppl 1):1–10.

Fuchs B, Gilbart MK, Hodler J, Gerber C. Clinical and structural results of open repair of an isolated one-tendon tear of the rotator cuff. *J Bone Joint Surg Am.* 2006;88:309–316.

Gerber C, Krushell RJ. Isolated rupture of the tendon of the subscapularis muscle: clinical features in 16 cases. *J Bone Joint Surg Br.* 1991;73:389–394.

Gerber C, Hersche O, Farron A. Isolated rupture of the subscapularis tendon. *J Bone Joint Surg Am.* 1996;78:1015–1023.

Kasper JC, Itamura JM, Tibone JE, Levin SL, Stevanovic MV. Human cadaveric study of subscapularis muscle innervation and guidelines to prevent denervation. *J Shoulder Elbow Surg.* 2008;17:659–662.

Kreuz PC, Remiger A, Erggelet C, Hinterwimmer S, Niemeyer P, Gächter A. Isolated and combined tears of the subscapularis tendon. *Am J Sports Med.* 2005;33:1831–1837.

Lyons RP, Green A. Subscapularis tendon tears. *J Am Acad Orthop Surg.* 2005;13:353–363.

Mall NA, Chahal J, Heard WM, et al. Outcomes of arthroscopic and open surgical repair of isolated subscapularis tendon tears. *Arthroscopy.* 2012;28:1306–1314.

Neviaser RJ, Neviaser TJ. Recurrentin stability of the shoulder after age 40. *J Shoulder Elbow Surg.* 1995;4:416–418.

Piasecki DP, Nicholson GP. Tears of the subscapularis tendon in athletes. Diagnosis and repair techniques. *Clin Sports Med.* 2008;27:731–745.

Yung SW, Lazarus MD, Harryman DT. Practical guidelines to safe surgery about the subscapularis. *J Shoulder Elbow Surg.* 1996;5:467–470.

Yoo JC, Rhee YG, Shin SJ, et al. Subscapularis tendon tear classification based on 3-dimensional anatomic footprint: a cadaveric and prospective clinical observational study. *Arthroscopy.* 2015;31:19–28.

9 Revision Repair

9-9A POSTERIOR CUFF

KYLE R. DUCHMAN, MD and BRIAN R. WOLF, MD, MS

Introduction

- Loss of structural integrity after primary rotator cuff repair is common.
- Revision rotator cuff repair presents several challenges that are often not present at the time of primary rotator cuff repair.
- Recognizing the reason for failure of the primary rotator cuff repair is essential for success in the revision setting.
- Appropriate patient selection and preoperative planning cannot be overlooked in order to achieve success after revision rotator cuff repair.

Modes of Failure

Failure after rotator cuff repair in the appropriately indicated patient depends on a variety of factors but can often be broadly categorized as biologic failure, technical error, traumatic failure, or the result of a complication from the primary surgery (George & Khazzam, 2012) (Box 9A.1). Of these factors, biology continues to be the most influential force. Despite technical advances and multiple local and systemic augmentation strategies (Duchman et al, 2016; Gulotta et al, 2011; Kovacevic & Rodeo, 2008; Moffat et al, 2008; Seeherman et al, 2008), rotator cuff repair fails to replicate the native tendon to bone interface (Aoki et al, 2001; Thomopoulos et al, 2010). In the revision setting, poor tissue quality and atrophy or fatty infiltration of the muscles further limits the biologic potential (Cummins & Murrell, 2003). Because of this, it is important to optimize the mechanical environment with a low-tension and high-surface-area repair. If this environment cannot be created because of local tissue loss or other factors, it may be necessary to consider options other than a standard revision rotator cuff repair.

The most common technical error is failure to accurately recognize the rotator cuff tear pattern. Most, but not all, rotator cuff tears can be categorized using descriptions popularized by Burkhart and include crescent, U-shaped, L-shaped, and reverse L-shaped tears (Burkhart, 2000). Crescent tears are the most common and most easily repaired. If the torn rotator cuff tissue is not reduced anatomically and according to tear pattern, then undue tension is the likely result. For example, trying to repair the tissue at the apex of a U-shaped tear to the tuberosity, as would be done in the typical crescent-shaped tear, will almost certainly fail. Additionally, there has been much debate about the optimal insertion angle of suture anchors during rotator cuff repair, including Burkhart's so-called deadman theory (Burkhart, 1995), which has more recently been called into question with several biomechanical studies (Clevenger et al, 2014; Green et al, 2014). The current evidence cannot deem a particular angle of anchor insertion as an error because results and theories have been variable. However, anchor pullout or migration, which may be visualized with plain radiographs or advanced imaging depending on the material of the anchor, may be indicative of technical error and explain a rotator cuff repair failure. As more evidence becomes available, suture technique and location of the suture relative to the musculotendinous junction are likely to become important technical considerations (Kullar et al, 2014; Montanez et al, 2016).

Traumatic failure after rotator cuff repair typically occurs within the first 3 to 6 months after surgery (Miller et al, 2011). Failure is often secondary to repetitive microtrauma caused by noncompliance with postoperative rehabilitation or overzealous physical therapy. In the revision setting, it is important to understand the patient's rehabilitative course after the initial surgery because this may provide clues to potential modes of failure. Additionally, any history of a fall or acute change in pain and function after a specific activity may suggest traumatic failure.

In general, complications after rotator cuff repair are rare, ranging from 5% to 10% (Berjano, 1998; Brislin et al, 2007; Mansat et al, 1997; Randelli et al, 2010). The most frequent complications, not including early failure, are stiffness and infection. Any of these complications can lead to an unsatisfactory outcome for the patient. Deep infection after rotator cuff repair is particularly problematic because underlying infection limits the reparative process and puts the articular cartilage at risk. Although rare, it is important to consider any and all of these complications during the workup of a patient with failure of a previous rotator cuff repair because management options, including the surgical approach and plan, may have to be altered to adequately address the complication at hand.

Patient Evaluation

HISTORY

An adequate history is essential when evaluating a patient with a suspected rotator cuff repair failure. Patients with failure of posterior rotator cuff repairs most frequently present with persistent anterolateral shoulder pain and

Box 9A.1 Modes of Failure of Rotator Cuff Repair

Biology

Poor tendon quality
- Muscle atrophy and fatty infiltration
- Decreased bone mineral density at the greater tuberosity

Technical Errors

Inadequate tissue mobilization
- Excessive tension on the repair
- Inadequate "time zero" strength of the repair construct

Traumatic Failure

Early, active range of motion
- Noncompliance with activity restrictions
- Falls or other specific injuries

Complications

Infection
- Loss of deltoid origin

functional deficits. When obtaining the history, it is important to consider the clinical picture before the primary rotator cuff repair, including physical therapy and diagnostic or therapeutic injections, and how they affected symptomatology. If available, imaging that was obtained before previous surgeries, procedure notes, and arthroscopic images can provide valuable information about the type(s) of procedure(s) performed as well as the size of the tear and quality of the tendon at the time of the primary procedure. These details will not only help delineate possible causes of failure that may ultimately guide treatment but also serve to expose any concomitant pathology that may or may not have been addressed.

PHYSICAL EXAMINATION

Physical examination of the patient with suspected rotator cuff repair failure should include general inspection of the shoulder, taking care to note the location and type(s) of incision(s) used for the primary repair. In the revision setting, it is particularly important to note the contour and appearance of the deltoid because loss or insufficiency of the deltoid origin at the acromion can occur, particularly in the setting of a prior open or mini-open rotator cuff repair (Bigliani et al, 1992) (Fig. 9A.1). Inspection of both the supra- and infraspinatus fossae should also be performed because atrophy may indicate suprascapular nerve pathology. Active and passive range of motion should be assessed in all planes. When evaluating a patient with a failed rotator cuff repair, active range of motion assessment provides crucial information. In the senior author's experience, patients with preserved active motion are more apt to benefit from revision repair than a patient with pseudoparalysis, which is supported by the literature (Lädermann et al, 2011). A variety of special tests have been described to assess the function of the posterior rotator cuff with variable diagnostic accuracy (Jain et al, 2017). Concomitant shoulder pathology, including acromioclavicular joint, biceps, and labral pathology, should be evaluated with provocative testing maneuvers because these areas may

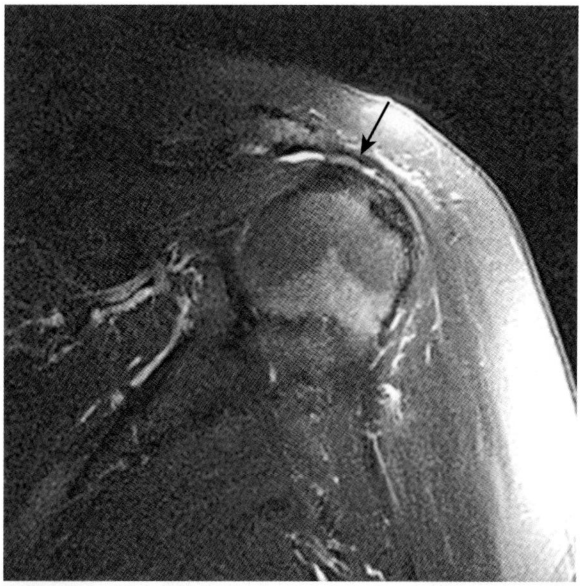

Fig. 9A.1 Coronal magnetic resonance images of a left shoulder in a patient who underwent a previous mini-open rotator cuff repair. Thinning of the deltoid origin on the acromion *(arrow)* and surrounding high signal consistent with fluid and edema are concerning for insufficiency of the deltoid origin.

serve as the source of ongoing pain after rotator cuff repair. Last, because cervical spine pathology can result in shoulder pain, a thorough examination of the cervical spine is warranted.

DIAGNOSTIC IMAGING

Standard radiographs, including anteroposterior, axillary, and scapular outlet (Y scapular) views, should be obtained. Superior humeral head migration may be indicative of a large or massive rotator cuff tear. An acromiohumeral distance less than 6 mm, which is measured off plain radiographs, may call into question the feasibility of rotator cuff repair (Deutsch et al, 1996; Goutallier et al, 2011) (Fig. 9A.2). Additionally, evaluation of the glenohumeral and acromioclavicular joint for degenerative changes may shed light on concomitant pathology. Close inspection of the axillary shoulder radiograph should be performed to rule out an os acromiale and further assessment of glenohumeral joint space. Advanced imaging modalities, including magnetic resonance imaging (MRI) and ultrasonography, are now easily accessible and routinely obtained. However, postsurgical changes often limit the ability of MRI to detect the presence of recurrent tears in the revision setting (Gaenslen et al, 1996; Motamedi et al, 2002), with limited additional benefit with the use of intraarticular contrast (Duc et al, 2006). In the revision setting, ultrasound evaluation of the rotator cuff repair may provide improved diagnostic accuracy (Prickett et al, 2003), although operator dependence may limit its applicability. Despite its limitations in detecting tears compared with ultrasonography, MRI can provide additional information, including fatty infiltration and atrophy of the supraspinatus and infraspinatus muscle bellies (Fuchs et al, 1999), that can help guide treatment and prognosticate outcomes (Burkhart et al, 2007; Iannotti et al, 1996).

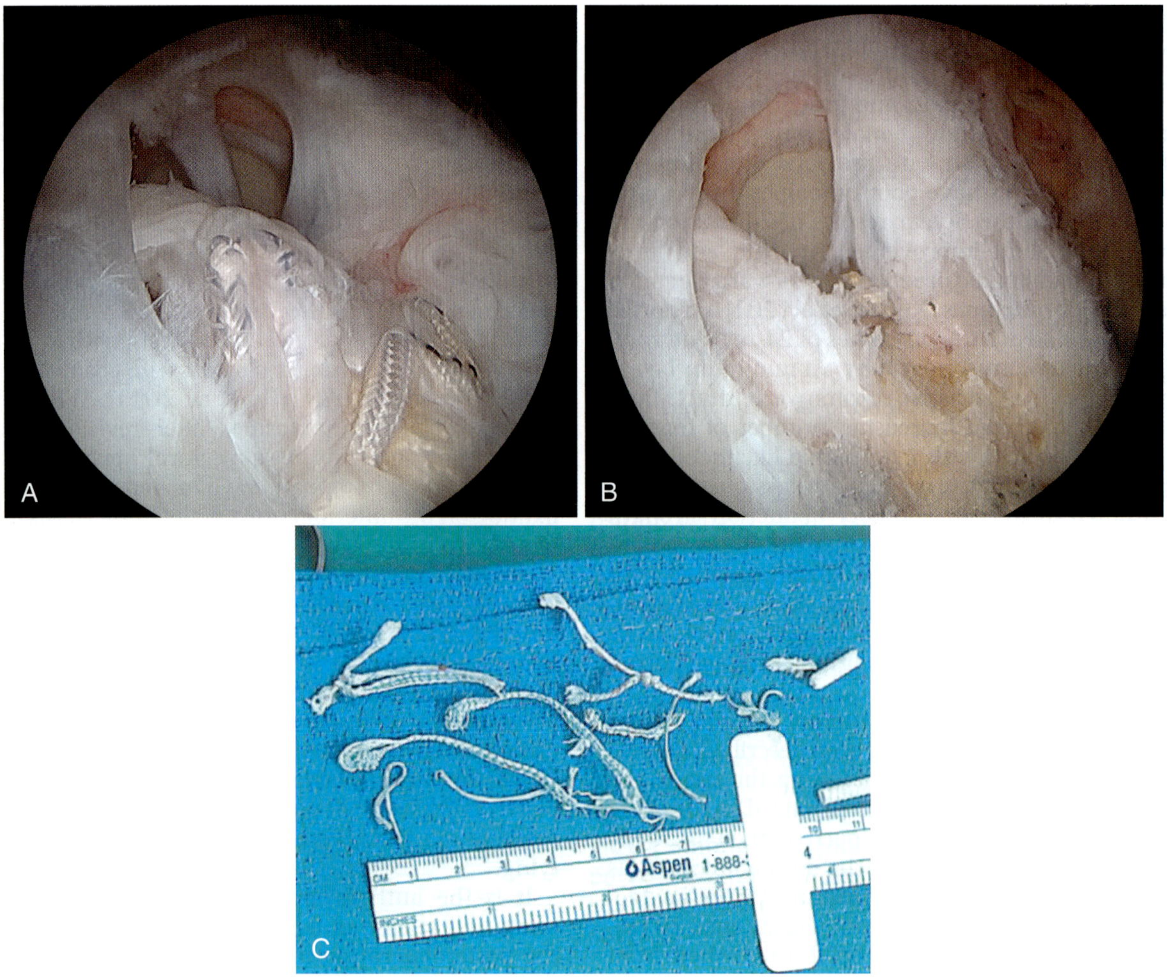

Fig. 9A.3 Arthroscopic view of a failed rotator cuff repair from a posterolateral view portal with multiple sutures noted at the greater tuberosity before (**A**) and after (**B**) suture and suture anchor device removal during greater tuberosity preparation. **C,** It is common for a large amount of suture material and anchors to be present from previous repair(s) that typically need to be removed for adequate footprint preparation.

If excessive tension is noted with attempted mobilization to the footprint, an anterior interval release can be performed. Specifically, the coracohumeral ligament should be identified and released using the radiofrequency wand. Additionally, the capsule beneath the torn and retracted rotator cuff can be released and mobilized under the tear and around the glenoid as needed. A posterior interval release, between the posterior border of the supraspinatus and infraspinatus, has been described and can be performed if necessary, although the senior author does not routinely use this release. These techniques typically allow adequate mobilization to the footprint on the greater tuberosity.

After mobilization of the tendon, the footprint itself is debrided of all soft tissue and previous suture material (Fig. 9A.3). Placing the shoulder into an adducted position assists in instrument access to the tuberosity. The footprint is then finally prepared with a bone-cutting shaver or arthroscopic bur. Bone quality should be accounted for and the cortex left intact, especially in osteoporotic female patients or when anchor fixation is of concern. Prior anchors are assessed. If prior anchors are loose, they can be removed. If the anchors are not loose, then it is preferred to leave them in place and work around or over prior implants. If metal anchors were used previously and are prominent, a bur can be used to remove prominent anchor material taking care to suction away all metal debris.

Revision repair of the rotator cuff can be done using either single- or double-row repair configurations. If a double-row repair is deemed feasible, then this is the authors' preference given the biomechanical advantages of double row repair. If the tear shape or interval slide requires margin convergence, we typically pass simple sutures with a suture passing device and tie arthroscopic knots before mobilizing the tear laterally as a single unit to the footprint (Fig. 9A.4). With adequate footprint preparation, we typically place a medial row of anchors 2 to 3 mm lateral to the articular margin, with the number of anchors used dictated by tear size. Anchors are placed through an accessory stab incision portal just off the lateral acromion. This anchor placement portal should be needle-localized to achieve the best access and angle to the anchor locations needed. Next, anchor sutures are passed through the tendon. We typically place sutures in a horizontal mattress pattern. All anchors and sutures are placed medially from anterior to posterior. Care must be taken to accurately judge medial suture placement to avoid placing sutures too medial, thus creating a repair construct with too much tension. Medial sutures are typically placed 3 to 5 mm lateral to the musculotendinous

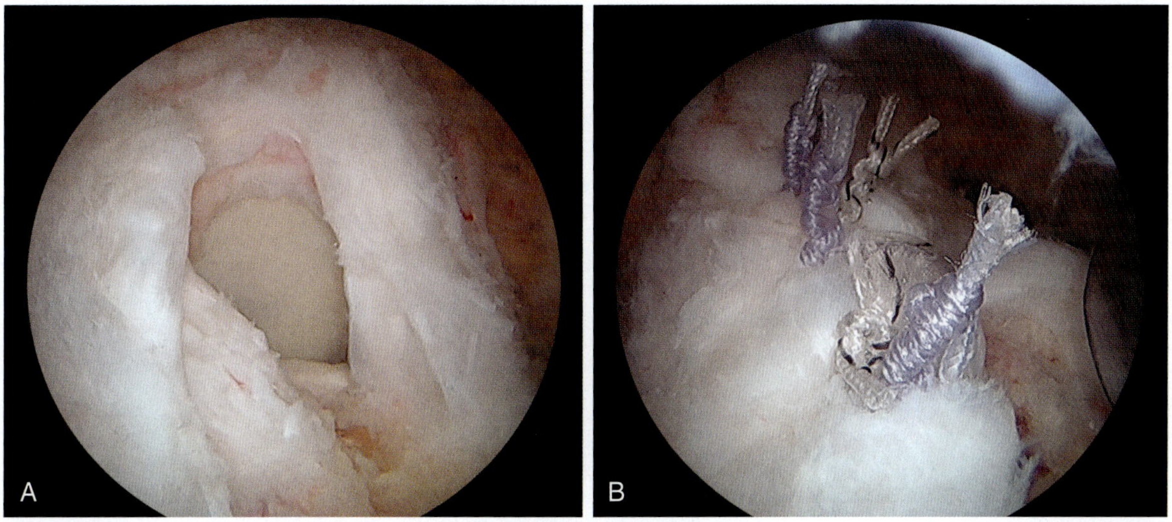

Fig. 9A.4 Arthroscopic view of a failed rotator cuff repair from a posterolateral view portal (**A**) after footprint preparation and tear debridement with a tear amenable to margin convergence repair (**B**).

junction and should never be placed medial to the musculotendinous junction. Arthroscopic knots are tied for the medial row, working sequentially from posterior to anterior. After tying medial row knots, we place at least two knotless lateral row anchors using the tag ends of the medial row knots in a suture bridge fashion to optimize footprint coverage and the surface area for healing (Nho et al, 2009). Alternatively, tape sutures that obviate the need for knot tying can be used.

Although double-row constructs have been recently popularized, single-row constructs can be helpful and appropriate in tear patterns not easily addressed with double-row suture configurations. For single-row repairs, it is still crucial to judge tissue mobility. Triple-loaded anchors are placed on the tuberosity at the point where the cuff tendon can be mobilized. Simple sutures are passed from anterior to posterior into the tendon, and knots are tied from posterior to anterior.

After completion of the rotator cuff repair, the subacromial space and acromion are visualized. Any acromial spurs that would be concerning for impingement on the rotator cuff repair are removed (Fig. 9A.5). Similarly, if large acromioclavicular spurs or symptomatic degenerative changes are present, a distal clavicle resection is performed using a 5.5-mm shaver through the anterior portal, taking care to maintain the integrity of the superior and posterior capsule of the acromioclavicular joint. Bony debris from any acromioplasty or clavicle resection should be meticulously debrided away. At the conclusion of the procedure, portals are closed with a nonabsorbable suture, and sterile dressings applied. If regional anesthesia was not performed, then a local anesthetic and pain medication cocktail can be injected. A shoulder abduction sling is applied in the operating room before the patient awakens from general anesthesia.

Postoperative Rehabilitation

The rationale behind rehabilitation protocols after primary and revision rotator cuff repair is based on limited evidence. An appropriate postoperative rotator cuff repair rehabilitation protocol balances tasks that allow adequate tendon-to-bone healing while also promoting long-term mobility and function. It must also be structured in a fashion that promotes patient compliance. Recently, the American Society of Shoulder and Elbow Therapists released a consensus statement on rehabilitation after arthroscopic rotator cuff repair (Thigpen et al, 2016). Although these guidelines are not specific to revision rotator cuff repair, the dialogue provides opportunity for extrapolation to the revision rotator cuff repair cohort. The ideal time to begin motion and the appropriate amount of tension or force to promote tendon-to-bone healing continue to be topics of debate (Galatz et al, 2009; Hettrich et al, 2014; Keener et al, 2014; Koh et al, 2014). In general, a period of immobilization is followed by protected passive range of motion exercises because there has been some concern with retear with early active motion (Kluczynski et al, 2015). Although the absolute necessity and duration of immobilization remains controversial, we prefer a 6-week period of immobilization in a shoulder abduction sling in the revision setting. This is followed by 6 weeks of protected passive range of motion exercises. At 12 weeks postoperatively, we initiate progressive strengthening exercises. Depending on progression through the previous stages, we consider work-hardening therapy and graduated return to work at 6 months postoperatively for patients performing manual labor tasks. Although this timeline serves as a guideline, it is important to consider the quality of the tissue and repair at the time of surgery, as well as the patient's general progression through the protocol, making adjustments accordingly.

Conclusion

Revision rotator cuff surgery poses several challenges that require a thoughtful diagnostic workup and careful indications to optimize patient outcomes. Although the outcomes of revision rotator cuff repair are consistently inferior to the outcomes of primary rotator cuff repair, improvements in pain and functional outcomes leave the

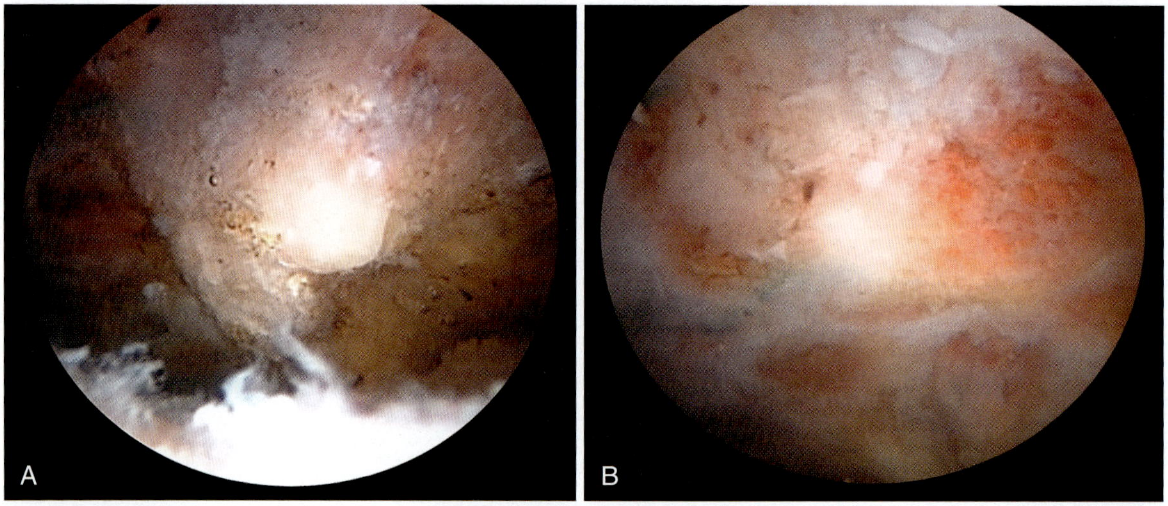

Fig. 9A.5 Residual acromial spur noted during revision rotator cuff repair before (**A**) and after (**B**) debridement with an arthroscopic shaver.

majority of patients satisfied after revision surgery. Previous work has helped identify several patient and tear characteristics, including more than one previous rotator cuff repair, age older than 65 years, grade 3 or 4 fatty infiltration of the rotator cuff musculature, deltoid origin compromise, and limited preoperative forward elevation, which confer inferior outcomes and where alternative procedures or physical therapy may be beneficial. Given the limited biologic potential to overcome technical shortcomings during revision rotator cuff repair, it is important to optimize healing with a low-tension, high-surface-area repair. In our hands, arthroscopy provides the best option for visualization and rotator cuff tendon mobilization. Last, there is a great deal of effort going into improving the biologic and mechanical environment for rotator cuff healing. Although the early results of biologic augmentation are promising and may expand the indications for revision rotator cuff repair in certain scenarios, more long-term results are required for these practices to be consistently implemented.

References

Aoki M, Oguma H, Fukushima S, Ishii S, Ohtani S, Murakami G. Fibrous connection to bone after immediate repair of the canine infraspinatus: the most effective bony surface for tendon attachment. *J Shoulder Elbow Surg*. 2001;10(2):123–128.

Athwal GS, Sperling JW, Rispoli DM, Cofield RH. Deep infection after rotator cuff repair. *J Shoulder Elbow Surg*. 2007;16(3):306–311.

Berjano P. Complications in arthroscopic shoulder surgery. *Arthroscopy*. 1998;14(8):785–788.

Bigliani L, Cordasco F, McIlveen S, Musso E. Operative treatment of failed repairs of the rotator cuff. *J Bone Joint Surg Am*. 1992;74(10): 1505–1515.

Brislin KJ, Field LD, Savoie FH. Complications after arthroscopic rotator cuff repair. *Arthroscopy*. 2007;23(2):124–128.

Burkhart SS. The deadman theory of suture anchors: observations along a south Texas fence line. *Arthroscopy*. 1995;11(1):119–123.

Burkhart SS. A stepwise approach to arthroscopic rotator cuff repair based on biomechanical principles. *Arthroscopy*. 2000;16(1):82–90.

Burkhart SS, Barth JR, Richards DP, Zlatkin MB, Larsen M. Arthroscopic repair of massive rotator cuff tears with stage 3 and 4 fatty degeneration. *Arthroscopy*. 2007;23(4):347–354.

Burkhart SS, Nottage WM, Ogilvie-Harris DJ, Kohn HS, Pachelli A. Partial repair of irreparable rotator cuff tears. *Arthroscopy*. 1994;10(4):363–370.

Clevenger TA, Beebe MJ, Strauss EJ, Kubiak EN. The effect of insertion angle on the pullout strength of threaded suture anchors: a validation of the deadman theory. *Arthroscopy*. 2014;30(8):900–905.

Cuff DJ, Pupello DR, Santoni BG. Partial rotator cuff repair and biceps tenotomy for the treatment of patients with massive cuff tears and retained overhead elevation: midterm outcomes with a minimum 5 years of follow-up. *J Shoulder Elbow Surg*. 2016;25(11):1803–1809.

Cummins CA, Murrell GA. Mode of failure for rotator cuff repair with suture anchors identified at revision surgery. *J Shoulder Elbow Surg*. 2003;12(2):128–133.

Deutsch A, Altchek DW, Schwartz E, Otis JC, Warren RF. Radiologic measurement of superior displacement of the humeral head in the impingement syndrome. *J Shoulder Elbow Surg*. 1996;5(3):186–193.

Djurasovic M, Marra G, Arroyo JS, Pollock RG, Flatow EL, Bigliani LU. Revision rotator cuff repair: factors influencing results. *J Bone Joint Surg Am*. 2001;83(12):1849–1855.

Duc SR, Mengiardi B, Pfirrmann CW, Jost B, Hodler J, Zanetti M. Diagnostic performance of MR arthrography after rotator cuff repair. *AJR Am J Roentgenol*. 2006;186(1):237–241.

Duchman KR, Goetz JE, Uribe BU, et al. Delayed administration of recombinant human parathyroid hormone improves early biomechanical strength in a rat rotator cuff repair model. *J Shoulder Elbow Surg*. 2016;25(8):1280–1287.

Duralde XA, Bair B. Massive rotator cuff tears: the result of partial rotator cuff repair. *J Shoulder Elbow Surg*. 2005;14(2):121–127.

Fuchs B, Weishaupt D, Zanetti M, Hodler J, Gerber C. Fatty degeneration of the muscles of the rotator cuff: assessment by computed tomography versus magnetic resonance imaging. *J Shoulder Elbow Surg*. 1999;8(6):599–605.

Gaenslen ES, Satterlee CC, Hinson GW. Magnetic resonance imaging for evaluation of failed repairs of the rotator cuff. Relationship to operative findings. *J Bone Joint Surg Am*. 1996;78(9):1391–1396.

Galatz LM, Charlton N, Das R, Kim HM, Havlioglu N, Thomopoulos S. Complete removal of load is detrimental to rotator cuff healing. *J Shoulder Elbow Surg*. 2009;18(5):669–675.

George MS, Khazzam M. Current concepts review: revision rotator cuff repair. *J Shoulder Elbow Surg*. 2012;21(4):431–440.

Goutallier D, Le Guilloux P, Postel J-M, Radier C, Bernageau J, Zilber S. Acromio humeral distance less than six millimeters: its meaning in full-thickness rotator cuff tear. *Orthop Traumatol Surg Res*. 2011;97(3):246–251.

Goutallier D, Postel J-M, Bernageau J, Lavau L, Voisin M-C. Fatty muscle degeneration in cuff ruptures: pre-and postoperative evaluation by CT scan. *Clin Orthop Relat Res*. 1994;304:78–83.

Green RN, Donaldson OW, Dafydd M, Evans SL, Kulkarni R. Biomechanical study: determining the optimum insertion angle for screw-in suture anchors—is deadman's angle correct? *Arthroscopy*. 2014;30(12):1535–1539.

Gulotta LV, Kovacevic D, Packer JD, Deng XH, Rodeo SA. Bone marrow–derived mesenchymal stem cells transduced with scleraxis improve rotator cuff healing in a rat model. *Am J Sports Med*. 2011;39(6):1282–1289.

Gupta AK, Hug K, Berkoff DJ, et al. Dermal tissue allograft for the repair of massive irreparable rotator cuff tears. *Am J Sports Med.* 2012;40(1):141–147.

Harryman DT 2nd, Mack L, Wang K, Jackins S, Richardson ML, Matsen FA 3rd. Repairs of the rotator cuff. Correlation of functional results with integrity of the cuff. *J Bone Joint Surg Am.* 1991;73(7):982–989.

Herrera MF, Bauer G, Reynolds F, Wilk RM, Bigliani LU, Levine WN. Infection after mini-open rotator cuff repair. *J Shoulder Elbow Surg.* 2002;11(6):605–608.

Hettrich CM, Gasinu S, Beamer BS, et al. The effect of mechanical load on tendon-to-bone healing in a rat model. *Am J Sports Med.* 2014;42(5):1233–1241.

Hsu AR, Ghodadra NS, Provencher CMT, Lewis PB, Bach BR. Biceps tenotomy versus tenodesis: a review of clinical outcomes and biomechanical results. *J Shoulder Elbow Surg.* 2011;20(2):326–332.

Iannotti J, Bernot M, Kuhlman J, Kelley M, Williams G. Postoperative assessment of shoulder function: a prospective study of full-thickness rotator cuff tears. *J Shoulder Elbow Surg.* 1996;5(6):449–457.

Jain NB, Luz J, Higgins LD, et al. The diagnostic accuracy of special tests for rotator cuff tear: the ROW cohort study. *Am J Phys Med Rehabil.* 2017;96(3):176–183.

Jost B, Pfirrmann CW, Gerber C. Clinical outcome after structural failure of rotator cuff repairs. *J Bone Joint Surg Am.* 2000;82(3):304–314.

Jost B, Zumstein M, Pfirrmann CW, Gerber C. Long-term outcome after structural failure of rotator cuff repairs. *J Bone Joint Surg Am.* 2006;88(3):472–479.

Keener JD, Galatz LM, Stobbs-Cucchi G, Patton R, Yamaguchi K. Rehabilitation following arthroscopic rotator cuff repair. *J Bone Joint Surg Am.* 2014;96(1):11–19.

Keener JD, Wei AS, Kim HM, et al. Revision arthroscopic rotator cuff repair: repair integrity and clinical outcome. *J Bone Joint Surg Am.* 2010;92(3):590–598.

Kluczynski MA, Isenburg MM, Marzo JM, Bisson LJ. Does early versus delayed active range of motion affect rotator cuff healing after surgical repair? A systematic review and meta-analysis. *Am J Sports Med.* 2015;44(3):785–791.

Koh KH, Lim TK, Shon MS, Park YE, Lee SW, Yoo JC. Effect of immobilization without passive exercise after rotator cuff repair. *J Bone Joint Surg Am.* 2014;96(6):e44.

Kovacevic D, Rodeo SA. Biological augmentation of rotator cuff tendon repair. *Clin Orthop Relat Res.* 2008;466(3):622–633.

Kullar RS, Reagan JM, Kolz CW, Burks RT, Henninger HB. Suture placement near the musculotendinous junction in the supraspinatus: implications for rotator cuff repair. *Am J Sports Med.* 2014;43(1):57–62.

Lädermann A, Denard PJ, Burkhart SS. Midterm outcome of arthroscopic revision repair of massive and nonmassive rotator cuff tears. *Arthroscopy.* 2011;27(12):1620–1627.

Lädermann A, Denard PJ, Burkhart SS. Revision arthroscopic rotator cuff repair: systematic review and authors' preferred surgical technique. *Arthroscopy.* 2012;28(8):1160–1169.

Mansat P, Cofield RH, Kersten TE, Rowland CM. Complications of rotator cuff repair. *Orthop Clin North Am.* 1997;28(2):205–213.

Mazzocca AD, Rios CG, Romeo AA, Arciero RA. Subpectoral biceps tenodesis with interference screw fixation. *Arthroscopy.* 2005;21(7):896.

Mihata T, Lee TQ, Watanabe C, et al. Clinical results of arthroscopic superior capsule reconstruction for irreparable rotator cuff tears. *Arthroscopy.* 2013;29(3):459–470.

Miller BS, Downie BK, Kohen RB, et al. When do rotator cuff repairs fail? Serial ultrasound examination after arthroscopic repair of large and massive rotator cuff tears. *Am J Sports Med.* 2011;39(10):2064–2070.

Moffat KL, Kwei AS-P, Spalazzi JP, Doty SB, Levine WN, Lu HH. Novel nanofiber-based scaffold for rotator cuff repair and augmentation. *Tissue Eng Part A.* 2008;15(1):115–126.

Montanez A, Makarewich CA, Burks RT, Henninger HB. The medial stitch in transosseous-equivalent rotator cuff repair: vertical or horizontal mattress? *Am J Sports Med.* 2016;44(9):2225–2230.

Motamedi AR, Urrea LH, Hancock RE, Hawkins RJ, Ho C. Accuracy of magnetic resonance imaging in determining the presence and size of recurrent rotator cuff tears. *J Shoulder Elbow Surg.* 2002;11(1):6–10.

Mulieri P, Dunning P, Klein S, Pupello D, Frankle M. Reverse shoulder arthroplasty for the treatment of irreparable rotator cuff tear without glenohumeral arthritis. *J Bone Joint Surg Am.* 2010;92(15):2544–2556.

Namdari S, Donegan RP, Chamberlain AM, Galatz LM, Yamaguchi K, Keener JD. Factors affecting outcome after structural failure of repaired rotator cuff tears. *J Bone Joint Surg Am.* 2014;96(2):99–105.

Nho SJ, Ghodadra N, Provencher MT, Reiff S, Romeo AA. Anatomic reduction and next-generation fixation constructs for arthroscopic repair of crescent, L-shaped, and U-shaped rotator cuff tears. *Arthroscopy.* 2009;25(5):553–559.

Parnes N, DeFranco M, Wells JH, Higgins LD, Warner JJ. Complications after arthroscopic revision rotator cuff repair. *Arthroscopy.* 2013;29(9):1479–1486.

Pauzenberger L, Grieb A, Hexel M, Laky B, Anderl W, Heuberer P. Infections following arthroscopic rotator cuff repair: incidence, risk factors, and prophylaxis. *Knee Surg Sports Traumatol Arthrosc.* 2017;25:595–601.

Paxton ES, Teefey SA, Dahiya N, Keener JD, Yamaguchi K, Galatz LM. Clinical and radiographic outcomes of failed repairs of large or massive rotator cuff tears. *J Bone Joint Surg Am.* 2013;95(7):627–632.

Petri M, Warth RJ, Horan MP, Greenspoon JA, Millett PJ. Outcomes after open revision repair of massive rotator cuff tears with biologic patch augmentation. *Arthroscopy.* 2016;32(9):1752–1760.

Piasecki DP, Verma NN, Nho SJ, et al. Outcomes after arthroscopic revision rotator cuff repair. *Am J Sports Med.* 2010;38(1):40–46.

Prickett WD, Teefey SA, Galatz LM, Calfee RP, Middleton WD, Yamaguchi K. Accuracy of ultrasound imaging of the rotator cuff in shoulders that are painful postoperatively. *J Bone Joint Surg Am.* 2003;85(6):1084–1089.

Randelli P, Castagna A, Cabitza F, Cabitza P, Arrigoni P, Denti M. Infectious and thromboembolic complications of arthroscopic shoulder surgery. *J Shoulder Elbow Surg.* 2010;19(1):97–101.

Russell RD, Knight JR, Mulligan E, Khazzam MS. Structural integrity after rotator cuff repair does not correlate with patient function and pain. *J Bone Joint Surg Am.* 2014;96(4):265–271.

Seeherman HJ, Archambault JM, Rodeo SA, et al. rhBMP-12 accelerates healing of rotator cuff repairs in a sheep model. *J Bone Joint Surg Am.* 2008;90(10):2206–2219.

Shamsudin A, Lam PH, Peters K, Rubenis I, Hackett L, Murrell GA. Revision versus primary arthroscopic rotator cuff repair: a 2-year analysis of outcomes in 360 patients. *Am J Sports Med.* 2014;43(3):557–564.

Tashjian RZ, Hollins AM, Kim H-M, et al. Factors affecting healing rates after arthroscopic double-row rotator cuff repair. *Am J Sports Med.* 2010;38(12):2435–2442.

Thigpen CA, Shaffer MA, Gaunt BW, Leggin BG, Williams GR, Wilcox RB. The American Society of Shoulder and Elbow Therapists' consensus statement on rehabilitation following arthroscopic rotator cuff repair. *J Shoulder Elbow Surg.* 2016;25(4):521–535.

Thomopoulos S, Genin GM, Galatz LM. The development and morphogenesis of the tendon-to-bone insertion—what development can teach us about healing. *J Musculoskelet Neuronal Interact.* 2010;10(1):35.

Tokish JM, Beicker C. Superior capsule reconstruction technique using an acellular dermal allograft. *Arthrosc Tech.* 2015;4(6):e833–e839.

Young SW, Zhu M, Walker CG, Poon PC. Comparison of functional outcomes of reverse shoulder arthroplasty with those of hemiarthroplasty in the treatment of cuff-tear arthropathy. *J Bone Joint Surg Am.* 2013;95(10):910–915.

9-9B SUBSCAPULARIS: PECTORALIS MAJOR TRANSFER

PHILIPP MORODER, MD; FABIAN PLACHEL, MD; SHEJLA ABDIC, BSC (HONS); and HERBERT RESCH, MD

Introduction

- The subscapularis is an important muscle for stability and function of the glenohumeral joint.
- A tear of the subscapularis tendon can cause pain and weakness in internal rotation.
- In large acute tears, early operative management with primary tendon reconstruction is indicated to restore cuff integrity and function.
- If repair is delayed, subscapularis tendon tears can become irreparable because of tendon retraction and muscle atrophy.
- In the case of irreparable anterior or anterosuperior rotator cuff tears, the pectoralis major tendon transfer (PMTT) is a valuable treatment option, especially for young and active patients.

As the largest of the four rotator cuff muscles in the shoulder, the subscapularis is a major internal rotator and plays a key role in stabilizing the shoulder joint (Piasecki & Nicholson, 2008). Along with the supraspinatus muscle, it makes up the anterosuperior portion of the rotator cuff. Tears of the subscapularis may either involve the entire tendon (complete tear) or parts of it (partial tear). The overall incidence of subscapularis tendon tears is difficult to determine but includes an approximate range of 3% to 27% of all rotator cuff tears (Mall et al, 2012). Compared with the general population, the prevalence of subscapularis tendon tears may be higher in athletes. Whereas "contact athletes" such as football players may be more likely to sustain traumatic injury, "throwing athletes" such as baseball players may be more inclined to injure the tendon because of overuse.

The mechanism of subscapularis tendon injury involves traumatic hyperextension or forced external rotation of an abducted shoulder (Deutsch et al, 1997). Clinical signs of such tears are anterior shoulder pain, weakness in internal rotation, and increased passive external rotation. A series of clinical tests has been proposed to facilitate the diagnosis of subscapularis tendon injury, including the "lift-off test" (Gerber et al, 1991), the "belly-press test" (Gerber et al, 1996), the "belly-off test" (Scheibel et al, 2005), and the "bear hug test" (Barth et al, 2006), to name a few.

Patient Selection

Although direct repair of a torn tendon is the typical treatment of choice, there are cases of long-standing chronic tears in which a repair is no longer possible because of massive tendon retraction and fatty degeneration of the muscle. A treatment option for an irreparable subscapularis or subscapularis plus supraspinatus tendon tear is the PMTT, as first described by Wirth and Rockwood (1997). In younger patients with active life styles, PMTT represents an especially feasible alternative to reverse shoulder arthroplasty, which is a procedure that can lead to a high complication and reoperation rate in patients younger than the age of 65 years (Ek et al, 2013). In our own long-term study of PMTT, we did not observe a correlation between the clinical outcome and age of the patient, which is why we believe that PMTT is an excellent option for younger patients with high functional demands and may be a viable treatment option in older adult patients as well (Moroder et al, 2017). Further surgical indication criteria are displayed in Box 9B.1.

Pectoralis Major Tendon Transfer

Over time, modifications to the original technique of PMTT have evolved. Originally, the pectoralis major tendon was directly transferred superiorly and reattached at the lesser tuberosity. This form of transfer is also termed *supracoracoidal pectoralis major transfer* or may be referred to as being above, over, or anterior to the conjoined tendon. An alternative is the subcoracoidal PMTT in which the tendon is passed underneath the coracoid process and behind the conjoined tendon before reinserting it at the lesser tuberosity (Resch et al, 2000). Based on the size of the rotator cuff tear, size of the pectoralis tendon and muscle, route of pectoralis transfer, or the surgeon's preferences, the pectoralis major tendon may be transferred partially by using the clavicular or sternocostal–abdominal portion alone or in its entirety.

Jost et al (2003) gave account on 28 patients who underwent 30 pectoralis major transfers for isolated irreparable subscapularis tears. They transferred the entire pectoralis major and passed it anteriorly to the conjoined tendon. Their results showed improvement in terms of the Constant score increasing significantly from 47% to 70%, but in cases of concomitant supraspinatus tears, the results were less favorable, which made the authors conclude that pectoralis major transfer may not be warranted in cases of irreparable subscapularis tears associated with irreparable supraspinatus tears.

The senior author of this chapter proposed the transfer of the cranial aspect of the pectoralis major tendon underneath the conjoined tendon before reinsertion at the lesser tuberosity (Resch et al, 2000). The reasoning behind this method is the assumption that rerouting the transfer underneath the conjoined tendon would reproduce the original force vector of the torn subscapularis muscle more closely. This assumption was later confirmed in a biomechanical study (Konrad et al, 2007).

The clinical outcome with this technique showed a high level of patient satisfaction, which resulted primarily from relief of pain but also improved subjective function with a postoperative increase of the Constant score by 40 points (Resch et al, 2000).

Box 9B.1 Surgical Indications and Contraindications for Pectoralis Major Tendon Transfer

Surgical Indications

The presence of an IASRCT combined with
1. Failed intraoperative attempt to close the tendon defect
2. Failed conservative treatment
3. Age younger than 75 years

Surgical Contraindications

1. >50% tear of the infraspinatus tendon
2. Cuff-arthropathy >grade 2 according to Hamada et al (1990)
3. Anterior migration of the humeral head
4. Pseudoparalysis

IASRCT, Irreparable anterosuperior rotator cuff tear.

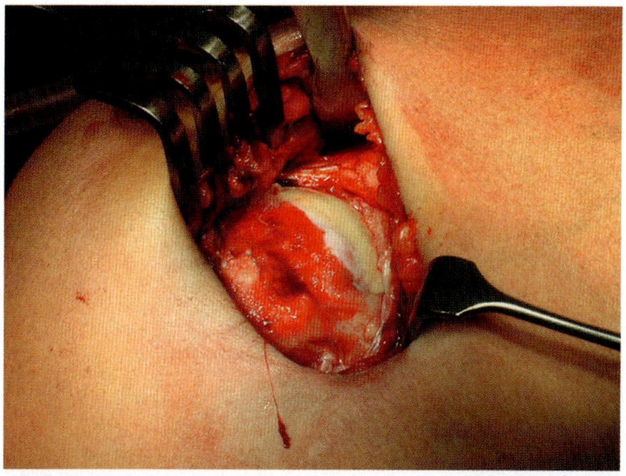

Fig. 9B.1 Using a deltopectoral approach, the lesser tuberosity is exposed, and the extent and reparability of the subscapularis tendon tear are evaluated.

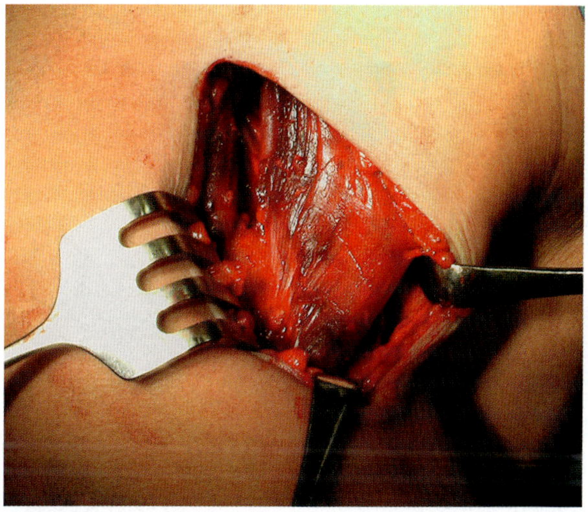

Fig. 9B.2 The upper and lower margins of the pectoralis major muscle are identified. The deltoid muscle is retracted laterally.

Several authors have since reproduced the method of subcoracoid pectoralis major transfer and reported similar results. Galatz et al (2003) performed a subcoracoid tendon transfer of the entire pectoralis major tendon in 14 patients. Compared with the technique by Resch et al (2000), the tendon was attached to the greater tuberosity. The authors reported good pain relief and an improved function of the affected shoulder. Gavriilidis et al (2010) used the clavicular part of the pectoralis major tendon in order to substitute for the subscapularis tendon. Their results showed significant improvement of pain level and activities of daily living at short-term follow-up. Magnetic resonance imaging (MRI) revealed a rupture of the transferred tendon in two of 13 patients. Lederer et al (2011) hypothesized that a tendon with a bone chip adherent to it would heal better than plain tendon tissue when fixated to bone. Their technique of fixation using bone chips led to improved transplant attachment with lower rerupture rate as seen on MRI. Nevertheless, both the bone chip and conventional fixation methods showed a similar overall increase in function and reduction of pain at short-term follow-up.

In their long-term follow-up study, Moroder et al (2017) observed that subcoracoidal PMTT results in significant clinical improvement in terms of pain and internal rotation even 10 years after surgery, with high patient satisfaction and minimal requirement for revision with reverse shoulder arthroplasty. Even though the authors noted a low general complication rate, they pointed out the risk for iatrogenic nerve injury when performing a subcoracoidal transfer. Klepps et al (2001) evaluated the subcoracoid pectoralis major transfer in human cadavers and defined the specific surgical anatomy relevant to the success of this method. Similar to Resch et al (2000), they found the best route of transfer of the pectoralis major to be superficial to the musculocutaneous nerve as opposed to deep because transferring the muscle deep to the musculocutaneous nerve increases the possibility of putting the nerve under tension. Klepps et al (2001) also support the method of partial-tendon transfer as opposed to routing the entire pectoralis major below the conjoined tendon because this may compress the musculocutaneous nerve from excessive bulkiness of the transferred muscle medial to the conjoined tendon. Because anatomical variations regarding the exact localization of the nerve branches and available space underneath the conjoined tendon exist, it is advisable to properly identify the musculocutaneous nerve before performing the transfer (Klepps et al, 2001; Ruiz-Iban et al, 2013).

Surgical Technique According to Resch

The patient is placed in a beach-chair position under general anesthesia. The deltopectoral approach is used to expose the anterior surface of the humeral head (Fig. 9B.1) and the pectoralis major muscle (Fig. 9B.2). An attempt is made to mobilize and directly repair the subscapularis tendon. Only in the presence of an irreparable tear is the PMTT performed. The often-dislocated biceps tendon is treated by means of a tenotomy. Upon exposing the insertion of the pectoralis major tendon on the humerus, approximately the superior half of the tendon is detached along with a thin bone chip (Fig. 9B.3). The dimension of the tendon to be used is based on the size of the defect to be repaired. The muscle fibers pertinent to the detached portion of the tendon are split from the remainder of the fibers by blunt dissection. Care must be taken to avoid splitting the

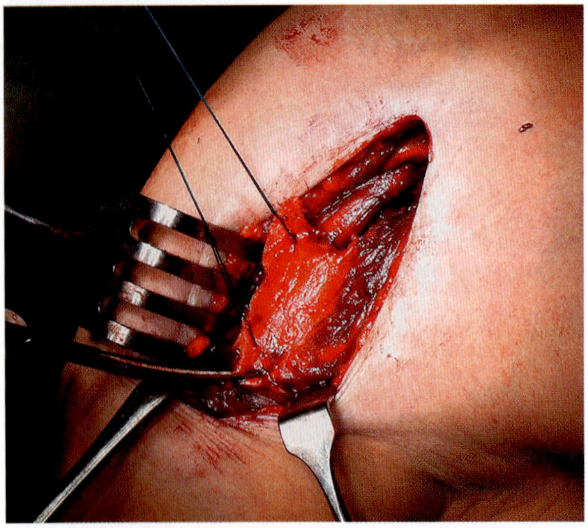

Fig. 9B.3 The upper half of the pectoralis major tendon is harvested, including a thin bone chip.

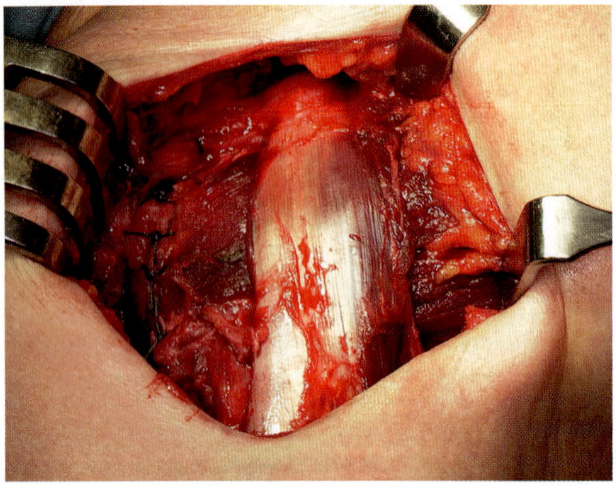

Fig. 9B.4 The detached portion of the tendon is passed underneath the conjoint tendon and fixed to the lesser tuberosity using transosseous, nonabsorbable sutures.

muscle farther than 8 cm medial from the insertion to avoid denervation. Because of the twisted insertion of the pectoralis major tendon on the humerus, the successful detachment of the cranial part of the tendon mainly involves harvesting of fibers from the sternocostal and abdominal part of the muscle. The use of this portion of the muscle more closely restores the force vector of the subscapularis muscle. Subsequently, the area medial to the conjoined tendon and caudal to the pectoralis minor is carefully dissected to identify the exact localization of the musculocutaneous nerve. A passage is created underneath the conjoined tendon by blunt dissection using the index finger. Using stay sutures, the muscle is transferred underneath the conjoined tendon while attention is paid to avoid nerve interposition or compression. In very muscular individuals, it may be necessary to reduce the volume of the attached muscle belly to avoid compression of the musculocutaneous nerve. The transferred tendon is then reattached to the previously decorticated lesser tuberosity with transosseous, nonabsorbable sutures (Fig. 9B.4). In the case of a large anterosuperior defect, the superior two-thirds of the pectoralis major tendon are harvested and attached to the lesser tuberosity as well as the anterior aspect of the greater tuberosity. The reason for harvesting the tendon with an adherent bone chip is to facilitate ingrowth. Upon transfer completion, the shoulder is immobilized in a sling for 4 weeks, and limited passive range of motion exercises for abduction, flexion, and internal rotation are begun on the first day postoperatively. After 6 weeks, active range of motion exercises may be started in all planes excluding external rotation, which remains limited for 8 weeks. After 12 weeks, full loading is permitted.

Acknowledgments

The study was performed at the Department of Traumatology and Sports Injuries of the Paracelsus Medical University, Salzburg, Austria.

References

Barth JR, Burkhart SS, De Beer JF. The bear-hug test: a new and sensitive test for diagnosing a subscapularis tear. *Arthroscopy*. 2006;22(10):1076–1084.

Deutsch A, Altchek DW, Veltri DM, Potter HG, Warren RF. Traumatic tears of the subscapularis tendon. Clinical diagnosis, magnetic resonance imaging findings, and operative treatment. *Am J Sports Med*. 1997;25(1):13–22.

Ek ET, Neukom L, Catanzaro S, Gerber C. Reverse total shoulder arthroplasty for massive irreparable rotator cuff tears in patients younger than 65 years old: results after five to fifteen years. *J Shoulder Elbow Surg*. 2013;22(9):1199–1208.

Galatz LM, Connor PM, Calfee RP, Hsu JC, Yamaguchi K. Pectoralis major transfer for anterior-superior subluxation in massive rotator cuff insufficiency. *J Shoulder Elbow Surg*. 2003;12(1):1–5.

Gavriilidis I, Kircher J, Magosch P, Lichtenberg S, Habermeyer P. Pectoralis major transfer for the treatment of irreparable anterosuperior rotator cuff tears. *Int Orthop*. 2010;34(5):689–694.

Gerber C, Hersche O, Farron A. Isolated rupture of the subscapularis tendon. *J Bone Joint Surg Am*. 1996;78(7):1015–1023.

Gerber C, Krushell RJ. Isolated rupture of the tendon of the subscapularis muscle. Clinical features in 16 cases. *J Bone Joint Surg Br*. 1991;73(3):389–394.

Hamada K, Fukuda H, Mikasa M, Kobayashi Y. Roentgenographic findings in massive rotator cuff tears. A long-term observation. *Clin Orthop Relat Res*. 1990;254:92–96.

Jost B, Puskas GJ, Lustenberger A, Gerber C. Outcome of pectoralis major transfer for the treatment of irreparable subscapularis tears. *J Bone Joint Surg Am*. 2003;85-A(10):1944–1951.

Klepps SJ, Goldfarb C, Flatow E, Galatz LM, Yamaguchi K. Anatomic evaluation of the subcoracoid pectoralis major transfer in human cadavers. *J Shoulder Elbow Surg*. 2001;10(5):453–459.

Konrad GG, Sudkamp NP, Kreuz PC, Jolly JT, McMahon PJ, Debski RE. Pectoralis major tendon transfers above or underneath the conjoint tendon in subscapularis-deficient shoulders. An in vitro biomechanical analysis. *J Bone Joint Surg Am*. 2007;89(11):2477–2484.

Lederer S, Auffarth A, Bogner R, et al. Magnetic resonance imaging-controlled results of the pectoralis major tendon transfer for irreparable anterosuperior rotator cuff tears performed with standard and modified fixation techniques. *J Shoulder Elbow Surg*. 2011;20(7):1155–1162.

Mall NA, Chahal J, Heard WM, et al. Outcomes of arthroscopic and open surgical repair of isolated subscapularis tendon tears. *Arthroscopy*. 2012;28(9):1306–1314.

Moroder P, Schulz E, Mitterer M, Plachel F, Resch H, Lederer S. Long-term outcome after pectoralis major transfer for irreparable antero-superior rotator-cuff tears. *J Bone Joint Surg Am*. 2017;99(3):239–245.

Piasecki DP, Nicholson GP. Tears of the subscapularis tendon in athletes—diagnosis and repair techniques. *Clin Sports Med*. 2008;27(4):731–745.

Resch H, Povacz P, Ritter E, Matschi W. Transfer of the pectoralis major muscle for the treatment of irreparable rupture of the subscapularis tendon. *J Bone Joint Surg Am*. 2000;82(3):372–382.

Ruiz-Iban MA, Murillo-Gonzalez JA, Diaz-Heredia J, Avila-Lafuente JL, Cuellar R. Pectoralis major transfer for subscapular deficiency: anatomical study of the relationship between the transferred muscle and the musculocutaneous nerve. *Knee Surg Sports Traumatol Arthrosc*. 2013;21(9):2177–2183.

Scheibel M, Magosch P, Pritsch M, Lichtenberg S, Habermeyer P. The belly-off sign: a new clinical diagnostic sign for subscapularis lesions. *Arthroscopy*. 2005;21(10):1229–1235.

Wirth MA, Rockwood CA Jr. Operative treatment of irreparable rupture of the subscapularis. *J Bone Joint Surg Am*. 1997;79(5):722–731.

10 Rotator Cuff Physical Therapy, Rehabilitation and Return to Sport

10-10A POSTOPERATIVE PHYSICAL THERAPY AND REHABILITATION

BROOKE M. DELVECCHIO, PT, DPT, OCS, PAUL E. WESTGARD, PT, DPT, OCS, SCS, CSCS, and HELEN BRADLEY, PT, MSc, SCS, CSCS

Introduction

- Rotator cuff tears (RCTs) are one of the most prevalent shoulder pathologies, occurring in 13% of people older than 50 years and more than 50% of people 80 years and older (van der Zwaal et al, 2011).
- Massive tears make up 20% of all RCTs and 80% of all reoccurring tears (Ladermann et al, 2015).
- Although RCTs can be asymptomatic, many people experience pain, muscle weakness, and loss of range of motion (ROM), resulting in altered glenohumeral kinematics.
- Current research supports initial conservative physical therapy management for full-thickness RCTs (Kuhn et al, 2013).
- In the past 10 years, the rate of arthroscopic rotator cuff repair (RCR) has increased by 600% (Colvin et al, 2012).
- The objective of postoperative rehabilitation is to restore overall function without compromising the integrity of the repaired tissue.

Factors Affecting Postoperative Outcomes

The mechanism of injury (acute vs. chronic, traumatic vs. overuse), type of surgery performed, and subsequent physical therapy following a repair are just a few factors that can affect the surgical outcome. There are several factors, preoperative and postoperative, that play a role in and affect the outcome of rehabilitation following a RCR (Chung et al, 2011; Warrender et al, 2011; Wessel et al, 2007). Table 10A.1 provides an outline of several important intrinsic and extrinsic prognostic factors that can be used to determine an expected level of success with rehabilitation; these factors are also associated with a higher rate of recurrent RCT (Kokmeyer et al, 2016).

Poor compliance with postoperative rehabilitation is a significant independent prognostic factor that can result in poor functional outcomes or recurring RCTs (Ahmad et al, 2015). Therefore patient education regarding the postoperative precautions, restrictions, and rehabilitative program is imperative for a successful outcome (Ahmad et al, 2015). Older age, typically more than 60 years, is associated with less optimal functional outcomes and longer healing and recovery times (Manaka et al, 2011). A systematic review performed by Fermont et al (2014) identified 12 significant prognostic factors that affect rehabilitation and long-term outcomes following RCR. The positive predictive prognostic factors that affect healing and subsequent rehabilitation and recovery after an RCR were found to be: age less than 60 years, male gender, high bone mineral density (BMD), absence of diabetes mellitus (DM), high level of preoperative activity, good preoperative shoulder ROM, absence of obesity, smaller sagittal tear size, less tendon retraction, low amount of fatty infiltration, single tendon involvement, and no other procedures being performed concurrently with the RCR (Fermont et al, 2014). Acute RCTs typically manifest with less fatty infiltration and less tendon retraction, so rehabilitation expectations are more favorable than for chronic progressive tears. Large RCTs are associated with greater tendon retraction, greater fatty infiltration, and increased muscle atrophy and have a higher failure rate than small RCTs (Le et al, 2014). It is important to consider both intrinsic and extrinsic prognostic factors for each patient in order to determine an accurate prognosis and to set appropriate expectations for the patient regarding duration of rehabilitation and return to functional and athletic activities. Table 10A.1 can be utilized as a guide to determine whether a moderate, intermediate, or conservative rehabilitation approach is most appropriate for a particular patient.

Subjective quantification of patient satisfaction should be measured at baseline and periodically throughout rehabilitation with the use of functional outcome measure forms specific to the shoulder. Outcome measures commonly used to assess subjective function and quality of life include the American Shoulder and Elbow Surgeons (ASES) score, the Disability of the Arm, Shoulder and Hand (DASH) score, the Western Ontario Rotator Cuff Index (WORC), the Constant-Murley score, the Single Assessment Numeric Evaluation (SANE), and the Medical Outcomes Study Instruments Short Form 12 (SF-12) and Short Form 36 (SF-36) (Kokmeyer et al, 2016).

Force Couples of the Rotator Cuff and Scapulothoracic Musculature

The rotator cuff is composed of the supraspinatus, infraspinatus, teres minor, and subscapularis muscles, which together with the glenohumeral joint capsule and ligaments

Table 10A.1 Shoulder Prognostic Spectrum to Recommend the Type of Postoperative Rehabilitation Program after Rotator Cuff Repair Surgery

	Moderate	Intermediate	Conservative
Age (years)	<50	50-60	>60
BMD	>−1	−2.4 to −1 (osteopenia)	<−2.5 (osteoporosis)
FI + atrophy	Stage 0	Stage 0–1	Stage 1–2
DM	+	+	−
BMI	<25	25–30	>30
Smoker	−	−	+
Tear size	Partial–small (1 tendon)	Small–medium (1–2 tendon)	Large–massive (2+ tendons)
Retraction	None	In-between	>Glenoid
Tissue quality	Good	Fair	Poor
Preoperative strength	Good	Fair	Poor

BMD, bone mineral density; *BMI*, body mass index; *FI*, fatty infiltration; *DM*, diabetes mellitus.
From Kokmeyer D, Dube E, Millett PJ. Prognosis driven rehabilitation after rotator cuff repair surgery. *The Open Orthopaedics Journal.* 2016; 10: 339-348.

provide a unique balance of dynamic control and stability to the glenohumeral joint, which inherently lacks bony stability. The rotator cuff musculature in concert with the scapulothoracic musculature generates force couples that enhance dynamic stability and promote normal scapulohumeral rhythm. Normal scapulohumeral rhythm has been defined by Inman et al as 2 degrees of glenohumeral motion for every 1 degree of scapular motion, which generally results in 120 degrees of glenohumeral motion in addition to 60 degrees of scapular rotation in order to achieve 180 degrees of shoulder elevation (Inman et al, 1944). The force couples provided by co-contraction of the rotator cuff musculature are important for approximation of the humeral head in the glenoid as well as to generate the appropriate amount of torque required for rotation of the joint, both of which are crucial to establish proper kinematics of the upper extremity with functional activities.

The anteroposterior force couple of the rotator cuff, which is established by opposing forces of the subscapularis and infraspinatus/teres minor muscles, is essential to creating the dynamic compression mechanism required to provide stability to the glenohumeral joint. This force couple, along with co-contraction of the supraspinatus, also counteracts the superior force generated by the deltoid with shoulder elevation and produces a dynamic caudal glide of the humeral head in the glenoid to allow for proper translation of the humerus, crucial for activities above shoulder level. The integrity of each force couple directly affects the kinematics of the glenohumeral joint; when a force couple is disrupted as a result of injury or weakness, the magnitude and direction of the force couple are also affected (Parsons et al, 2002). The result is decreased compression of the humeral head in the glenoid, and therefore decreased dynamic stability, leading to altered glenohumeral kinematics.

Proper kinematics of the scapulothoracic joint are essential to establish normal scapulohumeral rhythm. Function of the glenohumeral joint is affected when the force couple between the serratus anterior and middle/lower trapezius muscles is compromised by strength deficits or muscle dysfunction secondary to chronic compensation patterns. Decreased muscle activation of the rotational force couple created by the serratus anterior and middle/lower trapezius results in decreased stability and altered kinematics of the scapula during glenohumeral motion, causing inefficient mechanics of the shoulder complex as a whole, which in turn produces increased stress on the structures within and surrounding the glenohumeral joint (Paine & Voight, 2013).

Tissue Healing Timelines

Soft tissue and tendon healing consists of three main phases: inflammation, proliferation, and maturation. The inflammatory phase begins at the time of injury and lasts up to 5 days after trauma or surgical repair. In this phase, inflammatory cells remove tissue debris and form callus consisting of type I and III collagen fibers (Hsu et al, 2016). Proliferation begins after the inflammatory phase and can last up to 6 weeks; this phase is characterized by fibroblastic repair and sets the stage for deposits of collagen and extracellular matrix (Prentice, 2014; Hsu et al, 2016). During this repair phase, overly vigorous mechanical loading can reignite the inflammatory phase and result in weaker tissue. The maturation phase begins at weeks 6 to 8 after surgical repair and can last more than a year. In this phase, collagen fibers respond to gradually progressive stress and strain to realign in a position of maximum efficiency parallel to the lines of tension (Prentice, 2014). Larger rotator cuff tears have been shown to exhibit less fibroblastic activity and therefore more limited proliferation in comparison with smaller rotator cuff tears, a difference that slows the physiologic rate of tissue healing (Matthews et al, 2006).

Early Versus Delayed Range of Motion

There are many studies comparing early versus delayed ROM following an RCR. Some surgeons choose immobilization for a period ranging from 2 to 6 weeks postoperatively in order to protect the repaired tissue from overloading and from increased tension on the repair that may negatively affect the healing potential, whereas other surgeons select early passive mobilization in order to reduce risk of postoperative shoulder stiffness and to improve early function without overloading the surgical repair. A 2015 meta-analysis showed that an ROM protocol begun early postoperatively reduced postoperative stiffness; however, it found no difference between early and delayed ROM protocols regarding overall shoulder function (Chang et al, 2015). Early ROM protocols are most beneficial when utilized for the patient with a small to medium RCR and no intrinsic risks of improper healing as well as for those with preoperative presentation of restricted ROM (Chang et al, 2015). Delayed ROM protocols are favored for large to massive cuff tears as determined by tissue and repair integrity in order to ensure appropriate healing (Chang et al, 2015). Tendon healing responds well to controlled loading; overloading may result in an ineffective repair but underloading may not

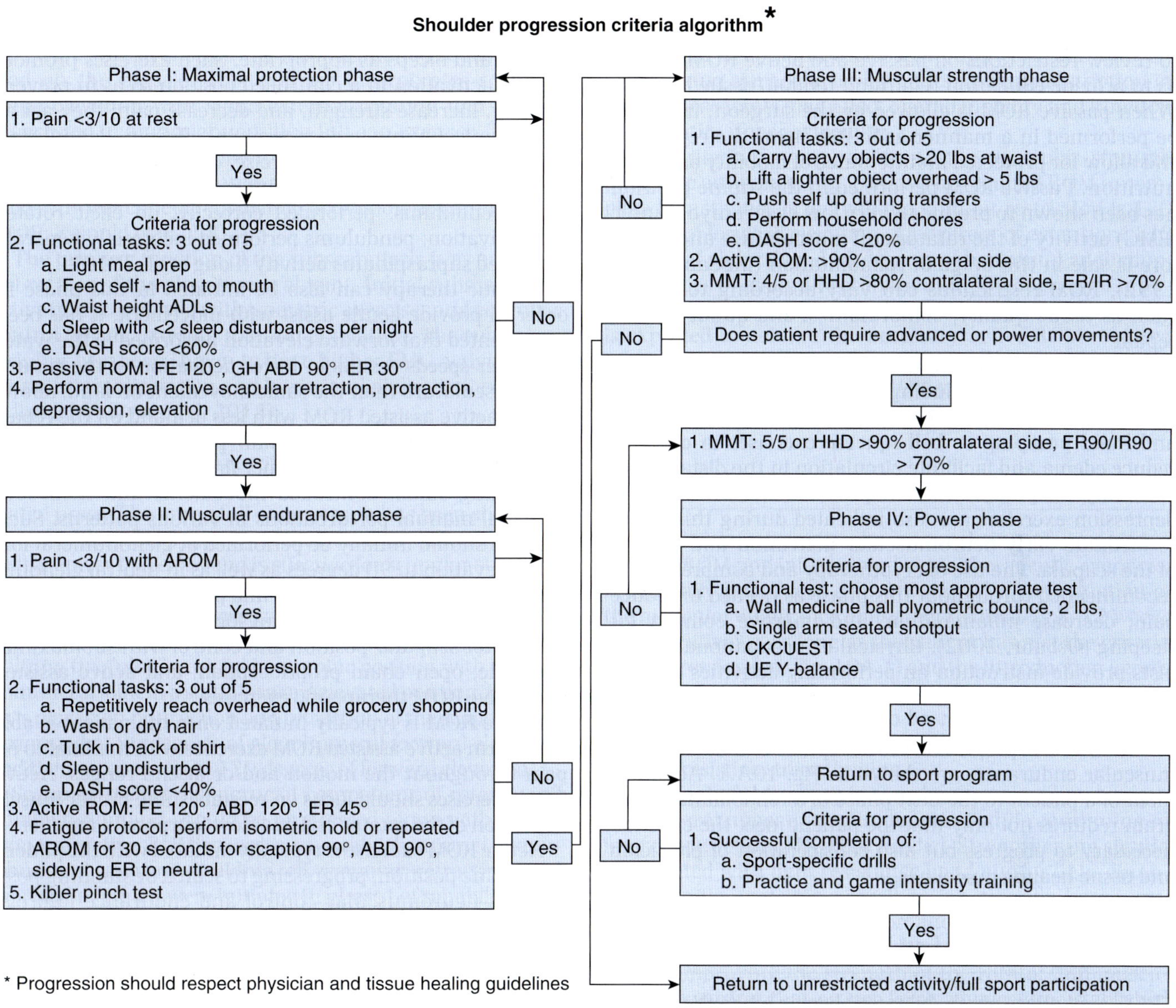

Fig. 10A.1 Shoulder progression criteria algorithm. *ABD,* abduction; *ADLs,* activities of daily living; *AROM,* active range of motion; *CKCUEST,* closed kinetic chain upper extremity stability test; *DASH,* Disability of the Arm, Shoulder and Hand (score); *ER,* external rotation; *FE,* forward elevation; *GH,* glenohumeral; *HHD,* hand held Dynamometer; *IR,* internal rotation; *med,* medicine; *MMT,* manual muscle test; *plyo,* plyometric; *ROM,* range of motion; *UE,* upper extremity.

stimulate the repair site enough for proper healing (Hsu et al, 2016). A proper rehabilitation protocol should be constructed according to an analysis of the risks and benefits, that is, considering both protection of tissue integrity and prevention of postoperative stiffness (Chang et al, 2015). Good communication between the physical therapist and surgeon is paramount to establish a proper rehabilitation program that achieves optimal results for each patient.

Guidelines for Rotator Cuff Repair Rehabilitation

As with all postoperative rehabilitation programs, it is important to consider physician recommendations in conjunction with prognostic factors (see Table 10A.1) as well as criterion-based and healing timeline–based progression to advance through the phases of rehabilitation. The phases of rehabilitation, as described here, and the algorithm shown in Fig. 10A.1 were developed with regard to healing timelines and criterion-based and function-based progression.

Phase I: Maximal Protection

The primary goals during the maximal protection phase are to protect the integrity of the repaired tissue, minimize pain and inflammation, and improve passive ROM without compromising the surgical repair. Postoperatively, the arm is placed in a sling with an abduction pillow, allowing the glenohumeral joint to assume an open-packed position in the scapular plane. On the basis of multiple factors, including the structural integrity of the RCR as determined by the orthopedic surgeon, ROM may begin early or is delayed.

During the initial rehabilitation visit, the physical therapist reviews postoperative restrictions and educates the kinematics should be emphasized with all resisted exercise throughout this phase in order to achieve proper glenohumeral kinematics with a resisted load.

Initial closed chain exercises are also begun in this phase to improve neuromuscular control, muscular strength, and proprioception of the glenohumeral joint. Closed chain exercises have been shown to increase compressive forces through the glenohumeral joint, resulting in greater muscle activation and stabilization (Uhl et al, 2003). Closed chain exercises are initiated in the standing position with the hands on a wall, then progressively advanced to a declined position and then quadruped and plank positions. Closed chain activities consist of weight shifts, static holds with and without manual perturbations to promote rhythmic stability, scapular protraction/retraction, double arm to single arm support, and initial push-ups.

If the patient's functional demands do not consist of repetitive overhead or power movements, the muscular strength phase may be his or her final stage of rehabilitation before discharge from physical therapy. In order for a patient who needs to progress to the muscular power phase to do so, criteria regarding strength, function, and ROM must be met (see Fig. 10A.1) The muscular power phase is used for patients who require their shoulders to function at a higher level, including those whose occupation requires repetitive or heavy overhead activity as well as recreational and competitive athletes.

Phase IV: Muscular Power

In order to transition to the muscular power phase, the patient must have a manual muscle test grade of 5/5 in all planes of glenohumeral range of motion on the repaired side or must demonstrate more than 90% of the strength of the uninvolved upper extremity on a handheld dynamometer test. The muscular power phase consists of advanced band and weight resistance, advanced closed chain and rhythmic stabilization, and plyometric exercises. The purpose of this phase is to prepare the patient for return to demanding occupation-specific or sport-specific activities. At this point in rehabilitation, the patient is expected to have full active ROM and may be given a home program consisting of stretching and mobility work as needed. Repetitions and sets of each exercise should be adjusted according to the American College of Sports Medicine (ACSM) recommendations most appropriate for each patient's rehabilitative goal (Ratamess et al, 2009). In this phase, resistance band exercises should progress to external and internal rotation at 45 and 90 degrees of abduction in order to improve muscle function in overhead positions. Closed chain stabilization exercises are progressed to advanced push-ups with plus on stable and variable surfaces; resisted proprioceptive neuromuscular facilitation, deceleration, and plyometric exercises are also introduced. Deceleration and plyometric exercises should focus on the posterior cuff musculature combined with trunk stabilization. Plyometric activity has been shown to improve force production of the elbow extensors and activation of the scapulothoracic musculature (Maenhout et al, 2016; Schulte-Edelmann et al, 2005).

References

Ahmad S, Ortho M, Haber M, Bokor DJ. The influence of intraoperative factors and postoperative rehabilitation compliance on the integrity of the rotator cuff after arthroscopic repair. *J Shoulder Elbow Surg*. 2015;24:229–235.

Alizadehkhaiyat O, Hawkes DH, Kemp GJ, Frostick SP. Electromyographic analysis of the shoulder girdle musculature during external rotation exercises. *Orthop J Sports Med*. 2015;3(11):1–9.

Ballantyne BT, O'Hare SJ, Paschall JL, et al. Electromyographic activity of selected shoulder muscles in commonly used therapeutic exercises. *Phys Ther*. 1993;73:668–677.

Blackburn TA, McLeod WD, White B, Wofford L. EMG analysis of posterior rotator cuff exercises. *J Athl Train*. 1990;25:40–45.

Chang KV, Hung CY, Han DS, et al. Early versus delayed passive range of motion exercise for arthroscopic rotator cuff repair: a meta-analysis of randomized controlled trials. *Am J Sports Med*. 2015;43:1265–1273.

Chung SW, Oh JH, Gong HS, Kim JY, Kim SH. Factors affecting rotator cuff healing after arthroscopic repair: osteoporosis as one of the independent risk factors. *Am J Sports Med*. 2011;39:2099–2107.

Colvin AC, Egorova N, Harrison AK, Moskowitz A, Flatow EL. National trends in rotator cuff repair. *J Bone Joint Surg Am*. 2012;94:227–233.

Cools AM, Dewitte V, Lanszweert F, et al. Rehabilitation of scapular muscle balance: Which exercises to prescribe? *Am J Sports Med*. 2007;35(10):1744–1751.

Ekstrom RA, Donatelli RA, Soderberg GI. Surface electromyographic analysis of exercises for the trapezius and serratus anterior muscles. *J Orthop Sports Phys Ther*. 2003;33(5):247–258.

Escamilla RF, Yamashiro K, Paulos L, et al. Shoulder muscle activity and function in common shoulder rehabilitation exercises. *Sports Med*. 2009;39(8):663–685.

Fermont AJM, Wolterbeek N, Wessel RN, Baeyens JP, de Bie RA. Prognostic factors for successful recovery after arthroscopic rotator cuff repair: A systematic literature review. *J Orthop Sports Phys Ther*. 2014;44(3):153–163.

Graichen H, Hinterwimmer S, von Eisenhart-Rothe R, Vogl T, Englmeier KH, Eckstein F. Effect of abducting and adducting muscle activity on glenohumeral translation, scapular kinematics and subacromial space width in vivo. *J Biomech*. 2005;38:755–760.

Hsu JE, Horneff JG, Gee AO. Immobilization after rotator cuff repair: What evidence do we have now? *Orthop Clin N Am*. 2016;47:169–177.

Inman VT, Saunders JB, Abbott LC. Observations on the function of the shoulder joint. *J Bone Joint Surg*. 1944;26(1):1–30.

Kelly BT, Roskin LA, Kirkendall DT, Speer KP. Shoulder muscle activation during aquatic and dry land exercises in nonimpaired subjects. *J Orthop Sports Phys Ther*. 2000;30(4):204–210.

Kokmeyer D, Dube E, Millet PJ. Prognosis driven rehabilitation after rotator cuff repair surgery. *Open Orthop J*. 2016;(suppl 1):339–348 (M10).

Kuhn JE, Dunn WR, Sanders R, et al. Effectiveness of physical therapy in treating atraumatic full-thickness rotator cuff tears: A multicenter prospective cohort study. *J Shoulder Elbow Surg*. 2013;22:1371–1379.

Ladermann A, Denard PJ, Collin P. Massive rotator cuff tears: Definition and treatment. *Int Orthop*. 2015;39:2403–2414.

Le BT, Wu XL, Lam PH, Murrell GA. Factors predicting rotator cuff retears: An analysis of 1000 consecutive rotator cuff repairs. *Am J Sports Med*. 2014;42(5):1134–1142.

Long JL, Thiele RAR, Skendzel JG, et al. Activation of the shoulder musculature during pendulum exercises and light activities. *J Orthop Sports Phys Ther*. 2010;40(4):230–237.

Maenhout A, Benzoor M, Werin M, Cools A. Scapular muscle activity in a variety of plyometric exercises. *J Electromyogr Kinesiol*. 2016;27:39–45.

Manaka T, Ito Y, Matsumoto I, Takaoka K, Nakamura H. Functional recovery period after arthroscopic rotator cuff repair: is it predictable before surgery? *Clin Orthop Relat Res*. 2011;469(6):1660–1666.

Matthews TJ, Hand GC, Rees JL, Athanasou NA, Carr AJ. Pathology of the torn rotator cuff tendon: Reduction in potential for repair as tear size increases. *J Bone Joint Surg Br*. 2006;88(4):489–495.

Moseley JB, Jobe FW, Pink M, et al. EMG analysis of the scapular muscle during a shoulder rehabilitation program. *Am J Sports Med*. 1992;20(2):128–134.

Namdari S, Yagnik G, Ebaugh DD, et al. Defining functional shoulder range of motion for activities of daily living. *J Shoulder Elbow Surg*. 2012;21:1177–1183.

Osbahr DC, Cawley PW, Speer KP. The effect of continuous cryotherapy on glenohumeral joint and subacromial space temperatures in the postoperative shoulder. *Arthroscopy*. 2002;18(7):748–54.

Paine R, Voight M. The role of the scapula. *Int J Sports Phys Ther.* 2013;8(5):617–629.

Parsons IM, Apreleva M, Fu FH, Woo SL. The effect of rotator cuff tears on reaction forces at the glenohumeral joint. *J Orthop Res.* 2002;20: 439–446.

Prentice WE. *Principles of Athletic Training: A Competency-Based Approach.* 15th ed. New York: McGraw-Hill; 2014:265–284.

Ratamess NA, Alvar VA, Evetoch TK, et al. American College of Sports Medicine Position Stand: Progression models in resistance training for healthy adults. *Med Sci Sports Exerc.* 2009;41(3):687–708.

Reinold MM, Wilk KE, Fleisig GS, et al. Electromyographic analysis of the rotator cuff and deltoid musculature during common shoulder external rotation exercises. *J Orthop Sports Phys Ther.* 2004;34:385–394.

Reinold MM, Macrina LC, Wilk KE, et al. Electromyographic analysis of the supraspinatus and deltoid muscles during 3 common rehabilitation exercises. *J Athl Train.* 2007;42(4):464–469.

Schulte-Edelmann JA, Davies GJ, Kernozek TW, Gerberding ED. The effects of plyometric training of the posterior shoulder and elbow. *J Strength Cond Res.* 2005;19(1):129–134.

Townsend H, Jobe FW, Pink M, Perry J. Electromyographic analysis of the glenohumeral muscles during a baseball rehabilitation program. *Am J Sports Med.* 1991;19:264–272.

Uhl TL, Carver TJ, Mattacola CG, et al. Shoulder musculature activation during upper extremity weight-bearing exercise. *J Orthop Sports Phys Ther.* 2003;33:109–117.

van der Zwaal P, Pekelharing JF, Thomassen BJ, Swen JW, van Ariel ER. Diagnosis and treatment of rotator cuff tears. *Ned Tijdschr Geneeskd.* 2011;155:A3163.

Warrender WJ, Brown OL, Abboud JA. Outcomes of arthroscopic rotator cuff repairs in obese patients. *J Shoulder Elbow Surg.* 2011;20:961–967.

Wessel RN, Rasenberg EIJ, Guldenmond NA, Lim TE. Artroscopisch rotator cuff repair nader geanalyseerd: een prospectieve studie bij 70 patiënten met een rotator cufflaesie. *Ned Tijdschr Orthop.* 2007;4:137–142.

10-10B RETURN TO SPORT

BROOKE M. DELVECCHIO, PT, DPT, OCS, PAUL E. WESTGARD, PT, DPT, OCS, SCS, CSCS, and HELEN BRADLEY, PT, MSc, SCS, CSCS

Introduction

- A loss of glenohumeral adduction, internal rotation, and total range of motion along with lower unilateral external rotation/internal rotation strength ratios is correlated with an increased risk of shoulder injury in the athlete.
- Following rotator cuff repair the rate of return to previous level of competition is higher for recreational athletes, lower for professional athletes, and significantly lower for professional overhead athletes.
- A gradual, progressive return to sport program should be used before an athlete returns to competition and should begin after the athlete is cleared by the surgeon and has achieved milestones for pain, range of motion, strength, scapulothoracic kinematics, and functional testing.
- The interval sports program should be individualized to the athlete and should be accompanied by a maintenance program of upper extremity, lower extremity, and trunk strength, flexibility, and plyometric training.

Risk Factors for Shoulder Injuries in the Athlete

Rotator cuff injuries are common in athletes in contact sports and sports that involve repetitive overhead motion (Plate et al, 2013). Several risk factors for shoulder injury have been identified in various sports. In contact sports like rugby and soccer, most shoulder injuries are the result of a direct traumatic injury to the upper extremity, as in falling onto an arm while being tackled (Horsley et al, 2013) or having the shoulder in an abducted and externally rotated position while tackling another player (Hart & Funk, 2015). In addition to traumatic injuries, there is also a higher chance of shoulder injuries in rugby players who demonstrate a lack of internal rotation range of motion (McDonough & Funk, 2014).

In sports that involve overhead motion, shoulder injuries are typically related to musculoskeletal adaptations from performing either high-intensity activities like throwing or repetitive, low-intensity motions like swimming and paddling. Increased prevalence of shoulder pain was observed in flatwater kayakers who exhibited reduced internal rotation range of motion and scapular dyskinesis (Johansson et al, 2016) as well as in handball players who had scapular dyskinesis, reduced total range of motion, reduced external rotation strength (Clarsen et al, 2014), and side-to-side muscle imbalance (Edouard et al, 2013). In swimmers (Bak & Magnusson, 1997), shoulder injury was correlated with increased repetitive upper extremity usage and exposure to swimming but was negatively correlated with participation in another sport. Also, shoulder internal rotation weakness (Bak & Magnusson, 1997) and reduced shoulder flexibility and latissimus dorsi tightness along with middle trapezius weakness were found in symptomatic young swimmers, whereas pectoralis minor tightness and decreased core endurance were associated with symptoms in swimmers 12 years and older (Tate et al, 2012). In addition, shoulder laxity along with internal and external rotation weakness, previous history of pain or injury, and competitive level were determined to be risk factors for shoulder pain and injury in swimmers (Hill et al, 2015). In sports that involve overhead serving, such as volleyball and tennis, the risk of injury increases with decreased eccentric internal and external rotation strength (Stickley et al, 2008) and possibly with shoulder rotation muscle imbalances (Cools et al, 2014).

Several risk factors for shoulder injury have been investigated among adolescent and professional throwing athletes.

Adolescent throwers appear to be at an increased risk of shoulder injury if they throw when fatigued or in pain, throw too hard, throw too often, or participate in showcases (Olsen et al, 2006). In addition, pitching more than 100 innings in a calendar year, playing catcher in addition to pitching (Fleisig et al, 2011), pitching on multiple teams during overlapping seasons, pitching in more than one game on the same day, and pitching on consecutive days all increase the risk of injury (Yang et al, 2014). Also, loss of passive internal rotation and horizontal adduction range of motion occurs in injured adolescents (Shanley et al, 2011, 2015). These changes are observed following an acute bout of throwing and over a season, possibly from transient soft tissue tightness in the posterior rotator cuff (Bailey et al, 2015; Shanley et al, 2012). Adolescent throwers also demonstrate greater internal rotation strength along with decreased strength in the supraspinatus (McHugh et al, 2016; Trakis et al, 2008; Tyler et al, 2014) and middle trapezius (Trakis et al, 2008) muscles.

Professional pitchers with an internal rotation deficit (Burkhart et al, 2003), total rotational range of motion loss (Wilk et al, 2011), and decreased external rotation range of motion (Wilk et al, 2015) are at a higher risk for a shoulder injury. Range of motion changes in older throwers can occur from transient soft tissue tightness (Shanley et al, 2012) but can also involve a permanent bony adaptation that causes humeral retroversion (Crocket, 2002). This torsion increases with the age of the thrower (Hibberd et al, 2014), leading to increased passive external rotation (Wilk et al, 2015), which is actually thought to be protective at the shoulder (Noonan et al, 2016) rather than being a risk factor for shoulder injury (Myers et al, 2011). In addition to the range of motion changes, the injured professional throwing athlete has been shown to demonstrate a preseason weakness in external rotation and scapular elevation (Byram et al, 2010).

Rotator Cuff Repair Outcomes in the Athlete

Shoulder injuries have detrimental effects on the ability of athletes to return to participating in their sports. Athletes who are unable to successfully return to play following a rotator cuff injury may require rotator cuff repair. The goal after rotator cuff surgery and subsequent rehabilitation is to return overhead athletes to their respective sports at the same level as prior to injury. Successful outcomes in the general public have been shown to be as high as 94% at 5 years and 83% at 10 years after such repair (Millett et al, 2011). In comparison, a systematic review found the overall rate of return of recreational and professional or competitive athletes to their sports after rotator cuff repair to be 84.7%, with 65.9% returning to previous level of play; however, only 49.9% of professional and competitive athletes returned to play at the same level (Klouche et al, 2015). Professional overhead throwing athletes are able to return to play at a rate of 73% (Namdari et al, 2011), but only 25% return to the same level of play as before injury (Mazoué et al, 2006); in comparison, 93% to 100% of recreational overhead throwing athletes return to the previous level of play (Liem et al, 2008; Plate et al, 2013). Professional athletes playing contact sports have a higher rate of return to play, as high as 90% (Plate et al, 2013; Tambe et al, 2009). Age also has an influence on the rate of return to play after rotator cuff repair, in that 86.8% of athletes younger than 70 years return to recreational sports (Antoni et al, 2016) but only 77% of athletes older than 70 years do so (Bhatia et al, 2015).

Decision-Making Process for Return to Sport

Following rotator cuff repair the athlete follows a postoperative rotator cuff repair protocol that will culminate in a return to play. The decision to clear an athlete to return to play is an important and critical component of the overall management of the injured athlete. These decisions can be difficult and quite complex, involving many variables that influence the final decision to clear an athlete to return to practice or competition. However, no matter how compelling these variables may be in regard to influencing the return to play decision, the ultimate goal is to return an injured athlete to play without exposing him or her to an increased risk of re-injury.

A collaborative consensus statement from several medical associations created a decision-making process for returning an injured athlete to full participation in his or her sport (Herring et al, 2012). This statement identifies four areas in the decision-making process: (1) establishment of a return to play process that includes an evaluation of the athlete's health status, participation risk, and extrinsic factors; (2) evaluation of the injured or ill athlete to establish a diagnosis, direct treatment, and decide when an athlete may safely return to play; (3) provision of treatment and rehabilitation of injured or ill athletes to optimize the safe and timely return to play; and (4) the safe and timely return of an injured or ill athlete to play.

In addition, a return to play model was developed in which three steps are needed prior to a return to play (Fig. 10B.1) (Creighton et al, 2010; Matheson et al, 2011; Shrier, 2015). First, a health status evaluation based on history, symptoms, signs, and results of laboratory and functional tests should be performed along with determination of the amount of stress the injured tissue can absorb. Second, an evaluation of participation risk is completed by comparison of the current type of sport and position played, limb dominance, level of competition, and the athlete's ability to protect the self with how much stress will be applied to the tissue during activity. Third, decision modifiers, such as timing and season, internal and external pressures on the athlete, masking of the injury with medication or injections, conflict of interests, and fear of litigation, help the clinician and athlete determine the acceptable level of risk of re-injury upon returning the athlete to the sport.

Evaluation for Return to Sport

The first step is to evaluate the readiness of the athlete to return to play by collecting patient-rated outcome measures to assess functional status. An outcome measure such

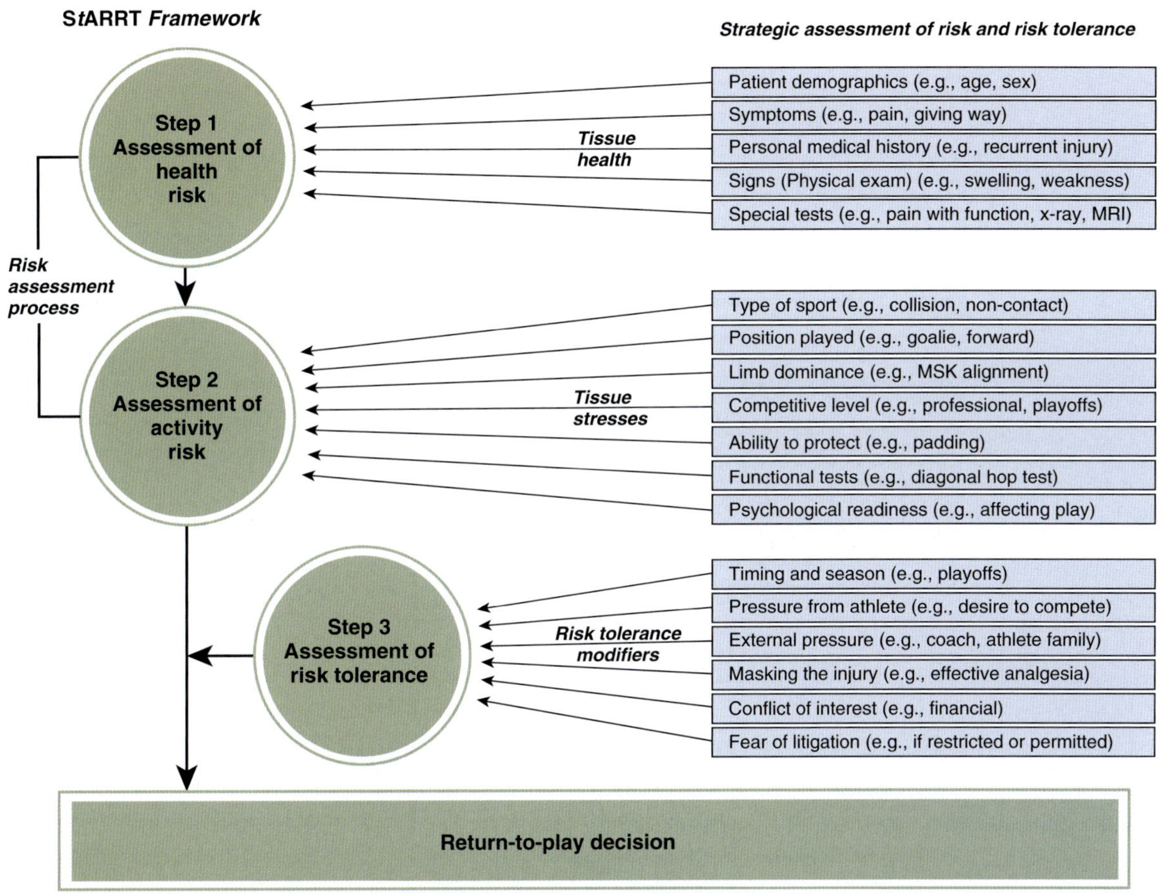

Fig. 10B.1 The Strategic Assessment of Risk and Risk Tolerance (StARRT) framework for return to play decisions. This framework illustrates that patients should be allowed to return to play when the risk assessment (steps 1 and 2) is below the acceptable risk tolerance threshold (step 3), and not allowed if the risk assessment is above the threshold. *MSK,* musculoskeletal; *MRI,* magnetic resonance imaging. (From Shrier I. Strategic Assessment of Risk and Risk Tolerance (StARRT) framework for return-to-play decision-making. *Br J Sports Med.* 2015;49[20]:1311-1315.)

as the Kerlan-Jobe Orthopaedic Clinic Shoulder and Elbow Score (Fig. 10B.2) provides clinically relevant information for overhead athletes that is similar to other regionally specific tools recommended after a rotator cuff repair, such as the American Shoulder and Elbow Surgeons scale, Penn Shoulder Score, and Western Ontario Rotator Cuff Index. (Alberta et al, 2010; Kraeutler et al, 2013).This score contains four questions related to pain, one question regarding interpersonal relationships associated with athletic performance, and five questions about function and athletic performance. Each item is scored on a visual analog scale and individual scores are added to create a score from 0 to 100, with a higher score representing higher levels of function and decreasing levels of symptoms. This tool has been shown to be a responsive, valid, and accurate assessment for overhead throwing athletes, and a score less than 90 could be a cause for concern.

Psychological factors are an important part of overall health of the athlete and have a role in a successful return to play (Roy et al, 2015). Emotions such as lack of confidence, apprehension, and fear may affect an athlete's return to play and can be sufficiently problematic as to interfere with performance and increase the chance of re-injury (ACSM, 2006). Also personal and situational factors, such as competing interests, kinesiophobia, age, and internal stressors and motivators, can have a major effect on a patient's psychological response to injury and the decision to return to sport even when the patient has excellent objective functional outcome scores (Tjong et al, 2015).

Clinician-rated impairments such as range of motion, strength, scapular position and movement, and functional testing should also be performed. Range of motion is measured in degrees with a goniometer; active range of motion is assessed in a seated or standing patient (Jain et al, 2013), and passive range of motion with the patient supine (Johansson et al, 2016; Reinold & Gill, 2010; Wilk et al, 2015) and the scapulae stabilized. All planes of motion should be evaluated with special attention to glenohumeral external and internal rotation in 90 degrees of glenohumeral abduction and glenohumeral horizontal adduction measurements along with comparison of dominant and nondominant measurements. A loss of more than 13 degrees (Shanley et al, 2015) to 25 degrees (Wilk et al, 2011) of internal rotation range of motion, a decrease of more than 5 degrees of external rotation motion (Wilk et al, 2015), and a loss of more than 5 degrees of total rotational motion have been shown to put the overhead throwing athlete at risk for injury. Similarly, losses of more than 10 degrees of internal rotation range of motion and more than 13.6 degrees of total rotational range of motion may increase the incidence of shoulder pain in flatwater kayakers (Johansson et al, 2016). When the range of motion deficits meet these criteria, intervention

Kerlan-jobe orthopaedic clinic shoulder and elbow score

Name________ Age ____ Sex ____ Dominant hand (R) ____ (L) ____ (Ambidextrous)
________ Date of examination ________ Sport ______ Position ______ Years played ______

Please answer the following questions related to your history of injuries to **YOUR ARM ONLY:**

	YES	NO
1. Is your arm currently injured?	☐	☐
2. Are you currently active in your sport?	☐	☐
3. Have you missed game or practice time in the last year due to an injury to your shoulder or elbow ?	☐	☐
4. Have you been diagnosed with an injury to your shoulder or elbow other than a strain or sprain?	☐	☐
If yes, what was the diagnosis? ______	☐	☐
5. Have you received treatment for an injury to your shoulder or elbow?	☐	☐
If yes, what was the treatment? (check all that apply) ☐ Rest ☐ Therapy ☐ Surgery (please describe): ______	☐	☐

Please describe your level of competition in your current sport:
(Use professional major league, professional minor league, intercollegiate, high school as the choices)

6. What is the highest level of competition you've participated at? ______
7. What is your current level of competition? ______
8. If your current level of competition is not the same as your highest level, do you feel it is due to an injury to your arm? ☐ ☐

Please check the ***ONE category only*** that best describes your current status:
☐ Playing without any arm trouble ☐ Playing, but with arm trouble
☐ Not playing due to arm trouble

Instructions to athletes:
The following questions concern your physical functioning during game and practice conditions. Unless otherwise specified, all questions relate to your **shoulder or elbow**. Please answer with an **X** along the horizontal line that corresponds to your current level.

1. How difficult is it for you to get loose or warm prior to competition or practice?
   Never feel loose during games or practice ●———● Normal warm-up time
2. How much pain do you experience in your shoulder or elbow?
   Pain at rest ●———● No pain with competition
3. How much weakness and/or fatigue (ie, loss of strength) do you experience in your shoulder or elbow?
   Weakness or fatigue preventing any competition ●———● No weakness, normal competition fatigue
4. How unstable does your shoulder or elbow feel during competition?
   "Peeping out" routinely ●———● No instability
5. How much have arm problems affected your relationship with your coaches, management, and agents?
   Left team, traded or waived, lost contract or scholarship ●———● Not at all

The following questions refer to your level of competition in your sport. Please answer with an **X** along the horizontal line that corresponds to your current level.

6. How much have you had to change your throwing motion, serve, stroke, etc, due to your arm?
   Completely changed, don't perform motion anymore ●———● No change in motion
7. How much has your velocity and/or power suffered due to your arm?
   Lost all power became linesse or distance athlete ●———● No change in velocity/power
8. What limitation do you have in endurance in competition due to your arm?
   Significant limitation (became relief pitcher, switched to short races for example) ●———● No endurance limitation in competition
9. How much has your control (of pitches, serves, strokes,etc) suffered due to your arm?
   Unpredictable control on all pitches, serves, strokes, etc. ●———● No loss of control
10. How much do you feel your arm affects your current level of competition in your sport (ie, is your arm holding you back from being at your full potential)?
   Cannot compete, had to switch sports ●———● Desired level of competition

Fig. 10B.2 Kerlan-Jobe Orthopaedic Clinic Shoulder and Elbow Score. (From Alberta FG, ElAttrache NS, Bissell S, et al. The development and validation of a functional assessment tool for the upper extremity in the overhead athlete. *Am J Sports Med*. 2010;38[5]:903-911.)

through the use of selective stretching, such as the modified sleeper and cross-body stretches, is advised (Wilk et al, 2013). These stretches have been recommended to decrease posterior shoulder stiffness (McClure et al, 2007), increase acromiohumeral distance (Maenhout et al, 2012), and decrease an internal rotation deficit (Lintner et al, 2007). Additionally, muscle energy techniques such as an isometric hold-relax stretch can be added to the sleeper and cross-body stretch (Moore et al, 2011), as can instrumented assisted soft tissue mobilization (Bailey et al, 2015) or joint mobilizations (Manske et al, 2010), to improve both glenohumeral internal rotation, horizontal adduction, and total rotational range of motion.

Strength should be assessed with isokinetic, isometric, and eccentric testing to determine absolute and relative strength ratios, with comparison of external and internal rotation strength values. Isokinetic testing has identified a relative muscular imbalance between the internal and external rotators on the dominant arm of elite junior tennis players (Ellenbecker & Roetert, 2003) but may not be time or cost effective in a clinical setting. Isometric rotational shoulder strength assessments with a handheld dynamometer have been shown to have excellent reliability (Cools, De Wilde, et al, 2014) and good to excellent reliability when combined with an accelerometer to measure eccentric rotator cuff strength (Johansson et al, 2015). An isokinetic external rotation/internal rotation ratio of 66% (Ellenbecker & Davies, 2000), an isometric external rotation/internal rotation ratio of 75% (Cools, Palmans, et al, 2014), and an eccentric external rotation/isometric internal rotation ratio of at least 1.0 (Cools, Vanderstukken, et al, 2015) are recommended as cutoff criteria for assessing risk of injury in the overhead throwing athlete. Scapular position and movement assessment should include static observation and measurement of posture, muscle strength, muscle length, dynamic movement, and symptom modification tests (Kibler et al, 2009). Even though cutoff values are not well defined, tests such as visual observation, acromial distance and Baylor/double square tests for protraction, pectoralis minor length test, scapular dyskinesis test, and inclinometry of scapular upward rotation may be of use in determining the presence or absence of scapular dyskinesis (Struyf et al, 2014).

If rotator cuff weakness and scapular dyskinesis are observed, an intervention program that follows a clinical reasoning algorithm (Ellenbecker & Cools, 2010) can guide the clinician in the treatment of scapular dyskinesis; in this program, flexibility deficits are addressed by stretching and mobilization techniques involving the pectoralis minor, and muscle performance issues are addressed by an appropriate muscular strengthening program of concentric, eccentric, and plyometric strengthening (Cools, Johansson, et al, 2015; Ellenbecker & Cools, 2010). Effort should be made to limit deltoid and upper trapezius muscle activation exercises while emphasizing activation of the supraspinatus, infraspinatus/teres minor, and subscapularis (Reinold et al, 2004, 2010) along with activation of the middle trapezius, lower trapezius, and serratus anterior (Schory et al, 2016).

Lastly, functional testing in the form of physical performance tests can be utilized to assess open and closed kinetic chain power. Tests such as the closed kinetic chain upper extremity stability test (CKCUEST), bilateral seated shotput test, unilateral seated shotput test, medicine ball throw, modified push-up test, and one-arm hop test have been examined but high-quality evidence related to their validity and reliability is lacking. Therefore they provide limited information regarding functional performance, although the CKCUEST, unilateral seated shotput test, and medicine ball throw may provide useful information as part of a larger athlete profile to determine whether the athlete has adequate strength, endurance, and power to return to sport participation (Tarara et al, 2016).

Interval Sport Programs

A gradual and progressive interval sport program is initiated after completion of earlier phases of rehabilitation and only after the athlete has been cleared by the surgeon and has achieved milestones for pain, range of motion, strength, scapulothoracic kinematics, and functional testing. Each session should start after a cardiovascular and dynamic warm-up involving a combination of activities in all three planes of movement along with static stretching of the major muscle groups required in the movements and mechanics of the sport (McCrary et al, 2015). The program can be performed up to three times per week with at least one rest day between sessions; a maintenance exercise program focusing on cardiovascular endurance and flexibility along with scapulothoracic, rotator cuff, lower extremity, and core strength should be performed on alternate days (Brumitt et al, 2011; Reinold et al, 2002). The program should be advanced when the athlete is able to complete the current level without pain or limitations; the volume of the training load should not be increased by more than 10% to 15%, because an increase in the ratio between acute workload (new level) and chronic workload (previous level) of 1.5 or higher equates to a 20% to 50% increase in injury risk (Blanch & Gabbett, 2016; Gabbett, 2016).

Throwing Program

A data-based interval throwing program for baseball players (Axe et al, 2009) can be used to gradually and progressively return a pitcher or positional player to practice and competition. The program is divided into four phases: return to throwing, return to pitching, intensified pitching, and a simulated game. The program begins with short throws at 50% effort and with longer tosses from level ground, followed by throwing from the pitching mound with fastballs thrown exclusively until 75% of the expected game volume is achieved. Finally, off-speed pitches are added, and when the athlete can throw without soreness, the program culminates with a simulated game.

Golf

A return to golf progression program (Fig. 10B.3) along with a comprehensive strength training program (Brumitt et al, 2011) should be completed before a golfer returns to full, unrestricted play. The return to golf progression is initiated with putting and chipping and gradually works through short-, medium-, and long-distance irons and woods. Once

HOWARD HEAD SPORTS MEDICINE
hhsm.com

Return to golf progression

The following recommendations are to assist in your return to golf. Prior to initiating this program, you need to receive clearance from your physician and pass any functional testing that your physician requires. Mild soreness should be treated with rest and ice. Contact your therapist if you have any concerns about symptoms experienced while golfing.

1st week:
Putting and green side chipping. (no sand)

2nd week:
Chipping and wedges under 60 yards. (no sand)

3rd week:
Short irons (7-sand wedge only)

4th week:
Long irons 6-4

5th week:
Rescue clubs and fairway woods, use tees!

6th week:
Driver, all clubs, using tees for driver, rescue and woods.

7th week:
9 holes, no divots or bunkers, no heavy rough or awkward lies, tee up on the fairway.

8th week:
18 holes, no restrictions

Name:____________
Date:____________

Fig. 10B.3 Return to golf progression. (Copyright 2010 Howard Head Sports Medicine.)

the athlete is able to work through all clubs and equal the approximate number of strokes expected in nine holes of golf without pain or soreness, he or she can play 9 holes of golf on a course. If the athlete can successfully complete a round of 9 holes without pain or soreness, he or she may then progress to playing 18 holes (Kim et al, 2004).

Swimming

An interval swimming program is used to gradually return a swimming athlete to the sport. The program focuses on freestyle stroke technique drills ranging from incremental yardage increases as the athlete progresses to interval work with larger yardage increases, culminating with a progression to other strokes or distance events (Spigelman et al, 2014).

Tennis

Similarly, an interval tennis program should be utilized before an athlete returns to full, unrestricted play. The program for tennis progresses from limited number of forehand and backhand ground strokes to overhead serves and culminates in a return to competitive matches occurring over a 4-week period (Wilk et al, 2009). In addition, a training program combining core strength, elastic resistance, and medicine ball exercises can improve serve velocity and increase shoulder external and internal range of motion (Fernandez-Fernandez et al, 2013).

Climbing

As rock climbing increases in popularity, a need for a return to sport program specific to rock climbing has been identified to help an athlete return to the previous level of climbing. A proposed return to climbing program consists of five phases with progressive increases in weight bearing through the upper extremity and performance of more complex climbing movements. Phase 1 of the program is initiated with basic technique training on a system board, two-handed assisted arm hang board drills at less than body weight, and easy vertical-only training wall practice. Phase 2 is a progression to more advanced technique training on a steeper system board, two-handed arm hang board and lock-off drills at full body weight, and introduction of a modified campus board with a progressive decrease in lower body assistance. Progressing to phase 3, the athlete starts two-handed arm hang board and advanced lock-off drills at more than body weight, and progresses to a modified campus board to increase upper extremity involvement. Phase 4 consists of progression to single arm assisted hang board and full campus board drills, and incorporates gentle cross-throughs, gaston moves, and dynamic movements along with a return to actual climbing at one or two grades below the athlete's skill level. Phase 5 is the progression to full-limit climbing using single arm and advanced dynamic techniques.

References

Alberta FG, ElAttrache NS, Bissell S, et al. The development and validation of a functional assessment tool for the upper extremity in the overhead athlete. *Am J Sports Med.* 2010;38(5):903–911.

Antoni M, Klouche S, Mas V, Ferrand M, Bauer T, Hardy P. Return to recreational sport and clinical outcomes with at least 2 years follow-up after arthroscopic repair of rotator cuff tears. *Orthop Traumatol Surg Res.* 2016;102(5):563–567.

Axe M, Hurd W, Snyder-Mackler L. Data-based interval throwing programs for baseball players. *Sports Health.* 2009;1(2):145–153.

Bailey LB, Shanley E, Hawkins R, et al. Mechanisms of shoulder range of motion deficits in asymptomatic baseball players. *Am J Sports Med.* 2015;43(11):2783–2793.

Bak K, Magnusson SP. Shoulder strength and range of motion in symptomatic and pain-free elite swimmers. *Am J Sports Med.* 1997;25(4): 454–459.

Bhatia S, Greenspoon JA, Horan MP, Warth RJ, Millett PJ. Two-year outcomes after arthroscopic rotator cuff repair in recreational athletes older than 70 years. *Am J Sports Med.* 2015;43(7):1737–1742.

Blanch P, Gabbett TJ. Has the athlete trained enough to return to play safely? The acute:chronic workload ratio permits clinicians to quantify a player's risk of subsequent injury. *Br J Sports Med.* 2016;50(8):471–475.

Brumitt J, Meira EP, Gilpin HE, Brunette M. Comprehensive strength training for a recreational senior golfer 11-months after a rotator cuff repair. *Int J Sports Phys Ther.* 2011;6(4):343–356.

Burkhart SS, Morgan CD, Kibler WB. The disabled throwing shoulder: Spectrum of pathology Part I: pathoanatomy and biomechanics. *Arthroscopy.* 2003;19(4):404–420.

Byram IR, Bushnell BD, Dugger K, Charron K, Harrell FE, Noonan TJ. Preseason shoulder strength measurements in professional baseball pitchers: identifying players at risk for injury. *Am J Sports Med.* 2010;38(7):1375–1382.

Clarsen B, Bahr R, Andersson SH, Munk R, Myklebust G. Reduced glenohumeral rotation, external rotation weakness and scapular dyskinesis are risk factors for shoulder injuries among elite male handball players: a prospective cohort study. *Br J Sports Med.* 2014;48(17):1327–1333.

Cools AM, De Wilde L, Van Tongel A, et al. Measuring shoulder external and internal rotation strength and range of motion: comprehensive intra-rater and inter-rater reliability study of several testing protocols. *J Shoulder Elbow Surg.* 2014;23(10):1454–1461.

Cools AM, Johansson FR, Borms D, Maenhout A. Prevention of shoulder injuries in overhead athletes: a science-based approach. *Braz J Phys Ther.* 2015;19(5):331–339.

Cools AM, Palmans T, Johansson FR. Age-related, sport-specific adaptions of the shoulder girdle in elite adolescent tennis players. *J Athl Train.* 2014;49(5):647–653.

Creighton DW, Shrier I, Shultz R, Meeuwisse WH, Matheson GO. Return-to-play in sport: a decision-based model. *Clin J Sport Med.* 2010;20(5):379–385.

Crockett HC, Gross LB, Wilk KE, Schwartz ML, Reed J, O'Mara J, Reilly MT, Dugas JR, Meister K, Lyman S, Andrews JR. Osseous adaptation and range of motion at the glenohumeral joint in professional baseball pitchers. *Am J Sports Med.* 2002;30(1):20–6.

Edouard P, Degache F, Oullion R, Plessis J-Y, Gleizes-Cervera S, Calmels P. Shoulder strength imbalances as injury risk in handball. *Int J Sports Med.* 2013;34(7):654–660.

Ellenbecker TS, Cools A. Rehabilitation of shoulder impingement syndrome and rotator cuff injuries: an evidence-based review. *Br J Sports Med.* 2010;44(5):319–327.

Ellenbecker T, Roetert EP. Age specific isokinetic glenohumeral internal and external rotation strength in elite junior tennis players. *J Sci Med Sport.* 2003;6(1):63–70.

Ellenbecker TS, Davies GJ. The application of isokinetics in testing and rehabilitation of the shoulder complex. *J Athl Train.* 2000;35(3):338–350.

Fernandez-Fernandez J, Ellenbecker T, Sanz-Rivas D, Ulbricht A, Ferrauti A. Effects of a 6-week junior tennis conditioning program on serve velocity. *J Sports Sci Med.* 2013;12(2):232–239.

Fleisig GS, Andrews JR, Cutter GR, et al. Risk of serious injury for young baseball pitchers: a 10-year prospective study. *Am J Sports Med.* 2011;39(2):253–257.

Gabbett TJ. The training-injury prevention paradox: should athletes be training smarter and harder? *Br J Sports Med.* 2016;50(5):273–280.

Hart D, Funk L. Serious shoulder injuries in professional soccer: return to participation after surgery. *Knee Surg Sports Traumatol Arthrosc.* 2015;23(7):2123–2129.

Herring SA, Kibler WB, Putukian M. The team physician and the return-to-play decision: a consensus statement-2012 update. *Med Sci Sports Exerc.* 2012;44(12):2446–2448.

Hibberd EE, Oyama S, Myers JB. Increase in humeral retrotorsion accounts for age-related increase in glenohumeral internal rotation deficit in youth and adolescent baseball players. *Am J Sports Med.* 2014;42(4):851–858.

Hill L, Collins M, Posthumus M. Risk factors for shoulder pain and injury in swimmers: a critical systematic review. *Phys Sportsmed.* 2015;43(4):412–420.

Horsley IG, Fowler EM, Rolf CG. Shoulder injuries in professional rugby: a retrospective analysis. *J Orthop Surg Res.* 2013;8(1):9.

Jain NB, Wilcox RB, Katz JN, Higgins LD. Clinical examination of the rotator cuff. *PM R.* 2013;5(1):45–56.

Johansson A, Svantesson U, Tannerstedt J, Alricsson M. Prevalence of shoulder pain in Swedish flatwater kayakers and its relation to range of motion and scapula stability of the shoulder joint. *J Sports Sci.* 2016;34(10):951–958.

Johansson FR, Skillgate E, Lapauw ML, et al. Measuring eccentric strength of the shoulder external rotators using a handheld dynamometer: reliability and validity. *J Athl Train.* 2015;50(7):719–725.

Kibler WB, Ludewig PM, McClure P, Uhl TL, Sciascia A. Scapular Summit 2009: Introduction. July 16, 2009, Lexington, Kentucky. *J Orthop Sports Phys Ther.* 2009;39(11):A1–A13.

Kim DH, Millett PJ, Warner JJP, Jobe FW. Shoulder injuries in golf. *Am J Sports Med.* 2004;32(5):1324–1330.

Kraeutler MJ, Ciccotti MG, Dodson CC, Frederick RW, Cammarota B, Cohen SB. Kerlan-Jobe Orthopaedic Clinic overhead athlete scores in asymptomatic professional baseball pitchers. *J Shoulder Elbow Surg.* 2013;22(3):329–332.

Liem D, Lichtenberg S, Magosch P, Habermeyer P. Arthroscopic rotator cuff repair in overhead-throwing athletes. *Am J Sports Med.* 2008;36(7):1317–1322.

Lintner D, Mayol M, Uzodinma O, Jones R, Labossiere D. Glenohumeral internal rotation deficits in professional pitchers enrolled in an internal rotation stretching program. *Am J Sports Med.* 2007;35(4):617–621.

Maenhout A, Van Eessel V, Van Dyck L, Vanraes A, Cools A. Quantifying acromiohumeral distance in overhead athletes with glenohumeral internal rotation loss and the influence of a stretching program. *Am J Sports Med.* 2012;40(9):2105–2112.

Manske RC, Meschke M, Porter A, Smith B, Reiman M. A randomized controlled single-blinded comparison of stretching versus stretching and joint mobilization for posterior shoulder tightness measured by internal rotation motion loss. *Sports Health.* 2010;2(2):94–100.

Matheson GO, Shultz R, Bido J, Mitten MJ, Meeuwisse WH, Shrier I. Return-to-play decisions: Are they the team physician's responsibility? *Clin J Sport Med.* 2011;21(1):25–30.

Mazoué CG, Andrews JR. Repair of full-thickness rotator cuff tears in professional baseball players. *Am J Sports Med.* 2006;34(2):182–189.

McClure P, Balaicuis J, Heiland D, Broersma ME, Thorndike CK, Wood A. A randomized controlled comparison of stretching procedures for posterior shoulder tightness. *J Orthop Sports Phys Ther.* 2007;37(3):108–114.

McCrary JM, Ackermann BJ, Halaki M. A systematic review of the effects of upper body warm-up on performance and injury. *Br J Sports Med.* 2015;49(14):935–942.

McDonough A, Funk L. Can glenohumeral joint isokinetic strength and range of movement predict injury in professional rugby league? *Phys Ther Sport.* 2014;15(2):91–96.

McHugh MP, Tyler TF, Mullaney MJ, Mirabella MR, Nicholas SJ. The effect of a high pitch volume on musculoskeletal adaptations in high school baseball pitchers. *Am J Sports Med.* 2016;44(9). 2246–2254.

Millett PJ, Horan MP, Maland KE, Hawkins RJ. Long-term survivorship and outcomes after surgical repair of full-thickness rotator cuff tears. *J Shoulder Elbow Surg.* 2011;20(4):591–597.

Moore SD, Laudner KG, McLoda TA, Shaffer MA. The immediate effects of muscle energy technique on posterior shoulder tightness: A randomized controlled trial. *J Orthop Sports Phys Ther.* 2011;41(6):400–407.

Myers JB, Oyama S, Rucinski TJ, Creighton RA. Humeral retrotorsion in collegiate baseball pitchers with throwing-related upper extremity injury history. *Sports Health.* 2011;3(4):383–389.

Namdari S, Baldwin K, Ahn A, Huffman GR, Sennett BJ. Performance after rotator cuff tear and operative treatment: a case-control study of major league baseball pitchers. *J Athl Train.* 2011;46(3):296–302.

Noonan TJ, Thigpen CA, Bailey LB, et al. Humeral torsion as a risk factor for shoulder and elbow injury in professional baseball pitchers. *Am J Sports Med.* 2016;44(9):2214–2219.

Olsen SJ, Fleisig GS, Dun S, Loftice J, Andrews JR. Risk factors for shoulder and elbow injuries in adolescent baseball pitchers. *Am J Sports Med.* 2006;34(6):905–912.

Plate JF, Haubruck P, Walters J, et al. Rotator cuff injuries in professional and recreational athletes. *J Surg Orthop Adv.* 2013;22(02):134–142.

Reinold MM, Escamilla RF, Wilk KE, Current concepts in the scientific and clinical rationale behind exercises for glenohumeral and scapulothoracic musculature. *J Orthop Sports Phys Ther.* 2009;39(2):105–117.

Reinold MM, Wilk KE, Reed J, Crenshaw K, Andrews JR. Interval sport programs: Guidelines for baseball, tennis, and golf. *J Orthop Sports Phys Ther.* 2002;32(6):293–298.

Reinold MM, Wilk KE, Fleisig GS, et al. Electromyographic analysis of the rotator cuff and deltoid musculature during common shoulder external rotation exercises. *J Orthop Sports Phys Ther.* 2004;34:385–394.

Reinold MM, Gill TJ, Wilk KE, Andrews JR. Current concepts in the evaluation and treatment of the shoulder in overhead throwing athletes, part 2: injury prevention and treatment. *Sports Health.* 2010;2(2):101–15.

Roy J, Mokhtar AH, Abdul Karim S, Ayathupady Mohanan S. Cognitive appraisals and lived experiences during injury rehabilitation: a narrative account within personal and situational backdrop. *Asian J Sports Med.* 2015;6(3):e24039.

Schory A, Bidinger E, Wolf J, Murray L. A systematic review of the exercises that produce optimal muscle ratios of the scapular stabilizers in normal shoulders. *Int J Sports Phys Ther.* 2016;11(3):321–336.

Shanley E, Kissenberth MJ, Thigpen CA, et al. Preseason shoulder range of motion screening as a predictor of injury among youth and adolescent baseball pitchers. *J Shoulder Elbow Surg.* 2015;24(7):1005–1013.

Shanley E, Rauh MJ, Michener LA, Ellenbecker TS, Garrison JC, Thigpen CA. Shoulder range of motion measures as risk factors for shoulder and elbow injuries in high school softball and baseball players. *Am J Sports Med.* 2011;39(9):1997–2006.

Shanley E, Thigpen CA, Clark JC, et al. Changes in passive range of motion and development of glenohumeral internal rotation deficit (GIRD) in the professional pitching shoulder between spring training in two consecutive years. *J Shoulder Elbow Surg.* 2012;21(11):1605–1612.

Shrier I. Strategic Assessment of Risk and Risk Tolerance (StARRT) framework for return-to-play decision-making. *Br J Sports Med.* 2015;49(20):1311–1315.

Spigelman T, Sciascia A, Uhl T. Return to swimming protocol for competitive swimmers: A post-operative case study and fundamentals. *Int J Sports Phys Ther.* 2014;9(5):712–725.

Stickley CD, Hetzler RK, Freemyer BG, Kimura IF. Isokinetic peak torque ratios and shoulder injury history in adolescent female volleyball athletes. *J Athl Train.* 2008;43(6):571–577.

Struyf F, Nijs J, Mottram S, Roussel NA, Cools AMJ, Meeusen R. Clinical assessment of the scapula: a review of the literature. *Br J Sports Med.* 2014;48(11):883–890.

Tambe A, Badge R, Funk L. Arthroscopic rotator cuff repair in elite rugby players. *Int J Shoulder Surg.* 2009;3(1):8–12.

Tarara DT, Fogaca LK, Taylor JB, Hegedus EJ. Clinician-friendly physical performance tests in athletes part 3: a systematic review of measurement properties and correlations to injury for tests in the upper extremity. *Br J Sports Med.* 2016;50(9):545–551.

Tate A, Turner GN, Knab SE, Jorgensen C, Strittmatter A, Michener LA. Risk factors associated with shoulder pain and disability across the lifespan of competitive swimmers. *J Athl Train.* 2012;47(2):149–158.

Tjong VK, Devitt BM, Murnaghan ML, Ogilvie-Harris DJ, Theodoropoulos JS. A qualitative investigation of return to sport after arthroscopic Bankart repair: beyond stability. *Am J Sports Med.* 2015;43(8):2005–2011.

Trakis JE, McHugh MP, Caracciolo PA, Busciacco L, Mullaney M, Nicholas SJ. Muscle strength and range of motion in adolescent pitchers with throwing-related pain: implications for injury prevention. *Am J Sports Med.* 2008;36(11):2173–2178.

Tyler TF, Mullaney MJ, Mirabella MR, Nicholas SJ, McHugh MP. Risk factors for shoulder and elbow injuries in high school baseball pitchers: the role of preseason strength and range of motion. *Am J Sports Med.* 2014;42(8):1993–1999.

Wilk KE, Hooks TR, Macrina LC. The modified sleeper stretch and modified cross-body stretch to increase shoulder internal rotation range of motion in the overhead throwing athlete. *J Orthop Sports Phys Ther.* 2013;43(12):891–894.

Wilk KE, Macrina LC, Fleisig GS, et al. Correlation of glenohumeral internal rotation deficit and total rotational motion to shoulder injuries in professional baseball pitchers. *Am J Sports Med.* 2011;39(2):329–335.

Wilk KE, Macrina LC, Fleisig GS, et al. Deficits in glenohumeral passive range of motion increase risk of shoulder injury in professional baseball pitchers: a prospective study. *Am J Sports Med.* 2015;43(10):2379–2385.

Wilk KE, Reinold MM, Olsen AD. Interval sport programs for the shoulder. In: Wilk KE, Reinold MM, Andrews JR, eds. *The Athlete's Shoulder.* 2nd ed. Philadelphia: Churchill Livingstone Elsevier; 2009:789–803.

Yang J, Mann BJ, Guettler JH, et al. Risk-prone pitching activities and injuries in youth baseball: Findings from a national sample. *Am J Sports Med.* 2014;42(6):1456–1463.

SECTION III

Acromioclavicular Joint Injury

SECTION OUTLINE

11 Acromioclavicular Joint Anatomy

PETER MACDONALD, BSC, MD, FRCS (C), GAUTAM DEEPAK TALAWADEKAR, and KATHERINE CABREJO-JONES, MD

Introduction

- The most widely used classification is Rockwood et al's, which is based on severity of injury.
- Clinical evaluation is especially important in assessing posterior dislocations and scapulothoracic dyskinesia.
- Imaging should always include standard shoulder views, including an axillary view in addition to bilateral Zanca views.
- Nonoperative treatment is the best approach for most acromioclavicular (AC) injuries and should include short-term immobilization and active physical therapy.
- Type III injuries are the most controversial in the literature, but there is a recent trend toward conservative treatment as well.
- Surgical treatment should be considered in late-presenting patients, high-level athletes, and overhead workers.

Articulating Surfaces

The AC joint consists of an articulation between the lateral end of the clavicle and the acromion of the scapula. Being a diarthrodial joint, the AC joint is surrounded by a capsule and has an intraarticular synovium and an articular cartilage interface. The distal clavicle articulates with the acromion via the medial facet, which is oriented posteriorly and laterally; the articular surface of the acromion is directed medially and anteriorly (Renfree & Wright, 2003; Tillman & Peterson, 1998). The average size of the joint surfaces in the adult AC joint has been found to be 9 mm (vertical) by 19 mm (anteroposterior [AP]) (Bosworth, 1949; Renfree & Wright, 2003). The average width of the AC joint ranges from 1 mm to 3 mm and decreases with advancing age, regardless of gender. It has two atypical features:

1. The articular surfaces of the joint are lined with fibrocartilage (as opposed to hyaline cartilage). The hyaline articular cartilage becomes fibrocartilage on the acromial side of the joint by the age of 17 years and on the clavicular side by the age of 24 years.
2. The joint cavity is partially divided by an articular disk, a wedge of fibrocartilage suspended from the upper part of the capsule. This disk varies in size and shape and is of mainly two types: a complete disk (very rare) and a meniscoid-like disk that only partially separates the articular surfaces and occupies the upper part of the articulation (Depalma, 1963; Renfree & Wright, 2003; Tillman & Peterson, 1998). The thickness of this disk varies, ranging from 1.5 to 4 mm. Beginning in the second decade of life, this structure undergoes rapid degeneration; by the fourth decade, this degeneration is significant.

Ligaments

The AC joint is supported by multiple ligaments, including the joint capsular ligaments, the coracoacromial (CC) ligament, and the coracoclavicular ligament. The AC joint capsule, although thin, provides considerable ligamentous support. The capsule, especially its superior and posterior parts, has been identified as the primary restraint to posterior translation of the clavicle (Klimkiewicz et al, 1999). There are four AC ligaments: superior, inferior, anterior, and posterior.

The superior AC ligament is a quadrilateral band composed of parallel fibers that interlace with the trapezius and deltoid aponeuroses, covering the superior part of the articulation and extending between the upper part of the lateral end of the clavicle and the adjoining part of the upper surface of the acromion. This ligament is thicker (2.0–5.5 mm) than the inferior and has a more defined insertion into the distal clavicle. Inferiorly, it is in contact with the articular disk when this is present.

The inferior AC ligament is the thinner of the two and covers the under part of the articulation and is attached to the adjoining surfaces of the two bones. Below this ligament lies the tendon of the supraspinatus. The CC ligament, which runs from the coracoid process to the acromion, is a strong triangular band, extending between the coracoid process and the acromion. It is attached, by its apex, to the summit of the acromion just in front of the articular surface for the clavicle and by its broad base to the whole length of the lateral border of the coracoid process. Superior to the ligament are the clavicle and undersurface of the deltoid and inferiorly is related to the tendon of the supraspinatus, a bursa being interposed. The ligament is sometimes described as consisting of two marginal bands and a thinner intervening portion, the two bands being attached, respectively, to the apex and the base of the coracoid process and joining together at the acromion. When the pectoralis minor is inserted into the capsule of the shoulder joint instead of into the coracoid process, it passes between these two bands, and the intervening portion of the ligament is then deficient.

Two other major ligaments supporting the AC joint are:

- Conoid: runs vertically from the coracoid process of the scapula to the conoid tubercle of the clavicle
- Trapezoid: runs from the coracoid process of the scapula to the trapezoid line of the clavicle

Collectively, the conoid and trapezoid ligaments are known as the coracoclavicular ligaments. They are a very strong structure, effectively suspending the weight of the upper limb from the clavicle (Fig. 11.1).

The conoid tubercle is located at the most posterior aspect of the clavicle, at the point where the middle third of the shaft curves into the lateral third. The trapezoid ridge extends anteriorly and laterally across the inferior surface of the lateral third of the clavicle. These landmarks represent the insertions of the corresponding ligaments (Klassen et al, 1997; Renfree & Wright, 2003). The conoid ligament is the posteromedial portion and the trapezoid ligament is the anterolateral portion of the CC ligament complex. Bursae can exist between these ligaments. The clavicular insertion of the conoid ligament is approximately twice as wide (medial to lateral) and thick (anterior to posterior) as its coracoid insertion, giving rise to its inverted cone shape. The trapezoid ligament is three times thicker at its clavicular end than at its coracoid end, but it shows less narrowing of its width compared with the conoid ligament. The coracoid origin of the trapezoid covered the posterior half of the coracoid dorsum; the conoid origin is more posterior on the base of the coracoid, limited anteriorly by the trapezoid insertion. The trapezoid ligament varies from 0.8 cm to 2.5 cm both in length and in width, and the conoid ligament varies from 0.7 cm to 2.5 cm in length and from 0.4 cm to 0.95 cm in width. Several studies have shown the center of the trapezoid and the conoid ligament insertion to be located 2.5 cm and 4.6 cm from the lateral edge of the clavicle, respectively (Boehm et al, 2003; Mazzocca et al, 2007; Renfree et al, 2003; Rios et al, 2007; Salzmann et al, 2008).

Neurovascular Supply

VESSELS

The arterial supply to the joint is via two vessels:

- The suprascapular artery arises from the subclavian artery at the thyrocervical trunk.
- The thoracoacromial artery arises from the axillary artery.

The veins of the joint follow the major arteries.

NERVES

The AC joint is innervated by articular branches of the suprascapular and lateral pectoral nerves. They both arise directly from the brachial plexus.

Movements and Function

The AC joint allows a degree of axial rotation and AP movement. Because no muscles act directly on the joint, all movement is passive and is initiated by movement at other joints. The motions of the AC joint are described as scapular movement with respect to the clavicle, including (Teece et al, 2008):

- Upward and downward rotation about an axis directed perpendicular to the scapular plane facing anteriorly and medially
- Internal and external rotation about an approximately vertical axis
- Anterior and posterior tipping or tilting about an axis directed laterally and anteriorly

The primary functions of the AC joint are:

1. To allow additional range of rotation for the scapula on the thorax

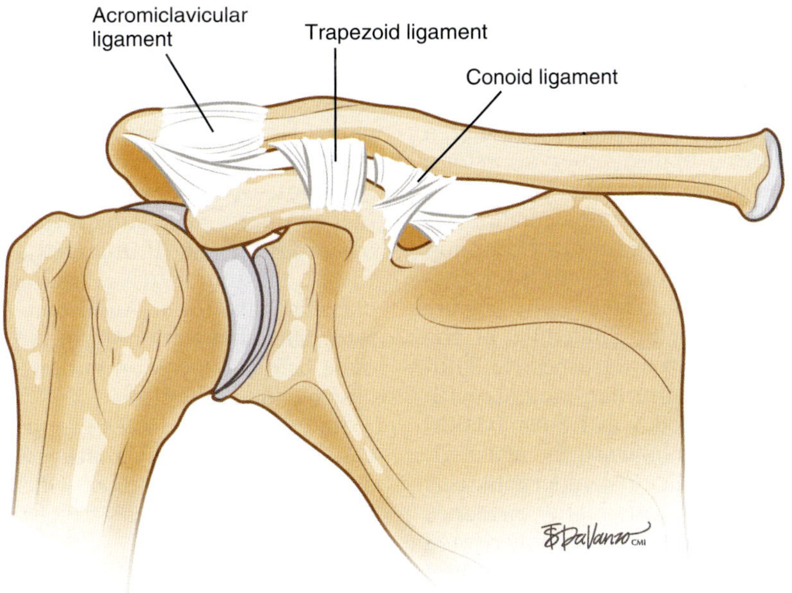

Fig. 11.1 The ligaments of the acromioclavicular joint. (Modified from TeachMeAnatomy. http://teachmeanatomy.info/upper-limb/joints/acromioclavicular. Copyright Jay F. Cox, 2006.)

2. To allow adjustments of the scapula (tipping and internal and external rotation) outside the initial plane of the scapula to follow the changing shape of the thorax as arm movement occurs

Applied Anatomy

1. The AC joint is extremely susceptible to both trauma and degenerative change because of its small and incongruent surfaces that result in large forces per unit area. Degenerative change is common from the second decade of life on, with the joint space itself commonly narrowed by the sixth decade.
2. The various procedures used for the operative management of AC joint dislocations are centered on the principle of reconstructing the strong conoid and trapezoid coracoclavicular ligaments in as physiological position as possible.

Etiology

An AC joint injury often occurs as a result of a direct blow to the tip of the shoulder from, for example, an awkward fall onto the dome of the shoulder, or impact with another player. This forces the acromion process downward, beneath the clavicle. The clavicle rests against the first rib, which blocks further downward displacement of the clavicle. If the clavicle is not fractured, the AC and coracoclavicular ligaments rupture. Other structures injured could include deltoid and trapezius muscles (Fig. 11.2, *A*).

Alternately, an AC joint injury may result from an upward force to the long axis of the humerus such as a fall that directly impacts on the wrist of a straightened arm. Most typically the shoulder is in an adducted and flexed position (Fig. 11.2, *B*).

Epidemiology

Dislocation of the AC joint is not infrequent, representing about 9% of all shoulder injuries, and should be considered whenever a young adult comes to clinical observation for a direct impact to the shoulder girdle. However, information about the basic epidemiologic features of this condition is scarce (Chillemi et al, 2013). It is the third most common injury seen in college hockey players and accounts for 41% of all shoulder injuries seen in elite college rugby players (Johansen et al, 2011). In the study by Chillemi et al, the incidence of pure AC dislocations, in a retrospective database search performed to identify all urban patients with an AC dislocation over a 5-year period, was 1.8 per 10,000 per year (Chillemi et al, 2013). Men between the age of 20 and 39 years were identified as significant demographic risk factors. AC joint injury has a significantly higher incidence rate for men compared with women; this is probably related to differences in lifestyle and hobbies, the men being more inclined to engage in high-risk activities. The other study that assessed the incidence of AC dislocation in a city-like population was by Nordqvist and Petersson (1995), who reported an incidence of 1.5 per 10,000 for males and of 0.2 for females.

In most cases, AC dislocation is the result of a direct and high-energy impact to the shoulder, which is a frequent occurrence in many sports as well as in road accidents. This explains why injuries to the AC joint are more common in the active population, highly exposed to forceful contacts. Sport activity, mainly cycling, represents the most common cause of AC dislocation, followed by road accidents. The principal mechanism of lesion regarding cycling is a direct impact to the joint when the arm is adducted or outstretched (putting the AC and CC ligaments in a position more susceptible to tears and strains) (Scott & Orr, 1973). Other sporting activities, namely soccer, rugby, and basketball, are associated with a higher risk of AC injuries because of tackling or wrong landing after a jump (Flik et al, 2005; Garraway et al, 2000; Headey et al, 2007; Mosiener & Wadsworth, 2010; Rios & Mazzocca, 2008). The second most common cause of AC dislocation is road accidents. In these cases, the tightening effect from safety belts may play a key role in the genesis of the injury, with or without an additional direct trauma to the shoulder.

Pallis et al (2012), in their epidemiologic study of 162 new AC joint injuries to determine the incidence and characteristics of AC joint injury at the United States Military Academy between 2005 and 2009, concluded that the majority of the AC joint injuries were low grade (145 sprains, 89%), and the injury occurred most commonly during athletics (91%). They also concluded that AC injuries resulted in at least 1359 total days lost to injury and an average of 18.4 days lost per athlete. The average time lost to injury for low-grade sprains was 10.4 days compared with high-grade injuries at 63.7 days. Of their patients with high-grade injuries, 71% elected to undergo coracoclavicular or AC reconstructions and the rate of surgical intervention in their study was 19 times higher for high-grade AC joint injuries than for low-grade injuries.

Classification

Acromioclavicular joint injuries were first described by Tossy et al in 1963. The injuries were divided into three categories depending on severity and were meant to guide treatment. Grade I was considered a sprain of the AC joint. Grade II was identified if the clavicle was displaced about 50% superiorly with regards to the acromion, and grade III included all complete separations of the AC joint. In 1967, Allman (1967) described a similar classification for a American Academy of Orthopaedic Surgeons instructional course lecture, the main difference being a special mention of a posteriorly dislocated clavicle for grade IIIs.

In 1989, Rockwood's group developed another classification based on Tossy's earlier work (Galatz et al, 2010). To date, it has been the most widely used classification in the literature and involves six types (Fig. 11.3).

TYPE I

Clinically the patient presents with pain and some edema at the AC joint but there is no gross deformity. On radiographs,

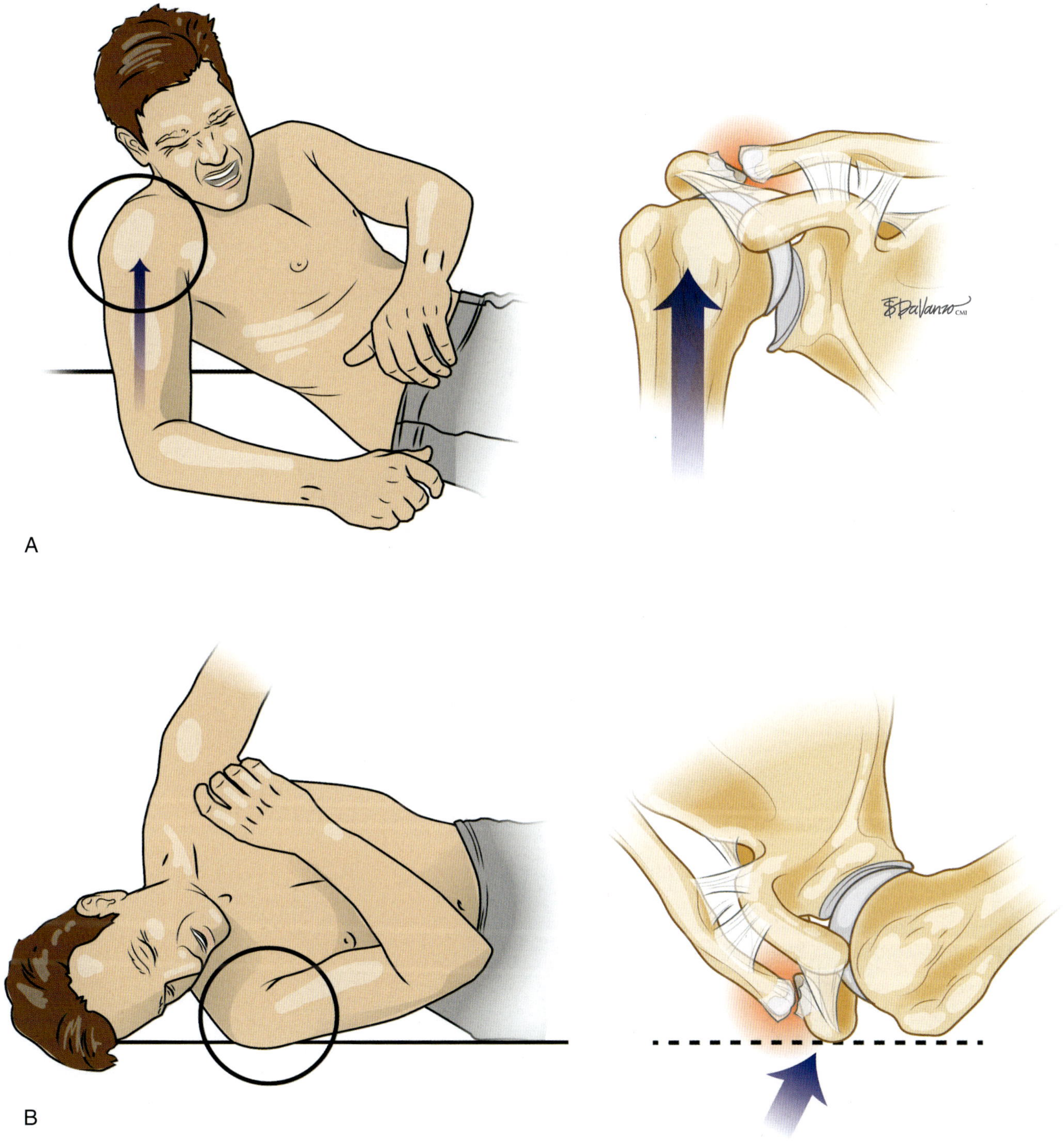

Fig. 11.2AB **The mechanism of injury.** (Modified from Oster DM. AC Joint Sprains: Shoulder Separation. http://www.davidostermd.com/David_M._Oster/AC_Joint_Sprain.html.)

the joint is normally positioned. The AC ligament is only sprained and the coracoclavicular ligament is intact.

TYPE II

Upon presentation, the distal end of the clavicle may be more prominent. The radiographs usually show widening of the AC joint. There may be superior displacement of the clavicle but typically less than 25% of the CC distance compared with the normal side. The AC ligament is torn, but the CC ligaments are only sprained.

TYPE III

Classically, in a type III injury, the distal end of the clavicle is completely displaced above the level of the acromion. On radiographs, the CC distance can be between 25% to 100% greater than on the opposite side. This type of dislocation can be associated with fractures of the acromion, distal clavicle, or coracoid process. A coracoid fracture may be suspected if the AC joint is completely displaced but the CC distance is normal, but this type of injury is quite rare. Normally, the AC and CC ligaments are torn, but the deltoid is intact.

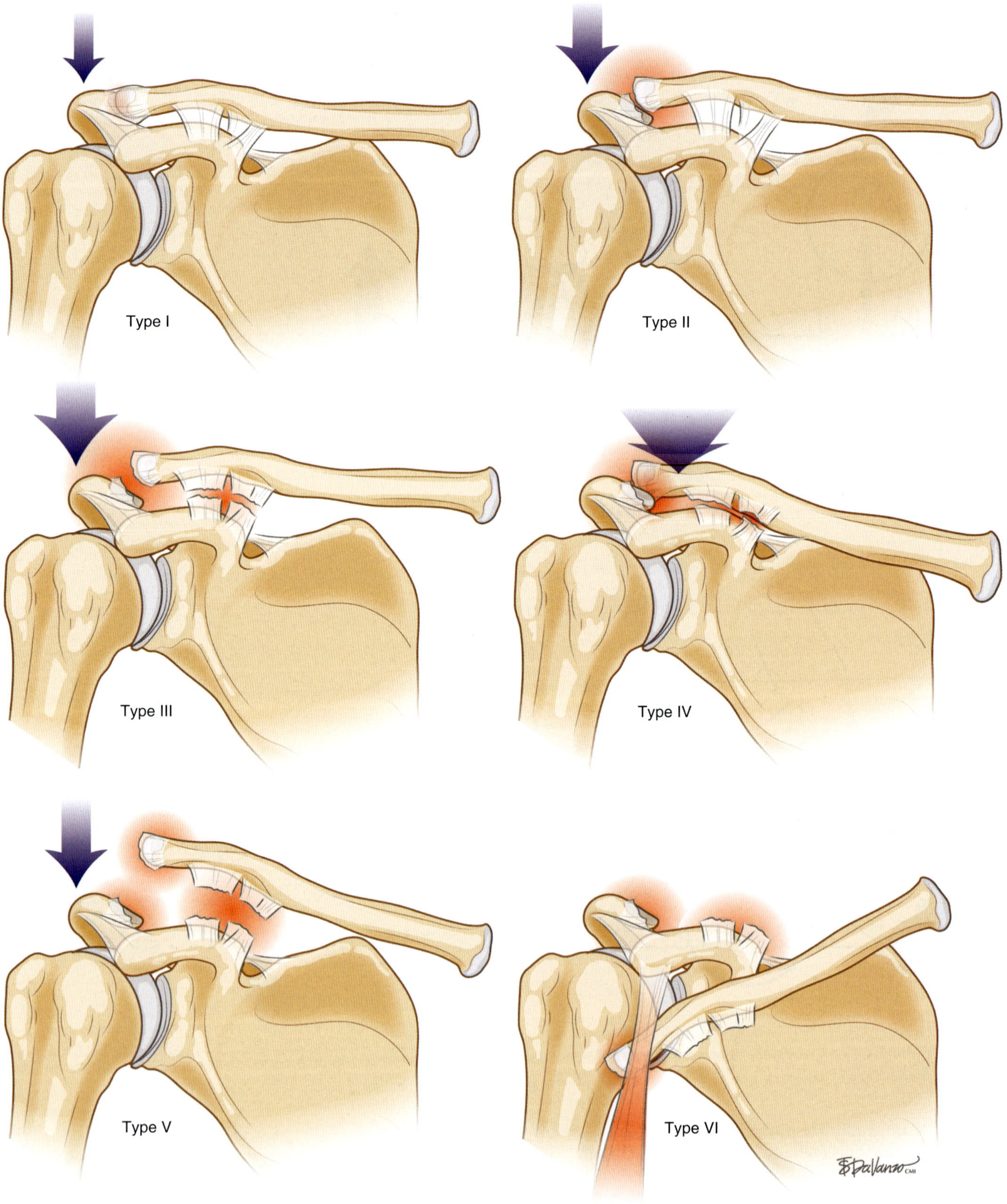

Fig. 11.3 Rockwood acromioclavicular joint injury classification. (Adapted from Rockwood CA, Young DC. Disorders of the acromioclavicular joint. In: Rockwood CA, Matsen F III, eds. *The shoulder*. Philadelphia: WB Saunders, 1990: 433, with permission).

TYPE IV

Allman did allude to this type of injury in 1967. The AC joint dislocation occurs posteriorly. The AP radiographs may underestimate the degree of displacement. To diagnose this type of dislocation, an axillary view is necessary. All the ligaments are torn as well as the deltoid and trapezius muscles.

TYPE V

This level of injury is the continuum of a type III. On the radiographs, the CC distance should be increased between 100% and 300%. Clinically, the patient usually has a very obvious deformity of the AC joint, and the distal clavicle is herniated through trapezius fascia. Thus, this type may not be easily reducible.

TYPE VI

This category includes both subcoracoid and subacromial dislocations. Only three subcoracoid dislocations have been described in the literature. Indeed, this very rare injury is usually associated with high-velocity trauma and multiple other injuries.

In 2014, The International Society of Arthroscopy, Knee Surgery and Orthopaedic Sports Medicine (ISAKOS) Upper Extremity Consensus suggested a subdivision of the type III injuries into stable (IIIa) and unstable (IIIb) categories. An unstable injury would be defined as overriding of the clavicle on the acromion on the cross-body adduction view and therapy-resistant scapular dysfunction and would probably warrant a surgical treatment (Beitzel et al, 2014). Clinical studies are still needed to evaluate the pertinence of these modifications.

Assessment

Completing a thorough history and physical examination with a patient suspected of having an AC injury is imperative. It is especially important to determine past upper extremity injuries or problems, occupation (overhead labor), and level of sport participation because these may influence the choice of treatment. In terms of the physical examination, the clinician needs to be able to see both AC joints as well as the scapulae and shoulder joints (Johansen et al, 2011). The initial assessment is performed with the arm hanging freely at the side (Beitzel et al, 2014). Asymmetry is noted in terms of swelling, deformity, and bruising. The AC joint will be tender to palpation. The examiner may try to reduce the joint by translating the shoulder joint superiorly with a hand under the elbow. If the AC joint injury is not obvious, the crossed-arm adduction and active compression test are used to identify an injury (Beitzel et al, 2014; Mazzocca et al, 2007). To differentiate between a type III and V injury, the evaluator can ask the patient to shrug his or her shoulders. If a type V injury is present, the AC joint may not reduce itself. A type IV injury might also be assessed by grasping the acromion in one hand and the clavicle in the other and translating it anteriorly and posteriorly. All these maneuvers can be very painful for the patient and be impossible to perform at the initial evaluation. Also, the sternoclavicular joint should be examined because biclavicular dislocations have been reported (Echo et al, 1988; Scapinelli, 2004). The scapulothoracic joint should also be assessed with regards to resting position, especially asymmetry of the medial scapular border, and dyskinesia with motion. Unless there is a clear indication for surgery, it is quite acceptable to start with conservative treatment and reassess the patient 3 to 6 weeks after the initial injury (Beitzel et al, 2014).

In terms of a chronic injury, the cross-arm adduction, active compression test, and palpation can still be used to elicit AC symptoms. However, concomitant pathology can make the diagnosis more difficult, and a diagnostic injection with xylocaine in the AC joint can become a very useful assessment tool.

Imaging

Classically, plain radiographs are always the first step in diagnostic imaging. Any patient with a suspected AC joint injury should get a standard shoulder series (AP, axillary, and Neer) and bilateral Zanca views (Beitzel et al, 2014; Headey et al, 2007; Stucken & Cohen, 2015). The CC distance can be measured and compared with the opposite side. An increase of 25% to 50% is indicative of complete CC disruption (type 3) (Bearden et al, 1973). A Zanca view is obtained by aiming the beam 10 to 15 degrees cephalad with 50% of the standard penetration strength, and its purpose is to clear the scapular spine to better assess the AC joint (Mazzocca et al, 2007). Weighted radiographs have fallen out of favor because they are quite uncomfortable for the patient and do not add diagnostic value. If a coracoid fracture is suspected, a Stryker notch view is added to view the coracoid in profile. It is done with the patient supine and holding her or his head with the affected arm and elbow pointing upward (Fig. 11.4). The axillary view is universally used to identify type IV injuries. However, one group performed a cadaveric study that showed this view had a high sensitivity but poor specificity, which could lead to a high number of false positives (Rahm et al, 2013). Although this was a small cadaveric study, it is a good reminder that it is always important to correlate the radiological findings with the clinical information.

During the long-term follow-up of the patient, one may see chronic changes secondary to the AC joint injury. AC arthritis, distal clavicle osteolysis, and ossification of the CC ligaments may all be present (Calvo et al, 2006). Although these changes may be present, they do not necessarily correlate with the clinical presentation and do not automatically warrant treatment.

Although these classic radiographs and measurements have been widely used to classify the injury, new evidence has suggested an overall lack of reliability for the Rockwood classification in terms of interobserver agreement (Cho et al, 2014; Kraeutler et al, 2012). The addition of three-dimensional computed tomography did not improve reliability of the classification and a more recent study also

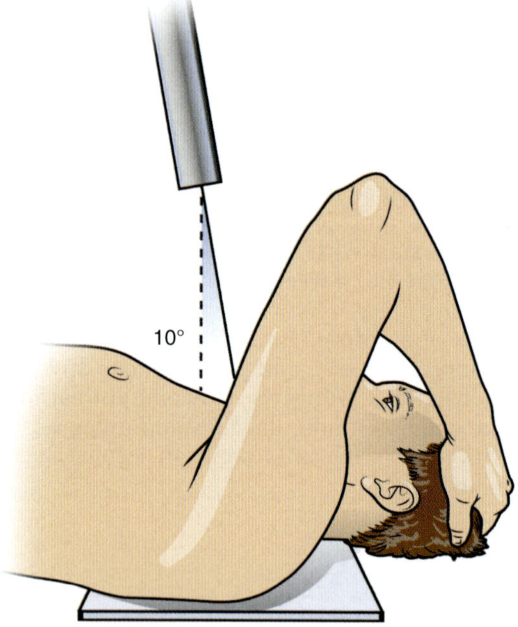

Fig. 11.4 **Stryker notch view for suspected coracoid process fracture.** (Adapted from Rockwood CA, Young DC. Disorders of the acromioclavicular joint. In: Rockwood CA, Matsen F III, eds. *The shoulder*. Philadelphia: WB Saunders, 1990: 433, with permission).

put into question intraobserver reliability (Cho et al, 2014). Furthermore, because there was a lack of reliability in the classification of the injury, especially for types III and V, the preferred treatment also differed significantly among surgeons (Kraeutler et al, 2012). Nevertheless, these remain small studies, and this needs to be further evaluated before we discard the classic methods of imaging and classifying AC joint injuries.

A few groups have studied other imaging modalities, including magnetic resonance imaging (MRI). It is difficult to describe AC joint injuries according to the original Rockwood classification when the patient is supine and gravity is eliminated from the equation. One group found a concordance of only 52% between radiographs and MRIs (Nemec et al, 2011). In addition, they modified the classification to accommodate for the details that were seen on MRI (e.g., sprain versus partial tear versus full tear). The pertinence of using more advanced imaging remains to be demonstrated in the current conservative treatment trends for grade I to III injuries. However, concomitant glenohumeral injuries (SLAP [superior labrum anterior and posterior], rotator cuff tear) may be present in up to 18% of patients and may be identified with the help of MRI (Tischer et al, 2009).

Nonoperative Treatment

The management of AC joint injuries has varied through time. The large majority of orthopedic surgeons treat type I and II injuries conservatively and type IV to VI injuries surgically. Although Mouhsine et al (2003) demonstrated that patients with type I and II injuries may have a high rate of complications in the long term, they did not recommend primary surgical treatment for these patients. They maintain that the severity of these injuries is underestimated and that a surprisingly high number of patients require secondary surgery but still do well after a distal clavicle excision.

Type III injuries have always been controversial. In 1974, a survey of orthopedic surgeons revealed that 60% preferred surgical treatment for Tossy's grade III AC joint injuries (Bradley & Elkousy, 2003; Nissen & Chatterjee, 2007). In 1992, a subsequent survey showed the pendulum had swung the other way, and 86.4% of surgeons opted for conservative treatment for Rockwood type III injuries. Recently, a new survey showed that the preferred treatment for acute type III AC joint injuries is still nonoperative treatment (81.6%–86.9%) (Nissen & Chatterjee, 2007). In 2008, a thorough literature review was performed by Ceccarelli et al (2008) to identify the best treatment for grade III injuries, but they were unable to conclude on one because of an insufficient number of randomized controlled trials (RCTs), systematic reviews, and meta-analyses.

In 2010, a Cochrane review was conducted to compare surgical versus conservative treatment in AC joint injuries. Only three trials were included, and the authors concluded that there was insufficient evidence to determine when surgical treatment was indicated. They found no significant difference among the different treatment groups except a higher rate of complications and longer delay before return to work in the surgical groups (Tamaoki et al, 2010). In 2015, the Canadian Orthopaedic Trauma Society published the results of a multicenter RCT comparing nonoperative treatment with surgical treatment with a hook plate construct (Canadian Orthopaedic Trauma Society, 2015). They included all patients having a type III to V injury without attempting to categorize them because there is sufficient evidence showing that the intraobserver reliability of the Rockwood classification is low. Their 83-patient cohort demonstrated that in regards to functional status (Disabilities of the Arm, Shoulder and Hand (DASH), Constant score), patients in the no operative group did better initially until about 6 months, but there was no difference at 1 year. Patients also returned to work earlier in the nonoperative group. The main advantage of the surgical group was cosmesis. Indeed, a significant number of patients were dissatisfied with the appearance of their shoulders in the nonoperative group. As expected, there were an appreciably higher number of complications in the surgical group. This study is in contradiction with the standard surgical management of type IV and V injuries because it supports conservative treatment for all fully displaced AC joint dislocations (Canadian Orthopaedic Trauma Society, 2015). It is clear, however, that not all patients do well with nonoperative management, and further studies need to identify negative prognostic factors to facilitate our decision process. Furthermore, although this is the most recent and well-done study of its type, it did not evaluate other surgical techniques, long-term results, or the impact of scapular dyskinesia.

Recently, a retrospective study showed that about 70% of patients have successful nonoperative treatment (Petri et al, 2016). They also established that patients who present more than 30 days after injury have a high risk of conservative treatment failure. Surprisingly, patients who underwent AC joint reconstruction were more likely to return to their previous intensity level of sport participation. In 2014, the ISAKOS

Upper Extremity Committee Consensus stated that because of the lack of clear evidence that surgical treatment is superior, all type III injuries should have a trial of conservative management but should be reevaluated within 3 to 6 weeks for AC joint instability (Beitzel et al, 2014). At this point, patients may receive surgical stabilization if they have persistent pain and inability to return to their sport or job. Even if an emphasis on initial nonoperative management is the current recommendation, the decision for treatment should be made on a case-by-case basis with regard to the patient's goals and specific demands such as manual labor and overhead throwing (Ceccarelli et al, 2008; Johansen et al, 2011; Murena et al, 2013; Stucken & Cohen, 2015; Tamaoki et al, 2010).

Moreover, scapular dyskinesia has been associated with type III AC dislocations. This may explain why these patients have persistent periscapular, scapulothoracic, and AC joint pain after an injury. Gumina et al (2009) showed that 70.6% of patients with chronic AC dislocation have scapular dyskinesia. On the other hand, only 11.7% of patients treated surgically presented scapular dyskinesia (Murena et al, 2013). Fortunately, rehabilitation can remediate this problem after conservative treatment. Seventy-eight percent of Gumina et al's original cohort no longer exhibited signs of scapular derangement and significantly increased their Constant scores after a 12-month rehabilitation (Carbone et al, 2015). On average, patients were 5 years postinjury, and the benefits may be even greater if started earlier.

When the nonoperative treatment avenue has been chosen, several options are available for the patient. Usually, a regular sling is used for comfort until the patient feels well enough to wean out of it (Canadian Orthopaedic Trauma Society, 2015; Johansen et al, 2011). A Kenny Howard brace may be used as opposed to a simple sling, but compliance is low because of its bulkiness (Bradley & Elkousy, 2003). In 2007, only about 10% of surgeons preferred this type of immobilization as opposed to symptomatic treatment (Nissen & Chatterjee, 2007). Usually, the higher the grade of injury, the longer the patient needs to wear the sling. Concomitantly, patients may benefit from nonsteroidal antiinflammatory drugs and ice. They are also encouraged to start range of motion (ROM) exercises as soon as possible, and ideally, all patients should be referred to a physiotherapist. Several protocols have been established based on Gladstone's original work (Cote et al, 2010; Gladstone et al, 1997; Petri et al. 2016). There are usually four phases (Table 11.1) progressing the patient from elimination of pain and simple ROM to strengthening and endurance. More recently, in light of the work of Gumina et al (2009), closed-chain scapular exercises have also been incorporated while rehabilitating AC joint injuries (Cote et al, 2010; Reid et al, 2012).

Table 11.1 Gladstone's Acromioclavicular Joint Injury Rehabilitation Guidelines*

Grade	Phase	Recommendations

I–II	I: Immediate motion	▪ Sling 3–10 days
		▪ ROM:
		  ▪ Flexion to tolerance
		  ▪ IR/ER at 0 degrees of abduction
		  ▪ Progress to scapula plane
		  ▪ PROM, pulley and pendulum exercises
		▪ Isometric exercises:
		  ▪ Multiangle, submaximal, subpainful
		  ▪ Pain relief modalities

	II: Intermediate	Criteria: ROM 65%–75% of contralateral side strength (4/5) of deltoid, trapezius
		▪ ROM:
		  ▪ Flexion (170 degrees or greater)
		  ▪ IR/ER performed at 90 degrees of abduction
		  ▪ Gentle horizontal abduction
		  ▪ Gentle self-capsular stretches
		▪ Isotonic strengthening exercises:
		  ▪ Dumbbells: flexion, abduction, extension
		  ▪ Tubing IR/ER
		  ▪ Biceps curls
		  ▪ Prone horizontal abduction
		  ▪ Manual resistance PNF
		▪ Restrictions: no overhead, shoulder press, bench press, pullovers, pec flies

	III: Advanced strengthening exercises	Criteria: no pain, full ROM, strength 70%–75% contralateral side
		▪ Strengthening and endurance program:
		  ▪ Isotonic shoulder flexion, abduction, extension
		  ▪ Shoulder shrugs
		  ▪ PNF tubing exercises
		  ▪ IR/ER tubing
		  ▪ Biceps curls
		  ▪ Scapula retraction
		  ▪ Push-ups
		  ▪ Seated rowing and prone rowing
		  ▪ Initiate light bench press, shoulder press (front)
		  ▪ "Throwers" IR/ER at 90 degrees of abduction
		  ▪ Initiate plyometrics (two-hand throws)
		▪ Restrictions: no pec deck, pullovers, wide-grip bench press

Continued

Table 11.1 Gladstone's Acromioclavicular Joint Injury Rehabilitation Guidelines—cont'd

Grade	Phase	Recommendations
	IV: Return to activity	Criteria: full and painless ROM, isokinetic tests fulfill criteria, satisfactory clinical examination ■ Initiate interval sports program ■ Continue all exercises in phase III ■ Progress resistance levels ■ Progress stretching ■ Remove restrictions ■ Fit for protective padding or bracing

III	I: Protection and immediate motion; 1–2 weeks	■ Sling 7–14 days (discontinue earlier if symptoms allow)
		■ Pain neuromodulation techniques
		■ ROM exercises:
		  ■ AAROM exercises
		  ■ ER/IR (0 degrees of abduction) progress to scapula plane
		  ■ Pulley, pendulum exercises
		■ Strengthening exercises:
		  ■ Isometric-multiangle, submaximal, subpainful
		  ■ Shoulder shrugs
		  ■ Flexion, abduction IR/ER at 0 degrees abduction, elbow flexion

	II: Intermediate; 3–4 weeks	Discontinue sling
		■ ROM exercises
		  ■ Flexion (160 degrees plus)
		  ■ IR/ER at 90 degrees of abduction)
		  ■ Shoulder extension
		■ Stretches as indicated
		■ Strengthening: isotonic exercises, light weights initially
		  ■ Shoulder flexion, abduction, extension
		  ■ Biceps curls
		  ■ IR/ER with tubing
		  ■ Scapula retraction
		  ■ Manual resistance
		  ■ Rhythmic stabilization drills
		■ Restrictions: no pullovers, pec deck, bench press, shoulder press, dips

III	III: Advanced strengthening exercises; 4–6 weeks	Criteria: must have full and pain-free ROM, no pain, strength 70%–75% contralateral side; ROM exercises continue
		■ Strengthening:
		  ■ Isotonic shoulder press (front), shrugs, flexion, abduction, extension
		  ■ Long lever and complex patterns (PNF, cables)
		  ■ IR/ER tubing
		  ■ Bench press (narrow grip)
		  ■ Push-ups
		  ■ Scapula retraction
		  ■ Seated rowing
		  ■ Prone rowing
		■ Plyometric training
		■ Restrictions: no pec deck, pullovers, wide grip bench, press, dips

III	IV: Return to activity; weeks 5–8	■ Sports-specific training ■ Continue with phase II exercises ■ Remove restrictions ■ RTS planning and assessment

*Divided into phases, progressed according to symptoms.

AAROM, Active assisted range of motion; *ER*, external rotation; *IR*, internal rotation; *PNF*, proprioceptive neuromuscular facilitation; *PROM*, passive range of motion; *ROM*, range of motion; *RTS*, return to sport.

These exercises were originally described by Burkhart et al (2003) for the treatment of disabled throwing shoulders and were successfully used in patients presenting scapular dyskinesia after an AC joint injury (Beitzel et al, 2014; Carbone et al, 2015). Patients who demonstrate little or no response to therapy after 6 weeks have a tendency to go on to need surgery, which is in accordance with the ISAKOS recommendations.

With regards to athlete, return to sport varies according to severity of symptoms. For type I, they can usually return after 2 to 4 weeks. For type II, athletes are usually able to return to play after 4 to 8 weeks. Occasionally, a cortisone injection may be used to relieve pain (Bradley & Elkousy, 2003). For type III, 6 to 12 weeks is recommended, although it may take longer (Reid et al, 2012). Return to sport should be delayed until full, painless ROM is obtained (Johansen et al, 2011).

If the patient presents with a chronic injury, a trial of conservative management can be attempted. Available modalities of treatment include a cortisone injection and physiotherapy. However, in the chronic setting, if these modalities fail, the patient should be counseled on surgical options such as AC joint reconstruction or distal clavicle excision.

References

Allman FL. Fractures and ligamentous injuries of the clavicle and its articulation. *J Bone Joint Surg Am*. 49(4):774–784.

Bearden JM, Hughston JC, Whatley GS. Acromioclavicular dislocation: method of treatment. *J Sports Med*. 1973;1(4):5–17.

Beitzel K, Mazzocca AD, Bak K, et al. Upper Extremity Committee of ISAKOS. ISAKOS upper extremity committee consensus statement on the need for diversification of the Rockwood classification for acromioclavicular joint injuries. *Arthroscopy*. 2014;30(2):271–278.

Boehm TD, Kirschner S, Fischer A, Gohlke F. The relation of the coracoclavicular ligament insertion to the acromioclavicular joint: a cadaver study of relevance to lateral clavicle resection. *Acta Orthop Scand*. 2003;74(6):718–721.

Bosworth BM. Complete acromioclavicular dislocation. *N Engl J Med*. 1949;241(6):221–225.

Bradley JP. Elkousy H. Decision making: operative versus nonoperative treatment of acromioclavicular joint injuries. *Clin Sports Med*. 2003;22(2):277–290.

Burkhart SS, Morgan CD, Kibler WB. The disabled throwing shoulder: spectrum of pathology part III: The SICK Scapula, scapular dyskinesis, the kinetic chain, and rehabilitation. *Arthroscopy*. 2003;19(6):641–661.

Calvo E, López-Franco M, Arribas IM. Clinical and radiologic outcomes of surgical and conservative treatment of type III acromioclavicular joint injury. *J Shoulder Elbow Surg*. 2006;15(3):300–305.

Canadian Orthopaedic Trauma Society. Multicenter randomized clinical trial of nonoperative versus operative treatment of acute acromio-clavicular joint dislocation. *J Orthop Trauma*. 2015;29(11):479–487.

Carbone S, Postacchini R, Gumina S. Scapular dyskinesis and SICK syndrome in patients with a chronic Type III acromioclavicular dislocation. Results of rehabilitation. *Knee Surg Sports Traumatol Arthrosc*. 2015;23(5):1473–1480.

Ceccarelli E, Bondì R, Alviti F, Garofalo R, Miulli F, Padua R. Treatment of acute grade III acromioclavicular dislocation: a lack of evidence. *J Orthop Traumatol*. 2008;9(2):105–108.

Chillemi C, Franceschini V, Dei Giudici L, et al. Epidemiology of isolated acromioclavicular joint dislocation. *Emerg Med Int*. 2013;2013:171609.

Cho CH, Hwang I, Seo JS, et al. Reliability of the classification and treatment of dislocations of the acromioclavicular joint. *J Shoulder Elbow Surg*. 2014;23(5):665–670.

Cote MP, Wojcik KE, Gomlinski G, Mazzocca AD. Rehabilitation of acromioclavicular joint separations: operative and nonoperative considerations. *Clin Sports Med*. 2010;29(2):213–228. vii.

Depalma AF. Surgical anatomy of the acromioclavicular and sternoclavicular joints. *Surg Clin North Am*. 1963;43(Dec):1541–1550.

Echo BS, Donati RB, Powell CE. Bipolar clavicular dislocation treated surgically. A case report. *J Bone Joint Surg Am*. 1988;70(8):1251–1253.

Flik K, Lyman S, Marx RG. American collegiate men's ice hockey: an analysis of injuries. *Am J Sports Med*. 2005;33(2):183–187.

Galatz LM, Hollis RF Jr, Williams GR Jr. Acromioclavicular joint injuries. In: Bucholz RW, Heckman JD, Court-Brown CM, Tornetta P, eds. *Rockwood and Green's Fractures in Adults*. 7th ed. Philadelphia: Lippincott Williams & Wilkins; 2010:1211–1242. I.

Garraway WM, Lee AJ, Hutton SJ, Russell EB, Macleod DA. Impact of professionalism on injuries in rugby union. *Br J Sports Med*. 2000;34(5):348–351.

Gladstone JN, Wilk KE, Andrews JR. Nonoperative treatment of acromioclavicular joint injuries. *Oper Tech Sports Med*. 1997;5(2):78–87.

Gumina S, Carbone S, Postacchini F. Scapular dyskinesis and SICK scapula syndrome in patients with chronic type III acromioclavicular dislocation. *Arthroscopy*. 2009;25(1):40–45.

Headey J, Brooks JHM, Kemp SPT. The epidemiology of shoulder injuries in English professional rugby union. *Am J Sports Med*. 2007;35(9): 1537–1543.

Johansen JA, Grutter PW, McFarland EG, Petersen SA. Acromioclavicular joint injuries: indications for treatment and treatment options. *J Shoulder Elbow Surg*. 2011;20(suppl 2):S70–S82.

Klassen J, Morrey BF, Ann KN. Surgical anatomy and the function of the acromioclavicular and coracoclavicular ligaments. *Oper Tech Sports Med*. 1997;5:60–64.

Klimkiewicz JJ, Williams GR, Sher JS, Karduna A, Des Jardins J, Iannotti JP. The acromioclavicular capsule as a restraint to posterior translation of the clavicle: a biomechanical analysis. *J Shoulder Elbow Surg*. 1999;8(2):119–124.

Kraeutler MJ, Williams GR Jr, Cohen SB, et al. Inter- and intraobserver reliability of the radiographic diagnosis and treatment of acromioclavicular joint separations. *Orthopedics*. 2012;35(10):e1483–e1487.

Mazzocca AD, Arciero RA, Bicos J. Evaluation and treatment of acromioclavicular joint injuries. *Am J Sports Med*. 2007;35(2):316–329.

Moslener MD, Wadsworth LT. Ice hockey: a team physician's perspective. *Curr Sports Med Rep*. 2010;9(3):134–138.

Mouhsine E, Garofalo R, Crevoisier X, Farron A. Grade I and II acromioclavicular dislocations: results of conservative treatment. *J Shoulder Elbow Surg*. 2003;12(6):599–602.

Murena L, Canton G, Vulcano E, Cherubino P. Scapular dyskinesis and SICK scapula syndrome following surgical treatment of type III acute acromioclavicular dislocations. *Knee Surg Sports Traumatol Arthrosc*. 2013;21(5):1146–1150.

Nemec U, Oberleitner G, Nemec SF, Gruber M, Weber M, Czerny C, Krestan CR. MRI versus radiography of acromioclavicular joint dislocation. *AJR Am J Roentgenol*. 2011;197(4):968–973.

Nissen CW, Chatterjee A. Type III acromioclavicular separation: results of a recent survey on its management. *Am J Orthop (Belle Mead NJ)*. 2007;36(2):89–93.

Nordqvist A, Petersson CJ. Incidence and causes of shoulder girdle injuries in an urban population. *J Shoulder Elbow Surg*. 1995;4(2):107–112.

Pallis M, Cameron KL, Svoboda SJ, Owens BD. Epidemiology of acromioclavicular joint injury in young athletes. *Am J Sports Med*. 2012;40(9):2072–2077.

Petri M, Warth RJ, Greenspoon JA, et al. Clinical results after conservative management for grade III acromioclavicular joint injuries: does eventual surgery affect overall outcomes? *Arthroscopy*. 2016;32(5): 740–746.

Rahm S, Wieser K, Spross C, Vich M, Gerber C, Meyer DC. Standard axillary radiographs of the shoulder may mimic posterior subluxation of the lateral end of the clavicle. *J Orthop Trauma*. 2013;27(11):622–626.

Reid D, Polson K, Johnson L. Acromioclavicular joint separations grades i-iii: a review of the literature and development of best practice guidelines. *Sports Med*. 2012;42(8):681–696.

Renfree KJ, Riley MK, Wheeler D, Hentz JG, Wright TW. Ligamentous anatomy of the distal clavicle. *J Shoulder Elbow Surg*. 2003;12(4):355–359.

Renfree KJ, Wright TW. Anatomy and biomechanics of the acromioclavicular and sternoclavicular joints. *Clin Sports Med*. 2003;22(2):219–237.

Rios CG, Arciero RA, Mazzocca AD. Anatomy of the clavicle and coracoid process for reconstruction of the coracoclavicular ligaments. *Am J Sports Med*. 2007;35(5):811–817.

Rios CG, Mazzocca AD. Acromioclavicular joint problems in athletes and new methods of management. *Clin Sports Med*. 2008;27(4):763–788.

Rockwood CA Jr. Fractures and dislocations of the shoulder. In: Rockwood CA Jr, Green DP, eds. *Fractures in Adults*. Philadelphia, PA: Lippincott; 1984:860–910.

Salzmann GM, Paul J, Sandmann GH, Imhoff AB, Schöttle PB. The coracoidal insertion of the coracoclavicular ligaments: an anatomic study. *Am J Sports Med*. 2008;36(12):2392–2397.

Scapinelli R. Bipolar dislocation of the clavicle: 3D CT imaging and delayed surgical correction of a case. *Arch Orthop Trauma Surg*. 2004;124(6): 421–424.

Scott JC, Orr MM. Injuries to the acromioclavicular joint. *Injury*. 1973;5(1): 13–18.

Stucken C, Cohen SB. Management of acromioclavicular joint injuries. *Orthop Clin North Am*. 2015;46(1):57–66.

Tamaoki MJ, Belloti JC, Lenza M, et al. Surgical versus conservative interventions for treating acromioclavicular dislocation of the shoulder in adults. *Cochrane Database Syst Rev*. 2010;8. CD007429.

Teece RM, Lunden JB, Lloyd AS, Kaiser AP, Cieminski CJ, Ludewig PM. Three-dimensional acromioclavicular joint motions during elevation of the arm. *J Orthop Sports Phys Ther*. 2008;38(4):181–190.

Tillman B, Peterson W. Clinical anatomy. In: Fu FH, Ticker JB, Imhoff AB, eds. *Analysis of Shoulder Surgery*. Stamford, CT: Appleton and Lange; 1998:1–29.

Tischer T, Salzmann GM, El-Azab H, Vogt S, Imhoff AB. Incidence of associated injuries with acute acromioclavicular joint dislocations types III through V. *Am J Sports Med*. 2009;37(1):136–139.

Tossy JD, Mead NC, Sigmond HM. Acromioclavicular separations: useful and practical classification for treatment. *Clin Orthop Rel Res*. 1963;28:111–119.

12 Surgical Treatment

12-12A SURGICAL TREATMENT: ARTHROSCOPIC

ERIK M. FRITZ, MD, BROOKE M. DELVECCHIO, PT, DPT, OCS, JONAS POGORZELSKI, MD, MHBA, and PETER J. MILLETT, MD, MSC

Introduction

- Injuries to the acromioclavicular (AC) joint are common shoulder injuries with an incidence of 1.8/1000 per year (Warth et al, 2013).
- The majority of AC injuries occur in athletes from contact sports as a result of collision or direct fall onto the shoulder.
- In general, concomitant lesions to the shoulder girdle may occur in up to approximately 20% of cases; shoulder arthroscopy during AC joint stabilization may help detect these lesions (Tischer et al, 2009).
- Rockwood and colleagues developed the classification scheme for AC joint injuries, recognizing the importance of the coracoclavicular (CC) ligaments in joint stability (Williams et al, 1989).
- Surgery is the treatment of choice for Rockwood injuries types IV through VI and for patients with persistent symptoms and AC joint instability after nonoperative treatment of lower grade AC joint injuries. Management of type III injuries is controversial, and types I and II are treated nonoperatively.
- Our preferred surgical technique involves a knotless fixation system because it can reduce irritation of the subcutaneous tissue.
- Following surgical treatment of AC joint injury, patients typically obtain good to excellent postoperative clinical outcomes; however, a complication rate of approximately 25% can negatively impact the outcomes (Clavert et al, 2015; Martetschlager et al, 2013; Woodmass et al, 2015).

Classification

Rockwood and colleagues developed the most commonly used classification system for AC joint injuries (Fig. 12A.1) on the basis of the work of Tossy et al (1963). In Rockwood type I injuries, the AC ligaments are sprained but there is no anatomic dislocation, and the trapezius and deltoid fascia remain intact. Type II injuries involve rupture of the AC joint ligaments, with the CC ligaments and the trapezius and deltoid fascia remaining intact. With type III injuries, the AC and CC ligaments are both ruptured, and the clavicle is superiorly displaced by 25% to 100% in comparison with the uninjured side; the trapezius and deltoid fascia are not disrupted. Type IV injuries are similar to type III, but with horizontal instability of the distal end of the clavicle and disruption of the trapezius and deltoid fascia. Type V injuries are again similar to type III, but the clavicle is superiorly displaced more than 100% in comparison with the uninjured side with disruption of the trapezius and deltoid fascia. Finally, type VI injuries, are rarely seen and involve rupture of both AC and CC ligaments with inferior displacement of the distal clavicle; the trapezius and deltoid fascia are disrupted (Tossy et al, 1963; Williams et al, 1989). Beitzel et al (2014) proposed a modification to the classic Rockwood classification in which type III injuries may be further subdivided into IIIA and IIIB; type IIIA injuries are stable and may respond well to conservative management, but type IIIB injuries are unstable and should be treated surgically.

Patient Examination and Diagnostics

AC joint injuries are rarely subtle and can often be diagnosed by inspection and palpation. Patients typically present holding the injured extremity at the elbow with the contralateral arm for pain relief. The AC joint is tender to palpation, and range of movement (ROM) is limited owing to pain. Imaging evaluation (Fig. 12A.2) should include standard axillary views, Y-views, and panoramic views. Although the axillary view can assist in determining posterior displacement (as in type IV injuries), the Y-view helps to detect further bony lesions of the shoulder. Panoramic views are useful to compare the injured AC joint with the uninjured side. Additional weighted stress views are often advocated to distinguish between types II and III; however, we do not routinely recommend this practice because it rarely alters treatment and causes unnecessary patient discomfort.

Surgical Treatment

INDICATIONS

Nonoperative management is usually the preferred initial treatment for Rockwood types I and II injuries. Treatment of type III has historically been controversial; however, a new subclassification provides evidence supporting nonoperative treatment of Rockwood type IIIA (horizontally stable) and surgical reconstruction of type IIIB (horizontally

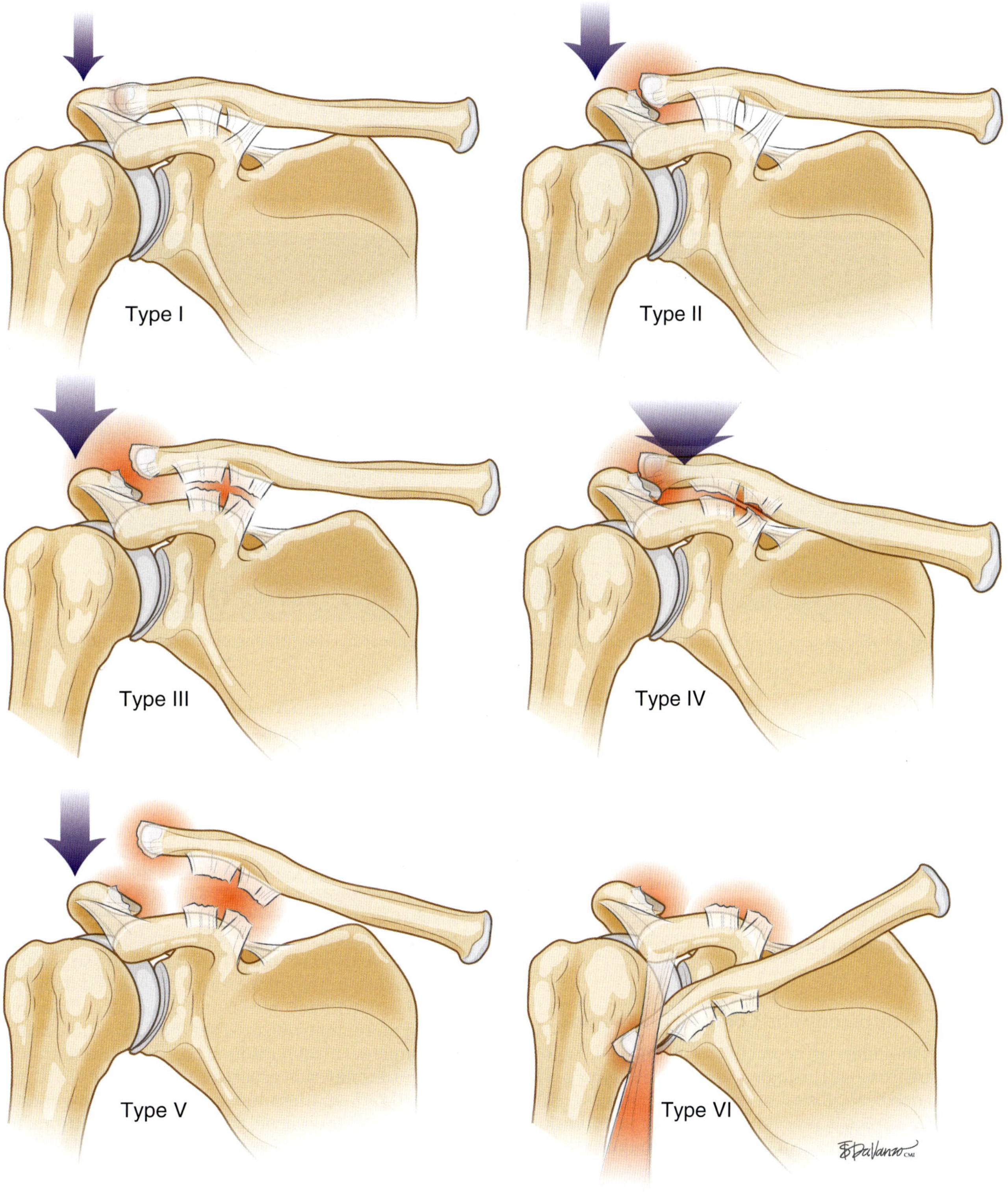

Fig. 12A.1 Rockwood classification of AC joint injuries (Williams et al, 1989). (Reprinted from Ponce BA, Millett PJ, Warner JJ. Acromioclavicular joint instability: Reconstruction indications and techniques. *Oper Tech Sports Med*. 2004;12(1):35-42.)

unstable) (Beitzel et al, 2014). Acute and chronic Rockwood type IV through VI injuries should also be treated surgically, as should symptomatic type IIIA injuries for which conservative management has failed (Beitzel et al, 2014; Petri et al, 2016).

PATIENT POSITIONING AND ANESTHESIA

Following induction of general endotracheal anesthesia, the patient is placed in the beach-chair position. Intraoperative fluoroscopy is positioned with the x-ray tube

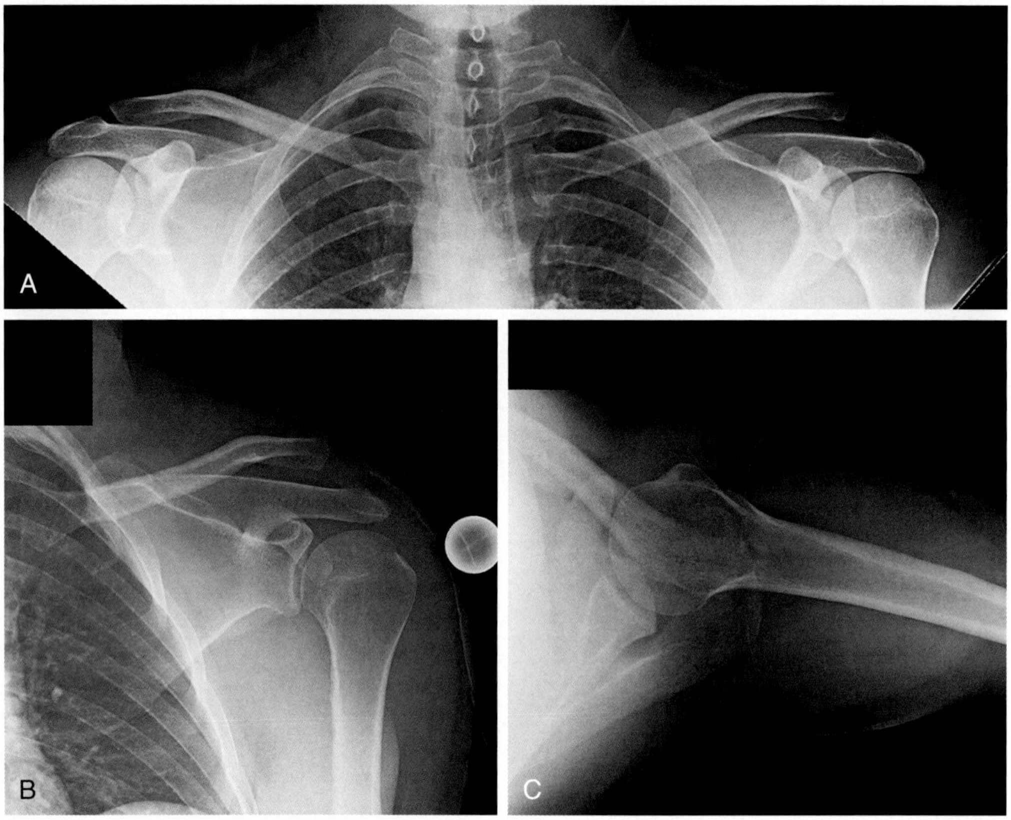

Fig. 12A.2 Left-sided Rockwood type V AC joint dislocation seen in the (**A**) unweighted panorama view, (**B**) anteroposterior view, and (**C**) axillary view.

anterior to the patient's shoulder; this positioning permits utilization of fluoroscopy throughout the procedure to assist with visualization of the bony structures, confirmation of AC joint reduction, and placement of hardware. The patient and fluoroscopy machine are then prepared and draped in sterile fashion with the operative extremity placed in a pneumatic arm holder. Single-shot intravenous antibiotics are administered prior to the incision.

OPERATIVE TECHNIQUE

See Video 12A.1.

Diagnostic Arthroscopy and Coracoid Preparation

Diagnostic shoulder arthroscopy is performed with a 30-degree arthroscope through a standard posterior portal. With spinal needle localization, an anterior portal is created lateral to the coracoid process, followed by insertion of a 5-mm cannula (Arthrex, Naples, FL) and an intraarticular diagnostic arthroscopy is performed. Next, a mechanical shaver and radiofrequency ablator are used to expose the inferior surface of the coracoid process as well as to address any intraarticular pathology. If necessary, a 70-degree arthroscope may be utilized to assist with visualization of the subcoracoid space.

Knotless Coracoclavicular Fixation

After sufficient exposure of the coracoid, an additional anteroinferolateral (AIL) portal is created inferior and lateral to the previously placed anterior portal. An 8.25-mm cannula (Arthrex) is then inserted through the portal, and attention is turned to the superior aspect of the lateral clavicle. A 2- to 3-cm incision is created over the distal end of the clavicle perpendicular to its long axis, approximately 3 cm medial to the AC joint. The skin and subcutaneous tissues are sharply dissected to expose the superior surface of the clavicle.

An acromioclavicular aiming guide (Arthrex) is then placed through the cannula and positioned on the inferior aspect of the coracoid, centered medial to lateral. The drilling sleeve of the guide is placed on the superior aspect of the clavicle, centered anterior to posterior. A 3.0-mm cannulated drill (Arthrex) is then drilled from the superior aspect of the clavicle to the inferior aspect of the coracoid process under direct arthroscopic visualization. Great care must be taken at this point to ensure that the cannulated drill enters in the superocentral portion of the clavicle and that it exits at the posteroinferior aspect of the coracoid; if it is drilled incorrectly, the patient has a higher chance of postoperative clavicular or coracoid fracture. Next, a 5.0-mm unicortical reamer (Arthrex) is used to create a small socket in the superior aspect of the clavicle; this socket ultimately allows the superior clavicle fixation device to sit flush within the bone, thus minimizing soft tissue irritation for the patient.

The central pin of the drill is removed, and a shuttling suture is passed through the drill cannula from the superior aspect of the clavicle and out the inferior aspect of the coracoid, and retrieved through the AIL portal. The cannula is removed and the shuttling suture is used to pass the double-loaded knotless CC fixation device (Knotless AC TightRope, Arthrex) from superior to inferior and out the AIL portal. A large cortical fixation button (DogBone, Arthrex) is secured to the fixation device; it is then passed through the AIL portal

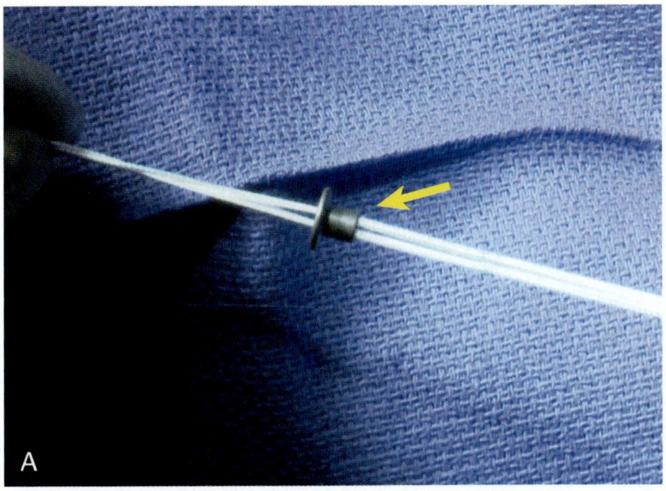

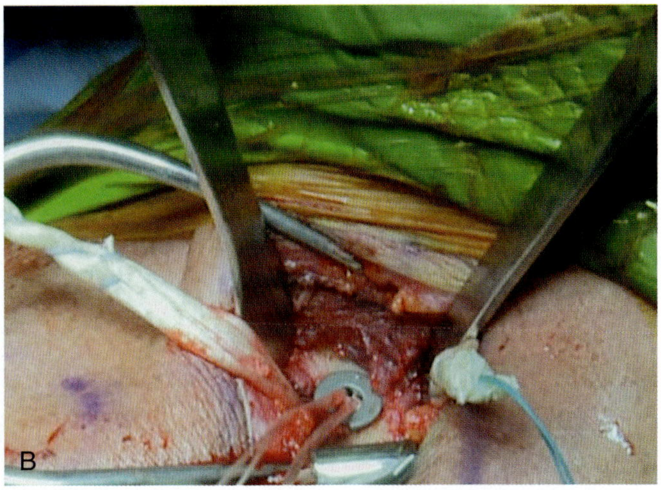

Fig. 12A.3 (**A**) The superior hardware of the knotless fixation device. (**B**) View of the superior knotless fixation device on the superior aspect of the clavicle; the ends of the tibialis anterior allograft have been successfully passed around the coracoid process.

while the knotless fixation device is tightened superiorly until the button sits flush on the inferior coracoid process. The knotless fixation is further tightened until the clavicle is reduced; intraoperative fluoroscopy is utilized at this point to confirm reduction. Also at this point, the suture ends may be cut or preserved for additional compression.

Allograft Coracoclavicular Ligament Reconstruction

Augmentation of the knotless CC fixation may be performed with an 8-mm double-diameter tibialis anterior or hamstring allograft. This is typically added in the patient who has a chronic acromioclavicular joint injury, in whom there is a lot of force on the reduction, or in whom there is considerable anteroposterior translation even after the CC ligaments have been reconstructed to reduce postoperative re-dislocations.

A switching stick is used to bluntly create two soft tissue tunnels from clavicle to coracoid. The first tunnel is created posterior to the clavicle and medial to the coracoid process under direct arthroscopic visualization; this recreates the anatomic orientation of the conoid ligament. A soft-tissue dilator (Arthrex) is placed over the switching stick, and the switching stick is removed. Subsequently, a rigid shuttling suture (Fiberstick, Arthrex) is passed through the dilator from superior to inferior and retrieved out the AIL portal. The process is repeated for the second tunnel, beginning anterior to the clavicle and exiting lateral to the coracoid process. This maneuver recreates the anatomic orientation of the trapezoid ligament. Next, the shuttling sutures are used to pass the allograft around both the clavicle and coracoid. The graft is first passed posterior to the clavicle, enters the subcoracoid space medial to the coracoid, and is retrieved out the AIL portal, thus re-creating the conoid ligament. With the second shuttling suture, the graft is next shuttled from inferior to superior; it is passed under the coracoid process and through the soft tissue lateral to the coracoid, and exits anterior to the clavicle (Fig. 12A.3), thus re-creating the trapezoid ligament.

At this point, both the graft and the CC fixation device are secured. The knotless CC fixation device can be retensioned, and an inferior force may be applied to the clavicle to ensure its reduction into anatomic position. The CC fixation device contains a self-locking mechanism, so no knots are required on the top of the clavicle; thus minimizing soft-tissue irritation for the patient. Next, the ends of the graft are placed over the superior aspect of the clavicle and secured with a simple overhand throw stitch using nonabsorbable sutures. The free ends of the graft are sharply cut. This completes the repair, and wound closure is performed to finish the surgery (Fig. 12A.4).

Postoperative Rehabilitation and Return to Sport

See Table 12A.1.

PRECAUTIONS

Precautions after AC joint reconstruction surgery include avoidance of passive and active traction to the shoulder girdle, of downward force on the repair for 6 weeks, and of heavy lifting or carrying for 12 weeks. Physical therapists and patients should avoid internal rotation behind the back and horizontal adduction for 8 weeks. AC joint mobilizations should not be performed for 8 weeks, and then only as indicated. Patients are not allowed to begin bench presses or full pushups until 12 weeks postoperatively.

PHASE I: PROTECTION

The patient is immobilized in a sling with abduction pillow for 4 to 6 weeks positioned in the scapular plane to unload the reconstructed AC joint. Full passive range of motion (PROM) of the glenohumeral joint is initiated postoperative day 1; it is not uncommon to restrict PROM forward elevation and abduction to 90 degrees for the first 2 postoperative weeks. The patient may also begin full active range of motion (AROM) of the cervical spine, elbow, wrist, and hand as well as neuromuscular re-education scapular exercises on postoperative day 1.

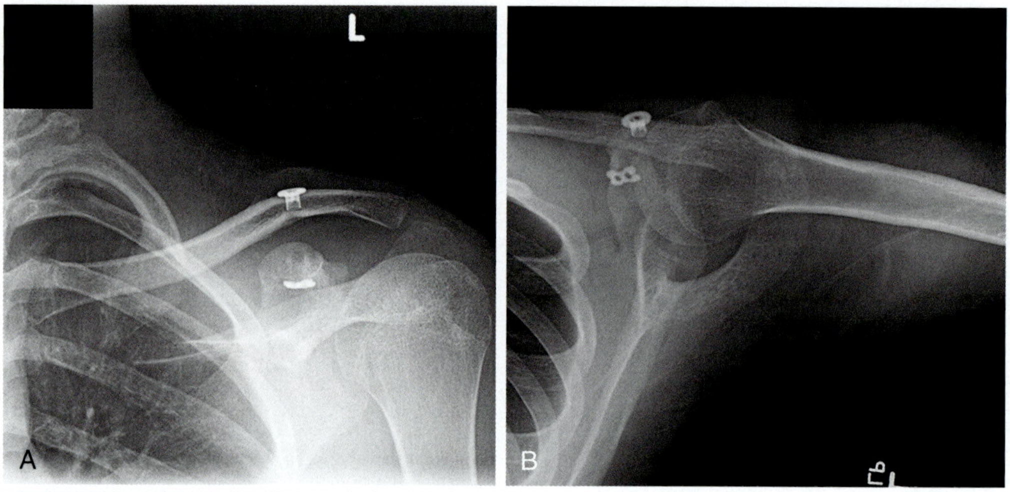

Fig. 12A.4 Postoperative radiography of previous Rockwood type V AC joint dislocation now fixed in anatomic position; **(A)** anteroposterior view, **(B)** axillary view.

Table 12A.1 Summary of Postoperative Rehabilitation Phases

Phase(s)	Approximate Time Postoperatively	Description
I: protection	First 4–6 weeks	Sling immobilization with abduction pillow Glenohumeral joint PROM
II: muscular endurance	Weeks 4–6 to weeks 8–10	Sling discontinued Glenohumeral joint AAROM and AROM
III: muscular strength	Weeks 8–10 to week 16	Week 8: resisted open kinetic chain exercise Week 10: resisted closed kinetic chain exercise Patient progresses to phase IV once strength has reached 90% of uninvolved upper extremity
IV and V: muscular power and return to sport	Weeks 16–20	Double and single arm plyometrics Sport-specific training initiated Once full restoration of strength and stability is achieved, patient returns to sport

AAROM, active assisted range of motion; *AROM,* active range of motion; *PROM,* passive range of motion.

PHASE II: MUSCULAR ENDURANCE

Active assisted range of motion (AAROM) and active range of motion (AROM) are initiated between 4 and 6 weeks postoperatively; PROM should be continued during this phase until full ROM is achieved. AAROM and AROM exercises focusing on the glenohumeral and scapulothoracic joint musculature are initiated with the patient in supine, prone, and sidelying positions in order to reduce load on the AC reconstruction. It is paramount to establish normal scapulohumeral rhythm throughout full AROM in all planes during this phase prior to progression to initial strengthening in phase III.

PHASE III: MUSCULAR STRENGTH

The rehabilitation goals of phase III consist of advancing muscular strength by means of resisted initial open and closed kinetic chain exercises, generally introduced at weeks 8 and 10, respectively. Introduced first are isotonic exercises to strengthen the rotator cuff and periscapular musculature (Figs. 12A.5 and 12A.6) using light band or dumbbell resistance with emphasis on controlled eccentric and concentric motion. Closed kinetic chain exercises are initiated in positions of low-load weight bearing through the upper extremities in a fixed position. Once scapular stability and strength of the involved upper extremity has improved to 90% of that of the uninvolved upper extremity in all planes, transition to phase IV is appropriate.

PHASE IV AND PHASE V: MUSCULAR POWER AND RETURN TO SPORT

The rehabilitation goals of phase IV consist of establishing muscular power to return to high-level occupations or athletics, generally introduced at week 16. Supervised throwing progressions and sport-specific training are also incorporated at this time. Patients are allowed to return to sport between 16 and 20 weeks postoperatively if they have achieved full restoration of strength and stability as assessed by functional testing and have received physician approval.

Outcomes

Surgical techniques for arthroscopic fixation of AC joint separations vary substantially, and so far, there is no gold standard of treatment. As recently as 2013, Beitzel et al (2013) identified 162 surgical techniques for AC joint reconstruction in a systematic review of the literature. The potential

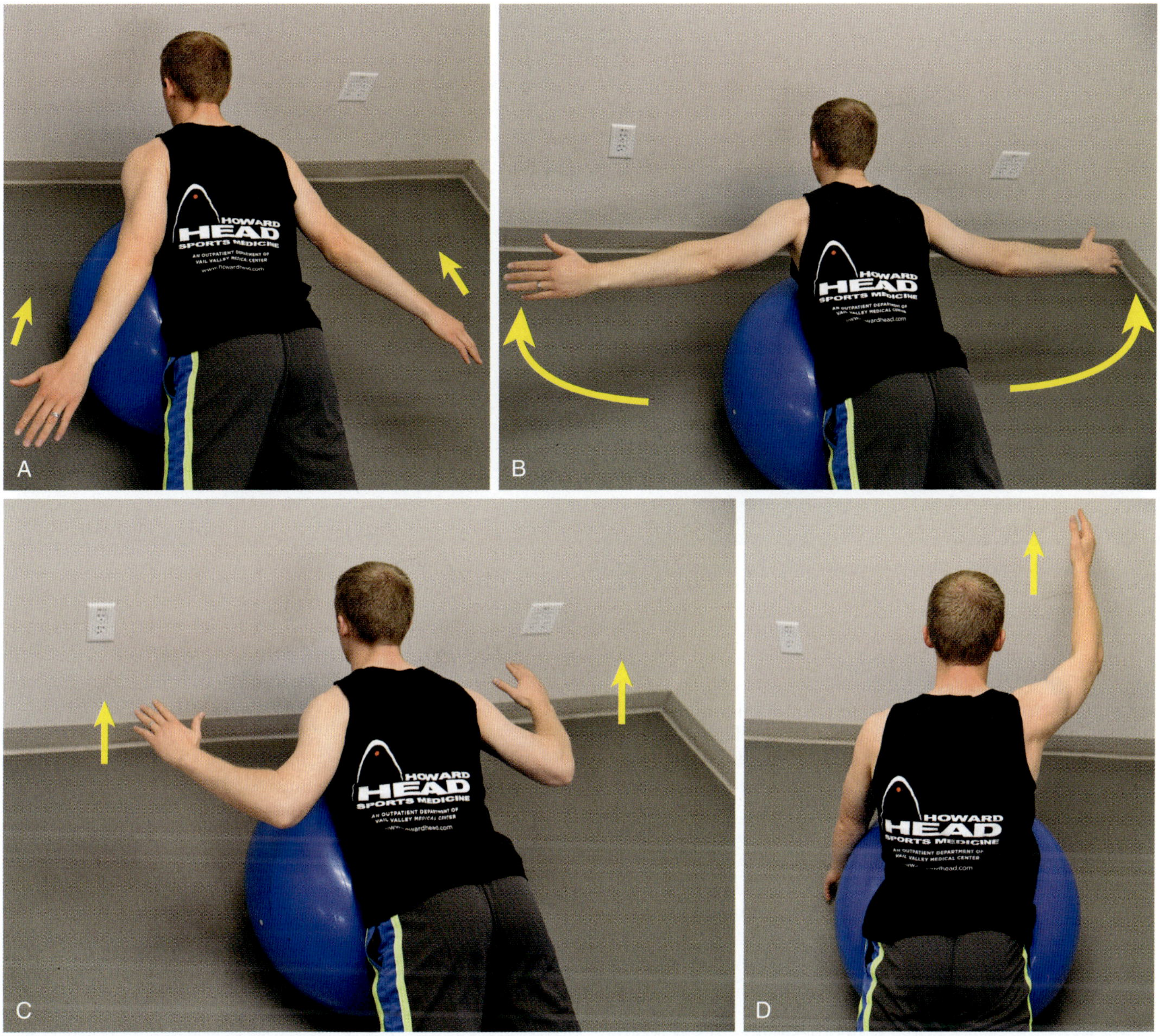

Fig. 12A.5 Scapular stabilization exercises on ball in kneeling or full plank position. Right shoulder is the operative side. (A) A: Middle and lower trapezius activation in conjunction with glenohumeral external rotation and extension. (B) T: Middle trapezius and rhomboid activation in conjunction with glenohumeral horizontal abduction. (C) W: Middle trapezius and rhomboid activation in conjunction with glenohumeral external rotation and horizontal abduction. (D) Single Arm Y: Lower trapezius and serratus anterior activation in conjunction with glenohumeral forward elevation.

advantages of arthroscopically assisted procedures include minimal invasiveness, better visualization, and ability to diagnose and treat concomitant glenohumeral pathologies that frequently occur with higher-grade AC injuries.

Thiel et al (2011) investigated outcomes for arthroscopic AC joint fixation with a knotted CC fixation device (AC TightRope, Arthrex). Twelve patients with Rockwood type IV or V injuries underwent surgical fixation, and final outcomes were obtained at approximately 2 years postoperatively. All patients had more than 110 degrees of total elevation and mean Simple Shoulder Test (SST) scores of 11 out of 12. Of the patients not lost to follow-up, all were satisfied and experienced no subjective functional deterioration. Radiographically, there were two failures of reduction and one loss of reduction (Thiel et al, 2011). Comparable results were found by Shin and Kim (2015), who also investigated clinical outcomes following arthroscopic AC joint fixation with a single knotted CC fixation device (AC TightRope, Arthrex). Eighteen patients were included with Rockwood type III, IV, and V injuries. Six patients experienced loss of reduction following surgery; however, Constant scores were not significantly different between patients with loss of reduction and those in whom reduction was maintained (95.6 vs. 98.4, respectively).

The previous studies demonstrate that as with other surgical techniques, it is not uncommon to see complications and loss of reduction following AC joint stabilization surgery. A systematic review performed by Woodmass et al (2015) found that loss of reduction occurs in 26.8% of patients who underwent arthroscopic fixation for AC joint

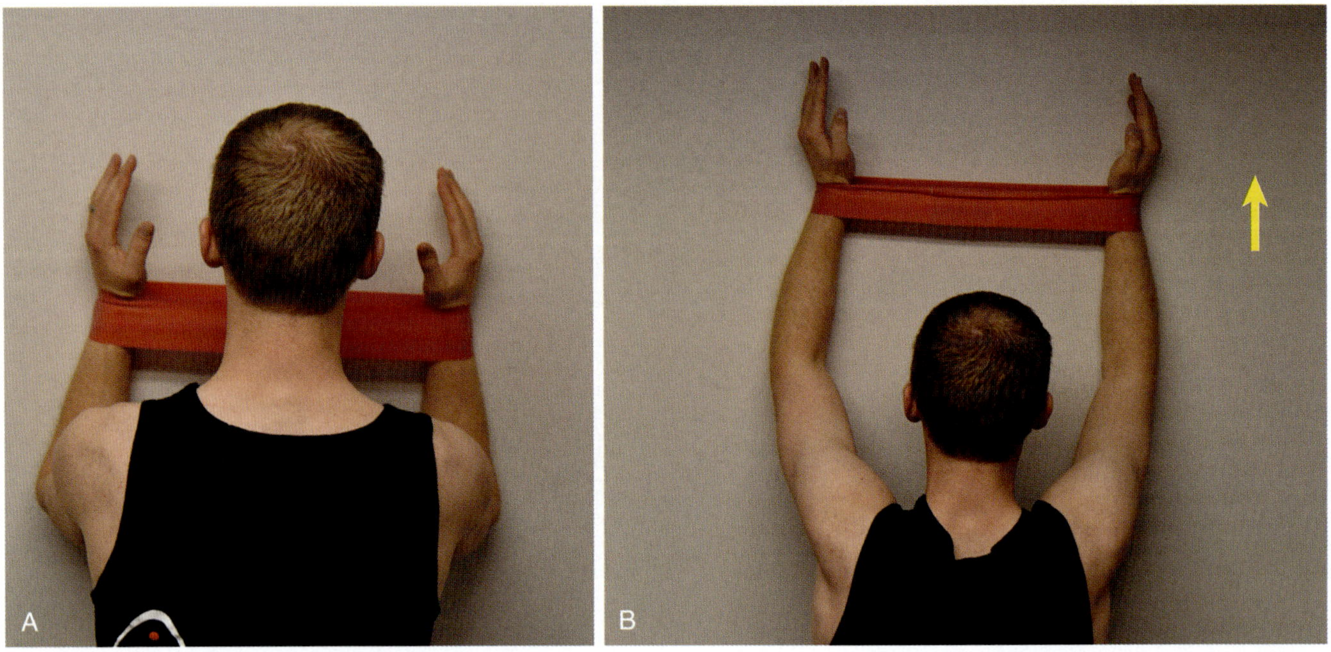

Fig. 12A.6 Forearm wallslide for serratus anterior. (**A**) Start position with resistance band at wrists to facilitate glenohumeral external rotation. (**B**) Slide arms up wall to facilitate combined activation of lower trapezius and serratus anterior to stabilize the scapula with glenohumeral forward elevation with external rotation.

injury. Clavert et al (2015) prospectively investigated outcomes for arthroscopic AC joint fixation with multiple techniques in 116 patients. They found an overall complication rate of 22.4%; the complications included loss of reduction, coracoid fracture, adhesive capsulitis, infection, and persistent pain. However, among patients who did not experience complications, good to excellent outcomes were reported (Constant score 91).

Given the frequency of loss of reduction with AC joint fixation, we believe that additional fixation can help reduce the risk of this complication. This is why our preferred surgical technique utilizes CC fixation along with tendon allograft augmentation; this technique was developed on the basis of outcome results at our own institution, where Millett et al (2015) reported 2-year outcomes following anatomic CC ligament reconstruction for AC joint dislocations in 31 patients. In this study, the arthroscopic surgical technique utilized a single knotted graft through two bone tunnels of the distal clavicle with no additional fixation. One-fifth of patients experienced complications including graft rupture, clavicle fracture, distal clavicle hypertrophy, and adhesive capsulitis. However, patients without complications experienced excellent postoperative outcomes with the following mean scores: American Shoulder and Elbow Surgeons (ASES) score 93.8, Single Assessment Numeric Evaluation (SANE) score 89.1, Quick Disabilities of Arm, Shoulder & Hand (QuickDASH) score 5.6, and patient satisfaction rating 9 out of 10.

References

Beitzel K, Cote MP, Apostolakos J, et al. Current concepts in the treatment of acromioclavicular joint dislocations. *Arthroscopy*. 2013;29(2):387–397.

Beitzel K, Mazzocca AD, Bak K, et al. ISAKOS upper extremity committee consensus statement on the need for diversification of the Rockwood classification for acromioclavicular joint injuries. *Arthroscopy*. 2014;30(2):271–272.

Clavert P, Meyer A, Boyer P, Gastaud O, Barth J, Duparc F. Complication rates and types of failure after arthroscopic acute acromioclavicular dislocation fixation: Prospective multicenter study of 116 cases. *Orthop Traumatol Surg Res*. 2015;101(suppl 8):S313–S316.

Martetschlager F, Horan MP, Warth RJ, Millett PJ. Complications after anatomic fixation and reconstruction of the coracoclavicular ligaments. *Am J Sports Med*. 2013;41(12):2896–2903.

Millett PJ, Horan MP, Warth RJ. Two-year outcomes after primary anatomic coracoclavicular ligament reconstruction. *Arthroscopy*. 2015;31(10):1962–1973.

Petri M, Warth RJ, Greenspoon JA, et al. Clinical results after conservative management for grade III acromioclavicular joint injuries: Does eventual surgery affect overall outcomes? *Arthroscopy*. 2016;32(5):740–746.

Shin S-J, Kim N-K. Complications after arthroscopic coracoclavicular reconstruction using a single adjustable–loop-length suspensory fixation device in acute acromioclavicular joint dislocation. *Arthroscopy*. 2015;31(5):816–824.

Thiel E, Mutnal A, Gilot GJ. Surgical outcome following arthroscopic fixation of acromioclavicular joint disruption with the tightrope device. *Orthopedics*. 2011;34(7):e267–e274.

Tischer T, Salzmann GM, El-Azab H, Vogt S, Imhoff AB. Incidence of associated injuries with acute acromioclavicular joint dislocations types III through V. *Am J Sports Med*. 2009;37(1):136–139.

Tossy JD, Mead NC, Sigmond HM. Acromioclavicular separations: Useful and practical classification for treatment. *Clin Orthop Relat.Res*. 1963;28:111–119.

Warth RJ, Martetschläger F, Gaskill TR, Millett PJ. Acromioclavicular joint separations. *Curr Rev Musculoskelet Med*. 2013;6(1):71–78.

Williams G, Nguyen V, Rockwood C. Classification and radiographic analysis of acromioclavicular dislocations. *Appl Radiol*. 1989;18:29–34.

Woodmass JM, Esposito JG, Ono Y, et al. Complications following arthroscopic fixation of acromioclavicular separations: A systematic review of the literature. *Open Access J Sports Med*. 2015;6:97–107.

12-12B SURGICAL TREATMENT: OPEN

TAYLOR WILEY, MD, FELIX DYRNA, MD, and AUGUSTUS D. MAZZOCCA, MS, MD

Introduction

Acromioclavicular (AC) joint injuries are encountered with great frequency in the practice of sports medicine. Although AC injuries encompass 9% of all shoulder injuries in the general population (Mazzocca et al, 2007), they are even more common in contact athletes, accounting for 40% of shoulder injuries in collegiate and professional football players (Thomas et al, 2011). AC injuries are not unique to football; they are the third most common injury in Division I college hockey (Flik et al, 2005). Epidemiologic studies estimate the incidence of complete dislocations (Rockwood types III–VI) at approximately 60,000 new cases yearly in the United States (Chillemi et al, 2013). In a study of a physically active United States Military Academy population, the vast majority (89%) of AC injuries sustained by cadets were low-grade (Rockwood type I or II) (Pallis et al, 2012). Males were twice as likely as females to sustain AC injuries, with male intercollegiate athletes being at the highest risk. With this prevalence in mind, it is important to understand the nonoperative (discussed elsewhere) and operative treatment options for AC injuries. This chapter reviews the operative indications, techniques, results, and complications of open operative management of AC injuries.

Indications for Surgery

Despite years of research on the subject, the optimal role of surgery in the treatment of AC joint injuries remains controversial. Surgery is clearly indicated for treatment of acute Rockwood type IV, V, and VI AC dislocations to prevent long-term shoulder pain and dysfunction (Bannister et al, 1989; Imatani et al, 1975; Larsen et al, 1986; Weinstein et al, 1995). Patients with persistent AC pain and instability after nonoperative treatment for type III AC injuries are indicated for surgical intervention as well. Significantly more debate exists regarding the treatment of acute type III injuries. The current trend is toward initial nonoperative management of type III injuries during season because many authors have obtained good to excellent results with this treatment approach (Bjerneld et al, 1983; Calvo et al, 2006; Hootman, 2004; Rolf et al, 2008; Schlegel et al, 2001; Spencer, 2007; Taft et al, 1987). However, up to 20% of patients with type III AC injuries treated nonoperatively have persistent pain and instability requiring delayed surgical treatment (Harris et al, 2000; Mouhsine et al, 2003). In addition, studies have shown improved clinical outcomes after early versus delayed reconstruction for type III dislocations (Ceccarelli et al, 2008; Dias et al, 1987; Millett et al, 2009; Rolf et al, 2008; Tamaoki et al, 2010). A more detailed addendum to the Rockwood classification suggested the separation of Rockwood grade III into grade IIIA and grade IIIB injuries regarding horizontal instability. Although grade IIIA injuries demonstrate horizontal instability, the posteriorly unstable grade IIIB injury demonstrates overriding of the clavicle on a cross-body adduction radiograph and would more likely result in a therapy-resistant scapular dysfunction (Beitzel et al, 2014). We recommend a patient-centered approach to type III injuries, in which the patient's occupation, hand dominance, job or sport requirements, and risk of reinjury are all considered. High-demand laborers and athletes (i.e., throwing, contact) should be considered for acute surgical intervention for Rockwood type III because of the risk of persistent pain and instability. Acute type III AC injuries in high-demand patients may be considered a relative indication for early operative intervention.

Goals of Surgery

Regardless of the technique, the main goal of treatment for AC injuries is to obtain a pain-free shoulder with unrestricted range of motion and full strength, without any limitations in activity. To obtain these goals, a set of crucial elements should be addressed during operative treatment of AC injuries: (1) correction of the superior displacement and anterior-to-posterior translation of the clavicle through anatomic reduction of the AC joint, (2) maintenance of AC joint stability during acute healing by supplementation of the coracoclavicular (CC) ligament reconstruction with a synthetic material or rigid implant or reconstructing the CC ligaments in a chronic case, and (3) meticulous deltotrapezial fascia closure.

Historical Perspective on Open Treatment Options

Since the first operative treatment for an AC joint injury was reported by Cooper in 1861, well over 150 different operative techniques for AC joint injuries have been described (Beitzel et al, 2013; Cooper, 1861; Rockwood, 1984). The vast number of procedures can be broken down broadly into three general categories: primary AC fixation, coracoclavicular fixation, and anatomic or nonanatomic ligament reconstruction. The first surgical approaches used Steinmann pins or K-wires to reduce the AC joint. These constructs resulted in a high failure rate of the stiff construct because of hardware failure or migration. This was followed by a time of distal clavicle resection as a treatment option, which did not result in improving the patient's outcome and satisfaction because pain caused by residual instability remained. Although a multitude of surgeries have been described, the modified Weaver-Dunn procedure has been the most popular technique until recently. In 1972, Weaver and Dunn first described open treatment of acute and chronic AC injuries using transfer of the coracoacromial ligament from the acromion to the clavicle (Weaver & Dunn, 1972). Their technique was modified to allow for distal clavicle resection

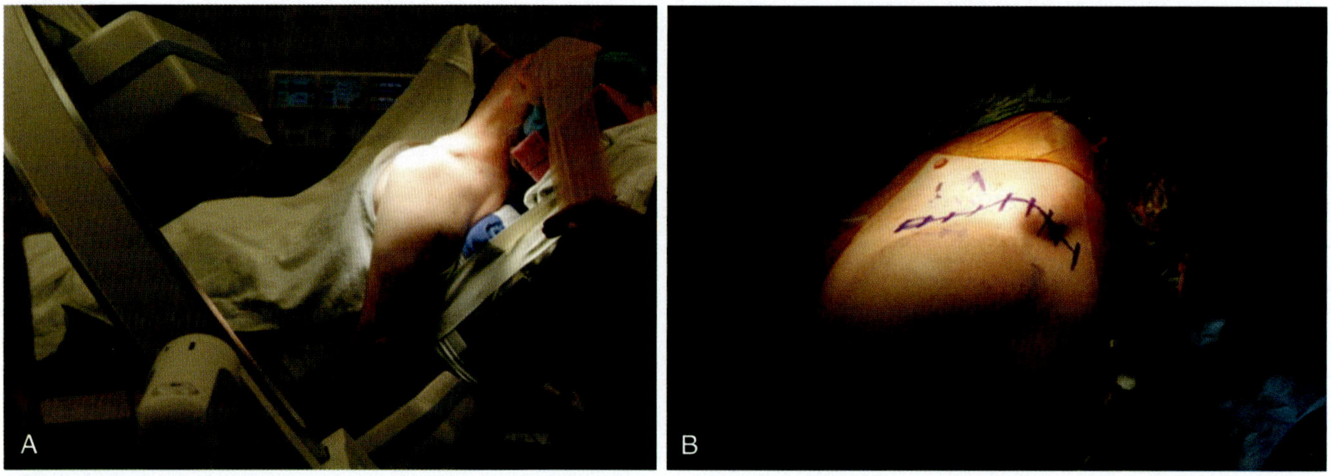

Fig. 12B.1 Patient positioned in a beach-chair position with additional scapular support, the head is turned medial to improve clavicle tunnel drilling. Surgical approach and anatomical landmarks are marked.

to prevent symptomatic arthrosis at the AC joint and later by the addition of coracoclavicular fixation (Neer, 1990; Sloan et al, 2004; Williams et al, 1989). A major challenge facing this operation has been maintenance of reduction, and this is likely secondary to the transferred CA ligament lacking the strength of the native CC ligaments and inadequately reproducing their normal anatomy. This deficiency led to the development of the anatomic coracoclavicular reconstruction (ACCR), which aims to recreate the anatomy of the coracoclavicular ligaments while using stronger graft materials (Carofino & Mazzocca, 2010).

Senior Author's Preferred Technique: Anatomic Coracoclavicular Reconstruction

ANATOMY AND BIOMECHANICS

The primary static stabilizers of the AC joint include the AC ligaments and coracoclavicular ligaments. The AC ligaments are the primary restraints to horizontal instability of the distal clavicle, with the superior ligament providing 56% of the resistance to posterior translation and the posterior ligament contributing 25%. The coracoclavicular ligaments are the primary restraint to vertical instability, with the conoid ligament specifically providing 60% of the resistance to superior translation of the clavicle (Fukuda et al, 1986). The trapezoid and conoid ligaments both originate posterior to the pectoralis minor insertion on the coracoid and traverse the coracoclavicular interspace. The conoid inserts onto the posteroinferior clavicle approximately 46 mm medial to the AC joint. The trapezoid inserts 26 mm medially to the AC joint and more centrally in the anteroposterior dimension (Rios et al, 2007).

The author's preferred technique for treatment of operative AC joint injuries is the ACCR. This surgical technique attempts to reconstruct the appropriate anatomy and biomechanics of the AC joint and coracoclavicular space, with the goal of restoring both vertical and horizontal stability to the AC joint. In the ACCR, the conoid and trapezoid ligaments are reconstructed using autograft or allograft tendon tissue, with reconstruction of the AC joint capsular ligaments. Fixation of the graft to the clavicle is performed using interference screws, but fixation of the graft to the coracoid can be performed one of two ways. The tendon graft may be passed around the coracoid base with the loop technique, or it may be fixed to the coracoid with an interference screw in the tenodesis technique. The tendon graft is supplemented with nonbiologic fixation in the form of high-strength nonabsorbable suture (no. 2 FiberWire, Arthrex). The biomechanical advantage of the anatomic coracoclavicular ligament reconstruction has been demonstrated in multiple studies. Thomas et al (2011) found that anatomic CC reconstruction with allograft had a significantly higher load to failure than modified Weaver-Dunn, anatomic suture, nonanatomic allograft, and GraftRope techniques. Although the ACCR can be performed via an arthroscopic approach (Warth et al, 2014), the open approach using a loop technique is the author's preference and will be described here.

POSITIONING

The importance of proper patient positioning should not be overlooked because it is a crucial step in this surgery. The patient is placed in the beach-chair position, with the torso and operative extremity brought to the edge of the surgical table (Fig. 12B.1). A small radiolucent bump placed at the medial border of the scapula will serve to stabilize the scapula and elevate the coracoid anteriorly. The patient's head should be secured in the beach-chair position, but it should not be firmly taped to the table as repositioning of the head is occasionally necessary during drilling of the medial clavicular bone tunnel. Before prepping and draping, the mini-C-arm should be trialed to ensure appropriate biplanar fluoroscopic imaging of the clavicle can be obtained. The operative arm is draped free to allow for easy maneuverability and reduction of the AC joint.

SURGICAL EXPOSURE

Beginning laterally at the posterior clavicle and gently angling toward the coracoid process, a curvilinear

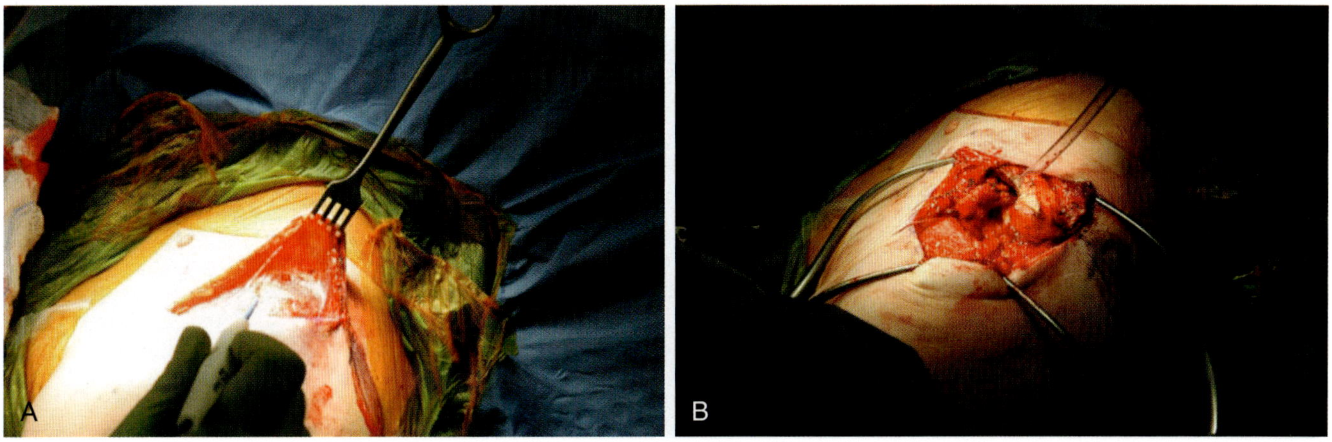

Fig. 12B.2 After curvilinear skin incision is made, full-thickness cutaneous flaps are elevated to expose the underlying deltotrapezial fascia. Deltotrapezial fascioperiosteal flaps are then elevated posteriorly and anteriorly from the midline of the clavicle to circumferentially expose the lateral end of the clavicle and the acromioclavicular joint laterally. Tagging sutures are placed during the approach to allow for retraction during dissection and effective soft tissue coverage over the repair upon closure.

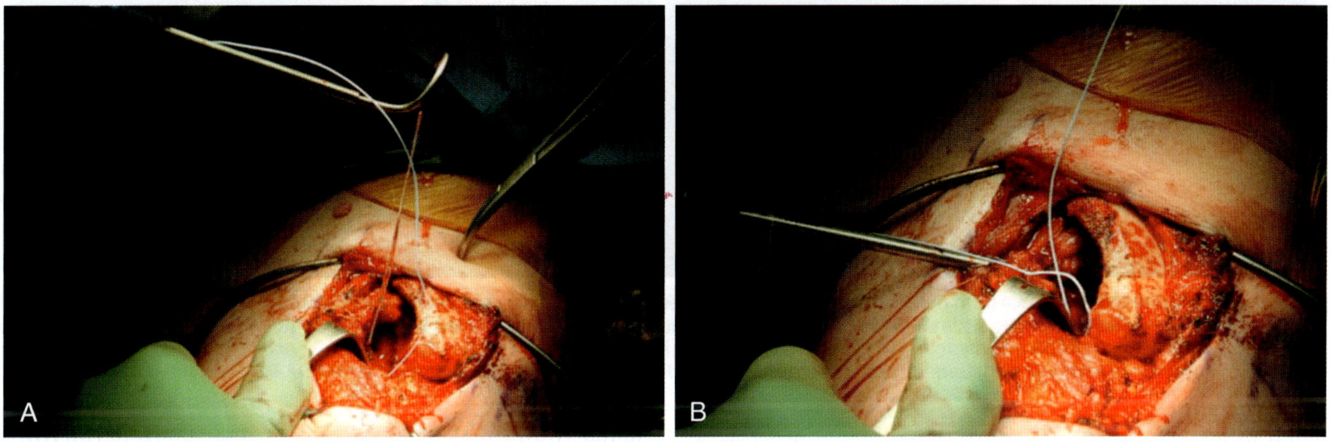

Fig. 12B.3 The coracoid process is first exposed with soft tissue dissection, with clear delineation of its medial and lateral margins. Loop the graft around the base of the coracoid with a Stanitsky aortic cross-clamp, or alternatively, a suture-passing device. The graft should be passed in a medial to lateral direction around the base of the coracoid process. A suture is fed around the base of the coracoid, and a loop is created at one of its free ends. The suture loop is then used to shuttle the tendon graft, along with a supplemental collagen coated no. 2 FiberWire suture, around the base of the coracoid.

skin incision is made along the Langer lines and centered approximately 3 cm medial to the AC joint. Full-thickness cutaneous flaps are elevated to expose the underlying deltotrapezial fascia (Fig. 12B.2). The raphe between the clavicular attachments of the deltoid and trapezius provides a relatively avascular plane for dissection. Deltotrapezial fascioperiosteal flaps are then elevated posteriorly and anteriorly from the midline of the clavicle to circumferentially expose the lateral end of the clavicle and the AC joint laterally. It is important to elevate the entirety of the deltoid origin circumferential from the clavicle, including the inferior aspect, to allow for a full-thickness robust repair at the time of wound closure. Tagging sutures may be placed during the approach to allow for retraction during dissection and effective soft tissue coverage over the repair upon closure.

GRAFT SELECTION AND PREPARATION

An allograft (typically peroneus longus) or autograft (typically semitendinosus or gracilis) tendon can be used for this procedure. A standard tendon sizer is used to size the tendon, which is usually 5 mm in size. The graft size determines the size of the drill holes. The tendon graft should be prepared with as much length as possible to allow for later reconstruction of the AC capsule–ligament complex. The free tendon ends are then bulleted, and a whip stitch is placed to allow for a tight passage through the bone tunnels.

CORACOID PREPARATION

As mentioned earlier, the tendon graft can be secured to the coracoid by either looping the graft around the base of the coracoid (loop technique) or by a tenodesis technique with the graft secured to the base of the coracoid with an interference screw. The loop technique is described here because it is our preferred technique. The coracoid process is first exposed with soft tissue dissection, with clear delineation of its medial and lateral margins (Fig. 12B.3). Importantly, the surgeon should not dissect too far into the posterior direction on the coracoid base because the suprascapular nerve is in close relationship. A Stanitsky aortic cross-clamp, or alternatively, a suture-passing device, is then passed in a

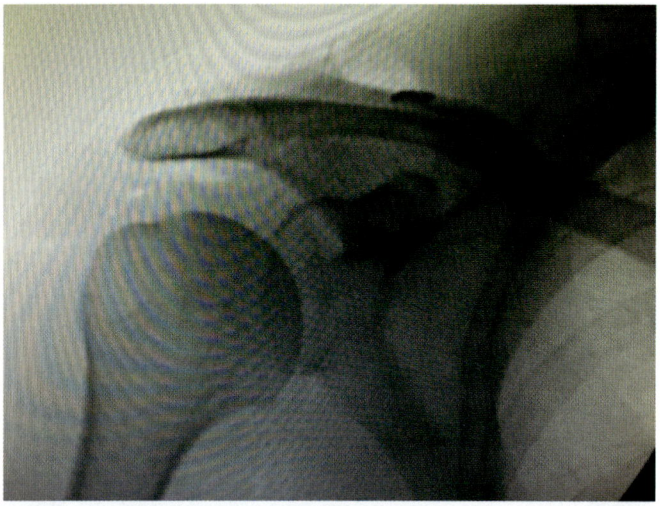

Fig. 12C.8 Postoperative radiograph after repair of a displaced AC separation utilizing a suture button construct.

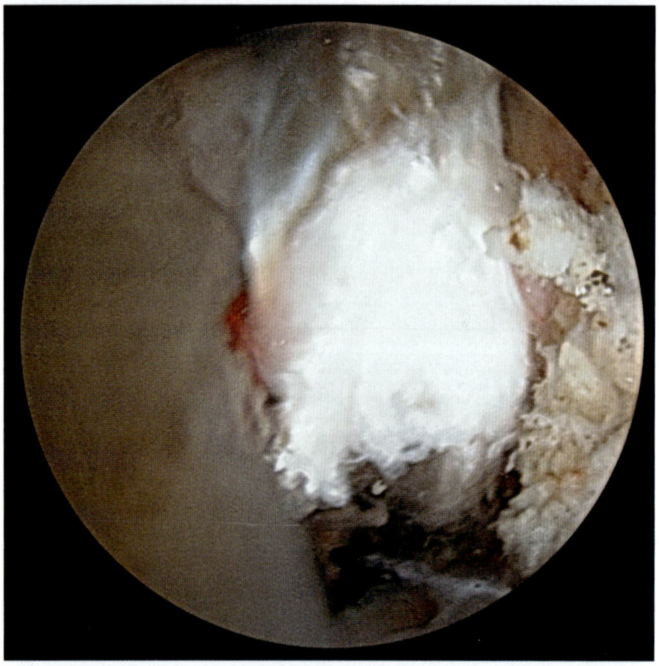

Fig. 12C.9 Arthroscopic view of a tendon allograft passed around the coracoid using an arthroscopic technique.

More research is required to determine the long-term survivorship of suture-only constructs, and clinical comparisons with anatomic reconstruction in the acute setting are also needed. One report has demonstrated a 33% rate of loss of reduction at 3 months for an arthroscopically assisted single-tunnel technique (Shin & Kim, 2015).

Arthroscopically assisted fixation has also been utilized in the treatment of chronic injuries, aiding in the surgeon's visualization and passage of the graft under or through the coracoid and clavicle and avoiding the larger incision associated with traditional open techniques (Baumgarten et al, 2006; Frank & Trenhaile, 2015) (Figs. 12C.9 and 12C.10). This approach may result in less iatrogenic injury to the deltotrapezial fascia, faster recovery, and less pain. Additionally, arthroscopy gives the surgeon the opportunity to treat

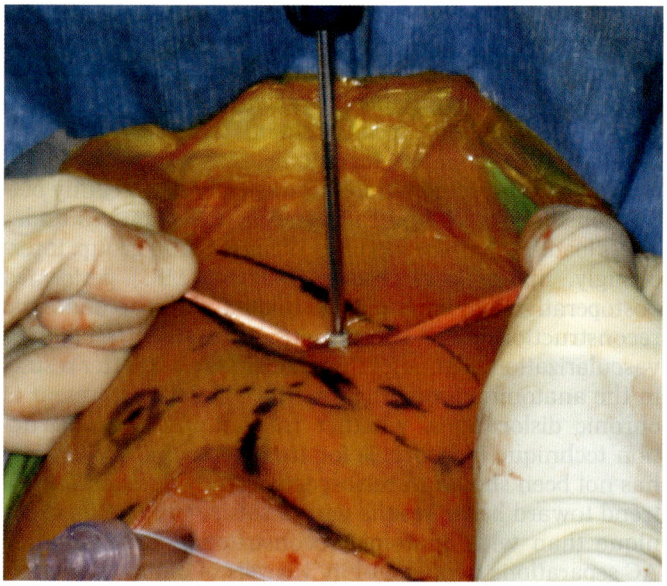

Fig. 12C.10 After a graft is passed subcoracoid, it can be secured through drill holes in the clavicle, as seen here. Others prefer to tie the graft itself around the clavicle.

concomitant injuries, which have been documented to be up to 30% in high-grade AC injuries (Pauly et al, 2013).

Conclusion

The treatment of AC injuries continues to evolve. Many surgical techniques for treating high-grade dislocations have been described. Newer techniques aim to reconstruct the CC ligaments anatomically in order to provide biologic healing without the complications associated with retained hardware. Arthroscopically assisted techniques continue to develop, particularly in the treatment of acute injuries. At this time, no gold standard treatment exists, and outcomes remain conflicted despite advancements in techniques.

References

Adamson G, Freedman JA, Lee TQ. Free tissue graft reconstruction of the acromioclavicular joint: a new technique. *Techn Shoulder Elbow Surg.* 2008;9:193–198.

Baumgarten KM, Altchek DW, Cordasco FA. Arthroscopically assisted acromioclavicular joint reconstruction. *Arthroscopy.* 2006;22:228.e1–228.e6.

Beitzel K, Obopilwe E, Chowaniec DM, et al. Biomechanical comparison of arthroscopic repairs for acromioclavicular joint instability: Suture button systems without biological augmentation. *Am J Sports Med.* 2011;39:2218–2225.

Bloom FA. Wire fixation in acromioclavicular dislocation. *J Bone Joint Surg.* 1945;27:273–276.

Bosworth BM. Acromioclavicular separation: New method of repair. *Surg Gynecol Obstet.* 1941;73:866–871.

Bundens WD, Cook JI. Repair of acromioclavicular separations by deltoid-trapezius imbrication. *Clin Orthop.* 1961;20:109–115.

Cadenat FM. The treatment of dislocations and fractures of the outer end of the clavicle. *Int Clin.* 1917:146–149.

Calvo E, Lopez-Franco M, Arribas IM. Clinical and radiologic outcomes of surgical and conservative treatment of type III acromioclavicular injury. *J Shoulder Elbow Surg.* 2006;15:300–305.

Cave, 1958.

Ceccarelli, 2008.

Cook, 1988.

Cooper ES. New method of treating long standing dislocations of the scapuloclavicular articulation. *Am J Med Sci*. 1861;41:389–392.
Cote, 2010.
Cox, 1981.
Debski RE, Parsons IM, Woo SLY, Fu FH. Effect of capsular injury on acromioclavicular joint mechanics. *J Bone Joint Surg*. 2001;83:1344–1351.
Deshmukh AV, Wilson DR, Zilberfarb JL, Perlmutter GS. Stability of acromioclavicular joint reconstruction: Biomechanical testing of various surgical techniques in a cadaveric model. *Am J Sports Med*. 2004;32:1492–1498.
Dias, 1987.
Dragoo, 2012.
Eskola, 1996.
Flatow, 1995.
Frank RM, Trenhaile SW. Arthroscopic-assisted acromioclavicular joint reconstruction using the TightRope device with allograft augmentation: Surgical technique. *Arthrosc Tech*. 2015;6:e293–e297.
Fukuda K, Craig EV, An KN, Cofield RH, Chao EYS. Biomechanical study of the ligamentous system of the acromioclavicular joint. *J Bone Joint Surg*. 1986;68-A:434–440.
Galatz, 2010.
Galpin RD. A comparative analysis of operative versus nonoperative treatment of grade III acromioclavicular separations. *Clin Orthop Rel Res*. 1985;193:150–155.
Gladstone, 1997.
Gonzalez-Lomas G, Javidan P, Lin T, Limpisvasti O, Lee TQ. Intramedullary acromioclavicular ligament reconstruction strengthens isolated coracoclavicular ligament reconstructions in acromioclavicular dislocations. *Am J Sports Med*. 2010;38:2113–2122.
Guy DK, Wirth MA, Griffin JL, Rockwood CA. Reconstruction of chronic and complete dislocations of the acromioclavicular joint. *Clin Orthop Relat Res*. 1998;347:138–149.
Habernek H, Weinstabl R, Schmid L, Fialka CA. Crook plate for treatment of acromioclavicular joint separation: Indication, technique, and results after one year. *J Trauma*. 1993;35:893–901.
Harris RI, Wallace AL, Harper GD, Goldberg JA, Sonnabend DH, Walsh WR. Structural properties of the intact and the reconstructed coracoclavicular ligament complex. *Am J Sports Med*. 2000;28:103–108.
Jari R, Costic RS, Rodosky MW, Debski RE. Biomechanical function of surgical procedures for acromioclavicular joint dislocations. *Arthroscopy*. 2004;20:237–245.
Klimkiewicz JJ, Williams GR, Sher JS, Karduna A, DesJardins JD, Iannotti JP. The acromioclavicular capsule as a restraint to posterior translation of the clavicle: A biomechanical analysis. *J Shoulder Elbow Surg*. 1999;8:119–124.
Lee KW, Debski RE, Chen C, Woo SL, Fuh SH. Functional evaluation of the ligaments at the acromioclavicular joint during anteroposterior and superoinferior translation. *Am J Sports Med*. 1997;25:858–862.
Lee SJ, Nicholas SJ, Akizuki KH, McHugh MP, Kremenic IJ, Ben-Avi S. Reconstruction of the coracoclavicular ligaments with tendon grafts: A comparative biomechanical study. *Am J Sports Med*. 2003;31:648–655.
Lindsey R, Gutowski W. The migration of a broken pin following fixation of the acromioclavicular joint: A case report and review of the literature. *Orthopedics*. 1986;9:413–416.
Lizaur A, Marco L, Cebrian R. Acute dislocation of the acromioclavicular joint: Traumatic anatomy and the importance of deltoid and trapezius. *J Bone Joint Surg*. 1986;68A:552–555.
Lowe GP, Fogarty MJ. Acute acromioclavicular joint dislocation: Results of operative treatment with the Bosworth screw. *Aus N Z J Surg*. 1977;47:664–667.
Martetschlager F, Horan MP, Warth RJ, Millett PJ. Complications after anatomic fixation and reconstruction of the coracoclavicular ligaments. *Am J Sports Med*. 2013;41:2896–2903.
Mazet R. Migration of a Kirschner wire from the shoulder region into the lung: Report of two cases. *J Bone Joint Surg*. 1943;25:477–483.
Mazzocca AD, Conway JE, Johnson S, et al. The anatomic coracoclavicular ligament reconstruction. *Op Tech Sports Med*. 2004;12:56–61.
Mazzocca AD, Santangelo SA, Johnson ST, Rios CG, Dumonski ML, Arciero RA. A biomechanical evaluation of an anatomical coracoclavicular ligament reconstruction. *Am J Sports Med*. 2006;34:236–246.
McFarland EG, Blivin SJ, Doehring CB, Curl LA, Silberstein C. Treatment of grade III acromioclavicular joint separations in professional throwing athletes: Results of a survey. *Am J Orthop*. 1997;26:771–774.
Milewski MD, Tompkins M, Giugale JM, Carson EW, Miller MD, Diduch DR. Complications related to anatomic reconstruction of the coracoclavicular ligaments. *Am J Sports Med*. 2012;40:1628–1634.
Motamedi AR, Blevins FT, Willis MC, et al. Biomechanics of the coracoclavicular ligament complex and augmentations used in its repair and reconstruction. *Am J Sports Med*. 2000:28:380–384.
Moushine, 2003.
Mumford, 1941.
Nicholas SJ, Lee SJ, Mullaney MJ, Tyler TF, McHugh MP. Clinical outcomes of coracoclavicular ligament reconstructions using tendon grafts. *Am J Sports Med*. 2007;35:1912–1917.
Norrell H, Llewellyn R. Migration of a threaded Steinmann pin from an acromioclavicular joint into the spinal canal: A case report. *J Bone Joint Surg Am*. 1965;47:1024–1026.
Pauly S, Kraus N, Greiner S, Scheibel M. Prevalence and pattern of glenohumeral injuries. *J Shoulder Elbow Surg*. 2013;22:760–766.
Rockwood, 1998.
Rokito AS, Oh YH, Zuckerman JD. Modified Weaver-Dunn procedure for acromioclavicular joint dislocations. *Orthopedics*. 2004;27:21–28.
Scheibel M, Droschel S, Gerhardt C, Kraus N. Arthroscopically assisted stabilization of acute high-grade acromioclavicular joint separations. *Am J Sports Med*. 2011;39:1507–1516.
Schlegel, 2001.
Shin SJ, Kim NK. Complications after arthroscopic coracoclavicular reconstruction using a single adjustable-loop-length suspensory fixation device in acute acromioclavicular joint dislocation. *Arthroscopy*. 2015;31:816–824.
Smith, 2011.
Spencer, 2007.
Tauber M, Gordon K, Koller H, et al. Semitendinosus tendon graft versus a modified Weaver-Dunn procedure for acromioclavicular joint reconstruction in chronic cases. *Am J Sports Med*. 2009;37:181–190.
Tibone, 1992.
Tienen TG, Oyen JF, Eggen P. A modified technique of reconstruction for complete acromioclavicular dislocation: A prospective study. *Am J Sports Med*. 2003;31:655–659.
Trainer, 2008.
Tsou PM. Percutaneous cannulated screw coracoclavicular fixation for acute acromioclavicular dislocations. *Clin Orthop Rel Res*. 1989;243:112–121.
Venjakob AJ, Salzmann GM, Gabel F, et al. Arthroscopically assisted 2-bundle anatomic reduction of acute acromioclavicular joint separations. *Am J Sports Med*. 2013;41:615–621.
Walz L, Salzmann GM, Fabbro T, Eichhorn S, Imhoff AB. The anatomic reconstruction of acromioclavicular joint dislocations using 2 TightRope devices: A biomechanical study. *Am J Sports Med*. 2008;36:2398–2406.
Weaver JK, Dunn HK. Treatment of acromioclavicular injuries, especially complete acromioclavicular separation. *J Bone Joint Surg Am*. 1972;54:1187–1194.
Weinstein DM, McCann PD, McIlveen SJ, Flatow EL, Bigliani LU. Surgical treatment of complete acromioclavicular dislocations. *Am J Sports Med*. 1995;23:324–331.
Williams et al, 1989.

12-12D POSTOPERATIVE REHABILITATION AND RETURN TO SPORT

HELEN BRADLEY, PT, BROOKE M. DELVECCHIO, PT, and PAUL E. WESTGARD, PT

Introduction

- There is no gold standard treatment protocol for the management of acromioclavicular (AC) joint injuries with regard to the surgical technique performed or the rehabilitation method used. This chapter considers an array of factors that should be considered when rehabilitating an after post AC reconstruction and returning them to peak sport performance.
- Clinicians need to have knowledge of anatomy and kinematics of the shoulder complex, tissue healing, exercise physiology, and kinetic chain concepts to optimize rehabilitation guidelines. Good communication between the physical therapist, patient-athlete, surgeon, coaches, and trainers is essential and helps to direct the course of rehabilitation. A rehabilitation guideline has been developed to aid in decision making.
- Criteria to progress through each phase of rehabilitation are proposed, which are focused on uniting time- and performance-based principles. This offers functional goals to accomplish before progressing to the next phase of rehabilitation and allows the patient to achieve a strong foundation in mobility, endurance, and strength before returning to sport performance.

Acromioclavicular (AC) joint injuries are common in the athletic population and account for 40% to 50% of all shoulder injuries seen in sports. An incidence of 9.2 injuries per 1000 person-years in young athletes has been reported (Pallis et al, 2012). AC joint separations usually occur after a direct blow to the acromion with the shoulder in an adducted position. Athletes, particularly those involved in contact sports as well as skiing and cycling, are at an increased risk of injury (Willimon et al, 2011).

The AC joint links the shoulder girdle to the axial skeleton. It subsequently coordinates normal movement of the glenohumeral, scapulothoracic, and sternoclavicular joints (Reid et al, 2012). Typically, with injury, the AC capsuloligamentous structures are disrupted initially followed by the coracoclavicular (CC) ligaments and the deltotrapezial fascia if there is sufficient force (Simovitch et al, 2009). AC joint separations are graded according to severity from grade I being a mild sprain to grade VI, which is severe dislocation with displacement. Nonsurgical management has typically been the gold standard for grade I to II AC joint injuries, classified by Rockwood (Rockwood, 1984), and surgical intervention has been indicated for grades IV to VI.

Grade III Acromioclavicular Joint Injuries

Controversy exists surrounding the best treatment option for grade III injuries, with valid arguments for both nonsurgical and surgical management. Often a period of conservative care involving physical therapy has been advocated to maximize functional recovery with reevaluation of symptoms at 6 to 12 weeks after injury. If continued disability and pain exist at this time, surgery has been promoted as the best plan of care. Conversely, a few studies have promoted early surgical management of grade III AC joint injuries to significantly improve outcomes when compared with individuals who underwent surgical treatment more than 3 months after injury (Rolf et al, 2007; Weinstein et al, 1995). This may also reduce complications after conservative care such as strength deficits; scapula dyskinesis; osteoarthritis of the AC joint; distal clavicle osteolysis; and failure to return to optimal function, including reduced sporting performance (Reid et al, 2012). For these reasons, early surgical intervention is occasionally considered for individuals at greater risk for functional disability, including high-level athletes (Warth et al, 2013). Management of AC joint injuries should be directed by severity of injury and symptoms, with consideration of individual needs and goals (Willimon et al, 2011).

Surgical Techniques

There is no gold standard technique for treating AC joint separation. Various types of surgical procedures have been described. The four main procedures include primary repair of AC joint with pins, screws, or rods; distal clavicle excision with soft tissue reconstruction (Weaver-Dunn method); anatomic coracoclavicular reconstruction (ACCR); and arthroscopic suture fixation. Some surgeons promote a combination of these techniques (Bontempo & Mazzocca, 2010). Many of these surgical fixation methods have been marred by technical shortcomings such as fixation failure, pin migration, nonunion, nerve injury, and in many cases the need for a second surgery to remove fixating hardware.

Recently, biomechanical and clinical studies have supported ACCR which typically includes the use of tendon grafts and cortical fixation to reconstruct the anatomy of the CC ligament. Anatomic restoration of the CC ligament improves joint kinematics and increases the ultimate failure load, making it a more robust reconstruction (Mazzocca et al, 2006).

Guidelines for Rehabilitation After Acromioclavicular Joint Reconstruction

The primary goal of a rehabilitation program is to return the athlete to full activities as quickly and safely as possible. However, postoperative rehabilitation needs to be tailored to the individual according to a criteria and functional based progression with consideration of tissue healing time frames and in conjunction with the referring physician.

Healing phases include the inflammatory phase, proliferation (repair) phase, and remodeling phase. The overall aim of rehabilitation is centered on the principle of gradual application of controlled stresses with consideration of the healing phases (Thigpin et al, 2016). Because of the vast array of surgical approaches and a lack of consensus for optimum surgical technique to treat AC joint injuries, there is limited research discussing rehabilitation after AC joint injury (Gladstone, 1997; Kibler & McCullen, 2003; Reid et al, 2012) or reconstruction (Cote et al, 2010; Culp & Romani, 2006) and no literature to support the efficacy of a specific rehabilitation protocol. Best practice requires that clinicians have a working knowledge of the healing continuum, kinetic chain concepts, exercise physiology, and anatomy and kinematics of the shoulder complex and are able to adapt treatment strategies accordingly to achieve an optimal outcome (Reid et al, 2012). Following a protocol that involves only time-based progressions lacks individuality and the need for clinical judgment. Time- and performance-based criteria need to be united. Current literature and professional opinion have been merged to inform the development of the suggested guidelines for rehabilitation after AC Joint Reconstruction (ACJR) (Table 12D.1) (Cote et al, 2010; Ellenbecker & Cools, 2010; Gladstone et al, 1997; Johnson et al, 2011; Kibler et al, 2013; Reid et al, 2012). This should provide clinicians who treat these injuries with the best evidence to enhance rehabilitation following surgical reconstruction.

Precautions After Acromioclavicular Joint Reconstruction

It is advised not to perform internal rotation behind the back and horizontal adduction movement to avoid stress on the AC joint for approximately 8 weeks. Thereafter it should be approached cautiously and within the patient's pain threshold (Reid et al, 2012). Heavy lifting or any other activity that would result in significant downward traction on the upper extremity is avoided for 3 months after surgery (Dimakopoulos & Panagopopulos, 2007). Bench presses and push-ups are also not advised until 3 months after surgery to avoid excessive loading of the AC joint.

Phase I: Protection Phase

The goals of this phase are to protect the surgical reconstruction, optimize the environment for tissue healing, decrease pain and inflammation, restore passive mobility to minimize stiffness, and initiate scapula or core activation exercises. These goals must be addressed without causing inappropriate stress to the AC joint.

The therapist should educate the patient on the rationale of the outlined rehabilitation protocol to ensure compliance and review a home exercise program involving active hand, wrist, and elbow range of motion (ROM). To reduce strain on the reconstruction, the arm is immobilized for 4 to 6 weeks in an abduction sling. The sling helps to elevate the proximal humerus and acromion, preventing additional stress on the reconstructed ligaments (Millett et al, 2009). Cryotherapy and other modalities to aid with pain relief, decrease swelling and muscle spasm, and minimize the inflammatory response are also advocated as needed. Normal active scapula movement (protraction, retraction, elevation, and depression) should be encouraged to facilitate early neuromuscular control of the scapula. The sidelying scapular clock exercise is a great starting point for this with progression to sitting or standing with the sling on. Isometric exercises of the muscles surrounding the shoulder girdle can also be initiated during this phase. These should be submaximal and nonpainful with the shoulder in a neutral position. Rhythmic stabilization, involving gentle manual resistance to the proximal forearm using oscillating perturbation in a neutral shoulder position, is appropriate to facilitate low contraction of the scapular and rotator cuff musculature and can be beneficial for early neuromuscular reeducation.

Addressing the kinetic chain early in rehabilitation will benefit the athlete for the long term; therefore, breathing and basic core exercises should be incorporated at this stage of rehabilitation. Core exercises in a hook-lying position with focus on lower extremity movement will ensure the surgical reconstruction is safe and not stressed. Using a stationary recumbent bike should be encouraged for the athlete to maintain cardiovascular conditioning.

Early passive ROM exercises are beneficial in preventing postoperative stiffness and help to nourish the articular cartilage, assist in collagen synthesis and organization, and neuromodulate the patient's pain (Sapega et al, 1976). Depending on the surgeons' preferred surgical technique and confidence in their repair, full supine passive shoulder ROM may be recommended immediately postoperatively (Martetschlanger et al, 2013; Millett et al, 2015; Willimon et al, 2011). The supine position is important because the weight of the scapula would be supported by the treatment table and would not pull on the surgical graft, which happens in gravity-dependent positions such as sitting or standing (Culp et al, 2006).

Conversely, some restrictions in passive ROM may be required. Sahara et al (2006) evaluated motion of the AC joint in regard to movements of the arm and showed that maximum posterior translation of the clavicle takes place when the arm is at 90 degrees of abduction. Furthermore, the closed pack position of the AC joint, indicating the position when the capsule and ligaments are maximally tight, is at 90 degrees of glenohumeral (GH) joint abduction. Some surgeons therefore restrict passive ROM for 4 to 6 weeks after surgery to less than 90 degrees of forward flexion (FF) and abduction to minimize stress on the ligaments (Beitzel & Mazzocca, 2014; Scheibel et al, 2011).

The criteria to progress to the next phase of rehabilitation are outlined in Fig. 12D.1. In addition, it is important to work with the individual surgeon to elicit her or his preferred time frames for progression and to understand the rationale in deciding any passive ROM restrictions.

Phase II: Muscle Endurance Phase

The goals of this phase of rehabilitation are to advance active shoulder motion, improve muscular endurance and neuromuscular control of the shoulder complex, and address any

Table 12D.1 Guidelines for Rehabilitation After Acromioclavicular Joint Reconstruction.

	Phase I: Protection	Phase II: Muscular Endurance	Phase III: Muscular Strength	Phase IV: Power	Phase V: Return to Sport
Precautions	Sling × 4-6 wk; avoid downward traction of shoulder × 12 wk	Avoid cross-body movement × 8 wk	Avoid bench press and push-up × 12 wk	No compensations observed, including scapular dyskinesis	Avoid irritation or pain with increasing demands of sport participation; use pad if needed
ROM	PROM within MD restrictions	AAROM progressing to AROM	Full AROM, C and T spine, IR/ER at 90 degrees	Full AROM	Full AROM should be present at this time
Soft tissue mobilization	Lymphatic drainage for swelling reduction	Joint mobilization (GH joint), massage, stretches as needed—pec minor, scalenes, UTM, posterior capsule	Capsular stretches as needed, including cross-body	Active release techniques, dry needling, IASTM as needed	Active release techniques, dry needling, IASTM as needed
Scapula	Active mobility (inf, sup, pro, ret); sidelying scapular clocks; isometrics—submaximal, pain free	CKC no loading—scapular clocks, wall plus, wall slides; scapular exercises—prone Ts, Is, Ys; sidelying ER	Diagonals, serratus punches, dynamic hugs, high rows	As needed; good scapular control should be present at this time	Integrated with sport-specific skills and drills
Strength	Isometrics in neutral shoulder position—submaximal, pain free	High reps, no to low weight; isotonic exercises	Mod to low reps, increasing resistance; isotonics with cords, dumbbells	Plyometrics—medicine ball tosses, tubing plyos, side-to-side throws	Integrated with sport-specific skills and drills
Proprioception and joint position sense	Gentle rhythmic stabilization in neutral shoulder position	PNF D2 flex/ext—no resistance (after week 8); continue with rhythmic stabilization	CKC exercises progressing load and to unstable surface; quadruped threading needle; wall push-ups. PNF with resistance	Plank moving body relative to fixed arm; push-ups on unstable surface	Integrated with sport-specific skills and drills
Core and kinetic chain exercises	Breathing reeducation; basic core exercises in supine and hook-lying positions involving LE movement only	Basic core exercises starting to involve UE and LE movement—dying bug; breathing assessment and exercises as needed	UE exercises in SL stance—chops, bird dog; kinetic chain exercises—diagonals, chops, PNF patterns in half-kneel position	Power, agility, and speed exercises with focus on appropriate transfer of energy through core and trunk to scapular and UE; perform throwing and catching in half-kneel position or SL; use medicine balls	Integrated with sport-specific skills and drills
CV conditioning	Recumbent bike—no loading of GH joint	Recumbent bike—no loading of GH joint	Stationary bike, pool jogging	Running, sprinting	Running, sprinting, sport-specific drills with cutting, stop and start, and agility if needed

AAROM, Active-assistive range of motion; *AROM,* active range of motion; *CKC,* closed kinetic chain; *C and T spine,* cervical and thoracic spine; *CV,* cardiovascular; *ER,* external rotation; *GH,* glenohumeral; *IASTM,* instrument-assisted soft tissue mobilization; *inf,* inferior; *Is,* prone extension; *LE,* lower extremity; *pec,* pectoralis; *MD,* physician; *plyos,* plyometrics; *PNF,* proprioceptive neuromuscular facilitation; *pro,* protraction; *PROM,* passive range of motion; *rep,* repetition; *ret,* retraction; *ROM,* range of motion; *SL,* single-leg; *sup,* superior; *Ts,* prone horizontal abduction with external rotation; *UE,* upper extremity; *UTM,* upper thoracic manipulation; *Ys,* prone flexion.

concerns with soft tissue mobility. Isotonic exercises should focus on high repetitions with low to no resistance. Gravity alone for resistance is often sufficient at this time.

Continuation of passive ROM is important during this phase until full passive ROM is achieved. However, active-assisted and active motion can be started at 4 to 6 weeks after surgery. Equipment to allow patients to progress active-assisted ROM at home can be used, including a foam roller (shoulder flexion; Fig. 12D.2),a stability ball (standing FF and circles), and a pole (supine L bar external rotation [ER] and FF). Active ROM can be started in supine, sidelying, or prone positions to reduce the effects of gravity, progressing to standing as endurance improves.

Progression of scapula control is of upmost importance during this phase. The scapula plays a key role in nearly every aspect of normal shoulder function. High-grade AC joint separations (grade III–VI) alter the strut function of the clavicle on the scapula and change the biomechanical screw axis of the scapulohumeral rhythm. (Gumina et al, 2009). This can manifest as scapular dyskinesis, which has been described as the loss of control of normal scapular physiology, mechanics, and motion (Kibler et al, 2012). Dyskinesis has been demonstrated in 70.6% of patients with high-grade AC joint symptoms (Gumina et al, 2009). Depending on the length of time between injury and surgery, individuals may have developed significant scapular dyskinesis before undergoing surgery. The upper, middle, and lower trapezius (UT, MT, and LT, respectively) muscles and the serratus anterior (SA) muscle are the greatest contributors to scapular stability and mobility (Speer et al, 1993). It has been hypothesized that compensation through increased activation of UT combined with decreased activation and control of the LT, MT, and SA contributes to abnormal scapular motion (Cools et al, 2007). Proper scapular kinesis

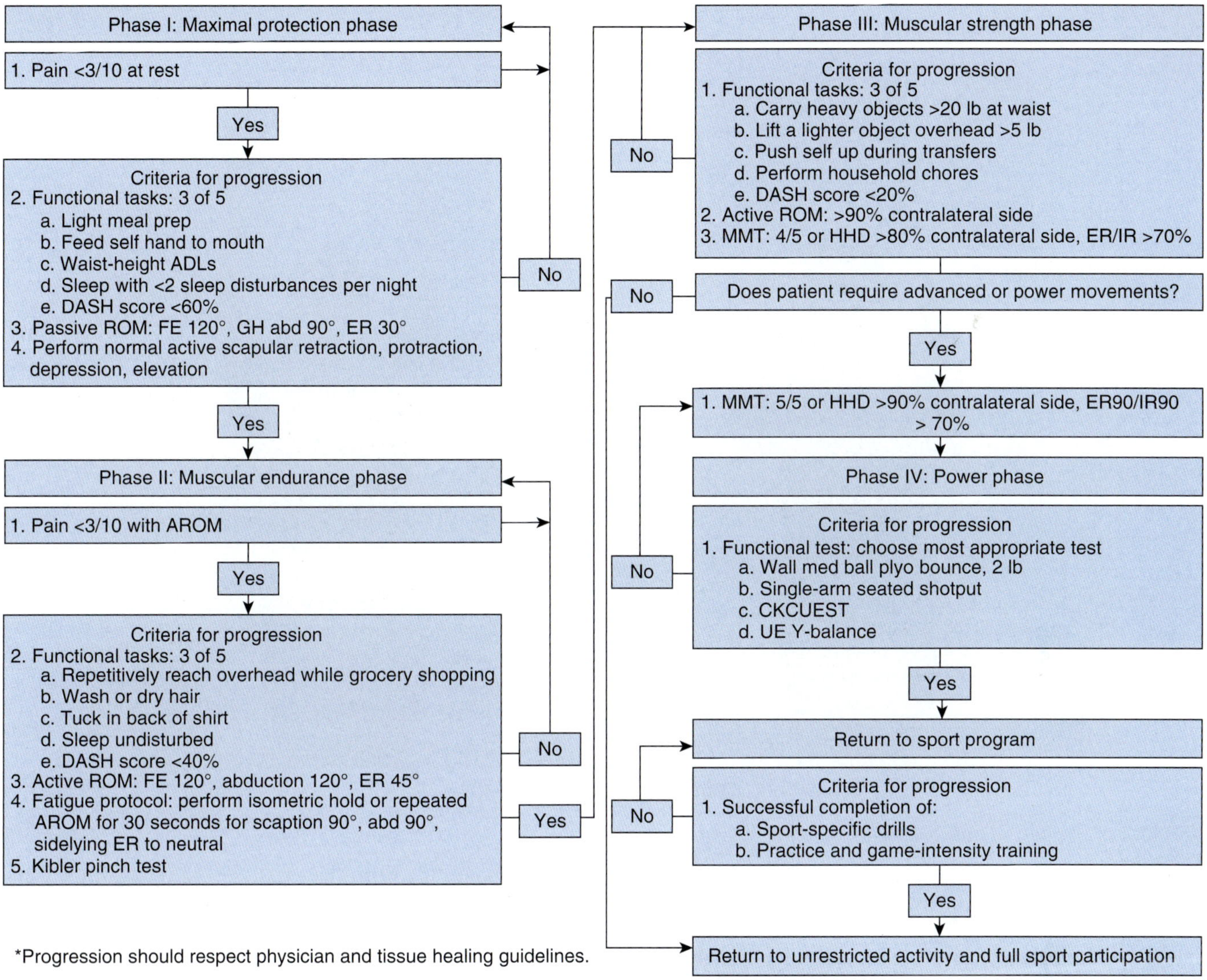

Fig. 12D.1 Acromioclavicular progression criteria algorithm.

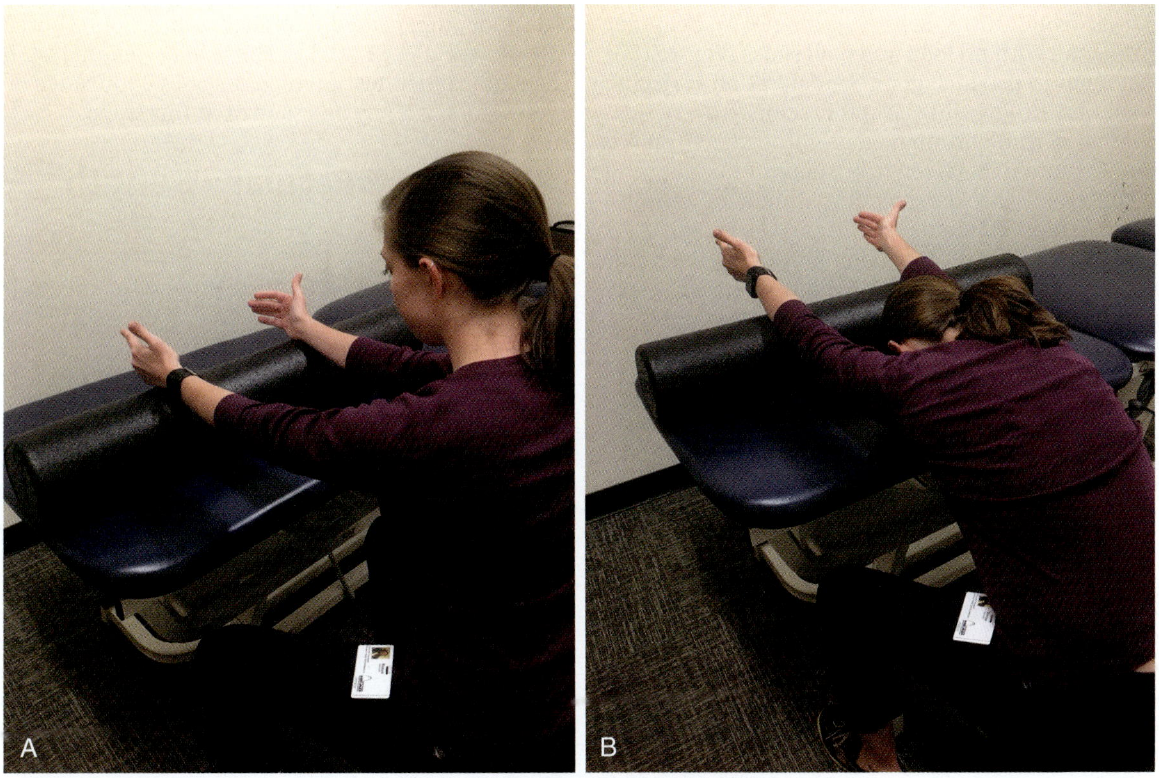

Fig. 12D.2 **A** and **B,** Foam roller roll-outs.

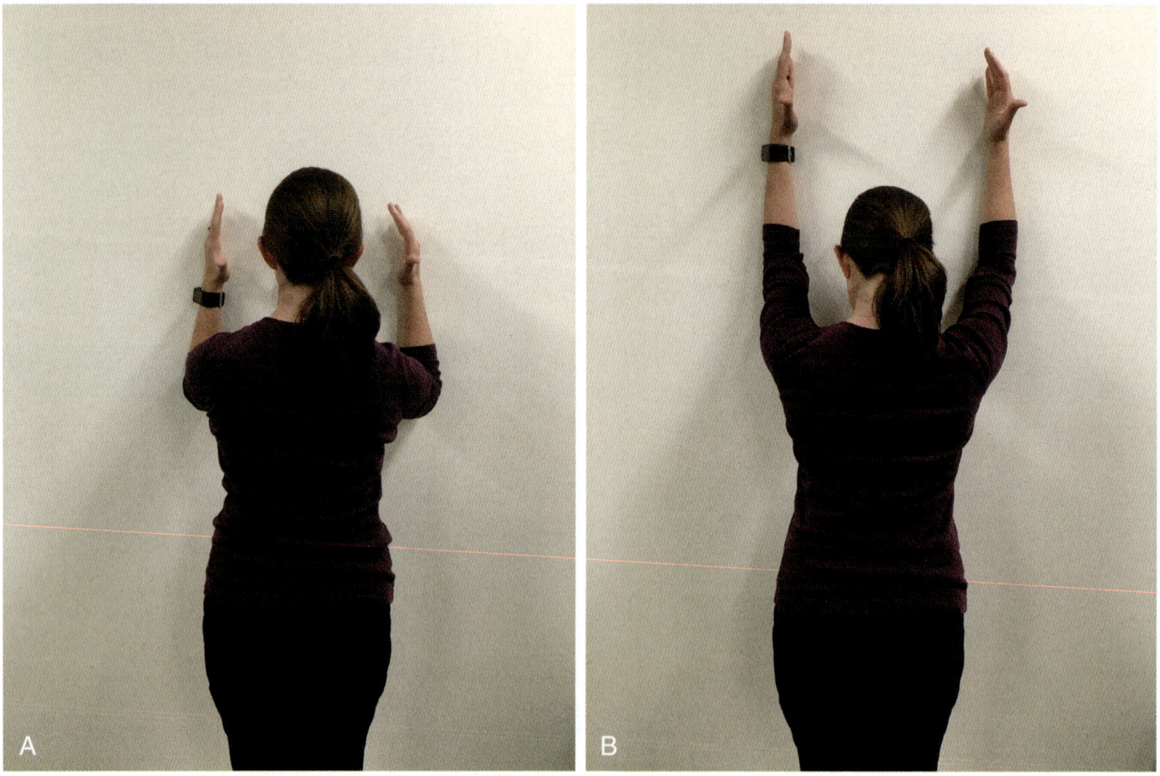

Fig. 12D.3 **A** and **B,** Wall slides.

should be trained early. Exercises focusing on periscapular control are appropriate during this phase of rehabilitation. Particular exercises that have been shown via electromyogram studies to accentuate periscapular control while minimizing UT muscle activation are sidelying ER, sidelying FF, prone horizontal abduction with ER, prone flexion, prone extension exercise (Cricchio & Frazer, 2011; Cools et al, 2007; Ekstrom, 2003; Schory et al, 2016). Scapular plus against a wall with no load and wall slides (Fig. 12D.3) have been shown to produce good SA activation (Cricchio & Frazer, 2011). Progressing scapular clocks from sidelying to against a wall can help to promote synchronized and rhythmic motion between the scapulothoracic and GH joint. These activate key scapular stabilizing muscles without putting high demands on the shoulder joint. At 8 weeks after surgery, when cross-body motions are permitted, proprioceptive neuromuscular facilitation (PNF) exercises, such as active D2 flexion/extension, should be started to help gain stability and control into functional patterns.

In addition to addressing scapular control, it is also important to assess for and address soft tissue dysfunctions. Not only can scapular dyskinesis contribute to muscle recruitment problems but also to flexibility dysfunctions, specifically in pectoralis minor, posterior GH joint capsule, and latissimus dorsi (Ellenbecker & Cools, 2010). Stretching and soft tissue mobilization techniques are recommended, including the unilateral corner stretch, GH joint accessory mobilization, and scapular orientation stretch (Mottram et al, 2009). Evaluating the athlete's breathing pattern in phase II is essential because of the importance of breathing to the proper positioning and functioning of the upper quadrant. Individuals with scapular dyskinesis can exhibit signs of faulty breathing mechanics (Clifton-Smith & Rowley, 2011). Dysfunction of the scalenes, UT, and pectoralis minor muscles can contribute to inefficient breathing patterns, specifically a thoracic breathing pattern (Chaitow et al, 2002).

Before progressing into phase III of rehabilitation, the patient needs to achieve adequate passive ROM as well as noncompensated shoulder and scapulothoracic active ROM (see Fig. 12D.1). The Kibler pinch test (isometric scapular pinch test), which assesses endurance of scapular retractors, is a key assessment at this stage.

Phase III: Muscular Strength Phase

With good muscle activation and endurance being established in phase II, the main goal of phase III is to increase the patient's strength through higher resistance and lower repetition. This can be done through a periodization format to load the reconstruction and stimulate healthy remodeling. Remodeling of repair tissue does not result in maximal tensile strength for a minimum of 12 weeks after reconstruction. Cote et al (2010) followed guidelines for progression of strengthening activities after ACJR based on tissue healing time frames of tendon healing in a bone tunnel, specific to ACCR. Research has shown construct failure through pull-out of the tendon from the tunnel occurred less than 12 weeks after surgery, but failure at the midsubstance of the tendon occurred at 12 weeks or more. This indicates adequate healing at the bone–tendon interface (Rodeo et al, 1993;

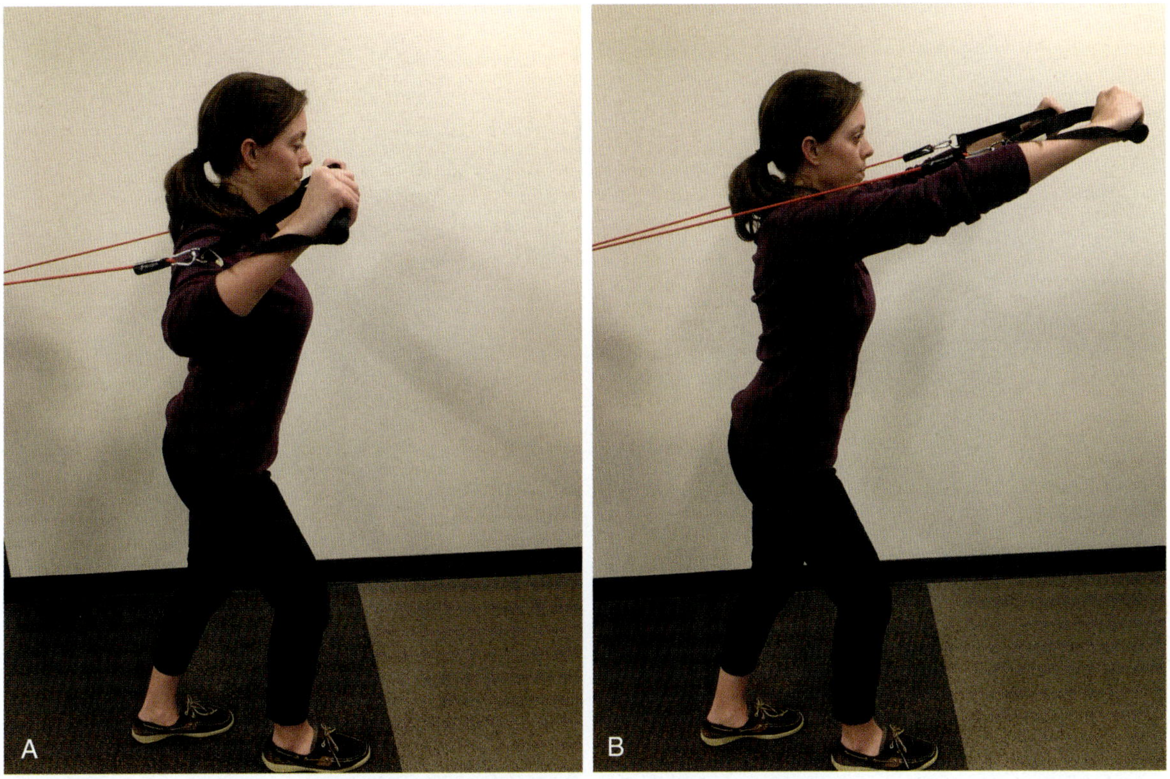

Fig. 12D.4 A and **B,** Bilateral serratus punch to 120 degrees.

St Pierre et al, 1995). As such, strengthening and significant loading of the reconstruction is delayed until 10 to 12 weeks after surgery.

A strengthening program for the entire shoulder girdle is used, with focus on rotator cuff and periscapular musculature. Exercises should include isotonic strengthening using sports cords or bands and dumbbells, with a focus on controlled concentric and eccentric contractions. Exercises showing optimal periscapular activation that should be added in this phase include dynamic hug, high rows, bilateral ER, bilateral serratus punch to 120 degrees of abduction (Fig. 12D.4), and diagonal patterns including chops and PNF exercises (Cricchio & Frazer, 2011; Reinold et al, 2009; Schory et al, 2016). Manual resistance including perturbation, medicine balls, dumbbells and cords can be gradually incorporated into these exercises to make them more challenging.

Closed chain exercises can be progressed to increase weight bearing through the upper extremities. Advancing from wall to table top or to quadruped position creates a gradual increase in loading and is excellent for scapular control. Some examples include push-up with a plus, which has demonstrated high electromyographic (EMG) activity for SA (Reinold et al, 2009); threading the needle, which also addresses thoracic mobility (Fig. 12D.5); and bird dog, which additionally challenges core stability. Placing an unstable base under the upper limbs such as a wobble board, stability ball, or BOSU enhances neuromuscular control at a reflex level, and the altering perturbation challenges proprioception and improves joint position sense (Jaggi & Lambert, 2010).

Another way to advance scapular muscle control and strength is by integrating kinetic chain concepts with exercise prescription. The kinetic chain model refers to the ability to transfer large forces through segmental links in the body with the theory of gaining proximal stability for distal mobility, power, and precision, all attributes that are required in sporting performance (Kibler & McMullen, 2003). The scapula serves as an efficient link between the core, which develops force, and the arm, which delivers the force (Kibler et al, 2012). Research has demonstrated maximal scapular muscle activation when muscles are activated in functional patterns and when muscles are activated in specific diagonal patterns using kinetic chain sequences (DeMay et al, 2011). DeMay and colleagues (2011) evaluated EMG activity during various exercises and found that unilateral rowing during single-leg squat position was most favorable for facilitating LT muscle activation (Fig. 12D.6). However, upright exercises in a squat or lunge position showed generally higher trunk muscle activation levels compared with a sitting or standing execution. Trunk and hip extension exercises help facilitate scapular retraction, and trunk and hip flexion exercises help facilitate scapular protraction (Kibler & McCullen, 2003). Using these principles, many rehabilitation exercises can be considered, including integration of ipsilateral and contralateral kinetic activation in single-leg squat, half-kneeling, and step-up positions while adding distal resistance (Kibler et al, 2013), for example, half-kneeling cable chop or single-leg lawnmower exercise (Fig. 12D.7) (Cote et al, 2010).

Kokmeyer and colleagues (2016) promoted the use of a hand-held dynamometer to determine a Limb Symmetry

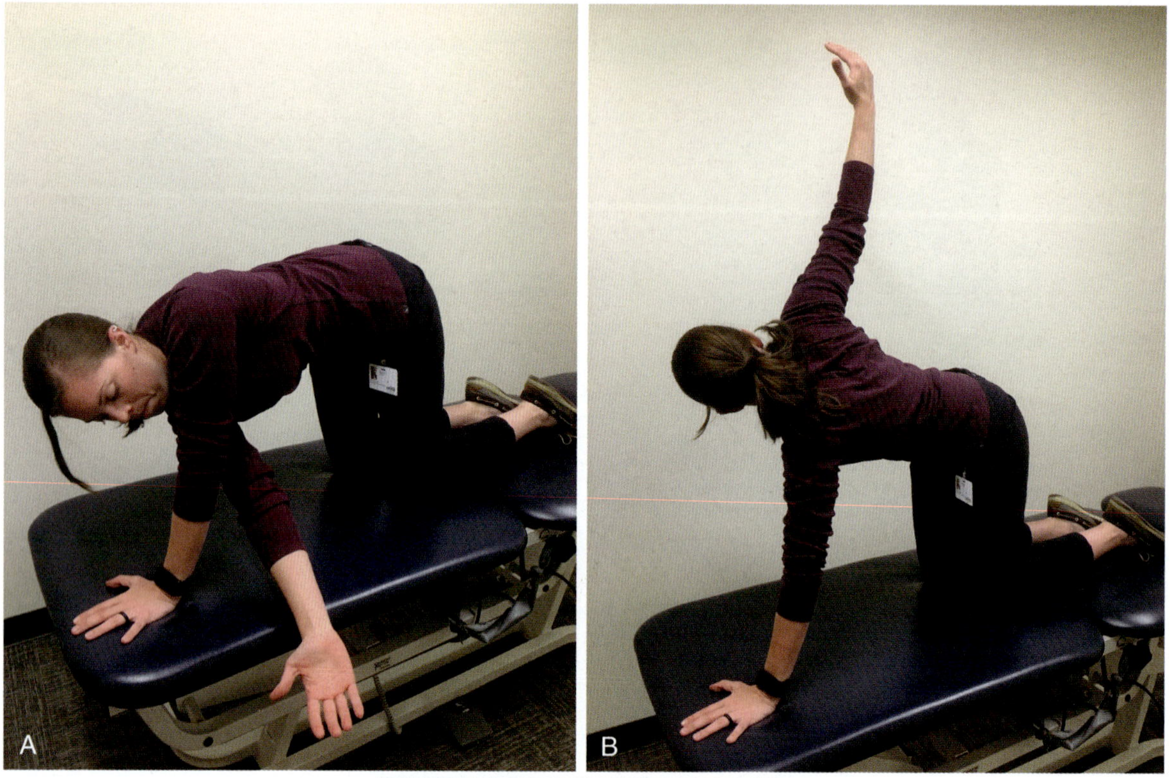

Fig. 12D.5 A and **B,** Threading the needle.

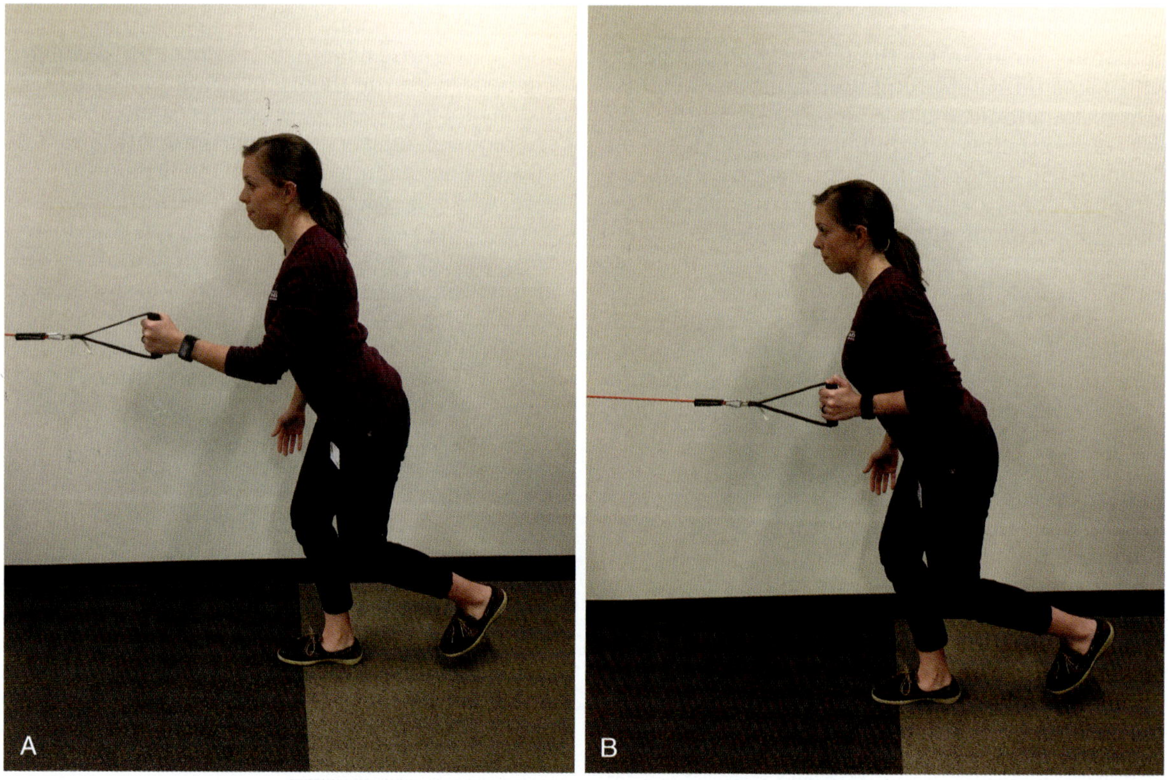

Fig. 12D.6 A and **B,** Unilateral row in single-leg squat position.

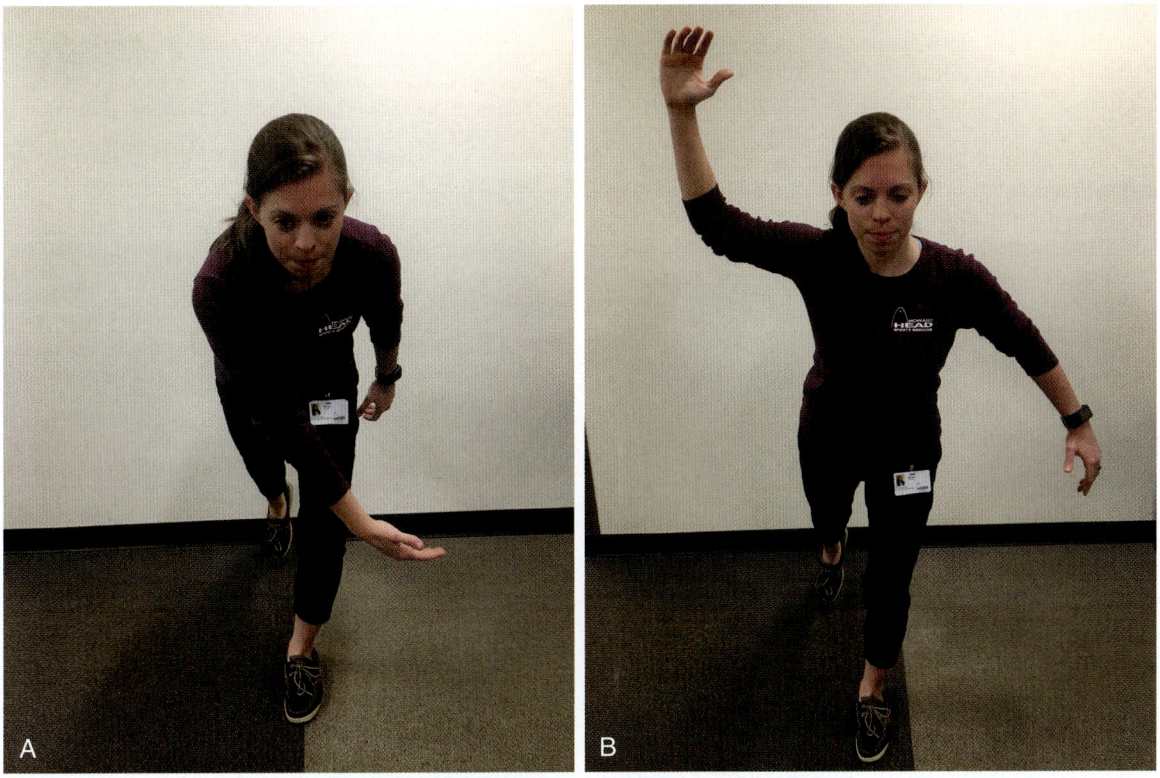

Fig. 12D.7 **A** and **B,** Single-leg lawnmower exercise.

Index (LSI). They suggested a 90% strength index or greater being a good baseline goal when evaluating an athlete's readiness to return to sport. The criteria to progress to phase IV require the athlete to have an LSI of 90% or greater.

Phase IV: Power Phase

The main goals for this phase are to incorporate speed and explosive strength and introduce patterns of movement biased toward the athlete's specific sporting demands. It is the role of the physical therapist to continue to develop and individualize the athlete's program. Repetition, speed, and load may be varied in relation to the desired task, facilitating feedforward processing (Griffin, 2003). Plyometric drills can help to transfer energy from the legs and trunk to the upper limbs. Examples of plyometric drills include two-hand chest passes, overhead soccer throws, and side-to-side throws (Wilk et al, 2002). Bouncing light-weight stability balls off a trampoline can be used to increase speed and endurance, and medicine balls can be used for strength training (Jaggi & Lambert, 2010).

Progressing closed kinetic chain exercises to incorporate loading of the upper extremity and moving the body relative to the fixed arm, such as a plank position with forward and backward movement, continues to challenge scapula and core strength (Reid et al, 2012).

Players preparing to return to sports such as rugby, football, and lacrosse should start a running conditioning program, which should include intermittent sprinting with jogging activities to replicate the types of physiological loads involved in match play (Helgeson et al, 2014).

Moving to phase V of rehabilitation requires the athlete to have no pain, ROM deficits, or scapular dyskinesis. A limited selection of functional tests has been identified in the literature for evaluating the readiness of an athlete to return to sport (see Fig. 12D.1). The most appropriate test reflective of the demands of the athlete's specific sport should be used and successfully passed before progressing to phase V.

Phase V: Return to Sport

The goal of this phase is to successfully return the athlete to full sports participation without compensation, risk of reinjury, or dysfunctional movement patterns. This usually occurs between 16 to 24 weeks after surgery depending on meeting the criteria in Fig. 12D.2 and the expectations of the surgeon. Loading is progressed toward normal participation levels by increasing volume and intensity. Progressive functional drills are performed to prepare the athlete to return to the skills and demands of the specific sport with awareness of good body mechanics, which protect the shoulder from excessive forces. The sport of interest should be scrutinized to determine the requirements and load involvement of the upper extremities. Good communication among coaches, trainers, and the physical therapist is vital at this time and will help with evaluating the demands on the athlete.

The rehabilitation program developed for players involved in contact sports should be consistent with the type of forces and mechanism players will encounter during practice and matches. These athletes can also have additional protection in the form of a donut or spider pad applied to the shoulder to help dissipate or absorb the force of a blow away from the AC joint (Gladstone et al, 1997).

There are currently no studies in the literature that have given evidence of objective measures to gauge return to sport for either the in- or off-season athlete. It is advised that clinical testing and sport-specific testing are undertaken before releasing an athlete to full play. This includes meeting all mobility and strength-based criteria in addition to sport-specific tests, such as simulated sporting activity, performing in sport practice, playing at a lower level, and the player feeling ready and confident (Helgeson et al, 2014). A slow reintroduction back into the sport using irritability as a guide to the athlete's progression is also recommended.

Conclusions

This rehabilitation program advances through five phases with criteria needing to be met to progress to the next phase. Phase 1 focuses on protection of the reconstruction and initiation of passive ROM. Phase II advances active-assisted and active ROM as tolerated with a focus on endurance and performance of movement without compensation. Scapular dyskinesis is addressed with appropriate exercise prescription. Phase III progresses muscular strength by incorporating bands, cords, dumbbells, and manual resistance as necessary, with consideration to the kinetic chain. Performing shoulder exercises in single-leg stance or half-kneeling positions can enhance scapular and core activation. Phase IV starts to prepare the athlete for return to play by addressing power, agility, and speed. Phase V focuses on returning the athlete back to preinjury sporting levels. Skills and drills appropriate for the athlete's specific sport are mastered. The criteria for progression through each phase are based on both functional and objective markers with consideration to tissue healing time frames. The ultimate goals are to allow the AC joint to heal and to return the athlete to competitive play as quickly and safely as possible without risk of further reinjury. The current review has blended current literature and expert opinion to inform the development of the ACJR rehabilitation guidelines (see Table 12D.1).

References

Beitzel K, Mazzocca AD. Open anatomic reconstruction of chronic acromioclavicular instability. *Oper Orthop Traumatol*. 2014;26(3): 237–224.

Bontempo NA, Mazzocca AD. Biomechanics and treatment of acromioclavicular and sternoclavicular joint injuries. *Br J Sports Med*. 2010;44(5):361–369.

Chaitow L, Bradley D, Gilbert C. *Multidisciplinary Approaches to Breathing Pattern Disorders*. London: Churchill Livingstone; 2002.

Clifton-Smith T, Rowley J. Breathing pattern disorders and physiotherapy: inspiration for our profession. *Phys The Rev*. 2011;16:75–86.

Cools AM, Dewitte V, Lanszweert F, et al. Rehabilitation of scapular muscle balance: which exercises to prescribe? *Am J Sports Med*. 2007;35(10):1744–1751.

Cote MP, Wojcik KE, Gomlinski G, Mazzocca AD. Rehabilitation of acromioclavicular joint separations: operative and nonoperative considerations. *Clin Sports Med*. 2010;29(2):213–228.

Cricchio M, Frazer C. Scapulothoracic and scapulohumeral exercises: a narrative review of electromyographic studies. *J Hand Ther*. 2011;24:322–333.

Culp LB, Romani WA. Physical therapist examination, evaluation and intervention following the surgical reconstruction of a grade III acromioclavicular joint separation. *Phys Ther*. 2006;86(6):857–869.

DeMay K, Danneels L, Cagnie B. Are kinetic chain rowing exercises relevant in shoulder and trunk injury prevention training? *Br J Sports Med*. 2011;45:320–321.

Dimakopoulos P, Panagopopulos A. Functional coracoclavicular stabilization for acute acromioclavicular joint disruption. *Orthopedics*. 2007;30(2):103–108.

Ekstrom RA, Donatelli RA, Soderberg GI. Surface electromyographic analysis of exercises for the trapezius and serratus anterior muscles. *J Orthop Sports Phys Ther*. 2003;33(5):247–258.

Ellenbecker TS, Cools A. Rehabilitation of shoulder impingement syndrome and rotator cuff injuries: an evidence-based review. *Br J Sports Med*. 2010;44(5):319–327.

Gladstone J, Wilk K, Andrews J. Nonoperative treatment of acromioclavicular joint injuries. *Oper Tech Sports Med*. 1997;5(2):78–87.

Griffin L. Neuromuscular training and injury prevention in sports. *Clin Orthop Relat Res*. 2003;409:53–60.

Gumina S, Carbone S, Postacchini F. Scapular dyskinesis and SICK scapula syndrome in patients with chronic type III acromioclavicular dislocation. *Arthroscopy*. 2009;25(1):40–45.

Helgeson K, Stoneman P. Shoulder injuries in rugby players: mechanisms, examination, and rehabilitation. *Phys Ther Sport*. 2014;15(4):218–227.

Jaggi A, Lambert S. Rehabilitation for shoulder instability. *Br J Sports Med*. 2010;44:333–340.

Johnson L, Polson K, Ried D. *Acromioclavicular Joint Separations Grade I-III: Best Practice Guidelines*. Auckland: New Zealand Academy of Sport; 2011:1–54.

Kibler WB, McMullen J. Scapular dyskinesis and its relation to shoulder pain. *J Acad Orthop Surg*. 2003;11(2):142–151.

Kibler WB, Sciascia A, Wilkes T. Scapular dyskinesis and its relation to shoulder injury. *J Acad Orthop Surg*. 2012;20(6):364–372.

Kibler WB, Ludewig PM, McClure PW. Clinical implications of scapular dyskinesis in shoulder injury: the 2013 consensus statement from the "Scapular Summit." *Br J Sports Med*. 2013;47(13):877–885.

Kokmeyer D, Dube E, Millett PJ. Prognosis driven rehabilitation after rotator cuff repair surgery. *Open Orthop J*. 2016;10:339–348.

Martetschlanger F, Horan M, Warth RJ, Millett PJ. Complications after anatomic fixation and reconstruction of the coracoclavicular ligaments. *Am J Sports Med*. 2013;41(12):2896–2903.

Mazzocca AD, Santangelo SA, Johnson ST. A biomechanical evaluation of an anatomical coracoclavicular ligament reconstruction. *Am J Sports Med*. 2006;34:236–246.

Millett PJ, Braun S, Gobezie R. Acromioclavicular joint reconstruction with coracoacromial ligament transfer using the docking technique. *BMC Musculoskel Disord*. 2009;10:6.

Millett PJ, Horan MP, Warth RJ. Two-year outcomes after primary anatomic coracoclavicular ligament reconstruction. *Arthroscopy*. 2015;31(10):1962–1973.

Mottram SL, Woledge RC, Morrissey. Motion analysis study of a scapular orientation exercise and subjects' ability to learn the exercise. *Man Ther*. 2009;14(1):13–18.

Pallis M, Cameron KL, Svoboda SJ. Epidemiology of acromioclavicular joint injury in young athletes. *Am J Sports Med*. 2012;40(9):2072–2077.

Reid D, Polson K, Johnson L. Acromioclavicular Joint separations grades I–III. *Sports Med*. 2012;42(8):681–696.

Reinold MM, Escamilla R, Wilk KE. Current concepts in the scientific and clinical rationale behind exercises for glenohumeral and scapulothoracic musculature. *J Orthop Sports Phys Ther*. 2009;39(2):105–117.

Rockwood CA. Injuries to the acromioclavicular joint. In: ed 2. Rockwood CA, Green DP, eds. *Fracture in Adults*. vol. 1. Philadelphia: JB Lippincott; 1984:860.

Rodeo SA, Arnoczky SP, Torzilli PA. Tendon-healing in a bone tunnel. A biomechanical and histological study in the dog. *J Bone Joint Surg Am*. 1993;75(12):1795–1803.

Rolf O, von Weyhern AH, Ewers A. Acromioclavicular dislocation Rockwood III-V: results of early versus delayed surgical treatment. *Arch Orthop Trauma Surg*. 2007;128(10):1153–1157.

Sahara W, Sugamoto K, Murai M, Tanaka H, Yoshikawa H. 3D kinematic analysis of the acromioclavicular joint during arm abduction using vertically open MRI. *J Orthop Res*. 2006;24:1823–1831.

Sapega AA. Biophysical factors in range of motion exercise. *Arch Phys Med Rehab*. 1976;57:122–126.

Scheibel M, Droschel S, Gerhardt C. Arthroscopically assisted stabilization of acute high-grade acromioclavicular joint separations. *Am J Sports Med*. 2011;39(7):1507–1516.

Schory A, Bidinger E, Wolf J, Murray L. A systematic review of the exercises that produce optimal muscle ratios of the scapular stabilizers in normal shoulders. *Int J Sports Phys Ther*. 2016;11(3):321–336.
Simovitch R, Sanders B, Ozbaydar M. Acromioclavicular joint injuries: diagnosis and management. *J Am Acad Orthop Surg*. 2009;17(4):207–219.
Speer KP, Garrett WE. Muscular control of motion and stability about the pectoral girdle. In: Matsen FA III, Fu FH, Hawkins RJ, eds. *The Shoulder: A Balance of Mobility and Stability*. Rosemont, IL: American Academy of Orthopaedic Surgeons; 1993:159–172.
St Pierre P, Olson EJ, Elliot JJ. Tendon-healing to cortical bone compared with healing to a cancellous trough. A biomechanical and histological evaluation in goats. *J Bone Joint Surg Am*. 1995;77(12):1858–1866.
Thigpin CA, Shaffer MA, Gaunt BW. The American Society of Shoulder and Elbow Therapists' consensus statement on rehabilitation following arthroscopic rotator cuff repair. *J Shoulder Elbow Surg*. 2016;25(4):521–535.
Warth RJ, Martetschlanger F, Gaskill TR. Acromioclavicular joint separations. *Curr Rev Musculoskel Med*. 2013;6(1):71–78.
Weinstein DM, McCann PD, McIlveen SJ. Surgical treatment of complete acromioclavicular dislocations. *Am J Sports Med*. 1995;23:324–331.
Wilk KE, Meister K, Andrews JR. Current concepts in the rehabilitation of the overhead throwing athlete. *Am J Sports Med*. 2002;30:136–151.
Willimon S, Gaskill T, Millett PJ. Acromioclavicular joint injuries: anatomy, diagnosis, and treatment. *Phys Sportsmed*. 2011;39(1):116–122.

SECTION **IV**

Clavicle Fractures

SECTION OUTLINE

13 Overview

JUSTIN L. HODGINS, MD and MICHAEL D. MCKEE, MD

Introduction

- Clavicle fractures are common and potentially devastating injuries in athletes that may result in complete loss of the competitive season.
- Approximately 20% to 45% of all clavicle fractures are attributed to sport-related activity with cycling and contact sports being the most common.
- A systematic approach is required when examining injured athletes. Isolated clavicle injuries can be diagnosed with standard radiographic views of the clavicle.
- Treatment recommendations rely heavily on patient-specific factors, including athlete age, type of sport, position, competitive level, future aspirations, and perceptions of surgical fixation.
- Nonoperative management is generally advocated for non- or minimally displaced fractures and most fractures in adolescent athletes.
- Excellent functional outcomes with early return to sport and minimal complications have been demonstrated with modern fixation techniques in displaced midshaft clavicle fractures.

Anatomy

The clavicle is the first bone to ossify during the fifth week of gestation, and it contains the last ossification center to fuse in the human body, the medial physis adjacent to the sternoclavicular (SC) joint (Gardner, 1968). During childhood, approximately 80% of clavicular growth occurs at the medial ossification center, which generally closes at age 23 to 25 years (Jit & Kulkarni, 1976; Ogden et al, 1979). The late fusion of the medial physis explains the pathophysiology behind adolescent physeal separation injuries.

The clavicle has an S-shaped morphology with an anterior apex medially and posterior apex laterally (Gardner, 1968; Lewonowski & Bassett, 1992). The long bone widens at its sternal and acromial ends, transitioning through a narrower middle third (Fig. 13.1). The clavicle is a subcutaneous structure and contains several fascial and muscular attachments that help create the predictable deformity seen with fractures.

The medial third of the clavicle has a flat superior border and articulates with the sternum through strong capsuloligamentous attachments. The extensive ligamentous supports between the SC joint and first rib are partly responsible for the undisplaced nature of most medial clavicle fractures. The sternocleidomastoid, pectoralis major, and sternohyoid muscles attach to the medial third of the clavicle. In displaced midshaft fractures, the medial fragment is pulled superiorly and posteriorly by the sternocleidomastoid muscles (Lazarus, 2002). Attached to the lateral third of the clavicle are the anterior fibers of the deltoid and trapezius muscles as well as the clavicular head of the pectoralis major. The pectoralis major and the weight of the arm provide the chief deforming force on the lateral clavicle fragment, causing inferomedial and anterior displacement in fractures of the middle third of the clavicle (Neer, 1963).

The clavicle widens along its acromial end and the lateral third contains the apex of the superior bow of the clavicle. The distal clavicle is securely anchored to the scapula by the acromioclavicular (AC) capsuloligament, and the coracoclavicular (CC) ligaments. The capsuloligamentous complex spans the AC joint, attaching to the distal clavicle approximately 6 mm medial to the AC joint (Postacchini et al, 2002). The AC ligament and joint capsule are the primary stabilizers to motion in the horizontal plane (Fukuda et al, 1986). The CC ligaments provide vertical stability consisting of the trapezoid and conoid ligaments, which originate from the base of the coracoid process and attach on the inferior surface of the distal clavicle. The trapezoid ligament originates approximately 2 cm lateral from the AC joint, and the more medial conoid ligament attaches approximately 4 cm from the AC joint (Renfree et al, 2003).

Sensory branches of the supraclavicular nerves and the platysma muscle transverse the subcutaneous plane superficial to the clavicle. The supraclavicular nerves lie deep to the platysma over the medial and middle thirds of the clavicle (Lazarus, 2002; Jupiter & Ring, 1999). The identification and protection of these cutaneous nerves is advocated to minimize dysesthesia or the formation of a painful neuroma during surgical fixation of clavicle fractures (Jupiter & Ring, 1999). Additionally, the patient should be warned of the possibility of dysesthesia or numbness in this nerve distribution.

Functionally, the clavicle acts as a strut connecting the shoulder girdle to the axial skeleton, and scapulothoracic motion depends on the stable relationship between the distal clavicle and scapula (Banerjee et al, 2011). The functional importance of restoring and maintaining the normal length and rotation of this strut after fracture has been demonstrated in various clinical and biomechanical studies (Basamania, 1999; Bosch et al, 1998; Chan et al, 1999; Kuhne, 1999; McKee et al, 2006). In addition, displacement and shortening of the clavicle result in alternations in scapular resting position and kinematics and has been associated with reductions in muscular strength and patient dissatisfaction (Lazarides & Zafiropoulos 2006; Ledger et al, 2005). The clavicle is also an important structural support protecting neurovascular and airway structures. The brachial plexus and the subclavian vessels

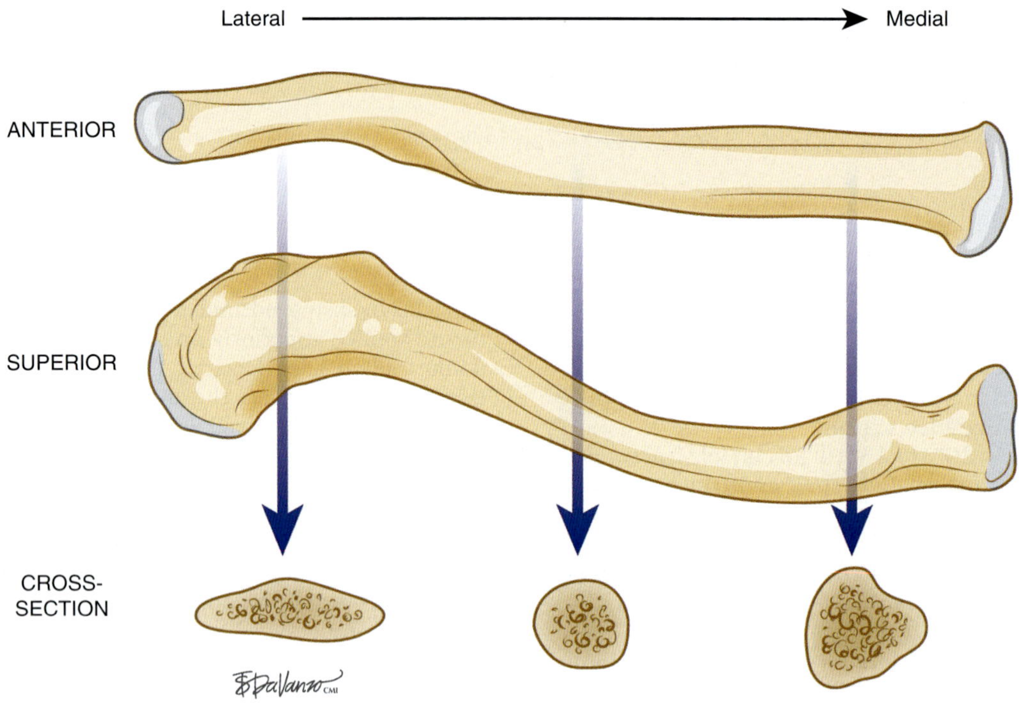

Fig. 13.1 Anatomy and cross-sectional geometry of the clavicle. (Adapted from Craig EV. Fractures of the shoulder: part II. Fractures of the clavicle. In Rockwood CA, Green DP, Bucholz RW, eds. *Rockwood and Green's Fractures in Adults.* 3rd ed, vol 1. Philadelphia: JB Lippincott; 1991:928-990.)

transverse toward the axillae under the middle third of the clavicle, and the carotid and jugular vessels are protected by the adjacent SC joint (Rumball et al, 1991). Similarly, the apex of the lungs lies immediately inferior to the medial clavicle and is at risk with displaced fractures and chest wall injuries.

The clavicle undergoes a complex three-dimensional motion that is intimately interconnected with the motion of the shoulder girdle through its articulation with the scapula. During arm elevation and abduction, the SC joint serves as a stable medial pivot point allowing clavicular elevation and rotation. With respect to the SC joint, the clavicle undergoes elevation of 11 to 15 degrees, retraction of 15 to 29 degrees, and posterior long-axis rotation of 15 to 31 degrees (Ludewig et al, 2004). Others suggest rotation being as high as 50 degrees and elevation in excess of 30 degrees with varying degrees of magnitude (Simpson & Jupiter, 1996). Clavicle rotation is relatively limited until humeral elevation exceeds 90 degrees; thus, the avoidance of over-the-shoulder motion during early rehabilitation can significantly limit rotational forces across fracture fixation (Fung et al, 2001).

Epidemiology

Fractures of the clavicle are common and potentially devastating injuries in athletes that often result in complete loss of the competitive season. Overall, clavicle fractures represent up to 5% of all fractures with an estimated incidence of 20 to 50 fractures per 100,000 population per year (Nordqvist & Petersson, 1994; Nowak et al, 2000; Robinson, 1998). Midshaft fractures are the most common, representing 69% to 82% of all clavicle fractures, with distal fractures comprising 10% to 30% and those of the medial third 2% to 4% (Nordqvist & Petersson, 1994; Postacchini et al, 2002; Robinson et al, 1998). Over two-thirds of clavicle fractures in adults are midshaft and these fractures are more likely to be displaced as compared with medial- and lateral-third fractures (Nordqvist & Petersson, 1994). In children and adolescents, 90% of fractures are midshaft injuries (Landin, 1983).

The incidence of clavicle fractures directly attributed to athletic trauma is less understood (Table 13.1). A study of 5953 patients over a single year reported a total of 195 clavicle fractures, of which 60 (30.8%) were sport related, the highest percentage of any fracture (Court-Brown et al, 2008). In a retrospective review of 1196 clavicle fractures in the United Kingdom, 21.4% of fractures were attributed to sport and 19.8% bicycle or motorcycle injury (Murray et al, 2013). A population-based epidemiologic study using the National Electronic Injury Surveillance System (NEISS) reported 9428 fractures of the clavicle through a representative sample of U.S. hospitals (Van Tassel et al, 2014). The authors estimated an overall incidence of 24.4 clavicle fractures per 100,000 person-years, with 45% of fractures attributed to sport-related activity, including cycling, football, soccer, and basketball. A study of U.S. high school sport-related fractures using the National High School Sports-Related Injury Surveillance System reported clavicle fractures comprised 8.9% of all fractures (Swenson et al, 2012).

Cycling and contact sports are the most common causes of clavicle fractures in athletics, although rugby, horseback riding, soccer, hockey, martial arts, snowboarding, and

Table 13.1 Epidemiology of Clavicle Fractures

	Clavicle Fractures (*n*)	Fractures Attributed to Sports (%)	Most Common Sports (%)
Court-Brown et al, 2008	195	60 (30.8)	Rugby (19.1) Horse riding (18.7) Hockey (16) Running (6.2) Martial arts (5.6) Football (4.4)
Murray et al, 2013	1196	201 (21.4)	
Van Tassel et al, 2014	9428	4135 (45.3)	Bicycling (16) Football (12) Soccer (5.6)
Nowak et al, 2000	187	94 (50.3)	Cycling (33.2) Skating or hockey (5.3) Soccer (4.8) Horse riding (4.8) Skiing (2.1)
Antabak et al, 2015	256	47 (18.4)	Football (11.7) Martial arts or wrestling (3.9) Hockey (1.2) Basketball (0.8) Gymnastics (0.8)

skiing have all been implicated (Court-Brown et al, 2008; Van Tassel et al, 2014). The NEISS study listed cycling (16%), football (12%), and soccer (5.6%) as the three most causative activities (Van Tassel et al, 2014). A smaller investigation in a Swedish population also listed cycling as the most common cause of clavicle fracture in both men and women, responsible for 62 of 187 (33%) fractures during a 2-year period (Nowak et al, 2000). However, the studies fail to differentiate competitive cycling injuries from those sustained while bicycling either recreationally or for personal transport. A study of clavicle fractures in professional football players using the National Football League (NFL) Injury Surveillance System identified 19 players with midshaft fractures over a 5-year period (Morgan et al, 2010). Similarly, when examining collegiate football players at the NFL Combine, 10 of 336 players had a history of clavicle fracture with the highest percentage in those playing wide receiver (Kaplan et al, 2005). Clavicle fractures have also been reported in men's collegiate lacrosse with an estimated occurrence of 0.02 per 1000 athletic exposures from 2004 to 2009, of which no athletes returned to play during the same season (Gardner et al, 2016).

The incidence of clavicle fractures is highest in the youngest part of the general population and typically those younger than the age of 20 years (Nordqvist & Petersson, 1994; Nowak et al, 2000; Robinson, 1998). For sport-related clavicle fractures, the highest incidence of fractures has been reported in athletes ages 10 to 19 years and 0 to 9 years (Van Tassel et al, 2014). These peaks coincide with those of organized sport during childhood and adolescence and the maximal number of athletic exposures. An estimated 45 million children and adolescents participate in organized sport in the United States, and as the competitive demands continue to increase, a rise in sports injuries has also been observed (Goldberg et al, 2007). In a study of 256 pediatric clavicle fractures over a 5-year period, sport-related fractures (18.4%) were second only to bicycle riding (18.7%) with football (11.7%) and martial arts (4%) the most common sports causes (Antabak et al, 2015). Previous studies have observed a predominance of clavicle fractures in men compared with women with male-to-female ratios reported at 2.6:1 (Robinson, 1998) and 2.2:1 (Nowak et al, 2000). When considering fractures attributed to sport activity alone, the male-to-female ratio significantly increases to 6.8:1 (Robinson, 1998), and males are estimated to sustain 74% of all clavicle fractures (Van Tassel et al, 2014).

Etiology

Most clavicle fractures result from a fall onto the shoulder or a direct blow to the shoulder girdle. Midshaft fractures were traditionally thought to occur from a fall on an outstretched hand, but biomechanical analysis has demonstrated that force transmitted directly through the shoulder, rather than the hand, which produces a force equal to the body weight, may exceed the critical buckling load of the clavicle and result in a midshaft fracture (Fig. 13.2) (Stanley et al, 1988). This compressive force to the clavicle is estimated to account for more than 85% of all clavicle fractures and up to 94% on midshaft injuries (Nordqvist & Petersson, 1994; Nowak et al, 2000; Robinson et al, 1998). The morphology of the clavicle and ligamentous supports also contribute to fracture patterns. The junction of the outer and middle thirds of the clavicle is the thinnest segment of the bone and is devoid of any protective muscular or ligamentous attachments, rendering it prone to fracture; therefore, midshaft fractures are the most common. No studies have proposed any definitive correlation between mechanism of injury and fracture location on the clavicle. When falling on an outstretched hand, the forces are not directly delivered to the clavicle and therefore are less likely to produce a fracture. This mechanism accounts for an estimated 2% to 5% of all midshaft fractures (Jeray, 2007).

In cycling, the axial load transmitted through the clavicle is proportionate to the velocity and weight of the rider, which often exceeds the critical buckling force needed for fracture. In contact sports such as football, rugby, lacrosse, and hockey, injuries are sustained by direct trauma to the shoulder by point contact with either another player during tackling or body checking or the playing surface. In a typical body check, the player lowers and drives the top of the shoulder into the other player's body. The force transmitted may injure the receiving player's clavicle depending on the vector, but the contact also forces the shoulder girdle of the attacking player downward and away from his or her own clavicle, potentially injuring the AC or CC ligaments (or both) (Gardner et al, 2016). Clavicle fractures are also more likely to occur when the critical force applied is absorbed quickly over a smaller surface area (Stanley et al, 1988). Improvements in protective shoulder equipment in contact sports help to dissipate energy over a larger area, slow the absorption of the impact, and reduce the incidence of injury.

The subcutaneous location of the clavicle, particularly the middle third, leaves it vulnerable to direct blows.

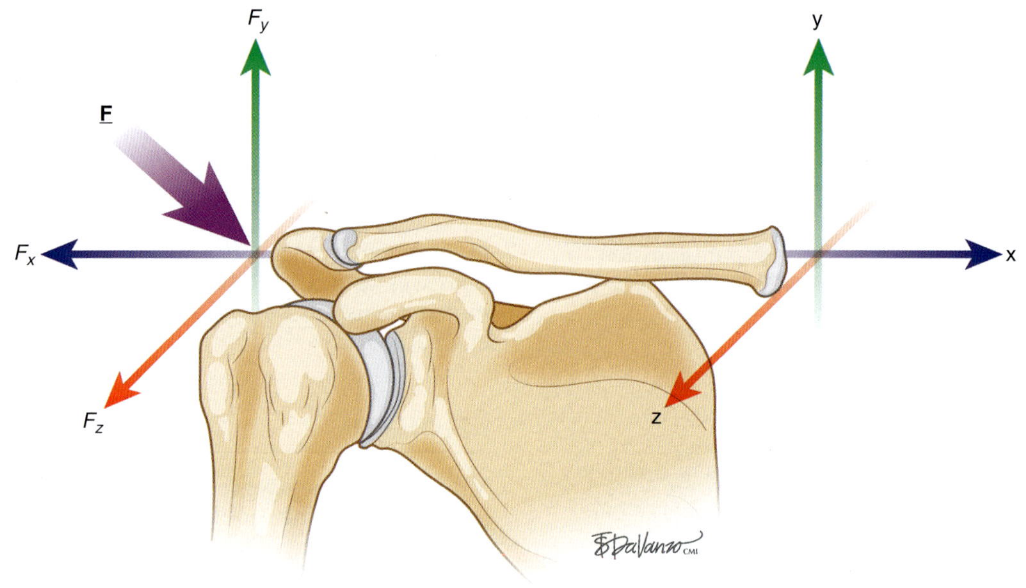

Fig. 13.2 Mechanism of clavicle fracture with a direct blow to the shoulder. The impact force vector *F* has three components; if F_y and F_z are both zero, then the blow will be directed purely along the clavicular axis (F_x). (Adapted from Stanley D, Trowbridge EA, Norris SH. The mechanism of clavicular fracture: A clinical and biomechanical analysis. *J Bone Joint Surg Br.* 1988;70:461-464.)

Violent contact from a hockey or lacrosse stick may produce a fracture, but this mechanism is more commonly seen as a result of seatbelt injuries during motor vehicle collisions and is estimated to account for 10% to 13% of midshaft fractures (Jeray, 2007). Alternatively, a direct force on the top of the shoulder during a sport collision may drive the midshaft clavicle against the first rib, resulting in a fracture.

Classification

A variety of classification systems have been proposed based on fracture location and complexity for clinical and research purposes (Allman, 1967; Craig, 2006; Neer, 1968; Nordqvist & Petersson, 1994; Robinson, 1998). Most modern classifications are primarily descriptive to facilitate communication among surgeons rather than predict clinical outcomes. The first widely accepted classification of clavicle fractures was introduced by Allman (1967). Fractures were classified based on the anatomic location of the fracture in descending order of incidence: group I (middle third), group II (medial third), and group III (lateral third). This simple system was easy to use but did not address fracture pattern.

Neer further subdivided lateral third fractures, recognizing the importance of an intact CC ligament in maintaining stability of the medial fragment (or shaft): type I (intact CC ligament), type II (CC detached from the medial fragment), and type III (intraarticular fractures of the AC joint with intact CC ligament) (Neer, 1968). Craig (2006) later combined and modified the Neer and Allman classifications for the most commonly used system for lateral clavicle fractures (Fig. 13.3). Type I fracture occurs lateral to the CC ligaments, spares the AC joint, and is often minimally displaced as the proximal fragment is stabilized by the CC ligaments and the distal fragment by the deltotrapezial fascia. Type II includes inherently unstable fractures as the proximal fragment is detached from the CC ligaments and the distal fragment remains attached to the scapula via the AC joint capsule. Type II fractures are further differentiated into those where the fracture occurs medial to the conoid ligament (type IIA) and those where the fracture lies between the conoid and trapezoid ligaments (type IIB). Determination of the precise location of the fracture and the integrity of the CC ligaments can be difficult to determine on plain radiographs (Banerjee et al, 2011). Type III fractures are minimally displaced as the CC ligaments remain intact but have an intraarticular component. Type IV fractures are rare fractures involving epiphyseal separation in pediatric patients (Neer, 1984). Type V injuries are comminuted and unstable as neither the proximal or distal fragments have ligamentous continuity with the coracoid (Neer, 1984).

The Edinburgh classification described by Robinson (1998) is the most recent and comprehensive system for clavicle fractures (Fig. 13.4). The primary classification is anatomically divided into fractures of the medial third (type I), middle third (type II), and lateral third of the clavicle (type III). Each type is then subdivided based on the magnitude of fracture displacement and includes subgroup A (<100% displacement) and subgroup B (>100% displacement). Type I (medial third) and type III (lateral third) fractures are additionally subdivided based on articular involvement into subgroup 1 (no articular involvement) and subgroup 2 (intraarticular extension). Similarly, type II (middle third) fractures are subcategorized according to the diaphyseal classification system of the Orthopaedic Trauma Association (OTA) by fracture comminution. Here, subgroup 1 consists of simple or wedge-type fracture patterns, and subgroup 2 includes those comminuted or segmental fractures.

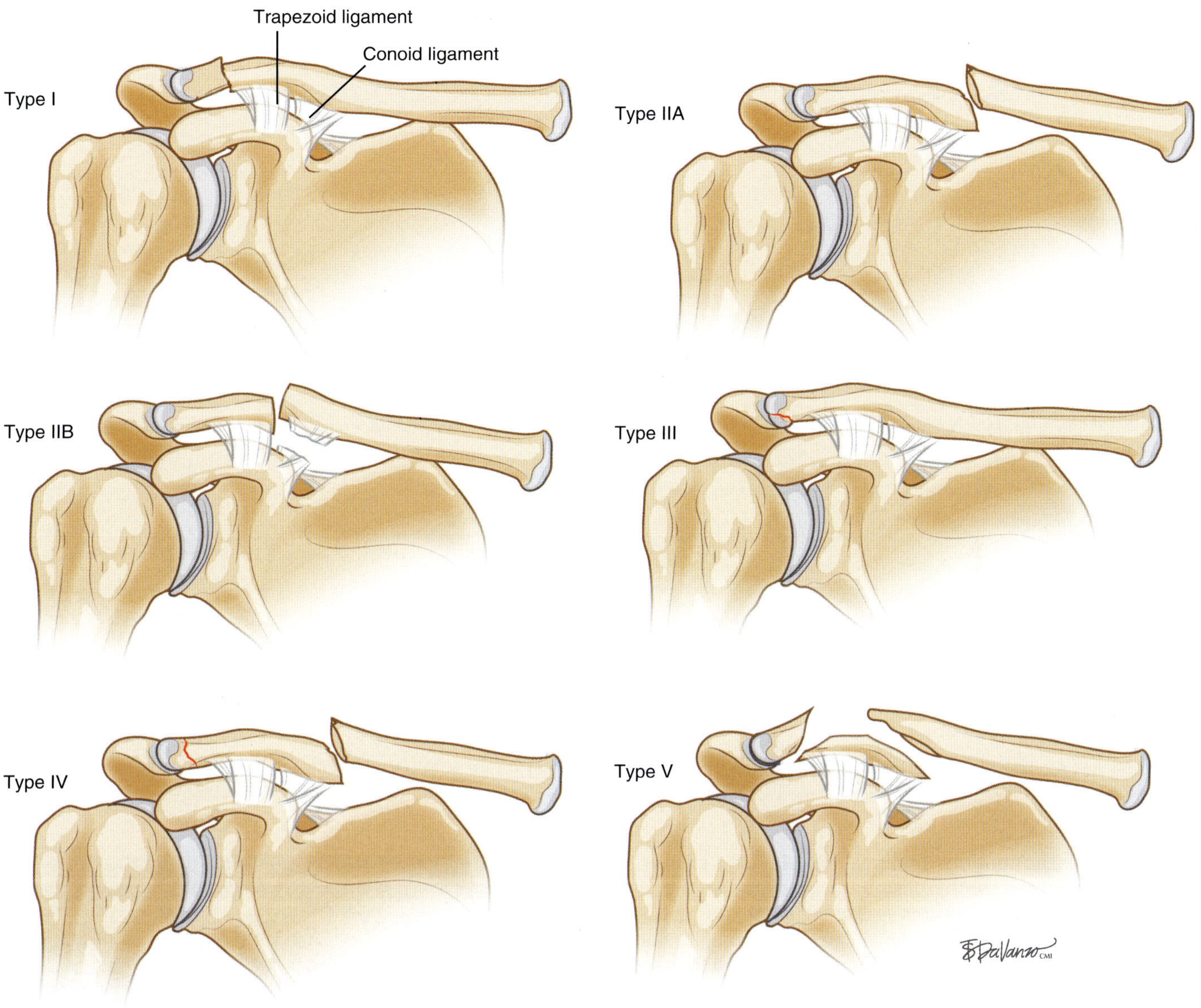

Fig. 13.3 Classification of distal clavicle fractures. (Adapted from Banerjee R, Waterman B, Padalecki J, Robertson W. Management of distal clavicle fractures. *J Am Acad Orthop Surg*. 2011;19(7):392-401.)

Direct comparisons of the various classification systems have shown the Craig classification system as most prognostic when predicting delayed or nonunion of lateral-third fractures (O'Neill et al, 2011). An investigation using shoulder fellowship–trained observers demonstrated overall fair agreement for the Neer classification but only slight agreement for the type IIB pattern, which is thought to be the most important determining factor for surgery (Bishop et al, 2015). Although complex, the Edinburgh classification has been shown to be most prognostic for middle-third fracture patterns and has demonstrated satisfactory levels of both inter- and intra-observer reliability testing (O'Neill et al, 2011; Robinson, 1998).

Assessment

Clinical assessment should follow a systematic approach when evaluating an injured athlete, adhering to the trauma principles of airway, breathing, and circulation (ABC's) and cervical spine precautions. In situations of high-energy trauma in contact sports, a complete examination should be performed to avoid missing associated injuries. In addition to midshaft clavicle injuries; fracture-dislocations of the SC and AC joints; or (in younger patients), physeal injuries may be present. Associated chest wall, scapular, or intrathoracic injuries including a pneumothorax or hemothorax rarely occur and require further investigation. In posteriorly displaced SC joint injuries, patients should be examined for evidence of dyspnea, dysphagia, tachypnea, and stridor. Injury to the subclavian vessels may manifest as an expanding hematoma at the fracture site (Kim & McKee, 2008). Although exceedingly rare in athletic trauma, injuries to the brachial plexus may manifest with ulnar nerve dysfunction because of its immediate location adjacent to the middle third of the clavicle. A thorough neurologic examination of the shoulder and the upper extremity should always be performed and documented.

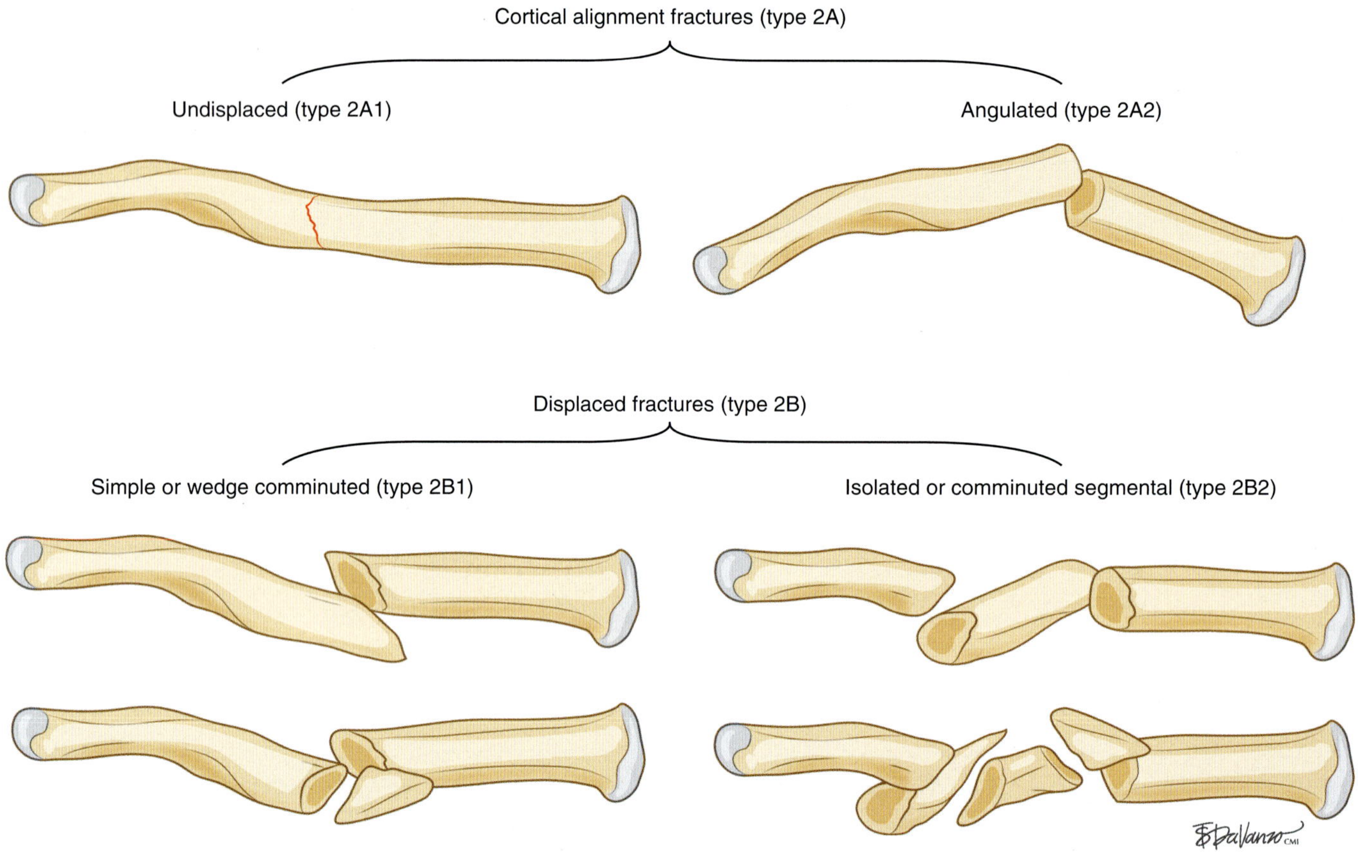

Fig. 13.4 **Robinson classification of midshaft clavicle fractures (type 2).** (Adapted from Robinson CM. Fractures of the clavicle in the adult. Epidemiology and classification. *J Bone Joint Surg Br.* 1998;80:476-484.)

Physical examination findings of clavicle fractures include tenderness, ecchymosis, and swelling at the site of injury. Displaced fractures are often associated with a painful bony prominence under the skin with crepitus and motion at the fracture site. Displaced lateral-third fractures may have an appearance similar to that of a high-grade AC joint separation. Prolonged skin tenting may lead to skin necrosis and a secondarily open fracture and requires expedited care.

The ipsilateral shoulder may demonstrate an asymmetric appearance with a typical droop or "ptosis" with associated scapular anterior rotation or winging and a shortened (McKee, 2006; Simpson & Jupiter, 1996). Shortening of the clavicle can be measured clinically with a tape measure. The distance measured from a mark at the midline of the suprasternal notch to the palpable ridge of the AC joint is compared with the contralateral side.

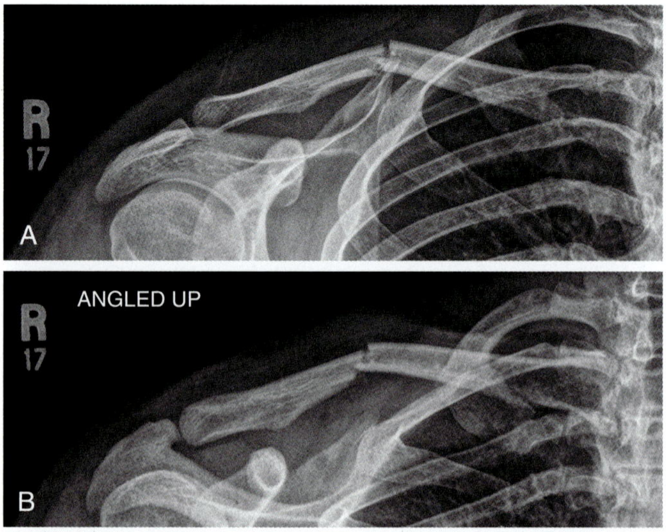

Fig. 13.5 Standard anteroposterior (**A**) and 45-degree cephalic tilt (**B**) radiographs of the clavicle demonstrating a midshaft clavicle fracture.

Imaging

Evaluation of an isolated clavicle injury begins with routine radiographs including a standard anteroposterior (AP) and 45-degree cephalic tilt film of the clavicle (Fig. 13.5). The AP view should evaluate the full length of the clavicle and include both the SC and AC joints. The 45-degree cephalic tilt film profiles the clavicle superior to the thorax and rib cage and may further help delineate fracture displacement, comminution, and angulation. Displacement without bony contact, particularly in transversely displaced fragments, and fracture shortening are associated with an increased incidence of non-union, delayed union, and symptomatic malunion with lower outcome scores after nonoperative treatment (Canadian Orthopaedic Trauma Society et al, 2007; Hill et al, 1997; Nowak et al, 2004, Robinson et al, 2004). The risk of symptomatic malunion, non-union, and functional limitations has been associated with overall fracture displacement greater than 1.5 cm (Eskola et al, 1986;

Robinson et al, 2004; Wick et al, 2001). This fracture displacement encompasses total shortening, distraction, and separation between the main fragments in any radiographic view.

Although shortening is considered a critical parameter in clinical decision making for midshaft fractures, no standardized method of radiographic measurement exists. Described techniques include standard 45-degree tilted radiographs, 20-degree uptilted AP panorama view, standard posteroanterior thorax view, and abduction lordosis view (Pandya et al, 2012). Comparative computed tomography (CT) scanning and posteroanterior thorax radiographs that show both clavicles may be helpful (Smekal et al, 2008). In addition, evidence suggest that plain unilateral radiographs are unreliable for determining critical shortening values of 1 to 2 cm, even among shoulder or sports medicine fellowship–trained orthopedic surgeons (Jones et al, 2014). Therefore additional views such as a posteroanterior chest radiograph for determining length of the contralateral clavicle or caudad views at varying angles may be beneficial (Jones et al, 2014). Although less commonly used than plain radiography, CT allows a three-dimensional reconstruction of the clavicle to evaluate total length, shortening, and comminution (Pandya et al, 2012). Benefits of CT visualization in midshaft fractures are weighted against cost, availability, and increased radiation exposure. In any event, radiographs should be used in combination with a careful clinical length measurement to aid in surgical decision making.

For injuries involving the medial third of the clavicle, the serendipity view has a 40-degree cephalic tilt directed at the SC joints, allowing comparison of both SC joints. The lateral fragment tends to sag with the weight of the arm while the medial fragment attached to the SC joint appears superiorly. The interpretation of medial clavicle fracture displacement using plain radiographs is often challenging, and CT is the preferred modality. Axial CT imaging allows visualization of bilateral SC joints and can delineate fracture displacement and the proximity of close neurovascular structures for surgical planning. CT scan can also differentiate medial physeal separations from true SC joint dislocations, which may have treatment and prognosis implications.

In lateral clavicle fractures, the Zanca view is centered over the AC joint with a 10- to 20-degree cephalic tilt and can be helpful in evaluating displacement and intraarticular involvement (Zanca, 1971). A single radiograph of bilateral clavicles including the AC joints can also be useful in assessing the overall fracture pattern and displacement. In high-energy sports injuries, radiographic assessment should include routine views of the shoulder girdle to identify associated scapular or glenoid fractures. An axillary view is particularly useful in identifying subtle injuries of the distal clavicle including posterior displacement.

Nonoperative Treatment

The goal of treatment is to restore shoulder function to the preinjury level as quickly as possible while avoiding long-term sequelae such as symptomatic malunion or non-union of the clavicle. Treatment recommendations rely heavily on patient-specific factors, including athlete age, type of sport, position, competitive level, future aspirations, and perceptions of surgical fixation. In general, nonoperative management is advocated for non- or minimally displaced fractures and most displaced fractures in adolescent athletes. Operative fixation is reserved for open or impending open fractures; those with associated neurovascular injuries; and more commonly, significantly displaced or comminuted fractures (Jeray, 2007; Kim & McKee, 2008; Pandya et al, 2012; van der Meijden et al, 2012). Varying degrees of clavicular shortening, displacement, and comminution have been associated with poorer functional outcomes and there is considerable debate on the degree of clavicle shortening required; ranging from >15 to >23 mm (Canadian Orthopaedic Trauma Society 2007; Hill et al, 1997; Jones et al, 2014; Lazarides & Zafiropoulos, 2006; Robinson et al, 2004; Zlowodzki et al, 2005). In addition, these data describe outcomes of the adult general population, and results must be extrapolated to competitive athletes in whom a variety of other patient-specific factors must be considered.

Nonoperative treatment consists of a period of rest, shoulder sling immobilization for 2 to 6 weeks, and early use of analgesia and cryotherapy. The athlete should avoid resisted or strength exercises on the affected extremity during this period but can begin shoulder range of motion (ROM) pendulum exercises in addition to hand, wrist, and elbow training. Passive and active shoulder elevation beyond 90 degrees should be avoided. Cardiovascular exercises such as stationary bicycle may be permitted to maintain fitness. After 4 to 6 weeks, graduated active-assisted motion within the scapular plane can begin progressing to full motion, and shoulder and periscapular isometric strengthening is initiated. Progressive strengthening and weight training may begin after radiographic and clinical union at approximately 6 to 10 weeks postinjury. Athletes may return to sport after full shoulder ROM and strength have been achieved, which is typically 0 to 6 weeks after clinical and radiographic healing has occurred. Therefore, the total missed playing time is approximately 6 to 12 weeks, depending on shoulder motion and strength, sport type, athlete confidence and comfort, and level of competition (Meisterling et al, 2013). In pediatric and adolescent athletes, this schedule may be accelerated with a briefer period of immobilization of 2 to 4 weeks followed by early ROM and strengthening and return to sport at 6 to 8 weeks postinjury (Bishop et al, 2005).

Questions remain concerning the optimal type and length of shoulder immobilization, but no superior results beyond a simple arm sling have been demonstrated (Lenza et al, 2009). When comparing evidence for figure-of-8 bracing versus arm sling, a Cochrane review failed to identify any benefits in healing time, fracture reduction, or function. The only statistically significant findings were higher pain scores for figure-of-8 bracing at 15 days and increased patient dissatisfaction (27% vs 7%) (Lenza et al, 2009). Additional modalities, including ultrasound and shockwave therapy, may be instituted, but no empirical evidence currently supports any advantages in clinical fracture healing, return to normal daily function, and return to sport for midshaft clavicle fractures (Griffin et al, 2014; Lubbert et al, 2008).

The literature regarding return to sport for the nonoperative treatment of clavicle fractures is sparse. In general, satisfactory outcomes can be achieved for non- or minimally displaced fractures in adults and some displaced fractures in adolescent athletes. Six NFL players with non- or minimally displaced clavicle fractures healed at an average time of 7.3 weeks (range, 6–8 weeks), but only a single player was able to return to play in the same season (the other 5 were placed on the injury reserve) (Morgan et al, 2010). All players progressed to radiographic union, and no subsequent sequelae were reported from these clavicle fractures. In this study, patients with displaced fractures did not do as well with nonoperative treatment, and there was a high refracture rate.

In adolescent athletes with midshaft clavicle injuries, fracture shortening and displacement have been shown not to have a significant impact on functional outcomes and sports participation (Robinson et al, 2015; Schulz et al, 2013). A review of 22 athletes ages 10 to 17 years with displaced midshaft fractures with an average radiographic shortening of 11.2 mm ± 6 mm failed to demonstrate any objective differences in ROM and strength between the injured and uninjured arms (Robinson et al, 2015). All patients went on to fracture union, of whom 15 participants were contact or overhead athletes, and the average time for return to competitive sport was 3.8 months. A similar investigation reported 16 adolescent patients ages 10 to 18 with displaced midshaft clavicle fractures with average shortening of 13.75 mm (Schulz et al, 2013). All patients achieved radiographic union, and all athletes returned to sport at the same level or higher and no differences in pain, strength, shoulder ROM, and subjective outcomes scores were identified. However, there is evidence that some adolescents with displaced fractures treated nonoperatively can develop non-union and symptomatic malunion, and operative intervention has been recommended in certain cases (Mehlman et al, 2009). Further prospective research is needed in this area.

Outcomes

Traditionally, nonoperative management was advocated for the treatment of most midshaft clavicle fractures (Neer, 1960; Rowe et al, 1968). However, more recent evidence suggests that a subgroup of displaced fractures treated nonoperatively have higher rates of nonunion and symptomatic malunion (Eskola et al, 1986; Hill et al, 1997; Kirmani et al, 2009; Lazarides & Zafiropoulos, 2006; Ledger et al, 2005; McKee et al, 1999; Nowak et al, 2004; Postacchini et al, 2010; Robinson, 1998; Robinson et al, 2004). Fracture displacement and comminution, particularly initial clavicle shortening of greater than 15 to 23 mm, has been associated with nonunion and unsatisfactory functional outcomes (Canadian Orthopaedic Trauma Society, 2007; Hill et al, 1997; Jones et al, 2014; Lazarides & Zafiropoulos, 2006; Robinson et al, 2004; Zlowodzki et al, 2005). In addition, recent clinical studies directly comparing operative versus nonoperative management for the treatment of displaced midshaft clavicle fractures have demonstrated improved functional outcomes with rigid plate fixation (Althausen et al, 2013; Canadian Orthopaedic Trauma Society, 2007; Judd et al, 2009; Kulshrestha et al, 2011; McKee et al, 2012; Mirzatolooei, 2011; Virtanen et al, 2012). However, the clinical advantages of plate fixation have been reported primarily in the general population, and there is a deficiency in studies evaluating the subgroup of athletes and the optimal time for return to sport.

In the first large series of 39 semiprofessional athletes who underwent plate fixation, radiographic union was achieved in 90% of athletes after 12 weeks, and 75% were very satisfied with their outcome (Verborgt et al, 2005). The ages of the athletes ranged from 17 to 34 years and included mountain bike racers, soccer players, swimmers, and cyclists. However, a high complication rate was reported, including a 5% refracture rate, 18% wound infections, and 75% transient neurologic symptoms. This study was also done before modern precontoured clavicular implants and plating techniques. More recently, a retrospective series of 29 athletes with displaced midshaft clavicle fractures reported all patients being able to return to sport after plate fixation, minimal disability, and a 100% patient satisfaction rate (Meisterling et al, 2013). The mean fracture displacement was 20 mm, ranging from 8 to 35 mm. The most common sport in the study was American football (11 of 30 fractures), and 67% of athletes were able to return to sport 12 weeks or less after surgery and 23% after 6 weeks or less. No refracture, loss of fixation, or non-union was reported, and only four minor complications occurred. The largest series reported on 54 athletes with displaced midshaft fractures with a mean age of 30.1 years and an average follow-up time of 22 months (Ranalletta et al, 2015). All athletes were able to return to sport with 94% returning to the same level, 74% returning after 6 and 12 weeks postsurgery, and 16.6% returning less than 6 weeks postsurgery. Excellent functional outcome scores were demonstrated and found to be independent of sport type (collision and noncollision) and level of competition (competitive and recreational) before surgery. The authors reported three major complications: one extrinsic compression of the subclavian vein, one nonunion, and one hardware loosening requiring revision.

Although most displaced adolescent clavicle fractures can be managed nonoperatively, emerging evidence supports excellent functional outcomes and return to sport with surgical treatment. In a retrospective review of 14 skeletally immature patients with displaced midshaft clavicle fractures and a mean age of 12.9 years, all fractures healed, and the mean postoperative quickDASH (Disabilities of the Arm, Shoulder and Hand) score was 7.0 (Namdari et al, 2011). However, 4 patients required a second procedure for hardware removal, and 8 had complaints of paresthesia at the surgical site. Similarly, a series of 19 adolescent patients with displaced midshaft injuries treated with plate fixation demonstrated excellent functional outcomes with 100% union rate at 3 months (Hosalkar et al, 2012). The mean age was 14.6 years, and all patients returned to full athletics at a mean time of 14 weeks (range, 12–17). No major complications were reported, and only a single patient had subsequent hardware removal. A retrospective review comparing operative versus nonoperative treatment in 42 adolescent patients reported a mean time for radiographic union of 8.7 weeks in the nonoperative group ($n = 25$) and 7.4 weeks in the operative group ($n = 17$) (Vander Have et al, 2010). The mean time for return to physical activities was 16 weeks in the nonoperative group compared with 12 weeks in the operative group. Symptomatic malunion occurred in 5 patients treated conservatively of whom 4 required corrective osteotomy and fixation. Many authors now advocate surgical treatment for adolescent athletes with completely displaced midshaft fractures with no cortical contact or a Z-shaped fracture pattern (Fanter et al, 2015; Pandya et al, 2012).

In elite contact and professional athletes, the threshold for undergoing operative fixation may be significantly less than compared with that of amateur or recreational athletes. For instance, when 7 NFL players with completely displaced clavicle fractures were treated nonoperatively, 4 players sustained a refracture within 1 year of the initial injury (Morgan et al, 2010). Two of these players were then treated with plate fixation and the remaining 2 conservatively. The average time lost from competition for the 4 players who sustained refracture was 1.5 seasons, and 3 of 4 players missed the entire subsequent season. Cadaveric investigations have demonstrated that clavicular deformity may lead to abnormal biomechanical stresses across the shoulder girdle providing the mechanical rationale for anatomic reduction in mitigating long-term disability (Andermahr et al, 2006; Hillen et al, 2012; Matsumura et al, 2010). Malunion may also affect the ability of the clavicle to resist axial loads, thereby lowering the critical force required for refracture. Therefore the authors recommended acute surgical management for all displaced or comminuted midshaft fractures in NFL players, which allows safe return to play at the earliest possible time while minimizing missed playing time.

In general, operative fixation provides the advantage of earlier return to play compared with nonoperative management. Although time to return is highly variable depending on sport type and patient factors, most athletes are able to return 6 weeks or less from clinical and radiographic union compared with a minimal of 6 to 12 weeks from the time of injury for nonoperative treatment (Kaplan et al, 2005; Meisterling et al, 2013; Morgan et al, 2010; Ranalletta et al, 2015). Persistent motion at the fracture site is often associated with significant pain during the first 6 weeks of nonoperative management, resulting in an inability to return to play and limitations in physical training.

The use of elastic intramedullary nailing (EIN) in athletes with midshaft clavicle fractures has also been reported. In a series of 12 high-performance athletes, the mean time to return to physical training was 5.9 days, and the mean time for return to competition was only 16.8 days (Jubel et al, 2003). Only simple transverse and oblique fracture patterns were included, and half (6 patients) were treated successfully with closed reduction and nail insertion. Excellent functional scores and no complications were reported, but all athletes required a subsequent surgery for hardware removal at a mean of 7.2 months. A similar report of 14 athletes treated with EIN for midshaft fractures described excellent functional results with early return to normal function and a loss of reduction in a single patient (Meier et al, 2006). However, other studies have reported more significant complications with elastic nailing. In a retrospective series of 34 patients who underwent intramedullary fixation, 70% experienced complications, including cortex perforation, nail breakage, nail dislocation, and hardware irritation (Frigg et al, 2009). An open reduction was required in 62% of the patients, and the reoperation rate was 36%. In addition, biomechanical testing has demonstrated superior resistance to cyclical loading in rigid plate fixation compared with intramedullary devices (Golish et al, 2008). Therefore plate fixation may provide a stronger construct, allowing for early rehabilitation protocols in overhead and contact athletes. Additionally, at the present time, the literature suggests that EIN should be reserved for stable fracture patterns (transverse, short oblique) where excessive shortening is not a concern.

References

Allman FL Jr. Fractures and ligamentous injuries of the clavicle and its articulation. *J Bone Joint Surg Am*. 1967;49:774–784.

Althausen PL, Shannon S, Minggen L, O'Mara TJ, Bray TJ. Clinical and financial comparison of operative and nonoperative treatment of displaced clavicle fractures. *J Shoulder Elbow Surg*. 2013;22:608–611.

Andermahr J, Jubel A, Elsner A, et al. Malunion of the clavicle causes significant glenoid malposition: a quantitative anatomic investigation. *Surg Radiol Anat*. 2006;28(5):447–456.

Antabak A, Matković N, Papeš D, et al. Clavicle fractures in children-circumstances and causes of injury. *Lijec Vjesn*. 2015;137(5-6):163–167.

Banerjee R, Waterman B, Padalecki J, Robertson W. Management of distal clavicle fractures. *J Am Acad Orthop Surg*. 2011;19(7):392–401.

Basamania CJ. Claviculoplasty. *J Shoulder Elbow Surg*. 1999;8(5):540.

Bishop JY, Jones GL, Lewis B, Pedroza A. MOON Shoulder Group. Intra- and interobserver agreement in the classification and treatment of distal third clavicle fractures. *Am J Sports Med*. 2015;43(4):979–984.

Bishop JY, Flatow EL. Pediatric shoulder trauma. *Clin Orthop Relat Res*. 2005;432:41–48.

Bosch U, Skutek M, Peters G, et al. Extension osteotomy in malunited clavicular fractures. *J Shoulder Elbow Surg*. 1998;7(4):402–405.

Canadian Orthopaedic Trauma Society. Nonoperative treatment compared with plate fixation of displaced midshaft clavicular fractures. A multicenter, randomized clinical trial. *J Bone Joint Surg Am*. 2007;89(1):1–10.

Chan KY, Jupiter JB, Leffert RD, et al. Clavicle malunion. *J Shoulder Elbow Surg*. 1999;8(4):287–290.

Court-Brown CM, Wood AM, Aitken S. The epidemiology of acute sports-related fractures in adults. *Injury*. 2008;39:1365–1372.

Craig EV. Fractures of the clavicle. In: Rockwood CA, Green DP, eds. *Fractures in Adults*. vol. 1. 6th ed. Philadelphia: Lippincott Williams & Wilkins; 2006:1216–1217.

Eskola A, Vainionpää S, Myllynen P, Pätiälä H, Rokkanen P. Outcome of clavicular fracture in 89 patients. *Arch Orthop Trauma Surg*. 1986;105:337–338.

Fanter NJ, Kenny RM, Baker CL, Baker CL Jr. Surgical treatment of clavicle fractures in the adolescent athlete. *Sports Health*. 2015;7(2):137–141.

Frigg A, Rillmann P, Perren T, Gerber M, Ryf C. Intramedullary nailing of clavicular midshaft fractures with the titanium elastic nail: problems and complications. *Am J Sports Med*. 2009;37(2):352–359.

Fukuda K, Craig EV, An KN, Cofield RH, Chao EY. Biomechanical study of the ligamentous system of the acromioclavicular joint. *J Bone Joint Surg Am*. 1986;68(3):434–440.

Fung M, Kato S, Barrance PJ, et al. Scapular and clavicular kinematics during humeral elevations: a study with cadavers. *J Shoulder Elbow Surg*. 2001;10:278–285.

Gardner E. The embryology of the clavicle. *Clin Orthop*. 1968;58:9–16.

Gardner EC, Chan WW, Sutton KM, Blaine TA. Shoulder injuries in men's collegiate lacrosse, 2004-2009. *Am J Sports Med*. 2016.

Goldberg AS, Moroz L, Smith A, Ganley T. Injury surveillance in young athletes: a clinician's guide to sports injury literature. *Sports Med*. 2007;37(3):265–278.

Golish SR, Oliviero JA, Francke EI, Miller MD. A biomechanical study of plate versus intramedullary devices for midshaft clavicle fixation. *J Orthop Surg Res*. 2008;3:28.

Griffin XL, Parsons N, Costa ML, Metcalfe D. Ultrasound and shockwave therapy for acute fractures in adults. *Cochrane Database Syst Rev*. 2014;(6):CD008579.

Hill JM, McGuire MH, Crosby LA. Closed treatment of displaced middle-third fractures of the clavicle gives poor results. *J Bone Joint Surg Br*. 1997;79(4):537–539.

Hillen RJ, Burger BJ, Pöll RG, van Dijk CN, Veeger DH. The effect of experimental shortening of the clavicle on shoulder kinematics. *Clin Biomech (Bristol, Avon)*. 2012;27(8):777–781.

Hosalkar HS, Parikh G, Bomar JD, Bittersohl B. Open reduction and internal fixation of displaced clavicle fractures in adolescents. *Orthop Rev (Pavia)*. 2012;4:e1.

Jeray KJ. Acute midshaft clavicular fracture [review]. *J Am Acad Orthop Surg*. 2007;15(4):239–248. Erratum in *J Am Acad Orthop Surg*. 2007;15(7):26A.

Jit I, Kulkarni M. Times of appearance and fusion of epiphysis at the medial end of the clavicle. *Indian J Med Res*. 1976;64(5):773–782.

Jones GL, Bishop JY, Lewis B, Pedroza AD. MOON Shoulder Group. Intraobserver and interobserver agreement in the classification and treatment of midshaft clavicle fractures. *Am J Sports Med*. 2014;42(5):1176–1181.

Jubel A, Andemahr J, Bergmann H, Prokop A, Rehm KE. Elastic stable intramedullary nailing of midclavicular fractures in athletes. *Br J Sports Med*. 2003;37(6):480–483.

Judd DB, Pallis MP, Smith E, Bottoni CR. Acute operative stabilization versus nonoperative management of clavicle fractures. *Am J Orthop*. 2009;38:341–345.

Jupiter JB, Ring D. Fractures of the clavicle. In: Iannotti JP, Williams GR, eds. *Disorders of the Shoulder: Diagnosis and Management*. Philadelphia: Lippincott Williams & Wilkins; 1999:709–736.

Kaplan LD, Flanigan DC, Norwig J, Jost P, Bradley J. Prevalence and variance of shoulder injuries in elite collegiate football players. *Am J Sports Med*. 2005;33:1142–1146.

Kim W, McKee MD. Management of acute clavicle fractures. *Orthop Clin North Am*. 2008;39(4):491–505. vii.

Kirmani SJ, Pillai SKG, Madegowda BR, Shahane SA. Vertical fragment in adult midshaft clavicle fractures: an indicator for surgical intervention. *Orthopedics*. 2009;32(10). pii.

Kuhne JE. Symptomatic malunions of the middle clavicle [abstract]. *J Shoulder Elbow Surg*. 1999;8(5):539.

Kulshrestha V, Roy T, Audige L. Operative versus nonoperative management of displaced midshaft clavicle fractures: a prospective cohort study. *J Orthop Trauma*. 2011;25:31–38.

Landin LA. Fracture patterns in children: analysis of 8682 fractures with special reference to incidence, etiology, and secular changes in Swedish urban populations. *Acta Orthop Scand*. 1983;54(suppl):1–109.

Lazarides S, Zafiropoulos G. Conservative treatment of fractures at the middle third of the clavicle: the relevance of shortening and clinical outcome. *J Shoulder Elbow Surg*. 2006;15(2):191–194.

Lazarus MD. Fractures of the clavicle. In: Bucholz RW, Heckman JD, eds. *Rockwood and Green's Fractures in Adults*. 5th ed. Philadelphia: Lippincott Williams & Wilkins; 2002:1041–1078.

Ledger M, Leeks N, Ackland T, Wang A. Short malunions of the clavcle: an anatomic and functional study. *J Shoulder Elbow Surg*. 2005;14(4):349–354.

Lenza M, Belloti JC, Andriolo RB, Gomes Dos Santos JB, Faloppa F. Conservative interventions for treatment middle third clavicle fractures in adolescents and adults. *Cochrane Database Syst Rev*. 2009;2:CD007121.

Lewonowski K, Bassett GS. Complete posterior sternoclavicular epiphysealaration. A case report and review of the literature. *Clin Orthop*. 1992;281:84–88.

Lubbert PH, van der Rijt RH, Hoorntje LE, van der Werken C. Low-intensity pulsed ultrasound (LIPUS) in fresh clavicle fractures: a multi-centre double blind randomised controlled trial. *Injury*. 2008;39(12):1444–1452.

Ludewig PM, Behrens SA, Meyer SM, Spoden SM, Wilson LA. Three-dimensional clavicular motion during arm elevation: reliability and descriptive data. *J Orthop Sports Phys Ther*. 2004;34:140–149.

Matsumura N, Ikegami H, Nakamichi N, et al. Effect of shortening deformity of the clavicle on scapular kinematics: a cadaveric study. *Am J Sports Med*. 2010;38(5):1000–1006.

McKee MD, Schemitsch EH, Stephen DJ, Kreder HJ, Yoo D, Harrington J. Functional outcome following clavicle fractures in polytrauma patients. *J Trauma Acute Care Surg*. 1999;47:616.

McKee MD, Pedersen EM, Jones C, et al. Deficits following non-operative treatment of displaced, mid-shaft clavicle fractures. *J Bone Joint Surg Am*. 2006;88:35–40.

McKee RC, Whelan DB, Schemitsch EH, McKee MD. Operative versus non-operative care of displaced midshaft clavicular fractures: a meta-analysis of randomized clinical trials. *J Bone Joint Surg Am*. 2012;94(8):675–684.

Mehlman CT, Yihua G, Bochang C, Zhigang W. Operative treatment of completely displaced clavicle shaft fractures in children. *J Pediatr Orthop*. 2009;29(8):851–855.

Meier C, Grueninger P, Platz A. Elastic stable intramedullary nailing for midclavicular fractures in athletes: indications, technical pitfalls and early results. *Acta Orthop Belg*. 2006;72:269–275.

Meisterling SW, Cain EL, Fleisig GS, Hartzell JL, Dugas JR. Return to athletic activity after plate fixation of displaced midshaft clavicle fractures. *Am J Sports Med*. 2013;41(11):2632–2636.

Mirzatolooei F. Comparison between operative and nonoperative treatment methods in the management of comminuted fractures of the clavicle. *Acta Orthop Traumatol Turc*. 2011;45:34–40.

Morgan RJ, Bankston LS Jr, Hoenig MP, Connor PM. Evolving management of middle-third clavicle fractures in the National Football League. *Am J Sports Med*. 2010;38(10):2092–2096.

Murray IR, Foster CJ, Eros A, Robinson CM. Risk factors for nonunion after nonoperative treatment of displaced midshaft fractures of the clavicle. *J Bone Joint Surg Am*. 2013;95(13):1153–1158. 3.

Namdari S, Ganley TJ, Baldwin K, et al. Fixation of displaced midshaft clavicle fractures in skeletally immature patients. *J Pediatr Orthop*. 2011;31:507–511.

Neer CS II. Non-union of the clavicle. *JAMA*. 1960;172:1006–1011.

Neer CS II. Fractures and dislocations of the shoulder. In: Rockwood Jr CA, Green DP, eds. *Fractures in Adults*. Philadelphia: JB Lippincott; 1984:711–712.

Neer CS II. Fractures of the distal third of the clavicle. *Clin Orthop Relat Res*. 1968;58:43–50.

Neer CS II. Fracture of the distal clavicle with detachment of the coracoclavicular ligaments in adults. *J Trauma*. 1963. 399–110.

Nordqvist A, Petersson C. The incidence of fractures of the clavicle. *Clin Orthop Relat Res*. 1994;300:127–132.

Nowak J, Holgersson M, Larsson S. Can we predict long-term sequelae after fractures of the clavicle based on initial findings? A prospective study with nine to ten years of follow-up. *J Shoulder Elbow Surg*. 2004;13:479–486.

Nowak J, Mallmin H, Larsson S. The aetiology and epidemiology of clavicular fractures. A prospective study during a two-year period in Uppsala, Sweden. *Injury*. 2000;31:353–358.

Ogden JA, Conlogue GJ, Bronson ML. Radiology of postnatal skeletal development: III. The clavicle. *Skeletal Radiol*. 1979;4(4):196–203.

O'Neill BJ, Hirpara KM, O'Briain D, McGarr C, Kaar TK. Clavicle fractures: a comparison of five classification systems and their relationship to treatment outcomes. *Int Orthop*. 2011;35:909–914.

Pandya NK, Namdari S, Hosalkar HS. Displaced clavicle fractures in adolescents: facts, controversies, and current trends. *J Am Acad Orthop Surg*. 2012;20(8):498–505.

Postacchini F, Gumina S, De Santis P, et al. Epidemiology of clavicle fractures. *J Shoulder Elbow Surg*. 2002;11:454–456.

Postacchini R, Gumina S, Farsetti P, Postacchini F. Long-term results of conservative management of midshaft clavicle fracture. *Int Orthop*. 2010;34:731–736.

Ranalletta M, Rossi LA, Piuzzi NS, Bertona A, Bongiovanni SL, Maignon G. Return to sports after plate fixation of displaced midshaft clavicular fractures in athletes. *Am J Sports Med*. 2015;43(3):565–569.

Renfree KJ, Riley MK, Wheeler D, Hentz JG, Wright TW. Ligamentous anatomy of the distal clavicle. *J Shoulder Elbow Surg*. 2003;12(4):355–359.

Robinson CM. Fractures of the clavicle in the adult. Epidemiology and classification. *J Bone Joint Surg Br*. 1998;80:476–484.

Robinson CM, Court-Brown CM, McQueen MM, Wakefield AE. Estimating the risk of nonunion following nonoperative treatment of a clavicular fracture. *J Bone Joint Surg Am*. 2004;86(7):1359–1365.

Robinson L, Gargoum R, Auer R, Nyland J, Chan G. Sports participation and radiographic findings of adolescents treated nonoperatively for displaced clavicle fractures. *Injury*. 2015;46(7):1372–1376.

Rowe CR. An atlas of anatomy and treatment of midclavicular fractures. *Clin Orthop Relat Res*. 1968;58:29–42.

Rumball KM, Da Silva VF, Preston DN, et al. Brachial plexus injury after clavicular fracture: case report and literature review. *Can J Surg*. 1991;34:264–266.

Schulz J, Moor M, Roocroft J, Bastrom TP, Pennock AT. Functional and radiographic outcomes of nonoperative treatment of displaced adolescent clavicle fractures. *J Bone Joint Surg Am*. 2013;95(13):1159–1165. 3.

Simpson NS, Jupiter JB. Clavicular nonunion and malunion: evaluation and surgical management. *J Am Acad Orthop Surg*. 1996;4:1–8.

Smekal V, Deml C, Irenberger A, et al. Length determination in midshaft clavicle fractures: validation of measurement. *J Orthop Trauma*. 2008;22(7):458–462.

Stanley D, Trowbridge EA, Norris SH. The mechanism of clavicular fracture: a clinical and biomechanical analysis. *J Bone Joint Surg Br.* 1988;70:461–464.

Swenson DM, Henke NM, Collins CL, Fields SK, Comstock RD. Epidemiology of United States high school sports-related fractures, 2008-09 to 2010-11. *Am J Sports Med.* 2012;40(9):2078–2084.

Vander Have KL, Perdue AM, Caird MS, Farley FA. Operative versus nonoperative treatment of midshaft clavicle fractures in adolescents. *J Pediatr Orthop.* 2010;30:307–312.

Van Tassel D, Owens BD, Pointer L, Moriatis Wolf J. Incidence of clavicle fractures in sports: analysis of the NEISS Database. *Int J Sports Med.* 2014;35(1):83–86.

van der Meijden OA, Gaskill TR, Millett PJ. Treatment of clavicle fractures: current concepts review. *J Shoulder Elbow Surg.* 2012;21(3):423–429.

Verborgt O, Pittoors K, Van Glabbeek F, Lercq G, Nuyts R, Somville J. Plate fixation of middle-third fractures of the clavicle in the semi-professional athlete. *Acta Orthop Belg.* 2005;71:17–21.

Virtanen KJ, Remes V, Pajarinen J, Savolainen V, Bjorkenheim JM, Paavola M. Sling compared with plate osteosynthesis for treatment of displaced midshaft clavicle fractures: a randomized clinical trial. *J Bone Joint Surg Am.* 2012;94:1546–1553.

Wick M, Müller EJ, Kollig E, Muhr G. Midshaft fractures of the clavicle with a shortening of more than 2 cm predispose to nonunion. *Arch Orthop Trauma Surg.* 2001;121:207–211.

Zanca P. Shoulder pain: involvement of the acromioclavicular joint: analysis of 1,000 cases. *Am J Roentgenol Radium Ther Nucl Med.* 1971;112(3):493–506.

Zlowodzki M, Zelle BA, Cole PA, Jeray K, McKee MD. Treatment of acute midshaft clavicle fractures: systematic review of 2144 fractures. *J Orthop Trauma.* 2005;19(7):504–508.

14 Surgical Treatment Options: Mid-Shaft Fracture

14-14A PERCUTANEOUS PINNING

CONNOR G. ZIEGLER, MD and ROBERT A. ARCIERO, MD

This chapter is adapted from Basamania CJ, Rockwood CA Jr. Fractures of the clavicle. In: Rockwood CA Jr, Matsen FA, Wirth MA, Lippitt SB, Fehringer EV, Sperling JW, eds. *Rockwood and Matsen's The Shoulder*. 5th ed. Philadelphia: Elsevier; 2017.

Introduction

Intramedullary (IM) pinning of clavicle fractures is a long-practiced technique with reported advantages over plate fixation, including reduced periosteal stripping, smaller skin incision, less risk to supraclavicular nerves, less bleeding, shorter surgical times, and healing via endochondral ossification (callus), which can be more easily assessed radiographically than direct bone healing (intramembranous ossification). A recent meta-analysis reported that IM fixation of midshaft clavicle fractures could achieve similar union rates and shoulder scores with superior surgical outcomes including significantly less time to union than plate fixation (Gao et al, 2016). These findings remained constant when conducting subanalyses in only randomized controlled trials (RCTs). Significantly less blood loss, shorter operative time, smaller surgical wounds, and fewer complications in the IM group were also reported (Gao et al, 2016).

Many surgeons may be reluctant to use IM clavicle fixation given past reports of major complications and perceived risk of pin migration. Randomized studies and a recent meta-analysis have reported both similar complication rates, as well as significantly lower overall and major complications with IM pinning versus plate fixation (Ferran et al, 2010; Gao et al, 2016; Liu et al, 2010). Nevertheless, there are numerous reports of IM device migration in clavicle fixation (Kettler et al, 2007; Lyons & Rockwood, 1990; Meier et al, 2006; Mueller et al, 2007; Wijdicks et al, 2013). Skin and soft tissue irritation resulting from migration, telescoping, or hardware protrusion represents one of the chief complications with IM fixation (Grassi et al, 2001; Strauss et al, 2007; Wijdicks et al, 2013). The dilemma of IM fixation, unlike plate fixation, is that nail removal is often intended after the fracture has healed. The challenge with this is that the device needs to have a low profile so it does not cause irritation, but it must be prominent enough to be easily retrieved. Unlike plate and screw constructs, IM fixation can be removed under light sedation and local anesthesia. With current techniques and implants, IM devices are reported to have a low rate of unplanned revision surgery and to be a safe and effective form of fixation (Gao et al, 2016; Millett et al, 2011).

Construct rigidity is a concern particularly when treating contact athletes who are at risk for refracture. In the setting of comminution, the cantilever effect for a pin extends to the medial-most portion of the pin, thereby providing fixation in bending loads. It also allows axial compression, which should enhance healing. However, Golish et al (2008) reported superior biomechanics to bending and torsional forces with plate versus IM fixation in a cadaveric midshaft clavicle fracture model (Golish et al, 2008). In contrast, Smith et al (2014) reported that failure torques of IM repair and plate repair were not significantly different; however, failure torque after IM device removal was significantly greater than after plate removal (Smith et al, 2014). Nevertheless, IM pinning is a viable fixation option in athletes, particularly considering recent data that suggest shorter time to union and lower rate of complications.

Management

The management of midshaft clavicle fractures should be individualized to the patient's goals and activity level. The primary surgical indications for open reduction internal fixation of midshaft clavicle fractures include shortening greater than 2 cm, 100% or greater fracture displacement, and fracture comminution (Canadian Orthopaedic Trauma Society, 2007). In athletes, prolonged recovery and deficit in shoulder strength are often poorly tolerated, making surgery the typically preferred treatment. For most midshaft fractures that do not have excessive comminution or obliquity to the fracture planes, IM fixation is an excellent option to minimize fragment stripping, avoid supraclavicular nerves, achieve relative stability, and improve cosmesis. Complex, comminuted fractures, however, are not appropriate for IM nailing, with reported difficulties achieving and securing accurate reduction (Meier et al, 2006; Verborgt et al, 2005). In such cases, surgeons should consider plate fixation. The primary IM options include smooth, threaded, and partially threaded devices. These can be rigid or flexible and, in the case of hybrid fixation, can have flexible and rigid components. Despite having less risk of migration than smooth devices, fully threaded devices are seldom used because of the risk of gapping at the fracture site, which can impede healing (Grassi et al, 2001). There are numerous reports of migration of smooth devices used in clavicle fixation (Lyons & Rockwood, 1990). If these devices are used, they need to be followed closely for any radiographic signs of migration. Although smooth pin fixation has declined in popularity, the use of smooth titanium elastic nails (TENs) gained popularity in the 2000s in treating clavicle fractures (Jubel et al, 2003, 2005; Kettler et al, 2007; Meier et al, 2006; Walz et al, 2006). One of the primary advantages in using a flexible nail is that it allows considerable length of fixation as compared with a rigid device. Despite this, there remains the risk of implant migration, and some studies show a rate of loosening or migration of 4% to 25% (Kettler et al, 2007; Meier et al, 2006; Mueller et al, 2007). The addition of a hybrid fixation has alleviated many of the problems associated with IM pinning with improved length and rotational control over other IM devices and the ability to place an interlocking screw for increased rigidity and rotational control (Leroux et al, 2014; Zehir et al, 2015).

Two important determinants of IM fixation are the diameter of the IM canal and the length of fixation. The IM canal determines the maximum size of the device. For the pin to travel the most effective length, it makes three-point contact with the walls of the canal: anterolaterally, then posteriorly at the apex of the posterior curve, and then again anteromedially when it contacts the anteromedial curve. An important relationship exists with a larger diameter IM fixation, whether it is a screw, pin, or smooth wire; namely, it will be stiffer but potentially allow less fixation length. There will also be greater stresses with short fixation, which could lead to increased risk of loosening, failure of the fixation, and healing. Significantly increased length of fixation with significantly more fixation in the lateral fragment has been reported using a 3.2-mm pin compared with a 4.0-mm pin (Harnroongroj et al, 2000). Another consideration in the diameter of pin fixation is that pin stiffness is directly proportional to the fourth power of the pin radius ($I = \pi r^4/4$). In other words, as the pin becomes larger, its stiffness increases considerably. Some micromotion is preferred to enhance endochondral bone formation. If the pin is too large, it will be excessively stiff, which may inhibit bone healing. Therefore the surgeon should pick the smallest pin that has stable fixation within the bone. In our experience, most midshaft clavicle fractures in female patients can be stabilized with a 2.5-mm pin, and most male patients receive a 3-mm pin. Seldom do we use a larger pin except in very large patients or in older patients who have age-related increases in their canal diameters. Because the clavicle has very little soft tissue coverage, any type of IM fixation that protrudes from the bone can cause soft tissue problems. It is imperative that the portion of any IM device outside of the bone have the lowest profile possible.

Another point to consider with IM pinning is that these devices frequently cannot be statically locked, thereby providing less rotational and length stability compared with other fixation techniques (Andermahr et al, 2007; Golish et al, 2008; Thumroj et al, 2005). However, there are implants now on the market that have an interlocking screw feature. Achieving good IM fit, typically achievable with a 3.0-mm pin, is desirable.

Surgical Technique: Intramedullary Nailing

The advantage of this technique is restoring length, alignment, and rotation with minimal soft tissue stripping, minimal blood loss, and small incisions. The IM device allows compression at the fracture site and load sharing, which are advantageous in the healing of other long-bone fractures. All cases are performed in an outpatient setting under general anesthesia with local anesthesia supplementation.

Patient Positioning

The procedure can be performed in a supine or modified beach-chair position on a radiolucent operating table. We prefer the modified beach-chair position for easier access to the posterior aspect of the shoulder. The torso of the patient is typically at about 45 degrees relative to the floor. A bump is placed under the ipsilateral scapula to help extend the arm and reduce scapula protraction. A large C-arm greatly facilitates pin placement. The C-arm base is brought in from the injured side (Fig. 14A.1). Standard prep and draping is performed, being mindful to include the entire shoulder girdle in the operative field all the way to the sternum. The arm should also be draped free, allowing movement of the arm to facilitate drilling of the lateral fragment and reduction of the fracture.

Intraoperative Imaging

The patient's torso should be approximately 45 degrees relative to the floor. The gantry of the C-arm should be situated such that the beam of the x-ray is parallel to the floor (see Fig. 14A.1). This gives the equivalent of a 45-degree cephalic tilt view of the medial clavicle, which allows the best view of the anterior curve of the clavicle. This orientation also gives a cephalic tilt view of the lateral fragment because placement of a retrograde IM fixation in the lateral fragment is crucial to obtaining anatomic reduction of the fracture. Furthermore, an "anteroposterior (AP) equivalent" view (Fig. 14A.2, *A*) can be obtained by extending the arm, and an "axillary equivalent" view can be obtained by forward flexing the arm (Fig. 14A.2, *B*). It should be noted that plain AP radiographs typically underestimate the length of the fracture because the clavicle is oblique to the x-ray beam.

Because of metallic or radiopaque devices on the operative table, the beam of the C-arm may need to be oriented in a posterolateral to anteromedial orientation. In this situation, there may be significant underestimation of the length of the fracture or overlap of the fragments because the clavicle is obliquely oriented relative to the beam of the x-ray. This underestimation will be exaggerated if the C-arm is oriented in an oblique fashion relative to the torso. If necessary, the patient's shoulder can be brought forward to obtain a better estimation of the true fracture length. It is also important that the entire length of the clavicle can be

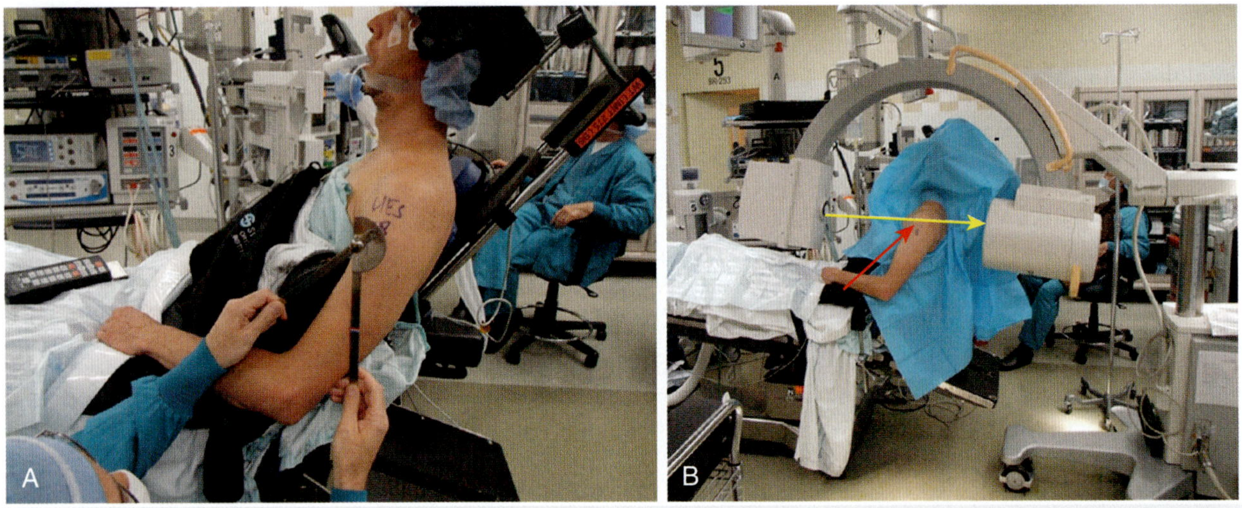

Fig. 14A.1 **A,** The patient is placed in the beach-chair position on the operating room table. **B,** The image intensifier is brought over the top of the patient and draped into the surgical field. The orientation of the image intensifier relative to the torso gives the equivalent of a 45-degree cephalic tilt view of the clavicle.

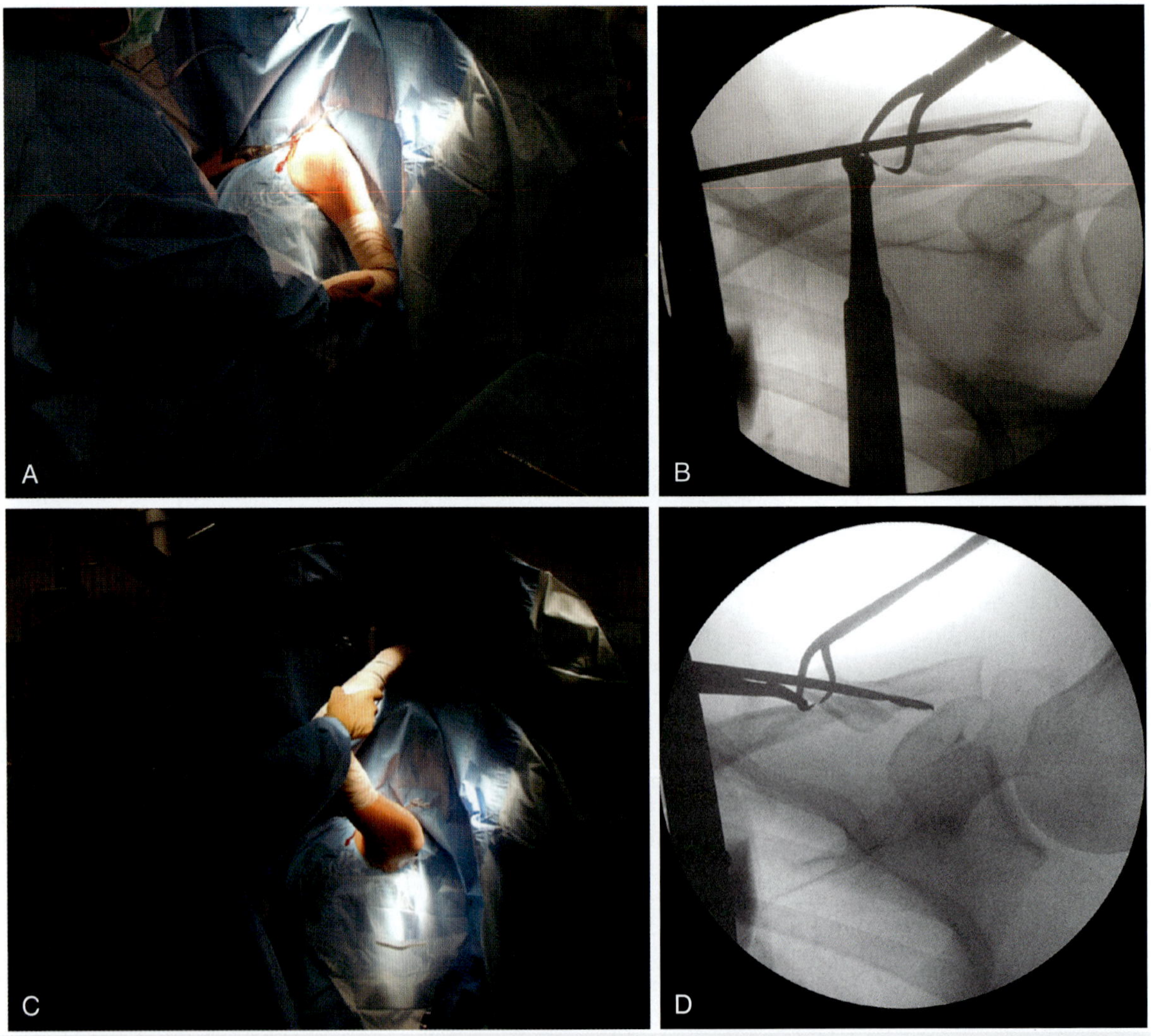

Fig. 14A.2 **A,** Extending the arm of the patient gives the equivalent of an anteroposterior view. **B,** C-arm image. Note the position of the drill bit relative to the equator of the clavicle. **C,** Forward flexing the arm gives the equivalent of a "near axillary" view. **D,** C-arm image. Note the exit point of the drill bit halfway between the conoid tubercle and the acromioclavicular joint.

viewed in one position. After these points are accomplished, the entire case can be completed with the use of a foot pedal to activate the C-arm, thereby negating the need to have a radiology technician. As mentioned, the patient's arm is draped free to allow movement during the case for better visualization and fracture reduction.

Surgical Method

A 2.5- to 3-cm incision is made in Langer lines over the palpable distal end of the medial fragment. The skin is more easily moved medially than laterally over the clavicle, and most patients have a skin crease in the same area where the incision is made, resulting in a more cosmetically pleasing scar. In fractures with a long oblique pattern, the incision is made slightly more medially and longer to allow elevation of the medial end of the distal fragment. The platysma muscle inserts on the skin near the clavicle, and damage to it may lead to dysfunction of facial expression. Scissors should be used to carefully free the platysma muscle from the overlying skin. Divide platysma muscle fibers longitudinally. Take care to prevent injury to the middle branch of the supraclavicular nerve, which is seen in approximately 50% of patients. It is usually found directly beneath the platysma muscle near the midportion of the clavicle. Injury to this nerve can cause dysesthesia in the anterior shoulder, deltoid, and anterior chest wall in 10% to 29% of cases (Mehta & Birch, 1997; Nathe et al, 2011). The incision should allow access to the less mobile lateral clavicle fragment, which is secured by the coracoclavicular ligaments and the more mobile medial fragment.

With acute fractures, the periosteum over the fracture site is disrupted and usually requires no further division. Any interposed soft tissue or hematoma should be carefully removed from the bone ends. Small butterfly fragments, usually found anteriorly and inferiorly, should be left attached to their soft tissue envelope. These can be cerclaged after primary fixation. The lateral end of the medial fragment is elevated into the incision. The medial medullary canal is identified with a 2-mm drill bit, which can be used to open the initial 1 to 2 cm of the canal. Palpating the medial aspect of the clavicle can help establish this orientation. The canal can be further opened with a 3.5-mm drill bit. Care must be taken to avoid penetration through the anteromedial cortex of the clavicle. Verify drill bit position periodically with fluoroscopy to assure the drill does not pass behind or inferior to the clavicle (see Fig. 14A.2) but attempt to keep fluoroscopy times to a minimum. When resistance is met, the drill bit is removed. A 3-mm awl can be used to further open the canal using a short back-and-forth motion but avoid a windshield wiper effect that can result in eccentric reaming. Advance the drill or awl as far past the fracture site as possible without undue force and without penetrating medially. A tap is then used to further open and prepare the canal.

Lateral Fragment Preparation

The lateral canal preparation can be somewhat more difficult, and proper placement is critical to the technique. The ideal exit point in the posterolateral clavicle is halfway between the conoid tubercle and the distal clavicle and at the equator of the clavicle. Although the exit point is at the equator in most patients, some patients may have an exaggerated downward lateral curve to their clavicle. In these cases, the exit point will be more superior; however, it should never be below the equator of the lateral clavicle because this will cause the distal fragment to be flexed upward relative to the medial fragment and may cause excessive rotation of the distal fragment relative to the medial fragment or problems passing the final fixation device past the spine of the scapula. Although it may seem daunting, it is similar to the importance of the piriformis fossa in intramedullary femoral nailing and can easily be achieved with proper drilling and C-arm use.

Locate the lateral fragment of the clavicle bone and maneuver the fragment to enable access to the medullary canal. Although good exposure is preferred, do not violate the coracoclavicular ligaments on the inferior border of the lateral third of the clavicle. If it is too difficult to access the canal because of the patient's head and neck, externally rotate the involved arm to bring the fragment into more of an AP orientation rather than a medial-lateral orientation. The medial end of the lateral fragment is usually located posterior and inferior to the lateral end of the medial fragment in most cases of lateral impact–mechanism fractures. In "seatbelt fractures," however, the medial end of the lateral fragment may be located anterior to the medial fragment. After the fragment is identified, it can be grasped with a towel clamp and carefully elevated into the incision. As with the medial fragment, a 2-mm drill is used to establish the orientation of the lateral canal. A 2-mm drill bit is used because the orientation can be changed without compromise of the canal. The orientation of the drill bit should be toward the mid-point of the posterior cortex of the lateral fragment. The surgeon can place the tip of his or her index finger at the "V" formed by the junction of the lateral clavicle and the spine of the scapula with the distal interphalangeal joint of his or her finger at the acromioclavicular (AC) joint and using this as an "aiming device." This orientation can be checked under fluoroscopy by extending the arm to allow more of an AP view of the distal fragment (see Fig. 14A.2, *A*). With this view, the drill bit should be aimed at the "equator" of the clavicle. After this orientation is established, the surgeon can forward-flex the arm to give more of an axillary view of the distal fragment (see Fig. 14A.2, *B*). With this view, the trajectory of the drill bit should be aimed toward the posterolateral cortex of the clavicle halfway between the conoid tubercle and the AC joint. The combination of these two aiming points represents the ideal exit point on the lateral fragment. Exiting too high may result in the fragments being flexed superiorly in relation to each other, and exiting too low can result in an apex inferior angulation. Exiting too far medially can cause an apex posterior angulation of the clavicle, and exiting too far laterally can result in an apex anterior angulation. After the orientation is verified, the canal is further opened with a 3.5-mm drill bit, which is passed through the posterolateral cortex. A small incision is then made over the palpable tip of the drill bit. The 3.5-mm drill bit is then removed, and the canal is tapped. Next, the clavicle pin is passed through the lateral fragment from medial to lateral and brought out through the posterior skin incision. The pin should exit just superior to the spine of the scapula.

Fracture Reduction and Final Fixation

After the clavicle pin is driven sufficiently out the posterolateral wound, the pin is unchucked, and the drill is reattached to the opposite (lateral) sharp end of the pin. With downward pressure on the medial fragment and upward force on the elbow to counteract the deformity caused by gravity, the pin can be advanced a short distance into the canal of the medial fragment, which will help temporarily hold the reduction. After reduction is verified under fluoroscopy, the pin is passed into the medial fragment and the reduction again checked with fluoroscopy. The fracture should be anatomically reduced. The final length of the pin can be estimated on fluoroscopy before cutting the pin. It is very important to check the diameters of the fragments after they are reduced. If the diameters are different, this means that there is a rotational deformity, which needs to be corrected. Loss of length caused by fracture comminution can also result in a discrepancy in fragment diameter. When satisfied with reduction, depending on the manufacturer, a locking or bolt mechanism used laterally on the pin can be placed. The pin is then cut flush with the locking mechanism, and any sharp edges are rasped flat. The pin is then advanced the remaining distance into the clavicle until it is seated in the medial-most aspect of the medial fragment with the lateral edge of the pin resting on the posterolateral clavicle cortex. In the case of a long oblique fracture, the fracture can be loosely held reduced with a small bone reduction clamp to prevent shortening of the fracture. In the case of significant comminution, the butterfly fragments can be provisionally fixed by passing #1 or 2 sutures around the clavicle and fragments to cerclage them together. Great care should be taken to keep the needle tip on bone when passing these sutures. If a longitudinal fracture is noted in the medial fragment, a cerclaged suture or wire can be passed around the clavicle to prevent fracture propagation. Fig. 14A.3 shows the preoperative and postoperative radiographs as well as clinical images of a typical case.

Postoperative Care

The patient's arm is placed in a sling for comfort and the sling may be removed as soon as he or she is comfortable and resumes simple activities of daily living. Restrictions are to refrain from lifting more than 10 lb with their operative hand; avoid repeated over-shoulder level motion to prevent excessive torque on the fixation; and cease all high-risk activities, including contact sports, for 6 weeks. They are seen back in the clinic 7 to 10 days postoperatively, and radiographs are taken at that time. A bilateral clavicle or Zanca view is helpful to compare symmetry, including clavicle-length restoration, with the contralateral side. The same weight-bearing restrictions are continued until the 6-week follow-up; however, the patient may begin full passive and active range of motion (ROM) and resume stationary bike training and running as tolerated in stable fracture patterns. Strengthening can begin at 4 weeks. In more comminuted and unstable fracture patterns, passive ROM while supine is initially started after the first postoperative visit, and active ROM can begin at 2 to 3 weeks postoperatively. If bridging callus is observed at 6 weeks and they are nontender at the fracture site, they are advanced to activities as tolerated. Weight and motion restrictions are continued for another 6 weeks if little to no callus is observed at 6 weeks postoperatively. Most patients are released for unrestricted activities at 3 months, and they can be scheduled for a routine deep implant removal if they wish beginning at 3 to 4 months after their index surgery.

Outcomes

The current high-quality level 1 evidence available is primarily focused on plate fixation versus nonoperative management of displaced midshaft clavicle fractures. These trials report a significantly lower incidence of nonunion and malunion with operative treatment compared with nonoperative treatment. In terms of function, both Constant and Disabilities of the Arm, Shoulder and Hand Score (DASH) are reported to be significantly better with open reduction internal fixation at longer than 1 year follow-up (Canadian Orthopaedic Trauma Society, 2007; Kulshrestha et al, 2011; Mirzatolooei, 2011; Smeeing et al, 2016; Zlowodzki et al, 2005). Gao et al (2016) performed a meta-analysis including 15 studies (RCT = 6 and non-RCT = 9) comprising 513 patients undergoing IM fixation and 521 undergoing plate fixation that were selected for final inclusion. Results demonstrated that IM fixation of a midshaft clavicle fracture achieved similar union rates and shoulder scores with superior surgical outcomes, including significantly less time to union than plate fixation. These findings remained constant when conducting subanalyses in only RCTs. Significantly less blood loss, shorter operative time, smaller surgical wounds, and fewer complications in the IM fixation group were also reported (Gao et al, 2016). However, these results should be interpreted with caution because few RCTs were identified, and these assessments were limited by the number of patients included. Another recent systematic review and meta-analysis of randomized and quasi-RCTs of IM versus plate fixation similarly reported no significant difference in functional outcomes between groups at 1 year (Hussain et al, 2016).

In a systematic review of complications after IM fixation for displaced midshaft clavicle fractures, reported rates for major complications, including bone healing problems and deep infections requiring implant removal, were no higher than 7% (Chen et al, 2010, 2012; Ferran et al, 2010; Judd et al, 2009; Smekal et al, 2011; Wijdicks et al, 2013; Witzel, 2007). In addition, only four refractures after pin removal were reported in a total of three studies (Chen et al, 2012; Judd et al, 2009; Smekal et al, 2011). Most complications were implant failures, breakages, irritations, or implant migrations. Reported rates of minor complications were as high as 31% (Wijdicks et al, 2013). Another recent systematic review (Robertson & Wood, 2016) reported similar complications as well as a rate of reintervention ranging from 67% to 100%, which largely represented planned implant removal (Grassi et al, 2001; Jubel et al, 2003;

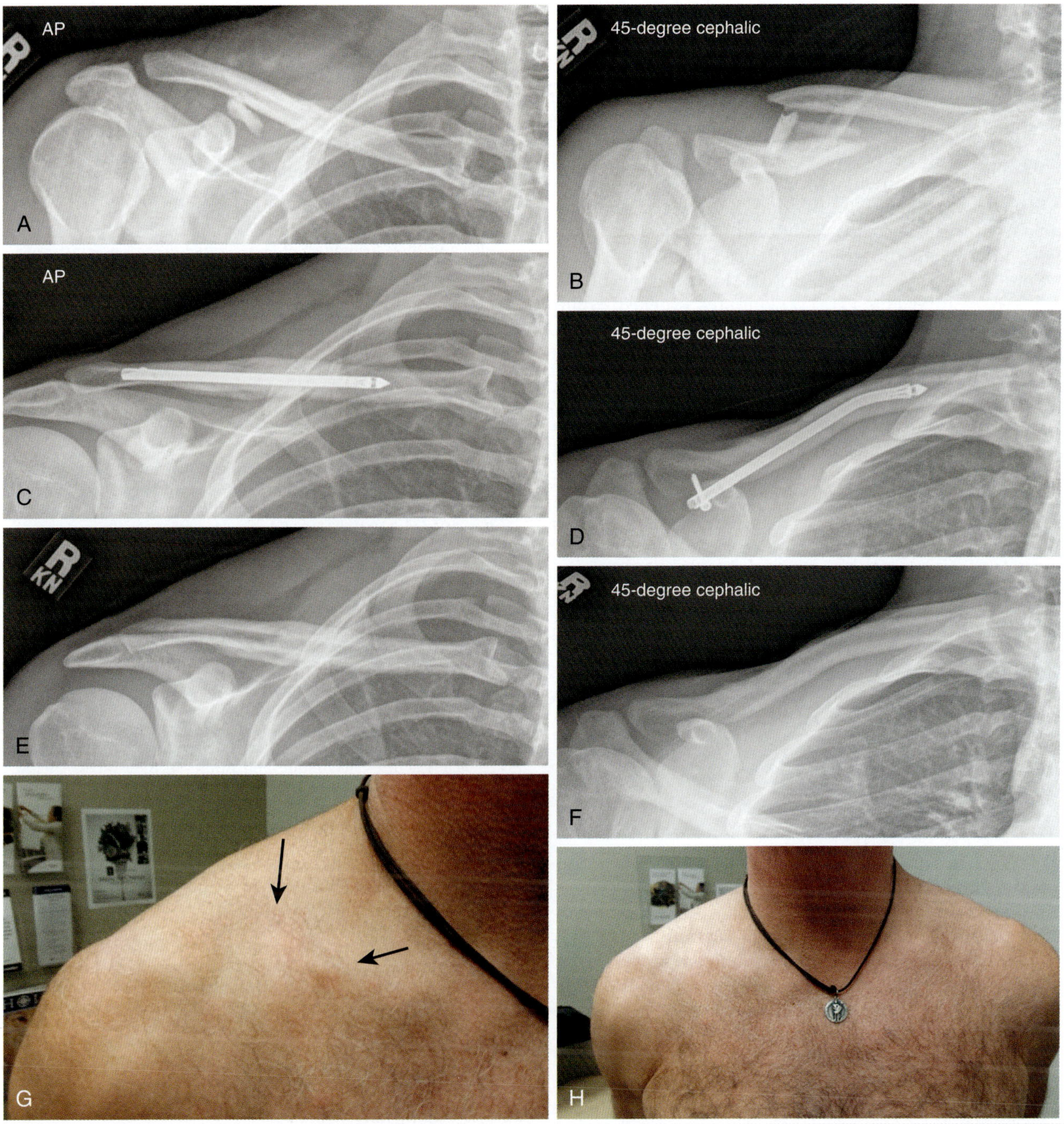

Fig. 14A.3 **A** to **H,** Before-and-after radiographs and clinical images. Note the cosmetic "necklace" incision in Langer lines. The implant used in this case was a hybrid device with an interlocking screw component. *AP,* Anteroposterior.

Morgan et al, 2010; Robertson & Wood, 2016). Hussain et al (2016) reported a 2.19 times greater risk of developing complications requiring nonroutine surgical intervention (e.g., refracture, symptomatic nonunion or malunion, hardware failure, or mechanical failure) compared with those receiving IM fixation; however, this result was not found to be statistically significant. Likewise, the same systematic review and meta-analysis reported that patients receiving plate fixation had a 2.11 times greater risk of adverse events not requiring surgery (i.e., infection, symptomatic hardware, inadequate cosmesis) compared with those receiving IM fixation, which was found to be statistically significant. In their review, all refractures occurred in the plating group (Hussain et al, 2016).

Considering refracture in an athletic population specifically, conservatively managed displaced midshaft fractures had a reported refracture rate of 57% compared with refracture in 5% with plate fixation and 8% after IM pin removal (Grassi et al, 2001; Morgan et al, 2010). Therefore although nonsurgical management can be considered for displaced midshaft clavicle fractures in high-level contact athletes, refracture can reportedly occur in more than half of cases and delayed surgical intervention may be required in more than a quarter (Morgan et al, 2010). Moreover, in nonoperatively treated midshaft clavicle fractures, refracture at the site of a united angular malunion in the absence of displacement has also been reported in adult athletes along with a significantly increased rate of refracture among pediatric patients with angulated fractures (Furey et al, 2017; Masnovi et al, 2014). It is recommended that clavicle refracture be reviewed with the athletic patient when discussing treatment options.

In athletes specifically, IM fixation of displaced midshaft clavicle fractures have reportedly resulted in faster return to sport, improved strength, and higher satisfaction scores (Jubel et al, 2003; Meier et al, 2006; Morgan et al, 2010; Witzel, 2007). Jubel et al (2003) evaluated IM elastic nailing for mid-third clavicle fractures in 12 top-performance athletes. The mean time to return to training was 5.9 days, and the mean time of return to competition was 16.8 days. A recent systematic review of primarily level II and III studies echoed similar results (Robertson & Wood, 2016). This review included 304 midshaft clavicle fractures, of which 197 were treated operatively. They reported significantly longer return times and return to preinjury level of sport for conservatively managed displaced midshaft fractures compared with those treated operatively, which was confirmed by meta-analysis of the study results. For the IM fixation subset specifically, the return to play rate was 99% and mean return time of 9.9 weeks compared with 98% and 9.3 weeks, respectively, with plating. Moreover, IM fixation and plating exhibited identical union rates (97%); however, the mean reported time to union for IM fixation was less than that for plating (7.9 vs 11.2 weeks) (Robertson & Wood, 2016).

Conclusions

Clavicle fractures are a common injury in athletes. Multiple factors need to be considered when choosing the appropriate management. These include both fracture characteristics and patient factors or goals. It is important to note that there is still a role for nonoperative management. However, in an athletic patient with a displaced, shortened, and comminuted clavicle fracture, the current literature supports operative treatment to prevent nonunion and symptomatic malunion and restore shoulder strength. Athletes are less likely to accept prolonged recovery and impaired shoulder function and are at increased risk for refracture, making surgery even more suitable in this group. Recent literature supports IM fixation as a viable treatment option with equivalent or improved outcomes compared to plating. To achieve optimal patient outcomes, surgeons treating clavicle fractures with IM fixation should be well versed in proper technique and understand key steps for success as highlighted in this chapter.

References

Andermahr J, Jubel A, Elsner A, et al. Anatomy of the clavicle and the intramedullary nailing of midclavicular fractures. *Clin Anat.* 2007;20(1):48–56.

Canadian Orthopaedic Trauma Society. Nonoperative treatment compared with plate fixation of displaced midshaft clavicular fractures. A multicenter, randomized clinical trial. *J Bone Joint Surg Am.* 2007;89(1):1–10.

Chen YF, Zeng BF, Chen YJ, et al. Clinical outcomes of midclavicular fractures treated with titanium elastic nails. *Can J Surg.* 2010;53(6):379–384.

Chen YF, Wei HF, Zhang C, et al. Retrospective comparison of titanium elastic nail (TEN) and reconstruction plate repair of displaced midshaft clavicular fractures. *J Shoulder Elbow Surg.* 2012;21(4):495–501.

Ferran NA, Hodgson P, Vannet N, Williams R, Evans RO. Locked intramedullary fixation vs plating for displaced and shortened mid-shaft clavicle fractures: a randomized clinical trial. *J Shoulder Elbow Surg.* 2010;19(6):783–789.

Furey MJ, Zdero R, McKee MD. Clavicular refracture at the site of angular malunion in young athletes. *J Orthop Trauma.* 2017;31(4):e130–e132.

Gao Y, Chen W, Liu YJ, Li X, Wang HL, Chen ZY. Plating versus intramedullary fixation for mid-shaft clavicle fractures: a systemic review and meta-analysis. *Peer J.* 2016;4:e1540.

Golish SR, Oliviero JA, Francke EI, Miller MD. A biomechanical study of plate versus intramedullary devices for midshaft clavicle fixation. *J Orthop Surg Res.* 2008;3:28.

Grassi FA, Tajana MS, D'Angelo F. Management of midclavicular fractures: comparison between nonoperative treatment and open intramedullary fixation in 80 patients. *J Trauma.* 2001;50(6):1096–1100.

Harnroongroj T, Jeerathanyasakun Y. Intramedullary pin fixation in clavicular fractures: a study comparing the use of small and large pins. *J Orthop Surg (Hong Kong).* 2000;8(2):7–11.

Hussain N, Sermer C, Prusick PJ, Banfield L, Atrey A, Bhandari M. Intramedullary nailing versus plate fixation for the treatment displaced midshaft clavicular fractures: a systematic review and meta-analysis. *Sci Rep.* 2016;6:34912.

Jubel A, Andemahr J, Bergmann H, Prokop A, Rehm KE. Elastic stable intramedullary nailing of midclavicular fractures in athletes. *Br J Sports Med.* 2003;37(6):480–483. discussion 484.

Jubel A, Andermahr J, Weisshaar G, Schiffer G, Prokop A, Rehm KE. [Intramedullary nailing (ESIN) in clavicular pseudoarthroses. Results of a prospective clinical trial]. *Unfallchirurg.* 2005;108(7):544–550.

Judd DB, Pallis MP, Smith E, Bottoni CR. Acute operative stabilization versus nonoperative management of clavicle fractures. *Am J Orthop (Belle Mead NJ).* 2009;38(7):341–345.

Kettler M, Schieker M, Braunstein V, Konig M, Mutschler W. Flexible intramedullary nailing for stabilization of displaced midshaft clavicle fractures: technique and results in 87 patients. *Acta Orthop.* 2007;78(3):424–429.

Kulshrestha V, Roy T, Audige L. Operative versus nonoperative management of displaced midshaft clavicle fractures: a prospective cohort study. *J Orthop Trauma.* 2011;25(1):31–38.

Leroux T, Wasserstein D, Henry P, et al. Rate of and risk factors for reoperations after open reduction and internal fixation of midshaft clavicle fractures: a population-based study in Ontario, Canada. *J Bone Joint Surg Am.* 2014;96(13):1119–1125.

Liu HH, Chang CH, Chia WT, Chen CH, Tarng YW, Wong CY. Comparison of plates versus intramedullary nails for fixation of displaced midshaft clavicular fractures. *J Trauma.* 2010;69(6):E82–E87.

Lyons FA, Rockwood CA Jr. Migration of pins used in operations on the shoulder. *J Bone Joint Surg Am.* 1990;72(8):1262–1267.

Masnovi ME, Mehlman CT, Eismann EA, Matey DA. Pediatric refracture rates after angulated and completely displaced clavicle shaft fractures. *J Orthop Trauma.* 2014;28(11):648–652.

Mehta A, Birch R. Supraclavicular nerve injury: the neglected nerve? *Injury.* 1997;28(7):491–492.

Meier C, Grueninger P, Platz A. Elastic stable intramedullary nailing for midclavicular fractures in athletes: indications, technical pitfalls and early results. *Acta Orthop Belg.* 2006;72(3):269–275.

Millett PJ, Hurst JM, Horan MP, Hawkins RJ. Complications of clavicle fractures treated with intramedullary fixation. *J Shoulder Elbow Surg.* 2011;20(1):86–91.

Mirzatolooei F. Comparison between operative and nonoperative treatment methods in the management of comminuted fractures of the clavicle. *Acta Orthop Traumatol Turc.* 2011;45(1):34–40.

Morgan RJ, Bankston LS Jr, Hoenig MP, Connor PM. Evolving management of middle-third clavicle fractures in the National Football League. *Am J Sports Med.* 2010;38(10):2092–2096.

Mueller M, Burger C, Florczyk A, Striepens N, Rangger C. Elastic stable intramedullary nailing of midclavicular fractures in adults: 32 patients followed for 1-5 years. *Acta Orthop.* 2007;78(3):421–423.

Nathe T, Tseng S, Yoo B. The anatomy of the supraclavicular nerve during surgical approach to the clavicular shaft. *Clin Orthop Relat Res.* 2011;469(3):890–894.

Robertson GA, Wood AM. Return to sport following clavicle fractures: a systematic review. *Br Med Bull.* 2016;119(1):111–128.

Smeeing DP, van der Ven DJ, Hietbrink F, et al. Surgical versus nonsurgical treatment for midshaft clavicle fractures in patients aged 16 years and older. *Am J Sports Med.* 2016;363546516673615.

Smekal V, Irenberger A, Attal RE, Oberladstaetter J, Krappinger D, Kralinger F. Elastic stable intramedullary nailing is best for mid-shaft clavicular fractures without comminution: results in 60 patients. *Injury.* 2011;42(4):324–329.

Smith SD, Wijdicks CA, Jansson KS, et al. Stability of mid-shaft clavicle fractures after plate fixation versus intramedullary repair and after hardware removal. *Knee Surg Sports Traumatol Arthrosc.* 2014;22(2):448–455.

Strauss EJ, Egol KA, France MA, Koval KJ, Zuckerman JD. Complications of intramedullary Hagie pin fixation for acute midshaft clavicle fractures. *J Shoulder Elbow Surg.* 2007;16(3):280–284.

Thumroj E, Kosuwon W, Kamanarong K. Anatomic safe zone of pin insertion point for distal clavicle fixation. *J Med Assoc Thai.* 2005;88(11):1551–1556.

Verborgt O, Pittoors K, Van Glabbeek F, Declercq G, Nuyts R, Somville J. Plate fixation of middle-third fractures of the clavicle in the semi-professional athlete. *Acta Orthop Belg.* 2005;71(1):17–21.

Walz M, Kolbow B, Auerbach F. [Elastic, stable intramedullary nailing in midclavicular fractures–a change in treatment strategies?]. *Unfallchirurg.* 2006;109(3):200–211.

Wijdicks FJ, Houwert RM, Millett PJ, Verleisdonk EJ, Van der Meijden OA. Systematic review of complications after intramedullary fixation for displaced midshaft clavicle fractures. *Can J Surg.* 2013;56(1):58–64.

Witzel K. [Intramedullary osteosynthesis in fractures of the mid-third of the clavicle in sports traumatology]. *Z Orthop Unfall.* 2007;145(5):639–642.

Zehir S, Akgul T, Zehir R. Results of midshaft clavicle fractures treated with expandable, elastic and locking intramedullary nails. *Acta Orthop Traumatol Turc.* 2015;49(1):13–17.

Zlowodzki M, Zelle BA, Cole PA, Jeray K, McKee MD. Treatment of acute midshaft clavicle fractures: systematic review of 2144 fractures: on behalf of the Evidence-Based Orthopaedic Trauma Working Group. *J Orthop Trauma.* 2005;19(7):504–507.

14-14B SURGICAL TREATMENT: ORIF WITH PLATE FIXATION

JEREMY N. TRUNTZER, MD, MALCOLM R. DEBAUN, MD and MICHAEL J. GARDNER, MD

Introduction

- Recent LEVEL I studies suggest that non-union rates are lower with open reduction and internal fixation (ORIF) for the midshaft clavicle than with nonoperative treatment, at the cost of higher complication rates.
- Beach-chair and supine positioning are most commonly used for operative treatment. Beach-chair positioning provides anterior and lateral access to the shoulder whereas supine positioning is helpful in patients with polytrauma.
- Plate position remains controversial. Superior plating has traditionally been considered a stronger construct. However, new data suggest that anteroinferior plating may actually provide better resistance to physiologic loading by resisting cantilever bending with less associated hardware irritation.
- Careful attention to avoid neurovascular structures is important for both superior and anteroinferior plating.
- Dual plating utilizing two 2.7-mm plates may offer comparable clinical and biochemical outcomes with less hardware irritation.

Indications

Fractures of the middle third of the clavicle have historically been treated nonoperatively, on the basis of several landmark studies by Neer (1960) and Rowe (1968) in the 1960s, which reported nearly universal healing although with minimal assessment of patient functional outcome. Later studies have found non-union rates between 15% and 26% after conservative treatment of displaced midshaft clavicle fractures, with a significant number of patients reporting unsatisfactory results (Hill et al, 1997; Virtanen et al, 2012; Zlowodzki et al, 2005). The evolution of modern surgical techniques has shifted the paradigm toward operative management. Although controversial, surgical fixation of midshaft clavicle fractures is often recommended over nonoperative treatment in the setting of displacement, comminution, or clavicle shortening greater than 20 mm (Canadian Orthopaedic Trauma Society, 2007; Fanter et al, 2015; McKee et al, 2006; Robinson, 1998; Robinson et al, 2013). Absolute indications for acute surgical management include skin tenting, open fracture, neurovascular compromise, polytrauma, or floating shoulder (Paladini et al, 2012).

Operative management of midshaft clavicle fractures can be performed with ORIF or with percutaneous intramedullary fixation. A meta-analysis by Houwert et al (2016) showed no differences in function or rate of union between the two surgical techniques. Fracture comminution, however, was identified as a relative contraindication to intramedullary fixation owing to poor ability to obtain length and rotational stability. Plate fixation provides several advantages over intramedullary techniques. Plate fixation is associated with lower rates of implant removal, provides a rigid construct with better torsional stability, and may be technically less demanding than intramedullary fixation. Disadvantages of plate fixation include a larger incision with more soft tissue disruption, higher potential for neurovascular complications, implant prominence, and increased refracture rates after plate removal (Leroux et al, 2014; Wijdicks et al, 2012).

Patient Positioning

Proper patient positioning is crucial to successful reduction and fixation of midshaft clavicle fractures. Generally one of two positions is employed, each with distinct advantages and disadvantages. The beach-chair position provides anterior and lateral access to the shoulder and is often most familiar to shoulder surgeons (Altamimi & McKee, 2008).

The image intensifier can be positioned at the head of the patient or across the table. The patient is seated at an angle of roughly 30 to 45 degrees with the ground, with the head carefully positioned in a headrest tilted 5 to 10 degrees toward the contralateral shoulder. Hyperextension of the shoulder should be avoided in order to prevent tension on the brachial plexus. To obtain the most useful view of the clavicle without the obstruction of thoracic structures, the intensifier beam is directed 20 to 60 degrees cephalad and centered over the area of interest. In the event of a vertical butterfly fragment, a 45-degree anteroposterior (AP) oblique view may be helpful (Renner, 2007). The supine position is advantageous in the patient with polytrauma because it allows combined surgical approaches for concurrent injuries without the need for repositioning, and for the patient with injuries, such as to the spine, for which minimal patient manipulation is desired (Fig. 14B.1A). However, the superior position requires a radiolucent table and limits access to the clavicle to an anterior or superior approach only.

Dissection

Surgical approach for clavicle fractures varies slightly according to anticipated fixation technique and plate

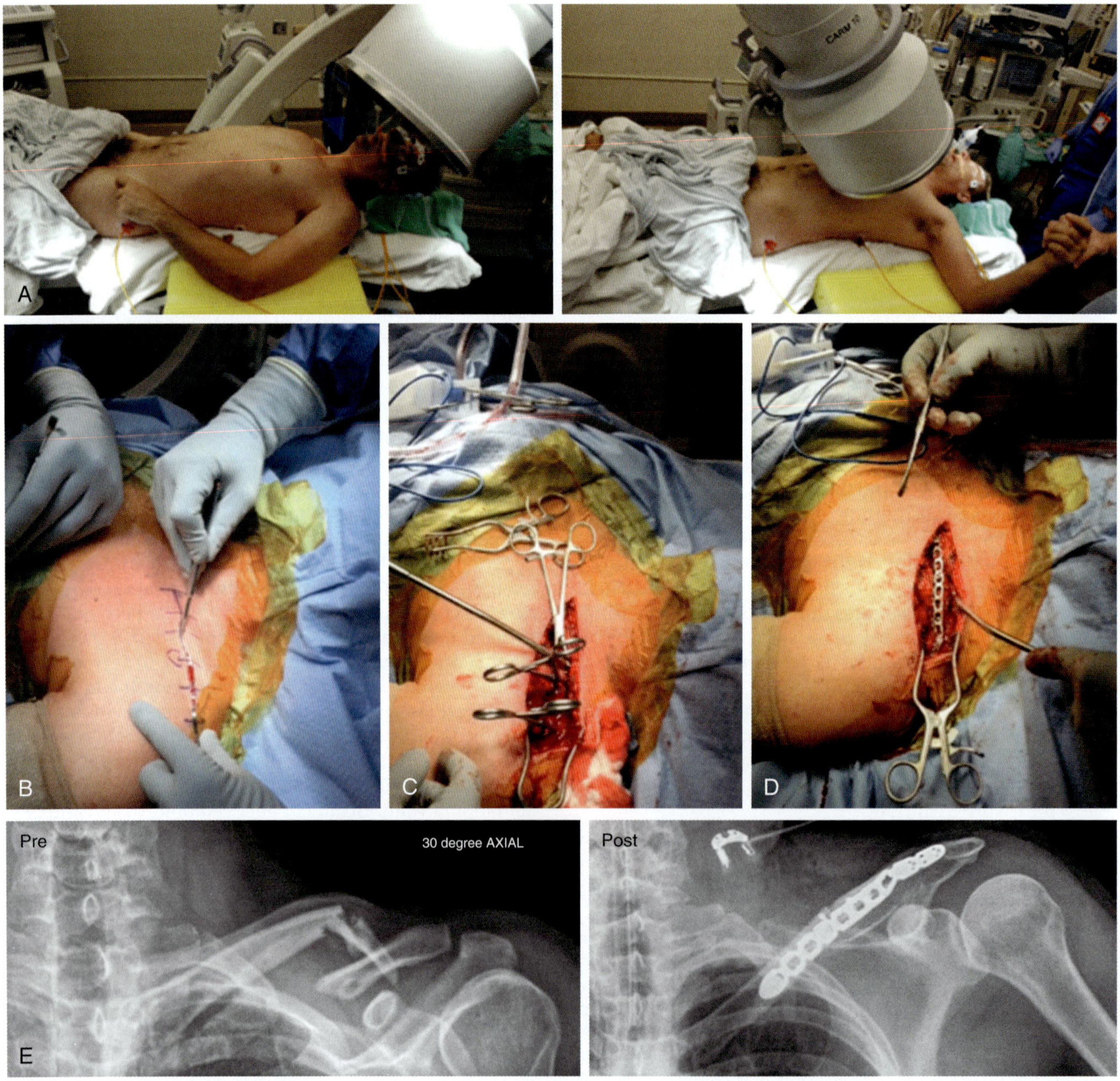

Fig. 14B.1 Operative technique for plate fixation of midshaft clavicle fracture. **A,** Patient is placed in the supine position. Image intensifier is positioned to allow for orthogonal views of the clavicle. **B,** Skin incision is made parallel and slightly inferior to the clavicle. **C,** Reduction of clavicle following lag screw placement with retractors. **D,** Placement of an anterior 3.5-mm precontoured clavicle plate. **E,** Preoperative *(left)* and postoperative (*right*) radiographs demonstrating restored length and alignment, and proper plate position.

location. The utilitarian incision for clavicle fractures, which allows for both superior and anterior plate placements, consists of a 4- to 5-cm transverse incision just in line or slightly inferior to the long axis of the clavicle and centered over the fracture site (Coupe et al, 2005; Jeray, 2007) (Fig. 14B.1B). In the case of more medial exposure requirements, the incision may be curved in order to follow the S shape of the clavicle; however, given the mobility of the skin in this area, such an incision is rarely necessary. Prior to incision, epinephrine may be injected subcutaneously to aid with hemostasis. Next, independent of plate location, superior and inferior subcutaneous flaps are created that include the underlying platysma. Several branches of the supraclavicular nerves cross this incision and can be identified and protected. However, such nerves may have to be sacrificed if they impede the ability to achieve adequate reduction and fixation or if extended manipulation of a multifragmentary fracture is anticipated, because stretching of the nerves, if preserved, could lead to painful neuroma. The pectoralis fascia is divided then elevated from the superior border of the clavicle. Progressing in a proximal direction may be helpful because the fascial layer thickens more proximally. When an anterior plate is planned, origins of the pectoralis major, pectoralis minor (medially), and deltoid may be extraperiosteally elevated off the anterior clavicle to expose the fracture surface. If possible, these structures should be repaired to provide a robust soft-tissue envelope over the implant to promote healing and minimize hardware irritation.

Another option is a vertical incision centered over the fracture that provides a theoretical advantage of less risk of superficial nerve injury (Wang, 2010). A minimally invasive technique has also been described but may limit direct visualization of the fracture in cases of comminution and make accurate plate positioning technically difficult (Jiang, 2012; Sohn, 2013).

Plate Fixation

The specific plate type and plating surface for clavicle fracture fixation remain controversial and often depend on surgeon preference, hardware availability, and patient factors. Traditional plating techniques include a 3.5-mm limited (bone) contact dynamic compression (LCDC) or DC plate, depending on fracture pattern (Ring et al, 2009) (Fig. 14B.1D). Historical results show good short- and long-term clinical outcomes (Kulshrestha et al, 2011; Robinson et al, 2013). However, to avoid the common complication of hardware irritation, both reconstruction plates and precontoured plates have come into favor (Altamimi & McKee, 2008). Multiple studies have shown lower rates of hardware removal with precontoured plates than with more traditional plate varieties and equivocal patient satisfaction scores (Campochiaro et al, 2012; Huang et al, 2007). In two matched-pair studies, precontoured plates placed superiorly had lower rates of plate prominence and hardware removal than noncontoured plates with equal range of movement (ROM) and subjective scores (Chandrasenan et al, 2009; VanBeek et al, 2011). Caution must be taken in the use of reconstruction plates in a bridging mode, because these plates are relatively malleable and have a higher rate of implant failure (Woltz et al, 2016).

Biomechanical studies have demonstrated superiority of locking plates over nonlocking LCDC plates and reconstruction plates for torsional and bending loading, especially for lateral and medial fracture patterns (discussed elsewhere) as well as in osteoporotic bone (Celestre et al, 2008; Demirhan et al, 2011; Eden et al, 2012). LCDC plates appear to provide better load-to-failure and torsional fracture rigidity than reconstruction plates (Drosdowech et al, 2011; Iannotti et al, 2002). Locking reconstruction plates do not appear to provide better biomechanics; however, caution is advised in the use of nonlocking constructs in patients with poor bone contact, comminution, or non-union and in elderly patients (Khan et al, 2008; Partal et al, 2010). Despite the biomechanical studies on traditional plates, clinical outcomes studies do not show significant differences in union rates between locking and nonlocking plate constructions in general populations (Lai et al, 2012).

Plate location remains controversial, likely because of variations in study technique and modeling for biomechanical studies as well as the lack of high-level clinical outcome studies (Formaini et al, 2013; Hulsmans et al, 2016). Early studies noted mechanically better constructs with a superior plate location (Iannotti et al, 2002; Kontautas et al, 2012). The ability to apply fixation to the tension side of the fracture with superior fixation was initially believed to explain such results. However, the theoretical benefits of anteroinferior plating, including greater screw length and purchase (Lo et al, 2010), safer screw trajectory away from neurovascular structures (Hussey et al, 2013), and—although controversial (Werner et al, 2011)—more soft tissue coverage and less prominent hardware (Formaini et al, 2013; Hulsmans et al, 2016; Wang et al, 2011; Zlowodzki et al, 2005) promoted a trend toward anteroinferior surface plating. Of note, injury to neurovascular structures may be reduced independent of plate location through the use of unicortical locking plates without sacrifice of biomechanical stability (Bravman et al, 2015), although evidence supporting this finding is limited so this technique should be used with caution. Additionally, biomechanical studies have shown that anteroinferior plating may provide a more stable construct against typical physiologic loading by resisting cantilever bending (Favre et al, 2011; Partal et al, 2010). Anteroinferior plating has also been found to provide a more stable construct in the context of an inferior cortical defect in vitro, a common presentation for wedge-type patterns (Harnroongroj & Vanadurongwan, 1996). Superior plating, however, may be recommended for a patient susceptible to axial compression based on deformation modes. Alternatively, dual plating utilizing two 2.7-mm plates has shown clinical and biomechanical outcomes comparable to those of single-plating techniques with a theoretical advantage of less hardware irritation and orthogonal stabilization vectors (Prasarn et al, 2015; Shannon et al, 2016) (Fig. 14B.2).

Technique (Authors' Preference)

Fixation technique is often dictated by fracture pattern, which is best accomplished by adherence to AO (Arbeitsgemeinschaft für Osteosynthesefragen/Association for the Study of Internal Fixation) principles (Video 14B.1).

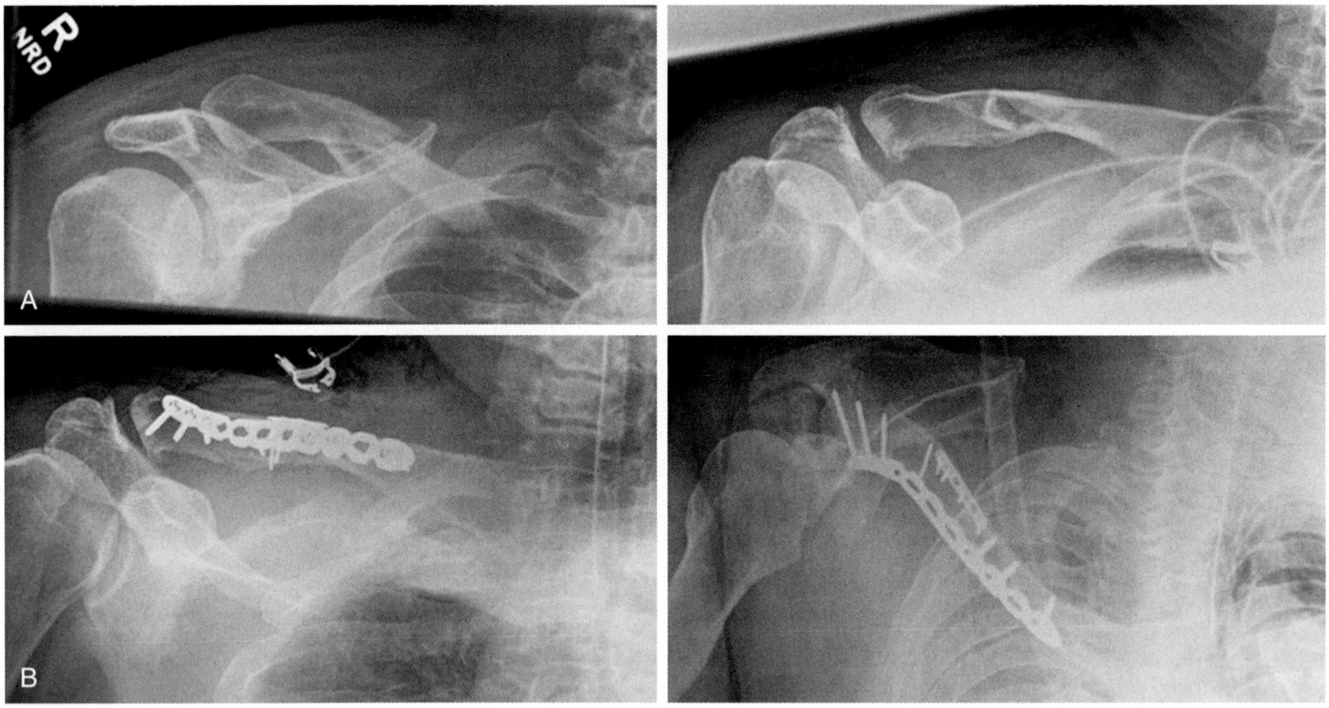

Fig. 14B.2 A 57-year-old man presented with a comminuted mid-shaft clavicle fracture and ipsilateral extraarticular scapula fracture following a bicycle collision. **A,** AP radiographs demonstrate the displacement and wedge fragment. **B,** Postoperative films demonstrate anterior precontoured plate and an adjunctive minifragment plate positioned superiorly.

The advent of dual plating, however, has provided more options, especially in the case of comminuted fracture patterns. In all cases, we prioritize adequate length to maximize stability and do not focus on number of cortices (Sanders et al, 2002). Simple fracture patterns (type AO 15.2 A1–3) are amenable to compression plating (3.5-mm LCDC plate) with lag screw fixation performed independently or through the plate in the presence of an oblique fracture orientation. Often even the shallowest of obliquities is amenable to a 2.0-mm lag screw, which can act like a permanent clamp and facilitate plate placement. Midshaft fractures, including a wedge fragment (type AO 15.2 B1–B3) are often treated with a bridge plate in either an anterior or superior position. In some cases, enough bony overlap of the wedge fragment (AO 15.2 B2) allows for utilization of lag screw(s) in combination with a neutralization plate, which provides the most torsional stability. Complex shaft fractures (AO 15.2 C1–C3) tend to be best treated with bridge plating, with the exception of segmental patterns (AO 15.2 C2) that involve large enough fragments for lag screw fixation that each segment may be treated independently.

Obtaining a reduction can often be challenging. The goal of limiting soft tissue stripping should be emphasized. We tend to use pointed reduction clamps on either side of the fracture for simple fractures and to use a derotation force to counter the deltoid and pectoralis muscle forces to facilitate reduction. For more complex patterns, we prioritize rotation and alignment over length initially. In these latter cases we often start with pointed reduction clamps and follow them with a properly contoured plate to help achieve reduction, with fixation established first on the medial side. A push-pull method has proven helpful to regain length when necessary. A small distractor can also be used in the case of marked comminution or with subacute fractures. We do not use K-wire fixation if possible, owing to their association with increased risk for neurovascular injury, frequent comminution, and relatively thick cortices.

Closure is completed in several layers, starting with the myofascial layer to provide a soft tissue envelope, using 0 or 2-0 Vicryl sutures (Ethicon US, LLC, Somerville, NJ). We then use buried 2-0 Monocryl sutures (Ethicon) to approximate the deep dermal layer, followed by 3-0 nylon sutures to approximate the subcuticular skin. Hypertrophy of scar is uncommon in this area.

Return to Sport

Despite the paucity of evidence-based rehabilitation protocols for clavicle injuries, the vast majority of athletes can expect excellent functional outcomes after plate fixation of midshaft clavicle fractures (Meisterling et al, 2013). In a series by Ranalletta et al (2015), 94% of athletes were able to return to the same level of sport as prior to surgery. Furthermore, the time to return to sport does not significantly differ between contact and noncollision sports. Around 20% of athletes can expect to return to sport less than 6 weeks after fixation, with the average time to return being 10 weeks (Meisterling et al, 2013; Ranalletta et al, 2015). An athlete should be allowed to return to play when there is clinical and radiographic evidence of fracture union, the shoulder has full range of motion, and strength is near 100%. For rehabilitation we recommend limiting elevation of the surgical arm in any plane more than 120 degrees for the first 4 postoperative weeks. Pendulum and isometric exercises should begin during the first postoperative week with a sling available for 2 weeks as needed for comfort. Gradual transition to active and light resistance exercises should start 4 weeks postoperatively if adequate healing has occurred and pain is minimal. Once fully healed, the athlete should be re-introduced to sport without any restrictions.

References

Altamimi SA, McKee MD. Nonoperative treatment compared with plate fixation of displaced midshaft clavicular fractures: Surgical technique. *J Bone Joint Surg Am*. 2008;9(suppl 2 Pt 1):1–8.

Bravman JT, Taylor ML, Baldini T, Vidal AF. Unicortical versus bicortical locked plate fixation in midshaft clavicle fractures. *Orthopedics*. 2015;38(5):e411–e416.

Campochiaro G, Tsatsis C, Gazzotti G, Rebuzzi M, Catani F. Displaced midshaft clavicular fractures: Surgical treatment with a pre-contoured angular stability plate. *Musculoskeletal Surg*. 2012;96(suppl 1):S21–S26.

Canadian Orthopaedic Trauma Society. Nonoperative treatment compared with plate fixation of displaced midshaft clavicular fractures: A multicenter, randomized clinical trial. *J Bone Jt Surg Am*. 2007;89(1):1–10.

Celestre P, Roberston C, Mahar A, Oka R, Meunier M, Schwartz A. Biomechanical evaluation of clavicle fracture plating techniques: Does a locking plate provide improved stability? *J Orthop Trauma*. 2008;22(4):241–247.

Chandrasenan J, Espag M, Dias R, Clark DI. The use of anatomic precontoured plates in the treatment of midshaft clavicle fractures. *J Bone Joint Surg Br*. 2009;91:179–180.

Coupe BD, Wimhurst JA, Indar R, Calder DA, Patel AD. A new approach for plate fixation of midshaft clavicular fractures. *Injury*. 2005;36(10):1166–1171.

Demirhan M, Bilsel K, Atalar AC, Bozdag E, Sunbuloglu E, Kale A. Biomechanical comparison of fixation techniques in midshaft clavicular fractures. *J Orthop Trauma*. 2011;25(5):272–278.

Drosdowech DS, Manwell SE, Ferreira LM, Goel DP, Faber KJ, Johnson JA. Biomechanical analysis of fixation of middle third fractures of the clavicle. *J Orthop Trauma*. 2011;25(1):39–43.

Eden L, Doht S, Frey SP, et al. Biomechanical comparison of the Locking Compression superior anterior clavicle plate with seven and ten hole reconstruction plates in midshaft clavicle fracture stabilisation. *Int Orthop*. 2012;36(12):2537–2543.

Fanter NJ, Kenny RM, Baker CL 3rd, Baker CL Jr. Surgical treatment of clavicle fractures in the adolescent athlete. *Sports Health*. 2015;7(2):137–141.

Favre P, Kloen P, Helfet DL, Werner CM. Superior versus anteroinferior plating of the clavicle: A finite element study. *J Orthop Trauma*. 2011;25(11):661–665.

Formaini N, Taylor BC, Backes J, Bramwell TJ. Superior versus anteroinferior plating of clavicle fractures. *Orthopedics*. 2013;36(7):e898–e904.

Harnroongroj T, Vanadurongwan V. Biomechanical aspects of plating osteosynthesis of transverse clavicular fracture with and without inferior cortical defect. *Clin Biomech (Bristol, Avon)*. 1996;11(5):290–294.

Hill JM, McGuire MH, Crosby LA. Closed treatment of displaced middle-third fractures of the clavicle gives poor results. *J Bone Joint Surg Br*. 1997;79(4):537–539.

Houwert RM, Smeeing DP, Ahmed Ali U, et al. Plate fixation or intramedullary fixation for midshaft clavicle fractures: A systematic review and meta-analysis of randomized controlled trials and observational studies. 2016;25(7):1195–1203.

Huang JI, Toogood P, Chen MR, Wilber JH, Cooperman DR. Clavicular anatomy and the applicability of precontoured plates. *J Bone Joint Surg Am*. 2007;89(10):2260–2265.

Hulsmans MH, van Heijl M, Houwert RM, Timmers TK, van Olden G, Verleisdonk EJ. Anteroinferior versus superior plating of clavicular fractures. *J Shoulder Elbow Surg*. 2016;25(3):448–454.

Hussey MM, Chen Y, Fajardo RA, Dutta AK. Analysis of neurovascular safety between superior and anterior plating techniques of clavicle fractures. *J Orthop Trauma*. 2013;27(11):627–632.

Iannotti MR, Crosby LA, Stafford P, Grayson G, Goulet R. Effects of plate location and selection on the stability of midshaft clavicle osteotomies: a biomechanical study. *J Shoulder Elbow Surg*. 2002;11(5):457–462.

Jeray KJ. Acute midshaft clavicular fracture. *J Am Acad Orthop Surg*. 2007;15(4):239–248.

Jiang H, Qu W. Operative treatment of clavicle midshaft fractures using a locking compression plate: comparison between mini-invasive plate osteosynthesis (MIPPO) technique and conventional open reduction. *Orthop Traumatol Surg Rese*. 2012;98(6):666–671.

Khan SA, Shamshery P, Gupta V, Trikha V, Varshney MK, Kumar A. Locking compression plate in long standing clavicular nonunions with poor bone stock. *J Trauma*. 2008;64(2):439–441.

Kontautas E, Pijadin A, Vilkauskas A, Domeika A. Biomechanical aspects of locking reconstruction plate positioning in osteosynthesis of transverse clavicle fracture. *Medicina (Kaunas, Lithuania)*. 2012;48(2):80–83.

Kulshrestha V, Roy T, Audige L. Operative versus nonoperative management of displaced midshaft clavicle fractures: A prospective cohort study. *J Orthop Trauma*. 2011;25(1):31–38.

Lai YC, Tarng YW, Hsu CJ, Chang WN, Yang SW, Renn JH. Comparison of dynamic and locked compression plates for treating midshaft clavicle fractures. *Orthopedics*. 2012;35(5):e697–e702.

Leroux T, Wasserstein D, Henry P, et al. Rate of and risk factors for reoperations after open reduction and internal fixation of midshaft clavicle fractures: A population-based study in Ontario, Canada. *J Bone Joint Surg Am*. 2014;96(13):1119–1125.

Lo EY, Eastman J, Tseng S, Lee MA, Yoo BJ. Neurovascular risks of anteroinferior clavicular plating. *Orthopedics*. 2010;33(1):21.

McKee MD, Pedersen EM, Jones C, et al. Deficits following nonoperative treatment of displaced midshaft clavicular fractures. *J Bone Joint Surg Am*. 2006;88(1):35–40.

Meisterling SW, Cain EL, Fleisig GS, Hartzell JL, Dugas JR. Return to athletic activity after plate fixation of displaced midshaft clavicle fractures. *Am J Sports Med*. 2013;41(11):2632–2636.

Neer CS 2nd. Nonunion of the clavicle. *JAMA*. 1960;172:1006–1011.

Paladini P, Pellegrini A, Merolla G, Campi F, Porcellini G. Treatment of clavicle fractures. *Transl Med UniSa*. 2012;2:47–58.

Partal G, Meyers KN, Sama N, et al. Superior versus anteroinferior plating of the clavicle revisited: A mechanical study. *J Orthop Trauma*. 2010;24(7):420–425.

Prasarn ML, Meyers KN, Wilkin G, et al. Dual mini-fragment plating for midshaft clavicle fractures: A clinical and biomechanical investigation. *Arch Orthop Trauma Surg*. 2015;135(12):1655–1662.

Ranalletta M, Rossi LA, Piuzzi NS, Bertona A, Bongiovanni SL, Maignon G. Return to sports after plate fixation of displaced midshaft clavicular fractures in athletes. *Am J Sports Med*. 2015;43(3):565–569.

Renner NL, Simmermacher RKJ. Scapula and clavicle. In: Rüedi TP, Buckley RE, Moran CG, eds. *AO Principles of Fracture Management*. 2nd ed. New York: Georg Thieme; 2007:557–572.

Ring D, Jupiter JB. Injuries to the shoulder girdle. In: Browner BD, Jupiter JE, Krettek C, Anderson P, eds. *Skeletal Trauma: Basic Science, Management, and Reconstruction*. 4th ed. vol. 2. Philadelphia: Saunders Elsevier; 2009.

Robinson CM. Fractures of the clavicle in the adult: Epidemiology and classification. *J Bone Joint Surg Br*. 1998;80(3):476–484.

Robinson CM, Goudie EB, Murray IR, et al. Open reduction and plate fixation versus nonoperative treatment for displaced midshaft clavicular fractures: A multicenter, randomized, controlled trial. *J Bone Joint Surg Am*. 2013;95(17):1576–1584.

Rowe CR. An atlas of anatomy and treatment of midclavicular fractures. *Clin Orthop Rel Res*. 1968;58:29–42.

Sanders R, Haidukewych GJ, Milne T, Dennis J, Latta LL. Minimal versus maximal plate fixation techniques of the ulna: The biomechanical effect of number of screws and plate length. *J Orthop Trauma*. 2002;16(3):166–171.

Shannon SF, Chen X, Torchia M, Schoch B. Extraperiosteal dual plate fixation of acute mid-shaft clavicle fractures: A technical trick. *J Orthop Trauma*. 2016;30(10):e346–e350.

Sohn HS, Kim BY, Shin SJ. A surgical technique for minimally invasive plate osteosynthesis of clavicular midshaft fractures. *J Orthop Trauma*. 2013;27(4):e92–e96.

VanBeek C, Boselli KJ, Cadet ER, Ahmad CS, Levine WN. Precontoured plating of clavicle fractures: Decreased hardware-related complications? *Clin Orthop Rel Res*. 2011;469(12):3337–3343.

Virtanen KJ, Remes V, Pajarinen J, Savolainen V, Bjorkenheim JM, Paavola M. Sling compared with plate osteosynthesis for treatment of displaced midshaft clavicular fractures: A randomized clinical trial. *J Bone Joint Surg Am*. 2012;94(17):1546–1553.

Wang J, Chidambaram R, Mok D. Is removal of clavicle plate after fracture union necessary? *Int J Shoulder Surg*. 2011;5(4):85–89.

Wang K, Dowrick A, Choi J, Rahim R, Edwards E. Post-operative numbness and patient satisfaction following plate fixation of clavicular fractures. *Injury*. 2010;41(10):1002–1005.

Werner SD, Reed J, Hanson T, Jaeblon T. Anatomic relationships after instrumentation of the midshaft clavicle with 3.5-mm reconstruction plating: An anatomic study. *J Orthop Trauma*. 2011;25(11):657–660.

Wijdicks FJ, Van der Meijden OA, Millett PJ, Verleisdonk EJ, Houwert RM. Systematic review of the complications of plate fixation of clavicle fractures. *Arch Orthop Trauma Surg*. 2012;132(5):617–625.

Woltz S, Duijff JW, Hoogendoorn JM, et al. Reconstruction plates for midshaft clavicular fractures: A retrospective cohort study. *Orthop Traumatol Surg Res*. 2016;102(1):25–29.

Zlowodzki M, Zelle BA, Cole PA, Jeray K, McKee MD. Treatment of acute midshaft clavicle fractures: Systematic review of 2144 fractures: On behalf of the Evidence-Based Orthopaedic Trauma Working Group. *J Orthop Trauma*. 2005;19(7):504–507.

15 Treatment Options: Distal Clavicle Fractures

ERIK M. FRITZ, MD, BROOKE M. DELVECCHIO, PT, DPT, OCS, JONAS POGORZELSKI, MD, MHBA, and PETER J. MILLETT

Background

- Distal fractures of the clavicle (DCFs) are defined as fractures of the lateral third of the clavicle and are classified by their relationship to the acromioclavicular (AC) and coracoclavicular (CC) ligaments.
- DCFs account for approximately 15% to 35% of all clavicle fractures.
- High-energy trauma and a direct fall onto the shoulder are among the most common causes of DCFs.
- In general, concomitant lesions are rare; however, injuries to the head, cervical spine, neurovascular structures, and the thorax must be excluded.
- Although stable fractures can be managed nonoperatively, unstable fractures normally require surgery.
- Operative treatment options include plate fixation with or without arthroscopically assisted CC fixation.

Classification

The most common and useful DCF classification for guidance of management and prognosis was proposed by Neer (1963, 1968) and expanded by Craig (1990), who classified DCFs into five types. Type 1 is lateral to the CC ligaments, minimally displaced, and usually stable. Type 2 is medial to the CC ligaments, displaced, and unstable owing to the tension of the trapezius muscle. It can also be further subclassified on the basis of injury to the CC ligaments; type 2A demonstrates intact CC ligaments, and type 2B is defined by a ruptured conoid ligament. Type 3 is intraarticular and stable with the CC ligaments intact. Type 4 is a periosteal sleeve avulsion with intact CC ligaments; it occurs in children and is stable. Type 5 is comminuted and unstable.

Patient Examination and Diagnostics

The inspection of the affected shoulder often shows a superior migration of the medial fragment, especially in unstable fractures. At the same time, palpation of the clavicle is painful and the patient often presents with the arm fixed in a relieving posture. The differential diagnosis includes an AC joint separation and is clinically difficult to distinguish from a distal clavicle fracture. Therefore a complete radiographic evaluation, including standard clavicle radiographs in two planes and an axillary lateral view (Fig. 15.1) of the affected shoulder, should be performed as first-line diagnostics when a lateral clavicle fracture is suspected. Magnetic resonance imaging (MRI) and computed tomography (CT) should be used only for suspicion of concomitant lesions and are not appropriate for a primary diagnosis.

Surgical Treatment

INDICATIONS

If the fracture is nondisplaced or minimally displaced, extraarticular, and stable, nonoperative management is usually the preferred treatment. In general, type 1, 3, and 4 fractures may be managed nonoperatively (Sambandam et al, 2014). Broadly accepted indications for operative management of clavicular fractures include open fracture, skin tenting that may lead to open fracture, and neurovascular compromise (van der Meijden et al, 2012). Additionally, unstable fractures (types 2 and 5) have a high risk for malunion and non-union and therefore should be treated surgically. Whenever there is evidence of CC ligament disruption (such as a superiorly displaced medial fragment), repair or reconstruction of the CC ligaments or CC fixation with cortical buttons and sutures should be performed to avoid a secondary dislocation of the clavicle.

PATIENT POSITIONING AND ANESTHESIA

After induction of general endotracheal anesthesia, the patient is placed in the beach-chair position. Intraoperative fluoroscopy is positioned with the x-ray tube anterior to the patient's shoulder; this positioning permits utilization of fluoroscopy throughout the procedure to assist with fracture visualization, fracture reduction, and hardware placement. The patient and fluoroscopy machine are then prepared and draped in sterile fashion with the operative extremity placed in a pneumatic arm holder. Intravenous antibiotics are administered prior to incision.

OPERATIVE TECHNIQUE WITHOUT CORACOCLAVICULAR RECONSTRUCTION

A longitudinal incision of approximately 8 cm is carried from medial to lateral, and the skin and subcutaneous tissues are sharply dissected to expose the fracture (Fig. 15.2). The fracture ends are dissected from soft tissue and hematoma. Subsequently, the fracture is reduced and can be held in place with wires, reduction forceps, or cerclage sutures to obtain satisfactory reduction. During this step, intraoperative fluoroscopy should be used to confirm appropriate anatomic reduction of the clavicle.

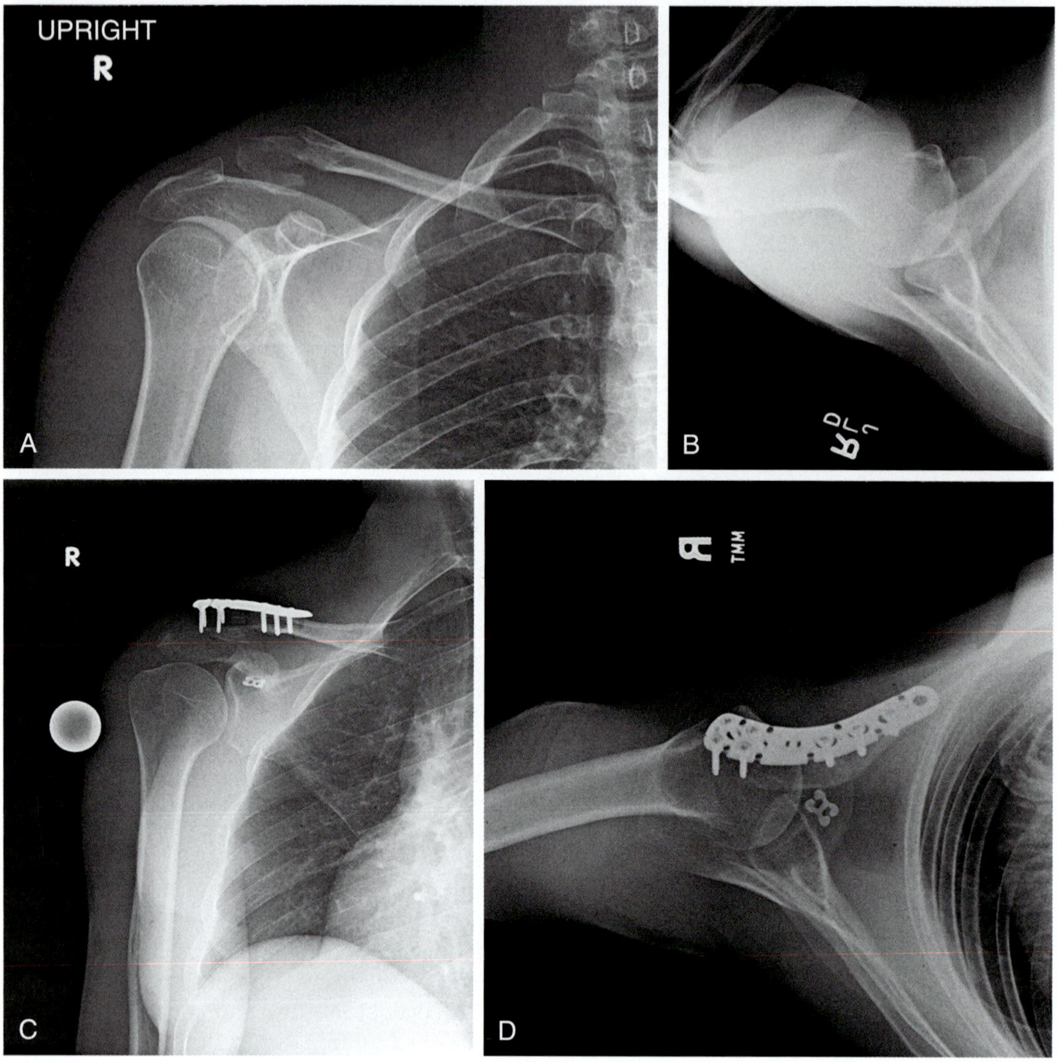

Fig. 15.1 A right-sided Neer type 5 distal clavicle fracture. **A,** Preoperative AP view. **B,** Preoperative axillary view. **C,** Postoperative AP view of the same shoulder after open reduction and internal fixation with a precontoured distal clavicle plate and integrated CC fixation with cortical buttons and suture tape. **D,** Postoperative axillary view of the same shoulder; note the cortical button underneath the coracoid process.

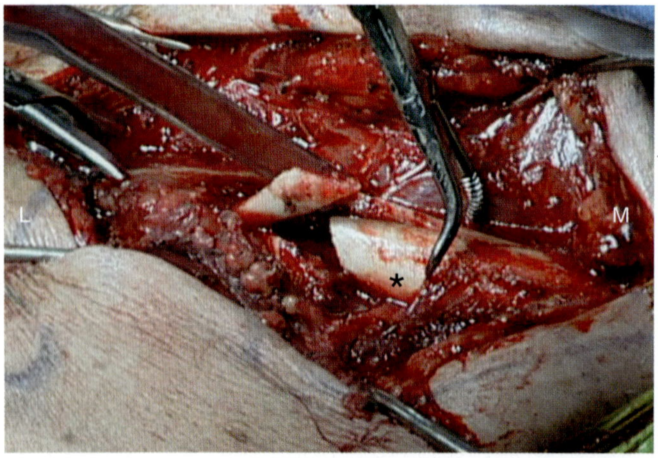

Fig. 15.2 Approach to right-sided clavicle fracture. *L*, lateral; *M*, medial; *, clavicle.

Reduction has been achieved, a precontoured distal clavicle plate is selected and placed over the superior aspect of the distal clavicle. Kirschner wires are applied to hold the plate in place while a drill guide is placed onto the lateral end of the plate. A guide sleeve is inserted into the desired drilling hole, and a 2-mm drill is used to drill through both cortices. Afterwards, the screw depth indicator is inserted into the sleeve to determine the screw length and a 2.7-mm locking screw of appropriate length is placed. This process is repeated for all required lateral drill holes according to the surgeon's preference. The center nonlocking drill holes are afterwards addressed by placement of a 2.5-mm drill guide into the appropriate plate slot and preparation of a hole using the 2.5-mm drill bit. If bicortical drilling is needed, a retractor should be placed under the clavicle to protect the neurovascular structures. The screw-depth device is used to determine the screw length, and 3.5-mm screws are inserted with the driver. The medial drill holes are finally addressed with locking screws in the same manner. Final fluoroscopic images are obtained to confirm correct

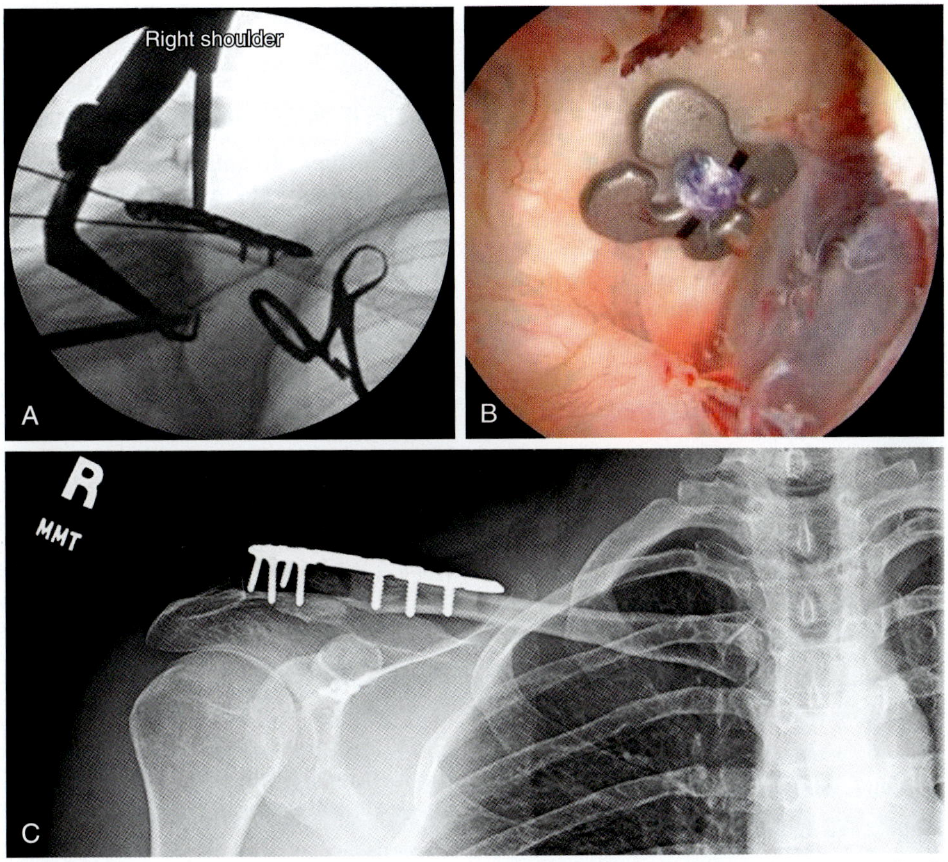

Fig. 15.3 Images of a right shoulder undergoing operative fixation of distal clavicle fracture and CC ligament fixation. **A,** Drilling through the plate and the bone of the clavicle and coracoid process under fluoroscopic guidance. **B,** Arthroscopic view of the cortical button fixation to the base of the coracoid process. **C,** Postoperative AP radiograph of the same shoulder demonstrating plate and cortical fixation button in place.

fracture reduction, placement of plates and screws, and screw length. The shoulder is then copiously lavaged and meticulously closed.

OPERATIVE TECHNIQUE WITH KNOTLESS CORACOCLAVICULAR FIXATION

(Video 15.1)

In cases with disruption of the CC ligaments, CC fixation may be added for additional stability with either an open or an arthroscopically assisted technique. For an arthroscopically assisted CC fixation technique, a standard diagnostic shoulder arthroscopy is performed and a 70-degree arthroscope is used through a posterior standard portal to visualize the undersurface of the coracoid through the rotator interval. Afterward, an anterior working portal is created lateral to the coracoid using spinal needle localization followed by insertion of a 5-mm cannula. If present, any concomitant intraarticular pathology is addressed. Next, a mechanical shaver and radiofrequency ablator are placed through the anterior cannula to debride the subcoracoid space and expose the base of the coracoid. Subsequently, an additional anteroinferolateral (AIL) portal is created inferior and lateral to the previously placed anterior portal, and an 8.25-mm cannula is inserted.

Once the coracoid is adequately exposed, the aforementioned open exposure and reduction of the clavicle is performed. The same recontoured distal clavicle plate as described earlier is placed on the superior aspect of the clavicle and is medially and laterally fixed with the corresponding screws. The center nonlocking drill holes are used to find the best available spot for the CC fixation. An acromioclavicular aiming guide is then placed through the 8.25-mm cannula, and the drilling sleeve on the guide is placed on the superior aspect of the clavicle, centered meticulously anterior to posterior, while the aiming arm is positioned on the undersurface of the coracoid, centered from medial to lateral. A 3.0-mm cannulated drill is then drilled through the clavicle and coracoid under direct arthroscopic vision. Great care must be taken to ensure that the cannulated drill enters in the superocentral portion of the clavicle and exits at the posteroinferiocentral aspect of the coracoid. The central pin is removed from the drill and a shuttle suture is passed through the cannulated drill, through the clavicle and coracoid, and into the subcoracoid recess. The shuttle suture is then retrieved out the AIL portal with a suture grasper. The drill is removed and the passing suture is used to shuttle the double-loaded knotless CC fixation device (Knotless AC TightRope, Arthrex) in an antegrade direction through the transosseous clavicle and coracoid tunnels. A large cortical fixation button (DogBone, Arthrex) is attached to the distal end of the knotless CC fixation device. The cortical button is then positioned on the base of the coracoid (Fig. 15.3) and the sutures are pulled from the superior side to secure the cortical fixation button on the undersurface of the coracoid. The knotless fixation device is inserted into the plate and pulled securely until the clavicle is reduced fully. The suture ends may be clipped at this point or preserved for additional compression. Intraoperative fluoroscopy is now used to confirm the reduction. Once the reduction is completed, the remaining drill holes are filled with corresponding screws. Final fluoroscopic images are taken to confirm correct fracture reductions, placement of plates and screws, screw length, and cortical button position. This completes the repair, and wound closure is performed to finish the procedure.

Postoperative Rehabilitation and Return to Sport

Precautions following plate fixation of the clavicle include avoidance of passive and active traction to the shoulder girdle, downward force on the repair for 6 weeks, and heavy lifting or carrying for 12 weeks. Physical therapists and patients should avoid internal rotation behind the back and horizontal adduction for 8 weeks, and patients are not allowed to begin heavy bench press or full push-ups until 16 weeks postoperatively.

PHASE I: PROTECTION (TABLE 15.1)

The patient is immobilized in a sling for 2 to 3 weeks to unload and support the shoulder complex. Full passive range of motion (PROM) of the glenohumeral joint and full active range of motion (AROM) of the cervical spine, elbow, wrist, and hand are initiated on postoperative day 1. Passive and active internal rotation behind the back and horizontal adduction motions should be avoided for up to 8 weeks. Active assisted range of motion (AAROM) is introduced within the first 2 weeks postoperatively according to patient tolerance in supported supine and standing positions. Manual therapy techniques, cryotherapy, and other modalities are utilized to reduce postoperative pain and swelling. Progression to each consecutive phase should take into consideration surgeon recommendations, bone healing timelines, and a clinically based criterion.

PHASE II: MUSCULAR ENDURANCE

AROM is typically introduced 2 to 3 weeks postoperatively; the patient can begin weaning from the sling at this time. PROM and AAROM are continued as necessary until full, pain-free AROM is achieved. It is paramount to establish normal scapulohumeral rhythm throughout all planes of AROM during this phase prior to progression to initial strengthening in phase III.

PHASE III: MUSCULAR STRENGTH

The rehabilitation goals of phase III consist of improving muscular strength by means of resisted isotonic open kinetic chain exercise, which is generally introduced at week 6. Initial closed kinetic chain exercise can be introduced after week 8 if sufficient bone healing has been demonstrated by imaging. Closed kinetic chain exercises are progressively advanced to allow for development of appropriate muscular stabilization and controlled load on the clavicle (Figs. 15.4 and 15.5). Once the patient has demonstrated proper bone healing, shoulder stability in closed chain positions, and strength of the involved upper extremity at 90% of the uninvolved upper extremity in all planes, transition to phase IV is appropriate.

PHASE IV AND PHASE V: MUSCULAR POWER AND RETURN TO SPORT

The rehabilitation goal of phase IV is to develop the muscular power required to return to high-demand work or athletic activity, which is typically introduced at week 16. Supervised throwing progressions and sport-specific training are incorporated at this time. Full return to sport after postoperative week 16 depends on proper healing, full restoration of strength, and stability as assessed by appropriate functional testing and the surgeon's approval.

Table 15.1 Summary of Postoperative Rehabilitation Phases

Phase	Approximate Time Postoperatively	Description
Phase I: protection	First 2-3 weeks	Sling immobilization Start with glenohumeral joint PROM Glenohumeral joint AAROM introduced within first 2 weeks Avoid passive or active IR behind back and horizontal adduction
Phase II: muscular endurance	Weeks 2-3 to week 6	Discontinue sling Glenohumeral joint AROM Avoid passive or active IR behind back and horizontal adduction Establish normal scapulohumeral rhythm prior to Phase III
Phase III: muscular strength	Weeks 6 to week 16	Week 6 resisted open kinetic chain exercise Week 8 resisted closed kinetic chain exercise Progress to phase IV once strength has reached 90% of uninvolved upper extremity
Phases IV and V: muscular power and return to sport	Weeks 16 and onward	Double and single arm plyometrics Sport specific training initiated Once full restoration of strength and stability is achieved, return to sport

AAROM, active assisted range of motion; *AROM*, active range of motion; *IR*, internal rotation; *PROM*, passive range of motion.

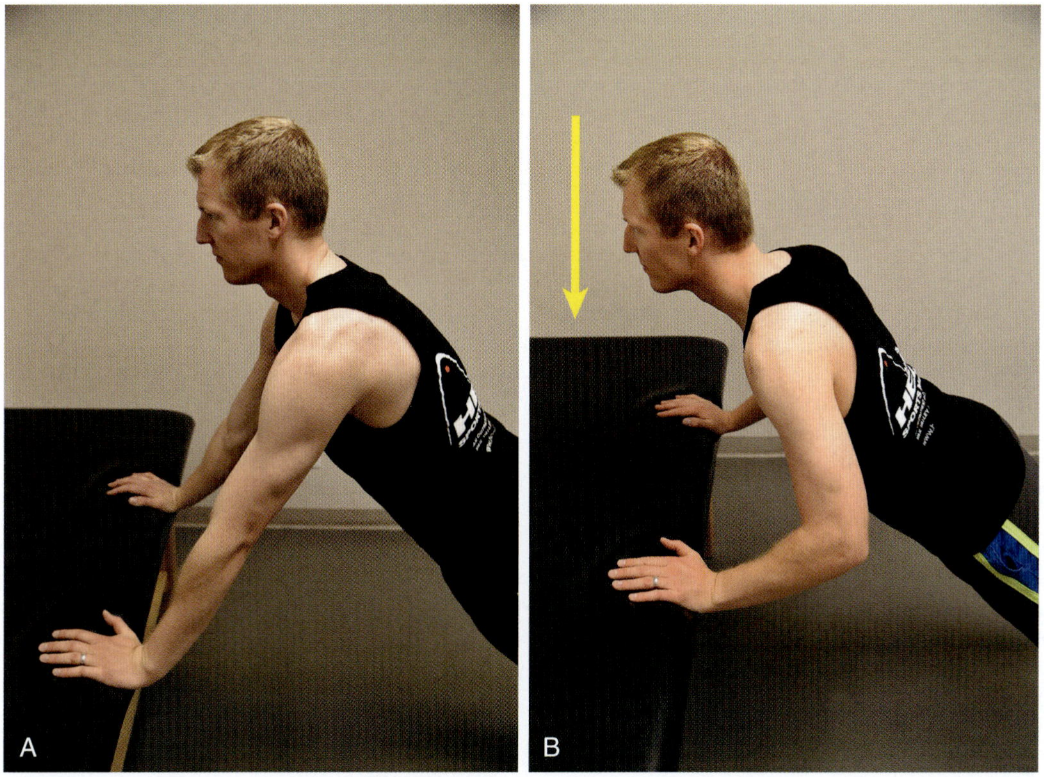

Fig. 15.4 Closed kinetic chain stabilization exercises performed on a table. **A,** Tall plank hold. Progression can incorporate weight shifts to the involved upper extremity and serratus anterior "plus" with scapular protraction. **B,** Shallow push-up from tall plank position. Progression can include serratus anterior "plus" with scapular protraction and advancement of the depth of the push-up.

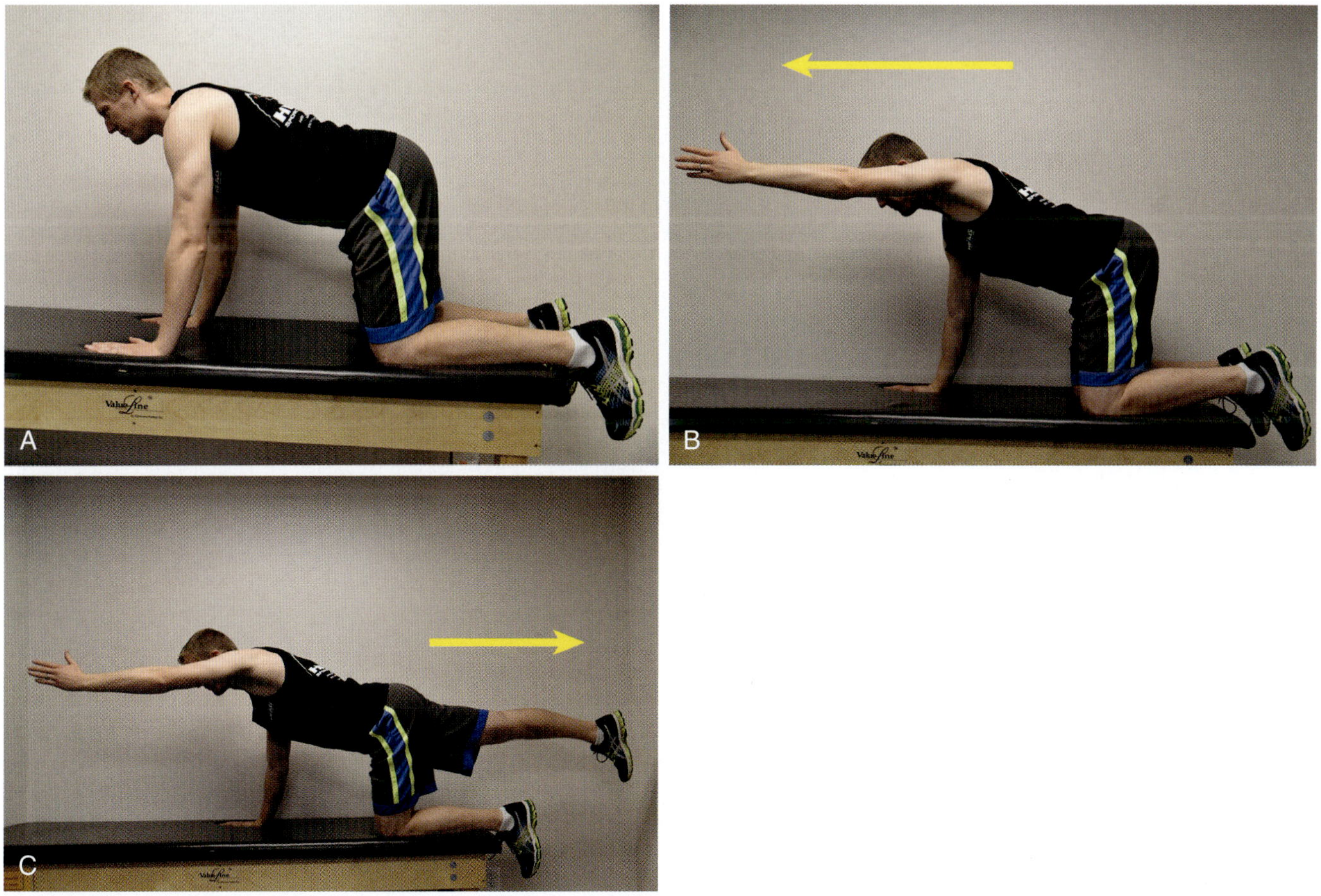

Fig. 15.5 "Birddog" exercise. Closed kinetic chain stabilization exercises in quadruped (hands-and-knees) position. Right shoulder is the operative side. **A,** Quadruped stability start position. **B,** Quadruped position with single upper extremity support. **C,** Quadruped position with concurrent alternate upper extremity and lower extremity raise to increase demand on the involved upper extremity and core stability.

Outcomes of Operative Management

PLATE FIXATION WITHOUT CORACOCLAVICULAR RECONSTRUCTION

Overall, clinical outcomes following plate fixation of DCFs are reliable and good. Lee et al (2013) evaluated 35 patients with Neer type 2 DCFs who underwent surgical fixation with precontoured locking compressive distal clavicular plates. All patients in the group achieved bony union over a mean of 4.1 months. At a mean follow-up of 24 months, there was no significant difference between injured and contralateral shoulders in Constant-Murley scores, UCLA scores, or CC distance (Lee et al, 2013). Shin et al (2016) also evaluated postoperative outcomes for DCFs. The researchers prospectively evaluated 25 patients with unstable Neer type 2 DCFs who underwent anatomic plate fixation. Bone union was achieved at an average of 12.8 weeks for all patients. At an average follow-up of 25 months, there was no difference in the Constant and UCLA scores between patients with type 2A and those with type 2B fractures. One patient experienced adhesive capsulitis and underwent arthroscopic capsular release; 13 patients underwent subsequent plate removal for cosmesis or patient preference. There were no infections or hardware failures (Shin et al, 2016). Finally, Kang et al (2012) prospectively analyzed outcomes of DCF fixation. They evaluated the treatment of 10 symptomatic non-unions of type 2 DCFs with modified locking T-plates and iliac bone autografts. They found that bony union was obtained at a mean of 14.7 weeks. At a minimum follow-up of 24 months, 9 of the 10 patients had regained full range of motion of their operative shoulders. Patients demonstrated significant improvement from preoperative to postoperative values in Constant score, Modified Shoulder Rating Scale score, and visual analog scale (Kang et al, 2012).

PLATE FIXATION WITH KNOTLESS CORACOCLAVICULAR RECONSTRUCTION

Clinical outcomes following DCF fixation with CC reconstruction have also been investigated. In general, the benefit is a stronger fixation construct, potentially leading to a lower risk of loss of reduction, and overall, clinical outcomes of plate fixation of DCFs with and without CC fixation are positive and reliable.

Hohmann et al (2012) investigated the outcomes of 31 Neer type 2 DCFs that were managed operatively using distal radius locking plates and a double-loaded knotless CC fixation device (TightRope, Arthrex). They reported that bony union was achieved at a mean of 6 ± 4 weeks; one patient experienced an infection, which resolved with antibiotics, and one patient experienced non-union with hardware failure requiring revision surgery. At final follow-up of 39 months, the mean Disabilities of the Arm, Shoulder, and Hand (DASH) score was 0.6 ± 2.1, and the mean Shoulder Pain and Disability Index value was 0.6 ± 2. Schliemann et al (2013) investigated 14 patients in whom unstable lateral clavicle fractures were treated with locked plate fixation and CC ligament reconstruction. In all cases, bony union was obtained within 6 to 10 weeks. Three patients required plate removal because of irritation. At a mean follow-up of 38 months, the Constant-Murley score for affected shoulders was 93.5, compared with 97.2 for unaffected shoulders; the mean AC joint instability score was 92 on the affected shoulders, compared with 96 on the unaffected shoulders. Finally, the mean CC distances were 21 mm at the time of injury, to 8.5 mm following surgery, and 12 mm at final follow-up (Schliemann et al, 2013).

References

Craig EV. Fractures of the clavicle. *Shoulder*. 1990;1:367–401.

Hohmann E, Hansen T, Tetsworth K. Treatment of Neer type II fractures of the lateral clavicle using distal radius locking plates combined with TightRope augmentation of the coraco-clavicular ligaments. *Arch. Orthop. Trauma Surg*. 2012;132(10):1415–1421.

Kang HJ, Kim HS, Kim SJ, Yoo JH. Osteosynthesis of symptomatic non-unions of type II fractures of the distal clavicle using modified locking T-plate and bone grafting. *J Trauma Acute Care Surg*. 2012;72(2): E14–E19.

Lee SK, Lee JW, Song DG, Choy WS. Precontoured locking plate fixation for displaced lateral clavicle fractures. *Orthopedics*. 2013;36(6):801–807.

Neer CS 2nd. Fracture of the distal clavicle with detachment of the coraco-clavicular ligaments in adults. *J Trauma*. 1963;3:99–110.

Neer CS 2nd. Fractures of the distal third of the clavicle. *Clin Orthop Relat Res*. 1968;58:43–50.

Sambandam B, Gupta R, Kumar S, Maini L. Fracture of distal end clavicle: a review. *J Clin Orthop Trauma*. 2014;5(2):65–73.

Schliemann B, Rosslenbroich SB, Schneider KN, Petersen W, Raschke MJ, Weimann A. Surgical treatment of vertically unstable lateral clavicle fractures (Neer 2b) with locked plate fixation and coraco-clavicular ligament reconstruction. *Arch Orthop Trauma Surg*. 2013; 133(7):935–939.

Shin SJ, Ko YW, Lee J, Park MG. Use of plate fixation without coracoclavicular ligament augmentation for unstable distal clavicle fractures. *J Shoulder Elbow Surg*. 2016;25(6):942–948.

van der Meijden OA, Gaskill TR, Millett PJ. Treatment of clavicle fractures: Current concepts review. *J Shoulder Elbow Surg*. 2012;21(3):423–429.

SECTION V

Sternoclavicular Joint Injury

SECTION OUTLINE

16 Overview

JOHN E. KUHN, MD

Anatomy, Epidemiology, and Etiology

Although injuries to the sternoclavicular joint are relatively rare in athletes, team physicians must be vigilant for such injuries because they represent one of the few potentially life-threatening injuries in sports. The sternoclavicular joint is a saddle-shaped, diarthrodial joint, with minimal osseous constraint and inherent stability in the joint. Motion at this joint is important for shoulder function. With forward elevation of the arm, the clavicle elevates 35 degrees and rotates posteriorly 45 degrees. With extension of the arm, the clavicle elevates 35 degrees and moves posteriorly 35 degrees. Because it is a relatively unconstrained joint, the ligamentous structures about the sternoclavicular joint are critical in allowing motion while preserving stability. The ligamentous structures include the anterior capsule, the posterior capsule, the interclavicular ligament, and the costoclavicular ligament (Fig. 16.1). Biomechanical studies have determined that the interclavicular ligament is important in keeping the clavicle elevated and the shoulder poised (Bearn, 1967). The anterior capsule and posterior capsules have been found to be the most important restraints to anterior displacement of the joint, and the posterior capsule to be the most important restraint to posterior displacement (Spencer et al, 2002).

The retrosternal contents, which lie immediately behind the sternoclavicular joint, include the subclavian and carotid arteries, the subclavian and jugular veins, and the trachea and esophagus. Because of these contents, when instability occurs in the posterior direction, the potential for life-threatening complications exists (Ponce et al, 2013).

Instability of the sternoclavicular joint is rare, with dislocations representing 3% of all shoulder dislocations (Cave, 1958) and anterior dislocations occurring more frequently than posterior (Finterbush & Pogrund, 1982; Nettles & Linscheid, 1968; Rockwood & Wirth, 1996).

As a result of the stout ligamentous structures that envelop this joint, dislocations require high-energy traumatic events to develop. Subluxations of the sternoclavicular joint may occur as a result of either a single traumatic event or the accumulation of repetitive microtraumatic events.

Classification, Assessment, and Imaging

Injuries to the sternoclavicular joint are classified by their severity and direction. As with the acromioclavicular joint, the capsule of the sternoclavicular joint may be sprained without displacement or instability. Subluxations of the joint may occur, and recurrent subluxation episodes may be symptomatic. Dislocations of the sternoclavicular joint

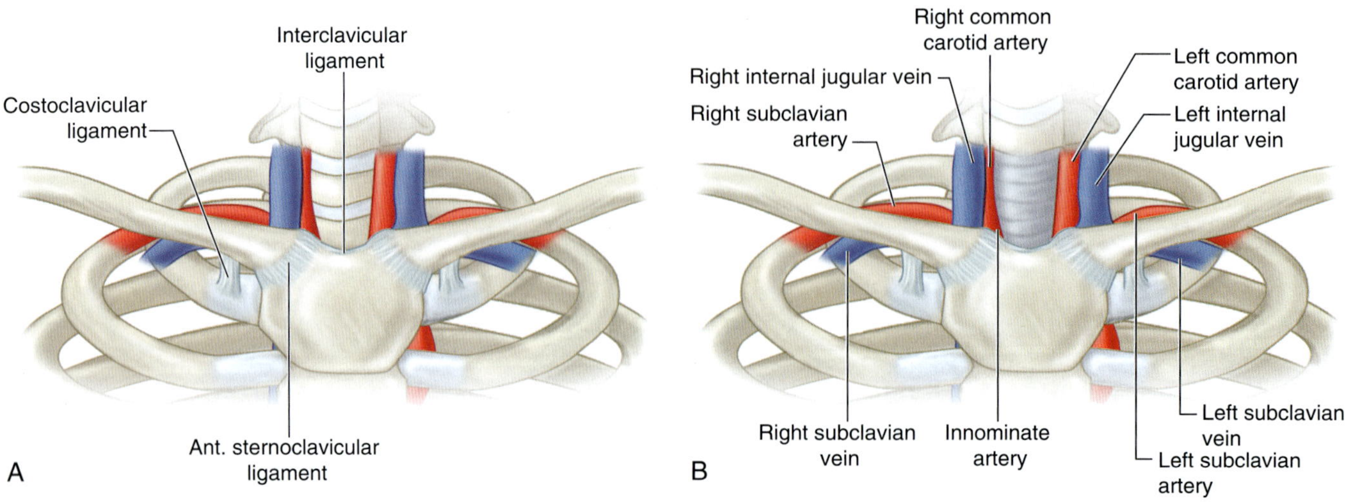

Fig. 16.1 Anatomy of the sternoclavicular joint. (**A** and **B**) The sternoclavicular joint is relatively unconstrained. Stability arises from the posterior capsule, anterior capsule, interclavicular ligament, and costoclavicular ligament. The mediastinal structures are immediately behind the sternoclavicular joint. *Ant.,* anterior. (From Kuhn JE, Mansour AA. Sternoclavicular joint reconstruction using semitendinosus graft. In Lee DH, Neviaser RJ, Eds. *Operative Techniques: Shoulder Elbow Surgery*. Philadelphia: Elsevier; 2011:414-415.)

may occur as well, and it is critically important to differentiate anterior dislocations of the clavicle head from posterior dislocations, because the latter may injure the retrosternal contents.

SUBLUXATION OF THE STERNOCLAVICULAR JOINT

In sports, subluxation of the sternoclavicular joint may manifest as a history of one traumatic event or of repetitive microtrauma (e.g., swimming backstroke). Patients with a history of repetitive microtrauma are predisposed to recurrent symptoms with their sport. The severity of symptoms is patient specific. Some patients find the subluxation events mildly symptomatic, whereas others will present with significant discomfort.

Patients without a history of trauma may present with the insidious onset of symptoms. These patients are usually younger than 25 years, are often female, and may have generalized ligamentous laxity or a collagen disorder. Instability is often bilateral and typically anterior. Alternatively, perimenopausal females are subject to the insidious onset of pain and swelling of the sternoclavicular joint, known as *pseudosubluxation* (Higgenbotham & Kuhn, 2005), which is arthritic and not true instability.

Patients with subluxation of the joint sometimes have tenderness and can often demonstrate the subluxation of the joint by forward elevation of the arm (Video 16.1). Imaging studies in these patients, including radiographs, CT, and magnetic resonance imaging (MRI), usually have normal findings. The dynamic nature of ultrasonography can detect subluxation of the sternoclavicular joint if it is not apparent on clinical examination.

ANTERIOR DISLOCATIONS OF THE STERNOCLAVICULAR JOINT

Anterior dislocations of the sternoclavicular joint are typically described as occurring from a blow to the front of the shoulder. The acromial end of the clavicle is pushed back, the clavicle pivots over the first rib, and the sternal portion of the clavicle is forced anteriorly (Fig. 16.2). These injuries always occur with relatively high-energy trauma, which in sports could occur in a contact sport or fall from a height.

Patients with anterior dislocations of the clavicle head have immediate and significant pain. They often walk off the field with the arm dangling, like someone with an anterior dislocation of the shoulder. They have swelling and tenderness to palpation of the sternal end of the clavicle. Patients are not comfortable trying to elevate, abduct, or extend the arm. Glenohumeral rotation of the adducted arm is tolerated well and can distinguish this injury from a glenohumeral joint dislocation.

As a result of the patient's discomfort and swelling in the joint, it can be extremely difficult to determine whether the dislocation is anterior or posterior, and imaging is usually required. Patients should be transported to the hospital immediately for imaging. Although a number of imaging options are available, computed tomography has been most helpful to assess sternoclavicular joint injuries. CT is the imaging technique of choice (Fig. 16.3). It is important to know that the physis of the medial clavicle does not close in some people until age 25, so in younger individuals, injury to this region may represent a physeal injury and not a dislocation. In addition, fracture of the medial clavicle, although rare, may manifest like a dislocation of the sternoclavicular joint (Lee et al, 2014).

POSTERIOR DISLOCATIONS OF THE STERNOCLAVICULAR JOINT

Posterior dislocations of the sternoclavicular joint always follow significant trauma and may occur as a result of direct trauma to the anterior chest wall or may occur from a blow to the back of the shoulder that allows the clavicle to pivot over the first rib, driving the head of the clavicle posteriorly (Fig. 16.2). Clinically these injuries are difficult to distinguish from anterior dislocations. Patients have significant pain and do not want to move the arm. They may exhibit symptoms related to injury to the mediastinal structures, such as dysphagia, hoarseness, decreased pulses in the arm on the involved side, swelling of the arm due to a reduction in venous return, and symptoms of thoracic outlet syndrome.

Examination of such patients demonstrates swelling and tenderness at the sternoclavicular joint. Occasionally examination of the affected arm may demonstrate signs of vascular compression (decreased pulses, swelling, bluish discoloration from lack of venous return). Again, it may be difficult to distinguish this injury from anterior dislocation, so patients should be transported to the hospital urgently so appropriate imaging can be obtained. CT demonstrates the posteriorly displaced head of the clavicle (Fig. 16.4). If vascular injury is suspected, an intravascular contrast agent should be added to the CT scan, because damage to the great vessels has been reported as a consequence of this injury. Posteriorly displaced physeal injuries and fractures are also at risk for mediastinal structure damage.

Conclusions

Sternoclavicular joint instability, like glenohumeral joint instability, is classified by severity (subluxation vs dislocation), direction (anterior or posterior), and mechanism of injury (traumatic or atraumatic). Posterior sternoclavicular joint dislocation represents an orthopedic emergency because of the potential for damage to the mediastinal contents. Athletes with suspected sternoclavicular joint dislocation should undergo emergency transportation to the hospital for assessment and imaging, and CT is required, with assessment of vasculature for posterior dislocations. Team physicians should be especially vigilant for this injury because it may be difficult to determine on the field whether the dislocation is anterior or posterior.

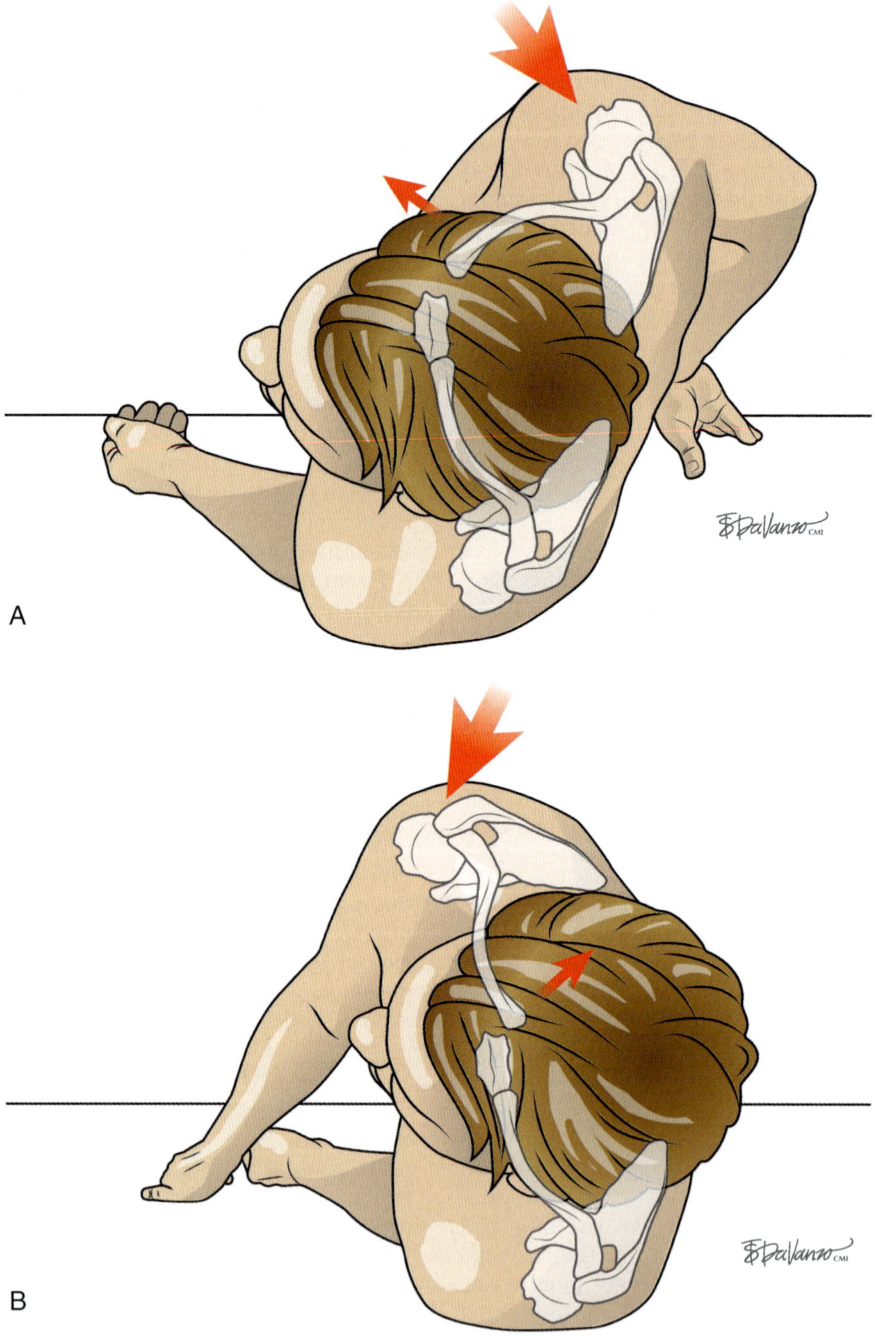

Fig. 16.2 Mechanism of injury for anterior and posterior sternoclavicular joint dislocations. The clavicle pivots over the first rib, so such anterior dislocations result from a impact to the anterior shoulder (**A**) and posterior dislocations result from impact to the posterior shoulder (**B**). (Modified from Spencer EE, Wirth MA, Rockwood CA, Jr. Disorders of the sternoclavicular joint; pathophysiology, diagnosis, and management. In Ianotti JP, Williams G. *Disorders of the Shoulder, Diagnosis & Management.* 2nd ed. Philadelphia: Lippincott Williams & Wilkins; 2007:1033.)

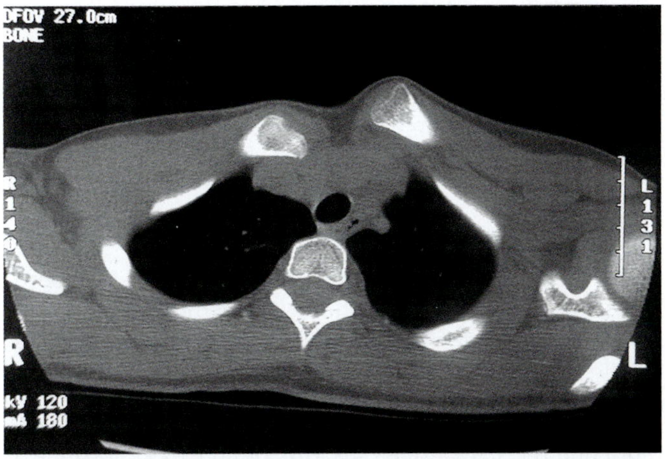

Fig. 16.3 Anterior dislocation of the sternoclavicular joint.

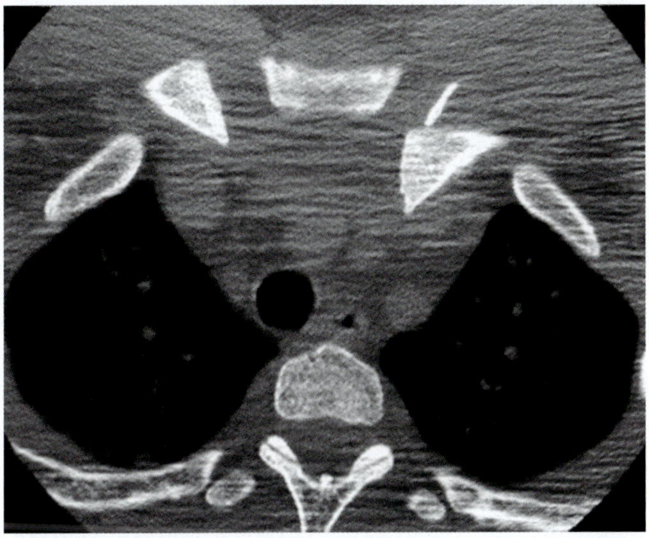

Fig. 16.4 Posterior physeal dislocation. Note that the epiphysis remains in continuity with the manubrium.

References

Bearn JG. Direct observations on the function of the capsule of the sternoclavicular joint in clavicular support. *J Anat*. 1967;101:159–170.

Cave EF. *Fractures and Other Injuries*. Chicago: Year Book Medical Publishers; 1958.

Finsterbush A, Pogrund H. The hypermobility syndrome: Musculoskeletal complaints in 100 consecutive cases of generalized joint hypermobility. *Clin Orthop Relat Res*. 1982;168:124–127.

Higginbotham T, Kuhn JE. Atraumatic disorders of the sternoclavicular joint. *J Am Acad Orthop Surg*. 2005;13:138–145.

Lee JT, Nasreddine AY, Black EM, Bae DS, Kocher MS. Posterior sternoclavicular joint injuries in skeletally immature patients. *J Pediatr Orthop*. 2014;34(4):369–375.

Nettles JL, Linscheid RL. Sternoclavicular dislocations. *J Trauma*. 1968;8:158–164.

Ponce BA, Kundukulam JA, Pflugner R, et al. Sternoclavicular joint surgery: how far does danger lurk below? *J Shoulder Elbow Surg*. 2013;22(7):993–999.

Rockwood CA, Wirth MA. Injuries to the sternoclavicular joint. In: Rockwood CA, Green DP, Bucholz RW, Heckman JD, eds. *Rockwood and Green's Fractures in Adults*. 4th ed. Philadelphia: Lippincott-Raven; 1996:1415–1471.

Spencer EE, Kuhn JE, Huston LJ, Carpenter JE, Hughes RE. Ligamentous restraints to anterior and posterior translation of the sternoclavicular joint. *J Shoulder Elbow Surg*. 2002;11(1):44–47.

17 Treatment

JOHN E. KUHN, MD

Indications for Surgery

Sternoclavicular joint injuries are rare, and indications for their surgery are also rare. Fractures of the medial end of the clavicle are usually not sports related, are the result of vehicular trauma, and rarely need surgery (Throckmorton & Kuhn, 2007). Generally, surgery is avoided in atraumatic subluxations of the sternoclavicular joint, because this disorder is generally found in patients with generalized ligamentous laxity and failures after surgery are common (Rockwood & Odor, 1989).

An acute traumatic anterior or posterior dislocation of the sternoclavicular joint should undergo an attempt at closed reduction in the operating room. Open reduction with repair or reconstruction of the sternoclavicular joint capsule is indicated for irreducible posterior dislocations because a chronically dislocated clavicular head can erode into the mediastinal contents, causing late complications (Ecke, 1984; Gangahar & Flogaites, 1978; Noda et al, 1997; Rayan, 1994; Wasylenko & Busse, 1981).

For these reasons, a chronic posterior dislocation of the sternoclavicular joint is an indication for open reduction and reconstruction of the stabilizing ligaments. As with most type III acromioclavicular joint dislocations, most chronically displaced anterior dislocations stabilize with scarring and may be minimally symptomatic. Surgery can be entertained in those few patients in whom anterior instability remains symptomatic.

Nonoperative Treatment

STERNOCLAVICULAR JOINT SPRAIN

The sternoclavicular joint, like the acromioclavicular joint, is subject to different severities of injury. Sprains of the sternoclavicular joint capsule may occur. The patient with such a sprain has tenderness and pain in extremes of motion but the joint is not dislocated. Sprains can be treated with nonsteroidal antiinflammatory drugs (NSAIDs), ice, and rest. A sling may be used for comfort. Decisions about return to play are based on the patient's comfort and ability to do sport-specific tasks with comfort. Unlike with the acromioclavicular joint, injecting a sternoclavicular joint to reduce pain and return to play is not recommended.

STERNOCLAVICULAR JOINT DISLOCATION

A dislocated sternoclavicular joint should undergo an attempt at closed reduction with the patient under general anesthesia. The patient is placed supine with a rolled towel under the spine. The chest is prepared, and an assistant provides longitudinal traction on the arm of the affected side. A towel clip is placed around the clavicle percutaneously and the clavicle is pulled laterally with pressure toward the operating room table for anterior dislocation, and pulled away toward the ceiling for posterior dislocation (Fig. 17.1). The reduction registers as a large clunk or pop; it is not subtle. If the reduction is not clearly felt, one can assume the attempt was unsuccessful. Post reduction computed tomography (CT) can be used to ensure a successful reduction.

It is important to have a thoracic surgeon available when one is performing a closed reduction of a posterior sternoclavicular joint. There are cases in which the dislocated clavicle has been providing tamponade for an injured great vessel. Upon reduction of the clavicle head, life-threatening hemorrhage is possible. Closed reduction is successful in approximately one-third of patients and is more likely to be successful if performed within 10 days after injury (Groh et al, 2011).

Once the dislocated clavicle head is reduced, a standard arm sling for anterior dislocations is applied, and a figure-of-eight brace or pillow sling is used to keep the scapula retracted for 6 weeks. After this time, physical therapy directed toward gradually restoring active motion is employed for 6 weeks; strengthening and sport-specific training can begin at 12 weeks, with return to sport when the patient's shoulder is ready. It is important to note that there is little data in the literature regarding the treatment of athletes with this condition. One case report of a posterior dislocation in a National Football League (NFL) player allowed return to play after 5 weeks with no apparent complications (Yang et al, 2015). In

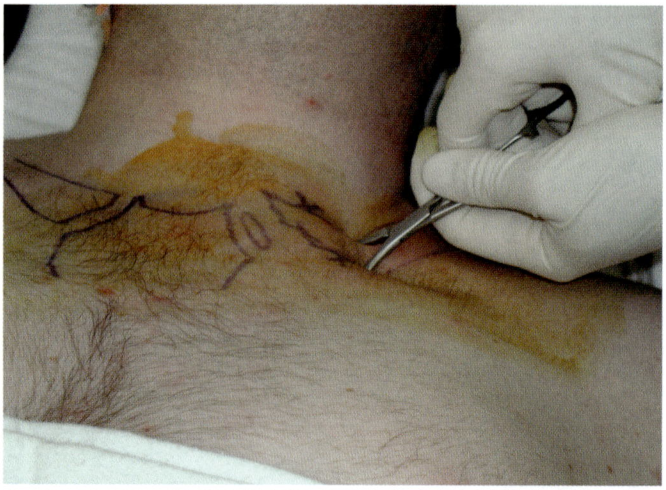

Fig. 17.1 Closed reduction of posterior sternoclavicular joint dislocation.

this report the literature was reviewed and summarized; most contact athletes with posterior sternoclavicular joint dislocations required open reduction and surgical repair or fixation (Yang et al, 2015).

If the reduction of an anterior dislocation is lost, the clavicular head can be left dislocated, because chronic, stable, anterior dislocations may do well with nonoperative treatment (De Jong & Sukul, 1990; Wirth & Rockwood, 1996). Clinicians should employ the same program for recovery as described for a successful reduction. Surgery should be performed for a failed reduction of a posterior dislocation, for a chronic posterior dislocation, and for a chronic anterior dislocation with symptoms related to instability.

Surgical Treatment

ACUTE INJURIES

If a closed reduction is unsuccessful and an open reduction is required, the torn ligamentous structures, if generally intact, can be repaired primarily. It is important to bring the posterior capsule back to the clavicle—typically using sutures passed through drill holes in the clavicle. Repairing the posterior capsule is of paramount importance because it is the primary restraint to posterior and anterior translation of the sternoclavicular joint (Spencer et al, 2002). Some writers have recommended using a figure-of-eight suture impregnated with para-aramid synthetic fiber (Kevlar, DuPont USA, Wilmington, DE); however the suture does not deform and could potentially cut through bone if the soft tissues do not heal (Adamcik et al, 2017). Other writers report success using plate fixation (Shuler & Pappas, 2008), or hook plate fixation (Liu et al, 2008); hardware that spans across the joint would require removal, however, as there is a tremendous amount of motion across the sternoclavicular joint. If the soft tissues are inadequate for primary repair, graft reconstruction of the anterior and posterior capsule is typically employed using techniques described here.

CHRONIC DISLOCATIONS

A variety of different techniques are employed to reconstruct the unstable sternoclavicular joint. They include transferring capsule and disk material into the end of the resected clavicle (Rockwood et al, 1997); using the subclavius tendon as described by Burrows (1951); using part of the sternocleidomastoid as local graft (Bae et al, 2006; Lee et al, 2010; Uri et al, 2014); and a variety of subtle variations of the figure-of-eight technique with autograft or allograft.* In a cadaveric biomechanical analysis, the mechanical properties of the figure-of-eight technique were found to be superior to those of the subclavius technique and the disk/capsule stabilization technique (Spencer & Kuhn, 2004). Interestingly, in this cadaver study, the subclavius

*Bak & Fogh, 2014; Guan & Wolf, 2013; Kawaguchi et al, 2015; Kusnezov et al, 2015; Martetschlager et al, 2016; Petri et al, 2016; Sabatini et al, 2015; Singer et al, 2013; Spencer & Kuhn, 2004; Willinger, 2016.

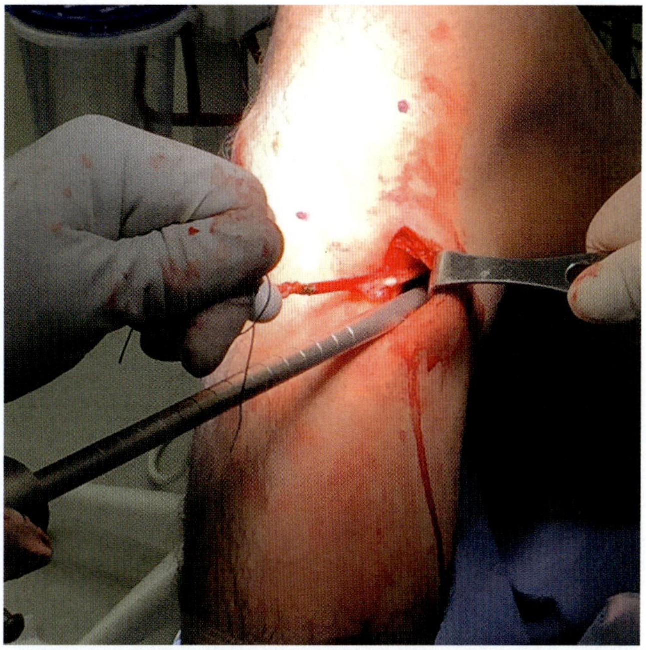

Fig. 17.2 Hamstring tendon autograft harvest for figure-of-eight reconstruction.

was found to be of inadequate length in 25% of the specimens (Spencer & Kuhn, 2004). As a result of its better biomechanical properties, the figure-of-eight technique is likely the most popular, and it has been used in more case series in the literature than other techniques (Bae et al, 2006; Bak & Fogh, 2014; Guan & Wolf, 2013; Kusnezov et al, 2015; Petri et al, 2016; Sabatini et al, 2015; Singer et al, 2013).

The Figure-of-Eight Graft for Sternoclavicular Joint Instability

The patient is placed prone on a flat operating room table, with a small rolled towel placed behind the spine to allow the shoulders to retract. The patient's entire chest is prepared and draped. If a semitendinosus autograft is going to be used, the patient's leg is prepared and draped as well. Generally, the semitendinosus is harvested first through a small incision medial to the tibial tubercle. The tendon is identified and a tendon stripper is used to harvest the tendon after release of any adhesions (Fig. 17.2). Each end of the tendon is cleaned and sutured with #2 permanent suture.

After the bony landmarks of the clavicle, manubrium, sternal notch, and sternocleidomastoid are marked, a curved incision is made following Langer's lines over the medial clavicle and sternoclavicular joint to the midline over the manubrium (Fig. 17.3). The platysma layer is incised in the same plane and reflected superiorly and inferiorly. The capsule of the sternoclavicular joint is incised and opened by reflection of the superior flap superiorly and the inferior flap inferiorly. It is important to find and protect the sternocleidomastoid muscle. Next any scar tissue in the joint space is removed. A towel clamp is placed on the clavicle, and lateral traction is

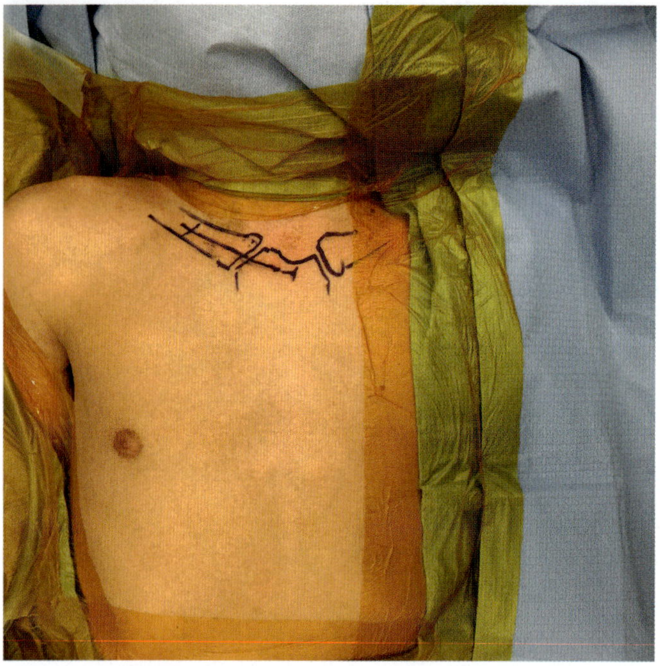

Fig. 17.3 Incision for figure-of-eight reconstruction.

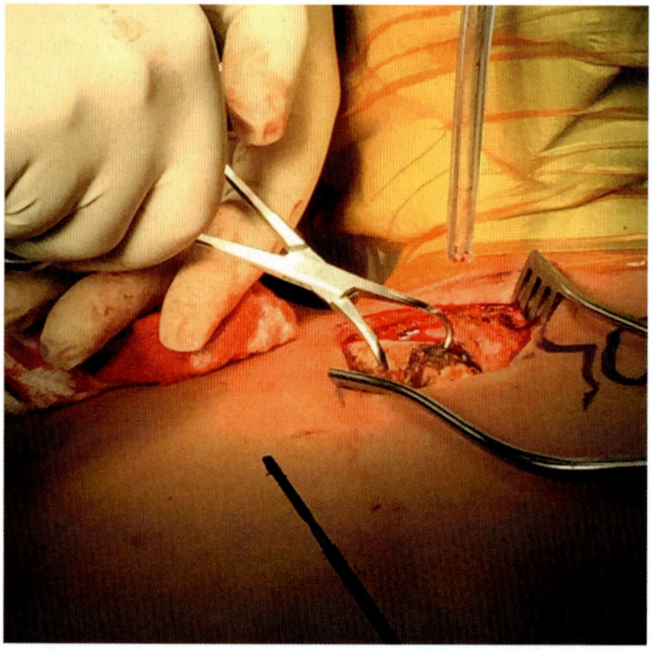

Fig. 17.4 The clavicle is exposed and reduced.

applied to reduce the joint (Fig. 17.4). It is notable that a lot of force may be required for highly displaced posterior dislocations.

If the standard figure-of-eight technique is to be employed, a thoracic surgeon makes an incision in the muscle above the sternal notch, using blunt dissection to develop the plane in the mediastinum behind the manubrium. With a ribbon retractor in place behind the manubrium, two drill holes are placed in parallel through the distal clavicle and through the manubrium (Fig. 17.5). The drill size can be determined by the size of the semitendinosus graft. A Hewson suture passer or wire loop is passed through the manubrial drill hole and into the incision above the sternal notch. A suture loop is then passed into each hole. Similarly suture loops are placed through the clavicle holes (Fig. 17.6). The suture loops are used to pass the tendon graft in a figure-of-eight fashion. The graft is passed such that there are parallel fibers posterior and crossed fibers anterior (Fig. 17.7). The graft is placed under slight, not excessive tension and tied to itself, then secured with #2 permanent suture (Fig. 17.8). Extra tendon material can be sutured to itself for additional strength. After the repair is completed, the platysma, subcutaneous tissue, and skin are closed in layers. A sterile dressing is applied.

A variety of modifications have been developed to avoid working behind the manubrium (Bak & Fogh, 2014; Guan & Wolf, 2013; Martetschlager et al, 2016; Sabatini et al, 2015). Most of these techniques were reserved for patients with anterior instability. Reported outcomes are also generally good (Table 17.1). These techniques do not reconstruct the posterior capsule well, however, a matter of concern because the posterior capsule is the primary restraint to anterior and posterior sternoclavicular joint translation (Spencer et al, 2002).

Postoperative Rehabilitation and Return to Sport

Immobilization is used for 4 to 6 weeks to allow graft healing into the bone tunnels. A standard arm sling is used for comfort but can be removed for desk work. After 4 to 6 weeks after surgery shoulder range of motion is begun, avoiding extremes of extension, and elevation until 10 weeks after surgery, at which time motion should be complete and unrestricted. After 12 weeks light strengthening of the shoulder is permitted, including the scapular-stabilizing serratus anterior and lower trapezius muscles. Return to running is allowed when shoulder motion is full. Return to sports that require heavy loading of the shoulder (contact sports, gymnastics, swimming, etc.) should be delayed for 6 months and should be allowed only if motion and strength have returned completely.

Outcomes of Surgical Treatment

The outcomes of the figure-of-eight graft technique and its variations are reported in Table 17.1. In general results are good, with at least 70% of patients returning to full unrestricted activity, including military duty and sports. Reported complications of this procedure include hematoma, low-grade infection, and persistent discomfort. Later complications include the development of osteoarthritis and the recurrence of symptoms in fewer than 15% of patients (Table 17.1).

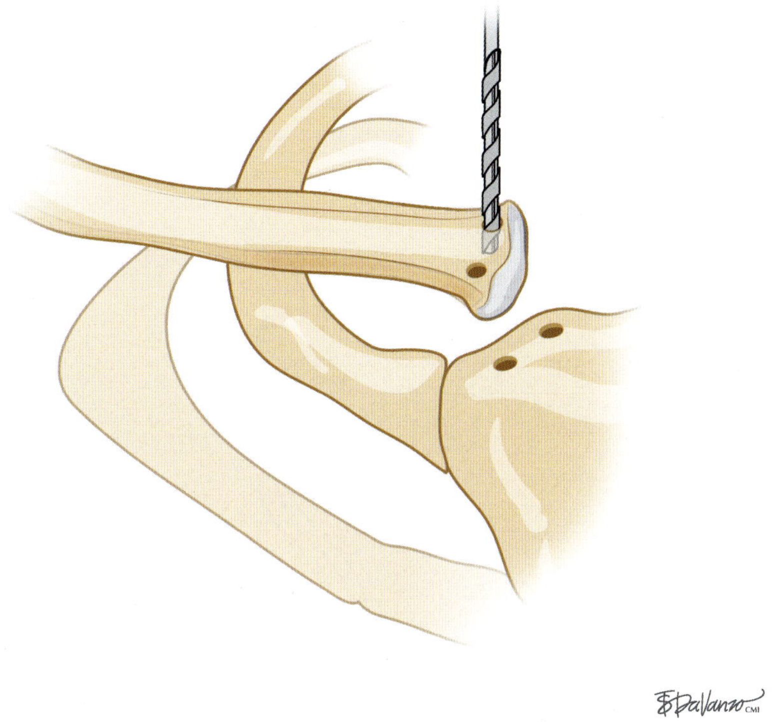

Fig. 17.5 **Drill holes are placed in manubrium and clavicle. Note the ribbon retractor placed behind the manubrium to protect vital structures.** (Modified from Zuckerman JD, ed. *Advanced Reconstruction: Shoulder*. Rosemont, IL: American Academy of Orthopaedic Surgeons; 2007.)

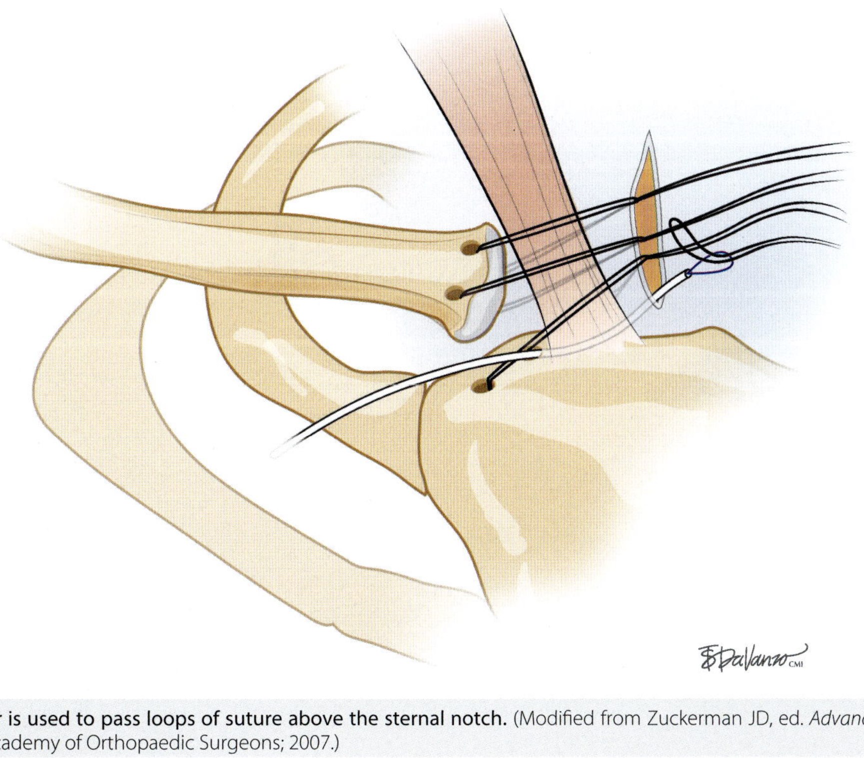

Fig. 17.6 **A suture passer is used to pass loops of suture above the sternal notch.** (Modified from Zuckerman JD, ed. *Advanced Reconstruction: Shoulder*. Rosemont, IL: American Academy of Orthopaedic Surgeons; 2007.)

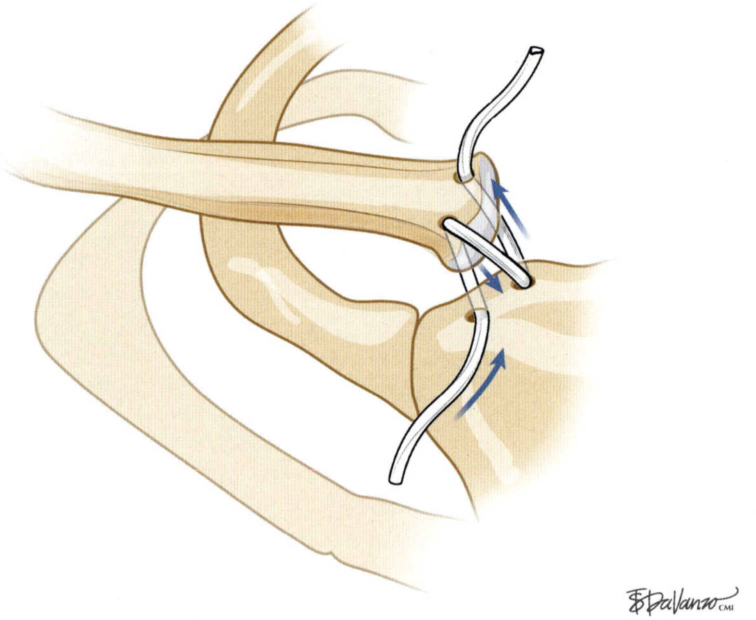

Fig. 17.7 The graft is passed in figure-of-eight fashion with parallel fibers posterior and cruciate fibers anterior. (Modified from Zuckerman JD, ed. *Advanced Reconstruction: Shoulder.* Rosemont, IL: American Academy of Orthopaedic Surgeons; 2007.)

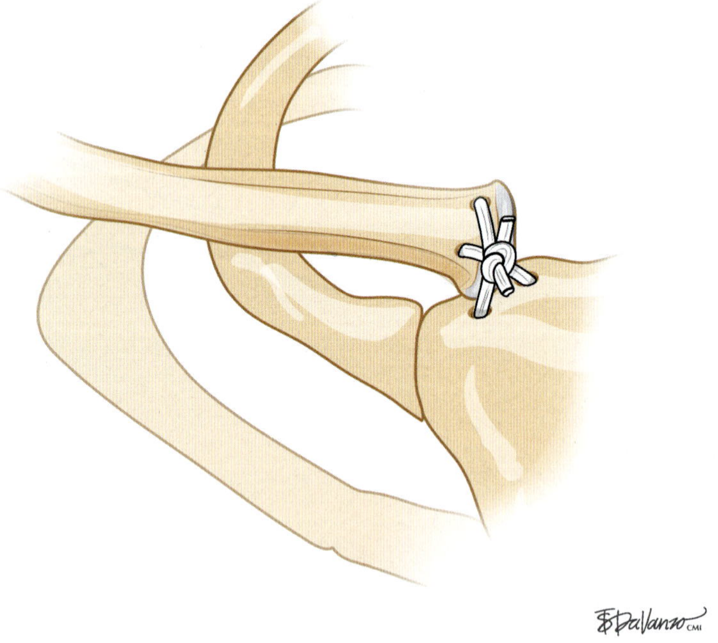

Fig. 17.8 The graft is secured to itself anteriorly. (Modified from Zuckerman JD, ed. *Advanced Reconstruction: Shoulder.* Rosemont, IL: American Academy of Orthopaedic Surgeons; 2007.)

Table 17.1 Results of Figure-of-Eight Graft Reconstruction for Sternoclavicular Joint Instability

Reference	Technique	Population	Direction	N	Follow-up	Outcomes
STANDARD TECHNIQUE						
Kusnezov et al, 2016	Figure-of-eight autograft through manubrium	Age 26.6 yr 1 F, 13 M Military	8 anterior, 6 posterior	14	27 months	10/12 (71.4%) on full active military duty 2/12 persistent instability, 2/12 required additional surgery
Petri et al, 2016	Figure-of-eight autograft through manubrium	Age 30 yr 9 F, 10 M 2 Bilateral	Not reported	21	24 months	No complications, no recurrence
Singer et al, 2013	Figure-of-eight autograft through manubrium	Age 22 yr 3 F, 3 M	3 anterior, 2 posterior, 1 both	6	22 months	All patients returned to full activity, including contact sports
MODIFIED TECHNIQUE						
Bak et al, 2014	Autograft figure-of-eight with intraarticular suture anchors in manubrium	Age 35 yr 17 F, 10 M	All anterior	27	54 months	2 failures; 68% had donor site morbidity, 40% had some discomfort
Guan & Wolf, 2013	Autograft hamstring figure-of-eight with bone tunnels connecting anterior drill holes	Age 22.2 yr 5 F, 1 M	All anterior	6	40 months	No instability, full motion, one case of osteoarthritis at 4 years All returned to preoperative activity and sport
Sabatini et al, 2015	Allograft figure-of-eight with interference screw	Age 40.1 yr 7 F, 3 M	9 anterior, 1 posterior	10	38 months	7 patients had symptoms with activity, 1 hematoma, 1 seroma, 1 failure

F, Female; *M*, Male.

Conclusion

Sternoclavicular joint injuries include fractures, sprains, and dislocations. Although most fractures and sprains can be treated nonoperatively, an attempt should be made to reduce a dislocated sternoclavicular joint in the operating room with the patient under anesthesia. Successful reductions are treated with immobilization and later rehabilitation. Unsuccessfully reduced anterior dislocations can be left in place and, if scar tissue produces stability, need no further treatment. Unsuccessfully reduced posterior dislocations should undergo open reduction with repair of the damaged capsule and/or reconstruction using tendon graft. Symptomatic chronic anterior dislocation and all chronic posterior dislocations should be treated with open reduction and reconstruction of the joint capsule. The figure-of-eight technique using tendon graft is popular and, in athletes, produces good outcomes with reasonably high rates of return to play.

References

Adamcik S, Ahler M, Gioutsos K, Schmid RA, Kocher GJ. Repair of sternoclavicular joint dislocations with FiberWire. *Arch Orthop Trauma. Surg.* 2017;137(3):341–345. http://dx.doi.org/10.1007/s00402-017.2632-z.

Bae DS, Kocher MS, Waters PM, Micheli LM, Griffey M, Dichtel L. Chronic recurrent anterior sternoclavicular joint instability. *J Pediatr Orthop.* 2006;26:71–74.

Bak K, Fogh K. Reconstruction of the chronic anterior unstable sternoclavicular joint using a tendon autograft: medium-term to long-term follow-up results. *J Shoulder Elbow Surg.* 2014;23:245–250.

Burrows HJ. Tenodesis of subclavius in the treatment of recurrent dislocation of the sterno-clavicular joint. *J Bone Joint Surg Br.* 1951;33:240–243.

De Jong KP, Sukul DMKS. Anterior sternoclavicular joint dislocation: A long-term follow-up study. *J Orthop Trauma.* 1990;4:420–423.

Ecke H. [Late lesions following luxation of the sternoclavicular joint] [in German]. *Hefte Unfallheilkd.* 1984;170:52–55.

Gangahar DM, Flogaites T. Retrosternal dislocation of the clavicle producing thoracic outlet syndrome. *J Trauma.* 1978;18:369–372.

Groh GI, Wirth MA, Rockwood CA Jr. Treatment of traumatic posterior sternoclavicular joint dislocations. *J Shoulder Elbow Surg.* 2011;20: 107–113.

Guan JJ, Wolf BR. Reconstruction for anterior sternoclavicular joint dislocation and instability. *J Shoulder Elbow Surg.* 2013;22:775–781.

Kawaguchi K, Tanaka S, Yoshitomi H, et al. Double figure-of-eight reconstruction technique for chronic anterior sternoclavicular joint dislocation. *Knee Surg Sports Traumatol Arthrosc.* 2015;23: 1559–1562.

Kusnezov N, Dunn JC, DeLong JM, Waterman BR. Sternoclavicular reconstruction in the young active patient: risk factor analysis and clinical outcomes at short-term followup. *J Orthop Trauma.* 2016;30(4):e111–e117.

Lee SU, Park IJ, Kim YD, Kim YC, Jeong C. Stabilization for chronic sternoclavicular joint instability. *Knee Surg Sports Traumatol Arthrosc.* 2010;18:1795–1797.

Liu H, Wang W, Ye H, Li X. [Clinical observation of sternoclavicular joint dislocation fixed by clavicular hook plate] [Chinese]. *Zhongguo Xiu Fu Chong Jian Wai Ke Za Zhi.* 2008;22(10):1193–1195.

Martetschlager F, Braun S, Lorenz S, Lenich A, Imhoff AB. Novel technique for sternoclavicular joint reconstruction using gracilis tendon autograft. *Knee Surg Sports Traumatol Arthrosc.* 2016;24:2225–2230.

Noda M, Shiraishi H, Mizuno K. Chronic posterior sternoclavicular dislocation causing compression of a subclavian artery. *J Shoulder Elbow Surg.* 1997;6:564–569.

Petri M, Greenspoon JA, Horan MP, Martetschlager F, Warth RJ, Millett PJ. Clinical outcomes after reconstruction for sternoclavicular joint instability. *J Shoulder Elbow Surg.* 2016;25:435–441.

Rayan GM. Compression brachial plexopathy caused by chronic posterior dislocation of the sternoclavicular joint. *J Okla State Med Assoc.* 1994;87:7–9.

Rockwood CA Jr, Groh GI, Wirth MA, Grassi FA. Resection arthroplasty of the sternoclavicular joint. *J Bone Joint Surg Am.* 1997;79(3):387–393.

Rockwood CA Jr, Odor JM. Spontaneous atraumatic anterior subluxation of the sternoclavicular joint. *J Bone Joint Surg Am.* 1989;71:1280–1288.

Sabatini JB, Shung JR, Clay TB, Oladeji LO, Minnich DJ, Ponce BA. Outcomes of augmented allograft figure-of-eight sternoclavicular joint reconstruction. *J Shoulder Elbow Surg.* 2015;24:902–907.

Shuler FD, Pappas N. Treatment of posterior sternoclavicular dislocation with locking plate osteosynthesis. *Orthopedics.* 2008;31:273.

Singer G, Ferlic P, Kraus T, Eberl R. Reconstruction of the sternoclavicular joint in active patients with the figure-of-eight technique using hamstrings. *J Shoulder Elbow Surg.* 2013;22:64–69.

Spencer EE, Kuhn JE, Huston LJ, Carpenter JE, Hughes RE. Ligamentous restraints to anterior and posterior translation of the sternoclavicular joint. *J Shoulder Elbow Surg.* 2002;11(1):43–47.

Spencer EE, Kuhn JE. Biomechanical analysis of reconstructions for sternoclavicular joint instability. *J Bone Joint Surg Am. 86A*. 2004:98–105.

Throckmorton T, Kuhn JE. Fractures of the medial end of the clavicle. *J Shoulder Elbow Surg.* 2007;16:49–54.

Uri O, Barmpagiannis K, Higgs D, Falworth M, Alexander S, Lambert S. Clinical outcome after reconstruction for sternoclavicular joint instability using sternocleidomastoid tendon graft. *J Bone Joint Surg Am.* 2014;96:417. 22.

Wasylenko MJ, Busse EF. Posterior dislocation of the clavicle causing fatal tracheoesophageal fistula. *Can J Surg.* 1981;24:626–627.

Willinger L1, Schanda J1, Herbst E1, Imhoff AB2, Martetschläger F1. Outcomes and complications following graft reconstruction for anterior sternoclavicular joint instability. *Knee Surg Sports Traumatol Arthrosc.* 2016;24(12):3863–3869. Epub 2015 Sep 3.

Wirth MA, Rockwood CA Jr. Acute and chronic traumatic injuries of the sternoclavicular joint. *J Am Acad Orthop Surg.* 1996;4. 268–278.

Yang JS, Bogunovic L, Brophy RH, Wright RW, Scott R, Matava M. A case of posterior sternoclavicular dislocation in a professional American football player. *Sports Health.* 2015:7(4):318–325.

SECTION **VI**

Biceps Labral Complex Injury

SECTION OUTLINE

18 Overview

SAMUEL A. TAYLOR, MD and STEPHEN J. O'BRIEN, MD, MBA

Important Points

- There is a shift away from SLAP (superior labrum anterior and posterior) repair toward biceps tenodesis.
- The biceps–labrum complex (BLC) can be divided into three anatomic locations: inside (the superior labrum and biceps anchor), junction (the intraarticular segment of the long head of the biceps tendon and the biceps pulley), and bicipital tunnel (the extraarticular segment of the biceps tendon and its fibro-osseous constraint).
- The bicipital tunnel commonly confines lesions hidden from standard diagnostic arthroscopy and should be considered when selecting an appropriate surgical technique.
- Lesions may occur in one location or more commonly along the BLC at multiple sites.
- Physical examination can be particularly useful in identifying BLC disease and ruling out (tenderness to palpation and O'Brien sign) bicipital tunnel disease.

Anatomy, Epidemiology, and Etiology

Our understanding of the anatomy and clinical relevance of the BLC continues to evolve as do our means for diagnosis and therapeutic interventions. Although the BLC has long been recognized as a clinically relevant pain generator in the shoulder, traditional teaching categorized pathology separately as biceps and labrum. As a result, there was an early focus on SLAP (superior labrum anterior and posterior) tears as the primary symptoms-producing culprit. New York State database reports, in fact, showed a 238% increase in SLAP repairs from 2002 to 2009 (Vogel et al, 2014). Furthermore, SLAP repairs amounted to 9.4% of all shoulder cases submitted by board-eligible surgeons to the American Board of Orthopaedic Surgeons (ABOS) during a similar chronologic window from 2003 to 2008 (Weber et al, 2012).

More recently, our attention has shifted from SLAP to a more comprehensive understanding of the BLC spurred in part by several important studies that identified high failure rates among SLAP repair patients. For example, the landmark paper by Provencher et al (2013) cited a 37% failure rate among an active duty military population and found that age older than 36 years was a risk factor for failure. Others have shown biceps tenodesis to be an effective salvage procedure for failed tenodesis (McCormick et al, 2014; Werner et al, 2014). Gottshalk et al (2014) reported on a series of 36 patients with type II and type IV SLAP tears who were treated primarily with open subpectoral biceps tenodesis. At 40 months of follow-up, American Shoulder and Elbow Surgeons (ASES) scores improved from 48 to 88, visual analog scale pain score is decreased from 6.4 to 1.5, and 90% of patients returned to play at their previous level.

Recent ABOS data reflect the changing indication landscape (Patterson et al, 2014). From 2002 to 2011, repairs of SLAP tears decreased from 69% to 45%, tenodesis increased from 2% to 19%, and tenotomy increased from 0.4% to 1.7%. For SLAP repairs in the setting of rotator cuff tear, repairs decreased from 60% to 15%, and tenodesis increased from 6% to 28% during the same time period.

Taylor et al (2015b) noted high rates of concomitant lesion along the BLC, especially hidden extraarticular disease within the bicipital tunnel. They suggested failure to recognize additional pathology along the BLC as an explanation for failed SLAP repairs. The authors evaluated 277 patients who underwent arthroscopic subdeltoid transfer of the long head of the biceps tendon to the conjoint tendon for chronic refractory BLC symptoms. Seventy percent of patients were found to have multiple BLC lesions, 45% with intraarticular pathology also demonstrated hidden bicipital tunnel disease, and 27% of patients had bicipital tunnel disease despite a normal-appearing intraarticular biceps tendon. The authors categorized lesion by location as "inside," "junction," or "bicipital tunnel." Such a scheme helps us better understand normal anatomy and pathologic processes.

Normal Anatomy

The BLC can be divided into three anatomic zones: inside, junction, and bicipital tunnel. "Inside" includes the glenoid labrum and biceps anchor. "Junction" includes the intraarticular portion of the long head of the biceps tendon and its stabilizing biceps pulley. "Bicipital tunnel" encompasses the extraarticular segment of the long head of the biceps tendon and its constraining fibro-osseous enclosure (Fig. 18.1).

INSIDE

The glenoid labrum is a collagenous structure that is approximately 4 mm thick and attaches to the glenoid circumferentially (Cooper et al, 1992). It functions to deepen the otherwise shallow glenoid fossa and increase its radius of curvature and also acts as an attachment site for capsule and ligamentous structures (O'Brien et al, 1990). The morphology of the superior labrum is distinct, with more of a meniscal-type attachment that consists of thin elastic tissue than that of the inferior portion of the labrum (Cooper et al,

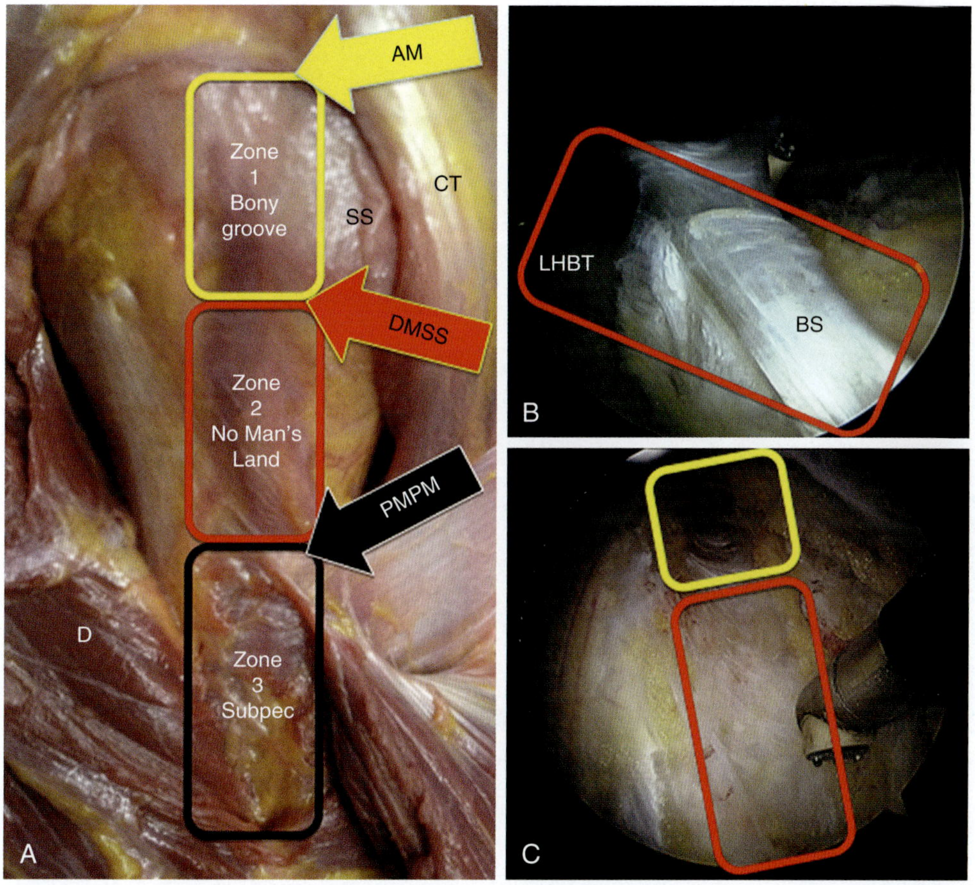

FIG. 18.1 A sift tissue sheath (**A** and **B**) consistently covers the long head biceps tendon (LHBT) to the level of the proximal margin of the pectoralis major tendon (PMPM) and contributes to the roof of the bicipital tunnel. The sheath is clearly visible during open procedures (**A**) and extraarticular arthroscopic procedures within the subdeltoid space (**B** and **C**). The fibro-osseous bicipital tunnel consists of three distinct anatomic zones (**A**). Zone 1 represents the traditional bony bicipital groove *(yellow box)* beginning at the articular margin (AM) and ending at the distal margin of the subscapularis tendon (DMSS). Zone 2 *(red box)* extends from the DMSS to the PMPM and represents a "no man's land" because it is not viewable from arthroscopy above or from subpectoral exposure below. Zone 3 is distal to the PMPM and represents the subpectoral (subpec) region. The sheath overlying zone 2 can be robust (**B**). *BS,* Bicipital sheath; *CT,* conjoint tendon; *D,* deltoid; *SS,* subscapularis. (With permission from Taylor SA, Fabricant PD, Bansal M, et al. The anatomy and histology of the bicipital tunnel of the shoulder. *J Shoulder Elbow Surg.* 2015;24:511-519.)

1992). It has been proposed that the more elastic nature of the anterosuperior labrum exists to accommodate tensile stresses within the rotator interval, which may also make this region more vulnerable to injury (Arai et al, 2010). The vascularity of the superior labrum arises from an anastomotic vascular network emanating from the anterior humeral circumflex, posterior humeral circumflex, and suprascapular arteries, without vascular contribution from the glenoid itself (Cooper et al, 1992). The most poorly vascularized region is the anterosuperior labrum, which may also contribute to vulnerability to injury and impaired healing capacity.

Several variations of normal labral anatomy have been described, including a synovial reflection at the superior aspect of the glenoid, which varies in depth that may result in a meniscoid superior labrum that appears as redundant labrum (2.6- to 7.3-mm overhang) with more of a recessed attachment (Rispoli et al, 2009). Other variations include a sublabral foramen and Buford complex. A sublabral foramen is quite common and reported to be present in 12% of patients (Williams et al, 1994). A Buford complex is identified as absent anterior-superior labrum in association with a cordlike middle glenohumeral ligament and is less common (1.5%). In each case, it is important that these normal variants are identified as such intraoperatively and not mistaken for pathology to avoid untoward morbidity associated with inappropriate attempted repair (meniscoid superior labrum or recessed attachment) or overtightening the rotator interval (sublabral foramen and Buford complex).

The biceps anchor includes attachment to both the supraglenoid tubercle as well as the superior glenoid labrum. The supraglenoid tubercle is approximately 5 mm medial to the superior glenoid rim. Vangsness et al (1994) examined 105 cadaveric specimens and found direct attachment to the supraglenoid tubercle only 50% of the time; the remaining specimens demonstrated primary attachment to the superior labrum and a variable pattern, which they further classified into four types. Type I attachment was entirely to the posterior labrum, type II attachment was predominantly posterior but included some anterior labral attachment, type III included equal attachment to the anterosuperior and posterosuperior labrum, and type IV represented a predominantly anterosuperior labral attachment. The majority of specimens demonstrated type I or type II (prominently posterior) attachment sites.

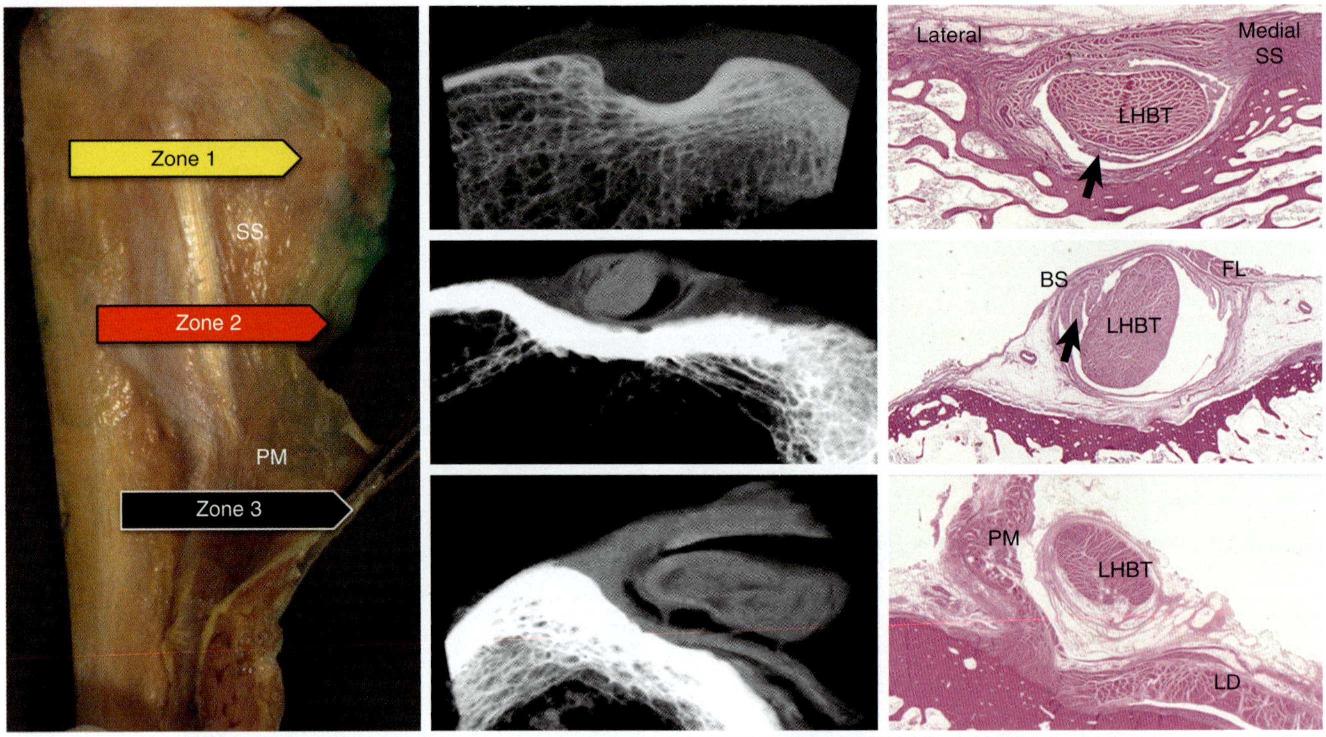

FIG. 18.2 Using a cadaveric model, the entire bicipital tunnel was harvested en bloc and fixed in formalin. Cross-sections were then taken from each of the three zones of the bicipital tunnel, including zone 1 *(yellow)*, zone 2 *(red)*, and zone 3 *(black)*. Plain radiographs were taken demonstrating the osseous architecture of the bicipital tunnel floor from each zone. Histologic evaluation demonstrated that zones 1 and 2 were consistently enclosed by dense connective tissue and contained synovium. Zone 3 had significantly more percent empty tunnel and lacked the same dense connective tissue boundaries. *BS*, Bicipital sheath; *FL*, falciform ligament; *LD*, latissimus dorsi; *LHBT*, long head biceps tendon; *PM*, pectoralis major tendon; SS, subscapularis. (With permission from Taylor SA, Fabricant PD, Bansal M, et al. The anatomy and histology of the bicipital tunnel of the shoulder. *J Shoulder Elbow Surg*. 2015;24:511-519.)

JUNCTION

The intraarticular segment of the long head of the biceps tendon measures approximately 2.5 to 3.4 cm in length (Denard et al, 2012; Taylor et al, 2015b) and is 6.6 mm in diameter (Denard et al, 2012; Lafrance et al, 2013). During normal shoulder motion, the long head of the biceps tendon experiences 19 mm of excursion (McGahan et al, 2013). The vascular supply to the long head of the biceps tendon emanates primarily from tributaries of the superior labrum proximally and ascending branches of the anterior humeral circumflex artery more distally (Cooper et al, 1992). As a result, there is a vascular watershed area that occurs 12 to 30 mm from the biceps anchor and has been proposed as a rationale for susceptibility of tendon rupture in this region (Cheng et al, 2010). Alpantaki et al (2005) evaluated the long head of the biceps tendon histologically and found a dense network of sensory and sympathetic neural elements that were most dense within the proximal intraarticular segment of tendon.

The biceps pulley is a structure along the articular margin consisting of the proximal portion of the bicipital groove (zone 1 of the bicipital tunnel) and a confluence of fibers from the superior glenohumeral ligament, coracohumeral ligament, subscapularis tendon, and supraspinatus tendon. The biceps pulley acts as a proximal tether to the long head of the biceps tendon to resist shear forces and prevent abnormal medial excursion (Arai et al, 2010; Braun et al, 2010; Kask et al, 2010).

BICIPITAL TUNNEL

Taylor et al (2015a, 2015b) described the bicipital tunnel and defined its anatomy and histology subsequently. The bicipital tunnel encompasses the extraarticular segment of the long head of the biceps tendon and its constraining fibro-osseous enclosure. The bicipital tunnel can further be divided into three anatomic zones that have diagnostic and therapeutic significance (Fig. 18.2).

Zone 1 (bicipital groove) of the bicipital tunnel refers to what was traditionally considered the bony bicipital groove. It begins at the articular margin and extends to the distal margin of the subscapularis. The floor of zone 1 is made up of a relatively deep osseous groove that can be quite variable among specimens (Pfahler et al, 1998) but has an average depth of 4.3 mm and an average width ranging from 8.8 mm proximally and 5.4 mm more distally (Cone et al, 1983). The roof of zone 1 is composed of what was formerly termed the *transverse humeral ligament* but has been more recently shown to be an expansion of the subscapularis attachment as well as contributions from the supraspinatus and coracohumeral ligament attachments (Cone et al, 1983; MacDonald et al, 2007; Taylor et al, 2015a). Synovial tissue is present in 100% of specimens in this area (Taylor et al, 2015a).

Zone 2 ("no man's land") is defined proximally by the distal margin of the subscapularis tendon and distally by the proximal margin of the pectoralis major tendon insertion on the humerus. It has been deemed "no man's land" because of its relative invisibility to arthroscopic evaluation from above and from subpectoral evaluation below. Within zone 2, the osseous floor is represented by more of a shallow trough and is covered by periosteum as well as an extension of fibers from the latissimus dorsi and subscapularis. The roof of the bicipital sheath that encloses zone 2 is made up of axially oriented dense connective tissue as well as histologically discrete perpendicularly oriented fibers emanating from the expansion of the pectoralis major attachment to the humerus traditionally referred to as the falciform ligament (Burkhead et al, 2009; Romeo et al, 2004; Taylor et al, 2015a; Yamaguchi et al, 1997). Importantly, synovium was identified and 67% of specimens within zone 2, which contrasts with previous reports that synovial reflection occurs more proximally (Burkhead et al, 2009). Furthermore, zone 2 is consistently a closed space that may harbor pathologic lesions and contains statistically similar percent empty tunnel to that of zone 1 (Taylor et al, 2015a, 2015b).

Zone 3 (sub-pectoral region) is marked anatomically by the superior margin of the pectoralis major tendon. Its osseous floor is relatively flat and architecture and covered by fibers of the latissimus dorsi and periosteum. The percent empty tunnel is significantly greater within zone 3 than in zones 1 and 2, suggesting that space-occupying lesions may be of less significance in this area. Partial extension of synovium was identified and 18% of specimens within zone 3 (Taylor et al, 2015a).

Classification of Pathology

Pathology of the BLC should similarly be thought of as divided into the aforementioned regions: inside, junction, and bicipital tunnel. The rationale for such division is related to clinical symptoms as well as our diagnostic capabilities. In general, whereas inside and junction lesions may readily be identifiable at arthroscopy, bicipital tunnel lesions are commonly invisible to this diagnostic modality.

INSIDE

SLAP tears were originally described by Andrews et al (1985) and subsequently classified as types I through IV by Snyder et al (1990). Type I SLAP tears are characterized by fraying and degenerative appearance of the superior labrum without destabilization of the biceps anchor. Type II SLAP tears are identified by visible detachment of the biceps anchor, leading to destabilization. Type III SLAP tears are marked by a bucket handle tear of the superior labrum with stable attachment of the biceps anchor. Type IV SLAP tears include a bucket handle tear of the superior labrum with extension into the biceps tendon anchor or the biceps tendon itself. Others have since modified Snyder's original classification (Maffet et al, 1995; Morgan et al, 1998; Nord et al, 2004; Pfahler et al, 2003).

Dynamic incarceration of the long head of the biceps tendon described by Verma et al (2005) may be pathologic or a variation of normal. This can be evaluated arthroscopically while viewing from the standard posterior portal when the arm is brought into a forward flexed, adducted, and internally rotated position whereby the long head of the biceps tendon is incarcerated between the humeral head and glenoid fossa.

Medial biceps chondromalacia occurs along the anteromedial aspect of the humeral head from attritional wear caused by abnormal friction between the long head of the biceps tendon and the chondral surface. Such an arthroscopic or imaging finding of medial biceps chondromalacia may suggest disease of the BLC.

JUNCTION

Tearing of the long head of the biceps tendon may occur within its intraarticular segment or more commonly near its articular margin secondary to the aforementioned vascular watershed region (Cheng et al, 2010). Other morphologic abnormalities resulting from pathologic processes include the hourglass biceps described by Boileau et al (2004) in which the intraarticular segment of the biceps tendon becomes hypertrophic and flattened resulting in proximal entrapment of the tendon and limited excursion.

Lesions of the biceps pulley may result in proximal instability of the long head of the biceps tendon with or without subscapularis tear. Biceps pulley lesions are uncommonly found in conjunction with SLAP tears (10%) and may be correlated with a history of a fall with the arm in an internally rotated position (Patzer et al, 2011).

Junctional biceps chondromalacia results from attritional wear of the humeral cartilage from rubbing of the long head of the biceps tendon but occurs below the biceps tendon near its articular margin, which differs in location from the aforementioned medial biceps chondromalacia. Other authors have termed this abnormal finding the "biceps tendon footprint"(Sistermann, 2005) or "humeral head abrasion" (Byram et al, 2011) or "biceps chondral print" (Patzer et al, 2010). This finding is been found in conjunction with biceps pulley lesions, SLAP tears, rotator cuff tears, and failed SLAP repairs (Byram et al, 2011; Morris et al, 2014; Patzer et al, 2010; Sistermann, 2005).

BICIPITAL TUNNEL

The extraarticular bicipital tunnel commonly harbors hidden pathology. Taylor et al (2015b) identified a prevalence of 47% bicipital tunnel lesions among 277 chronically symptomatic patients. Several authors have recently recognized the limitations of diagnostic arthroscopy to identify bicipital tunnel disease (Festa et al, 2014; Gilmer et al, 2015; Moon et al, 2015; Taylor et al, 2015a, 2015b). Moon et al (2015) found that 79% of arthroscopically identified proximal long head biceps tendon tears extended distally into the bicipital tunnel and were frequently accompanied by tenosynovitis. Festa et al (2014) reported that arthroscopy only allowed visualization of 31% of the extraarticular long head of the biceps tendon and 54% of the long head of the biceps tendon in the bicipital groove (zone 1). Gilmer et al (2015) looked at the long head of the biceps tendon in 62 patients who underwent open subpectoral biceps tenodesis and reported that arthroscopy failed to identify pathology 33% of the time and underestimated the actual pathology 56% of the time. Taylor et al (2015b) reported in a cadaveric study that diagnostic arthroscopy only visualized 78% of the long head of the biceps tendon relative to the inferior margin of the subscapularis (zone 1) and only 55% of the tendon relative to the proximal margin of the pectoralis major tendon (zone 2). As a result, diagnostic arthroscopy fails to identify any pathology existing in zone 2 (Fig. 18.3).

A wide array of pathology exists within the bicipital tunnel inherent to the biceps tendon itself (partial tearing, adhesion, and scar) or resulting from the bicipital tunnel itself (incarcerated loose bodies, abrasive osteophytes, bony or soft tissue stenosis, pathologic inflamed vincula, and synovitis) (Taylor et al, 2015b).

In patients with suspected BLC disease, it is important to consider hidden extraarticular bicipital tunnel disease as a source of the patient's symptoms. Failure to consider this may lead to persistent symptoms and the need for reoperation.

Clinical Assessment

Accurate clinical assessment of patients with suspected BLC disease relies on an accurate patient history, comprehensive physical examination, advanced imaging, and in many instances use of diagnostic injections.

PHYSICAL EXAMINATION

Patient history and physical examination are paramount, particularly with respect to the identification of hidden bicipital tunnel disease. Many different physical examination maneuvers have been described in the literature. We favor employment of the "three-pack" examination (tenderness to palpation of the bicipital tunnel, active compression test [O'Brien sign], and throwing test) in addition to more traditional tests (full can, empty can, Speed, and Yergason tests) (Fig. 18.4).

In a recent prospective study, Taylor et al (2017) correlated the aforementioned preoperative physical examination maneuvers with intraoperative findings in 145 consecutive chronically symptomatic patients who underwent arthroscopic subdeltoid transfer of the long head of the biceps tendon to the conjoined tendon compared with asymptomatic match control participants. The authors found that the three-pack tests were very sensitive (73%–98%) but less specific (46%–79%) than the more traditional tests for lesions in all three zones (inside, junction, bicipital tunnel) (Fig. 18.5).

Conclusion

The biceps and labrum should no longer be considered separate entities but rather should be thought of as one unit termed the *biceps–labrum complex*. The BLC can be divided into three zones: inside, junction, and bicipital tunnel. Lesions may occur in one location or more commonly along the BLC at multiple sites. Physical examination can be particularly useful in identifying BLC disease and ruling out (tenderness to palpation and O'Brien sign) bicipital tunnel disease.

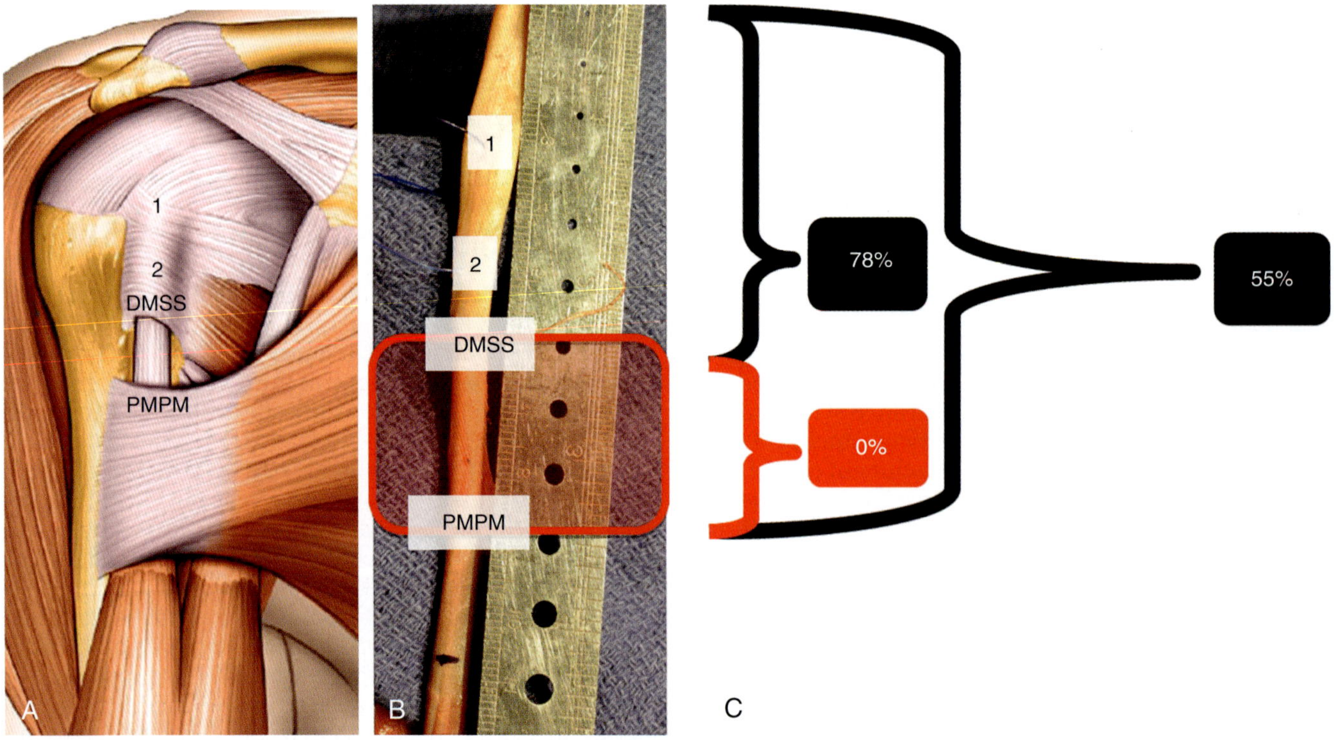

FIG. 18.3 Using a cadaveric model, percutaneous tagging sutures were placed into the long head biceps tendon (LHBT) with the tendon at rest (**A1** and **B1**) and after maximum tendon excursion applied by arthroscopic grasper (**A2** and **B2**). The specimens were dissected and the distal margin of the subscapularis (DMSS) and the proximal margin of the pectoralis major (PMPM) were marked on the LHBT and used to calculate the percentage of tendon that can be visualized during glenohumeral arthroscopy (**C**), which was 78% relative to the DMSS and 55% relative to the PMPM. Zone 2 of the bicipital tunnel was named "no man's land" because it cannot be visualized from above or below. (With permission from Taylor SA, Khair MM, Gulotta LV, et al. Diagnostic glenohumeral arthroscopy fails to fully evaluate the biceps-labral complex. *Arthroscopy*. 2015;31(2):215-224.)

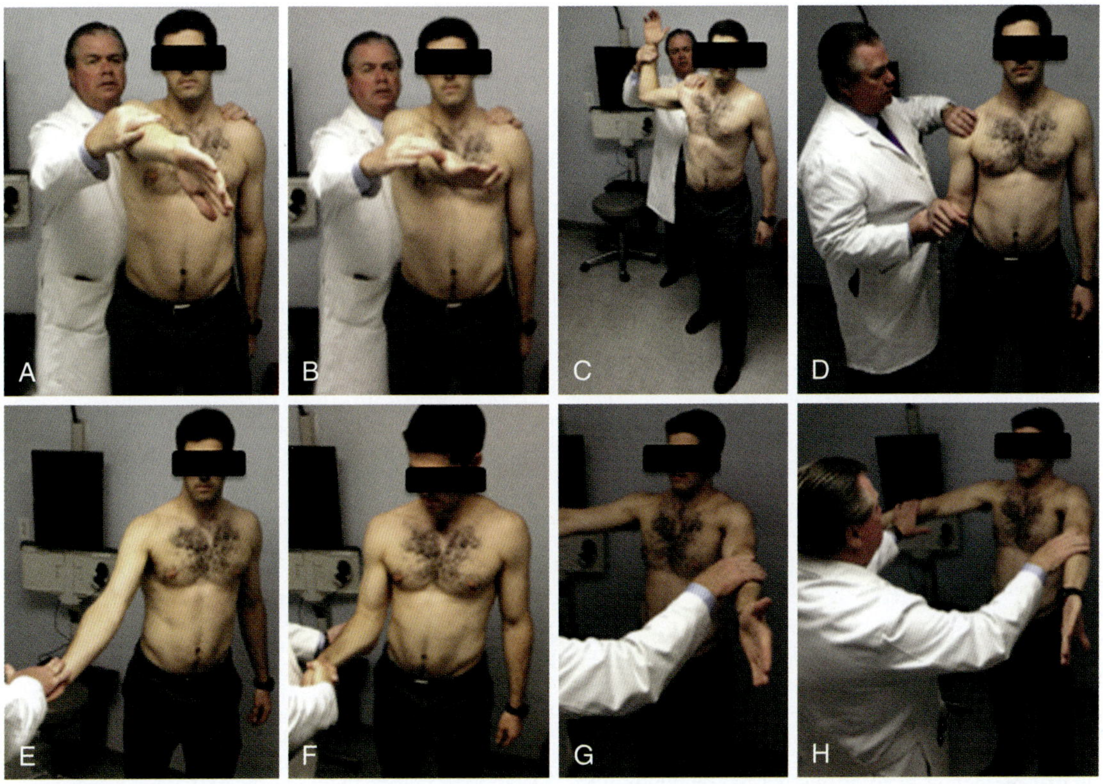

FIG. 18.4 The three-pack examination includes the active compression test (**A** and **B**), the throwing test (**C**), and palpation of the bicipital tunnel (**D**). Traditional physical examination maneuvers include Speed (**E**), Yergason (**F**), full can (**G**), and empty can (**H**). (With permission from Taylor SA, Newman AM, Dawson C, et al. The 3-pack examination is critical for comprehensive evaluation of the biceps-labrum complex lesions: a prospective clinical series. *Arthroscopy*. 2017;33(1):28-38.)

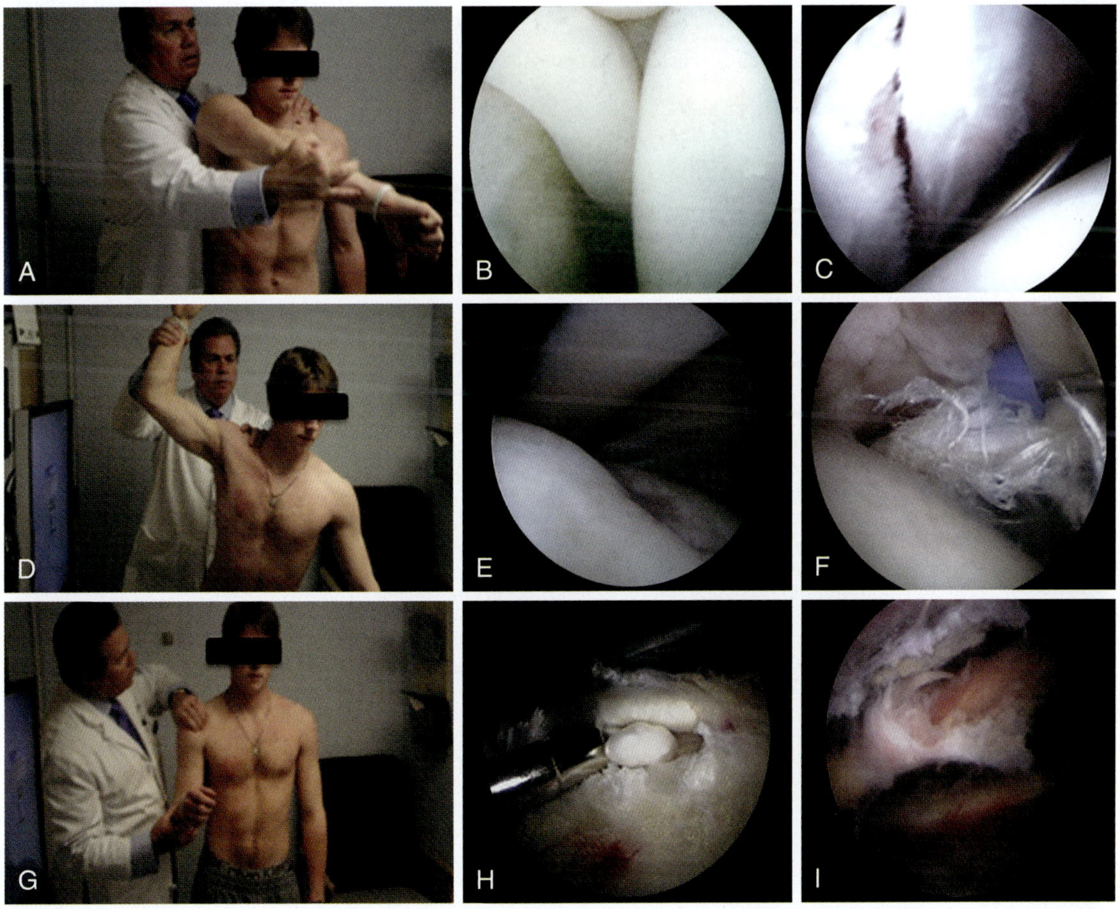

FIG. 18.5 The active compression test (O'Brien sign). The right shoulder viewed from standard posterior viewing portal (**A**) is particularly useful for picking up inside lesions such as incarceration of the biceps (**B**) and labral tears (**C**). The throwing test left shoulder viewed from a standard posterior viewing portal (**D**) is helpful for junctional lesions such as junctional biceps chondromalacia (**E**) and partial tears of the biceps tendon (**F**). Palpation of left shoulder viewed from an anterolateral subdeltoid viewing portal (**G**) is very sensitive for bicipital tunnel disease, which is a diverse set of lesions such as loose bodies (**H**) and adhesion or scar (**I**). (With permission from Taylor SA, Newman AM, Dawson C, et al. The 3-pack examination is critical for comprehensive evaluation of the biceps-labrum complex lesions: a prospective clinical series. *Arthroscopy*. 2017;33(1):28-38.)

References

Alpantaki K, McLaughlin D, Karagogeos D, Hadjipavlou A, Kontakis G. Sympathetic and sensory neural elements in the tendon of the long head of the biceps. *J Bone Joint Surg Am*. 2005;87:1580–1583.

Andrews J, Carson W, Mcleod W. Glenoid labrum tears related to the long head of the biceps. *Am J Sports Med*. 1985;13:337–341.

Arai R, Mochizuk T, Yamaguchi K, et al. Functional anatomy of the superior glenohumeral and coracohumeral ligaments and the subscapularis tendon in view of stabilization of the long head of the biceps tendon. *J Shoulder Elbow Surg*. 2010;19:58–64.

Boileau P, Ahrens PM, Hatzidakis AM. Entrapment of the long head of the biceps tendon: the hourglass biceps—a cause of pain and locking of the shoulder. *J Shoulder Elbow Surg*. 2004;13:249–257.

Braun S, Millett PJ, Yongpravat C, et al. Biomechanical evaluation of shear force vectors leading to injury of the biceps reflection pulley: a biplane fluoroscopy study on cadaveric shoulders. *Am J Sports Med*. 2010;38:1015–1024.

Burkhead W, Habermeyer P, Walch G. The biceps tendon. In *The Shoulder*. 4th ed. Elsevier, 2009:1309–1360.

Byram IR, Dunn WR, Kuhn JE. Humeral head abrasion: an association with failed superior labrum anterior posterior repairs. *J Shoulder Elbow Surg*. 2011;20:92–97.

Cheng NM, Pan WR, Vally F, Le Roux CM, Richardson MD. The arterial supply of the long head of biceps tendon: anatomical study with implications for tendon rupture. *Clin Anat*. 2010;23:683–692.

Cone RO, Danzig L, Resnick D, Goldman AB. The bicipital groove: radiographic, anatomic, and pathologic study. *AJR Am J Roentgenol*. 1983;141:781–788.

Cooper DE, Arnoczky SP, O'Brien SJ, Warren RF, DiCarlo E, Allen AA. Anatomy, histology, and vascularity of the glenoid labrum. An anatomical study. *J Bone Joint Surg Am*. 1992;74:46–52.

Denard PJ, Dai X, Hanypsiak BT, Burkhart SS. Anatomy of the biceps tendon: implications for restoring physiological length-tension relation during biceps tenodesis with interference screw fixation. *Arthroscopy*. 2012;28:1352–1358.

Festa A, Allert J, Issa K, Tasto JP, Myer JJ. Visualization of the extra-articular portion of the long head of the biceps tendon during intra-articular shoulder arthroscopy. *Arthroscopy*. 2014;30(11):1413–1417.

Gilmer BB, DeMers AM, Guerrero D, Reid JB, Lubowitz JH, Guttmann D. Arthroscopic versus open comparison of long head of biceps tendon visualization and pathology in patients requiring tenodesis. *Arthroscopy*. 2015;31(1):29–34.

Gottschalk MB, Karas SG, Ghattas TN, Burdette R. Subpectoral biceps tenodesis for the treatment of type II and IV superior labral anterior and posterior lesions. *Am J Sports Med*. 2014;42:2128–2135.

Kask K, Põldoja E, Lont T, et al. Anatomy of the superior glenohumeral ligament. *J Shoulder Elbow Surg*. 2010;19:908–916.

Lafrance R, Madsen W, Yaseen Z, Giordano B, Maloney M, Voloshin I. Relevant anatomic landmarks and measurements for biceps tenodesis. *Am J Sports Med*. 2013;41:1395–1399.

MacDonald K, Bridger J, Cash C, Parkin I. Transverse humeral ligament: does it exist? *Clin Anat*. 2007;20:663–667.

Maffet MW, Gartsman GM. Moseley B. Superior labrum-biceps tendon complex lesions of the shoulder. *Am J Sports Med*. 1995;23:93–98.

McCormick F, Nwachukwu BU, Solomon D, et al. The efficacy of biceps tenodesis in the treatment of failed superior labral anterior posterior repairs. *Am J Sports Med*. 2014;42:820–825.

McGahan PJ, Patel H, Dickinson E, Leasure J, Montgomery W. The effect of biceps adhesions on glenohumeral range of motion: a cadaveric study. *J Shoulder Elbow Surg*. 2013;22:658–665.

Moon SC, Cho NS, Rhee YG. Analysis of "hidden lesions" of the extra-extraarticular biceps after subpectoral biceps tenodesis: the subpectoral portion as the optimal tenodesis site. *Am J Sports Med*. 2015;43(1):63–68.

Morgan CD, Burkhart SS, Palmeri M, Gillespie M. Type II SLAP lesions: three subtypes and their relationships to superior instability and rotator cuff tears. *Arthroscopy*. 1998;14:553–565.

Morris BJ, Byram IR, Lathrop RA, Dunn WR, Kuhn JE. Mapping the articular contact area of the long head of the biceps tendon on the humeral head. *Anat Res Int*. 2014;2014:814721.

Nord KD, Masterson JP, Mauck BM. Superior labrum anterior posterior (SLAP) repair using the Neviaser portal. *Arthroscopy*. 2004;20(suppl 2):129–133.

O'Brien SJ, Neves MC, Arnoczky SP, et al. The anatomy and histology of the inferior glenohumeral ligament complex of the shoulder. *Am J Sports Med*. 1990;18:449–456.

Patterson BM, Creighton RA, Spang JT, Roberson JR, Kamath GV. Surgical trends in the treatment of superior labrum anterior and posterior lesions of the shoulder: analysis of data from the American Board of Orthopaedic Surgery Certification Examination Database. *Am J Sports Med*. 2014;42(8):1904–1910.

Patzer T, Kircher J, Lichtenberg S, Sauter M, Magosch P, Habermeyer P. Is there an association between SLAP lesions and biceps pulley lesions? *Arthroscopy*. 2011;27:611–618.

Patzer T, Lichtenberg S, Kircher J, Magosch P, Habermeyer P. Influence of SLAP lesions on chondral lesions of the glenohumeral joint. *Knee Surg Sports Traumatol Arthrosc*. 2010;18:982–987.

Pfahler M, Branner S, Refior HJ. The role of the bicipital groove in tendopathy of the long biceps tendon. *J Shoulder Elbow Surg*. 1998;8:419–424.

Pfahler M, Haraida S, Schulz C, et al. Age-related changes of the glenoid labrum in normal shoulders. *J Shoulder Elbow Surg*. 2003;12(1):40–52.

Provencher MT, McCormick F, Dewing C, McIntire S, Solomon D. A prospective analysis of 179 type 2 superior labrum anterior and posterior repairs: outcomes and factors associated with success and failure. *Am J Sports Med*. 2013;41:880–886.

Rispoli DM, Athwal GS, Sperling JW, Cofield RH. The macroscopic delineation of the edge of the glenoid labrum: an anatomic evaluation of an open and arthroscopic visual reference. *Arthroscopy*. 2009;25:603–607.

Romeo AA, Mazzocca AD, Tauro JC. Arthroscopic biceps tenodesis. *Arthroscopy*. 2004;20:206–213.

Sistermann R. The biceps tendon footprint. *Acta Orthop*. 2005;76:237–240.

Snyder SJ, Karzel RP, Del Pizzo W, Ferkel RD, Friedman MJ. SLAP lesions of the shoulder. *Arthroscopy*. 1990;6:274–279.

Taylor SA, Fabricant PD, Bansal M, et al. The anatomy and histology of the bicipital tunnel of the shoulder. *J Shoulder Elbow Surg*. 2015a;24:511–519.

Taylor SA, Newman AM, Dawson C, et al. The 3-pack examination is critical for comprehensive evaluation of the biceps-labrum complex lesions: a prospective clinical series. *Arthroscopy*. 2017;33(1):28–38.

Taylor SA, Khair MM, Gulotta LV, et al. Diagnostic glenohumeral arthroscopy fails to fully evaluate the biceps-labral complex. *Arthroscopy*. 2015b;31(2):215–224.

Vangsness CT, Jorgenson SS, Watson T, Johnson DL. The origin of the long head of the biceps from the scapula and glenoid labrum. An anatomical study of 100 shoulders. *J Bone Joint Surg Br*. 1994;76:951–954.

Verma NN, Drakos M, O'Brien SJ. The arthroscopic active compression test. *Arthroscopy*. 2005;21:634.

Vogel LA, Moen TC, Macaulay AA, et al. Superior labrum anterior-to-posterior repair incidence: a longitudinal investigation of community and academic databases. *J Shoulder Elbow Surg*. 2014;23:e119–e126.

Weber SC, Martin DF, Seiler JG, Harrast JJ. Superior labrum anterior and posterior lesions of the shoulder: incidence rates, complications, and outcomes as reported by American Board of Orthopedic Surgery. Part II candidates. *Am J Sports Med*. 2012;40:1538–1543.

Werner BC, Pehlivan HC, Hart JM, et al. Biceps tenodesis is a viable option for salvage of failed SLAP repair. *J Shoulder Elbow Surg*. 2014;23:e179–e184.

Williams MM, Snyder SJ, Buford D. The Buford complex—the middle glenohumeral ligament and absent anterosuperior labrum complex: a normal anatomic capsulolabral variant. *Arthroscopy*. 1994;10:241–247.

Yamaguchi K, Riew KD, Galatz LM, Syme JA, Neviaser RJ. Biceps activity during shoulder motion: an electromyographic analysis. *Clin Orthop Relat Res*. 1997:122–129. Mar.

19 Treatment

19-19A LABRAL REPAIR

DUSTIN L. RICHTER, MD, JOURDAN CANCIENNE, MD, and
STEPHEN F. BROCKMEIER, MD

Introduction

- Superior labrum anterior and posterior (SLAP) tear is are commonly a result of a traction injury and is often seen in overhead athletes. It may occur as an isolated lesion or may be associated with other concomitant pathology such as internal impingement or partial-thickness articular-sided rotator cuff tear.
- Type II SLAP tear, characterized by a detached biceps tendon anchor, is the most common type of SLAP tear to require surgical repair.
- Indications for arthroscopic repair of SLAP lesions continue to evolve. The strongest indication for, and the situation with the best-expected outcome following repair, is an active younger patient with consistent history, physical examination, and imaging findings, in whom nonoperative management has failed and who has no identifiable concomitant pathologic abnormality (i.e., biceps, rotator cuff).
- Portal placement is critical for an effective anatomic repair. The most important suture in the SLAP repair is the suture loop placed posterior to the biceps at the corner of the glenoid to resist torsional peel-back.
- Current literature suggests that repair of type II SLAP lesions provides significant improvement in patient-reported outcome scores and satisfaction. However, this improvement may not translate to return to preinjury activity levels, especially in elite overhead athletes.

Anatomy and Background

The long head of the biceps tendon originates from the supraglenoid tubercle on the scapula and is an intraarticular structure continuous with the superior glenoid labrum (Tuoheti et al, 2005). In a cadaveric study, the bicipital insertion on the labrum was classified as entirely or predominantly posterior in 55% of cases, split equally between anterior and posterior in 37%, and predominantly anterior in 8% (Vangsness et al, 1994). Several anatomic variants of both the anterosuperior labrum and the long head of the biceps have been described in the literature (Dierickx et al, 2009; Rao et al, 2003; Wahl & MacGillivray, 2007). Proximally, the long head of the biceps receives its blood supply from the anterior humeral circumflex artery, whereas the labrum is supplied separately by branches of the suprascapular, circumflex scapular, and posterior circumflex humeral arteries. The anterosuperior labrum and glenoid represent a vascular watershed region without a robust blood supply, a feature that can lead to both tearing and difficulty healing after surgical repair (Abrassart et al, 2006; Bicos, 2008; McDonald et al, 2013).

The term "superior labrum anterior to posterior" (SLAP) describes the superior aspect of the glenoid labrum, starting posteriorly and extending anteriorly, including the origin of the long head of the biceps. Andrews et al, in 1985, first described disruption of the long head of the biceps (LHB) anchor and superior labrum from the glenoid. Snyder et al, in 1990, coined the term SLAP lesion and designated the first four anatomic classifications (Fig. 19A.1) Type II SLAP tears are the most commonly repaired of the various types. These lesions occur when the superior labrum detaches medially from the glenoid bone—leaving the superior glenoid neck uncovered for at least 5 mm from the corner of the glenoid. This creates a gap between the articular cartilage and the labral attachment onto the bone.

Since the original description and classification, there has been a substantial amount of research focusing on the anatomy, pathogenesis, clinical diagnosis, and arthroscopic treatment of the SLAP tear (Burkhart et al, 2003; Cooper et al, 1992; Kim SJ et al, 2012; Kim TK et al, 2003; Kuhn et al, 2003). Once thought to be unique to overhead athletes, SLAP lesions are increasingly being diagnosed and recognized as a major source of shoulder pain and dysfunction in cohorts of older, nonthrowing patients (Erickson et al, 2015; Kuhn et al, 2003) Furthermore, SLAP lesions are typically encountered with concomitant shoulder pathology. In a review of 2375 shoulder arthroscopies with 140 SLAP lesions, Snyder et al (1990) noted that 29% of these lesions were accompanied by a partial-thickness tear of the rotator cuff, 11% by a full-thickness tear of the rotator cuff, and 22% by an anterior Bankart lesion; isolated SLAP lesions were present in only

6% of cases. Maffet et al (1995) noted a similar occurrence of isolated SLAP lesions (11.8%) in a review of 712 shoulder arthroscopies.

Later research has reported an overall decrease in the rate of isolated arthroscopic SLAP repairs, whereas the rates of biceps tenodesis and tenotomy have increased (Patterson et al, 2014). Despite this decrease, there remain a significant number of patients who present with symptomatic, isolated SLAP lesions and who are candidates for repair. This chapter provides a current and comprehensive review of SLAP tears, including evaluation and diagnosis, nonoperative management, surgical indications and technique, rehabilitation, and expected outcomes.

Diagnosis

Patient presentation can be variable, but common symptoms include pain localized to either the posterior or the anterior glenohumeral joint line. The pain is often provoked by certain activities and is sometimes associated with mechanical catching in the joint and "dead-arm" episodes. In the overhead athlete population, pain can often be accompanied by fatigue, disordered shoulder mechanics, and diminished performance (Barber et al, 2007; Keener & Brophy, 2009) Throwing athletes may have pain in the late cocking phase and may note a decrease in velocity. Physical examination findings can be variable, and no single finding has been shown to be acceptably specific for the diagnosis of a SLAP lesion. When a SLAP lesion is suspected on the basis of history and examination, magnetic resonance imaging (MRI) with or without arthrography can further assist in the diagnosis.

Nonoperative Treatment

Initially, SLAP lesions should be treated conservatively with antiinflammatory medication, rest, and stretching exercises. Nonoperative management of SLAP lesions also relies on the successful identification and treatment of associated pathology. Scapular dyskinesia and glenohumeral internal rotational deficit (GIRD) should be identified and addressed with targeted therapy, including improved posterior capsular flexibility in patients with GIRD. The so-called sleeper stretch has up to a 90% success rate in resolving GIRD (Abrams & Safran, 2010; Burkhart et al, 2003). If several months of conservative treatment do not alleviate symptoms, surgical treatment should be considered.

Surgical Indications

Indications for arthroscopic repair of SLAP lesions continue to evolve and depend on several patient factors. Patients with consistent history, examination, and imaging findings who meet the following criteria may be best served by surgical repair:

- Failure of conservative measures
- Younger age (<35 years)
- Type II SLAP tear
- Absence of biceps tendon pathologic abnormality
- Member of active athletic population/overhead athlete

SLAP Repair Technique

See Video 19A.1.

Arthroscopic SLAP repair is most commonly carried out with the patient in the beach-chair position. Portal placement is extremely important to allow for an effective anatomic repair. An anterior portal (often cannulated) placed high and slightly lateral provides a good angle for anchor placement. Once the diagnosis of a SLAP tear that is amenable to repair is confirmed, proceeding with the repair typically includes the use of accessory portals—namely the portal of Wilmington and/or the Neviaser portal (Werner et al, 2016).

The SLAP tear site is then prepared. To facilitate healing, an arthroscopic rasp is used to mobilize the tear site and a high-speed bur can be used to remove cartilage and allow punctate bleeding to improve healing. The position and number of anchors for a SLAP repair can vary, but for most SLAP lesions the tear extends from the biceps anchor posteriorly, requiring one or two anchors placed posterior to the biceps anchor. We prefer small-diameter, biocomposite, absorbable, tap-in anchors because they are easier to control during insertion, limit the size of the perforation of the glenoid rim bone, and may diminish the risk of subsequent chondral injury due to anchor migration and prominence. We also favor knotless anchor constructs in this region to limit the potential for abrasion or irritation related to knot prominence (Fig. 19A.2).

The high and lateral portal is used for superior labral anchor placement at the 11 o'clock/1 o'clock position. Posterior anchors are best placed through either a portal of Wilmington or posterolateral portal. For most SLAP tears, posterior anchors alone are sufficient to stabilize the biceps-labral complex and normalize the peel-back phenomenon. After anchor placement, the suture limb closest to the labrum is passed through the labrum and tied in a simple configuration, with care being taken to keep the knot away from the articular surface.

Postoperative Protocol

Patient compliance is crucial for successful outcomes, particularly in the early post-operative period. Our rehabilitation program is divided into four phases, which have previously been described (Werner et al, 2016). Phase I (0–6 weeks) involves sling use and gentle passive range of motion. Phase II (7–12 weeks) includes weaning from the sling and isotonic rotator cuff strengthening. Phase III (13–20 weeks) focuses on full active and passive, painless range of motion with restoration of strength. No throwing or overhead sport progression is allowed until week 16. Phase IV (21–26 weeks) is the advanced strengthening phase with the progression of interval sports programs.

With successful rehabilitation, return to sport often takes at least 6 months from the time of surgery. Throwing athletes may take a year or longer to return, given the stresses placed on the anterior shoulder and eccentric load on the long head of the biceps tendon that their sport involves.

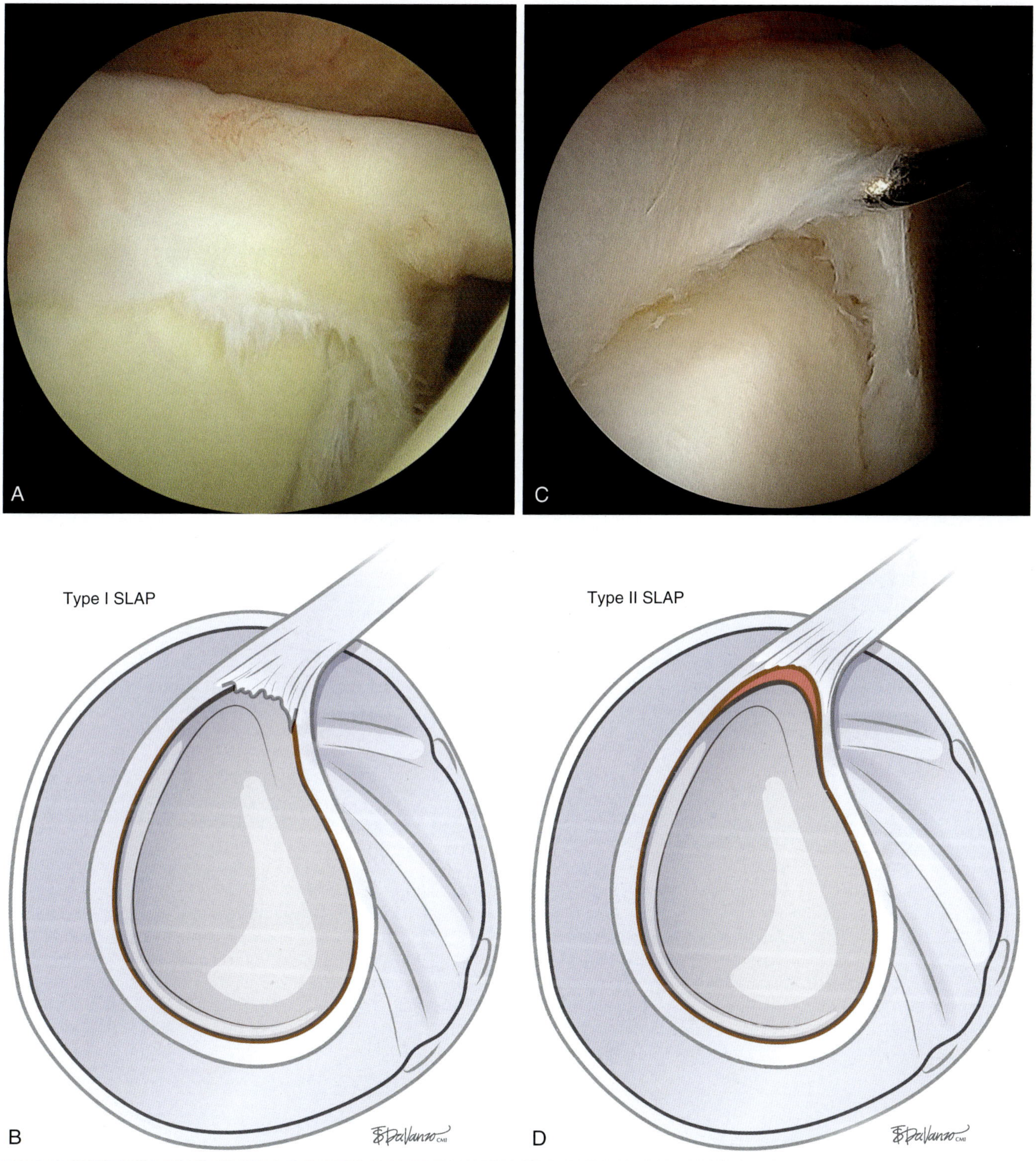

Fig. 19A.1 Arthroscopic image (**A**) and illustration (**B**) of a type I SLAP tear characterized by biceps and labral fraying with an intact biceps tendon anchor. Operative management for type I SLAP tears most commonly is labral debridement. Arthroscopic image (**C**) and illustration (**D**) of a type II SLAP tear characterized by labral fraying and a detached biceps tendon anchor. Operative management for type II SLAP tears (in a younger patient) most commonly is a SLAP repair. Arthroscopic image

Continued

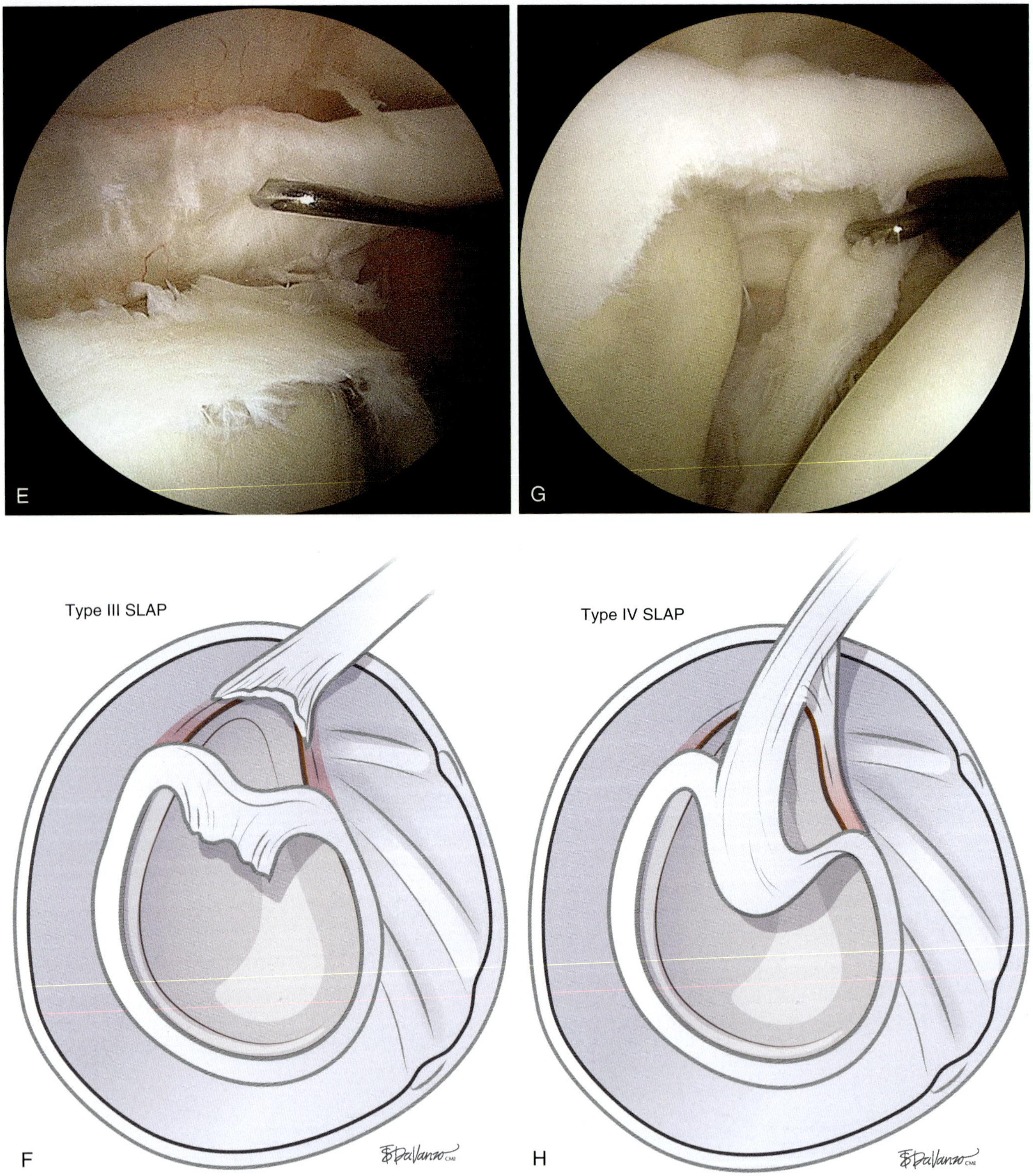

Fig. 19A.1, cont'd (**E**) and illustration (**F**) of a type III SLAP tear characterized by a bucket-handle tear of the superior labrum with an intact biceps tendon anchor. Operative management for type III SLAP tears is debridement of the flaps. Arthroscopic image (**G**) and illustration (**H**) of a type IV SLAP tear characterized by a bucket-handle tear of the superior labrum that extends into the biceps tendon root (detached anchor that remains attached to the bucket-handle tear). Operative management for type IV SLAP tears depends on the extent of biceps tendon involvement, which is treated with either excision of the bucket-handle tear or biceps tenodesis or tenotomy.

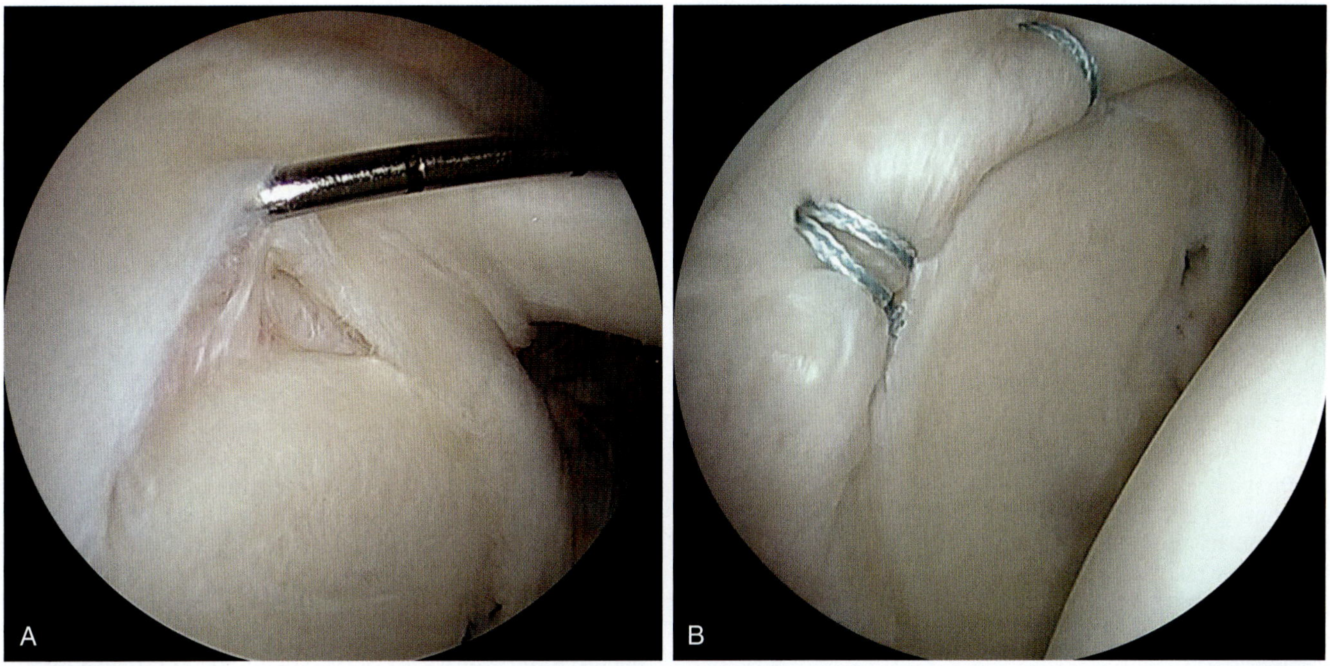

Fig. 19A.2 (**A**) Arthroscopic image from a left shoulder standard posterior viewing portal, demonstrating detachment of the superior labrum and an uncovered superior glenoid neck, consistent with a type II SLAP tear. (**B**) Arthroscopic repair of the type II SLAP tear using a knotless anchor technique.

Pearls and Pitfalls

- Definitive diagnosis of SLAP lesions requires arthroscopy with direct visualization, probing, and dynamic testing for the peel-back sign.
- SLAP repairs are best performed arthroscopically with the use of suture anchors. Portal placement is critical for effective anatomic repair.
- The most important suture in the SLAP repair is the suture loop placed posterior to the biceps at the corner of the glenoid to resist torsional peel-back.
- Anchor placement anterior to the biceps tendon is described but may overconstrain the shoulder.
- Knots should be tied away from the articular surface or use of knotless constructs should be considered to avoid abrasion and chondral injury.

Discussion

The arthroscopic treatment of isolated SLAP lesions has produced variable and conflicting clinical results and outcomes. Several writers have reported substantially better patient outcome scores and satisfaction; however, these scores have not necessarily correlated with return to preinjury activity or play, particularly in elite athletes. Cohen et al (2006), investigated the treatment of isolated type II SLAP lesions repaired with a bioabsorbable tack. They retrospectively studied 41 patients who underwent arthroscopic fixation with a mean follow-up of 3.7 years. They reported mean L'Insalata and American Shoulder and Elbow Society (ASES) scores of 86.7 and 86.8, respectively, with 71% of the cohort reporting good to excellent results. However, less than half of the 29 athletes in the cohort had returned to their preinjury playing level. SH Kim et al (2002) evaluated 34 patients at a mean of 33 months following arthroscopic repair of an isolated SLAP lesion with suture anchors. These researchers reported that 94% of the patients had satisfactory UCLA shoulder scores and 91% had regained their preinjury level of shoulder function. However, patients who participated in overhead sports had significantly lower shoulder scores and a significantly lower percentage of return to preinjury level of shoulder function than those who did not participate in overhead activity.

Brockmeier et al (2009) were one of the first groups to prospectively evaluate outcomes of repair of SLAP tears using modern arthroscopic techniques. They reported on a cohort of 47 patients with symptomatic type II SLAP tears who were treated with arthroscopic suture anchor fixation and followed for a minimum of 2 years. At an average of 2.7-year follow-up, 87% of patients rated their outcomes as good or excellent; however, only 74% of athletes were able to return to their preinjury level of competition. Interestingly, these investigators also demonstrated that patients with a distinct traumatic etiology had a greater likelihood of a successful return to sports (Brockmeier et al, 2009).

Neri et al (2011) used the Kerlan-Jobe Orthopaedic Clinic (KCOC) shoulder and elbow score and the ASES scoring system to evaluate 23 collegiate or professional overhead athletes more than 1 year after repair of type II SLAP lesions. At an average 3- to 8-month follow-up, 57% of patients had returned to pain-free play, 26% were playing with pain, and 17% were not playing because of pain; 96% of the patients had good to excellent ASES scores, but only 52% of the cohort had good to excellent KCOC scores. The group concluded that the rate of return to preinjury level of competition for elite overhead athletes after type II SLAP repairs was low despite high ASES scores and that the inability to return to play correlated with the presence of a partial-thickness rotator cuff tear. Maier et al (2013), compared the functional outcome and return to sport for arthroscopic repair of isolated type II SLAP lesions using suture anchors and for repair using transglenoidal sutures. They performed a matched-pair retrospective analysis of 24 competitive amateur athletes and reported constant scores of 91 and 81 in the suture anchor and transglenoidal suture groups, respectively; 67% of the total cohort was able to return to overhead sport without restrictions, whereas 58% achieved their preinjury sports level. The group concluded that suture anchor repair resulted in superior objective and subjective shoulder function; regardless of the technique used, however, nearly half of the athletes did not return to their preinjury level of sport. Finally, Park et al (2013) reviewed data from 24 elite overhead athletes with a mean follow-up of 45 months and reported average ASES scores of 87. However, only 50% of the athletes had returned to play after the operation, substantiating concerns that return to play after type II SLAP repairs remains problematic in elite overhead athletes.

Provencher et al (2013) conducted the largest study to date on type II SLAP repairs. The group prospectively collected clinical outcomes of 179 SLAP tear repairs in young, active patients at a mean follow-up of 40 months. Average outcome scores were 88 for ASES, 82% for the Western Ontario Shoulder Instability (WOSI) score, and 85% for the Single Assessment Numeric Evaluation (SANE) score. These researchers reported that 37% of the cohort met repair failure criteria, with 28% electing to undergo revision surgery. Age of 36 years or older was the only significant risk factor associated with a higher incidence of repair failure.

Other writers have investigated concomitant procedures that might improve outcomes of isolated SLAP repair. Coleman et al (2007) evaluated the effect of performing an acromioplasty at the time of a type II SLAP repair. They compared the clinical results in 34 patients who underwent an isolated type II SLAP repair with those in 16 patients who underwent a type II SLAP repair with an acromioplasty. Clinical outcome scores of the two groups were similar, with the combined group reporting slightly more "good" or "excellent" satisfaction ratings and significantly less postoperative clinical impingement.

Given the lack of conclusive evidence and often cited poor functional results for isolated SLAP tears in the young, active population, other writers have compared the outcomes of SLAP repair with those of biceps tenodesis. Boileau et al (2009) compared 10 patients who underwent repair with 15 patients who underwent arthroscopic biceps tenodesis for isolated type II SLAP tears. These investigators reported that 87% of the patients in the biceps tenodesis group were able to return to the previous level of sports participation, compared with only 20% of the SLAP repair group. They concluded that biceps tenodesis should be considered an effective alternative to SLAP repair in type II lesions that affords patients the ability to return to a preinjury level of sports participation (Fig. 19A.3).

Conclusion

Isolated superior labral tears are an uncommon but significant source of shoulder pain. Arthroscopic SLAP repair is indicated for type II SLAP lesions in active younger patients with consistent history, physical examination, and imaging findings and no identifiable concomitant pathologic biceps tendon abnormality. Current evidence suggests that repair

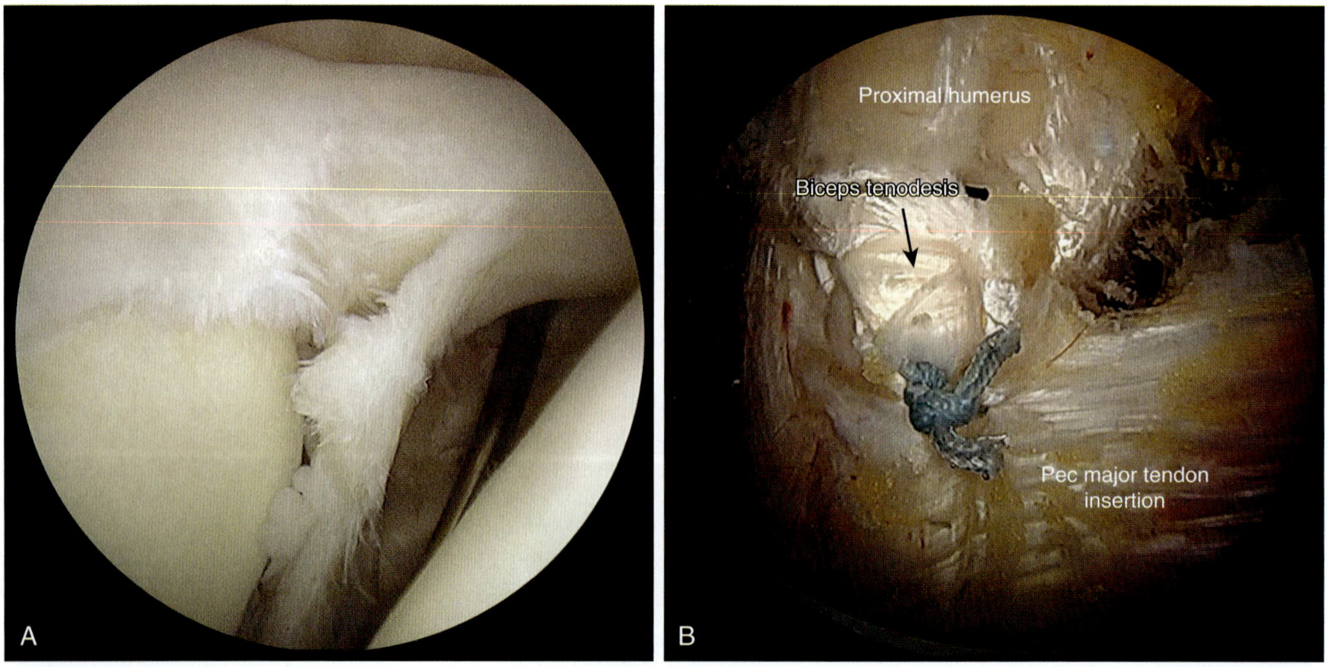

Fig. 19A.3 (**A**) Arthroscopic image from a left shoulder standard posterior viewing portal, demonstrating a bucket-handle tear of the superior labrum with detachment of the biceps tendon anchor, consistent with a type IV SLAP tear. (**B**) Arthroscopic suprapectoral biceps tenodesis in a right shoulder using a tenodesis screw for management of a type IV SLAP tear. *Pec,* pectoralis.

of type II SLAP lesions provides significant improvement in patient-reported outcome scores and satisfaction. However, such improvement may not correlate with rates of return to preinjury activity levels, especially in elite overhead athletes and older patients. The management of these injuries and their surgical indications and treatment continue to evolve.

References

Abrams GD, Safran MR. Diagnosis and management of superior labrum anterior posterior lesions in overhead athletes. *Br J Sports Med.* 2010;44(5):311–318.

Abrassart S, Stern R, Hoffmeyer P. Arterial supply of the glenoid: an anatomic study. *J Shoulder Elbow Surg.* 2006;15(2):232–238.

Andrews JR, Carson Jr WG, McLeod WD. Glenoid labrum tears related to the long head of the biceps. *Am J Sports Med.* 1985;13:337–341.

Barber A, Field LD, Ryu R. Biceps tendon and superior labrum injuries: decision-making. *J Bone Joint Surg Am.* 2007;89:1844–1855.

Bicos J. Biomechanics and anatomy of the proximal biceps tendon. *Sports Med Arthrosc.* 2008;16(3):111–117.

Boileau P, Parratte S, Chuinard C, et al. Arthroscopic treatment of isolated type II SLAP lesions: biceps tenodesis as an alternative to reinsertion. *Am J Sports Med.* 2009;37:929–936.

Brockmeier SF, Voos JE, Williams 3rd RJ, et al. Outcomes after arthroscopic repair of type-II SLAP lesions. *J Bone Joint Surg Am.* 2009;91(7):1595–1603.

Burkhart SS, Morgan CD, Kibler WB. The disabled throwing shoulder: spectrum of pathology part I: pathoanatomy and biomechanics. *Arthroscopy.* 2003;19(4):404–420.

Cohen DB, Coleman S, Drakos MC, et al. Outcomes of isolated type II SLAP lesions treated with arthroscopic fixation using a bioabsorbable tack. *Arthroscopy.* 2006;22:136–142.

Coleman SH, Cohen DB, Drakos MC, et al. Arthroscopic repair of type II superior labral anterior posterior lesions with and without acromioplasty: a clinical analysis of 50 patients. *Am J Sports Med.* 2007;35:749–753.

Cooper DE, Arnoczky SP, O'Brien SJ, et al. Anatomy, histology, and vascularity of the glenoid labrum: an anatomical study. *J Bone Joint Surg Am.* 1992;74:46–52.

Dierickx C, Ceccarelli E, Conti M, et al. Variations of the intraarticular portion of the long head of the biceps tendon: a classification of embryologically explained variations. *J Shoulder Elbow Surg.* 2009;18(4):556–565.

Erickson J, Lavery K, Monica J, et al. Surgical treatment of symptomatic superior labrum anterior-posterior tears in patients older than 40 years: a systematic review. *Am J Sports Med.* 2015;43:1274–1282.

Keener JD, Brophy RH. Superior labral tears of the shoulder: pathogenesis, evaluation, and treatment. *J Am Acad Orthop Surg.* 2009;17:627–637.

Kim SH, Ha KI, Kim SH, et al. Results of arthroscopic treatment of superior labral lesions. *J Bone Joint Surg Am.* 2002;84-A:981–985.

Kim SJ, Lee IS, Kim SH, et al. Arthroscopic repair of concomitant type II SLAP lesions in large to massive rotator cuff tears: comparison with biceps tenotomy. *Am J Sports Med.* 2012;40:2786–2793.

Kim TK, Queale WS, Cosgarea AJ, et al. Clinical features of the different types of SLAP lesions: an analysis of one hundred and thirty-nine cases. *J Bone Joint Surg Am.* 2003;85-A:66–71.

Kuhn JE, Lindholm SR, Huston LJ, et al. Failure of the biceps superior labral complex: a cadaveric biomechanical investigation comparing the late cocking and early deceleration positions of throwing. *Arthroscopy.* 2003;19(4):373–379.

Maffet MW, Gartsman GM, Moseley B. Superior labrum-biceps tendon complex lesions of the shoulder. *Am J Sports Med.* 1995;23:93–98.

Maier D, Jaeger M, Ogon P, et al. Suture anchors or transglenoidal sutures for arthroscopic repair of isolated SLAP-2 lesions? A matched-pair comparison of functional outcome and return to sports. *Arch Orthop Trauma Surg.* 2013;133:227–235.

McDonald LS, Dewing CB, Scupe PG, et al. Disorders of the proximal and distal aspects of the biceps muscle. *J Bone Joint Surg.* 2013;95:1235–1245.

Neri BR, ElAttrache NS, Owsley KC, et al. Outcome of type II superior labral anterior posterior repairs in elite overhead athletes: effect of concomitant partial-thickness rotator cuff tears. *Am J Sports Med.* 2011;39:114–120.

Park JY, Chung SW, Jeon SH, et al. Clinical and radiological outcomes of type 2 superior labral anterior posterior repairs in elite overhead athletes. *Am J Sports Med.* 2013;41:1372–1379.

Patterson BM, Creighton RA, Spang JT, et al. Surgical trends in the treatment of superior labrum anterior and posterior lesions of the shoulder: analysis of data from the American Board of Orthopaedic Surgery Certification Examination Database. *Am J Sports Med.* 2014;42:1904–1910.

Provencher MT, McCormick F, Dewing C, et al. A prospective analysis of 179 type 2 superior labrum anterior and posterior repairs: outcomes and factors associated with success and failure. *Am J Sports Med.* 2013;41:880–886.

Rao AG, Kim TK, Chronopoulos E, et al. Anatomical variants in the anterosuperior aspect of the glenoid labrum: a statistical analysis of seventy-three cases. *J Bone Joint Surg Am.* 2003;85-A(4):653–659.

Snyder SJ, Karzel RP, Del Pizzo W, et al. SLAP lesions of the shoulder. *Arthroscopy.* 1990;6:274–279.

Tuoheti Y, Itoi E, Minagawa H, et al. Attachment types of the long head of the biceps tendon to the glenoid labrum and their relationships with the glenohumeral ligaments. *Arthroscopy.* 2005;21(10):1242–1249.

Vangsness Jr CT, Jorgenson SS, Watson T, et al. The origin of the long head of the biceps from the scapula and glenoid labrum. An anatomical study of 100 shoulders. *J Bone Joint Surg Br.* 1994;76(6):951–954.

Wahl CJ, MacGillivray JD. Three congenital variations in the long head of the biceps tendon: a review of pathoanatomic considerations and case reports. *J Shoulder Elbow Surg.* 2007;16(6):e25–e30.

Werner BC, Holzgrefe RE, Brockmeier SF. Arthroscopic surgical techniques for the management of proximal biceps injuries. *Clin Sports Med.* 2016;35:113–135.

19-19B LABRAL TEAR, SPINOGLENOID CYST, AND SUPRASCAPULAR NEUROPATHY

AYDIN BUDEYRI, MD, FEBOT, RAFFAELE GAROFALO, MD, and SUMANT "BUTCH" KRISHNAN, MD

Introduction

- Tears of the posterosuperior glenoid labrum have been recognized as a source of shoulder pain and functional disability (Chen et al, 2003; Harrison et al,, 2016; Hirayama & Takemitsu, 1981; Iannotti & Ramsey, 1996; Piatt et al, 2002).
- These tears could be due to developing "paralabral" cysts secondary to extravasation of glenohumeral joint fluid through the tear. Magnetic resonance imaging (MRI) has been used to confirm a direct relationship between these posterosuperior glenoid labral tears and associated paralabral cysts (Chen et al, 2003; Tirman et al, 1994; Tung et al, 2000).

- Patients usually have symptoms from the labral tear and also from accompanying cysts, which manifest as pain accompanied by weakness, especially with overhead sports activities (Piatt et al, 2002).
- Previous peer-reviewed publications have also documented another source for both pain and weakness in this cohort: compression of the suprascapular nerve exactly at the spinoglenoid notch by the paralabral cyst (Chen et al, 2003; Iannotti & Ramsey, 1996; Piatt et al, 2002).
- The location of the paralabral cyst determines the potential extent of suprascapular nerve dysfunction. Not all cysts may be caused by labral tears, and not every cyst is associated with weakness and/or neuropathic findings on electromyography (EMG). Hence, all potential causes of pain and weakness must be evaluated to determine the specific treatment to each patient (Harrison et al, 2016; Hill et al, 2014).
- Traditionally, surgical treatment of spinoglenoid notch cysts with open suprascapular nerve decompression has been successful (Chen et al, 2003; Harrison et al, 2016). However, open techniques do not necessarily address the inciting posterosuperior labral tear.
- Consequently, arthroscopic management of this pathology has become prevalent as arthroscopic surgical techniques have evolved. Nevertheless, there is at present no large comprehensive series published that documents the long-term outcomes and/or return of nerve function or muscular tropism following all-arthroscopic management (Andrews et al, 1985; Chen et al, 2003; Gupta et al, 2015; Hirayama & Takemitsu, 1981; Iannotti & Ramsey, 1996; Moore et al,1997; Piatt et al, 2002; Tirman et al, 1994; Tung et al, 2000).

Pathology

Glenoid paralabral cysts can develop as a result of lesions within the glenoid labrum or the glenolabral interface and/or because of myxoid degeneration of glenohumeral capsule. Such injuries can create a one-way valve mechanism that allows egress but prevents ingress of glenohumeral joint synovial fluid. Once that fluid is forced through the tear and trapped around the glenohumeral joint, a ganglion cyst may form, although the exact pathophysiology of this cyst formation remains unknown. Several reviews using MRI studies demonstrated an association between the labral tear and a ganglion cyst in 52% to 100% of cases (Gupta et al, 2015; Tirman et al, 1994; Tung et al, 2000). Paralabral cysts that are located on the spinoglenoid notch have been associated with posterosuperior glenoid labral tears, which have also been described as "SLAP" tears (superior labrum anterior and posterior tears). When ganglion cysts develop in the suprascapular fossa, pressure from those tears compresses the inferior branch of the suprascapular nerve, generating pain as well as weakness of the infraspinatus muscle (Chen et al, 1999; Harrison et al, 2016; Iannotti & Ramsey, 1996; Moore et al, 1997; Piatt et al, 2002).

LABRAL TEARS

The glenoid labrum is a fibrocartilaginous ring that surrounds and deepens the glenoid. The superior labrum can be meniscoid in appearance and attached to the glenoid peripherally, or it can be firmly attached to the glenoid both centrally and peripherally. The long head of the biceps attaches to the posterosuperior labrum and supraglenoid tubercle, which lies 5 mm medial to the superior glenoid rim. The primary site of attachment of the biceps to the labrum is variable. SLAP lesions have been identified as an underlying reason for pain in the shoulder since the mid-1980s (Andrews et al, 1985; Dini et al, 2016; Harrison et al, 2016).

The predominant mechanisms for the etiology of SLAP lesions are traction on the overhead or abducted arm, shearing stress or compression on the outstretched arm such as from a fall, and repetitive overhead rotational movements of the arm during sporting activities. Because natural degenerative processes in the glenoid labrum set in with age, isolated SLAP lesions are not commonly diagnosed as the primary source of shoulder pain in patients older than 40 years (Bhatia et al, 2012).

The classification for SLAP tears developed by Snyder et al (1990) is as follows: A type I lesion manifests as a frayed and degenerating superior labrum while showing an uninvolved biceps anchor; a type II tear involve removal of the biceps anchor; a type III tear involves a bucket-handle tear of the superior labrum with intact biceps tendon component; and a type IV lesion is characterized by the bucket-handle tear along with a displaced biceps tendon root. The clinical symptomatology related to the SLAP lesion can be variable. However, when a SLAP type II tear is associated with a ganglion cyst and also involves the suprascapular fossa, the patient may experience pain and weakness because of suprascapular nerve compression (Hashiguchi et al, 2016; Piatt et al, 2002;).

ANATOMIC DETAILS OF THE SPINOGLENOID NOTCH AND THE SUPRASCAPULAR NERVE

The suprascapular nerve begins within the upper part of the brachial plexus (i.e., C5, C6, and a variable contribute of C4 root). This nerve courses through the posterior cervical triangle laterally and reaches to the suprascapular notch, passing in an inferior position to the transverse scapular ligament and medial to the coracoid process base. On exit from the suprascapular notch, the nerve travels across the floor of the suprascapular fossa posterolaterally and also around the posterior glenoid neck (Kim et al, 2017).

At the posterolateral corner of the suprascapular fossa, it reaches the spinoglenoid notch, which is located 1.8 to 2.1 cm medial to the superior glenoid rim (Bigliani et al, 1990; Dini et al, 2016; Plancher & Petterson, 2016Warner et al, 1992). The suprascapular nerve provides sensory fibers of the coracoacromial ligament and the acromioclavicular and glenohumeral joints. In 15% of the healthy population, it may also provide a cutaneous branch functioning for the sensation of the lateral arm. Its main function is to serve as a motor nerve to the supraspinatus and infraspinatus muscles (Antoniou et al, 2001; Plancher & Petterson, 2016).

A spinoglenoid ligament, as a variation, has been identified coursing around the top of the spinoglenoid notch (Kaspi et al, 1988). Work with cadavers demonstrated a spinoglenoid ligament to be a stout structure in all studied specimens (Plancher et al, 2005). Beyond the spinoglenoid notch, the suprascapular nerve turns around the bottom of the scapular spine acutely and travels along the scapular body while providing some motor branches for the infraspinatus muscle (Bigliani et al, 1990; Ghodadra et al, 2009).

Within the confines of the suprascapular notch, the suprascapular nerve is vulnerable. Narrowing of the notch may impair the nerve's functioning. The suprascapular nerve more vulnerable to compression by cyst formation within the spinoglenoid notch with medial extension of paralabral cysts (Bigliani et al, 1990). Within the spinoglenoid notch, any ganglion cyst may cause compression of the inferior section of suprascapular nerve in the infraspinatus fossa. Some researchers have classified this combined pathology as a GLEN lesion: ganglion cyst origination at the superior labrum and entrapping the inferior section of the suprascapular nerve (Iannotti & Ramsey, 1996).

Trapping of suprascapular nerve at the spinoglenoid notch, just under the spinoglenoid ligament, may also happen without cyst formation. Many researchers have suggested that the nerve is damaged as a result of the anatomic structure of the spinoglenoid notch and trauma caused by continuous overhead activities (Bryan & Wild, 1989; Ferretti et al, 1998). In particular, it has been postulated that a section of the spinoglenoid ligament inserts on the posterior capsule and becomes taut b adduction and internal rotation. This position corresponds with the follow-through phase of throwing and similar overhead activities (Plancher et al, 2005).

Clinical Presentation

No single clinical symptom or physical finding can serve as a definite diagnosis for a spinoglenoid ganglion cyst. Most patients are either overhead athletes (young active people) or overhead laborers (Bedi et al, 2010; Gupta et al, 2015; Hashiguchi et al, 2016; Lichtenberg et al, 2004). Patients may experience posterior and posterolateral shoulder pain with concomitant weakness in external rotation (Plancher & Petterson, 2016; Tung et al, 2000). There have also been a few reports of isolated shoulder weakness with little or no pain accompanied by infraspinatus fossa atrophy (Fig. 19B.1). This weakness may not be proportional to other findings of the physical examination.

Extreme adduction and internal rotation activities may trigger pain at the posterior shoulder that may be secondary in nature to the tightening of the spinoglenoid ligament. The diagnosis should be distinguished from primary acromioclavicular pathologies (Plancher et al, 2005). In patients who have incidents of isolated infraspinatus nerve involvement, there may be signs of coexisting labral pathology, so a careful evaluation for posterosuperior and/or SLAP tears should be performed. The tests for SLAP lesions remain unclear and debatable at best. The active compression test (also known as the O'Brien test) has been reported as the most predictive test for evaluating a SLAP type II lesion, whereas the modified Jobe relocation test is highly specific for assessment of posterior SLAP lesions (Burkhart et al, 2003).

Patients who present with the clinical symptoms of the suprascapular neuropathy require a careful overall neurovascular evaluation, including tests specific to distal cervical root impairment between C5 and T1.

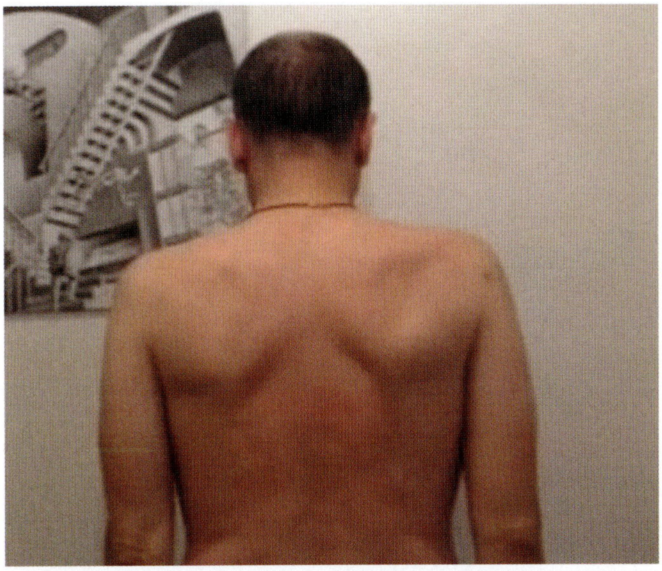

Fig. 19B.1 Clinical photograph of right-sided infraspinatus muscle atrophy in a patient with a documented positive result on EMG analysis for suprascapular neuropathy at the spinoglenoid notch.

Diagnostic Studies

Conventional radiography positions are the true scapular-plane anteroposterior, outlet/scapular, Y, axillary, and Stryker notch views. They are utilized at the initial evaluation of any patient who presents with shoulder pain in order to rule out an osseous etiology of suprascapular nerve entrapment. The Stryker notch view ensures evaluation of the suprascapular notch and may sometimes reveal a complete ossification of the foramen (Dini et al, 2016; Plancher & Petterson, 2016).

MRI without contrast enhancement remains the next best modality for examining patients who have shoulder pain believed to be associated with labral tears, paralabral cysts, and possible suprascapular neuropathies. High-resolution MRI is able to show the distinction between intraneural ganglion cysts and paralabral (extraneural) cysts in the glenohumeral joint (Hill et al, 2014). Suprascapular intraneural ganglion cysts have a pathomechanism similar to that of their paralabral counterparts, starting from a tear within the glenoid labrum (Prasad et al, 2015). However, some writers have indicated that MRI does not provide the specificity needed to identify SLAP lesions that were subsequently identified during surgery. The use of MRI with intraarticular gadolinium contrast media can be very useful for accurately identifying both labral tears and paralabral cysts. MRI examinations also ensure accurate examination of rotator cuff integrity and muscle trophicity (Sherman et al, 2004; Tung et al, 2000).

A ganglion cyst has a characteristic appearance on MRI (Sherman et al, 2004; Tung et al, 2000). The lesion appears to be round and homogeneous but may contain thin septations. It appears with increased signal on a T2-weighted image and looks dark on a T1-weighted image (Fig. 19B.2). A heterogenous or irregular appearance may indicate that the lesion is a tumor rather than a cyst. In patients in whom there is suspicion of suprascapular neuropathy, the most important tests for the diagnosis and confirmation

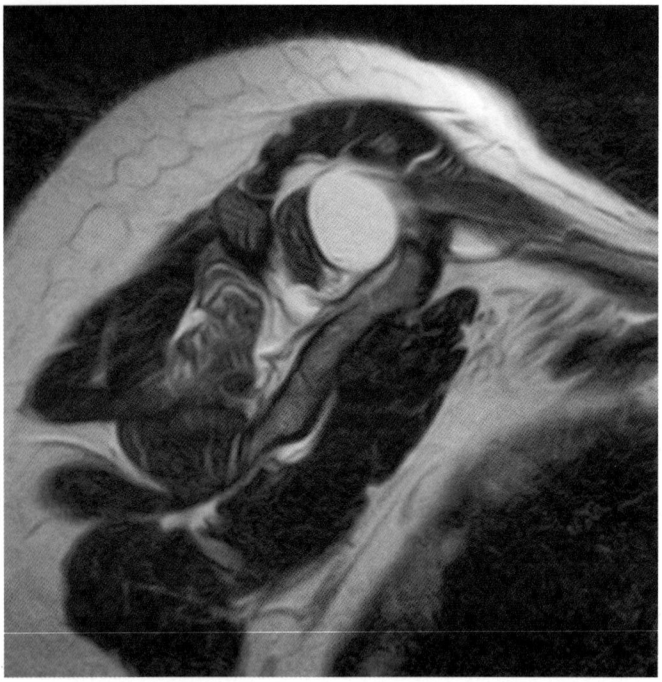

Fig. 19B.2 A T2-weighted sagittal MRI study demonstrating a paralabral cyst extending superiorly into the suprascapular fossa; only the nerve section going toward the infraspinatus is affected. The atrophy in the infraspinatus muscle is apparent.

are bilateral electromyography (EMG) with nerve conduction velocity (NCV) studies of the suprascapular nerve. The EMG/NCV study should include the whole upper extremity and cervical spine so as to exclude other probable causes of neuropathy (Kim et al, 2017). Even though these two studies have intrarater and interrater variabilities, they may be useful to localize the nerve compression site. Possible positive findings are increased latency, increased fibrillation potential, and decreased amplitude. Normal values for the motor nerve conduction velocity study have been established for the suprascapular nerve. Unfortunately, there is no clear evidence to support the level of sensitivity and specificity provided by EMG studies in detecting the presence or absence of suprascapular neuropathy. This situation has led to later research to evaluate the use of diagnostic injections of local anesthesia in the suprascapular notch as a potential diagnostic test for this problem (Gupta et al, 2015; Hashiguchi et al, 2016).

Treatment Options

The appropriate managements of combined posterosuperior labral tears, paralabral cysts, and/or suprascapular neuropathy are based on the severity of the symptoms, etiology of the pathology, and experience of the surgeon.

CONSERVATIVE MANAGEMENT

Nonsurgical management is preferred for spinoglenoid and suprascapular fossa cysts that are found incidentally and appear to be normal on EMG/NCV study (Buschbacher et al, 2009). Nonsurgical management is also preferred for most patients who present with a suprascapular neuropathy without any evidence of a compressing lesion. Such patients usually have an overuse-type etiology. Conservative modalities include avoidance of overhead activities, administration of nonsteroidal antiinflammatory drugs, injection therapies, and physical therapy focusing on shoulder motion as well as on muscle strengthening of the scapular stabilizers. This approach is widely accepted as appropriate standard initial treatment (Dini et al, 2016).

Duration of symptoms and etiology of entrapment are important in the decision about how long any nonsurgical treatment option should be pursued. Although pain relief and restoration of shoulder function are reliably achieved among a majority of patients, muscle bulk and motor strength may not be regained once significant atrophy has settled in. In one study, the outcomes of a conservative treatment protocol were reported in 15 patients suffering from suprascapular neuropathy without any mass lesion. After a minimum of 6 months' follow-up, 80% of the patients were reported to achieve a good to excellent clinical result. Most of the patients were not restricted in activity by the impaired shoulder, but persistent atrophy and weakness on isokinetic testing were reported to be prevalent. This pattern suggests that the nonsurgical treatment provides benefit mostly in the form of compensatory muscle action and less for nerve recovery (Martin et al, 1997). Consequently, some investigators have suggested that operative interventions should be undertaken as soon as suprascapular neuropathy is confirmed. This management strategy helps prevent further muscle damage in the setting of a compressed nerve (Post, 1999).

Observation is also usually indicated for an isolated paralabral cyst that is causing pain but no nerve dysfunction or weakness, because spontaneous resolution is believed to occur in 10% to 17% of cases (Moore et al, 1997; Piatt et al, 2002). Treatment of the cyst is generally recommended if the pain persists after several months of observation or if weakness develops.

OPERATIVE TREATMENT

When there is no lesion taking up space, procedural management may be considered if nonsurgical treatment fails. In contrast to the situation described previously, when there is a significantly compressing lesion, such as spinoglenoid or paralabral, suprascapular neuropathy at the spinoglenoid notch is evidently secondary to the compression of the nerve. Usually this compression is caused by the cystic lesion in association with a posterosuperior labral tear. Sterile aspiration guided by ultrasound, computerized tomography, or MRI is the least invasive method for the decompression of the cyst (Chiou et al, 1999; Fehrman et al, 1995). This treatment appears to be reliable in draining the cyst and carries little risk to the patient. However, image-guided drainage does not address the intraarticular pathology, and the rate of persistent or recurrent symptoms is high. Cyst recurrence has been reported in such cases (Chiou et al, 1999; Fehrman et al, 1995; Romeo et al, 2010).

The historical standard for the management of paralabral cysts resulting in suprascapular nerve entrapment with conclusive EMG findings has been an open excision as described in previous research (Savoie et al, 2016; Takagishi & Saitoh, 1994).The disadvantages of this technique include difficulty in evaluating the glenohumeral joint and identifying or treating intraarticular lesions that might play a part in casing the creation of the cyst. Hence, several arthroscopic methods have been described to treat this pathology, and the short-term results are encouraging (Bedi et al, 2010; Chen et al, 2003; Gupta et al, 2015; Hashiguchi et al, 2016; Iannotti & Ramsey, 1996; Lichtenberg et al, 2004; Moore et al, 1997; Piatt et al, 2002). Several small series have reported that abnormalities seen in the EMG study had resolved 6 to 9 months after decompression with clinical improvement (Abboud et al, 2006; Iannotti & Ramsey, 1996).

THE AUTHORS' PREFERRED SURGICAL TECHNIQUE—ALL-ARTHROSCOPIC

The patient can be placed in a beach-chair or lateral position (Video 19B.1). A standard "high" posterior viewing portal is used to begin the intraarticular arthroscopy and then a single anterior portal is created "high" in the rotator interval to reach just posterior to the biceps. With both portals used as viewing and also repair portals ("two-portal technique"), the following three surgical goals must be reached:

1. *Posterior glenohumeral joint capsulotomy immediately adjacent to the labral tear.* This "transcapsular" approach to the cyst allows for direct visual confirmation of the location of the cyst relative to the labral tear, which is confirmed by correlation with the sagittal plane MR images (Fig. 19B.3).
2. *Decompression of the paralabral cyst and excision of the entire cyst wall.* Cystic fluid can be visualized decompressing into the glenohumeral joint, and the remaining cyst wall is meticulously excised within the substance of the infraspinatus muscle to prevent recurrence of compression. Special care must be taken to avoid injury to infraspinatus section of the suprascapular nerve at the spinoglenoid notch (Fig. 19B.4).
3. *Anatomic repair of the posterosuperior labrum.* The glenoid rim is prepared to a bleeding surface, and a standard suture anchor repair of the labrum is performed. We prefer to use absorbable anchors with nonabsorbable sutures to repair the labral tear (Fig. 19B.5).

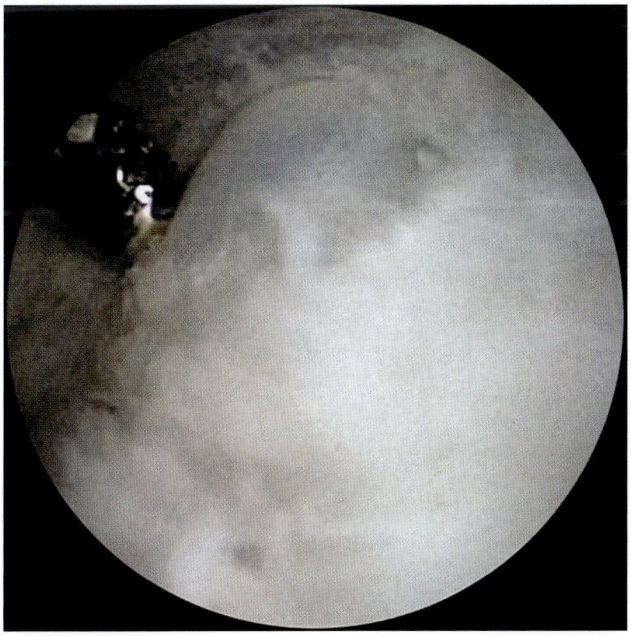

Fig. 19B.3 Posterior glenohumeral capsulotomy adjacent to the labral tear. The paralabral cyst is identified, with the shaver introduced through a high posterior portal. The arthroscope is in the "high" anterior portal.

POSTOPERATIVE CARE

After surgery, a Velpeau sling is used for 6 weeks. No motion of the shoulder is allowed for 3 weeks. Beginning Week 4

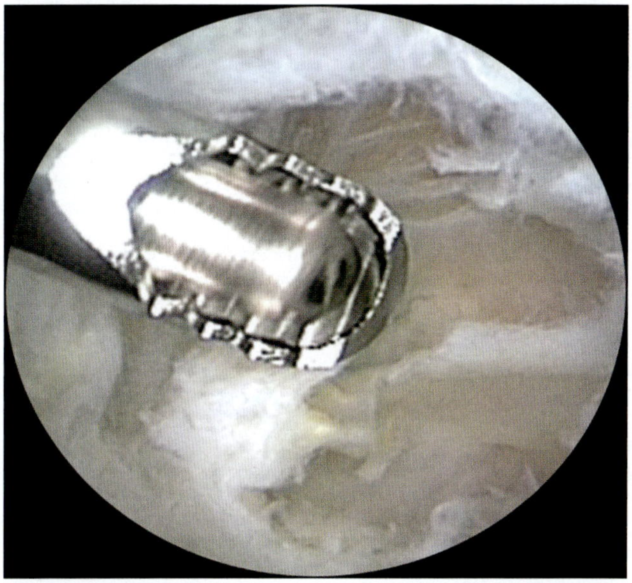

Fig. 19B.4 Arthroscopic view of decompression of the paralabral cyst and excision of the cyst wall.

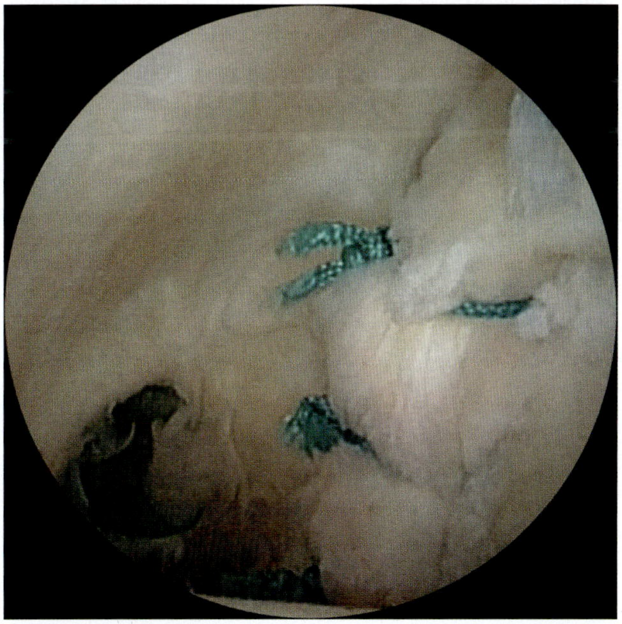

Fig. 19B.5 Posterosuperior labral repair with absorbable anchors and nonabsorbable suture.

and continuing to week 6, supine passive motion is limited to 90 degrees of forward flexion, full external rotation and no internal rotation; passive motion during weeks 5 and 6 is forward flexion to 90 degrees, full external rotation, and no internal rotation. Active motion is allowed at week 7. Resistance exercises begin at week 10. No overhead throwing motion for overhead athletes is allowed until week 12. Full activity (including contact sports, overhead sports, and full work capacity) is allowed at 6 months after surgery.

References

Abboud JA, Silverberg D, Glaser DL, et al. Arthroscopy effectively treats ganglion cysts of the shoulder. *Clin Orthop Related Res.* 2006;444:129–133.

Andrews JR, Carson Jr WG, McLeod WD. Glenoid labrum tears related to the long head of the biceps. *Am J Sports Med.* 1985;13:337–341.

Antoniou J, Tae SK, Williams GR, et al. Suprascapular neuropathy: variability in the diagnosis, treatment and outcome. *Clin Orthop.* 2001:131–138.

Bedi A, Dodson C, Altcheck DW. Symptomatic SLAP tear and paralabral cyst in a pediatric athlete: a case report. *J Bone Joint Surg Am.* 2010;92:721–725.

Bhatia S, Chalmers PN, Yanke AB, Romeo AA, Verma NN. Arthroscopic suprascapular nerve decompression: transarticular and subacromial approach. *Arthrosc Tech.* 2012;1(2):e187–e192.

Bigliani LU, Dalsey RM, McCann PD. An anatomical study of the suprascapular nerve. *Arthroscopy.* 1990;6:301–305.

Bryan WJ, Wild Jr JJ. Isolated infraspinatus atrophy: a common cause of posterior shoulder pain and weakness in throwing athletes. *Am J Sports Med.* 1989;17:130–131.

Burkhart SS, Morgan CD, Kibler WB. The disabled throwing shoulder: Spectrum of pathology part II: evaluation and treatment of SLAP lesions in throwers. *Arthroscopy.* 2003;19(5):531–539.

Buschbacher RM, Weir SK, Bentley JG, Cottrell E. Normal motor nerve conduction studies using surface electrode recording from supraspinatus, infraspinatus, deltoid, and biceps. *PM R.* 2009;1(2):101–106.

Chen AL, Ong BC, Rose DJ. Arthroscopic management of spinoglenoid cysts associated with SLAP lesions and suprascapular neuropathy. *Arthroscopy.* 2003;19:E15–E21.

Chiou HJ, Chou YH, Wu JJ, et al. Alternative and effective treatment of shoulder ganglion cyst: ultrasonographically guided aspiration. *J Ultrasound Med.* 1999;18:531–535.

Dini AA, O'Brien MJ, Savoie III FH. Suprascapular nerve release: general principles. In: Kelly JD IV, ed. *Elite Techniques in Shoulder Arthroscopy: New Frontiers in Shoulder Preservation.* vol. 5. Philadelphia: Springer International Publishing; 2016:271–281.

Fehrman DA, Orwin JF, Jennings R. Suprascapular nerve entrapment by ganglion cysts: A report of six cases with arthroscopic findings and review of the literature. *Arthroscopy.* 1995;11:727–734.

Ferretti A, De Carli A, Fontana M. Injury of the suprascapular nerve at the spinoglenoid notch: the natural history of infraspinatus atrophy in volleyball players. *Am J Sports Med.* 1998;26:759–763.

Ghodadra N, Nho SJ, Verma NN, et al. Arthroscopic decompression of the suprascapular nerve at the spinoglenoid notch and suprascapular notch through the subacromial space. *Arthroscopy.* 2009;25(4):439–445.

Gupta R, Kapoor L, Shagotar S. Arthroscopic decompression of paralabral cyst around suprascapular notch causing suprascapular neuropathy. *J Clin Orthop Trauma.* 2015;6(3):184–186.

Harrison R, Lutton D, Cuomo F. Arthroscopic suprascapular nerve decompression. In: Scuderi GR, Tria AJ, eds. *Minimally Invasive Surgery in Orthopedics.* 2nd ed. vol. 2. Philadelphia: Springer International; 2016:173–180.

Hashiguchi H, Iwashita S, Ohkubo A, Takai S. SLAP repair with arthroscopic decompression of the spinoglenoid cyst. *SICOT J.* 2016;2:1–9.

Hill LJ, Jelsing EJ, Terry MJ, Strommen JA. Evaluation, treatment, and outcomes of suprascapular neuropathy: a 5-year review. *PM R.* 2014;6(9):774–780.

Hirayama T, Takemitsu Y. Compression of the suprascapular nerve by a ganglion at the suprascapular notch. *Clin Orthop.* 1981;155:95–96.

Hashiguchi H, Iwashita S, Ohkubo A, Takai S. SLAP repair with arthroscopic decompression of spinoglenoid cyst. *SICOT J.* 2016;1:1–6.

Iannotti JP, Ramsey ML. Arthroscopic decompression of a ganglion cyst causing suprascapular nerve compression. *Arthroscopy.* 1996;12:739–745.

Kaspi A, Yanai J, Pick CG. Entrapment of the distal suprascapular nerve: Anatomical study. *Int Orthop.* 1988;12:273–275.

Kim SJ, Choi YR, Jung M, Park JY, Chun YM. Outcomes of arthroscopic decompression of spinoglenoid cysts through a subacromial approach. *Arthroscopy.* 2017;33(1):62–67.

Lichtenberg S, Magosh P, Habermeyer P. Compression of the suprascapular nerve by a ganglion cyst of the spinoglenoid notch: the arthroscopic solution. *Knee Surg Sports Traumatol Arthrosc.* 2004;12:72–79.

Martin SD, Warren RF, Martin TL, Kennedy K, O'Brien SJ, Wickiewicz TL. Suprascapular neuropathy: results of non-operative treatment. *J Bone Joint Surg Am.* 1997;79:1159–1165.

Moore TP, Fritts HM, Quick DC, Buss DD. Suprascapular nerve entrapment caused by supraglenoid cyst compression. *J Shoulder Elbow Surg.* 1997;6:455–462.

Piatt BE, Hawkins RJ, Fritz RC, et al. Clinical evaluation and treatment of spinoglenoid notch ganglion cysts. *J Shoulder Elbow Surg.* 2002;11:600–604.

Plancher KD, Peterson RK, Johnston JC, Luke TA. The spinoglenoid ligament: anatomy, morphology, and histological findings. *J Bone Joint Surg Am.* 2005;87:361–365.

Plancher KD, Petterson SC. Distal suprascapular nerve compression: spinoglenoid ligament release. In: Kelly JD IV, ed. *Elite Techniques in Shoulder Arthroscopy: New Frontiers in Shoulder Preservation.* vol IV. Philadelphia: Springer International Publishing; 2016:283–302.

Post M. Diagnosis and treatment of suprascapular nerve entrapment. *Clin Orthop Relat Res.* 1999;368:92–100.

Prasad NK, Spinner RJ, Smith J, et al. The successful arthroscopic treatment of suprascapular intraneural ganglion cysts. *Neurosurg Focus.* 2015;39(3):E11.

Romeo AA, Ghodadra NS, Salata MJ, Provencher MT. Arthroscopic suprascapular nerve decompression: indications and surgical technique. *J Shoulder Elbow Surg.* 2010;19(2):118–123.

Savoie III FH, Zunkiewicz M, Field LD, Replogle WH, O'Brien MJ. A comparison of functional outcomes in patients undergoing revision arthroscopic repair of massive rotator cuff tears with and without arthroscopic suprascapular nerve release. *Open Access J Sports Med.* 2016;7:129–134.

Sherman PM, Sehrman DA, Orwinanders TG, De Lone DR. A benign soft tissue mass simulating a glenoid labral cyst on unenhanced magnetic resonance imaging. *Mil Med.* 2004;169:376–378.

Snyder SJ, Karzel RP, Pizzo WD, Ferkel RD, Friedman MJ. SLAP lesions of the shoulder. *Arthroscopy.* 1990;6(4):274–279.

Takagishi K, Saitoh A, Tonegawa M, et al. Isolated paralysis of the infraspinatus muscle. *J Bone Joint Surg Br.* 1994;76:584–587.

Tirman PF, Feller JF, Janzen DL, et al. Association of glenoid labral cysts with labral tears and glenohumeral instability: radiologic findings and clinical significance. *Radiology.* 1994;190:653–658.

Tung GA, Entzian D, Stern JB. MR imaging and MR arthrography of paraglenoid labral cysts. *AJR Am J Roentgenol.* 2000;174:1707–1715.

Warner JP, Krushell RJ, Masquelet A, Gerber C. Anatomy and relationships of the suprascapular nerve: anatomical constraints to mobilization of the supraspinatus and infraspinatus muscles in the management of massive rotator cuff tears. *J Bone Joint Surg Am.* 1992;74:36–45.

SECTION **VII**

Pectoralis Major Injury

SECTION OUTLINE

20 Overview

LIONEL E. LAZARO, MD and FRANK A. CORDASCO, MD

Introduction

- Injuries to the pectoralis major (PM) occur infrequently, typically in young male athletes (Bak et al, 2000; Cordasco & Delos, 2013; Cordasco et al, 2017; Guity et al, 2014; Haley & Zacchilli, 2014; Kang et al, 2014).
- This injury most often develops during high loads, with the arm extended, abducted, and externally rotated, while transitioning from eccentric to concentric contractions of the PM (Cordasco et al, 2017; Garrigues et al, 2012; Kang et al, 2014; Wolfe et al, 1992).
- Although some of these injuries can be successfully treated nonoperatively, rupture of the tendon can result in significant functional deficits limiting high level athletics.
- An accurate and timely diagnosis is of paramount importance in order to achieve definitive treatment and the best possible outcomes after surgical repair (Bak et al, 2000; Cordasco et al, 2017; De Castro Pochini et al, 2014; Elmaraghy & Devereaux, 2012; Garrigues et al, 2012; Haley & Zacchilli, 2014; Hanna et al, 2001; Kang et al, 2014; Kretzler & Richardson, 1989; Mcentire et al, 1972; Park & Espiniella, 1970; Pavlik et al, 1998; Wolfe et al, 1992; Zeman et al, 1979).
- This chapter first reviews the anatomy of the PM and then discusses the epidemiology, classification, clinical assessment, and advanced imaging modalities for injuries of the PM.

Anatomy

The musculotendinous anatomy of the PM is complex and can be misinterpreted (Fung et al, 2009; Elmaraghy & Devereaux, 2012). The PM consists mainly of two heads (the clavicular head and sternocostal head) with a broad origin, which insert as a bilaminar conjoined tendon along the lateral lip of the bicipital grove (Cordasco & Delos, 2013; Elmaraghy & Devereaux, 2012; Haley & Zacchilli, 2014). The clavicular head originates from the medial and middle third of the clavicle and courses parallel essentially as a uniform structure that forms the vast majority of the anterior tendon lamina, which then inserts more distally (Elmaraghy & Devereaux, 2012; Haley & Zacchilli, 2014). The sternocostal head originates from the sternum and the costal cartilage of the first six ribs. This muscle unit can be divided into six or seven segments, with the inferior segments attaching to the fascia of the external oblique muscles and inserting proximally through the posterior tendon lamina (Cordasco & Delos, 2013; Elmaraghy & Devereaux, 2012; Haley & Zacchilli, 2014). The orientation of the PM heads has been described as a Asian fan where each superior and inferior adjacent segment overlaps at the musculotendinous junction and inserts into a bilaminar tendon that fuses laterally and attaches to the humerus (Elmaraghy & Devereaux, 2012) (Fig. 20.1).

The tendon of the PM, from the myotendinous junction to the humeral insertion, can measure 5 to 15 mm medial to lateral (Haley & Zacchilli, 2014; Lee et al, 2000). The overall tendon fiber length, including the intramuscular portion, can measure 5 to 6 cm medial-lateral (length) and 4 to 7.2 cm proximal-distal (width) (Carey & Owens, 2010; Fung et al, 2009; Haley & Zacchilli, 2014; Klepps et al, 2004). The footprint is at the lateral lip of the bicipital grove 4 cm distal to the greater tuberosity (Carey & Owens, 2010; Haley & Zacchilli, 2014) and 4.7 cm proximal deltoid insertion (Klepps et al, 2004). It measures 4.8 to 7.7 cm in width (proximal-distal) and 1.4 to 5.6 mm in thickness (Carey & Owens, 2010; Fung et al, 2009; Haley & Zacchilli, 2014; Klepps et al, 2004; Lee et al, 2000). The clavicular head and the superior segments of the sternocostal head constitute the anterior and inferior tendon laminal fibers. The middle portion of the sternocostal head constitutes the inferior U-shaped insertion to the anterior and posterior laminar fibers. The lower portion of the sternocostal head constitutes the more proximal segment of the posterior lamina fibers, inserting 11 mm more proximal in the humerus than the anterior layer (Elmaraghy & Devereaux, 2012; Fung et al, 2009) (Fig. 20.2).

The PM unit is innervated by the C5 to T1 nerve roots through the medial and lateral pectoral nerves. The lateral pectoral nerve (C5–C7) is the main nerve supplying the PM and arises from the lateral cord of the brachial plexus. Its course is anterior to the axillary artery and medial to the pectoralis minor and pierces the deep surface of the proximal PM 12.5 cm medial to the humeral insertion (Haley & Zacchilli, 2014; Klepps et al, 2004). The medial pectoral nerve (C8–T1) innervates the lower sternocostal segments and arises from the medial cord of the brachial plexus. It pierces the pectoralis minor muscle near the midclavicular line and then pierces the undersurface of the PM, with two or three branches, 11.9 cm medial to the humeral insertion and 2 cm proximal to the inferior edge (Haley & Zacchilli, 2014; Klepps et al, 2004) (Fig. 20.3). The previously described safe zone is lateral to the pectoralis minor for a distance of 8.5 cm from the humeral insertion (Haley & Zacchilli, 2014; Klepps et al, 2004). The blood supply to the PM derives mainly from the pectoral branch of the thoracoacromial artery with additional supply from the clavicular branch and internal mammary branch (Candiani et al, 1991). Venous drainage is through the axillary vein and internal mammary venous complex.

The PM functions as a strong adductor, forward elevator (clavicular head) and internal rotator of the glenohumeral joint (Haley & Zacchilli, 2014; Petilon et al, 2005; Quinlan

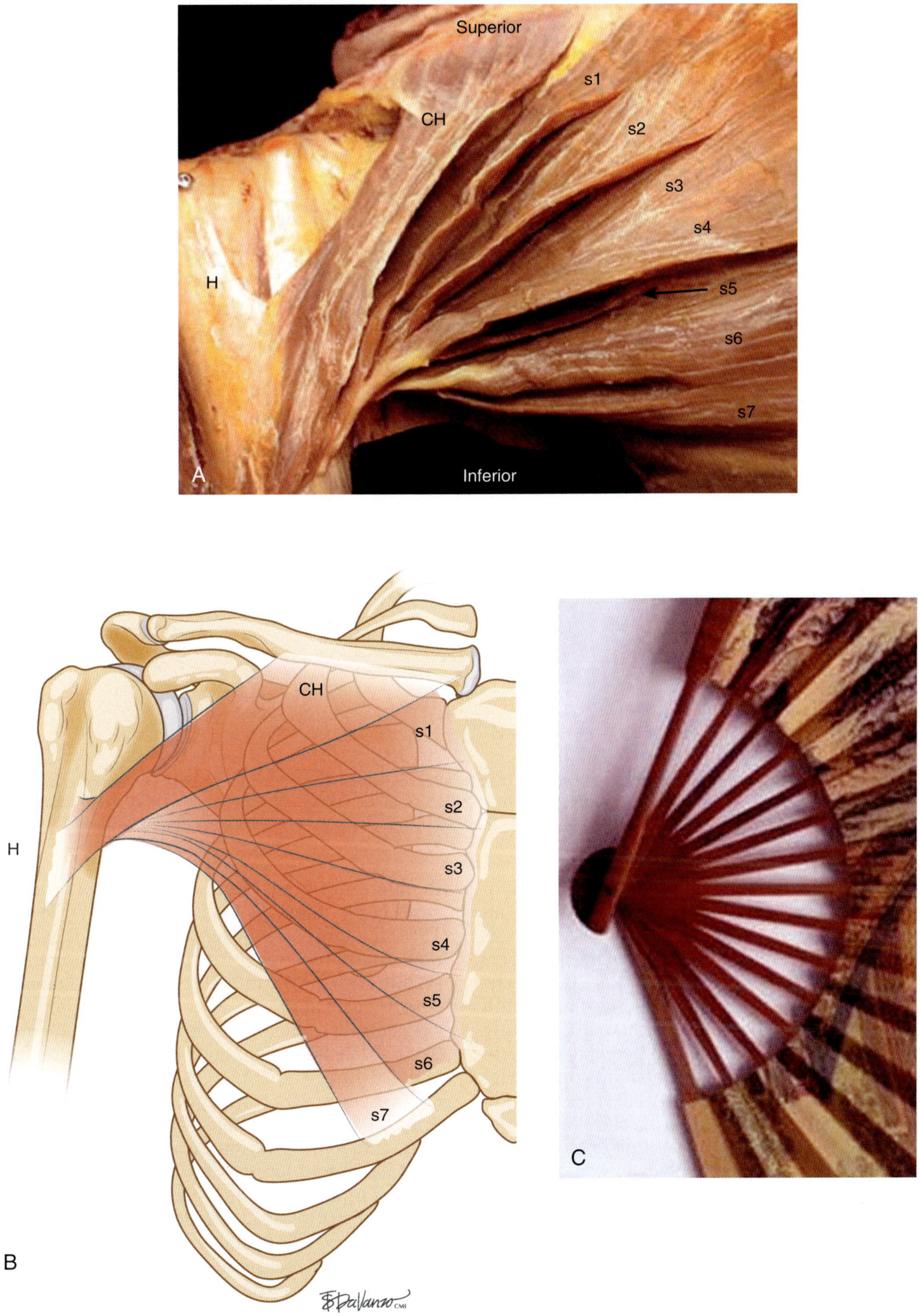

FIG. 20.1 A, Gross dissection of the muscle segments of the two heads of the pectoralis major: clavicular head (one segment) and sternocostal head (seven segments). Each muscle segment overlaps the segment below it (**B**), analogous to an Asian fan (**C**). *CH,* Clavicular head; *H,* humerus; *s1–s7,* sternal segments of the sternocostal head. (Reprinted from Elmaraghy A, Deveraux MW. A systematic review and comprehensive classification of pectoralis major tears. *J Shoulder Elbow Surg.* 2012;21:412-422 and Fung L, Wong B, Ravichandiran K, Agur A, Rindlisbacher T, Elmaraghy A. Three-dimensional study of pectoralis major muscle and tendon architecture. *Clin Anat.* 2009;22(4):500-508.)

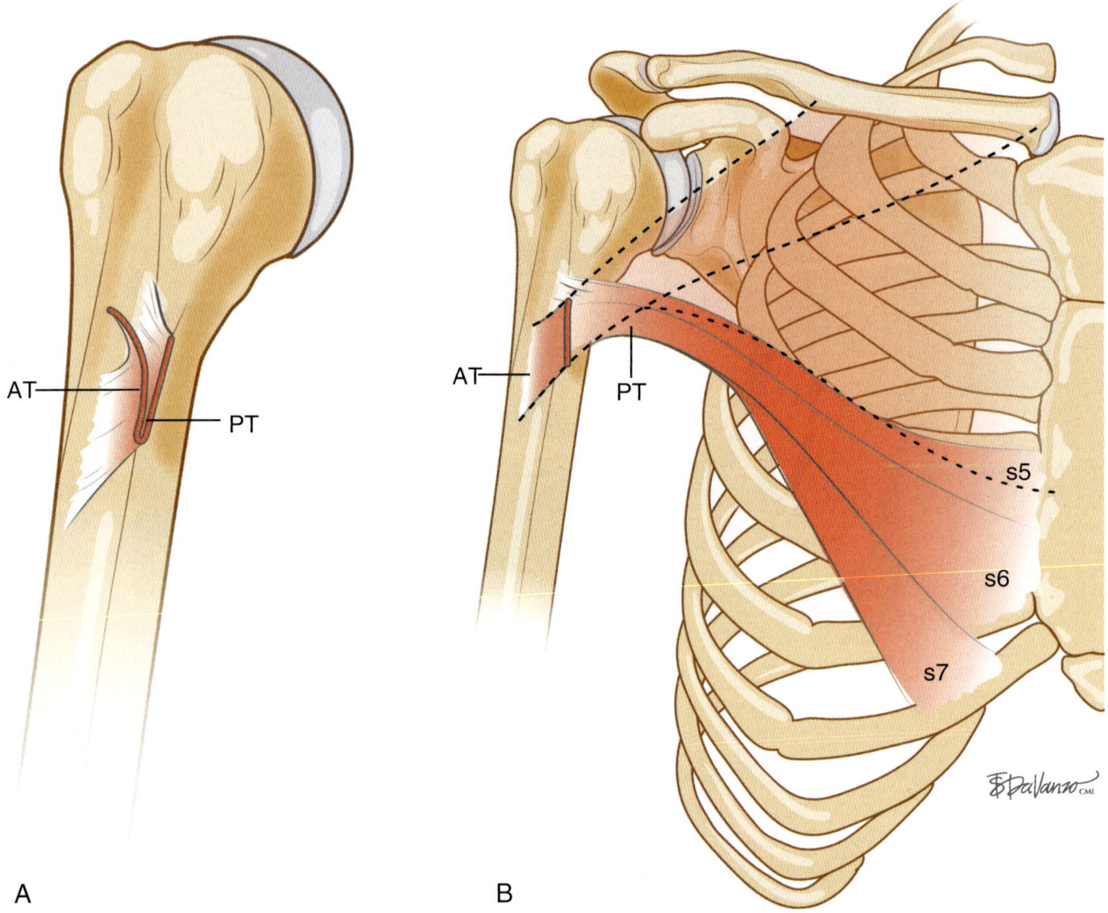

FIG. 20.2 A, The anterior part of the tendon inserts more anterior and distal relative to the posterior tendon. **B,** The posterior tendon is formed by the most inferior two or three segments (s5–s7) of the sternocostal head. *AT,* Anterior Portion of the Tendon; *PT,* Posterior Portion of the Tendon. (Reprinted from Elmaraghy A, Deveraux MW. A systematic review and comprehensive classification of pectoralis major tears. *J Shoulder Elbow Surg.* 21;2012:412-422.)

et al, 2002). The PM can work as either a flexor or extensor of the shoulder, depending on arm position. With an extended shoulder, the upper fibers of the PM function as flexors, and when the shoulder is flexed, the inferior fibers function as shoulder extensors (Rockwood, 2004). The PM muscle has significant variation in muscle fiber length across segments (Elmaraghy & Devereaux, 2012; Fung et al, 2009; Haley & Zacchilli, 2014). This composition produces disproportionately high fiber excursion in the inferior sternocostal segments between 0 and 30 degrees of shoulder extension (Haley & Zacchilli, 2014; Wolfe et al, 1992). When maximal force is applied in a position of mechanical disadvantage (shoulder abduction and extension), the inferior segments of the sternocostal head are at risk for injury. Previous reports describe a predictable anatomic sequence of rupture of the PM tendon, with the inferior segments tearing first followed by the rest of the sternocostal head and the clavicular head (Petilon et al, 2005; Wolfe et al, 1992).

Epidemiology and Etiology

Pectoralis major injury was first described by Patissier in 1822 (Patissier, 1822). In 2012, a meta-analysis of the literature from 1822 to 2010 reported a total of 365 cases of PM injury, with the majority (76%) reported after 1990 (Elmaraghy & Devereaux, 2012). U.S. Army population studies reported a rate of PM rupture of 1 per 13,317 (White et al, 2007) and 60 per 100,000 (Balazs et al, 2016) person-years at risk.

Pectoralis major tears mainly occur in men between 30 to 40 years and a majority (75%) are related to sports activity (Bak et al, 2000; Cordasco et al, 2017; Elmaraghy & Devereaux, 2012; Haley & Zacchilli, 2014; Provencher et al, 2010; White et al, 2007). Although jujitsu, wrestling, and gymnastics are commonly implicated with PM injuries, weight lifting is by far the most common mechanism of injury, accounting for 50% of the reported cases (Bak et al, 2000; De Castro Pochini et al, 2010; Elmaraghy & Devereaux, 2012; Haley & Zacchilli, 2014; Provencher et al, 2010). Several studies report that tears at the tendon insertion are the most common injury (59%–65%), followed by injury to the musculotendinous junction (24%–29%) (Bak et al, 2000; Elmaraghy & Devereaux, 2012; Haley & Zacchilli, 2014). The senior author has reported that 60% of injuries in his series were muscle–tendon junction tears (Cordasco et al, 2016). The majority (56%–91%) of the reported PM injuries were described as

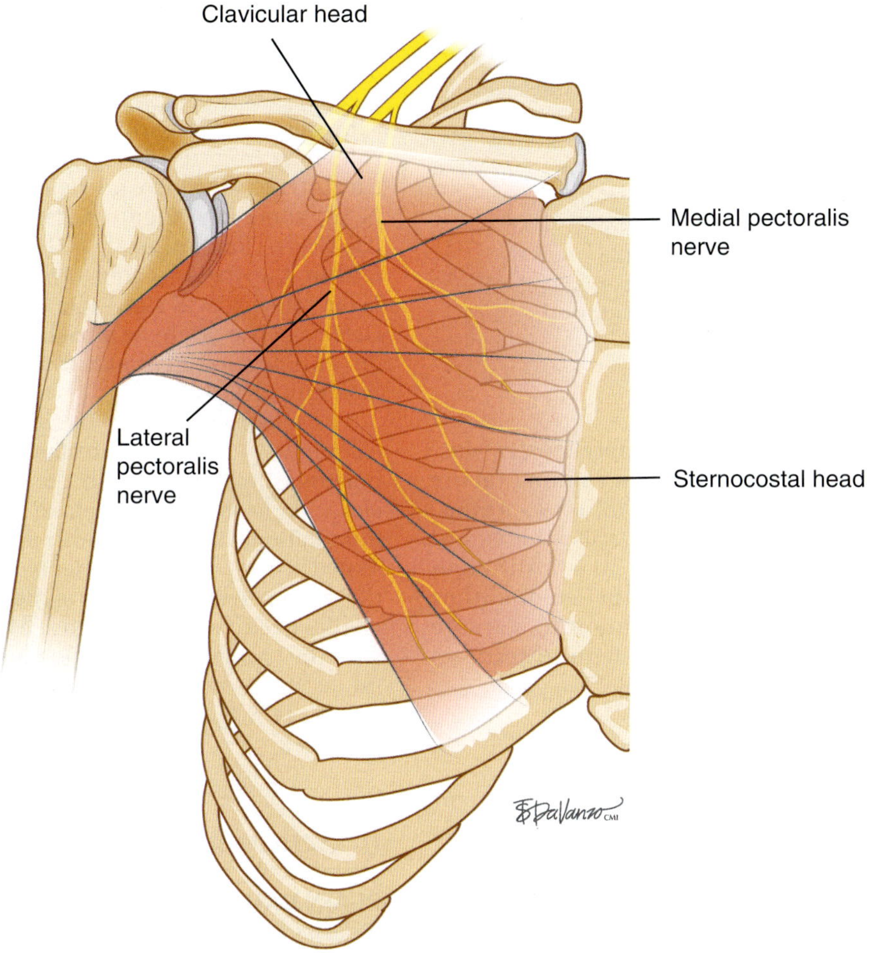

FIG. 20.3 **Illustration demonstrating the nerve supply to the pectoralis major muscle.** (Reprinted with permission from Kim DH, Hudson AR, Kline DG. Anatomy and function in the upper extremity. In Atlas *of Peripheral Nerve Surgery*. Elsevier, Philadelphia 2nd ed. 2013.)

complete tears or avulsions (Bak et al, 2000; Elmaraghy & Devereaux, 2012; Provencher et al, 2010). In the senior author's series, isolated sternocostal head tears were more common than complete tears (57.5%) (Cordasco et al, 2017). The PM tear pattern and location is likely the result of multiple factors. These factors include intrinsic components (patient's age, activity level, and tendon quality) and mechanical characteristics (arm position at the time of injury, velocity and mechanism of injury) (Elmaraghy & Devereaux, 2012).

Animal studies demonstrated a negative effect of anabolic steroid on rat tendons, increasing stiffness and diminishing the ability to absorb energy (Inhofe et al, 1995). The reported rate of anabolic steroid use in patients that suffered a PM rupture range between 36% to 90% (Aärimaa et al, 2004; De Castro Pochini et al, 2014). In the senior author's series, all of the athletes denied anabolic steroid use and the authors suspected that this was the result of under-reporting (Cordasco et al, 2017). The proposed explanation for increased risk of tendon ruptures in patients using anabolic steroids has been associated with the increased stiffness of the tendon coupled with a disproportionate gain in muscle and maximal force production (Aärimaa et al, 2004; Bak et al, 2000; De Castro Pochini et al, 2014; Petilon et al, 2005; Provencher et al, 2010).

The reported PM ruptures in the elderly are predominantly in female residents of nursing homes and the injuries were likely caused during patient transfer and positioning (Beloosesky et al, 2002, et al, 2003a, 2003b).

Classification

Pectoralis tears can occur at the tendon substance, the muscle belly, or within the musculotendinous junction. Tietjen, in 1980, described the first classification system of PM injuries (Tietjen, 1980). This classification system mainly provided an anatomic description based on the pattern (contusion or sprain, partial tear, or complete tear) and location of complete tears (muscle origin, muscle belly, musculotendinous junction, and tendon insertion). Bak et al (2000) modified the classification system to differentiate bony avulsions at the insertion site from tendon substance ruptures. A review of the literature revealed that Tietjen's classification system (Table 20.1) failed to accurately catch the location and extent of the injury (Elmaraghy & Devereaux, 2012). Elmaraghy and

Table 20.1 Tietjen's Classification System of Pectoralis Major Injuries

Type	Description	Recommended Treatment
I	Sprain or contusion	Nonoperative
II	Partially torn	Nonoperative
III	Complete tears	Nonoperative
IIIA	Origin	Nonoperative
IIIB	Muscle mass	Nonoperative
IIIC	Myotendinous junction	Operative in presence of limited function
IIID	Tendon	Operative

Devereaux (2012) proposed a more comprehensive classification system that also includes injury timing (acute vs chronic), recognition of all possible injury locations, and a standardized terminology to describe the extent (thickness and width) of the tear (Fig. 20.4). Although this classification system is interesting, the senior author has found the original Tietjen classification to be more relevant from a clinical perspective with respect to treatment.

Assessment

Patients usually are able to describe the mechanism of injury and often recall a tearing sensation with or without an audible pop. They commonly localize the pain to the axillary and chest wall area and complain of weakness, swelling, ecchymosis, and asymmetry.

Acute presentations commonly include swelling and ecchymosis at the axillary and chest wall area extending into the biceps brachii. The ecchymosis may last up to 6 weeks (Beloosesky et al, 2003a), and swelling can resolve by 3 weeks (Wolfe et al, 1992). When swelling dissipates, thinning or loss of the axillary fold may become apparent. Muscle retraction with resultant fullness may be obvious, but the morphologic appearance will occasionally reveal only subtle asymmetries. Side-to-side comparison and examination of the axillary fold are performed by resting the palms over the iliac crest while attempting adduction (isometric contraction) (Haley & Zacchilli, 2014). This often reveals either thinning or complete loss of the axillary fold (Provencher et al, 2010; Wolfe et al, 1992). It is important to understand that having a complete tear of the sternocostal head can still give the impression of an intact tendon because of an intact fascia or intact clavicular head (Zeman et al, 1979). Passive abduction and active adduction can also accentuate the defect (Joseph et al, 2003).

Shoulder adduction and internal rotation may demonstrate weakness and pain and limitation in range of motion. Patients often reveal tenderness to palpation over the humeral insertion and along the axillary fold (Haley & Zacchilli, 2014). In the chronic setting, a prominent skin fold, webbing, and a prominent distal insertion of the anterior deltoid have been described (De Castro Pochini et al, 2010; Haley & Zacchilli, 2014; Wolfe et al, 1992). Palpation of the axillary fold, especially in patients with athletic constitution, can be performed for 5 to 6 cm proximally and can help discern tears of complete versus incomplete width (Haley & Zacchilli, 2014). The presence of an apparent defect differentiates a partial thickness from a full-thickness tear. In cases with rupture of the sternocostal head and an intact clavicular head, some investigators described the "triangle sign" (De Castro Pochini et al, 2014). Evident retracted stump within the axillary fold during forward elevation has been called the "S sign" (De Castro Pochini et al, 2010). Defects at the origin or muscle belly should be assessed by direct palpation in a lateral to medial direction (Haley & Zacchilli, 2014).

The senior author has found components of the physical examination to be helpful. Observation of bilateral resisted horizontal adduction with the humerus in 90 degrees of elevation in the scapular plane and bilateral resisted internal rotation with the humerus adducted while the athlete is seated in front of the examiner have both been useful to identify asymmetries. Palpation of the posterior aspect of the clavicular head component of the PM while the athlete is supine with the humerus in abduction and elevation has been useful, as in cases of isolated sternocostal head avulsion the stump of the tendon or muscle–tendon junction tear can be identified.

Imaging Modalities

PLAIN RADIOGRAPHS

Radiographs are not essential for the diagnosis of PM ruptures. They usually are obtained to assess for avulsion fractures, present in 2% to 4% (Bak et al, 2000; Elmaraghy & Devereaux, 2012; Haley & Zacchilli, 2014) of PM ruptures and glenohumeral dislocation that had been previously reported simultaneously with PM rupture (Arciero & Cruser, 1997). Some investigators previously described loss of the PM soft tissue shadow on radiographs, but this finding has poor sensitivity (Arciero & Cruser, 1997; Bak et al, 2000; Bakalim, 1965; Berson, 1979; Park & Espiniella, 1970).

ULTRASONOGRAPHY

Pavlik et al, in 1998, was first to describe the use of ultrasonography to diagnose PM tears (Pavlik et al, 1998). This modality is quick, widely available, and relatively inexpensive but is extremely operator dependent (Haley & Zacchilli, 2014). In skillful hands, ultrasonography can provide an accurate and quick dynamic evaluation (Rehman & Robinson, 2005; Weaver et al, 2005). Some investigators raised the concern of false-negative results using sonography in complete PM tears (Lee et al, 2013).

MAGNETIC RESONANCE IMAGING

Magnetic resonance imaging (MRI) is the preferred imaging modality and is particularly helpful in establishing diagnosis in the acute phase when the physical examination is limited

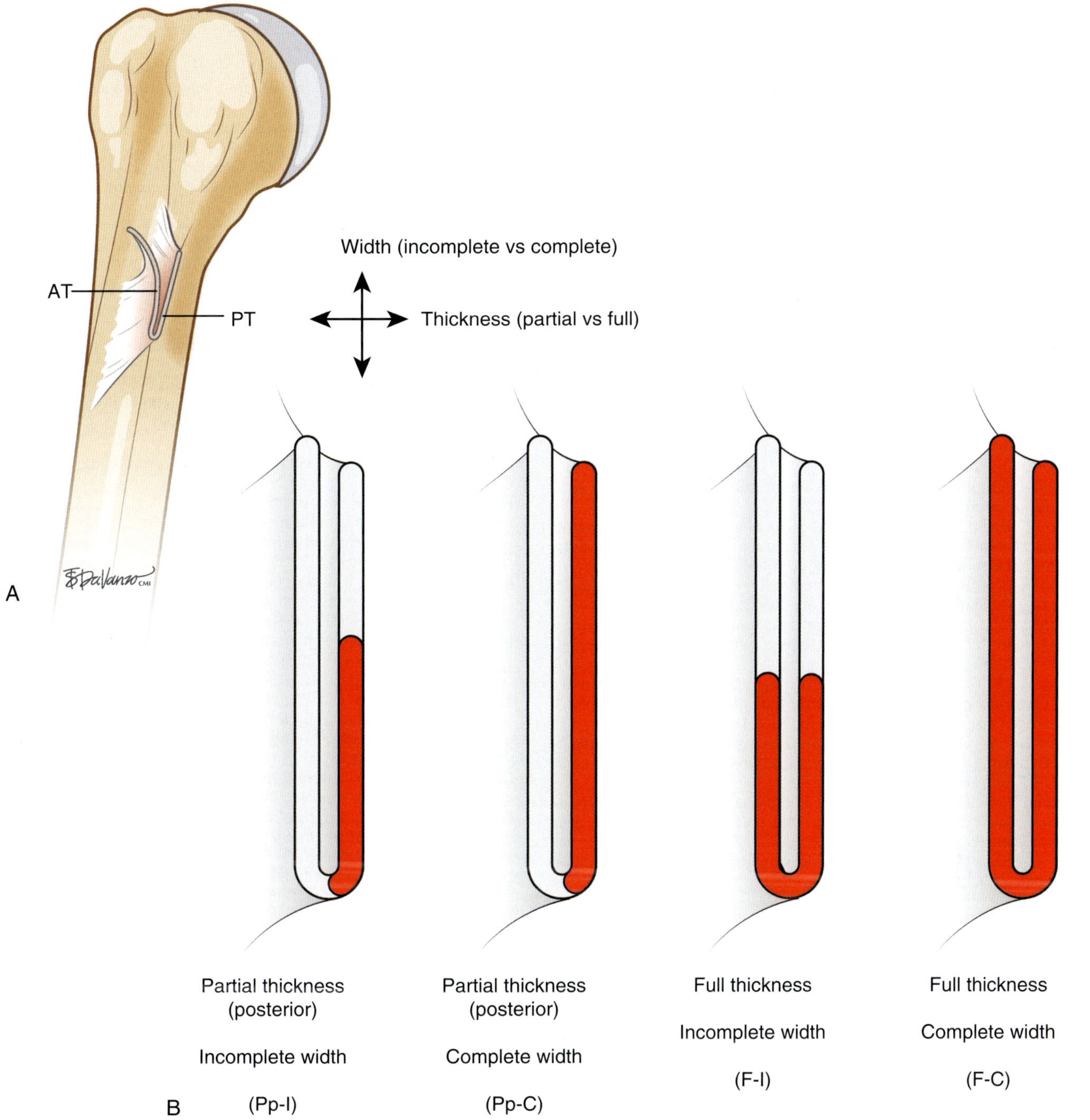

FIG. 20.4 Illustration demonstrating the pectoralis major tendon tear pattern classification as described by Elmaraghy and Devereaux (2012) using the terms *width* and *thickness* to describe the tendon involvement. **A,** The bilaminar tendinous insertion, with the anterior tendon inserting more anterior and distal relative to the posterior part of the tendon. **B,** The variable involvement of the tendon laminae (anterior and posterior) that can be torn. *AT,* Anterior Portion of the Tendon; *PT,* Posterior Portion of the Tendon. (Reprinted from Elmaraghy A, Devereaux MW. A systematic review and comprehensive classification of pectoralis major tears. *J Shoulder Elbow Surg.* 21;2012:412-422.)

by swelling and pain (Miller et al, 1993). MRI is helpful to determine injury location, to differentiate between partial and complete tears, and to reveal degree of retraction (Carrino et al, 2000; Egan & Hall, 1987; Ohashi et al, 1996). MRI can also help distinguish between acute and chronic tendon injuries. An acute injury demonstrates higher signal intensity than chronic injuries, which exhibit retraction of the muscle coupled with scarring and fibrosis (Connell et al, 1999). Several MRI sequences have been recommended to better identify the PM injury. Independent view (small field of view) of each side is recommended instead of a wide field of view (including both in the same images), when comparison is desired (Connell et al, 1999). Some authors recommended axial sequences, including fast spin echo (Connell et al, 1999), short-tau inversion recovery (STIR) (Carrino et al, 2000), or fat-suppressed T2 (Carrino et al, 2000). Others recommend oblique coronal fast spin echo to evaluate the severity of the tear (Connell et al, 1999). In 2000, Lee et al (Lee et al, 2000) described that the superior edge of the tendon insertion is located 1 to 1.5 cm distal to the quadrilateral space and 5 to 10 mm superior to the lateral head of the triceps.

At our institution, we first obtain axial fast-spin echo, and then the oblique coronal images are plotted from the axial images parallel to the long axis of the PM tendon unit. We also obtain coronal inversion recovery in a similar fashion.

References

Äärimaa V, Rantanen J, Heikkilä J, Helttula I, Orava S. Rupture of the pectoralis major muscle. *Am J Sports Med.* 2004;32(5):1256–1262.

Arciero RA, Cruser DL. Pectoralis major rupture with simultaneous anterior dislocation of the shoulder. *J Shoulder Elbow Surg.* 1997;6(3):318–320.

Bak K, Cameron EA, Henderson IJ. Rupture of the pectoralis major: a meta-analysis of 112 cases. *Knee Surg Sports Traumatol Arthrosc.* 2000;8(2):113–119.

Bakalim G. Rupture of the pectoralis major muscle. A case report. *Acta Orthop Scand.* 1965;36(3):274–279.

Balazs GC, Brelin AM, Donohue MA, et al. Incidence rate and results of the surgical treatment of pectoralis major tendon ruptures in active-duty military personnel. *Am J Sports Med.* 2016;44(7):1837–1843.

Beloosesky Y, Grinblat J, Hendel D, Sommer R. Pectoralis major rupture in a 97-year-old woman. *J Am Geriatr Soc.* 2002;50(8):1465–1467.

Beloosesky Y, Grinblat J, Katz M, Hendel D, Sommer R. Pectoralis major rupture in the elderly: clinical and sonographic findings. *Clin Imaging.* 2003a;27(4):261–264.

Beloosesky Y, Grinblat J, Weiss A, Rosenberg PH, Weisbort M, Hendel D. Pectoralis major rupture in elderly patients: a clinical study of 13 patients. *Clin Orthop Relat Res.* 2003b;(413):164–169.

Berson BL. Surgical repair of pectoralis major rupture in an athlete. Case report of an unusual injury in a wrestler. *Am J Sports Med.* 1979;7(6):348–351.

Candiani P, Campigliq GL, Quattrone P, Lovaria A. Computerized angiographic study of the vascular supply of the pectoralis major muscle. *Acta Chir Plast.* 1991;33(4):185–193.

Carey P, Owens BD. Insertional footprint anatomy of the pectoralis major tendon. *Orthopedics.* 2010;33(1):23.

Carrino JA, Chandnanni VP, Mitchell DB, Choi-Chinn K, DeBerardino TM, Miller MD. Pectoralis major muscle and tendon tears: diagnosis and grading using magnetic resonance imaging. *Skeletal Radiol.* 2000;29(6):305–313.

Connell DA, Potter HG, Sherman MF, Wickiewicz TL. Injuries of the pectoralis major muscle: evaluation with MR imaging. *Radiology.* 1999;210(3):785–791.

Cordasco FA, Delos D. Pectoralis major. In: *Disorders of the Shoulder: Sports Injuries, Part IV Muscle and Tendon Rupture.* Vol. 2. Philadelphia: Lippincott Williams & Wilkins; 2013:576.

Cordasco FA, Mahony GT, Tsouris N, Degen RM. Pectoralis major tendon tears: functional outcomes and return to sport in a consecutive series of 40 athletes. *J Shoulder Elbow Surg.* 2017;26(3):458–463.

de Castro Pochini A, Andreoli CV, Belangero PS, et al. Clinical considerations for the surgical treatment of pectoralis major muscle ruptures based on 60 cases: a prospective study and literature review. *Am J Sports Med.* 2014;42(1):95–102.

de Castro Pochini A, Ejnisman B, Andreoli CV, et al. Pectoralis major muscle rupture in athletes: a prospective study. *Am J Sports Med.* 2010;38(1):92–98.

Egan TM, Hall H. Avulsion of the pectoralis major tendon in a weight lifter: repair using a barbed staple. *Can J Surg.* 1987;30(6):434–435.

Elmaraghy A, Devereaux MW. A systematic review and comprehensive classification of pectoralis major tears. *J Shoulder Elbow Surg.* 2012;21:412–422.

Fung L, Wong B, Ravichandiran K, Agur A, Rindlisbacher T, Elmaraghy A. Three-dimensional study of pectoralis major muscle and tendon architecture. *Clin Anat.* 2009;22(4):500–508.

Garrigues GE, Kraeutler MJ, Gillespie RJ, O'Brien DF, Lazarus MD. Repair of pectoralis major ruptures: single-surgeon case series. *Orthopedics.* 2012;35(8):e1184–e1190.

Guity M, Sharafat Vaziri A, Shafiei H, Farhoud A. Surgical treatment of pectoralis major tendon rupture (outcome assessment). *Asian J Sports Med.* 2014;5(2):129–135.

Haley CA, Zacchilli MA. Pectoralis major injuries: evaluation and treatment. *Clin Sports Med.* 2014;33(4):739–756.

Hanna CM, Glenny AB, Stanley SN, Caughey MA. Pectoralis major tears: comparison of surgical and conservative treatment. *Br J Sports Med.* 2001;35(3):202–206.

Inhofe PD, Grana WA, Egle D, Min KW, Tomasek J. The effects of anabolic steroids on rat tendon. An ultrastructural, biomechanical, and biochemical analysis. *Am J Sports Med.* 1995;23(2):227–232.

Joseph TA, Defranco MJ, Weiker GG. Delayed repair of a pectoralis major tendon rupture with allograft: a case report. *J Shoulder Elbow Surg.* 2003;12(1):101–104.

Kang RW, Mahony GT, Cordasco FA. Pectoralis major repair with cortical button technique. *Arthrosc Tech.* 2014;3(1):e73–e77.

Klepps S, Auerbach J, Calhon O, Lin J, Cleeman E, Flatow E. A cadaveric study on the anatomy of the deltoid insertion and its relationship to the deltopectoral approach to the proximal humerus. *J Shoulder Elbow Surg.* 2004;13(3):322–327.

Kretzler HH Jr, Richardson AB. Rupture of the pectoralis major muscle. *Am J Sports Med.* 1989;17(4):453–458.

Lee J, Brookenthal KR, Ramsey ML, Kneeland JB, Herzog R. MR imaging assessment of the pectoralis major myotendinous unit: an MR imaging-anatomic correlative study with surgical correlation. *AJR Am J Roentgenol.* 2000;174(5):1371–1375.

Lee SJ, Jacobson JA, Kim SM, et al. Distal pectoralis major tears: sonographic characterization and potential diagnostic pitfalls. *J Ultrasound Med.* 2013;32(12):2075–2081.

McEntire JE, Hess WE, Coleman SS. Rupture of the pectoralis major muscle. A report of eleven injuries and review of fifty-six. *J Bone Joint Surg Am.* 1972;54(5):1040–1046.

Miller MD, Johnson DL, Fu FH, Thaete FL, Blanc RO. Rupture of the pectoralis major muscle in a collegiate football player. Use of magnetic resonance imaging in early diagnosis. *Am J Sports Med.* 1993;21(3):475–477.

Ohashi K, Khoury GY, Albright JP, Tearse DS. MRI of complete rupture of the pectoralis major muscle. *Skeletal Radiol.* 1996;25(7):625–628.

Park JY, Espiniella JL. Rupture of pectoralis major muscle. A case report and review of literature. *J Bone Joint Surg Am.* 1970;52(3):577–581.

Patissier P. *Malaides des bouchers. Traite des maladies des artisans.* Paris: Chez J-B Baillere Libraire; 1822:162–165.

Pavlik A, Csépai D, Berkes I. Surgical treatment of pectoralis major rupture in athletes. *Knee Surg Sports Traumatol Arthrosc.* 1998;6(2):129–133.

Petilon J, Carr DR, Sekiya JK, Unger DV. Pectoralis major muscle injuries: evaluation and management. *J Am Acad Orthop Surg.* 2005;13(1):59–68.

Provencher MT, Handfield K, Boniquit NT, Reiff SN, Sekiya JK, Romeo AA. Injuries to the pectoralis major muscle: diagnosis and management. *Am J Sports Med.* 2010;38(8):1693–1705.

Quinlan JF, Molloy M, Hurson BJ. Pectoralis major tendon ruptures: when to operate. *Br J Sports Med.* 2002;36(3):226–228.

Rehman A, Robinson P. Sonographic evaluation of injuries to the pectoralis muscles. *AJR Am J Roentgenol.* 2005;184(4):1205–12114.

Rockwood CE. *The Shoulder.* 3rd ed. Philadelphia: Saunders; 2004.

Tietjen R. Closed injuries of the pectoralis major muscle. *J Trauma.* 1980;20(3):262–264.

Weaver JS, Jacobson JA, Jamadar DA, Theisen SE, Ebrahim F, Kalume-Brigido M. Sonographic findings of pectoralis major tears with surgical, clinical, and magnetic resonance imaging correlation in 6 patients. *J Ultrasound Med.* 2005;24(1):25–31.

White DW, Wenke JC, Mosely DS, Mountcastle SB, Basamania CJ. Incidence of major tendon ruptures and anterior cruciate ligament tears in US Army soldiers. *Am J Sports Med.* 2007;35(8):1308–1314.

Wolfe SW, Wickiewicz TL, Cavanaugh JT. Ruptures of the pectoralis major muscle. An anatomic and clinical analysis. *Am J Sports Med.* 1992;20(5):587–593.

Zeman SC, Rosenfeld RT, Lipscomb PR. Tears of the pectoralis major muscle. *Am J Sports Med.* 1979;7(6):343–347.

21 Treatment

LIONEL E. LAZARO, MD and FRANK A. CORDASCO, MD

Introduction

- The pectoralis major (PM) muscle functions as a potent flexor, adductor, and internal rotator of the shoulder, as well as a dynamic stabilizer of the glenohumeral joint (Cordasco & Delos, 2013; Petilon et al, 2005; Quinlan et al, 2002).
- Although the PM is not required for activities of daily living (Mosconi & Kamath, 2003), rupture of the tendon or muscle–tendinous junction leads to significant functional deficits and limitations of athletic performance or labor-intensive activities (Cordasco & Delos, 2013; Cordasco et al, 2017; De Castro Pochini et al, 2010; Haley & Zacchilli, 2014; Kang et al, 2014; Schepsis et al, 2000; Zeman et al, 1979).
- Nonoperative treatment is reserved for partial tears, contusions, rupture at the muscle belly, and complete tears in older adult and low-demand patients (Haley & Zacchilli, 2014).
- Although patients with low functional demand can recover reasonable function during activities of daily living (Beloosesky et al, 2003; Haley & Zacchilli, 2014; Kang et al, 2014; McEntire et al, 1972; Scott et al, 1992; Wolfe et al, 1992), athletes and laborers are unable to return to their preinjury levels of activity (Haley & Zacchilli, 2014; Kang et al, 2014; Schepsis et al, 2000; Zeman et al, 1979).
- For young active athletes, surgical treatment provides optimal strength, cosmesis, satisfaction, and return to sports (Antosh et al, 2009; Bak et al, 2000; Cordasco & Delos, 2013; Cordasco et al, 2017; De Castro Pochini et al, 2010; De Castro Pochini et al, 2014; Haley & Zacchilli, 2014; Hanna et al, 2001; Kretzler & Richardson, 1989; McEntire et al, 1972; Park & Espiniella, 1970; Pavlik et al, 1998; Quinlan et al, 2002; Schepsis et al, 2000; Wolfe et al, 1992; Zeman et al, 1979).
- Advanced imaging is recommended to facilitate the timely diagnosis of acute injuries and is recommended when there is concern regarding injuries to the PM muscle or tendon (Carrino et al, 2000; Connell et al, 1999; Cordasco et al, 2017; Haley & Zacchilli, 2014; Lee et al, 2000; Miller et al, 1993; Weaver et al, 2005).
- The chronicity of the injury should be taken into account, but it should not preclude surgical repair given that successful outcomes can still be achieved (Hanna et al, 2001; Quinlan et al, 2002; Schepsis et al, 2000).

Surgical Treatment

When the history, physical examination, and appropriate PM specific imaging confirm the diagnosis, the athlete is indicated for surgery. The patient is positioned in the beach-chair position, and the repair is performed though either a deltopectoral or anterior axillary approach (Cordasco & Delos, 2013; Haley & Zacchilli, 2014; Kang et al, 2014; Provencher et al, 2010). Meticulous dissection and retraction is required to avoid injury to the pectoralis nerves, especially inferior and medial to the coracoid (Provencher et al, 2010). The long head of the biceps sits medial to the PM insertion, and the surgeon should remain cognizant of this during surgical fixation.

Various repair techniques to reattach the tendon back to its footprint have been described in the literature (Kang et al, 2014; Metzger et al, 2012; Petilon et al, 2005; Rabuck et al, 2012; Sherman et al, 2012) (Fig. 21.1). These techniques include tendon to tendon, bone trough (Fig. 21.1, *A*), suture anchors (Fig. 21.1, *B*) and cortical button repairs (Fig. 21.1, *C*). Although atypical, when enough healthy tissue remains attached to the insertion site, direct suturing of the tendon ends has been described for intratendinous tears (Äärimaa et al, 2004; Dodds & Wolfe, 2002; Haley & Zacchilli, 2014). For the majority of tears, sutures are passed through the ruptured tendon using either a modified Krakow or modified Mason Allen suture technique, which is then securely repaired to bone with either a transosseous method or more commonly with suture anchors or buttons.

The bone trough technique has been described using a 5-cm vertical trough that is created at the footprint which is lateral to the bicipital groove. Four 2-mm drill holes are placed 1 cm lateral to the trough. Nonabsorbable sutures, fixed to the ruptured tendon, are then passed into the trough and into the drill holes, and are then tied over the bone bridge (Haley & Zacchilli, 2014; Schepsis et al, 2000). For both the suture anchor and the cortical button techniques, the footprint is cleared from soft tissue and lightly abraded to prepare for tendon to bone healing without structurally compromising the cortex. With the suture anchor technique, two or three anchors preloaded with high-strength suture are applied within the footprint. One of the suture limbs of each anchor is secured to the tendon and then is tied to the other limb (Haley & Zacchilli, 2014; Rabuck et al, 2012). For the cortical button technique, three 3.2-mm unicortical drill holes are made within the footprint with an adequate bone bridge between sites. The button is designed to flip in the intramedullary canal, which allows unicortical

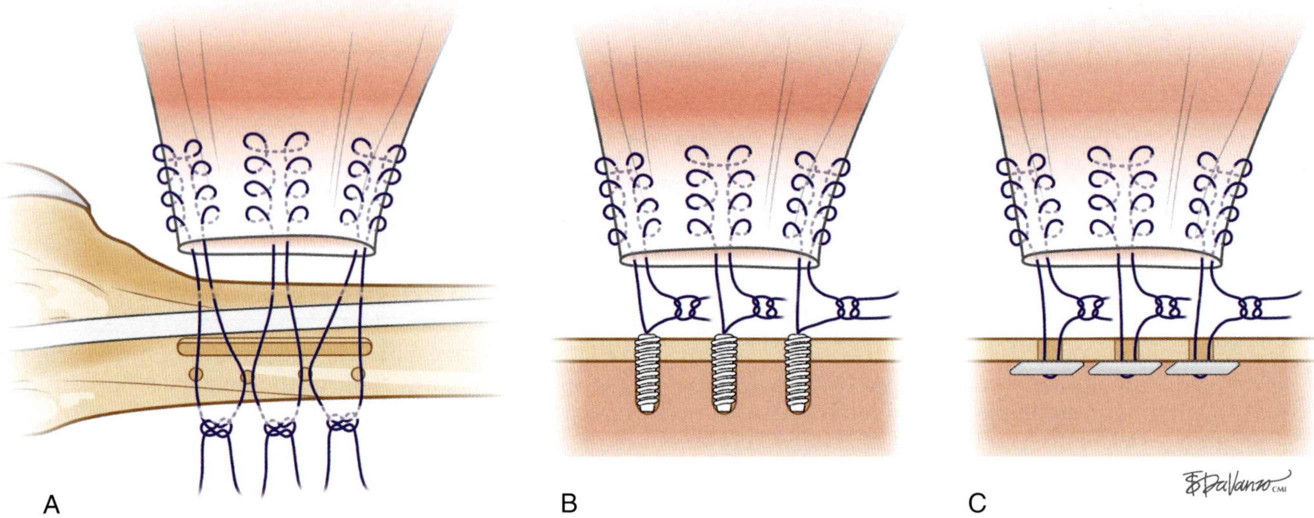

Fig. 21.1 Illustrations depict the different techniques use to secure the repair to the footprint: bone trough technique (**A**), suture anchor technique (**B**), and unicortical button technique (**C**) (authors' preferred repair). (Reprinted with permission from Haley CA, Zacchilli MA. Pectoralis major injuries: evaluation and treatment. *Clin Sports Med.* 2014;33(4);739-756.)

engagement on the near cortex. The titanium buttons are preloaded with one or two high-strength nonabsorbable sutures. One limb of each suture is secured to the tendon. Some buttons serve as suture anchors, and the limbs are simply tied to one another pushing the tendon to the footprint; other buttons are of the tensioning variety and may be used to pull the tendon to the footprint (Kang et al, 2014; Metzger et al, 2012; Sherman et al, 2012).

Several biomechanical cadaver studies have been done to evaluate the different techniques of PM tendon repair. Hart et al (2011) compared bone trough and suture anchor techniques and found no difference on ultimate load to failure. The mode of failure was fracture in 50% of the bone trough group and suture breakage in 100% of the suture anchor group. Rabuck et al (2012) compared the three techniques (bone trough, suture anchor, and button techniques) and found a slightly higher load to failure on the bone trough group (596 N) compared with the suture anchor group (383 N). The modes of failure were suture breakage in nine specimens and fracture in one specimen for the bone trough, suture breakage in all cortical button specimens, and failure of the suture eyelet in five specimens and suture breakage in the other four specimens in the suture anchor group. Sherman et al (2012) compared the three repair techniques and found no differences in load to failure, elongation, linear stiffness, initial excursion, cyclic elongation, or footprint restoration. All three techniques failed at the suture tendon interface. They reported a significantly greater stiffness and maximal load (1455 N) in the intact tendon specimens.

There is general agreement that all three repair techniques described here are adequate to repair a PM tendon rupture. Although some investigators favor suture anchor and cortical button repairs, given that there is less dissection laterally on the humerus compared with the bone trough technique (Haley & Zacchilli, 2014).

There is a lack of general agreement on the definition of acute versus chronic in PM injuries. Flint et al (2014), in their systematic review, defined chronic injuries as those beyond 6 weeks. As with several other surgical interventions, chronicity of the injury may increase risk of surgical morbidity because it requires greater surgical exposure and dissection of scar tissue to mobilize the retracted muscle (Cordasco & Delos, 2013; Elmaraghy & Devereaux, 2012; Haley & Zacchilli, 2014). Moreover, in some chronic injuries, the tendon length is insufficient to allow for primary repair with minimal tension and requires reconstruction or augmentation with either autograft or allograft. Extended chronicity of the injury should not preclude surgical intervention given that good outcomes can still be achieved (Cordasco & Delos, 2013; Cordasco et al, 2017; Haley & Zacchilli, 2014; Hanna et al, 2001; Kretzler & Richardson, 1989).

Postoperative Rehabilitation

After surgical repair, patients are instructed to remain in a sling for 4 to 6 weeks, with the arm in internal rotation and adducted (Berson, 1979; Egan and Hall, 1987; Park & Espiniella, 1970). By week 6, passive motion in all planes is allowed with the assistance of the physical therapist. At the 8-week postoperative phase, periscapular and isometric strengthening exercises are added. After week 12, the patient should have near full range of motion and light resistance, and strengthening exercises are started (Haley & Zacchilli, 2014; Petilon et al, 2005; Provencher et al, 2010; Schepsis et al, 2000). Additional strengthening and sport-specific rehabilitation progress for the next 12 weeks with a goal of unrestricted activity by 6 months postoperatively, when full range of motion and strengthening are achieved (Cordasco et al, 2017; Haley & Zacchilli, 2014; Provencher et al, 2010; Schepsis et al, 2000).

Complications

Unremitting weakness is the most prevalent complaint after nonoperative management of PM injuries, principally in active patients (Bak et al, 2000; De Castro Pochini et al, 2010; Haley & Zacchilli, 2014; Hanna et al, 2001; Kretzler & Richardson, 1989; Park & Espiniella, 1970; Schepsis et al, 2000; Zeman et al, 1979). Other reported complications of nonoperative treatment include myositis ossificans, hematoma, abscess formation, and asymmetric appearance (Haley & Zacchilli, 2014; Patissier, 1822; Purnell, 1988). Surgical repair of PM injuries allows patients to return to their preinjury activity levels, and complications are relatively uncommon but include infection, hypertrophic scar, stiffness, and rerupture (Balazs et al, 2016; Haley & Zacchilli, 2014; Nute et al, 2017). The two largest studies, using health care management databases regarding active-duty military personnel surgically treated for PM injuries, reported relatively high complication rates (Balazs et al, 2016; Nute et al, 2017). Balazs et al (2016) reviewed 214 patients and reported a 14% complication rate, with surgical site infection (12 superficial and 6 deep) notably the most common (8%). Reoperation was needed in 3% of the patients: 4 patients for infection and 3 patients for repair failure. Nute et al (2017) reviewed 257 patients and reported a 12% complication rate that required second surgery (5.8% to revise retears and 4.7% for wound complications). The senior author has reported the largest single surgeon continuous series reported to date (40 athletes, including 4 National Football League players), treated with the same surgical repair technique. There were no surgical site infections, and there was a 7.5% (3/40) reoperation rate (Cordasco et al, 2017). Two patients had repair failure because of recurrent trauma and noncompliance within 3 weeks of surgery, and the other developed refractory biceps tendon symptoms that required long head biceps tenodesis several months after repair. If the two noncompliant patients were excluded, the reoperation rate would be 2.5% (1/40), and there would be no reruptures in the series. Garrigues et al (2012) evaluated 19 patients and reported no second surgery or wound complications.

Outcomes and Return to Sport

The literature supports surgical repair of PM injuries over nonoperative treatment, especially in young, athletic, and active patients. Surgical repair reliably returns patient strength, allowing return to preinjury level of activity with excellent patient satisfaction and improved cosmesis (Balazs et al, 2016; Cordasco & Delos, 2013; Cordasco et al, 2017; Garrigues et al, 2012; Haley & Zacchilli, 2014; Kang et al, 2014; Nute et al, 2017).

In 1822, Patissier (Patissier, 1822) reported the first case of PM rupture. McEntire in 1972 was the first to report better functional outcome with surgical repair over nonoperative treatment. Several other small series confirmed McEntire's findings. Zeman et al (1979) reported excellent outcomes and full return to strenuous athletic activity in all four patients surgically treated, and those treated nonoperatively (five patients) were unable to return to the preinjury levels of activity. Kretzler and Richardson (1989) reported return of full strength in 81% (13/16) of patients treated with surgical repair. Wolfe et al (1992) demonstrated improved peak adduction torque and work production in those treated surgically, but those treated without surgery had pronounced residual deficits. Schepsis et al (2000) reported significantly better subjective (pain, satisfaction, and cosmesis) and objective (isokinetic testing) functional outcome measures in the surgical patients compared with nonoperative treatment.

In 2000, Bak et al in their meta-analysis reported significantly better functional outcome in the surgical group (57 patients) compared with the nonoperative group (15 patients). After this meta-analysis, Hanna et al (2001) reported complete return of peak torque (99%) and work performance (97%) after surgical repair compared with the contralateral uninjured side. The nonoperative group (12 patients) revealed marked residual deficits (44%) on both peak torque and work performance. In 2014, de Castro Pochini et al (2014) reported good to excellent outcomes in 90% of the surgical repair group (30 patients) and in 28% of the nonoperative group (30 patients). Peak torque deficit was seen in 14% of the surgical group and 42% of the non-operative group. Balazs et al (2016) identified 214 patients, all active-duty military personnel, who underwent surgical repair of PM tendon ruptures; 95% were able to return to military duty. Nute et al (2017) reviewed 257 patients, also active-duty military personnel, who were surgically treated for PM tendon rupture and reported a 94% return to full preoperative level of military function. The senior author reported the largest continuous, single-surgeon series of PM repairs in athletes (Cordasco et al, 2016). Good to excellent outcomes were obtained in 83% of the athletes, and all returned to their preinjury levels of function at an average of 5.5 months (range, 4.5–6.5 months) postoperatively. Isokinetic assessment revealed 90% return in strength compared with the uninjured side. Average preinjury bench press of 396-lb (range, 170–500 lb) was restored to 241 lb postoperatively (range, 150–550 lb) (Cordasco et al, 2016). Garrigues et al (2012) reviewed 19 patients after surgical repair of PM rupture and reported good to excellent outcomes in 96% of patients.

The current literature provides results from studies with various designs (meta-analyses, large health care management databases, and high-volume single-surgeon series). Meta-analyses and health care management databases with data pooled from multiple surgeons and medical centers as well as single-surgeon high-volume series have value for different reasons and may be used to improve outcomes (Cordasco, 2017).

Authors' Preferred Repair Technique

The athlete is indicated for PM repair after an appropriate history, clinical examination, and PM-specific magnetic

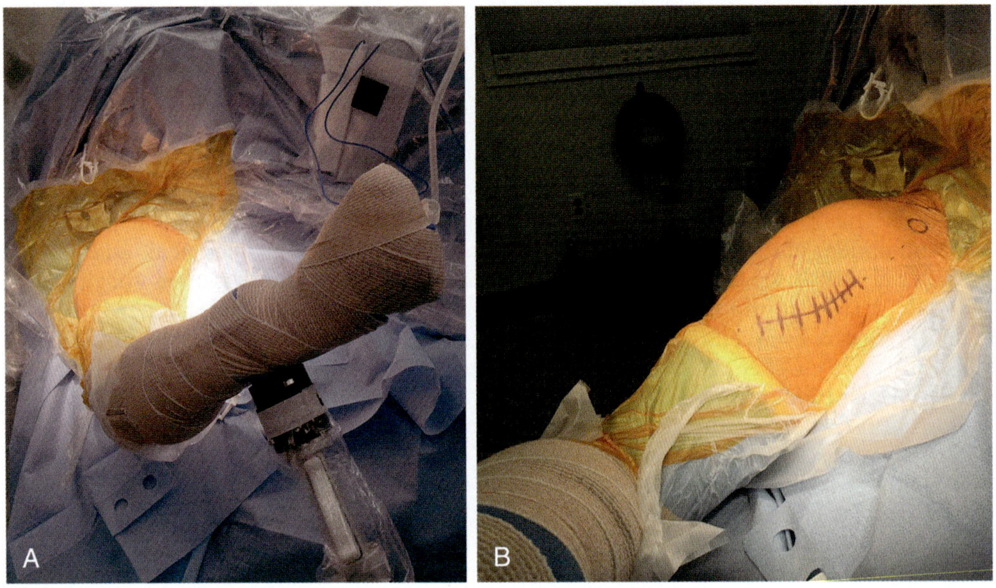

Fig. 21.2 A, The beach-chair position with arm holder. **B,** The planned incision at the distal segment of the standard deltopectoral approach to the shoulder.

resonance imaging (MRI) to define the injury. We obtain both axial fast-spin echo and coronal inversion recovery images, and then the oblique coronal images are plotted from the axial images parallel to the long axis of the PM tendon unit. The MRI can be used to determine whether there is a complete tear or an isolated sternocostal head tear. The senior author's series found the majority of tears (57.5%) were isolated sternocostal head injuries (Cordasco, 2017). The location of the tear using the Tietjen classification should be noted on MRI. In the senior author's experience, the majority of tears (60%) occurred at the muscle–tendon junction (type IIIC). There was a difference in the location of tears between the complete and isolated sternocostal groups (Cordasco, 2017). Whereas in the complete tear group the majority (71%) of intratendon injuries were type IIID tears, the isolated sternocostal head injury group had predominantly (83%) type IIIC muscle tendon injuries (Cordasco, 2017).

The athlete is placed in the beach-chair position after combined regional and general anesthesia, and an arm positioner is used (Fig. 21.2). A distal deltopectoral approach is used for exposure followed by blunt dissection to identify the torn, retracted PM tendon. Adhesions are freed, and the tendon is mobilized. As soon as the subcutaneous tissues are elevated, it will be quite evident if a complete tear is present. The entire PM insertion will be torn, and the surgical exposure will reveal a hematoma medial to the deltoid in the acute setting. In general, each torn head is secured with two sets of locking #2 fiber-wire sutures (Arthrex, Naples, FL) applied in a modified Krackow configuration, with four suture limbs for each head (Fig. 21.3). The deltoid is retracted to expose the footprint of the PM tendon lateral to the bicipital groove. The remnant tissue at the humeral insertion site is debrided while the long head of the biceps is protected. The 3.2-mm guide pin (Arthrex) is used to develop four unicortical drill holes. These are placed in a staggered fashion, leaving a sufficient bone bridge to avoid the potential risk of fractures (Fig. 21.4). Drill holes are angled to increase intramedullary length to flip the unicortical buttons. The corresponding ends of each of the #2 fiber-wire sutures are loaded through the cortical buttons, which are then deployed into the intramedullary canal. The arm is positioned in adduction and neutral position, and the repair is then performed in an anatomic fashion with the sternocostal head reduced to the footprint more posterior and proximal than the clavicular head. Sutures are tensioned with the sternocostal head reduced first, followed by the clavicular head, and secured by standard knots. Fluoroscopy is used to confirm appropriate button position. Layered closure is then performed, and the arm is placed in a sling in an adducted position.

In cases of isolated sternocostal head tears, the initial approach is modified in that the deltopectoral interval appears intact as the clavicular head remains attached. In these cases, the senior author has found it useful to approach the sternocostal head inferior to the clavicular head by elevating the subcutaneous tissues and developing the inferior flap. The deltopectoral interval is left intact, and the sternocostal head, after it has been identified and mobilized, can be repaired posteriorly and superiorly to the footprint by retracting the clavicular head superiorly. In the majority of cases, the clavicular head insertion can be left intact, and the deltopectoral interval does not need to be compromised. Generally, two buttons are used to secure isolated sternocostal head tendon tears.

Pearls, pitfalls and risks and key points can be reviewed in Box 21.1.

Patients are instructed to stay in the sling for 4 to 6 weeks followed by progressive range of motion exercises for up to 12 weeks. Additional strengthening and sport-specific rehabilitation is started after 3 months. Months 4 and 5 are sport specific and position specific with respect to the return-to-sport program. Estimated return to full activities is at 5 to 6 months after operatively but is predicated on a demonstration of adequate strength and successful progression through the rehabilitation program (Fig. 21.4).

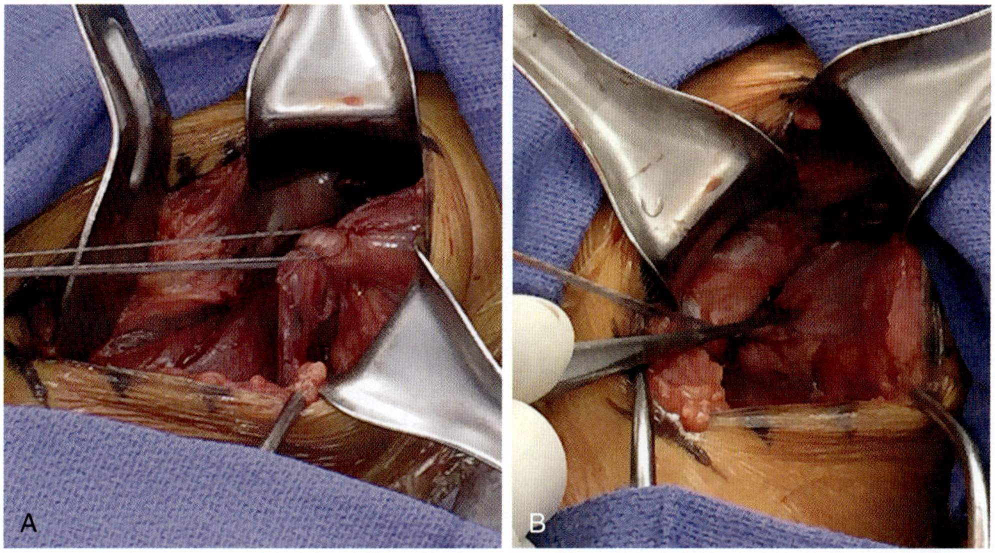

Fig. 21.3 Intraoperative photos. **A,** A modified Krackow configuration with four suture limbs passed through the muscle–tendon junction of the sternoclavicular head. **B,** The sternoclavicular head reapproximated to the footprint at the lateral lip of the bicipital groove.

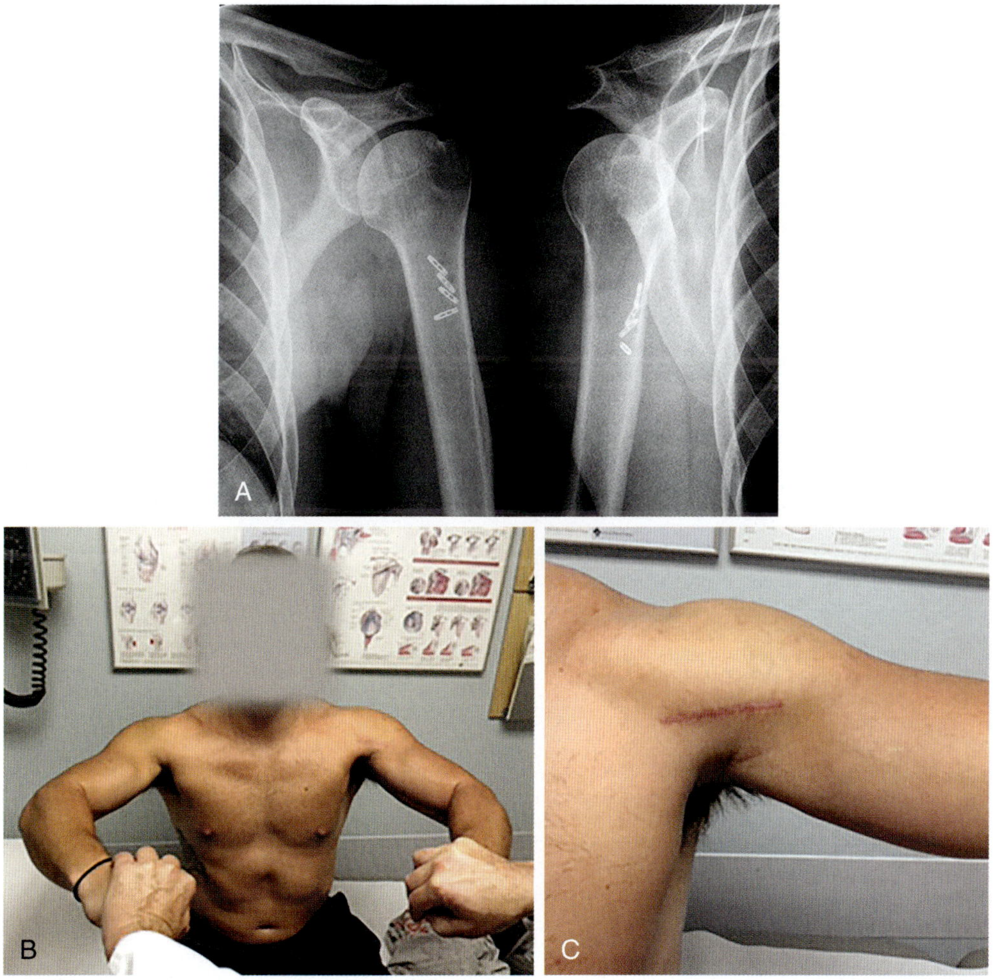

Fig. 21.4 **A,** Anteroposterior and lateral views demonstrating the unicortical buttons placed in a staggered fashion. **B** and **C,** Clinical pictures of a 22-year-old collegiate hockey player defenseman 5.5 months after surgery.

Box 21.1 Tips, Pearls, Pitfalls and Risks, and Key Points

Pearls

- To facilitate flipping the button in the intramedullary canal, the drill is angled slightly when preparing the unicortical drill hole.
- The arm is adducted and in neutral rotation when completing the repair.
- The sternoclavicular head inserts posterior and superior relative to the clavicular head insertion site. The sternocostal head is repaired first in complete tears.
- In isolated sternocostal head injuries, the approach is performed inferior to the clavicular head leaving the deltopectoral interval intact.
- Fluoroscopy is used to verify the correct position of the unicortical buttons.

Pitfalls and Risks

- Maintain a sufficient bone bridge between drill holes to minimize fracture risk.
- Remain cognizant of the potential to constrain the long head biceps within the bicipital groove as it relates to fixation of the tendon to the footprint.

Key Points

- Surgical repair of pectoralis major rupture in athletes leads to better functional outcomes than nonoperative management.
- Tendon-to-bone repair with tensioning button fixation at the footprint is successful.
- The success rate with repair is high (80%–90%).
- The patient satisfaction rate is high (90%–95%).
- The return-to-sport rate is high (90%).
- The complication and reinjury rates are low (<5%–10%).
- Athletes generally return to contact sports between 5 and 6 months.

References

Äärimaa V, Rantanen J, Heikkilä J, Helttula I, Orava S. Rupture of the pectoralis major muscle. *Am J Sports Med.* 2004;32(5):1256–1262.

Antosh IJ, Grassbaugh JA, Parada SA, Arrington ED. Pectoralis major tendon repairs in the active-duty population. *Am J Orthop (Belle Mead NJ).* 2009;38(1):26–30.

Bak K, Cameron EA, Henderson IJ. Rupture of the pectoralis major: a meta-analysis of 112 cases. *Knee Surg Sports Traumatol Arthrosc.* 2000;8(2):113–119.

Balazs GC, Brelin AM, Donohue MA, et al. Incidence rate and results of the surgical treatment of pectoralis major tendon ruptures in active-duty military personnel. *Am J Sports Med.* 2016;44(7):1837–1843.

Beloosesky Y, Grinblat J, Weiss A, Rosenberg PH, Weisbort M, Hendel D. Pectoralis major rupture in elderly patients: a clinical study of 13 patients. *Clin Orthop Relat Res.* 2003b;(413):164–169.

Berson BL. Surgical repair of pectoralis major rupture in an athlete. Case report of an unusual injury in a wrestler. *Am J Sports Med.* 1979;7(6):348–351.

Carrino JA, Chandnanni VP, Mitchell DB, Choi-Chinn K, DeBerardino TM, Miller MD. Pectoralis major muscle and tendon tears: diagnosis and grading using magnetic resonance imaging. *Skeletal Radiol.* 2000;29(6):305–313.

Connell DA, Potter HG, Sherman MF, Wickiewicz TL. Injuries of the pectoralis major muscle: evaluation with MR imaging. *Radiology.* 1999;210(3):785–791.

Cordasco FA. Outcomes of Pectoralis Major Tendon Repair: Does Study Design Matter? Commentary on an article by Drew W. Nute, MD, et al. "Return to Function, Complication, and Reoperation Rates Following Primary Pectoralis Major Tendon Repair in Military Service Members". *J Bone Joint Surg Am.* 2017;99(1).

Cordasco FA, Delos D. Pectoralis major. In: *Disorders of the Shoulder: Sports Injuries, Part IV Muscle and Tendon Rupture.* vol. 2. Lippincott Williams & Wilkins; Philadelphia: 2013:576.

Cordasco FA, Mahony GT, Tsouris N, Degen RM. Pectoralis major tendon tears: functional outcomes and return to sport in a consecutive series of 40 athletes. *J Shoulder Elbow Surg.* 2017;26(3):458–463.

de Castro Pochini A, Andreoli CV, Belangero PS, et al. Clinical considerations for the surgical treatment of pectoralis major muscle ruptures based on 60 cases: a prospective study and literature review. *Am J Sports Med.* 2014;42(1):95–102.

de Castro Pochini A, Ejnisman B, Andreoli CV, et al. Pectoralis major muscle rupture in athletes: a prospective study. *Am J Sports Med.* 2010;38(1):92–98.

Dodds SD, Wolfe SW. Injuries to the pectoralis major. *Sports Med.* 2002;32(14):945–952.

Egan TM, Hall H. Avulsion of the pectoralis major tendon in a weight lifter: repair using a barbed staple. *Can J Surg.* 1987;30(6):434–435.

Elmaraghy A, Deveraux MW. A systematic review and comprehensive classification of pectoralis major tears. *J Shoulder Elbow Surg.* 2012;21:412–422.

Flint JH, Wade AM, Giuliani J, Rue JP. Defining the terms acute and chronic in orthopaedic sports injuries: a systematic review. *Am J Sports Med.* 2014;42(1):235–241.

Garrigues GE, Kraeutler MJ, Gillespie RJ, O'Brien DF, Lazarus MD. Repair of pectoralis major ruptures: single-surgeon case series. *Orthopedics.* 2012;35(8;):e1184–e1190.

Haley CA, Zacchilli MA. Pectoralis major injuries: evaluation and treatment. *Clin Sports Med.* 2014;33(4):739–756.

Hanna CM, Glenny AB, Stanley SN, Caughey MA. Pectoralis major tears: comparison of surgical and conservative treatment. *Br J Sports Med.* 2001;35(3):202–206.

Hart ND, Lindsey DP, McAdams TR. Pectoralis major tendon rupture: a biomechanical analysis of repair techniques. *J Orthop Res.* 2011;29(11):1783–1787.

Kang RW, Mahony GT, Cordasco FA. Pectoralis major repair with cortical button technique. *Arthrosc Tech.* 2014;3(1):e73–e77.

Kretzler HH Jr, Richardson AB. Rupture of the pectoralis major muscle. *Am J Sports Med.* 1989;17(4):453–458.

Lee J, Brookenthal KR, Ramsey ML, Kneeland JB, Herzog R. MR imaging assessment of the pectoralis major myotendinous unit: an MR imaging-anatomic correlative study with surgical correlation. *AJR Am J Roentgenol.* 2000;174(5):1371–1375.

McEntire JE, Hess WE, Coleman SS. Rupture of the pectoralis major muscle. A report of eleven injuries and review of fifty-six. *J Bone Joint Surg Am.* 1972;54(5):1040–1046.

Metzger PD, Bailey JR, Filler RD, Waltz RA, Provencher MT, Dewing CB. Pectoralis major muscle rupture repair: technique using unicortical buttons. *Arthrosc Tech.* 2012;1(1):e1119–e1125.

Miller MD, Johnson DL, Fu FH, Thaete FL, Blanc RO. Rupture of the pectoralis major muscle in a collegiate football player. Use of magnetic resonance imaging in early diagnosis. *Am J Sports Med.* 1993;21(3):475–477.

Mosconi T, Kamath S. Bilateral asymmetric deficiency of the pectoralis major muscle. *Clin Anat.* 2003;16(4):346–349.

Nute DW, Kusnezov N, Dunn JC, Waterman BR. Return to function, complication, and reoperation rates following primary pectoralis major tendon repair in military service members. *J Bone Joint Surg.* 2017;99(1):25–32.

Park JY, Espiniella JL. Rupture of pectoralis major muscle. A case report and review of literature. *J Bone Joint Surg Am.* 1970;52(3):577–581.

Patissier P. *Malaides des bouchers. Traite des maladies des artisans.* Paris: Chez J-B Baillere Libraire; 1822:162–165.

Pavlik A, Csépai D, Berkes I. Surgical treatment of pectoralis major rupture in athletes. *Knee Surg Sports Traumatol Arthrosc.* 1998;6(2):129–133.

Petilon J, Carr DR, Sekiya JK, Unger DV. Pectoralis major muscle injuries: evaluation and management. *J Am Acad Orthop Surg.* 2005;13(1):59–68.

Provencher MT, Handfield K, Boniquit NT, Reiff SN, Sekiya JK, Romeo AA. Injuries to the pectoralis major muscle: diagnosis and management. *Am J Sports Med.* 2010;38(8):1693–1705.

Purnell R. Rupture of the pectoralis major muscle: a complication. *Injury.* 1988;19(4):284.

Quinlan JF, Molloy M, Hurson BJ. Pectoralis major tendon ruptures: when to operate. *Br J Sports Med.* 2002;36(3):226–228.

Rabuck SJ, Lynch JL, Guo X, et al. Biomechanical comparison of 3 methods to repair pectoralis major ruptures. *Am J Sports Med.* Jul 2012;40(7):1635–1640.

Schepsis AA, Grafe MW, Jones HP, Lemos MJ. Rupture of the pectoralis major muscle. Outcome after repair of acute and chronic injuries. *Am J Sports Med.* 2000;28(1):9–15.

Scott BW, Wallace WA, Barton MA. Diagnosis and assessment of pectoralis major rupture by dynamometry. *J Bone Joint Surg Br*. 1992;74(1): 111–113.

Sherman SL, Lin EC, Verma NN, et al. Biomechanical analysis of the pectoralis major tendon and comparison of techniques for tendo-osseous repair. *Am J Sports Med*. Aug 2012;40(8):1887–1894.

Weaver JS, Jacobson JA, Jamadar DA, Theisen SE, Ebrahim F, Kalume-Brigido M. Sonographic findings of pectoralis major tears with surgical, clinical, and magnetic resonance imaging correlation in 6 patients. *J Ultrasound Med*. 2005;24(1):25–31.

Wolfe SW, Wickiewicz TL, Cavanaugh JT. Ruptures of the pectoralis major muscle. An anatomic and clinical analysis. *Am J Sports Med*. 1992;20(5):587–593.

Zeman SC, Rosenfeld RT, Lipscomb PR. Tears of the pectoralis major muscle. *Am J Sports Med*. 1979;7(6):343–347.

SECTION **VIII**

Injuries of the Throwing Shoulder

SECTION OUTLINE

22

Epidemiology, Mechanism of Injury, History and Physical Examination, Imaging, Workup, and Indications for Surgery

NEIL BAKSHI, MD and MICHAEL T. FREEHILL, MD

Introduction

The overhead throwing motion is an intricate, highly coordinated musculoskeletal sequence placing multidirectional and supraphysiologic forces on the shoulder. In fact, the angular velocity during pitching represents the fastest human movement recorded (Fleisig et al, 1995). This repetitive and highly demanding action results in adaptive structural changes permitting the shoulder to effectively perform overhead athletic motions but potentially at the expense of normal kinematics at the glenohumeral joint. Abnormal kinematics coupled with altered motion could result in a variety of pathologic changes and injuries at the shoulder including scapular dyskinesia, glenohumeral internal rotation deficit (GIRD), superior labral anterior and posterior (SLAP) tears, and rotator cuff tears (Burkhart et al, 2003; Dines et al, 2009; Grossman et al, 2005; Kuhn et al, 2003; Myers et al, 2006; Ryu et al, 2002; Walch et al, 1992; Wilk et al, 2011). Because of the increasing prevalence of injury in this athletic population, it is important to understand the pathogenesis and biomechanics of throwing, how to evaluate and further workup these athletes, and subsequently how to determine the best treatment options.

Mechanism of Injury

To understand the pathology most often encountered in the throwing shoulder, a firm understanding of the biomechanics of the phases of throwing is essential. The overhead throwing motion requires the transfer of kinetic energy from the lower extremities, through the trunk, and into the pitching extremity to generate the optimal velocity on the ball. Although the pitching motion can vary among players, it is classically divided into six phases originally described by Dillman et al (1993) (Fig. 22.1).

The two phases most commonly associated with shoulder pathology are the late cocking (early acceleration) and the deceleration phases. The extremes of motion and forces borne by the shoulder in these phases is expected but can lead to altered anatomy and kinematics, resulting in injury. The repetitive loading of the posterior shoulder during deceleration can lead to posteroinferior capsular hypertrophy, thickening, and contracture. This can lead to GIRD (nonthrowing–throwing shoulder internal rotation at 90 degrees of abduction). Although there is no unanimous agreement on a threshold number for diagnosis, differences greater than 18 degrees should cause alert (Burkhart et al, 2003; Ruotolo et al, 2006; Wilk et al, 2011). Perhaps more important is the difference in total range of motion (ROM) between shoulders.

Walch et al (1992) described the pathologic contact between the posterosuperior glenoid labrum and the articular-sided rotator cuff and greater tuberosity during late cocking known as "internal impingement" in tennis players. Although numerous publications have determined internal impingement to be a normal phenomenon in overhead throwers (Halbrecht et al, 1999; Valadie et al, 2000), the presence of GIRD causes the humeral head to shift more posterior and superior (Grossman et al, 2005). This can accentuate the internal impingement, potentially leading to partial articular-sided rotator cuff tears (PASTA) or SLAP tears. Secondary to the significant distractive forces across the glenohumeral joint during deceleration, which are resisted by tensile forces in the rotator cuff and biceps tendon, these same injuries could occur via abrasion, delamination, and degeneration (Andrews & Angelo, 1988; Fleisig et al, 1995).

Burkhart et al (2003a, 2003b) described the constellation of findings known as the "SICK scapula" and believe its presence to be the cause of SLAP lesions and PASTA tears. However, Jobe et al (1989) theorized that anterior capsuloligamentous laxity is the central contributing factor to the development of pathologic internal impingement. This theory suggests that with late cocking, the humeral head translates anteriorly, resulting in increased tension on the rotator cuff and its abrasion on the superior glenoid (Jobe et al, 1989). This theory is supported by a cadaveric study demonstrating that excessive shoulder external rotation results in significantly increased anterior-inferior glenohumeral ligament length (30% increase in length) (Mihata et al, 2004). Thus, it is important to have an understanding of all the potential mechanisms that could lead to pathologic lesions in the throwing shoulder.

History

Obtaining a detailed history is critical to narrowing the differential diagnosis. Important questions regarding retraction, depression, elevation, and rotation with closed chain exercises. Additionally, stretching of the pectoralis minor is performed. When the affected scapula is 50% or more improved in position from its initial pathologic position and the thrower is asymptomatic, an interval throwing program is initiated. The scapular program is continued until the scapula is symmetric with the other side. At that time, return to sport and unrestricted throwing are allowed, and the thrower is encouraged to maintain an every-other-day scapular muscle strengthening program to prevent recurrence. In a compliant overhead athlete, the 50% repositioned scapula can be attained within 2 to 3 weeks, with complete scapular symmetry with the contralateral side being attained by 3 months. Of the 96 overhead athletes treated for this syndrome and followed up for more than 1 year, all successfully returned to asymptomatic throwing at their preinjury levels of performance by 4 months (Burkhart et al, 2003a, 2003b).

GLENOHUMERAL INTERNAL ROTATION DEFICIT

Nonoperative rehabilitation is the frontline treatment for GIRD with emphasis on posterior capsular stretching. Sleeper and cross-body adduction stretches are critical and have been shown to improve shoulder internal rotation and horizontal adduction (Yamauchi et al, 2016). The importance of a consistent stretching program and frequent monitoring cannot be understated because multiple studies have demonstrated significant changes in shoulder ROM after a single start, as well as after a single season (Case et al, 2015; Freehill et al, 2014; Lintner et al, 2007). Fortunately, 90% of throwers with symptomatic GIRD will respond positively to a posterior capsular stretching program and improve GIRD to an acceptable level (Burkhart et al, 2003a). In cases of refractory GIRD, arthroscopic posterior capsular release has been described with good results. Codding et al (2015) reported 10 of 13 overhead athletes with symptomatic GIRD were able to return to their prior level of play after arthroscopic posterior-inferior capsular release. However, with associated pathology addressed at the same time as posterior capsular release, Van Kleunen et al (2012) reported very poor results with only 6 of 17 athletes (35%) returning to their preinjury levels of performance.

PATHOLOGIC INTERNAL IMPINGEMENT

Pathologic internal impingement can present as signs and symptoms of rotator cuff or superior labral pathology. Treatment should be initiated with nonoperative management, including throwing cessation or rest, ice, anti-inflammatory medications, and physical therapy targeted at posterior capsular stretching and strengthening of the rotator cuff and periscapular musculature stabilization and rebalancing. When symptoms improve, throwers are to follow a regimented interval throwing program before return to play. Operative intervention is reserved for athletes with refractory symptoms despite nonoperative treatment for 4 to 6 months and would address the particular structural abnormality that is not allowing a return to throwing.

SLAP Tears

Nonoperative treatment is the initial management as described earlier for internal impingement. Secondary to "fair" results in this population, only after exhausting appropriate and focused conservative management should surgical intervention be considered. Sayde et al (2012) performed a systematic review regarding type 2 SLAP repairs and reported that only 63% of overhead athletes return to their prior level of performance. Neri et al (2011) described 23 elite overhead athletes with concomitant type 2 SLAP tears and partial-thickness rotator cuff tears and reported that only 57% of the athletes were able to return to their preinjury levels of competition if both the SLAP tear was repaired and the cuff tear debrided. Technical factors in SLAP repair of throwers include staying posterior to the biceps and ensuring the most posterior aspect of the lesion has been addressed. A trans–rotator cuff approach can be used safely if needed in this population (O'Brien et al, 2002). Additionally, it is important to not overconstrain the labrum, and thus polydioxanone (PDS) suture could potentially be a better option than heavy nonabsorbable suture (Fig. 22.3).

Rotator Cuff Tears

Rotator cuff pathology is common in overhead throwing athletes, yet most are asymptomatic. Connor et al (2003) reported on 20 asymptomatic overhead athletes, 8 of whom (40%) were found to have partial- or full-thickness rotator cuff tears in their dominant shoulders. None of the athletes interviewed 5 years later had any subjective symptoms or required any evaluation or treatment for shoulder-related problems during the study period. Again, the same conservative management program described for internal impingement should be initiated. When surgical intervention is required, there is a drastic difference between the results of debridement versus repair. Reynolds et al (2008) reported on 67 pitchers who underwent debridement of small partial-thickness rotator cuff tears in overhead athletes, and 76% were able to return to pitching at the professional level. Andrews et al (1985) reported 85% good to excellent with debridement of partial-thickness tears in 34 overhead athletes with average 13-month follow-up. However, Mazoué and Andrews (2006) reported only 2 (1 pitcher and 1 position player) of 16 professional baseball players (17%) were able to return to a high competitive level of baseball after mini-open rotator cuff repair for full thickness.

Conclusion

Shoulder injuries in throwing athletes can occur secondary to altered motion and kinematics coupled with the supraphysiologic forces involved in the overhead throwing action. A thorough history and physical examination are critical to help narrow the differential diagnosis and assist in planning a comprehensive diagnostic workup. An exhaustive and focused nonoperative treatment plan should be performed before attempting surgical intervention because studies have demonstrated only fair results in this patient population.

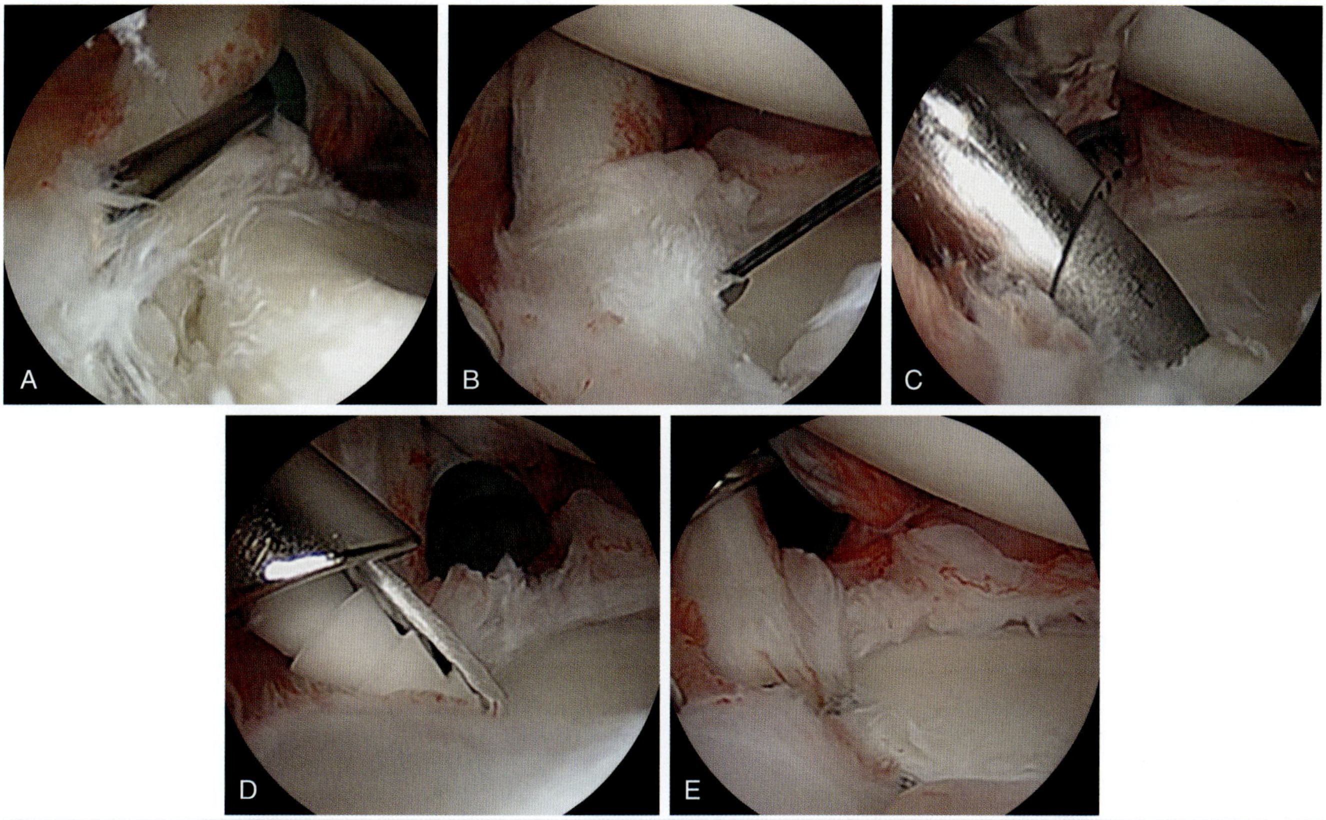

Fig. 22.3 A 20-year-old collegiate pitcher who exhausted conservative management with an inability to return to competitive pitching. Examination, advanced imaging, and findings at arthroscopy were consistent with a type 2 superior labral anterior and posterior tear. Two knotless anchors were placed through a trans–rotator cuff approach for stable repair of the more posterior aspect of the lesion.

References

Andrews JR, Angelo RL. Shoulder arthroscopy for the throwing athlete. *Tech Orthop.* 1988;3:75–81.

Andrews JR, Broussard TS, Carson WG. Arthroscopy of the shoulder in the management of partial tears of the rotator cuff: a preliminary report. *Arthroscopy.* 1985;1:117–122.

Bennett GE. Elbow and shoulder lesions of baseball players. *Am J Surg.* 1959;98:484–492.

Bhatnagar A, Bhonsle S, Mehta S. Correlation between MRI and arthroscopy in diagnosis of shoulder pathology. *J Clin Diagn Res.* 2016;10(2): RC18–RC21.

Brantigan CO, Roos DB. Diagnosing thoracic outlet syndrome. *Hand Clin.* 2004;20(1):27–36.

Burkhart SS, Morgan CD, Kibler WB. The disabled throwing shoulder: spectrum of pathology. Part I: pathoanatomy and biomechanics. *Arthroscopy.* 2003a;19(4):404–420.

Burkhart SS, Morgan CD, Kibler WB. The disabled throwing shoulder: spectrum of pathology. Part III: the SICK scapula, scapular dyskinesis, the kinetic chain, and rehabilitation. *Arthroscopy.* 2003b;19(6):641–661.

Case JM, Mannava S, Fallin JH, Stone AV, Freehill MT. Acute changes in glenohumeral range-of-motion following in-season minor league pitching starts. *Phys Sportsmed.* 2015;43(4):360–365.

Codding J, Dahm DL, McCarty 3rd LP, May JH, Tucker LH, Buss DD. Arthroscopic posterior-inferior capsular release in the treatment of overhead athletes. *Am J Orthop (Belle Mead NJ).* 2015;44(5):223–227.

Connor PM, Banks DM, Tyson AB, Coumas JS, D'Alessandro DF. Magnetic resonance imaging of the asymptomatic shoulder of overhead athletes: a 5-year follow-up study. *Am J Sports Med.* 2003;31(5):724–727.

Dillman CJ, Fleisig GS, Andrews JR. Biomechanics of pitching with emphasis upon shoulder kinematics. *J Orthop Sports Phys Ther.* 1993;18(2):402–408.

Dines JS, Frank JB, Akerman M, et al. Glenohumeral internal rotation deficits in baseball players with ulnar collateral ligament insufficiency. *Am J Sports Med.* 2009;37(3):566–570.

Fleisig GS, Andrews JR, Dillman CJ, Escamilla RF. Kinetics of baseball pitching with implications about injury mechanisms. *Am J Sports Med.* 1995;23(2):233–239.

Freehill MT, Archer KR, Diffenderfer BW, Ebel BG, Cosgarea AJ, McFarland EG. Changes in collegiate starting pitchers' range of motion after single game and season. *Phys Sportsmed.* 2014;42(1):69–74.

Grossman MG, Tibone JE, McGarry MH, et al. A cadaveric model of the throwing shoulder: a possible etiology of superior labrum anterior-to-posterior lesions. *J Bone Joint Surg Am.* 2005;87(4):824–831.

Halbrecht JL, Tirman P, Atkin D. Internal impingement of the shoulder: comparison of findings between the throwing and nonthrowing shoulders of college baseball players. *Arthroscopy.* 1999;15(3):253–258.

Jobe FW, Kvitne RS, Giangarra CE. Shoulder pain in the overhand or throwing athlete. The relationship of anterior instability and rotator cuff impingement. *Orthop Rev.* 1989;18(9):963–975.

Kuhn JE, Lindholm SR, Huston LJ, et al. Failure of the biceps superior labral complex: a cadaveric biomechanical investigation comparing the late cocking and early deceleration positions of throwing. *Arthroscopy.* 2003;19(4):373–379.

Levigne C, Garret J, Grosclaude S, et al. Surgical technique arthroscopic posterior glenoidplasty for posterosuperior glenoid impingement in throwing athletes. *Clin Orthop Relat Res.* 2012;470(6):1571–1578.

Lintner D, Mayol M, Uzodinma O, Jones R, Labossiere D. Glenohumeral internal rotation deficits in professional pitchers enrolled in an internal rotation stretching program. *Am J Sports Med.* 2007;35(4):617–621.

Lombardo SJ, Jobe FW, Kerlan RK, Carter VS, Shields Jr CL. Posterior shoulder lesions in throwing athletes. *Am J Sports Med.* 1977; 5(3):106–110.

Magee T. 3-T MRI of the shoulder: is MR arthrography necessary? *AJR Am J Roentgenol.* 2009;192(1):86–92.

Mazoué CG, Andrews JR. Repair of full-thickness rotator cuff tears in professional baseball players. *Am J Sports Med.* 2006;34:182–189.

Meister K, Day T, Horodyski M, Kaminski TW, Wasik MP, Tillman S. Rotational motion changes in the glenohumeral joint of the adolescent/Little League baseball player. *Am J Sports Med.* 2005;33(5):693–698.

Mihata T, Lee Y, McGarry MH, Abe M, Lee TQ. Excessive humeral external rotation results in increased shoulder laxity. *Am J Sports Med.* 2004;32(5):1278–1285.

Myers JB, Laudner KG, Pasquale MR, Bradley JP, Lephart SM. Glenohumeral range of motion deficits and posterior shoulder tightness in throwers with pathologic internal impingement. *Am J Sports Med.* 2006;34(3):385–391.

Neri BR, ElAttrache NS, Owsley KC, Mohr K, Yocum LA. Outcome of type II superior labral anterior posterior repairs in elite overhead athletes: effect of concomitant partial-thickness rotator cuff tears. *Am J Sports Med.* 2011;39(1):114–120.

O'Brien SJ, Allen AA, Coleman SH, Drakos MC. The trans-rotator cuff approach to SLAP lesions: technical aspects for repair and a clinical follow-up of 31 patients at a minimum of 2 years. *Arthroscopy.* 2002;18(4):372–377.

O'Brien SJ, Pagnani MJ, Fealy S, McGlynn SR, Wilson JB. The active compression test: a new and effective test for diagnosing labral tears and acromioclavicular joint abnormality. *Am J Sports Med.* 1998;26:610–613.

Ozaki J, Tomita Y, Nakagawa Y, Tamai S. Surgical treatment for posterior ossifications of the glenoid in baseball players. *J Shoulder Elbow Surg.* 1992;1(2):91–97.

Reynolds SB, Dugas JR, Cain EL, et al. Debridement of small partial-thickness rotator cuff tears in elite overhead throwers. *Clin Orthop Relat Res.* 2008;466:614–621.

Ruotolo C, Price E, Panchal A. Loss of total arc of motion in collegiate baseball players. *J Shoulder Elbow Surg.* 2006;15(1):67–71.

Ryu RK, Dunbar WH, Kuhn JE, et al. Comprehensive evaluation and treatment of the shoulder in the throwing athlete. *Arthroscopy.* 2002;18(9 suppl 2):70–89.

Savoie 3rd FH, Field LD, Atchinson S. Anterior superior instability with rotator cuff tearing: SLAC lesion. *Orthop Clin North Am.* 2001;32(3):457–461, ix.

Sayde WM, Cohen SB, Ciccotti MG, Dodson CC. Return to play after Type II superior labral anterior-posterior lesion repairs in athletes: a systematic review. *Clin Orthop Relat Res.* 2012;470(6):1595–1600.

Sodha S, Srikumaran U, Choi K, Borade AU, McFarland EG. Clinical assessment of the dynamic labral shear test for superior labrum anterior and posterior lesions. *Am J Sports Med.* 2017;45(4):775–781.

Valadie 3rd AL, Jobe CM, Pink MM, Ekman EF, Jobe FW. Anatomy of provocative tests for impingement syndrome of the shoulder. *J Shoulder Elbow Surg.* 2000;9(1):36–46.

Van Kleunen JP, Tucker SA, Field LD, Savoie 3rd FH. Return to high-level throwing after combination infraspinatus repair, SLAP repair, and release of glenohumeral internal rotation deficit. *Am J Sports Med.* 2012;40(11):2536–2541.

Walch G, Boileau P, Noel E, et al. Impingement of the deep surface of the supraspinatus tendon on the posterosuperior glenoid rim: an arthroscopic study. *J Shoulder Elbow Surg.* 1992;1(5):238–245.

Walch G, Liotard JP, Boileau P, et al. Postero-superior glenoid impingement. Another impingement of the shoulder [in French]. *J Radiol.* 1993;74(1):47–50.

Waldt S, Burkart A, Lange P, Imhoff AB, Rummeny EJ, Woertler K. Diagnostic performance of MR arthrography in the assessment of superior labral anteroposterior lesions of the shoulder. *AJR Am J Roentgenol.* 2004;182(5):1271–1278.

Wiener SN, Seitz Jr WH. Sonography of the shoulder in patients with tears of the rotator cuff: accuracy and value for selecting surgical options. *AJR Am J Roentgenol.* 1993;160(1):103–107 [discussion: 109–110].

Wilk KE, Macrina LC, Fleisig GS, et al. Correlation of glenohumeral internal rotation deficit and total rotational motion to shoulder injuries in professional baseball pitchers. *Am J Sports Med.* 2011;39(2):329–335.

Wright RW, Paletta Jr GA. Prevalence of the Bennett lesion of the shoulder in major league pitchers. *Am J Sports Med.* 2004;32(1):121–124.

Yamauchi T, Hasegawa S, Nakamura M, et al. Effects of two stretching methods on shoulder range of motion and muscle stiffness in baseball players with posterior shoulder tightness: a randomized controlled trial. *J Shoulder Elbow Surg.* 2016;25(9):1395–1403.

23 Surgical Management of Capsulolabral and Rotator Cuff Injuries in Throwing Athletes

SETH L. SHERMAN, MD, B. ISRAEL YAHUACA, MD, DEREK STOKES, JEFFREY FREYDER, MD, and PATRICK A. SMITH, MD

Introduction

- Surgical management of the throwing shoulder has unique challenges specific to the high demands of the overhead throwing motion.
- Repetitive throwing places the shoulder in extreme positions under tremendous stress that rival some of the fastest movements in competitive sport.
- There exists a delicate balance separating physiologic adaptation (i.e., capsular laxity, increased humeral external rotation) during normal throwing motion and pathophysiologic changes (i.e., anterior instability, posterior capsular contracture, decreased humeral internal rotation) that may occur in the injured throwing shoulder.
- There are consistent injury patterns that occur in the throwing shoulder, including anteroinferior labral tears, posterosuperior labral tears and biceps tendon pathology, posteroinferior capsular contracture, and partial-thickness articular rotator cuff tears.
- In throwers with chronic insidious pain or instability, surgery is only indicated after failure of conservative management (i.e., optimizing the "kinetic chain," improvement of scapular dyskinesia, and correction of pathologic humeral rotational deficits).
- Acute traumatic injuries in throwers may require earlier operative management. However, the vast majority are similarly treated with an initial course of conservative management and close observation before surgical intervention is offered.
- Preoperative planning includes detailed history and physical examination, review of imaging studies, and confirmation of the correct diagnosis during examination under anesthesia and diagnostic arthroscopy.
- The goal of surgical management is to recognize and treat pathologic structures while maintaining native joint laxity and range of motion (ROM), which are critical for return to throwing.
- Successful return to competitive throwing after shoulder surgery requires a combination of thoughtful preoperative planning, meticulous surgical technique, and a comprehensive goal-oriented postsurgical rehabilitation program.

Surgical Considerations

PREOPERATIVE PLANNING

Successful surgical management of the throwing shoulder must begin in the clinic setting. Carefully performed history, physical examination, and review of imaging studies gives the surgeon a working diagnosis before operative intervention. This may aid in selection of surgical approach (i.e., arthroscopic vs open) and arthroscopic surgical position (i.e., beach chair vs lateral decubitus) and allows for anticipation of procedure length and any special equipment needs before surgery. In general, the vast majority of surgical interventions in the throwing shoulder can be successfully performed using arthroscopic intervention. This includes capsulolabral and rotator cuff debridement or repair, removal of loose bodies, and synovectomy. Rarely, other procedures may be indicated, including subacromial decompression, distal clavicle excision, decompression of paralabral cysts, suprascapular nerve decompression, or debridement of small capsular exostosis (i.e., Bennett lesion). Open or mini-open approaches are considered for the management of humeral avulsion of the glenohumeral ligament (HAGL) lesions, for complex type IV tears or failed prior repair of the SLAP (superior labrum anterior and posterior) lesion when the surgeon selects to perform subpectoral biceps tenodesis, or for the rare case of complete subscapularis tears with retraction. Open approaches commonly performed in the athletic population are rarely performed in throwers but rather in the setting of complex shoulder instability, particularly when performing open Bankart and capsular shift procedures for contact or collision throwing athletes (i.e., football quarterback) with increased Injury Severity Index (ISI) scores or for athletes with substantial glenoid or humeral bone loss requiring reconstructive procedures.

ANESTHESIA AND SURGICAL POSITION

Shoulder surgery in throwing athletes is typically performed under general anesthesia with an interscalene nerve block. Open procedures are performed in the beach-chair or modified beach-chair position. Arthroscopic procedures may be performed in either the beach-chair or lateral decubitus position, based mainly on surgeon experience and preference (Li et al, 2015). With either approach, careful attention is placed on protective padding for critical structures (i.e., axillary roll for lateral decubitus, pillows under knees, and peroneal padding for beach chair). Cerebral perfusion is improved with the lateral decubitus position, and there is less risk of hypotension or bradycardia during the procedure (Li et al, 2015; Peruto et al, 2009). For arthroscopic management of the majority of conditions of the throwing shoulder, the authors prefer the lateral decubitus position (Li et al, 2015). Advantages of this setup include the use of traction, providing excellent 360-degree access to the glenohumeral joint, including easier access to the inferior labrum and the 6 o'clock position. A relative disadvantage is that repeat dynamic examination under anesthesia (EUA) is more cumbersome, requiring removal and replacement of the traction setup (Li et al, 2015; Peruto et al, 2009). Additionally, if open surgery is required, the patient may need to be repositioned. However, the majority of the time, this requires only minor readjustment of the torso without repeat preparation and draping. The beach-chair position provides anatomic orientation and easier access for repetitive dynamic EUA (Li et al, 2015; Peruto et al, 2009). This position may be favored for work limited to the anterior or superior quadrants, rotator cuff, biceps tendon, and Acromioclavicular (AC) joint. However, access to the posterior and inferior quadrants for labral repair or debridement requires substantial technical expertise to gain adequate exposure for appropriate treatment (Li et al, 2015).

EXAMINATION UNDER ANESTHESIA

Examination under anesthesia is a critical component of the workup and management of the throwing athlete. This should be performed after the induction of general anesthesia and before sterile preparation and draping so that both limbs may be examined. It is important to examine the normal nonoperative extremity to gain better appreciation for the athlete's native joint laxity and physiologic parameters for ROM (Cofield et al, 1993; Oliashirazi et al, 1999). Understanding baseline nonpathologic degrees of humeral internal and external rotation will assist in detecting abnormalities in the throwing shoulder, including residual glenoid internal rotation contracture (GIRD) secondary to posterior capsular contracture (Oliashirazi et al, 1999). Laxity testing on the noninvolved extremity includes assessment for sulcus sign and multidirectional load and shift of the humeral head (Oliashirazi et al, 1999). Comparison with the operative extremity allows the surgeon to detect pathologic instability patterns (anterior, posterior, inferior, combined instability) that require surgical attention versus symmetric global hyperlaxity where surgical stabilization may be contraindicated (Oliashirazi et al, 1999).

ARTHROSCOPIC PORTAL PLACEMENT AND DIAGNOSTIC ARTHROSCOPY

Standard arthroscopic portals are typically used for the management of the throwing shoulder. A posterior viewing portal is established with a #11 blade scalpel. In the lateral decubitus position, the posterior portal is placed generally 1 cm medial and inferior to the posterolateral corner of the acromion. In the beach-chair position, this is typically positioned two fingerbreadths inferior and medial to the posterolateral tip of the acromion. Standard anteroinferior portal is placed next using inside-out technique and a switching stick and dilator set. A transparent cannula is placed superior to the subscapularis under direct visualization, aiming toward the anterior pouch to avoid iatrogenic damage to the glenoid and humeral head. A high rotator interval portal is established using an outside-in technique with an 18-gauge needle for localization, coming just anterior to the leading edge of the supraspinatus tendon. Cannula size is per surgeon preference, ranging from 5.75 to 8 mm. The arthroscopic camera sheath may be switched out for a posterior cannula with attached inflow, allowing for "sheathless" arthroscopy and easy alternation of viewing portal and instrument utilization from any portal. Additional portals such as port of Wilmington and percutaneous transsubscapularis and 7 o'clock portals can be used based on location of pathology and surgeon preference.

Diagnostic arthroscopy is a critical component in the successful surgical treatment of the throwing shoulder (Burkhart et al, 2003a, 2003b; Craig, 1996; McFarland et al, 2001; Shaffer & Huttman, 2014). Differentiating normal variants from pathologic entities allows the surgeon to treat relevant pathology and to maintain the integrity and physiologic laxity of native structures. Diagnostic arthroscopy is systematic, reproducible, and goal oriented. It should be hypothesis driven to confirm or refute clinical suspicion based on preoperative workup and EUA findings. It is also helpful to identify relevant abnormalities (i.e., chondral lesions, synovitis, small loose bodies) that may not have eluded diagnostic imaging tests.

Diagnostic arthroscopy begins with the superior labrum–biceps complex. Care must be taken to differentiate sublabral recess or meniscoid appearing normal SLAP variants from pathologic tears. The superior and posterosuperior labrum should be probed and carefully evaluated. Type I, III, and IV SLAP tears are often easily identified. Type II tears are a more challenging diagnostic entity. The arm should be freely mobile and a "peel-back test" performed, visualizing the posterosuperior labrum–biceps and rotator cuff from different vantage points. During this test, the operative arm is taken out of suspension and manually placed at 90 degrees of abduction and 90 degrees of external rotation while visualizing the SLAP–biceps complex. (Fig. 23.1, *A*) This mimics the late cocking and early acceleration phase of the throwing cycle. A positive peel-back test occurs when the SLAP–biceps is unstable and drops medially over the edge of the glenoid, exposing the SLAP footprint (Burkhart et al, 2003a, 2003b). Contact between the posterosuperior glenoid and posterior articular surface of the rotator cuff is also noted during the peel-back test. Partial tears of the undersurface of the infraspinatus tendon may be recognized during this maneuver. In the throwing shoulder, the peel-back test is of major significance because the goal of SLAP repair is to stabilize the SLAP–biceps complex, thereby eliminating the "peel-back mechanism" (Burkhart et al, 2003a, 2003b).

The intraarticular biceps tendon itself should be carefully probed for tears, tenosynovitis, and instability. It is noted that diagnostic arthroscopy does not visualize the entire extent of the extraarticular biceps and may not be able to detect all relevant biceps pathology. The surgeon must rely on presurgical history, physical examination, imaging studies, and clinical suspicion to determine relevant treatment

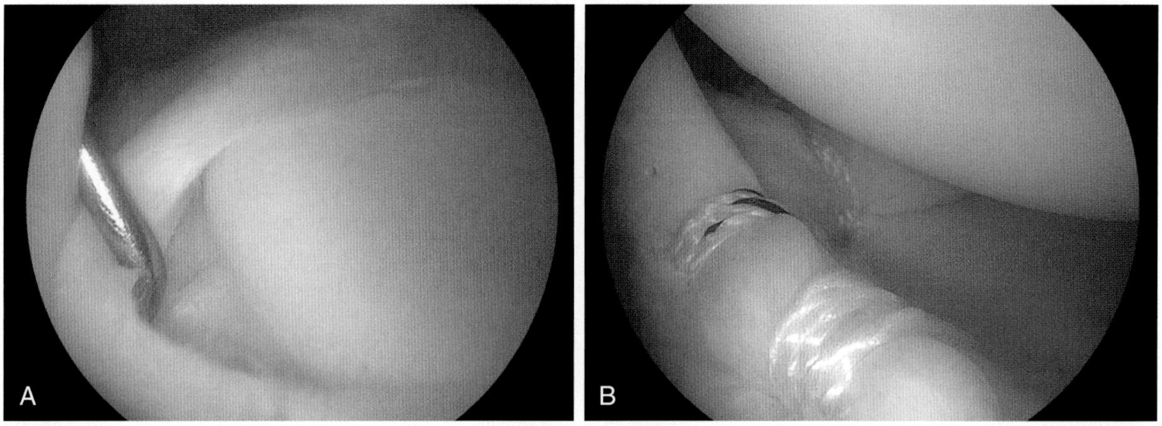

Fig. 23.1 SLAP (superior labrum anterior and posterior) tear demonstrating peel-back mechanism before (A) and after (B) SLAP repair.

of any "hidden lesions" of the extraarticular biceps tunnel. Next, the glenoid and humeral cartilage surfaces should be inspected and palpated. The joint should be evaluated for synovitis or loose bodies. Care should be taken to evaluate for the presence or absence of glenoid or humeral bone loss, which should be appropriately recorded and measured using standard techniques. The anterior, inferior, and posterior labrum are methodically visualized and probed from anterior and posterior viewing portals. The entire capsulolabral complex is evaluated for presence of labral and capsular tears, noting tissue quality and mobility. The drive-through test is commonly performed in the setting of instability. Although different methods have been used, our preference is to have the surgical assistant apply traction under direct arthroscopic visualization to assess the distance from the humeral head to the glenoid (McFarland et al, 2001). Successful instability repair should eliminate the drive-through at the conclusion of the procedure (Burkhart et al, 2003b). When there is index of suspicion for posteroinferior capsular contracture from EUA, thickening and fibrotic change of the capsule is confirmed with diagnostic arthroscopy, particularly while evaluating for posterior tightness as the arm is brought into internal rotation.

The undersurface of the rotator cuff is inspected for partial articular or full-thickness tears, particularly at the junction between the supraspinatus and infraspinatus. Internal impingement that occurs with the arm placed in abduction/external rotation can demonstrate the pathogenesis rotator cuff tear that requires treatment to provide symptom relief. The rotator cuff should be probed for evidence of intrasubstance delamination. If there is suspicion for a high-grade partial articular tear, the tear can be tagged with a PDS (polydioxanone) suture using spinal needle localization for further classification and visualization in the subacromial space. Additional diagnostic arthroscopy of the subacromial space can help to evaluate for and rule out signs of external impingement (i.e., subacromial bursitis, Coracoacromial (CA) ligament fraying, ossification or thickening, downsloping acromion) or acromioclavicular joint pathology.

Surgical Decision Making

The surgical treatment of the throwing shoulder is "a la carte." The treating surgeon must understand common injury patterns in order to identify and treat the spectrum of pathologic entities that are typically encountered during these cases. Information learned from preoperative planning, EUA, and diagnostic arthroscopy allows the surgeon to create a problem list and to design and implement a patient-specific surgical plan. It is important to recognize that our evidence-based treatment algorithms for the throwing shoulder may not mirror treatment pathways in nonthrowing athletes, particularly when considering the ultimate goal of effective return to competitive throwing. Treatment strategies that often lead to success in nonthrowing athletes (i.e., rotator cuff repair for high-grade partial tears) have not had the same excellent outcome for return to throwing. This has led to a separate set of guiding principles and surgical strategies in this unique and challenging population. Specific treatments for each of the involved pathologic entities are described in the relevant section below.

Internal Impingement

SLAP–BICEPS COMPLEX

SLAP tears are a common finding in disabled throwing shoulders. Although the cause of these tears remains controversial, it is well established that unstable SLAP tears contribute to pain, instability, and loss of velocity or accuracy in throwing athletes (Burkhart et al, 2003a, 2003b; Knesek et al, 2013). The treatment of symptomatic SLAP tear depends on the intraoperative classification (Burns et al, 2011). Type I and III SLAP tears are stable injury patterns that are less common in the throwing population and can be treated with arthroscopic debridement (Snyder et al, 1990). Type II SLAP tears are the most common pattern in throwing athletes (Knesek et al, 2013). This is an unstable tear pattern that should be treated with arthroscopic stabilization if true peel-back pathology is demonstrated. Type IV SLAP tears are also fairly uncommon in throwing athletes. This injury involves an unstable SLAP tear that extends into the proximal biceps anchor. In high-demand athletes, this lesion should be addressed with surgical repair if possible versus SLAP repair combined with biceps tenodesis. Type V-X SLAP tears occur in conjunction with pathologic instability (Knesek et al, 2013). In high-demand athletes with symptomatic instability, stabilization of the SLAP extension should be performed alongside combined anterior, posterior, or inferior capsulolabral repair as indicated.

SLAP repair is performed with the standard portals described earlier, including the Nevaiser portal per surgeon preference. The tear is mobilized so that it can be reduced to the footprint on the glenoid without undue tension. The footprint is debrided to a bleeding bed with use of shaver, rasp, or curette. Standard suture shuttling technique is performed to pass either simple or mattress suture through the SLAP tear. Our preference is for the use of simple or cinch stitch with 1.5-mm smooth polyethylene tape secured with two or three knotless biocomposite 2.9-mm anchors (Fig. 23.1, *B*). Knot tying is less desired to avoid iatrogenic damage to the humeral surface from prominent knots. The anchors are drilled and delivered from the anterosuperior portal. Anchors are spaced at least 5 mm apart, stabilizing the superior and posterosuperior labrum as indicated. Typically, the anterior-most anchor is placed just posterior to the biceps anchor to avoid incarceration of the biceps anchor or inadvertent tightening of the superior or middle glenohumeral ligaments and rotator interval. This is critical to avoid overconstraint and subsequent postoperative loss of motion.

At present, the indications for biceps tenodesis in throwing athletes are evolving and remain controversial. In this population, biceps tenodesis should be reserved for treatment of an irreparable biceps tear or pulley injury with subluxation associated with type II or IV SLAP tears and for patients with persistent symptoms associated with a failed SLAP repair (Boileau et al, 2009; Burns et al, 2011). Biceps tenosynovitis or hidden lesions of the extraarticular biceps are challenging to diagnose and manage. Throwers with biceps groove pain but normal-appearing SLAP–biceps complex at arthroscopy should be treated with aggressive conservative management. If symptoms persist and the thrower is unable to return to her or his prior level of activity after index arthroscopy and prolonged rehabilitation, biceps tenodesis may be considered if diagnostic or therapeutic ultrasound-guided injections suggest an extraarticular biceps location of the athlete's pain.

There is no consensus on the type or location of biceps tenodesis in throwing athletes. There is concern regarding stress riser and fracture risk with larger drill holes for biceps docking, which should be avoided in high-velocity athletes. Our preference is for open subpectoral biceps tenodesis. Intraarticular tenotomy is performed with a basket device. A small axillary incision is placed, and the fascia along the inferior border of the pectoralis major is incised, mobilizing the interval between the pectoralis major and the short head of the biceps. The long head of the biceps is retrieved from the biceps groove using a right-angle hemostat. Blunt neurovascular retractors are placed. All but 15 mm of tendon from the musculotendinous junction is excised, and a locking whipstitch suture is then placed in the remaining tendon. The suture limbs are loaded onto a biceps button. A 3.5-mm-diameter drill hole is placed in the biceps groove at the level of the inferior border of the pectoralis major. The biceps is docked with either unicortical or bicortical button fixation per surgeon preference. Alternatively, the anterior cortex may be overreamed to the diameter of the tendon, and the biceps may be docked within the endosteal space and secured with bicortical button fixation. Fibrin glue and impervious dressing are used for the wound, given the proximity to the axilla.

ROTATOR CUFF

Partial articular tears of the rotator cuff are commonly encountered in the dysfunctional throwing shoulder with internal impingement (Andrews et al, 1985b). The vast majority are chronic insidious tears or intrasubstance delamination (Mithöfer et al, 2004), located at the junction between the supraspinatus and infraspinatus. Acute traumatic high-grade partial or full-thickness tears may also occur on rare occasion. The decision to repair versus debride rotator cuff tears in the throwing shoulder differs from the treatment of a nonthrower. A systematic review of a series of 25 studies found that although recreational athletes return to the same level pre injury, only half of professional and competitive athletes return to an equivalent level of play (Klouche et al, 2016). As such, caution is recommended before moving forward with surgical repair in this population. Rotator cuff debridement is certainly recommended for low-grade partial articular tears and may be a desirable first-line option for throwers with tears up to 75% of the width of the tendon involvement (Economopoulos & Brockmeier, 2012; Rudzki & Shaffer, 2008) (Fig. 23.2). Gentle debridement is performed with a motorized shaver while taking the arm through a controlled ROM arc. Aggressive debridement or conversion of partial- to full-thickness tears is not routinely recommended in this population.

When surgical repair of a high-grade partial articular tear is selected in a thrower, a transtendinous approach is favored over takedown and repair of a full-thickness tear (Fox & Romeo, 2002). The goal of the transtendinous repair is to restore the deficient medial footprint of the rotator cuff while maintaining native length–tension relationship of the intact lateral tendon. Our preference is for knotless repair using two 2.4-mm biocomposite anchors for medial row compression placed through percutaneous transtendinous portals, tying on the bursal side with a double pulley technique, and a 4.75-mm biocomposite anchor placed lateral to the intact lateral row in the subacromial space to more evenly distribute forces across the repair. This technique is

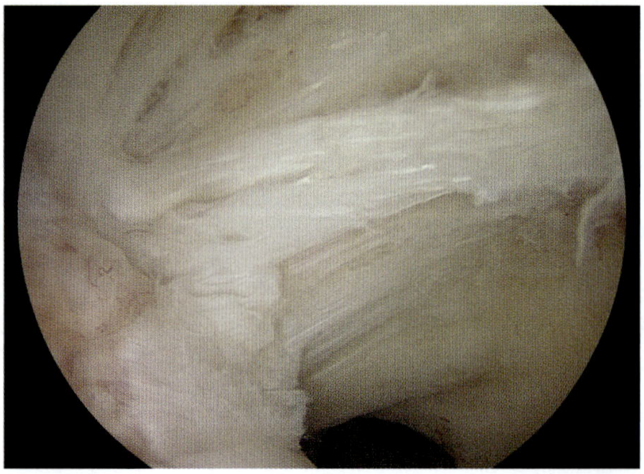

Fig. 23.2 Partial articular rotator cuff tear after debridement in a baseball pitcher.

low profile and provides anatomic restoration of the footprint without changing the length–tension relationship of the rotator cuff (Fig. 23.3).

Conway (2001) described a soft-tissue-only repair technique in throwers with partial-thickness tears including significant intrasubstance delamination at the posterior supraspinatus and anterior infraspinatus. In this technique, spinal needles are used to reduce the delaminated tear and to shuttle nonabsorbable sutures through the tendon. The sutures are tied in the subacromial space, reapproximating the tear. This series, demonstrating good results including return to throwing, is one of the few in the literature demonstrating consistent success with rotator cuff repair in throwing athletes (Conway, 2001).

Full-thickness tears in throwing athletes should be repaired. However, results regarding return to throwing are generally unfavorable. The goals of surgical repair is again anatomic footprint restoration without overconstraint (Burkhart et al, 1997). Our preference is for knotless transosseous equivalent repair using 2-mm polyethylene tape with at least two medial row and two lateral row biocomposite suture anchors. This approach is low profile with excellent biomechanical strength and decreased gap formation (Burkhart et al, 1997). Care is taken not to pass sutures too far medial in the rotator cuff, which may lead to excessive strain and construct failure (Park & Elattrache, 2008). Additionally, medial anchors should be placed at the lateral aspect of the bare area in the location of the native rotator cuff insertion. Overmedialization of the footprint in this region may alter rotator cuff function and reduce the chance of a successful outcome (Curtis et al, 2006; Minagawa et al, 1998).

POSTERIOR CAPSULAR CONTRACTURE

Indications for posterior capsular release include throwing athletes with a known history of GIRD that has been refractory to conservative management (i.e., sleeper stretching) or detection of internal rotation deficits and posteroinferior capsular fibrosis and thickening during EUA and diagnostic arthroscopy. This is used as an adjunct surgical treatment to restore internal rotation in throwers being treated for other pathology associated with internal impingement. Surgeon preference is to use a small thermal hooked device

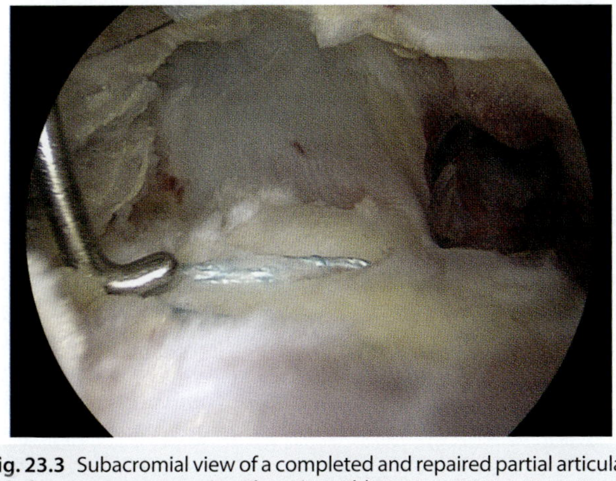

Fig. 23.3 Subacromial view of a completed and repaired partial articular-sided supraspinatus tear in a throwing athlete.

for posteroinferior capsular release. In the lateral decubitus position, capsular release is performed parallel and adjacent to the posterior labrum–capsular junction. A radiofrequency device allows for time-zero hemostasis with decreased chance of postsurgical scarring and the ability to detect proximity to the axillary nerve via muscular contraction as compared with other mechanical techniques (Tokish & Cook, 2013).

Shoulder Instability

In the throwing shoulder, there is a narrow separation between adaptive physiologic laxity and disabling pathologic instability. Failure to recognize native joint mechanics or normal variants may lead to inadvertent tightening of capsulolabral structures, overconstraint of joint motion, and inability to return to competitive throwing. Similarly, failure to address pathologic instability with capsulolabral repair may lead to persistent symptoms of pain or instability with throwing and surgical failure. Unlike the treatment of the contact or collision nonthrowing athletes, unidirectional or combined labral repair in throwers should include the labrum and only enough of the capsular reflection necessary for tissue integrity to avoid the detrimental effects of overtightening (Greiwe & Ahmad, 2010). Surgical management is decided on by a combination of preoperative planning, EUA, and diagnostic arthroscopic findings demonstrating symptomatic instability and associated true tears of the capsulolabral complex. Labral tears in throwers are more common posteriorly, particularly in the posterior and superior quadrant as opposed to the anterior; unless frank subluxation has occurred. Rarely, if ever, is a capsular plication indicated as a primary procedure for multidirection laxity in a thrower when the labrum is completely intact.

The vast majority of instability cases in throwing athletes can be managed with arthroscopic management (Fig. 23.4, *A*). Standard arthroscopic portals are used along with accessory portals as indicated for anchor placement (i.e., port of Wilmington, transsubscapularis, 7 o'clock). The capsulolabral complex is mobilized to allow for a tension-free repair using an elevator. The glenoid rim is prepared with bur, rasp, or curette to healthy bleeding bed. In general, arthroscopic repair proceeds from inferior to superior and from posterior to anterior. Standard suture shuttling technique is used to pass simple or cinch stitch 1.5-mm polyethylene tape, which is anchored to the glenoid with 2.9-mm biocomposite knotless anchors. Care is taken to place the anchors on the rim and not on the face of the glenoid to avoid overconstraint. In contrast to collision athletes, anchors are typically placed at the same level of the tissue passage and not advanced superiorly to avoid aggressive capsular shift which may overconstrain the throwing motion (Payne & Altchek, 1995). Similarly, the tape is passed at the capsulolabral junction to reapproximate the labral but not increase the size of the "bumper" (Fig. 23.4, *B*). In rare cases of early humeral bone loss and engaging Hill-Sachs lesion, arthroscopic remplissage may be considered. However, this may overconstrain in external rotation and should be used with extreme caution in throwing athletes. Surgeons should have a high index of suspicion evaluating for the presence of HAGL or

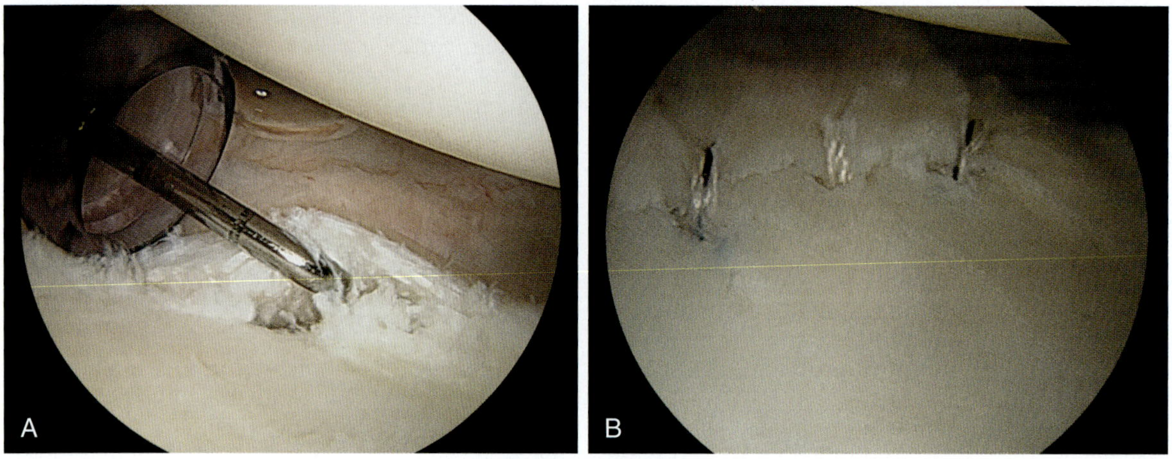

Fig. 23.4 Posteroinferior labral tear before (**A**) and after (**B**) surgical repair.

reverse HAGL lesions. Although not frequently encountered, when present, they can be detrimental to shoulder function. Wolf et al (1995) found HAGL lesions in 9.3% of patient with glenohumeral instability. Reverse HAGL lesions can usually be managed arthroscopically at the time of labral repair using knotless suture anchors placed through a percutaneous spinal needle localized portal (Smith et al, 2014). Anterior HAGL may be easiest to manage by mini-open deltopectoral approach and elevation of the inferior border of the subscapularis, followed by bony preparation of the humeral footprint and repair of the avulsion of the anterior inferior glenohumeral ligament with knotted or knotless suture anchor fixation followed by subscapularis repair (Arciero & Mazzocca, 2005).

Open surgical stabilization is reserved for complex or recurrent instability patterns. The instability severity index score (ISI) is a preoperative score that is helpful in selecting patients for arthroscopic versus open stabilization procedures. A score of 7 or greater corresponds to recurrence rate with arthroscopic surgery of at least 70% (Streubel et al, 2014). Open surgical management is considered particularly in athletes with ISIS scores of 7 or greater (i.e., age younger than 20 years [2 points], competitive forced overhead athlete [3 points]}, shoulder hyperlaxity [1 point], and visible Hill-Sachs lesion in external rotation [2 points]) (Streubel et al, 2014). Other indications for open surgery include large or retracted subscapularis tears or for the management of athletes with substantial glenoid or humeral bone loss requiring reconstructive procedures (i.e., Latarjet, distal tibial allograft glenoid reconstruction, osteochondral allograft transplantation to Hill-Sachs lesion). Although fairly common in the contact and collision athletes (Tjoumakaris et al, 2014), these open surgical options are less often used in throwing athletes because there is little evidence regarding return to competitive throwing to guide decision making.

Treatment of Concomitant Pathology

In addition to commonly encountered patterns of injury to the capsulolabral complex and rotator cuff, other pathologic structures in the throwing shoulder may contribute to pain and dysfunction and should be addressed at the time of arthroscopic surgery. Intraarticular synovitis and loose bodies may be treated with arthroscopic synovectomy and loose body removal, respectively. Unstable chondral flaps may be gently debrided, with care taken not to violate the underlying subchondral bone layer when exposed. Chondral restorative treatments (i.e., microfracture) are generally avoided in the first-line treatment of throwing athletes. A Bennett lesion is a posteroinferior glenoid exostosis. This may be excised if necessary with a shaver or bur with associated posteroinferior capsulolabral repair as needed for bony exposure (Yoneda et al, 2002). Paralabral cysts should be recognized on advanced imaging studies and adequately decompressed during surgical treatment of the labrum (Sandow & Ilic, 1998). In rare cases, entrapment of the suprascapular nerve may require decompression at the spinoglenoid, suprascapular notch, or both locations (Piasecki et al, 2009). External impingement may be addressed with standard treatments such as subacromial bursectomy, debridement of thickened or frayed CA ligament, and acromioplasty. Symptoms relating to the acromioclavicular joint may be treated with arthroscopic distal clavicle excision.

Outcomes

A summary of surgical outcomes of capsulolabral and rotator cuff injuries in throwing athletes can be found in Table 23.1.

Conclusion

Surgical management of the throwing shoulder has a unique and challenging set of management principles. Supraphysiologic stress and extreme shoulder ROM required for normal throwing motion are contributory issues. When an athlete has failed comprehensive conservative treatment, the goal of surgery is to recognize and treat pathologic entities while respecting native and adaptive changes to avoid overconstraint and postoperative ROM loss. Consistent injury patterns must be recognized through careful preoperative planning, including imaging, EUA, and diagnostic arthroscopy. Surgical treatment of capsulolabral and rotator cuff injury is guided by our best available evidence regarding successful return to throwing. This treatment algorithm may differ from the management of nonthrowing athletes. The potential for successful return to sport requires thoughtful presurgical planning, meticulous surgical technique, and a comprehensive goal-oriented rehabilitation program. Despite our best efforts, return to throwing rates remain variable even after well-executed surgery. This reinforces the principle that surgery is only indicated for persistent disabling symptoms and functional limitations after focused rehabilitation directed at correction of underlying biomechanical abnormalities, especially related to the scapula and abnormal throwing mechanics. Counseling the athlete regarding realistic goals and expectations is a critical component of surgical management in throwing athletes.

Table 23.1 Outcomes of Surgical Management in Throwing Athletes

Author(s)	Year	Design and LOE	Group	Treatment	Results	Commentary
ROTATOR CUFF REPAIR						
Reynolds et al	2008	Retrospective; LOE, 4	82 competitive pitchers	Partial-thickness rotator cuff debridement	55% returned to previous level of play at 11 months	The majority of overhead throwing athletes are able to return to competitive pitching after debridement of small partial-thickness rotator cuff debridement.
Andrews et al	1985b		36 patients (23 pitchers)	Debridement of PTaRCT	85% of patients returned satisfactorily to their preoperative athletic activity (76% had excellent results)	
Conway	2001		9 baseball players	Repair of intratendinous rotator cuff tears	89% returned to the same or higher level of play	
Mazoue et al	2006	Case series; LOE, 4	16 professional baseball players	Mini-open repair of a full-thickness rotator cuff tear	8% of pitchers returned to play 50% of position players returned to play	It is difficult for a professional baseball player to return to a competitive level of player after a mini-open repair of a full-thickness rotator cuff tear.
Namdari et al	2011	Case-control; N/A	33 elite pitchers	Rotator cuff tear repair	73% returned to play	Pitchers who underwent operative treatment tended to decline gradually in performance leading up to their operations and to improve gradually over the next two or three seasons after surgery before plateauing or declining.
SLAP REPAIR						
Morgan et al	1998		44 pitchers, 37 competitive	SLAP repair	87% returned to previous level of play	
Kim et al	2002		18 overhead athletes	SLAP repair	22% returned to previous level of play	
Reinold et al	2003		130 athletes (105 pitchers)	SLAP repair with or without thermal therapy in throwers	87% returned to previous level of play	
Neri et al	2011	Cohort study; LOE, 3	23 elite pitchers	Type II SLAP repair	57% returned to play pain-free	
Van Kleunen et al	2012	Case series; LOE, 4	17 high-level baseball players	Arthroscopic SLAP repair and infraspinatus repair	35% RTP at the same or superior level; 30% RTP at a lower level; 35% failure to RTP	The prognosis for a combination SLAP and infraspinatus tear is more guarded than a SLAP tear in isolation
Neuman et al	2011	Case series; LOE, 4	30 overhead athletes	Arthroscopic type II SLAP repair	Athletes' perception: RTP at 84.1% of preinjury level of function; significant drop in ASES to KJOC scores	Arthroscopic SLAP repairs show good results and high satisfaction; outcomes are less reliable in throwers
Fedoriw et al	2014	Case series; LOE, 4	40 professional pitchers	Surgical SLAP repair	48% RTP; 7% RPP in pitchers 85% RTP; 54% RPP in position players	Rate of returns after SLAP repairs are lower in pitchers than position players.

Continued

Table 23.1 Outcomes of Surgical Management in Throwing Athletes—cont'd

Author(s)	Year	Design and LOE	Group	Treatment	Results	Commentary
Chalmers et al	2014	Controlled laboratory study; LOE, N/A	11 pitchers	BT and SLAP repair	BT restored normal pattern of muscular activation than SLAP repair	SLAP repair may alter pitching biomechanics.
INSTABILITY AND POSTERIOR RELEASE						
McClincy et al	2015	Retrospective comparative study; LOE, 3	48 overhead athletes	Arthroscopic posterior capsulolabral reconstruction	60% RPP; no statistical difference between throwers and nonthrower comparison group	
Jobe et al	1991		25 overhand athletes	Anterior capsulolabral reconstruction	92% good or excellent ratings; 68% RTP	
Montgomery et al	1994		32 athletes	Anterior capsulolabral repair with modifications	96% good or excellent scores; 81% RPP; 13% RTP at a lower level	
Bigliani et al	1994		63 athletic patients; including 10 elite pitchers	Anterior-inferior capsular shift in athletes	50% of elite pitchers·RPP	

ASES, American Shoulder and Elbow Surgeons; *BT*, Biceps Tendon; *KJOC*, Kerlan-Jobe Orthopedic Clinic; *LOE*, level of evidence; *PTaRCT*, Partial Thickness articular-sided Rotator Cuff Tear; *RPP*, return to prior performance; *RTP*, return to play; *SLAP*, superior labrum anterior and posterior.

References

Andrews JR, Carson WG Jr, McLeod WD. Glenoid labrum tears related to the long head of the biceps. *Am J Sports Med*. 1985a;13(5):337–341.

Andrews JR, Broussard TS, Carson WG. Arthroscopy of the shoulder in the management of partial tears of the rotator cuff: a preliminary report. *Arthroscopy*. 1985b;1(2):117–122.

Arciero RA, Mazzocca AD. Mini-open repair technique of HAGL (humeral avulsion of the glenohumeral ligament) lesion. *Arthroscopy*. 2005;21(9):1152.

Boileau P, Parratte S, Chuinard C, Roussanne Y, Shia D, Bicknell R. Arthroscopic treatment of isolated type II SLAP lesions: biceps tenodesis as an alternative to reinsertion. *Am J Sports Med*. 2009;37(5):929–936.

Burkhart SS, Diaz Pagàn JL, Wirth MA, Athanasiou KA. Cyclic loading of anchor-based rotator cuff repairs: confirmation of the tension overload phenomenon and comparison of suture anchor fixation with transosseous fixation. *Arthroscopy*. 1997;13(6):720–724.

Burkhart SS, Morgan CD, Kibler WB. The disabled throwing shoulder: spectrum of pathology part I: pathoanatomy and biomechanics. *Arthroscopy*. 2003a;19(4):404–420.

Burkhart SS, Morgan CD, Kibler WB. The disabled throwing shoulder: spectrum of pathology part II: evaluation and treatment of SLAP lesions in throwers. *Arthroscopy*. 2003b;19(5):531–539.

Burns JP, Bahk M, Snyder SJ. Superior labral tears: repair versus biceps tenodesis. *J Shoulder Elbow Surg*. 2011;20(suppl 2):S2–S8.

Chalmers PN, Trombley R, Cip J, et al. Postoperative restoration of upper extremity motion and neuromuscular control during the overhand pitch: evaluation of tenodesis and repair for superior labral anterior-posterior tears. *Am J Sports Med*. 2014;42(12):2825–2836.

Cofield RH, Nessler JP, Weinstabl R. Diagnosis of shoulder instability by examination under anesthesia. *Clin Orthop Relat Res*. 1993;(291):45–53.

Conway JE. Arthroscopic repair of partial-thickness rotator cuff tears and SLAP lesions in professional baseball players. *Orthop Clin North Am*. 2001;32(3):443–456.

Craig EV. Shoulder arthroscopy in the throwing athlete. *Clin Sports Med*. 1996;15(4):673–700.

Curtis AS, Burbank KM, Tierney JJ, Scheller AD, Curran AR. The insertional footprint of the rotator cuff: an anatomic study. *Arthroscopy*. 2006;22(6):609. e1.

Economopoulos KJ, Brockmeier SF. Rotator cuff tears in overhead athletes. *Clin Sports Med*. 2012;31(4):675–692.

Fedoriw WW, Ramkumar P, McCulloch PC, Lintner DM. Return to play after treatment of superior labral tears in professional baseball players. *Am J Sports Med*. 2014;42(5):1155–1160.

Fox JA, Romeo AA. PASTA lesion-trans-tendon technique for repair. *Operative Tech Orthop*. 2002;12(3):191–196.

Greiwe RM, Ahmad CS. Management of the throwing shoulder: cuff, labrum, and internal impingement. *Orthop Clin North Am*. 2010;41(3): 309–323.

Jobe FW, Giangarra CE, Kvitne RS, Glousman RE. Anterior capsulolabral reconstruction of the shoulder in athletes in overhand sports. *Am J Sports Med*. 1991;19(5):428–434.

Kim SH, Ha KI, Kim SH, Choi HJ. Results of arthroscopic treatment of superior labral lesions. *J Bone Joint Surg Am*. 2002;84-A(6):981–985.

Klouche S, Lefevre N, Herman S, Gerometta A, Bohu Y. Return to sport after rotator cuff tear repair: a systematic review and meta-analysis. *Am J Sports Med*. 2016;44(7):1877–1887.

Knesek M, Skendzel JG, Dines JS, Altchek DW, Allen AA, Bedi A. Diagnosis and management of superior labral anterior posterior tears in throwing athletes. *Am J Sports Med*. 2013;41(2):444–460.

Li X, Eichinger JK, Hartshorn T, Zhou H, Matzkin EG, Warner JP. A comparison of the lateral decubitus and beach-chair positions for shoulder surgery: advantages and complications. *J Am Acad Orthop Surg*. 2015;23(1):18–28.

Mazoué CG, Andrews JR. Repair of full-thickness rotator cuff tears in professional baseball players. *Am J Sports Med*. 2006;34(2):182–189.

McClincy MP, Arner JW, Bradley JP. Posterior shoulder instability in throwing athletes: a case-matched comparison of throwers and non-throwers. *Arthroscopy*. 2015;31(6):1041–1051.

McFarland EG, Neira CA, Gutierrez MI, Cosgarea AJ, Magee M. Clinical significance of the arthroscopic drive-through sign in shoulder surgery. *Arthroscopy*. 2001;17(1):38–43.

Minagawa H, Itoi E, Konno N, et al. Humeral attachment of the supraspinatus and infraspinatus tendons: an anatomic study. *Arthroscopy*. 1998;14(3):302–306.

Mithöfer K, Fealy S, Altchek DW. Arthroscopic treatment of internal impingement of the shoulder. *Tech Shoulder Elbow Surg*. 2004; 5:66–75.

Montgomery WH 3rd, Jobe FW. Functional outcomes in athletes after modified anterior capsulolabral reconstruction. *Am J Sports Med*. 1994;22(3):352–358.

Morgan CD, Burkhart SS, Palmeri M, Gillespie M. Type II SLAP lesions: three subtypes and their relationships to superior instability and rotator cuff tears. *Arthroscopy*. 1998;14(6):553–565.

Namdari S, Baldwin K, Ahn A, Huffman GR, Sennett BJ. Performance after rotator cuff tear and operative treatment: a case-control study of major league baseball pitchers. *J Athl Train*. 2011;46(3):296–302.

Neri BR, ElAttrache NS, Owsley KC, Mohr K, Yocum LA. Outcome of type II superior labral anterior posterior repairs in elite overhead athletes: effect of concomitant partial-thickness rotator cuff tears. *Am J Sports Med*. 2011;39(1):114–120.

Neuman BJ, Boisvert CB, Reiter B, Lawson K, Ciccotti MG, Cohen SB. Results of arthroscopic repair of type II superior labral anterior posterior lesions in overhead athletes: assessment of return to preinjury playing level and satisfaction. *Am J Sports Med.* 2011;39(9):1883–1888.

Oliashirazi A, Mansat P, Cofield RH, Rowland CM. Examination under anesthesia for evaluation of anterior shoulder instability. *Am J Sports Med.* 1999;27(4):464–468.

Park MC, ElAttrache NS. Treating full-thickness cuff tears in the athlete: advances in arthroscopic techniques. *Clin Sports Med.* 2008;27(4):719–729.

Payne LZ, Altchek DW. The surgical treatment of anterior shoulder instability. *Clin Sports Med.* 1995;14(4):863–883.

Peruto CM, Ciccotti MG, Cohen SG. Shoulder arthroscopy positioning: lateral decubitus versus beach chair. *Arthroscopy.* 2009;25(8):891–896.

Piasecki DP, Romeo AA, Bach BR, Nicholson GP. Suprascapular neuropathy. *J Am Acad Orthop Surg.* 2009;17(11):665–676.

Reinold MM, Wilk KE, Hooks TR, Dugas JR, Andrews JR. Thermal-assisted capsular shrinkage of the glenohumeral joint in overhead athletes: a 15- to 47-month follow-up. *J Orthop Sports Phys Ther.* 2003;33(8): 455–467.

Reynolds SB, Dugas JR, El Cain, McMichael CS, Andrews JR. Débridement of small partial-thickness rotator cuff tears in elite overhead throwers. *Clin Orthop Relat Res.* 2008;466(3):614–621.

Rudzki JR, Shaffer B. New approaches to diagnosis and arthroscopic management of partial-thickness cuff tears. *Clin Sports Med.* 2008;27(4):691–717.

Sandow MJ, Ilic J. Suprascapular nerve rotator cuff compression syndrome in volleyball players. *J Shoulder Elbow Surg.* 1998;7(5):516–521.

Shaffer B, Huttman D. Rotator cuff tears in the throwing athlete. *Sports Med Arthrosc.* 2014;22(2):101–109.

Smith PA, Nuelle CW, Bradley JP. Arthroscopic repair of a posterior bony humeral avulsion of the glenohumeral ligament with associated teres minor avulsion. *Arthrosc Tech.* 2014;3(1):e89–e94.

Snyder SJ, Karzel RP, Del Pizzo W, Ferkel RD, Friedman MJ. SLAP lesions of the shoulder. *Arthroscopy.* 1990;6(4):274–279.

Streubel PN, Krych AJ, Simone JP, et al. Anterior glenohumeral instability: a pathology based surgical treatment strategy. *J Am Acad Orthop Surg.* 2014;22(5):283–294.

Tokish JM, Cook JB. Management of the throwing shoulder. In: Cole BJ, Sekiya JK, eds. *Surgical Techniques of the Shoulder, Elbow and Knee in Sports Medicine.* Philadelphia: WB Saunders; 2013.

Tjoumakaris FP, Austin LS, Bradley JP. Arthroscopic and open posterior instability repair in NFL linemen. *Oper Tech Sports Med.* 2014;22(1):18.

Van Kleunen JP, Tucker SA, Field LD, Savoie FH 3rd. Return to high-level throwing after combination infraspinatus repair, SLAP repair, and release of glenohumeral internal rotation deficit. *Am J Sports Med.* 2012;40(11):2536–2541.

Wolf EM, Cheng JC, Dickson K. Humeral avulsion of the glenohumeral ligaments as a cause of anterior shoulder instability. *Arthroscopy.* 1995;11(5):600–607.

Yoneda M, Nakagawa S, Hayashida K, Fukushima S, Wakitani S. Arthroscopic removal of symptomatic Bennett lesions in the shoulder of baseball players: arthroscopic Bennett-plasty. *Am J Sports Med.* 2002;30(5):728–736.

24 Throwing Programs and Return to Sport

TERRANCE A. SGROI, PT, DPT, SCS, MTC, PATRICK VIGNONA, MSPT, SCS, MDT, and MICHAEL LEVINSON

Return to a throwing sport after elbow or shoulder injury can be a daunting task. Return to play rates after ulnar collateral ligament reconstruction have been favorable but lower than once thought (Erickson et al, 2015; Ford et al, 2016; Keller et al, 2014). Many studies show a high return rate to major league baseball, but return to similar performance and workload is not as high (Jones et al, 2013). Return to throwing after surgical treatment for superior labral lesions is even more debilitating and sometimes unattainable (Fedoriw et al, 2014; Van Kleunen et al, 2012).

When helping guide patients back to throwing activities, a criteria-based algorithm should be followed that encompasses all aspects of the throwing motion and accounts for the physical characteristics of the athlete.

Phase 1

PROGRESSION CRITERIA

- 0/10 pain Numeric Rating Pain Score (NRPS)
- No joint swelling
- Normalized range of motion (ROM)
  - Shoulder external rotation + internal rotation (total rotational motion)
    - 176 to 180 degrees (Wilk et al, 2011): within 5 degrees of uninvolved side
  - Shoulder horizontal adduction
    - 42 to 44 degrees (Wilk et al, 2012)
  - Elbow ROM
    - 4 to 6 degrees lack of extension is within normal for throwing athletes (Wright et al, 2006)
- Normalized strength
  - 5/5 strength of rotator cuff
  - 4/5 or > mid trap, low traps, and rhomboids

Phase 2

PROGRESSION CRITERIA

Isokinetic Shoulder Testing

- 65% external rotation (ER)/internal rotation (IR) ratio at 180 degrees/sec, 61% ER/IR ratio at 300 degrees / sec (Ivey et al, 1985; Wilk et al, 1993)
- 85% shoulder symmetry at both 180 and 300 degrees/ sec

Balance

- Stand on balance leg with stride leg in 90 degrees of hip flexion and 90 degrees of knee flexion for 60 seconds without loss of balance
- Y-balance: anterior reach (within 4 cm side to side), posterolateral and posteromedial reach (within 6 cm side to side) (Garrison et al, 2013)

Core and Hip Strength

- Front and side plank for 90 seconds without pelvic drop
- Single-leg glute bridge for 30 seconds without contralateral pelvic drop

Phase 3

PROGRESSION CRITERIA

Fatigue Superset

- (Superset) Double-arm overhead wall taps: 45 sec, 2000-g ball
  - **Faults:** asymmetrical shrug
- (Superset) 90 degree/90 degree wall taps: 45 sec, 1000-g ball
  - **Faults:** leading with the elbow, elbow drop below shoulder height
- (Superset) 12, 2, 3 o'clock wall taps: 45 sec, 1000-g ball
  - **Faults:** increase in scapular winging, elbow dropping below shoulder height
- Eccentric ball catches over shoulder, 1000-g ball
  - 3 sets of 20 repetitions, 45-sec rest between sets
  - **Faults:** trunk flexion <45 degrees, irregular arm path (not smooth, not across the body)
- Posterior shoulder endurance test (Moore et al, 2013)
  - 10 reps prone horizontal abduction with ER using 2% of body weight at 30 beats per minute
  - **Faults:** elevation of entire upper torso; verbal report of inability to continue

The purpose of phase 3 is to test the endurance of the athlete's shoulder. Very few studies have examined shoulder endurance in overhead athletes (Moore et al, 2013; Myers et al, 2015). To pass phase 3, the athlete cannot display more than one fault of the above program. They are to remain on phase 3 until able to complete all tasks with adequate control and endurance. After phase 3 is successfully completed, the athlete may progress to a structured interval throwing program.

Phase 4

INTERVAL THROWING PROGRAM

An interval throwing program transitions the thrower back to the playing field. None of the exercises performed in rehabilitation or training can truly reproduce the forces and loads of throwing. The program prepares the thrower for the workloads required for competition. This interval throwing program is designed to minimize the chance of reinjury and can be adapted for pitchers and all position players.

The program:

- Progresses throwing volume, intensity, distance, and rest
- Consists of long tosses to improve arm strength and short tosses of higher intensity to reproduce the demands of each position
- Is designed to be progressed individually based on any symptoms the player may have
- Proper mechanics should be emphasized.
- Throwing velocity should only be sufficient to reach to target.

Dull pain or soreness is common during this program. However, one should never attempt to throw through sharp pain. If this pain persists, one should consult with a physician.

Finally, when beginning the throwing program, players should continue their training program to maintain strength, flexibility, and endurance because there is a tendency to "break down" as one begins advancing the throwing distance.

Instructions (Nonoperative, Mild Injury)

- Warm-up and stretching to be performed before throwing
- If the athlete has sharp pain during throwing, **STOP** immediately until pain ceases. Contact a physician or physical therapist if there is continued pain.
- Crow hop or side step should be used for flat ground throwing.
- Program to be performed every other day. Minimum of 1 day of rest between steps.
- If step is performed pain free, it is ok to progress to the next step.
- Do not continue with throwing if pain and soreness are noticed. Stop the step for that day and return to the same step after an additional rest day.
- Phases 1 to 6: 50% effort
- Phases 7 to 10: 75% effort
- Phases 10+ 100% effort

Instructions (Severe Tendon or Ligament Injury or Postoperative Elbow or Shoulder

- Phases 1 to 12: Advance no more than one phase every **3 days** with 2 days of active rest after each workout.
- Phase 12 +: Advance no more than one phase every other day with 1 day of active rest between phases.

PHASE 1 (50%)

DISTANCE (FT)	NUMBER OF THROWS	REST (MIN)
30	20	5
30	20	10
45	10	

PHASE 2 (50%)

DISTANCE (FT)	NUMBER OF THROWS	REST (MIN)
30	20	5
30	20	10
45	20	

PHASE 3 (50%)

DISTANCE (FT)	NUMBER OF THROWS	REST (MIN)
45	20	5
45	20	10
60	10	

PHASE 4 (50%)

DISTANCE (FT)	NUMBER OF THROWS	REST (MIN)
45	20	5
45	20	10
60	20	

PHASE 5 (50%)

DISTANCE (FT)	NUMBER OF THROWS	REST (MIN)
60	20	5
60	20	10
75	10	

PHASE 6 (50%)

DISTANCE (FT)	NUMBER OF THROWS	REST (MIN)
60	20	5
60	20	5
75	20	

PHASE 7 (75%)

DISTANCE (FT)	NUMBER OF THROWS	REST (MIN)
75	20	5
75	20	10
90	10	

PHASE 8 (75%)

DISTANCE (FT)	NUMBER OF THROWS	REST (MIN)
75	20	5
75	20	10
90	20	

PHASE 9 (75%)

DISTANCE (FT)	NUMBER OF THROWS	REST (MIN)
90	20	5
90	20	10
120	10	

PHASE 10 (75%)

DISTANCE (FT)	NUMBER OF THROWS	REST (MIN)
90	20	5
90	20	10
120	20	

PHASE 11 (100%)

DISTANCE (FT)	NUMBER OF THROWS	REST (MIN)
120	20	10
120	20	

PHASE 12 (100%)

DISTANCE (FT)	NUMBER OF THROWS	REST (MIN)
120	20	10
120	20	10
120	20	

PHASE 13 (OPTIONAL)

DISTANCE (FT)	NUMBER OF THROWS	REST (MIN)
150	20	5
150	20	

PHASE 14 (OPTIONAL)

DISTANCE (FT)	NUMBER OF THROWS	REST (MIN)
150	20	10
150	20	10
150	20	

PHASE 15 (OPTIONAL)

DISTANCE (FT)	NUMBER OF THROWS	REST (MIN)
180	20	10
180	20	

PHASE 16 (OPTIONAL)

DISTANCE (FT)	NUMBER OF THROWS	REST (MIN)
180	20	10
180	20	10
180	20	

After phase 16, position players progress to position specific drills and then to simulated games. Pitchers progress to the following pitching program.

Pitching Program

PHASE 5

Video Analysis and Return to Competition

PHASE 1: WINDING UP OFF FLAT GROUND (75%)

DISTANCE	NUMBER OF THROWS	REST (MIN)
60 ft, 6 in (warm-up throws)	20	5
60 ft, 6 in	20	5
60 ft, 6 in	20	

PHASE 2 (75%-100%)

DISTANCE	NUMBER OF THROWS	REST (MIN)
60 ft, 6 in (warm-up throws)	20	5
60 ft, 6 in	20	5
60 ft, 6 in	20	5
60 ft, 6 in	20	

PHASE 3: OFF THE MOUND (100%)

NUMBER OF THROWS	REST (MIN)
Warm-up throws: 20 fastballs at 50% intensity	5
20 fastballs at 50%	

PHASE 4

NUMBER OF THROWS	REST (MIN)
Warm-up throws: 20 fastballs at 50%	5
20 fastballs at 50%	5
20 fastballs at 50%	

PHASE 5

NUMBER OF THROWS	REST (MIN)
Warm-up throws: 20 fastballs at 50%	5
20 fastballs at 50%	5
20 fastballs at 50%	5
20 fastballs at 50%	

PHASE 6

NUMBER OF THROWS	REST (MIN)
Warm-up throws: 20 fastballs at 50%	5
20 fastballs at 50%	5
15 fastballs at 75%	5
15 fastballs at 75%	

PHASE 7

NUMBER OF THROWS	REST (MIN)
Warm-up throws: 20 fastballs at 50%	5
20 fastballs at 50%	5
20 fastballs at 75%	5
20 fastballs at 75%	

PHASE 8

NUMBER OF THROWS	REST (MIN)
Warm-up throws: 20 fastballs at 50%	5
20 fastballs at 75%	5
20 fastballs at 75%	5
20 fastballs at 75%	5
15 fastballs at 100%	

PHASE 9

NUMBER OF THROWS	REST (MIN)
Warm-up throws: 20 fastballs at 50%	5
20 fastballs at 75%	5
20 fastballs at 75%	5
20 fastballs at 100%	5
15 fastballs at 100%	

PHASE 10

NUMBER OF THROWS	REST (MIN)
Warm-up throws: 20 fastballs at 50%	10
20 fastballs at 100%	10
15 breaking balls and changeups	10
20 fastballs at 100%	10
15 fastballs at 100%	

PHASE 11

NUMBER OF THROWS	REST (MIN)
Warm-up throws: 20 fastballs at 75%	5
20 fastballs at 100%	10
6 breaking balls and changeups	10
20 fastballs at 100%, 6 breaking balls and changeups	

PHASE 12

NUMBER OF THROWS	REST (MIN)
Warm-up throws: 20 fastballs at 75%	5
20 fastballs at 100%	
10 breaking balls and changeups	10
15 fastballs at 100%	
10 breaking balls and changeups	10
15 fastballs at 100%	
10 breaking balls and changeups	

PHASE 13

Warm-up throws 20 fastballs at 75%
20 breaking balls and changeups

Batting practice: 50–60 pitches

PHASE 14

Warm-up throws: 15 fastballs at 75%
15 breaking balls and changeups

Batting practice: 70–80 pitches

PHASE 15

Simulated game: The simulated game is to be designed specifically for each individual pitcher.

- Patient-reported outcome scale
  - Kerlan Jobe Orthopedic Clinic Shoulder and Elbow Score (KJOC)
  - Score of 85 or greater (Domb et al, 2010; Franz et al, 2013)
- Video analysis (240 frames per second lateral and anterior view)
  - Key positions
    - Relaxed balance position
    - Arm in throwing position at front foot strike
    - Stride length >75% of pitcher height
    - Presence of hip and shoulder separation
    - ≥90 degrees of shoulder abduction at ball release
    - Presence of front knee extension from moment of foot strike to ball release
- When all the above criteria have been met, the athlete may progress to throwing bullpen session and clearance for gradual return to full competition.

References

Domb BG, Davis JT, Alberta FG, et al. 2010. Clinical follow-up of professional baseball players undergoing ulnar collateral ligament reconstruction using the new Kerlan-Jobe Orthopaedic Clinic overhead athlete shoulder and elbow score (KJOC Score). *Am J Sports Med.* 2010;38(8):1558–1563.

Erickson BJ, Chalmers PN, Bush-Joseph CA, Verma NN, Romeo AA. Ulnar collateral ligament reconstruction of the elbow: a systematic review of the literature. *Orthop J Sports Med.* 2015;3(12). 2325967115618914.

Fedoriw WW, Ramkumar P, McCulloch PC, Lintner DM. Return to play after treatment of superior labral tears in professional baseball players. *Am J Sports Med.* 2014;42(5):1155–1160.

Ford GM, Genuario J, Kinkartz J, Githens T, Noonan T. Return-to-play outcomes in professional baseball players after medial ulnar collateral ligament injuries: comparison of operative versus nonoperative treatment based on magnetic resonance imaging findings. *Am J Sports Med.* 2016;44(3):723–728.

Franz JO, McCulloch PC, Kneip CJ, Noble PC, Lintner DM. The utility of the KJOC score in professional baseball in the United States. *Am J Sports Med.* 2013;41(9):2167–2173.

Garrison JC, Arnold A, Macko MJ, Conway JE. Baseball players diagnosed with ulnar collateral ligament tears demonstrate decreased balance compared to healthy controls. *J Orthop Sports Phys Ther.* 2013;43(10):752–758.

Ivey FM Jr, Calhoun JH, Rusche K, Bierschenk J. Isokinetic testing of shoulder strength: normal values. *Arch Phys Med Rehabil.* 1985;66(6):384–386.

Jones KJ, Conte S, Patterson N, ElAttrache NS, Dines JS. Functional outcomes following revision ulnar collateral ligament reconstruction in Major League Baseball pitchers. *J Shoulder Elbow Surg.* 2013;22(5):642–646.

Keller RA, Steffes MJ, Zhuo D, Bey MJ, Moutzouros V. The effects of medial ulnar collateral ligament reconstruction on Major League pitching performance. *J Shoulder Elbow Surg.* 2014;23(11):1591–1598.

Moore SD, Uhl TL, Kibler WB. Improvements in shoulder endurance following a baseball-specific strengthening program in high school baseball players. *Sports Health.* 2013;5(3):233–238.

Myers NL, Toonstra JL, Smith JS, Padgett CA, Uhl TL. Sustained isometric shoulder contraction on muscular strength and endurance: a randomized clinical trial. *Int J Sports Phys Ther.* 2015;10(7):1015–1025.

Van Kleunen JP, Tucker SA, Field LD, Savoie FH 3rd. Return to high-level throwing after combination infraspinatus repair, SLAP repair, and release of glenohumeral internal rotation deficit. *Am J Sports Med.* 2012;40(11):2536–2541.

Wilk KE, Andrews JR, Arrigo CA, Keirns MA, Erber DJ. The strength characteristics of internal and external rotator muscles in professional baseball pitchers. *Am J Sports Med.* 1993;21(1):61–66.

Wilk KE, Macrina LC, Fleisig GS, et al. Correlation of glenohumeral internal rotation deficit and total rotational motion to shoulder injuries in professional baseball pitchers. *Am J Sports Med.* 2011;39(2):329–335.

Wilk KE, Macrina LC, Arrigo C. Passive range of motion characteristics in the overhead baseball pitcher and their implications for rehabilitation. *Clin Orthop Relat Res.* 2012;470(6):1586–1594.

Wright RW, Steger-May K, Wasserlauf BL, O'Neal ME, Weinberg BW, Paletta GA. Elbow range of motion in professional baseball pitchers. *Am J Sports Med.* 2006;34(2):190–193.

25 Prevention in Youth Sports (Early Sports Specialization): Injuries of the Throwing Shoulder

JULIE AGEL, MA, ATC

Introduction

- Eighty-seven percent of their parents report worrying about injury, making this a public health concern.
- Education of everyone responsible for protecting the health of the young athlete, including the parents, coach, and sport's governing body, is critical.
- Specific to youth athletes is the additional concern of growth plate disruption.
- Sports inherently have risk of injury. Some of this risk is unavoidable, and some of this risk is modifiable.

Sports inherently have risk of injury. Some of this risk is unavoidable, and some of this risk is modifiable. As early as 1993, the American College of Sports Medicine (ACSM) reported that up to half of sports-related injuries are preventable (Anonymous, 1993).

Upper extremity injuries range from mild soft tissue inflammation to fractures. Throwing sports, with their repetitive nature, add the complexity of overuse injuries. Specific to youth athletes is the additional concern of growth plate disruption.

Thirty-six million kids, ages 5 to 18 years, are estimated to play organized sports each year. Eighty-seven percent of their parents report worrying about injury, making this a public health concern (http://www.statisticbrain.com/youth-sports-statistics). Youth sport participation continues to rise, with one survey by the National Council of Youth Sports (http://www.ncys.org/pdfs/2008/2008-ncys-market-research-report.pdf) showing steep rises from 1987 to 2005 coupled with large increases in the number of girls participating.

The reasons children participate vary widely: Some participate because they are having fun, some because their friends do it, some because their parents want them to, and some because they believe it is a pathway to professional sports with its associated fame and fortune. The pressure on these children to excel at sports, particularly in one chosen sport, has created a group of injuries, primarily overuse in nature, that are believed to be the result of this push to specialize in one sport early in life.

Early sports specialization, defined in a recent consensus statement (LaPrade et al, 2016), include youth who participate in organized sports for more than 8 months of the year, participate in just one sport, and are prepubertal. Although there is no evidence that participating in only one sport year round starting at an early age will make an individual a better athlete, the expansion of travel and representative side teams for young athletes continues to push this trend.

Baseball (Popchak et al, 2015), specifically pitchers, is the throwing sport that has attracted the most attention in both the scientific and lay media, but other throwing sports have similar concerns, particularly in field sports (javelin, hammer, and discus), football (quarterbacks), and softball. In all of these sports, repetitive motions in one shoulder in one direction with large amounts of force are required, and large amounts of practice time are common. As an example, 53 youth windmill softball pitchers underwent three-dimensional high-speed video analysis (Werner et al, 2005). These young pitchers were found to generate forces around their elbows and shoulders similar to those of college pitchers. This puts them at high risk for overuse injuries, particularly around the biceps labrum complex, with the added worry about deformation of their bones and growth plate injuries.

In response to the well-documented rising trend of ulnar collateral ligament reconstructions in youth baseball pitchers, which reports more than 2 million participants (http://www.littleleague.org/Page56014.aspx) in the Little League system (most recent numbers available are through 2006), organizations such as the American Sports Medicine Institute have partnered with Major League Baseball and USA Baseball to provide guidance through programs such as Pitch Smart (http://m.mlb.com/pitchsmart) to reduce the risk of injury. This program provides education for coaches, players, and parents about potential risk factors. It also contains guidelines by age group for allowable pitch counts and rest days.

Outside of Pitch Smart, little exists in the way of formal prevention programs for injuries to the throwing shoulder in youth sports. There is no corollary to the FIFA Marc 11+ (http://f-marc.com/11plus/home) (Leonard & Hutchinson, 2010; Mautner & Blazuk, 2015; Shanley & Thigpen, 2013) program, designed as a warm-up program based on core stability and eccentric hamstring strength and known to reduce injury for upper extremity throwing shoulder prevention (Soligard et al, 2008).

A comprehensive list of available injury research prevention in youth sports covers 31 studies, including 17 randomized controlled clinical trials, across a variety of sports, but only three included sports with throwers, and they focused exclusively on lower extremity injuries (Emery et al, 2008).

There are anecdotal recommendations available on numerous websites, but none are based on science. Guidelines for youth discus throwers are available online (Rothery, 2016) that divide youth athletes by age, but nothing in those guidelines discusses limitations to practice or competition. Similarly, a variety of recommendations are available about softball pitching but nothing that has been formally developed and evaluated. In 2011, the National Athletic Trainers Association published a position statement on Prevention of Pediatric Overuse Injuries (Valovich McLeod et al, 2011) that recommended greater injury surveillance to identify risk factors and modifications of sport training and conditioning programs in conjunction with coaching education.

To prevent injuries to the throwing shoulder, the most important first step during a preparticipation examination or injury evaluation is a good participation history upon presentation. A clear understanding of the cumulative amount of time spent participating in a given sport, particularly in the same position or practicing the same skill, is critical. Asking questions about level of competition, time spent in competition, and frequency of competition provides invaluable information.

Sports participation has been shown to be hugely important for the maintenance of healthy lives both physically and mentally (Women's Sports Foundation, 2009). Sports participation can be done with an appropriate mix of structured and free play. Early warning signs of too much competition should be part of any physical examination; these signs include excessive complaints of aches and pains, too many visits, and reluctance to attend sporting events. Sports participation should be encouraged, but the level and amount of time spent in competition should be carefully monitored to reduce the risk of injury to throwing shoulders. A conversation with both the athlete and the responsible adult is critical if the time spent participating in structured sports appears excessive. Rest is a critical component of successful sports participation. Free play is another critical part of successful sports participation and is important for social as well as physical reasons.

Growth plate injuries are specific to youth and need careful monitoring because their impact is lifelong. Growth plate injuries are believed to result from skeletally immature bone having excessive repetitive motion (Mair et al, 2004). It is important to screen athletes who are at risk for physeal injury to rule out growth plate injury or changes at the time of examination.

Conditioning programs are often absent or inadequate in youth sports. Pre- or in-season conditioning is not something that many youth teams focus on nor do they have the coaching staff to properly supervise. The Marc11+ program takes 20 minutes a day. Recommendations for preseason conditioning may provide an avenue for injury prevention. As young athletes learn new skills that require motor control and strength in positions they are unaccustomed to, conditioning can help reduce the risk of injury. Throwing sports are a particular risk factor because most youths do not have much experience with overhead activities, particularly in the extreme ranges of motion required for throwing, especially with a weighted object (e.g., ball, discus) in one's hand. A conditioning program that focuses on shoulder strengthening above 90 degrees and eccentric as well as concentric motion bilaterally will impact injury rates due to unidirectional motion. In addition, many youth teams may have a policy of not cutting athletes so that some young athletes may be in a sport that is not appropriate for their body type. For young athletes, a recommendation for a different sport may be the most helpful way to reduce injury.

The most important factors in prevention of injuries to the throwing shoulder are proper technique and appropriate control over the amount of time spent practicing and competing in the sport. Coaching, parent, and athlete education are critical components in successful reduction in the risk of injuries to the throwing shoulder. Educational opportunities are plentiful. Each sport's governing body has educational programs. Coaching associations offer certifications that all include safe sports participation lectures and youth sports parents are often required to sign forms indicating that they will assist their children in safe sports participation. The National Alliance for Youth Sports (http://www.nays.org) was started because of concern about the damage to youths from volunteer coaches.

Injury prevention has to start on the level of the individual athlete, with parents and youths understanding the need to recognize limits. Although large-scale randomized controlled trials can be conducted to determine if a given strategy may reduce rates of injury over time, nothing is more important than sitting with an individual child and fully understanding her or his level of participation and fitness for the sport. Youth sports are unlikely to have access to appropriate medical care that can supervise formal prevention programs, so individual plans have the most benefit.

References

Anonymous. Current comment from the American College of Sports Medicine. August 1993—"The prevention of sport injuries of children and adolescents." *Med Sci Sports Exerc.* 1993;25(suppl 8):1–7.

Emery C, Roy T-O, Hagel B, Macpherson A, Nettel-Aguirre A. Injury prevention in youth sport. In: Caine D, Purcell L, eds. *Injury in Pediatric and Adolescent Sports: Epidemiology, Treatment and Prevention.* New York: Springer; 2008:208.

LaPrade RF, Agel J, Baker J, Brenner JS, et al. AOSSM Early Sport Specialization Consensus Statement. *Orthop J Sports Med.* 2016;4(4):1–8.

Leonard J, Hutchinson MR. Shoulder injuries in skeletally immature throwers: review and current thoughts. *Br J Sports Med.* 2010;44(5):306–310.

Mair SD, Uhl TL, Robbe RG, Brindle KA. Physeal changes and range-of-motion differences in the dominant shoulders of skeletally immature baseball players. *J Shoulder Elbow Surg.* 2004;13(5):487–491.

Mautner K, Blazuk J. Overuse throwing injuries in skeletally immature athletes—diagnosis, treatment, and preventions. *Curr Sports Med Rep.* 2015;14(3):209–214.

Popchak A, Burnett T, Weber N, Boninger M. Factors related to injury in youth and adolescent baseball pitching, with an eye toward prevention. *Am J Phys Med Rehabil.* 2015;94(5):395–409.

Rothery C. Discus: basics for little athletics. Greenwith, Australia: Golden Grove Little Athletics; 2016. http://www.goldengrovelac.org.au/forms/discusbasics.pdf.

Shanley E, Thigpen C. Throwing injuries in the adolescent athlete. *Int J Sports Phys Ther.* 2013;8(5):630–640.

Soligard T, Myklebust G, Steffen K, et al. Comprehensive warm-up programme to prevent injuries in young female footballers: cluster randomised controlled trial. *BMJ.* 2008;337:a2469.

Valovich McLeod TC, Decoster LC, Loud KJ, et al. National Athletic Trainers' Association position statement: prevention of pediatric overuse injuries. *J Athl Train.* 2011;46(2). 206-220.

Werner SL, Guido JA, McNeice RP, Richardson JL, Delude NA, Stewart GW. Biomechanics of youth windmill softball pitching. *Am J Sports Med.* 2005;33(4):552–560.

Women's Sports Foundation. Women's Sports & Fitness Facts & Statistics. Women's Sports Foundation; 2009. https://www.womenssportsfoundation.org/sitecore/content/home/research/articles-and-reports/athletes/~/media/PDFs/WSF%20Research%20Reports/WSF%20FACTS%20March%202009.pdf.

PART **2**

ELBOW

PART OUTLINE

SECTION **IX**

Elbow Instability

SECTION OUTLINE

26 Medial: Ulnar Collateral Ligament Injury

26-26A EPIDEMIOLOGY, ANATOMY, MECHANISM OF INJURY, HISTORY, PHYSICAL EXAMINATION, AND IMAGING

CHRISTOPHER S. AHMAD, MD and JUSTIN L. HODGINS, MD

Introduction

- Injury to the medial ulnar collateral ligament (MUCL) of the elbow is a debilitating condition primarily affecting throwing athletes.
- The MUCL complex provides the primary restraint to valgus stress in the elbow together with dynamic muscular support and the posterior bony articulations.
- Most MUCL injuries are the result of the cumulative valgus stress placed on the medial elbow during repetitive overhead throwing maneuvers, and clear associations have been made with overuse and risk of injury.
- Careful history and physical examination, including the presence of tenderness along the MUCL and a positive moving valgus stress test result, are sensitive and specific for MUCL injury
- Athletes with suspected MUCL injury should undergo either plain magnetic resonance imaging (MRI) or MR arthrographic studies to characterize the ligament

Epidemiology

Overuse injuries are common in overhead athletes, particularly in elite baseball, where throwing places tremendous valgus torque across the elbow and MUCL. As such, competitive baseball exhibits the highest incidence of MUCL injury and surgical reconstruction (Cain et al, 2010; Conte et al, 2015). However, MUCL injury has also been reported in other overhead throwing sports, including javelin, tennis, and American football (Dodson et al, 2006; Jobe et al, 1986; Waris, 1946). Before popularization by Dr. Frank Jobe, the first description of MUCL rupture was a review of 17 elite javelin throwers in 1946 (Waris, 1946). Although rare, MUCL injury has been reported in professional football (Dodson et al, 2010). A review of the National Football League Injury Surveillance System (NFLISS) from 1994 to 2008 identified 10 MUCL injuries in quarterbacks, primarily as a result of acute trauma. Other than these few accounts, MUCL tears and subsequent reconstruction are injuries exclusive to competitive baseball, and in particular, elite pitchers.

Clear associations have been demonstrated between the number of innings pitched in a calendar year and the chance of sustaining a serious elbow injury in youth baseball (Fleisig et al, 2011). The competitive culture of youth baseball may encourage talented players to participate on multiple teams and showcases, therefore throwing more frequently and with greater intensity at younger ages. A prospective cohort study of 481 youth pitchers over 10 years of play identified that players who pitched more than 100 innings per calendar year had a 3.5 times greater chance of sustaining a serious injury (Fleisig et al, 2011). A similar investigation of adolescent pitchers described overuse as the main cause of player injury, noting a 500% increased risk for surgery for players pitching more than 8 months per year and a 400% increased risk for those throwing more than 80 pitches per game (Kerut et al, 2008; Olsen et al, 2006). These trends have led to the implementation of injury prevention programs with emphasis on public education to the risks of overuse throwing injuries and the importance of adhering to pitch-count guidelines.

Despite these public health campaigns, reports suggest that the number of MUCL injuries and reconstructions continue to rise, with an estimated 10-fold increase in the first decade of the 21st century (Cain et al, 2010; Dugas, 2010; Fortenbaugh et al, 2009). Evidence also suggests an increase in the frequency of MUCL injury and reconstruction in younger athletes. A large review of high school baseball pitchers identified a 50% increase in MUCL reconstruction in players ages 15 to 19 reported by a single surgeon (Petty et al, 2004). Similarly, a database of a large privately insured U.S. population demonstrated significant increases in MUCL reconstructions in patients ages 15 to 19 years from 2007 to 2011 (Erickson et al, 2015). The estimated annual incidence of MUCL reconstruction was 3.96 per 100,000 patients for the overall population, and there was a significant increase in the number of procedures performed over time. A subsequent investigation using a New York State database demonstrated a threefold increase in the incidence of MUCL reconstruction from 2002 to 2011, in particular in patients ages 17 to 19 years (Hodgins et al, 2016).

Debate still exists regarding the relationship between pitch type and risk of medial elbow injury in youth baseball. Previously, the altered kinematics required to generate the throwing motion of breaking balls (curveball, slider) was linked to an increased risk in shoulder and elbow pain in adolescent pitchers (Lyman et al, 2002). A follow-up study evaluating the risk factors for shoulder and elbow injuries requiring surgery in adolescent pitchers failed to identify a correlation between injury and onset of throwing breaking-type pitches but indicated a 250% increased risk for those who could throw a fast ball faster than 85 mph (Olsen et al, 2006). Furthermore, biomechanical testing using three-dimensional motion analysis has demonstrated that the curveball produces less elbow torque than does the fastball in youth pitchers (Dun et al, 2008).

A major concern now exists regarding the increasing number of MUCL injuries and surgeries being performed within Major League Baseball (MLB), with the phenomenon being described as an "epidemic" of MUCL reconstruction (Bruce & Andrews, 2014). Studies using data from the MLB Disabled List (DL) have shown that medial elbow injuries represent 16% to 22% of all player injuries (Conte et al, 2001; Posner et al, 2011). The most recent investigation of both minor and major league baseball players estimated that as many as 10% of all players and 16% of pitchers have undergone MUCL reconstruction (Conte et al, 2015). The prevalence of MUCL reconstruction in nonpitching position players was substantially lower (3%). The rate of MUCL reconstruction was also higher among MLB pitchers compared with minor league players and was highest in older players. A separate study identified higher pitch velocity as the most predictive factor for MUCL reconstruction in MLB pitchers and increased player weight and younger age as secondary predictors (Chalmers et al, 2016).

Anatomy

The MUCL complex provides the primary restraint to valgus stress in the elbow and consists of an oblique, posterior, and anterior bundle (Dugas et al, 2007; Floris et al, 1998; Jobe, 1986) (Fig. 26A.1). The oblique or transverse ligament has its origin and insertion on the ulna and together with the posterior capsular thickening provides minimal stability to the elbow (Floris et al, 1998). The anterior bundle of the MUCL is the strongest component of the complex and the main restraint to valgus stress (Callaway et al, 1997; Hotchkiss & Weiland, 1987; O'Driscoll et al, 1992). It originates on the anterior-inferior surface of the medial humeral epicondyle and inserts on the sublime tubercle of the ulna (Hechtman et al, 1998). The anterior bundle is functionally composed of anterior and posterior bands that provide reciprocal function in resisting valgus stress between 20 and 120 degrees of elbow flexion (Farrow et al, 2011). The anterior band is active at lesser degrees up to 90 degrees, and the posterior band provides assistive restraint from 60 degrees to higher degrees of flexion (Floris et al, 1998).

In addition to the MUCL complex, dynamic muscular support and the bony articulations of the posterior elbow compartment contribute to medial stability. The fibers of the flexor carpi ulnaris (FCU) are intimately attached to the origin of the medial epicondyle and optimally positioned directly in line with the MUCL for contractile support (Conway et al, 1992). Cadaver biomechanical testing has demonstrated the FCU as the primary dynamic contributor to valgus stability in the elbow and the flexor digitorum superficialis as a secondary stabilizer (Conway et al, 1992; Park & Ahmad, 2004). Clinical electromyographic analysis has also demonstrated reduced forearm flexor muscle activity in pitchers with MUCL injuries, further suggesting the role of protective dynamic muscle activity (Sisto et al, 1987). The importance of the flexor-pronator mass is also appreciated

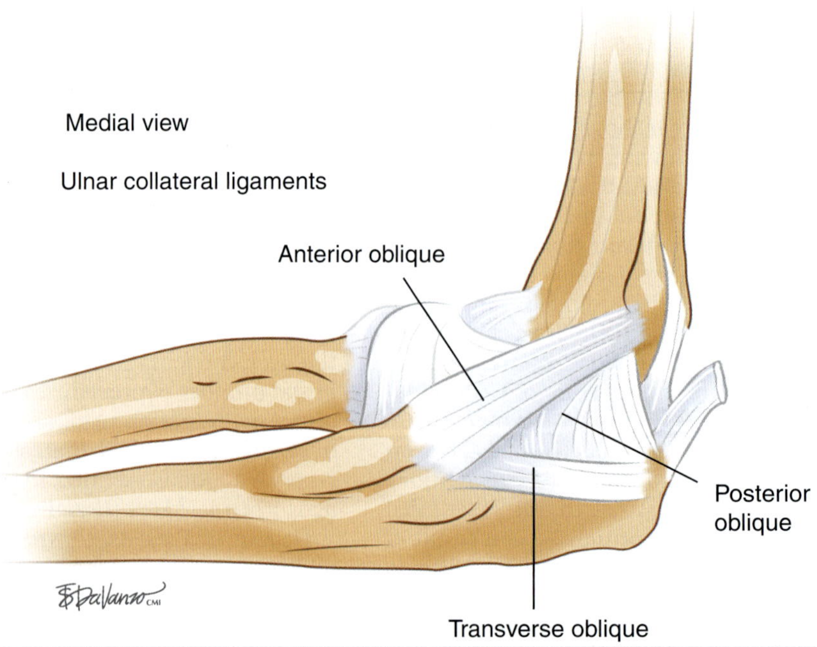

Fig. 26A.1 Normal anatomy of the medial ulnar collateral ligament complex. (Adapted from Conway JE, Jobe FW, Glousman RE, Pink M. Medial instability of the elbow in throwing athletes. Treatment by repair or reconstruction of the ulnar collateral ligament. *J Bone Joint Surg Am.* 1992;74(1): 67-83.)

by several authors, who advocate limiting dissection using muscle splitting techniques during MUCL reconstruction and recognize the importance of dynamic muscular rehabilitation during the postoperative period (Smith et al, 1996; Thompson et al, 2001).

The bony articulations of the posterior compartment share an intricate relationship with the soft tissues of the medial elbow. As the MUCL complex is stressed during valgus loading, the lateral radiocapitellar articulation undergoes compensatory compression. Biomechanical analysis has demonstrated that sequential partial resection of the posteromedial aspect of the olecranon results in a stepwise increase in elbow valgus angulation (Kamineni et al, 2003). Therefore both the olecranon and the MUCL contribute to valgus stability. This has also been observed clinically, where 25% of professional baseball players who underwent olecranon debridement eventually required MUCL reconstruction in a large series (Andrews & Timmerman, 1995). Testing in the cadaver model has also shown that strain in the MUCL is increased with increasing posteromedial resection of the olecranon beyond 3 mm, further suggesting that aggressive olecranon debridement may place the MUCL at risk for future injury (Kamineni et al, 2004).

Mechanism of Injury

The majority of MUCL injuries are the result of the cumulative valgus stress placed on the medial elbow during repetitive overhead throwing maneuvers (Jobe et al, 1986). Biomechanical studies have shown the valgus torque generated in the late cocking and acceleration phases of throwing can exceed 64 N-m and up to 60 N-m with a tennis serve, but the ultimate tensile strength of cadaveric MUCL specimens is only 33 N-m (Fleisig et al, 1995, 2003; Werner et al, 1993). The repetitive near-tensile failure loads result in microtrauma to the anterior band of the MUCL, leading to attenuation and ultimately failure. When the forearm flexors are fatigued or injured, the elbow loses the dynamic muscular supports, placing additional stress on the MUCL. Therefore flexor-pronator conditioning is an essential component of MUCL injury prevention programs.

Although rare, MUCL injury can occur as a result of direct trauma in contact athletes.

A total of 10 MUCL injuries were documented in professional quarterbacks over a 14-year period in the National Football League (NFL), where 70% of injuries were the result of traumatic contact and only 20% associated with a throwing motion (Dodson et al, 2010). The nature of these acute traumatic MUCL tears was attributed to the high contact loads experienced at the elbow by football players as opposed to the chronic repetitive injuries seen in baseball pitchers. Fundamental differences also exist in the passing motion of football quarterbacks compared with baseball pitching because the increased weight of the football prevents the extreme angular velocities and torque across the elbow seen in pitching (Fleisig et al, 1996; Kelly et al, 2002; Wick et al, 1991). Kinematic testing has also demonstrated reduced rotational velocities over a narrower shoulder range of motion during the football pass, thereby reducing valgus stress on the medial elbow (Fleisig et al, 1996; Kelly et al, 2002; Wick et al, 1991).

History and Physical Examination

A thorough history and physical examination are critical in evaluating MUCL injuries, as treatment recommendations rely heavily on a variety of patient- and injury-specific factors. Player age, type of sport, position, competitive level, future aspirations, willingness of the player to change sport or position, and perceptions of surgery should be considered (Anakwenze et al, 2014). Specifically for throwing athletes, any recent changes in throwing accuracy, velocity, and stamina before injury should be documented. The time of onset of symptoms in relation to ball release is also important because up to 85% of pitchers experience pain during the acceleration phase of throwing compared with fewer than 25% during the deceleration phase of throwing with MUCL injury (Conway et al, 1992) (Fig. 26A.2). Players may report a sudden event with sharp pain in the medial elbow accompanied with a "pop"; others may have a gradual progression of pain associated with changes in pitching speed and control. Duration of symptoms, prior episodes, and the exact location of the pain should be documented.

Injury risk factors should be assessed, such as a history of overuse (particularly in skeletally immature athletes), prior elbow surgery (arthroscopic posteromedial decompression), or change in pitching mechanics. Symptoms of valgus extension overload (VEO), including posteromedial elbow pain during either the acceleration phase or more commonly the deceleration phase of throwing, should be assessed because MUCL insufficiency may be overshadowed in these athletes. Limited extension and mechanical catching may also be present with VEO as a result of impinging osteophytes, chondromalacia, or loose bodies. Ulnar neuritis associated with MUCL insufficiency can manifest as paresthesia radiating from the elbow to the ring and small fingers. Cold intolerance, numbness or tingling in the hand, and difficulties with grip strength or dropping objects may also be present (Dugas & Weiland, 2000).

Physical examination should include a detailed evaluation of the entire upper extremity and assess problems within the core and kinetic chain. Careful attention should be given to the ipsilateral shoulder as it is not uncommon for elbow and shoulder pathology to coincide in elite throwing athletes. The presence of a glenohumeral internal rotation deficit (GIRD) and reduced total rotational motion (TRM) have been identified as independent risk factors for MUCL injury (Garrison et al, 2012). The scapula should be assessed with respect to muscle tone and scapulothoracic rhythm because scapular dysfunction is often present in throwing athletes (Kibler & Sciascia, 2004). The presence of a flexion contracture with a lack of full elbow extension is also common in mature throwers and may be asymptomatic and should be compared with the contralateral limb.

The medial aspect of the elbow should be inspected for swelling and ecchymosis and palpated for tenderness along the course of the MUCL from its origin to insertion. Chronic tears may not have associated tenderness, and in acute tears, tenderness often abates with rest. Local MUCL tenderness should be distinguished from flexor-pronator injury. The absence of pain with resisted wrist flexion and pronation and the presence of pain posterior to the flexor-pronator origin can help to differentiate (Chen et al, 2001). Ulnar nerve examination should include motor and sensory

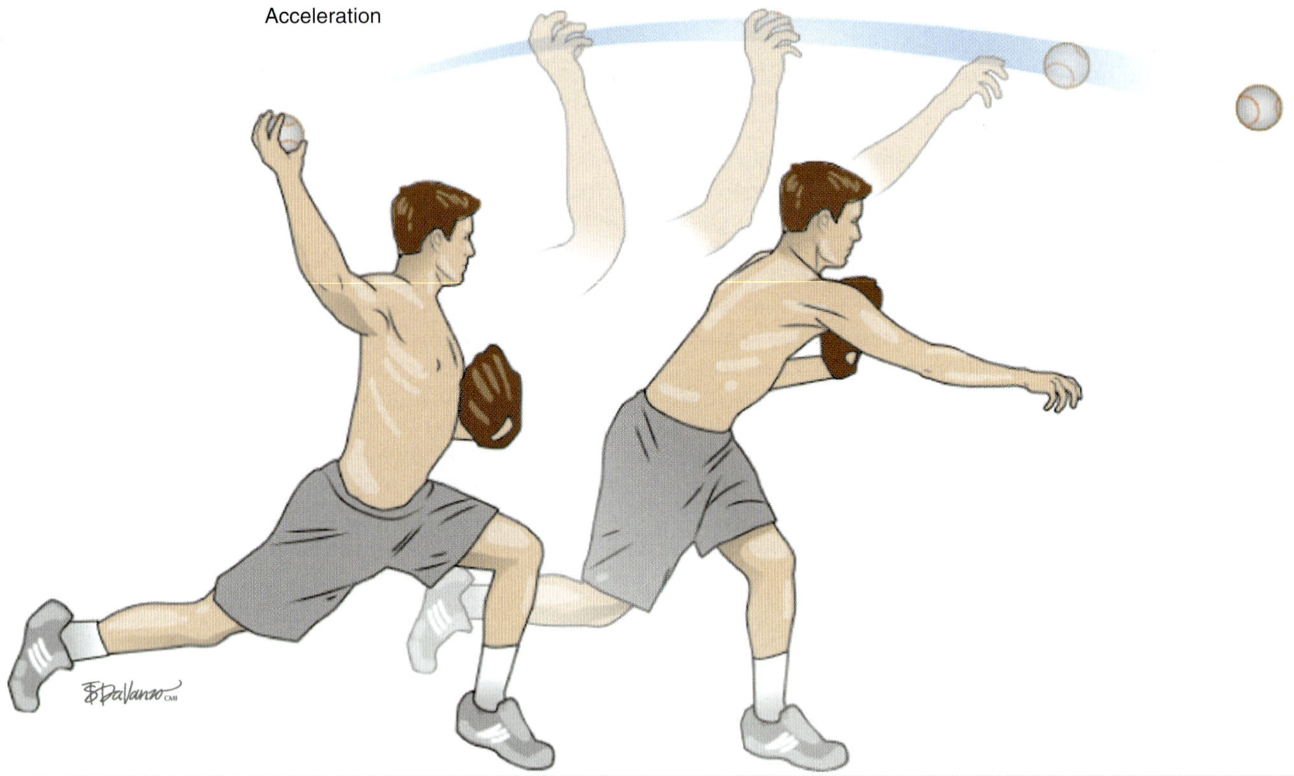

Fig. 26A.2 **Symptoms of ulnar collateral ligament insufficiency occur primarily during the late cocking and early acceleration phases of the throwing motion.** (Adapted from Ahmad CS, ElAttrache NS. Treatment of medial ulnar collateral ligament injuries in athletes. In *Morrey's The Elbow and Its Disorders*. 4th edition. Philadelphia: WB Saunders; 2008:659.)

testing and provocative maneuvers such as the Tinel test for direct nerve irritation and dynamic instability with elbow motion. The presence of a palmaris longus tendon should be determined if MUCL reconstruction is anticipated.

Valgus instability is assessed with the elbow flexed between 20 and 30 degrees to unlock the olecranon from its fossa (Anakwenze et al, 2014). The valgus stress test may be performed with the patient upright or lying supine as the examiner applies a valgus force, attempting to elicit painful opening of the medial ulnohumeral joint. Isolated anterior band injury can produce opening at 30 to 40 degrees of elbow flexion, but a global MUCL injury may demonstrate opening at 80 to 90 degrees of flexion (Floris et al, 1998). The milking maneuver is performed by the examiner pulling on the patient's thumb to create valgus stress with the patient's forearm supinated and elbow flexed beyond 90 degrees. A positive test result elicits pain, instability, and apprehension and indicates injury to the posterior band of the MUCL (Chen et al, 2001). The moving valgus stress test is the most sensitive and specific for MUCL pathology and is performed by applying a valgus torque while the elbow is repeatedly flexed and extended (Field et al, 1995) (Fig. 26A.3). The test result is considered positive if pain is reproduced at the MUCL and is usually maximal between 70 and 120 degrees of elbow flexion in an attempt to recreate the early acceleration and late cocking phases of throwing.

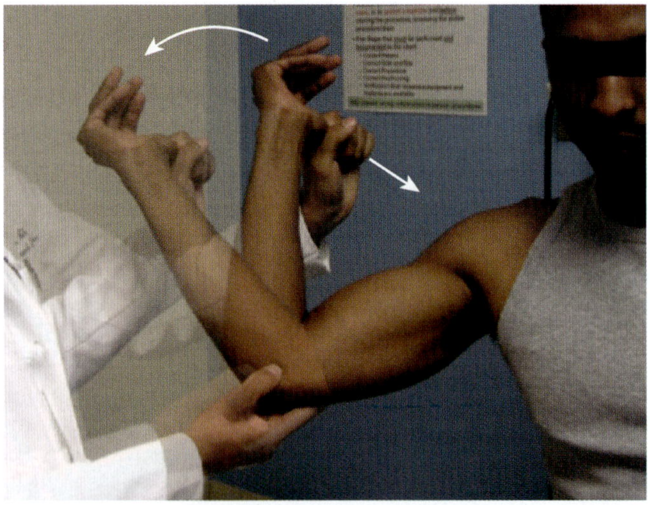

Fig. 26A.3 **Moving valgus stress test. The examiner flexes and extends the elbow while applying a valgus force. Reproducible pain at the medial ulnar collateral ligament (MUCL) in the arc between 80 and 120 degrees indicates MUCL injury.** (Reprinted with permission from Ahmad CS: Elbow Injuries and the Throwing Athlete, in Galatz LM (ed): *Orthopaedic Knowledge Update: Shoulder and Elbow 3*. Rosemont, IL, American Academy of Orthopaedic Surgeons, 2008, pp 451-460.)

Imaging

Standard anteroposterior, lateral, and oblique radiographs of the elbow are first obtained when evaluating for MUCL injury. In the presence of chronic injury, ossification along the path of the MUCL may be noted (Fig. 26A.4). The presence of olecranon osteophytes, posteromedial joint space narrowing, and loose bodies suggest underlying VEO, arthritis, or both. Radiographs can also identify other abnormalities, including bone deficiencies at the sublime tubercle or medial epicondyle from prior

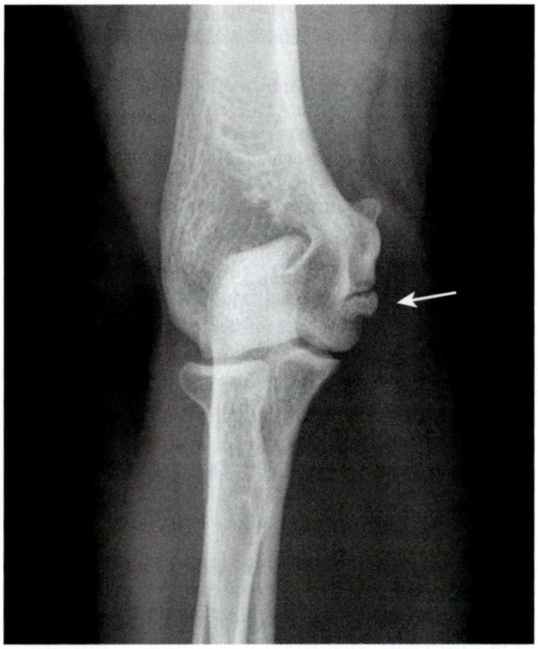

Fig. 26A.4 Anteroposterior radiograph of the elbow demonstrating ossification of the medial ulnar collateral ligament origin *(arrow)*.

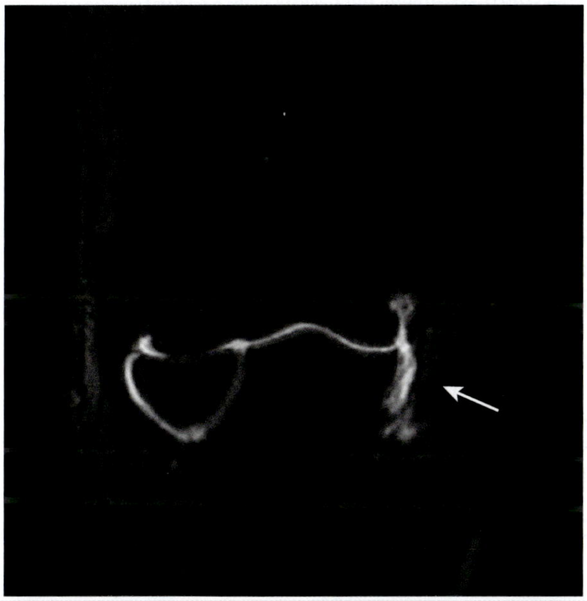

Fig. 26A.5 Magnetic resonance imaging arthrogram demonstrating medial ulnar collateral ligament discontinuity and dye extravasation *(arrow)*.

fracture, altered epicondylar morphology, or enthesopathy at the sublime tubercle, each potentially influencing treatment and reconstruction technique (Anakwenze et al, 2014). Computed tomography with three-dimensional reconstruction can further delineate osseous pathology around the elbow and help plan for future osteophyte resection.

All patients with suggestive history and positive examination findings undergo MRI to characterize the MUCL. Conventional MRI studies are capable of identifying ligament thickening from chronic injury and large full-thickness tears. MR arthrography, enhanced with intraarticular gadolinium contrast, improves the diagnostic ability for partial-thickness tears (Cotton et al, 1997; Hill et al, 2000). Therefore when standard MRI is inconclusive, the preferred imaging modality is MR arthrography using a high-field closed magnet with narrow slice images (Fig. 26A.5). The "T-sign" is seen where a pathologic volume of contrast dye leaks down along the sublime tubercle but is contained under the superficial fibers of a partially torn MUCL (Timmerman et al, 1994). However, anatomical studies have characterized the insertion of the MUCL at 2.8 mm, on average, from the articular surface of the ulna, and thus some T-signs may be normal (Dugas et al, 2007). MRI can also identify concomitant edema and injury to the flexor-pronator origin as well as posteromedial ulnohumeral chondromalacia (Shahabpour et al, 2008).

References

Ahmad CS. Elbow injuries and the throwing athlete. In: Galatz LM, ed. *Orthopaedic Knowledge Update: Shoulder and Elbow 3*. Rosemont, IL: American Academy of Orthopaedic Surgeons; 2008:451–460.

Ahmad CS, ElAttrache NS. Treatment of medial ulnar collateral ligament injuries in athletes. In: *Morrey's The Elbow and Its Disorders*. 4th ed. Philadelphia: WB Saunders; 2008:659.

Anakwenze O, Iyengar J, Ahmad C. Treatment of medial collateral ligament injuries of the elbow with use of the "Tommy John" operation: indications and results. *JBJS Rev*. 2014;2(6):e3.

Andrews JR, Timmerman LA. Outcome of elbow surgery in professional baseball players. *Am J Sports Med*. 1995;23:407.

Bruce JR, Andrews JR. Ulnar collateral ligament injuries in the throwing athlete. *J Am Acad Orthop Surg*. 2014;5:315–325.

Cain EL Jr, Andrews JR, Dugas JR, et al. Outcome of ulnar collateral ligament reconstruction of the elbow in 1281 athletes: results in 743 athletes with minimum 2-year follow-up. *Am J Sports Med*. 2010;38(12):2426–2434.

Callaway GH, Field LD, Deng XH, et al. Biomechanical evaluation of the medial collateral ligament of the elbow. *J Bone Joint Surg Am*. 1997;79:1223.

Chalmers PN, Erickson BJ, Ball B, Romeo A, Verma NN. Fastball pitch velocity helps predict ulnar collateral ligament reconstruction in major league baseball pitchers. *Am J Sports Med*. 2016;44(8):2130–2135.

Chen FS, Rokito AS, Jobe FW. Medial elbow problems in the overhead-throwing athlete. *J Am Acad Orthop Surg*. 2001;9(2):99–113.

Conte SA, Fleisig GS, Dines JS, et al. Prevalence of ulnar collateral ligament surgery in professional baseball players. *Am J Sports Med*. 2015;43(7):1764–1769.

Conte S, Requa RK, Garrick JG. Disability days in Major League Baseball. *Am J Sports Med*. 2001;29(4):431–436.

Conway JE, Jobe FW, Glousman RE, Pink M. Medial instability of the elbow in throwing athletes. Treatment by repair or reconstruction of the ulnar collateral ligament. *J Bone Joint Surg Am*. 1992;74:67.

Cotton A, Jacobson J, Brossmann J, et al. Collateral ligaments of the elbow: conventional MR imaging and MR arthrography with coronal oblique plane and elbow flexion. *Radiology*. 1997;204:806.

Dodson CC, Thomas A, Dines JS, et al. Medial ulnar collateral ligament reconstruction of the elbow in throwing athletes. *Am J Sports Med*. 2006;34:1926–1932.

Dodson CC, Slenker N, Cohen SB, Ciccotti MG, DeLuca P. Ulnar collateral ligament injuries of the elbow in professional football quarterbacks. *J Shoulder Elbow Surg*. 2010;19(8):1276–1280.

Dugas JR. Valgus extension overload: diagnosis and treatment. *Clin Sports Med*. 2010;29(4):645–654.

Dugas JR, Ostrander RV, Cain EL, Kingsley D, Andrews JR. Anatomy of the anterior bundle of the ulnar collateral ligament. *J Shoulder Elbow Surg*. 2007;16(5):657–660.

Dugas JR, Weiland AJ. Vascular pathology in the throwing athlete. *Hand Clin*. 2000;16:477–485.

Dun S, Loftice J, Fleisig GS, Kingsley D, Andrews JR. A biomechanical comparison of youth baseball pitches: is the curveball potentially harmful? *Am J Sports Med*. 2008;36(4):686–692.

Erickson BJ, Nwachukwu BU, Rosas S, et al. Trends in medial ulnar collateral ligament reconstruction in the United States: a retrospective review of a large private-payer database from 2007 to 2011. *Am J Sports Med*. 2015;43(7):1770–1774.

The posterolateral portal is used as the "viewing portal," and the posteromedial portal becomes the "working portal" when addressing the pathology associated with posteromedial impingement. The soft tissue is cleared with a 4.5-mm arthroscopic shaver and decompression of the osteophytes is done with a hooded 5.5-mm arthroscopic bur (Fig. 26B.3). The elbow is placed in near full extension to assist in debridement of the osteophyte while flexing of the elbow allows for evaluation of the humeral articular cartilage. Often, a "kissing lesion" on the trochlea can be seen and may need to be debrided. Radiographs or computed tomography (CT) scans (or both) are used preoperatively to evaluate the posteromedial osteophytes and should be present and viewed in the operating room before and during the operation. Overzealous resection of the osteophytes can preload the UCL. Care should be taken to resect only pathologic bone while leaving normal bone. Often, a fibrous union can be seen on radiographs or CT. A banana blade can be used to enter the fibrous union and dislodge the pathological osteophyte. Furthermore, axial traction with the elbow at 90 degrees of flexion can be used to assist in resection of the osteophyte. This technique creates a few millimeters of space between the olecranon and humerus, which helps define the underlying articular cartilage of the trochlea. After completion of the decompression, the arthroscope is placed in the posteromedial portal and the posterior compartment is evaluated for any loose bodies and any bony pieces that came loose from the decompression.

The skin portals are closed with #3-0 Ethilon (Ethicon, Somerville, NJ) suture, and a full-length compressive, sterile dressing is applied. The patient is placed in a simple sling and educated on range of motion (ROM) exercises of the shoulder, wrist, and hand. Often, a medium Hemovac drain is placed through the anterolateral portal for the first 24 hours. Gentle active and active-assisted exercises are begun immediately with passive ROM started on postoperative day 5. Aggressive early ROM exercises can cause drainage through the posterior portals and a sinus can potentially develop or even a postoperative wound infection. Motion exercises are progressed through week 3 until further strengthening and eccentric exercises are started. At 6 weeks, an interval-throwing program is started with return to full time activities by 12 to 16 weeks.

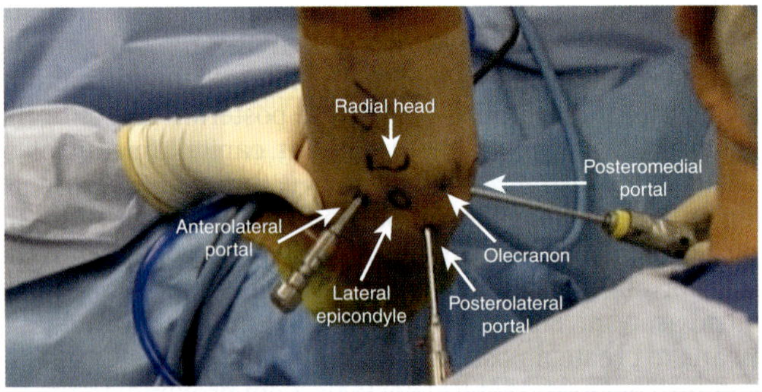

Fig. 26B.2 Portal placement.

OPEN DECOMPRESSION

The standard operative setup and approach to the elbow used for a UCL reconstruction as previously described is used for an open decompression and excision of posteromedial osteophytes. Before drilling the ulnar and humeral tunnels and after the ulnar nerve has been completely mobilized, a 1- to 2-cm vertical arthrotomy is made posterior to the posterior band of the UCL from the medial epicondyle to the tip of the olecranon. This allows for retraction and complete visualization of the posteromedial olecranon osteophytes from the medial side. A one-quarter inch osteotome is used to excise the osteophytes in addition to a 4.0-mm round bur (Stryker) for fine-tuning the posteromedial olecranon. The ulnar nerve is protected with army-navy retractors, and the elbow is placed in approximately 30 degrees of flexion with a valgus stress. Copious bulb irrigation is used to clear the joint of bone debris and improve visualization. The elbow is brought through an ROM to ensure adequate motion and elimination of bony impingement. The arthrotomy is closed with #1 absorbable braided suture before continuing with UCL reconstruction. The postoperative course is dictated by the UCL reconstruction protocol.

Posteromedial Impingement Outcomes

Both arthroscopic and open decompression of posteromedial impingement have reported favorable results in the literature (Andrews & Carson, 1985, 1995; Cain, 2010;

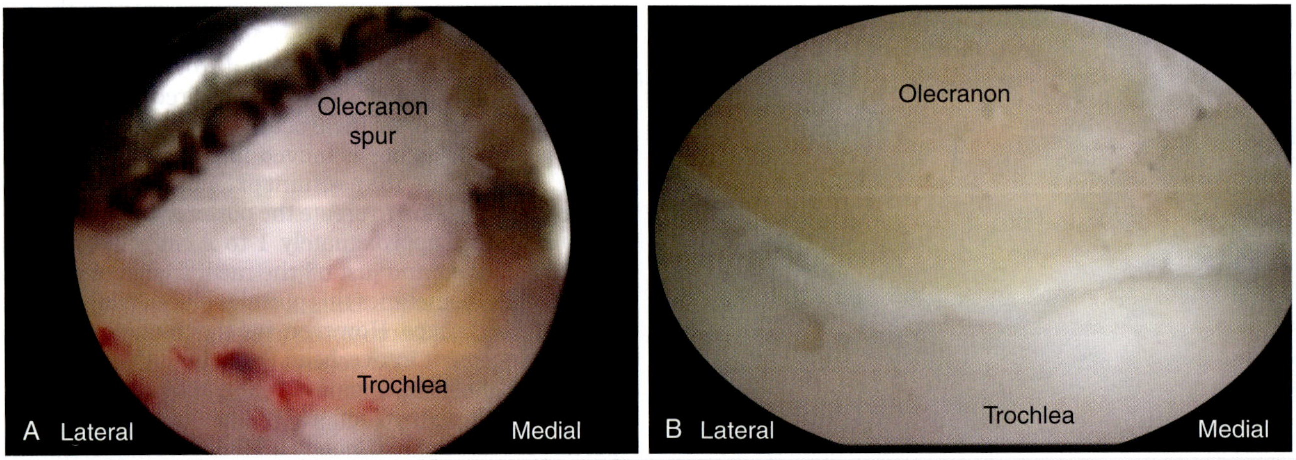

Fig. 26B.3 Before (A) and after (B) pictures of an arthroscopic decompression of a posteromedial osteophyte.

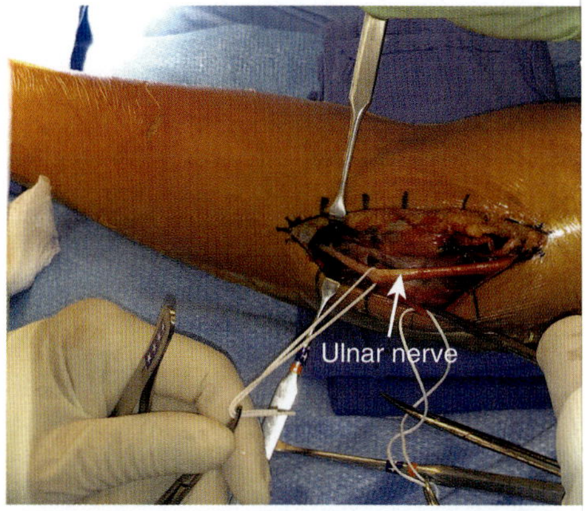

Fig. 26B.9 Ulnar nerve circumferentially freed and |
sel loop.

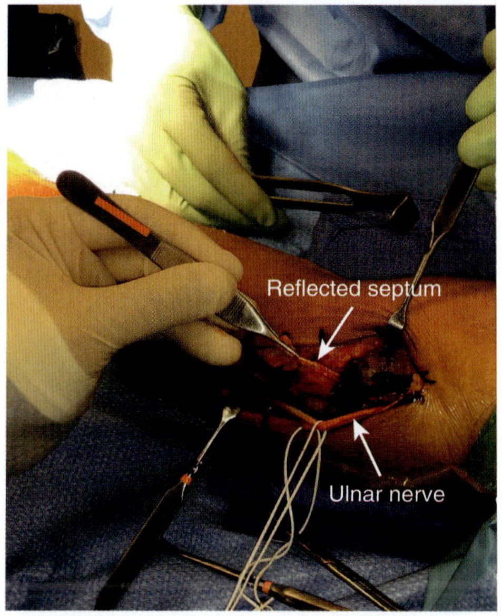

Fig. 26B.10 Medial intermuscular septum reflecte
sling.

The medial antebrachial cutaneous a
are retracted posteriorly, and the media
septum is transected 4 cm from the me
The transected portion of the septum is
for later use as a sling during ulnar ner
(Fig. 26B.10). It should be noted that the
the medial intermuscular septum should
to the medial epicondyle. Vessels in thi
coagulated to prevent hematoma formati

With the medial antebrachial cutane
nerves still retracted posteriorly, the UCL i
origin of the flexor digitorum sublimis (FD
the sublime tubercle of the ulna, exposing
The dissection of the FDS away from the
and UCL should proceed in a distal to pro
being careful not to detach the flexor-pron
the medial epicondyle. A small Hohmann re
on the radial side of the ulna to retract the
away from the UCL. The anterior band of t

Cohen et al, 2011; Rahusen et al, 2009; Reddy et al, 2000; Wilson et al, 1983). The first reported description of posteromedial impingement was reported by Wilson et al (1983) on five pitchers who underwent an open decompression. All five were able to return to pitching for a minimum of one full season at maximum effectiveness with an average time to return of 11 weeks (Wilson et al, 1983). One of the five patients required a second operation for recurrent symptoms. Open management of posteromedial impingement still remains the senior author's preference when performed in conjunction with a UCL reconstruction or ulnar nerve transposition. Cain et al (2010) reported no difference in return-to-play outcomes for players who had a concomitant open posteromedial olecranon excision during the index UCL reconstruction (86%) versus those without excision (82%) ($P = 0.21$).

As arthroscopic techniques have continued to advance, the management of posteromedial impingement is more commonly treated arthroscopically (Andrews & Timmerman, 1995; Cain et al, 2010; O'Holleran & Altchek, 2006; Rahusen et al, 2009; Reddy et al, 2000). In a large series Reddy et al (2000) reported that 47 of 55 (85%) professional athletes returned to previous level of play after arthroscopic treatment of posteromedial impingement and 87% reported "good" to "excellent" results (Reddy et al, 2000). Furthermore, Rahusen et al (2009) reported on 16 patients treated for posterior impingement of the elbow with an increase in Modified Andrews' Elbow Scoring System (MAESS) scores from 69 (average score) preoperatively to 93 (excellent score) postoperatively. Cohen et al (2011) reported on a series of 9 pitchers (5 professional and 4 recreational) with posteromedial elbow impingement treated arthroscopically. On the basis of Andrews-Carson scale, the subjective and objective outcomes were considered excellent in 7 patients and good in 2. Last, Hepler et al (1998) found a postoperative satisfaction rate of 91% in patients treated arthroscopically for posteromedial impingement.

Although arthroscopic techniques have demonstrated good to excellent results, the reoperation rate after an isolated arthroscopic debridement of posteromedial osteophytes has been reported to be as high at 41% (Andrews & Timmerman, 1995). Furthermore, Cain et al (2010) reported 10 of 53 (19%) patients who underwent posteromedial decompression returned for a secondary procedure on average at 25.4 months (range, 4.5–72.4) from the index procedure. Return-to-play for this cohort was 71% (38 of 53). In addition, Andrews and Timmerman (1995) reported that after removal of a posteromedial osteophyte, 25% of patients eventually required an UCL reconstruction. The authors suspected the reason for this was either loss of the posteromedial buttress or failure to initially appreciate the severity of the underlying associated UCL injury.

Ulnar Collateral Ligament Reconstruction Surgical Technique

The senior author's preferred graft choice for UCL reconstruction is the ipsilateral palmaris tendon. If the tendon is absent or insufficient, the contralateral gracilis tendon is used. The senior author prefers to harvest the gracilis tendon using a minimally invasive popliteal incision. The following surgical technique describes UCL reconstruction with ipsilateral palmaris autograft using the modified Jobe technique.

GRAFT HARVEST AND PREPARATION

The patient is placed in the supine position on the operating room table, and the operative extremity is placed on a hand table. A nonsterile tourniquet is placed on the extremity, and it is prepped and draped in standard fashion. Coban (3M, Maplewood, MN) is wrapped around the hand, being sure not to cover the incision sites for palmaris harvest. An Ioban (3M) drape is placed on the remaining exposed skin of the operative extremity. The extremity is exsanguinated, and the tourniquet is inflated to 250 mm Hg.

Two 1-cm incisions are then made over the palmaris tendon on the volar aspect of the forearm. The distal incision should be made over a wrist crease to improve cosmesis. The proximal incision should be created 2 to 3 cm proximal to the first incision. Blunt dissection is used to expose the palmaris tendon through both incisions. Care must be taken to coagulate bleeding vessels within these incisions because a hematoma can form in this area and compress the median nerve. The palmaris tendon is isolated by placing a curved hemostat beneath the tendon through each incision (Fig. 26B.4). The median nerve must be protected during retrieval of the palmaris tendon as it lies just deep to the palmaris tendon. The wrist is then flexed, and the tendon is transected using a scalpel through the distal incision. The tendon should be transected as distally as possible to ensure adequate graft length. The tendon is retrieved through proximal incision, and a 0 Ti-Cron (Covidien, New Haven, CT) suture is used to place a locking stitch that will be used for graft passage (Fig. 26B.5).

Tension is pulled on the transected tendon so that it is easier to palpate in the proximal forearm. A third transverse incision is made over the musculotendinous junction of the palmaris, approximately 15 cm proximal to

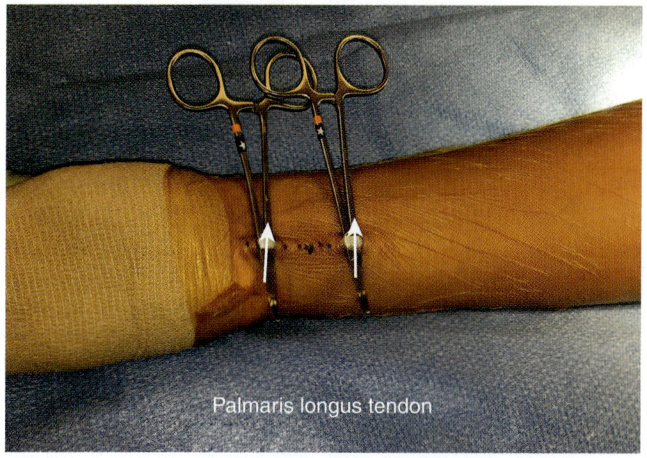

Fig. 26B.4 Palmaris longus tendon isolated in both distal wrist incisions.

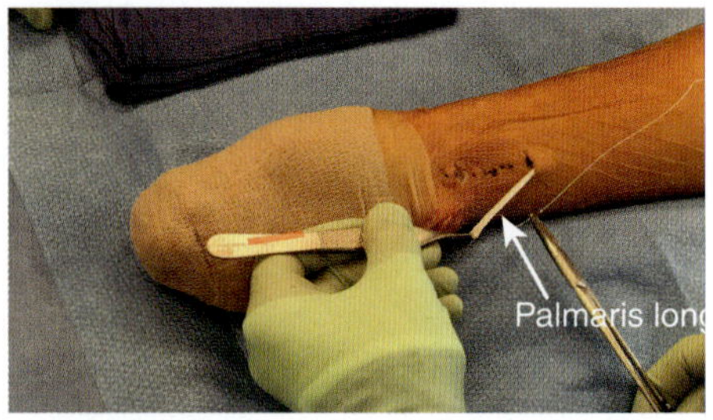

Fig. 26B.5 Transected palmaris longus tendon r
proximal wrist incision.

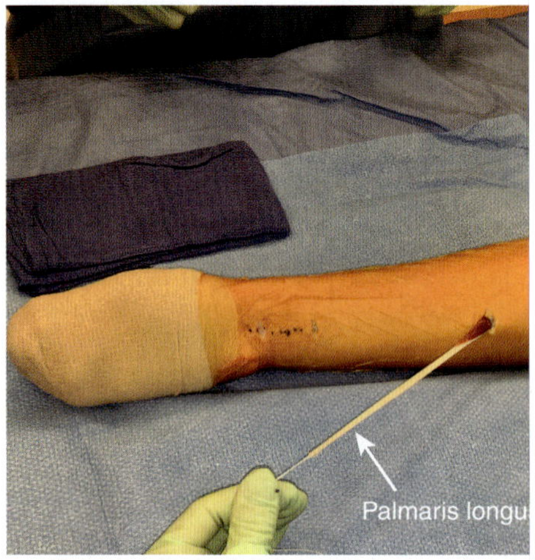

Fig. 26B.6 Palmaris longus tendon retrieved thro
incision.

the proximal wrist incision. Blunt disse
down to the forearm fascia, and any bl
coagulated. The forearm fascia is split l
a curved hemostat is placed beneath t
culotendinous junction. The palmaris t
through the third incision using the
Tension is pulled on the tendon to inc
(Fig. 26B.6). Muscle fibers are removed
portion of the palmaris tendon. The ten
and a 0 Ti-Cron (Covidien) suture is us
ing passing stitch in this end of the tend
graft length is 13 cm, but it should be
possible. When the graft harvest is con
longitudinal fascial split in the third inci
2.0 Vicryl (Ethicon). If this fascial split is
cular herniation can occur. Skin incisio
simple, interrupted 3.0 Prolene (Ethicon
taken to the back table and placed in a b

ULNAR COLLATERAL LIGAMENT RECONSTRUCTION

An incision is made, centered over the med
incision forms a 160-degree angle, with
extending 3 cm from the central aspect of
dyle and the distal limb extending 6 cm di
Blunt dissection is carried out down to the

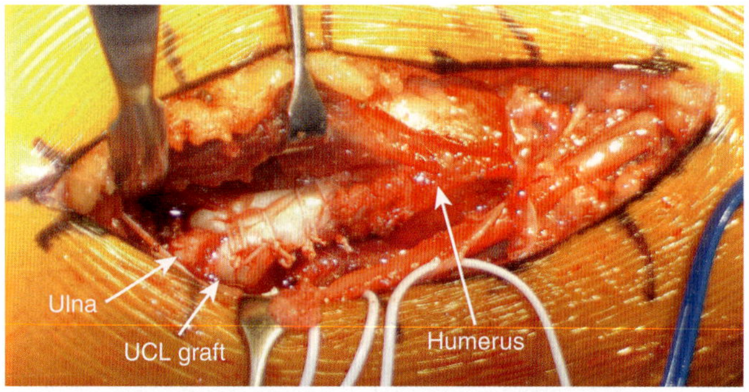

Fig. 26B.12 Ulnar collateral ligament (UCL) graft sutured to the native UCL.

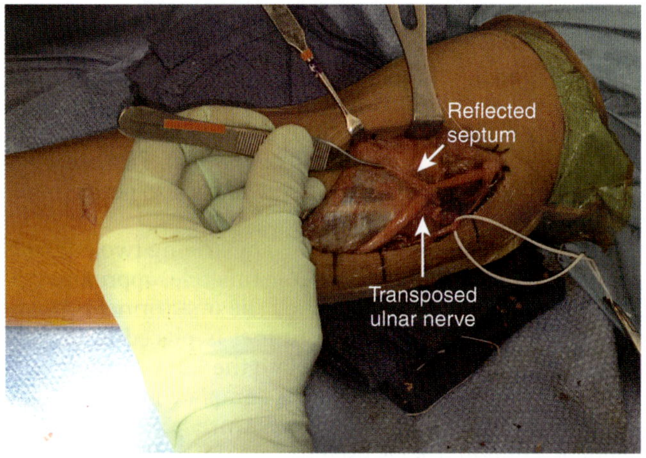

Fig. 26B.13 Transposed ulnar nerve beneath the septum formed by the portion of the intermuscular septum that was previously reflected.

with 0 Ti-Cron (Covidien) to prevent the ulnar nerve from subluxating posteriorly into the cubital tunnel.

The FCU fascia is closed with 0 Ti-Cron (Covidien). Care must also be taken while closing the FCU fascia, so as not to strangulate the ulnar nerve. A 2-cm opening between the two heads of the FCU should be left for passage of the ulnar nerve back into its muscular bed in the forearm. Another 0 Ti-Cron (Covidien) is used to sew a small portion of the medial portion of the triceps over the graft on the posterior aspect of the humerus. This minimizes bleeding and prevents anterior subluxation of the medial head of the triceps. A Hemovac drain is placed, and the tourniquet is deflated. When meticulous hemostasis is obtained, the skin is closed with 2.0 Vicryl followed by 3.0 running Prolene. Sterile dressing is applied, and a posterior splint is placed with the arm in 90 degrees of flexion. The splint will remain on for 5 days. After the splint is removed, the extremity is placed in a hinged elbow brace, which is removed during physical therapy sessions to perform aggressive ROM exercises.

Ulnar Collateral Ligament Reconstruction Outcomes

Overall, UCL reconstruction has been successful in allowing patients to return to play. Cain et al (2010) reported results on 743 patients undergoing UCL reconstruction with at least 2-year follow-up. Eighty-three percent of patients returned to the same level of play or higher. When considering Major League Baseball players, 75.5% returned to the same level of play. Minor league baseball players demonstrated a 73% return to the same level of play or higher. Eighty-seven percent of collegiate baseball players returned to play either collegiate or professional baseball after UCL reconstruction. Eighty-three percent of high school athletes returned to previous level of competition. Additionally, there was a 20% overall complication rate in the study. Sixteen percent of all patients undergoing UCL reconstruction experienced transient ulnar nerve neuropraxia, with the vast majority resolving by 6 weeks.

Osbahr et al (2014) reported 10-year results on the same cohort of patients. Ninety percent of pitchers were able to return to the same level of play or higher. Overall, baseball players who returned to play were able to continue their careers for an average of 3.6 years. Ninety-three percent of patients were satisfied with their results after their playing careers were finished. Only 3% experienced persistent elbow pain.

References

Andrews JR, Carson WG. Arthroscopy of the elbow. *Arthroscopy*. 1985;1(2):97–107.

Andrews JR, Timmerman LA. Outcome of elbow surgery in professional baseball players. *Am J Sports Med*. 1995;23(4):407–413.

Cain EL Jr, Andrews JR, Dugas JR, et al. Outcome of ulnar collateral ligament reconstruction of the elbow in 1281 athletes: results in 743 athletes with minimum 2-year follow-up. *Am J Sports Med*. 2010;38(12):2426–2434.

Cohen SB, Valko C, Zoga A, Dodson CC, Ciccotti MG. Posteromedial elbow impingement: magnetic resonance imaging findings in overhead throwing athletes and results of arthroscopic treatment. *Arthroscopy*. 2011;27(10):1364–1370.

Field LD, Altchek DW. Evaluation of the arthroscopic valgus instability test of the elbow. *Am J Sports Med*. 1996;24(2):177–181.

Hepler M, Steinman S, Rosenwasser M. Elbow arthroscopy in the treatment of posterior olecranon impingement. *Arthroscopy*. 1998;14:430.

O'Holleran JD, Altchek DW. The thrower's elbow: arthroscopic treatment of valgus extension overload syndrome. *HSS Journal*. 2006;2(1):83–93.

Osbahr DC, Cain EL, Raines BT, Fortenbaugh D, Dugas JR, Andrews JR. Long-term outcomes after ulnar collateral ligament reconstruction in competitive baseball players: minimum 10-year follow-up. *Am J Sports Med*. 2014:42(6):1333–1342.

Rahusen FTG, Brinkman J, Eygendaal D. Arthroscopic treatment of posterior impingement of the elbow in athletes: a medium-term follow-up in sixteen cases. *J Shoulder Elbow Surg*. 2009;18(2):279–282.

Reddy AS, Kvitne RS, Yocum LA, ElAttrache NS, Glousman RE, Jobe FW. Arthroscopy of the elbow: a long-term clinical review. *Arthroscopy*. 2000;16(6):588–594.

Wilson FD, Andrews JR, Blackburn TA, McCluskey G. Valgus extension overload in the pitching elbow. *Am J Sports Med*. 1983;11(2):83–88.

26-26C PREVENTION IN YOUTH SPORTS (EARLY SPORTS SPECIALIZATION)

OSAMA ELATTAR, MD and BRIAN BUSCONI, MD

Introduction

- Over the past few decades, there has been a continuous rise in the number of participants in overhead throwing sports. As a result, there has been a concomitant increase in the incidence of overuse elbow injuries.
- Common overuse injuries encountered in the throwing elbow include
- (1) ulnar collateral ligament tears; (2) ulnar neuritis; (3) flexor-pronator strain, tear, or tendinitis; (4) medial epicondyle apophysitis or avulsion; (5) valgus extension overload syndrome with olecranon osteophytes; (6) olecranon stress fractures; (7) osteochondritis dissecans (OCD) of the capitellum; and (8) loose bodies (Andrews, 1995; Ireland, 1988).
- Of extra concern is the apparent rise in elbow injuries to youth baseball pitchers. The number of ulnar collateral ligament (UCL) reconstructions ("Tommy John" surgeries) is increasing, especially in young baseball pitchers (Fleisig, 2006a; Petty, 2004).
- With the absence of national database documenting the total number of elbow surgeries in baseball pitchers, the experience at the Andrews Sports Medicine and Orthopedic Center supports the belief of increased rates of elbow injuries to youth pitchers (Table 26C.1) (Fleisig et al, 2012).
- The increase in the number of surgeries and percent of surgeries in young baseball pitchers may represent a true increase in injury incidence, improved diagnostics, or a combination of these two factors (Lynch et al, 2008).
- For youth baseball elbow injuries, there are four main risk factors recognized in the literature: number of pitches thrown, pitch type, pitching mechanics, and physical condition of the player (American College of Sports Medicine, American Dietetic Association, Dietitians of Canada, 2000).
- Of these four factors, the number of pitches thrown has the strongest correlation to youth pitching injuries (Collins & Comstock, 2008). Prevention of injury to the UCL is focused on addressing the risk factors for injury.

Youth Sports Participation and Specialization

In the United States, there has been an increase in sports participation across all age groups over the past 15 years. Concomitantly, there has been an increase in early year-round training in a single sport. Between the ages of 6 and 18 years, about 27 million U.S. youths participate in team sports, and 60 million participate in some form of organized athletics (DiFiori et al, 2014). In 1997, 9% of children younger than 7 years of age participated in organized sporting activities, compared with 12% in 2008 (Malina, 2010). Additionally, there has been an increase in high school sports participation in many sports, including baseball, soccer, softball, tennis, and swimming.

Despite the advantages of maximizing healthy physical activities in the preadolescent and adolescent age groups, the debate continues about when, how, and why a young person should become a "single-sport athlete."

Single-sport specialization has become increasingly popular among many coaches and parents with many factors contributing to this trend, including the desire to pursue scholarships, potential professional status, the ability to label a young athlete as elite at an early age, and public perception of the value of elite athletic competition and financial rewards for elite athletes.

The American Orthopaedic Society for Sports Medicine (AOSSM) Consensus meeting defined early sports specialization, or early single-sport specialization by the following three criteria (LaPrade et al, 2016):

1. Participation in intensive training or competition in organized sports more than 8 months per year (essentially year round) (Jayanthi et al, 2015)
2. Participation in one sport to the exclusion of participation in other sports (limited free play overall) (Jayanthi et al, 2013)
3. Involving prepubertal (seventh grade or roughly age 12 years) children

The degree of sports specialization can be defined as low, moderate, or high based on the number of definition components to which a young athlete may respond in a positive way (Jayanthi et al, 2015) (Table. 26C.2).

Early sports specialization, or early single-sport specialization, has not been proven as a requirement for adult elite performance. Additionally, it is believed that early sports specialization might potentially damage the long-term physical and mental health of the athlete. Furthermore, early youth sport specialization has been associated with increased rates of overuse injury, burnout, loss of motivation, decreased athletic development over time, and dropout from sports (DiFiori et al, 2014; Jayanthi et al, 2013, 2015). On the other hand, multisport participation has been proposed to result in better long-term performance and an increase in lifetime enjoyment of physical activity and recreational sports participation (Bahr, 2014).

Quantity of Pitching

In the past, young baseball pitchers would pitch for their school team or youth league team, averaging 20 scheduled games per year. They did not have the chance to play extensive schedules, despite the passion for playing baseball, motivation to throw breaking pitches, and having parents who pushed them. Nowadays, it is common for young pitchers to play more than 70 games a year and to play more than 8 consecutive months (Fleisig et al, 2011; Register-Mihalik et al, 2012).

A young baseball player can play for travel team and pitch for his or her school or a local league. Approximately 25% of all Little League pitchers also pitch for travel teams (Register-Mihalik et al, 2012).

In recent times, with extended competitive baseball, there has been a rapid increase in elbow injuries in youth baseball pitchers. With increasing demand on youth athletes to pitch more, there is less time for repair of bony and soft tissues in the elbow.

Olsen et al (2006) conducted a retrospective study of 140 adolescent baseball pitchers (aged 14–20 years). They compared 95 pitchers previously operated on for shoulder or elbow injury from pitching with an age-matched control group (45 active pitchers) with no history of pitching injury. The elbow surgery group was significantly taller and heavier than the control group and threw faster. There were no differences in number of years pitching or age began pitching between the two groups. The injured group self-reported pitching more months per year, innings per game, and pitches per game. Multivariate analysis revealed significant risk factors. Adolescent pitchers who pitched competitively more than 8 months per year were approximately five times (odds ratio [OR], 5.05) more likely to sustain an elbow or shoulder injury requiring surgery. Pitching more than 80 pitches per game almost quadrupled the chance of injury and surgery (OR, 3.83). Most startling was the finding that a pitcher who regularly pitched with her or his arm fatigued was 36 times as likely to be in the surgery group (OR, 36.18) (Olsen, 2006). Recent prospective studies have also identified overuse as the principal risk factor for pitching injury (Fleisig et al, 2011).

In 2006, USA Baseball published pitching safety guidelines. Little League Baseball enacted pitch limit regulations the following year. The guidelines are stratified for different age groups and require a set amount of rest based on the number of pitches thrown (Table 26C.3) (USA Baseball Medical and Safety Advisory Committee, 2013).

The importance of overuse as the chief risk factor for injury in youth baseball players cannot be overstated. "More" is not always "better," and the prospective data strongly correlate extensive pitching with risk of elbow injury. However, young pitchers must pitch enough to develop the technique, strength, and experience needed to improve their skill. Today's young pitchers and the adults around them, including parents and coaches, must find a reasonable balance between too much and too little. The bottom line is that even with all of the advances in medicine and research, the best tools for prevention of elbow injuries are common sense, awareness of pitch count, and avoiding (physical and mental) fatigue (Fleisig et al, 2009b).

Table. 26C.1 Ulnar Collateral Ligament Reconstructions

Year	Total (*n*)	Youth and High School	
1994	6	0	0
1995	21	2	10
1996	31	1	3
1997	23	1	4
1998	43	5	12
1999	65	12	18
2000	93	17	18
2001	93	17	18
2002	110	19	17
2003	172	45	26
2004	174	35	20
2005	153	42	27
2006	140	36	26
2007	125	38	30
2008	103	33	32
2009	121	34	28
2010	131	41	31
Total	1607	374	23

Adapted from Andrews Sports Medicine and Orthopedic Center and Fleisig GS, Andrews JR. Prevention of elbow injuries in youth baseball pitchers. *Sports Health*. 2012;4(5):419-424.

Pitch Type

For generations, there was a long-standing belief that curveball pitches are particularly deleterious to youth pitchers. The theory was that to impart the necessary spin to the ball to cause a break, the pitcher must put his or her arm in a position that increases strain on the elbow (Tutko & Bruns, 1976). It was thought that with the skeletal immaturity

Table 26C.2 Degree of Sports Specialization and Risk of All-Cause Injuries

Degree of Specialization	Risk of Injury	Risk of Serious Overuse Injury	Risk of Acute Injury
Low specialization (none or one of the following): Year-round training (>8 months per year) Chooses a single main sport Quit all sports to focus on one sport	Low	Low	Moderate
Moderately specialized (two of the following): Year-round training (>8 months per year) Chooses a single main sport Quit all sports to focus on one sport	Moderate	Moderate	Low
Highly specialized (three of three of the following): Year-round training (>8 months per year) Chooses a single main sport Quit all sports to focus on one sport	High	High	Low

From Jayanthi NA, LaBella CR, Fischer D, Pasulka J, Dugas LR. Sports-specialized intensive training and the risk of injury in young athletes: a clinical case-control study. *Am J Sports Med*. 2015;43:794-801.

and poor mechanics in youth pitchers, the growth plates at the UCL origin and insertion cannot withstand such increased strain, making youth pitchers prone to injury. With this theory, several experts over the years recommended avoiding throwing curveball pitches until achieving puberty and skeletal maturity.

Several biomechanical studies have compared fastball and curveball motion, forces, and torques. Dun et al (2008) and Nissen et al (2009) found greater forearm supination with the curveball than the fastball, yet they found significantly less varus torque in the curveball than in the fastball in youth baseball pitchers. Fleisig et al (2006a) found no significant varus torque difference between fastballs and curveballs in collegiate pitchers. Furthermore, a cadaveric study showed that changes in supination did not affect tension in the UCL during elbow varus torque (Pribyl et al, 1999).

Several retrospective and prospective studies have investigated the relationship between curveball pitching at a young age and elbow pain or injury. A retrospective study by Olsen et al (2006) compared adolescent pitchers with elbow surgery to a healthy control group; they found no significant difference in how old the pitch groups were when they began throwing breaking balls. A 10-year prospective study by the American Sports Medicine Institute (ASMI) found no difference between the surgery group (n = 25) and the successful, healthy outcomes group (n = 143) in terms of age and throwing curveballs. They concluded that pitchers who threw curveballs before 13 years old were no more likely to be injured than pitchers who began after 13 years (P = 0.41) (Fleisig et al, 2011).

Table. 26C.3 Limits for Number of Pitches Thrown in Games*

Age (yr)	2006 USA Baseball Guidelines	2008 Little League Baseball Regulations
DAILY LIMITS		
17–18	N/A	105/day
15–16	N/A	95/day
13–14	75/game	95/day
11--12	75/game	85/day
9–10	50/game	75/day
7–8	N/A	50/day
WEEKLY LIMITS		
17–18	N/A	26–50 pitches → 1 day of rest 51–75 pitches → 2 days of rest 76–105 pitches → 3 days of rest
15–16	N/A	
13–14	125/wk; 1000/season; 3000/yr	**21–40 pitches → 1 day of rest**
11–12	100/wk; 1000/season; 3000/yr	**41–60 pitches → 2 days of rest** **>60 pitches → 3 days of rest**
9–10	75/wk; 1000/season; 2000/yr	
7–8	N/A	

*The entries in bold type indicate regulations governing ages 7 to 16 years.
N/A, Not applicable.
Adapted from USA Baseball Medical and Safety Advisory Committee. *Position Statement for Youth Baseball Pitchers.* Durham, NC: USA Baseball Medical and Safety Advisory Committee; 2013; and Little League Baseball. Protecting Young Pitching Arms. http://www.Littleleague.org/Assets/old_assets/media/pitch_count_publication_2008.pdf.

Thus, the theory that curveball pitching increases the risk of elbow injury for youth pitchers has been disputed by biomechanical and clinical research studies. Curveball pitching might not be the risk for elbow injury itself; the issue might be an overenthusiastic adult who has a child throwing too much. The answer for when a young pitcher is ready to throw curveball pitches is when good mechanics for the fastball and changeup have been mastered. Suggested recommendations for the skill progression of a young baseball player are as follows (Fleisig et al, 2009b):

1. Basic skills of baseball, including throwing, catching, hitting, and running
2. Fastball pitching mechanics
3. Changeup pitching mechanics
4. Breaking pitches

Biomechanics of Pitching and Mechanical Flaws

Pitching involves a kinetic chain of events in which the pelvis rotates and then upper trunk to face the target while the abducted arm externally rotates at the shoulder (Fleisig et al, 1995, 1999). Peak values of shoulder internal rotation torque and elbow varus torque are produced near the time of maximum external rotation to decelerate shoulder external rotation, prevent elbow valgus opening, and initiate shoulder internal rotation (Fig. 26C.1) (Aguinaldo & Chambers, 2009; Dun et al, 2008; Fleisig et al, 1995, 1999, 2006a, 2006b; Keeley et al, 2008; Matsuo et al, 2006; Nissen et al, 2009; Sabick et al, 2005).

In this position, 50% of the varus torque is provided by UCL tension (Fleisig et al, 1995). Repetitive tensile load can lead to UCL tear (partial or complete). Despite the significantly less torque produced by youth pitchers as compared with adults (Fleisig et al, 1999), youth pitchers have open epiphyses, more compliant connective tissue, and underdeveloped muscles. As result, tensile load in the UCL can lead to bony avulsion at a growth plate near the origin or insertion of the anterior bundle of the UCL (Keeley et al, 2008).

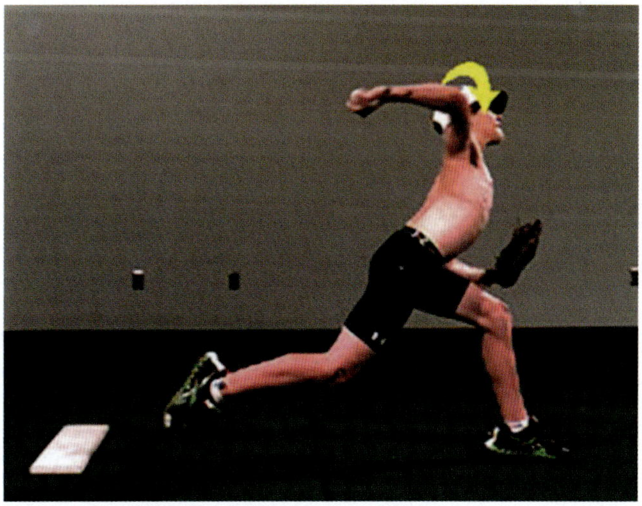

Fig. 26C.1 **Maximum elbow varus torque.** (From Aguinaldo AL, Chambers H. Correlation of throwing mechanics with elbow valgus load in adult baseball pitchers. *The American Journal of Sports Medicine.* 2009;37(10):2043-8.)

Elbow varus torque is generated not only by tension in the medial elbow but also by compression on the lateral elbow, with nearly one third of varus torque produced by compression between the radial head and humeral capitellum; this can lead to OCD, osteochondral chip fractures, or avascular necrosis (AVN) (Fleisig et al, 1995).

With rapid extension of the elbow from the arm-cocked position, posteromedial impingement can occur from combined varus torque and elbow extension velocity. Repetitive pitching can result in chondromalacia, osteophytes, and loose bodies at the posteromedial aspect of the olecranon tip (Fleisig et al, 1995).

Multiple previous studies have compared youth and adult pitchers and have shown similar motions and timing between the two age groups. The differences were in increased elbow and shoulder forces, velocities, and torques at higher levels (Fleisig et al, 1999). Furthermore, youth pitchers have greater pitch-to-pitch biomechanics inconsistency (Fleisig et al, 2009a). Similar to an adult pitcher, a young pitcher swings her or his arms apart and up during the leg stride. At the time of front foot contact, the pitcher abducts the throwing shoulder to about 90 degrees and flexes the elbow to about 80 degrees. The degree of elbow flexion at the time of maximum shoulder external rotation varies greatly from 57 to 100 degrees. From the arm-cocked position, elbow flexion and shoulder internal rotation are initiated. Shortly before ball release, maximum elbow extension velocity of approximately 2000 degrees per second is achieved (Dun et al, 2008; Keeley et al, 2008; Nissen et al, 2007; Sabick et al, 2004).

Improper pitching mechanics can lead to increased elbow varus torque with subsequent increased risk of elbow injury (Fortenbaugh et al, 2009). Specific mechanical flaws associated with increased varus torque include:

- Hand under the ball during the stride phase (Davis et al, 2009)
- Late arm rotation (measured as insufficient shoulder external rotation at the instant of front foot contact) (Fleisig, 1994)
- Excessive shoulder external rotation (Aguinaldo & Chambers, 2009; Sabick et al, 2004)
- Excessive elbow flexion (Aguinaldo & Chambers, 2009)
- Improper shoulder abduction and trunk tilt (Matsuo et al, 2006)

Young pitchers should first work on learning proper fastball biomechanics consistency in their motions. Proper mechanics for adult pitchers can be used as desired motions for young pitchers. For beginner leagues where young children are just learning how to play, the use of lighter baseballs might be beneficial (Fleisig, 2006b).

Davis et al (2009) identified five parameters that can be evaluated on video analysis such as leading with the hips, hand-on-top position, arm in throwing position (elbow at maximum height at stride foot contact), closed-shoulder position, and stride foot toward home plate. Youth pitchers that perform three or more of these parameters correctly display lower elbow valgus load, thus decreasing the stress on the UCL.

Finally, maintaining glenohumeral range of motion (ROM) and scapular functioning is essential to injury prevention. Loss in internal rotation ROM is partially caused by posterior shoulder tightness. Stretching of the posterior shoulder structures will improve ROM and decrease the risk of injury. Stretching of the posterior shoulder can be accomplished through a regular stretching program such as the sleeper stretch, modified sleeper stretch, and cross-body stretch (Laudner et al, 2008; McClure et al, 2007; Oyama et al, 2013). In addition to a regular stretching program, a strengthening program that focuses on scapular stabilization and shoulder strength should be performed regularly. The most common programs used in baseball are the Thrower's Ten or the Advanced Thrower's Ten (Wilk et al, 2009, 2011). Maintaining normal ROM, scapular control, and shoulder strength will decrease the stress on the medial elbow and decrease the risk of UCL tear.

Correcting pitching mechanical flaws can reduce the stress on the elbow, reduce the stress on the shoulder, or increase ball velocity. Improving biomechanics can increase a pitcher's chance of staying healthy and succeeding.

Strength and Conditioning

The physical conditioning, nutrition, hydration, and playing environment are potential risk factors. The strength and physical conditioning for youth baseball players should focus on coordination, athleticism, and developing general fitness, with concentration on functional strength for pitching added for the more advanced athletes (Fleisig et al, 2009b, 2012).

If a young baseball player does want to participate in a physical conditioning program, the alternative is a functional movement screening and training program. A functional movement training program includes not only strength training but also flexibility, ROM, coordination balance, and proprioception (Kiesel et al, 2007). On the other hand, for a youth pitcher who is relatively fit and athletic, a strength and conditioning program may not be needed. Biomechanical data suggest that good mechanics is a higher priority than strength for youth pitchers; more focus should be added to physical conditioning after the body matures (Fleisig et al, 1999, 2009a). For a youth pitcher with relatively good fitness, playing baseball, playing other sports and activities, and participating in physical education at school should be a sufficient physical fitness program.

Other Risk Factors

The pitcher–catcher combination has been suggested as a risk factor. With repetitive pitching, microscopic tears in the elbow or shoulder may occur. Although these tears require rest for recovery, the quantity of throws by a catcher may inhibit this recovery by adding cumulative load. This theory is supported by the ASMI 10-year longitudinal study. A pitcher who also played catcher was 2.7 times more likely to sustain a serious injury than a pitcher who did not also catch. However, this trend was not statistically significant ($P = 0.09$) because of limited sample size of the pitcher–catcher group ($n = 35$) (Fleisig et al, 2011)

Physical maturity is another potential risk factor for youth pitchers. Children who develop early are physically bigger, faster, and stronger; these children are usually overrepresented in key sports positions such as baseball pitcher (Hirose, 2009; Matthys et al, 2012). Overuse may be particularly risky for early developers. Muscles of young athletes develop secondary to growth spurts. Strong muscles with open growth plates may increase the risk of physeal plate injuries in a young pitcher's elbow or shoulder (Kelly & Pappas, 1997).

Summary

With the continuous increase in youth baseball pitchers elbow injuries, the adult community needs to take steps to prevent these injuries. USA Baseball, Little League Baseball, Baseball Canada, ASMI, the AAOSM, and the American Academy of Pediatrics have published or implemented guidelines and rules for prevention of youth pitching injuries (American Academy of Pediatricians, 2012; ASMI, 2012; Baseball Canada, 2012; Little League Baseball, 2012; Mueller et al, 2001; Stop Sports Injuries, 2012). The focus has been mostly on increasing the awareness of overuse as the most important risk factor and on the prevention of overuse injuries. In addition to monitoring of throwing limits, allowing the appropriate amount of time for recovery is recommended.

Throwing curveballs has also been suggested as a risk factor, but the existing research has been unable to prove an association between curveball and elbow injury. Many organizations and leading clinicians still believe this is a risk factor and discourage pitching curveballs before reaching skeletal maturity. Other suggested risk factors include poor pitching mechanics and poor fitness.

The recommendations for preventing elbow injuries in youth baseball pitchers are as follows (USA Baseball Medical and Safety Advisory Committee, 2013):

1. Watch and respond to signs of fatigue (e.g., decreased ball velocity, decreased accuracy, upright trunk during pitching, dropped elbow during pitching, or increased time between pitches). If a youth pitcher complains of fatigue or looks fatigued, rest is recommended.
2. No overhead throwing of any kind for at least 2 to 3 months per year (4 months is preferred). No competitive baseball pitching for at least 4 months per year.
3. Do not pitch more than 100 innings in games in any calendar year.
4. Follow limits for pitch counts and days of rest.
5. Avoid pitching on multiple teams with overlapping seasons.
6. Learn good throwing mechanics as soon as possible. The first steps should be (1) basic throwing, (2) fastball pitching, (3) changeup pitching.
7. Avoid using radar guns.
8. A pitcher should not also be a catcher for his or her team. The pitcher–catcher combination results in many throws and may increase the risk of injury.
9. If a pitcher complains of pain in his elbow or shoulder, discontinue pitching until evaluated by a sports medicine physician.
10. Inspire youth pitchers to have fun playing baseball and other sports. Participation and enjoyment of various physical activities will increase the youth's athleticism and interest in sports.

Early Sport Specialization Recommendations

Early sports specialization has been identified as damaging for the future physical and mental health of the athlete. Current recommendations for athletes who are involved in early sports specialization are as follows (Myer et al, 2016):

- Children who participate in more hours per week than their age, for more than 16 hours per week in intense training, and who are specialized in sport activities should be closely monitored for indicators of burnout, overuse injury, or potential decrements in performance due to overtraining (Jayanthi et al, 2011).
- All youth (including inactive youth) can benefit from periodized strength and conditioning (e.g., integrative neuromuscular training [INT]) to help them prepare for the demands of competitive sport participation.
- Youth who specialize in a single sport should plan periods of isolated and focused INT to enhance diverse motor skill development and reduce injury risk factors.

The consensus meeting emphasized that we need to reset expectations of when competitive events occur and the level of difficulty or skill expected at each age level. They have added the following recommendations (LaPrade et al, 2016):

- A public health message that multisport participation will not diminish the athletic capabilities of athletes; we need better and more effective messaging with improved data
- A focused effort toward the importance of physical education as an opportunity for noncompetitive play and to put it back into school curriculums
- Increased emphasis on the economic impact of a lack of physical fitness to health care costs as presented in obesity and various medical comorbidities
- Recognition that each sport has its own distinct loading pattern and a distinct overuse injury to go with it
- Identification of the optimal level of exposure to maximize training effect with minimal risk of injury
- Early sport specialization has not been shown to be beneficial for high-caliber athletic performance at the national team, Olympic, and professional levels and in fact may be detrimental

References

Aguinaldo AL, Chambers H. Correlation of throwing mechanics with elbow valgus load in adult baseball pitchers. *Am J Sports Med.* 2009;37:2043–2048.

American Academy of Pediatricians. Policy statement: baseball and softball. *Pediatrics.* 2012;129:e842–e856.

American College of Sports Medicine. American Dietetic Association, Dietitians of Canada. Joint position statement: nutrition and athletic performance. *Med Sci Sports Exerc.* 2000;32:2130–2145.

American Sports Medicine Institute. Position Statement for Youth Baseball Pitchers. http://www.asmi.org/asmiweb/position_statement.htm.

Andrews JR, Timmerman LA. Outcome of elbow surgery in professional baseball players. *Am J Sports Med.* 1995;23:407–413.

Bahr R. Demise of the fittest: are we destroying our biggest talents? *Br J Sports Med.* 2014;48(17):1265–1267.

Baseball Canada. Rules governing pitch count. http://www.baseball.ca/files/2012%20Pitch%20Count%201%20pager.pdf.

Collins CL, Comstock RD. Epidemiological features of high school baseball injuries in the United States, 2005-2007. *Pediatrics.* 2008;121:1181–1187.

Davis JT, Limpisvasti O, Fluhme D, et al. The effect of pitching biomechanics on the upper extremity in youth and adolescent baseball pitchers. *Am J Sports Med.* 2009;37:1484–1491.

DiFiori JP, Benjamin HJ, Brenner J, et al. Overuse injuries and burnout in youth sports: a position statement from the American Medical Society for Sports Medicine. *Br J Sports Med.* 2014;48:287–288.

Dun S, Loftice J, Fleisig GS, Kingsley D, Andrews JR. A biomechanical comparison of youth baseball pitches: is the curveball potentially harmful? *Am J Sports Med.* 2008;36:686–692.

Fleisig GS. *The Biomechanics of Baseball Pitching [dissertation].* University of Alabama at Birmingham; 1994.

Fleisig GS, Andrews JR, Cutter GR, et al. Risk of serious injury for young baseball pitchers: a 10-year prospective study. *Am J Sports Med.* 2011;39:253–257.

Fleisig GS, Andrews JR, Dillman CJ, Escamilla RF. Kinetics of baseball pitching with implications about injury mechanisms. *Am J Sports Med.* 1995;23:233–239.

Fleisig GS, Andrews JR. Prevention of elbow injuries in youth baseball pitchers. *Sports Health.* 2012;4(5):419–424.

Fleisig GS, Barrentine SW, Zheng N, Escamilla RF, Andrews JR. Kinematic and kinetic comparison of baseball pitching among various levels of development. *J Biomech.* 1999;32:1371–1375.

Fleisig GS, Chu Y, Weber A, Andrews JR. Variability in baseball pitching biomechanics among various levels of competition. *Sports Biomech.* 2009a;8:10–21.

Fleisig GS, Kingsley DS, Loftice JW, et al. Kinetic comparison among the fastball, curveball, change-up, and slider in collegiate baseball pitchers. *Am J Sports Med.* 2006a;34:423–430.

Fleisig GS, Phillips R, Shatley A, et al. Kinematics and kinetics of youth baseball pitching with standard and lightweight balls. *Sports Engineering.* 2006b;9:155–163.

Fleisig GS, Weber A, Hassell N, Andrews JR. Prevention of elbow injuries in youth baseball pitchers. *Curr Sports Med Rep.* 2009b;8:250–254.

Fortenbaugh D, Fleisig GS, Andrews JR. Baseball pitching biomechanics in relation to injury risk and performance. *Sports Health.* 2009;1:314–320.

Hirose N. Relationship among birth-month distribution, skeletal age and anthropometric characteristics in adolescent elite soccer players. *J Sports Sci.* 2009;27:1159–1166.

Ireland ML, Andrews JR. Shoulder and elbow injuries in the young athlete. *Clin Sports Med.* 1988;7:473–494.

Jayanthi N, Dechert A, Durazo R, Luke A. Training and specialization risks in junior elite tennis players. *J Med Sci Tennis.* 2011;16:14–20.

Jayanthi N, Pinkham C, Dugas L, Patrick B, Labella C. Sports specialization in young athletes: evidence-based recommendations. *Sports Health.* 2013;5:251–257.

Jayanthi NA, LaBella CR, Fischer D, Pasulka J, Dugas LR. Sports-specialized intensive training and the risk of injury in young athletes: a clinical case-control study. *Am J Sports Med.* 2015;43:794–801.

Keeley DW, Hackett T, Keirns M, Sabick MB, Torry MR. A biomechanical analysis of youth pitching mechanics. *J Pediatr Orthop.* 2008;28:452–459.

Kelly AM, Pappas AM. Shoulder and elbow injuries and painful syndromes. *Adolesc Med.* 1997;29:225–230.

Kiesel K, Plisky P, Voight M. Can serious injury in professional football be predicted by a preseason functional movement screen? *N Am J Sports Phys Ther.* 2007;2:147–158.

LaPrade RF, Agel J, Baker J, Brenner JS, et al. AOSSM Early Sport Specialization Consensus Statement. *Orthop J Sports Med.* 2016;4(4). 2325967116644241.

Laudner KG, Sipes RC, Wilson JT. The acute effects of sleeper stretches on shoulder range of motion. *J Athl Train.* 2008;43(4):359–363.

Little League Baseball. Protecting Young Pitching Arms. http://www.Littleleague.org/Assets/old_assets/media/pitch_count_publication_2008.pdf.

Lynch JR, Waitayawinyu T, Hanel DP, Trumble TE. Medial collateral ligament injury in the overhand-throwing athlete. *J Hand Surg Am.* 2008;33:430–437.

Malina RM. Early sport specialization: roots, effectiveness, risks. *Curr Sports Med Rep.* 2010;9:364–371.

Matsuo T, Fleisig GS, Zheng N, Andrews JR. Influence of shoulder abduction and lateral trunk tilt on peak elbow varus torque for college baseball pitchers during simulated pitching. *J Appl Biomech.* 2006;22:93–102.

Matthys SP, Vaeyens R, Coelho-E-Silva MJ, Lenoir M, Philippaerts R. The contribution of growth and maturation in the functional capacity and skill performance of male adolescent handball players. *Int J Sports Med.* 2012;33(7):543–549.

McClure P, Balaicuis J, Heiland D, Broersma ME, Thorndike CK, Wood A. A randomized controlled comparison of stretching procedures for posterior shoulder tightness. *J Orthop Sports Phys Ther.* 2007;37(3):108–114.

Mueller FO, Marshall SW, Kirby DP. Injuries in Little League Baseball from 1987 through 1996: implications for prevention. *Phys Sportsmed.* 2001;29:41–48.

Myer GD, Jayanthi N, DiFiori JP, et al. Sports specialization, part II: alternative solutions to early sport specialization in youth athletes. *Sports Health.* 2016;8:65–73.

Nissen CW, Westwell M, Ounpuu S, et al. Adolescent baseball pitching technique: a detailed three-dimensional biomechanical analysis. *Med Sci Sports Exerc.* 2007;39:1347–1357.

Nissen CW, Westwell M, Õunpuu S, Patel M, Solomito M, Tate J. A biomechanical comparison of the fastball and curveball in adolescent baseball pitchers. *Am J Sports Med.* 2009;37:1492–1498.

Olsen SJ, Fleisig GS, Dun S, Loftice J, Andrews JR. Risk factors for shoulder and elbow injuries in adolescent baseball pitchers. *Am J Sports Med.* 2006;34:905–912.

Oyama S, Yu B, Blackburn JT, Padua DA, Li L, Myers JB. Effect of excessive contralateral trunk tilt on pitching biomechanics and performance in high school baseball pitchers. *Am J Sports Med.* 2013;41(10):2430–2438.

Petty DH, Andrews JR, Fleisig GS, et al. Ulnar collateral ligament reconstruction in high school baseball players: clinical results and injury risk factors. *Am J Sports Med.* 2004;32:1158–1164.

Pribyl CR, Hurley DK, Wascher DC, McNally TP, Firoozbakhsh K, Weiser MW. Elbow ligament strain under valgus load: a biomechanical study. *Orthopedics.* 1999;22:607–612.

Register-Mihalik JK, Oyama S, Marshall SW, Mueller FO. Pitching practices and self-reported injuries among youth baseball pitchers: a descriptive study. *Athl Training Sports Health Care.* 2012;4:11–20.

Sabick MB, Kim YK, Torry MR, Keirns MA, Hawkins RJ. Biomechanics of the shoulder in youth baseball pitchers: implications for the development of proximal humeral epiphysiolysis and humeral retrotorsion. *Am J Sports Med.* 2005;33:1716–1722.

Sabick MB, Torry MR, Lawton RL, Hawkins RJ. Valgus torque in youth baseball pitchers: a biomechanical study. *J Shoulder Elbow Surg.* 2004;13(3):349–355.

Stop Sports Injuries. http://www.stopsportsinjuries.org.

Tutko T, Bruns W. *Winning Is Everything and Other American Myths.* New York: MacMillan Publishing; 1976:151.

USA Baseball Medical and Safety Advisory Committee. *Position Statement for Youth Baseball Pitchers.* Durham, NC: USA Baseball Medical and Safety Advisory Committee; 2013.

Wilk KE, Obma P, Simpson CD, Cain EL, Dugas JR, Andrews JR. Shoulder injuries in the overhead athlete. *J Orthop Sports Phys Ther.* 2009;39(2):38–54.

Wilk KE, Yenchak AJ, Arrigo CA, Andrews JR. The advanced throwers ten exercise program: a new exercise series for enhanced dynamic shoulder control in the overhead throwing athlete. *Phys Sportsmed.* 2011;39(4):90–97.

26-26D REHABILITATION AND RETURN TO SPORT

JOSHUA W. MAJOR, MD, MPH, CHRISTOPHER CAMP, MD, JOHN ZAJAC, PT, MS, OCS, SCS, CSCS, NASM-CES/PES, JOSHUA S. DINES, MD, and LUCAS S. McDONALD, MD, MPH

The views expressed in this chapter are those of the authors and do not reflect official policy or position of the Department of the Navy, the Department of Defense, or the United States Government.

Introduction

- Ulnar collateral ligament (UCL) injury is common in overhead athletes.
- There is a highly variable (53%–80%) return to sport after UCL reconstruction.
- Postinjury treatment varies widely.
- Factors affecting valgus elbow instability, including leg and core stability, glenohumeral internal rotation deficit (GIRD), and scapular dyskinesis, should be treated.
- Rehabilitation programs vary by institution and by treating physician.
- Rehabilitation should be sport specific based on injury pattern.
- Postinjury UCL rehabilitation protocols should include a progressive, sequential plan that achieves early full range of motion (ROM), restores strength and neuromuscular control to the entire upper extremity kinetic chain, and gradually incorporates sport-specific activities to return the athlete to sport.
- The authors recommend a four-phase postinjury rehabilitation program containing the following components:
  - Progression of increasingly demanding exercises to achieve early full ROM
  - The Thrower's Ten Program (a strengthening program)
  - An interval throwing program
  - Return to activity

Specific surgical treatment methods and rehabilitation programs after UCL injury vary, with return-to-play rates ranging between 53% and 90% (Dodson et al, 2006; Erikson et al, 2014; Makhni et al, 2014; Osbahr et al, 2014; Park et al, 2014; Rohrbough et al, 2002). Improvements outside of the operating room have evolved, with particular progress in rehabilitation strategies (Fleisig et al, 2011; Fleisig & Andrews, 2012; Olsen et al, 2006) to improve overall outcomes. Outcomes are maximized by instituting well-studied, standardized rehabilitation programs (Bernas et al, 2009; Ellenbecker et al, 2009).

Evaluation of UCL injury is complex and requires a comprehensive, multifaceted approach. All athletes with suspected UCL injuries should undergo a thorough evaluation of all factors that contribute to valgus instability. Surgical treatment of UCL injuries without addressing underlying contributing factors may increase the risk of recurrent injury. Deficiencies in core and leg strength, including the gluteus medius, hip flexors and extensors, and hamstrings; the presence of capsular stiffness with GIRD; and scapular dyskinesis should be identified and addressed as part of the pre- and postoperative rehabilitation process (Kibler et al, 2006). Sequential activation patterns from proximal muscle groups occur in athletic movements performed with various sports, including baseball (both pitching and batting), golf, and tennis (Chow et al, 2003; Shaffer et al, 1993; Watkins et al, 1989). Advanced stability and neuromuscular control of the lumbopelvic–hip complex decreases the risk of athletic injury (Myer et al, 2008). Kinetic chain deficiencies including core and trunk instability are screened for using exercises, including the single-leg squat and single-leg stance. An inability to perform a single-leg squat without recruiting additional muscle groups by rotating the trunk around the leg or a forward or lateral trunk tilt indicates a loss of dynamic control (Kibler et al, 2006). A positive Trendelenburg sign during single-leg stance suggests gluteus medius weakness.

At the onset of UCL injury rehabilitation programs, emphasis is placed on whole-body kinetic chain work to develop core and trunk stability through multiplane exercises such as balance exercises and lunges to ensure adequate ROM and strength (Kibler et al, 2006). In early rehabilitation phases, supine exercises without weights or resistance minimize loading of the upper extremities. Gradual loading through the ulnohumeral joint begins in the intermediate and advanced stages of rehabilitation (Ellenbecker et al, 2015).

Glenohumeral internal rotation deficit is common in overhead throwing athletes and may contribute to throwing injuries. Glenohumeral internal rotation deficit was defined by Burkhart et al (2003a, 2003b) as a loss of internal rotation of the throwing shoulder of 20 degrees or more compared with the nonthrowing shoulder. This is evaluated by stabilizing the scapula, placing the arm in 90 degrees of abduction in the scapular plane, and then internally and externally rotating the arm. Most throwers exhibit an obvious motion disparity with excessive external rotation and limited internal rotation at 90 degrees of abduction. Wilk and colleagues (2002, 2011a) developed the total rotational motion (TRM) concept, measured at 90 degrees of abduction with external rotation added to internal rotation. They found that TRM in the throwing shoulder is within 5 degrees of the nonthrowing shoulder and that athletes with TRM deficit greater than this may be more susceptible to injury. Treatment for GIRD should be initiated for a side-to-side difference greater than 5 degrees. Stretches to treat GIRD include the modified sleeper stretch and modified sidelying cross-body stretch (McClure et al, 2007; Wilk et al, 2013). The modified sleeper stretch is performed with the athlete in a sidelying position on the affected extremity, with the trunk stretched posteriorly 20 to 30 degrees (Fig. 26D.1). The contralateral arm is used to stretch the posterior capsule while preventing subacromial impingement and pain (Wilk et al, 2013). The modified sidelying cross-body stretch is also performed in the sidelying position

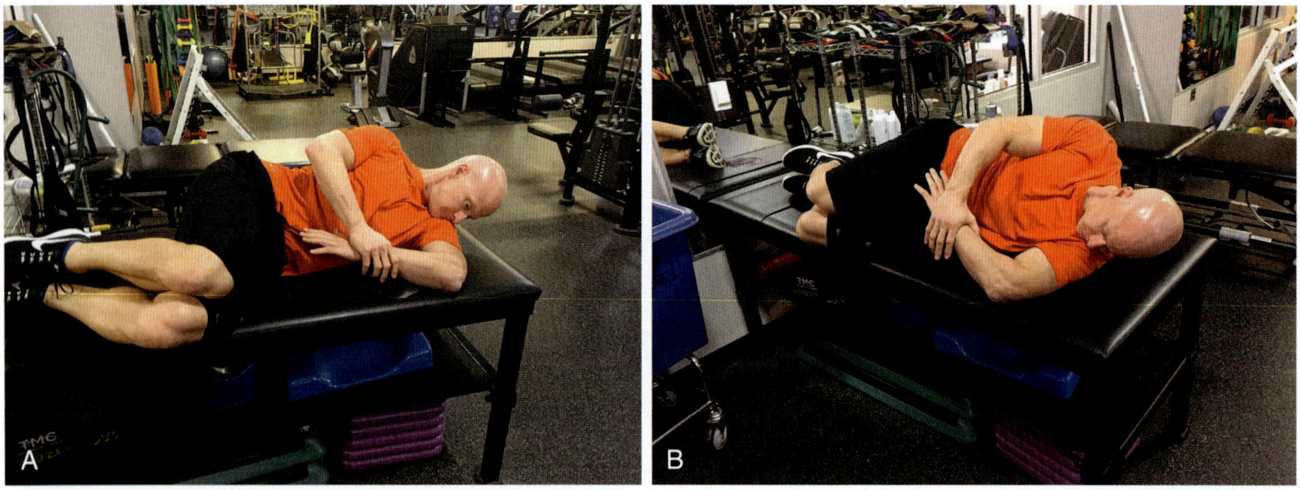

Fig. 26D.1 **A** and **B,** A demonstration of the modified sleeper stretch performed in the sidelying position on the affected extremity with the trunk stretched posteriorly 20 to 30 degrees. The contralateral arm is used to stretch the posterior capsule.

with the affected extremity facing the table (Fig. 26D.2). The opposite hand horizontally adducts the affected shoulder, and the scapula is stabilized to resist scapular protraction. The unaffected forearm is placed on top of the affected forearm, preventing external rotation of the humerus. These modifications allow superior localization and optimal stretching of the posterior capsule (McClure et al, 2007; Wilk et al, 2013). This stretch has been shown to be more effective than the sleeper stretch (McClure et al, 2007; Wilk et al, 2013). Each stretch should be repeated three times for 30 seconds each.

The open book and corner stretches improve flexibility of the pectoralis minor and the short head of the biceps (Fig. 26D.3). The open book stretch is performed lying in a lateral position on the unaffected extremity with the knees and hips flexed 90 degrees and the arms stretched in front of the body. The chest is then opened, laying the affected extremity on the opposite side and looking toward it, stretching both the pectoralis major and the short head of the biceps (Cools et al, 2014; Kibler & Sciascia, 2008). The corner stretch stretches the pectoralis minor muscle and is performed facing into a corner (or door frame) with the shoulders abducted and elbows flexed at 90 degrees then slowly leaning forward, increasing the stretch (Fig. 26D.4) (Borstad, 2006). Each stretch should be held for 30 seconds and repeated three times.

The biomechanical model for throwing is an open-ended chain of segments progressing in a proximal-to-distal sequence; therefore, the emphasis for UCL injury rehabilitation starts proximally and works distally, with an important focus on the scapular stabilizers (Kibler & Sciascia, 2008; Redler et al, 2016). The lower trapezius and rhomboid muscles are scapular stabilizers, and the serratus anterior functions as a scapular external rotator. When the scapula is stabilized by the trapezius and rhomboid muscles, there is a 23% to 24% increase in maximal rotator cuff activation, and maximal rotator cuff strength can only be obtained through a stabilized, retracted scapula (Kibler et al, 2006). A properly stabilized scapula directs distal muscle activity toward precision and control rather than power activation (Hirashima et al, 2002; Kibler et al, 2006). The scapula should be adjusted to its position of optimal function through recreation of posterior tilt, external rotation, and upward elevation, and pericapsular strengthening should take advantage of the synergistic activity of the proximal trunk and hip muscle activation (Kibler & Sciascia, 2008; Kibler et al, 2006). Primary exercises for scapular retraction include rowing exercises such as the lawn mower pull and low row exercises, which include horizontal abduction with the humerus in external rotation and a neutral plane (Kibler & Sciascia, 2008; Mosley et al, 1992).

Currently, no validated comprehensive rehabilitation program for treatment of elbow UCL injury exists. Rehabilitation programs vary by institution and treating physician, and specific postoperative rehabilitation guidelines are often based on the operative technique used. The Andrews Sports Medicine Institute rehabilitation program progresses through four phases, emphasizing early ROM and a gradual return to competitive throwing an average of 32 weeks after UCL reconstruction (Table 26D.1) (Wilk et al, 2015). The rehabilitation program used at the Hospital for Special Surgery is outlined in Table 26D.2. The rehabilitation program described for acute UCL repairs at Tulane/Mississippi Sports Medicine and Orthopaedic Center (MSMOC) uses the four-phase program described by Wilk with accelerated milestones described in Table 26D.3 (Savoie et al, 2015). The acute phase (phase I) emphasizes decreasing inflammation and initiating immediate motion to attain full (preinjury) elbow extension. Modalities including laser therapy, high-voltage stimulation, and cryotherapy may reduce both inflammation and pain. After subsidence of the acute phase, the tissue is prepared for stretching before treatment with additional modalities, including moist heat, whirlpool, and ultrasound. Athletes with persistent difficulty restoring terminal extension should use low-load, long-duration stretching. Patients should perform at least 60 minutes of rehabilitation daily (Ellenbecker et al, 2009; Wilk et al, 2015). Additionally, scapular activation and strengthening exercises are initiated in the immediate postoperative phase. Similarly, pain-free, submaximal isometric exercises are incorporated for elbow and wrist flexor and extensor muscle groups as well as the pronator and supinator muscles.

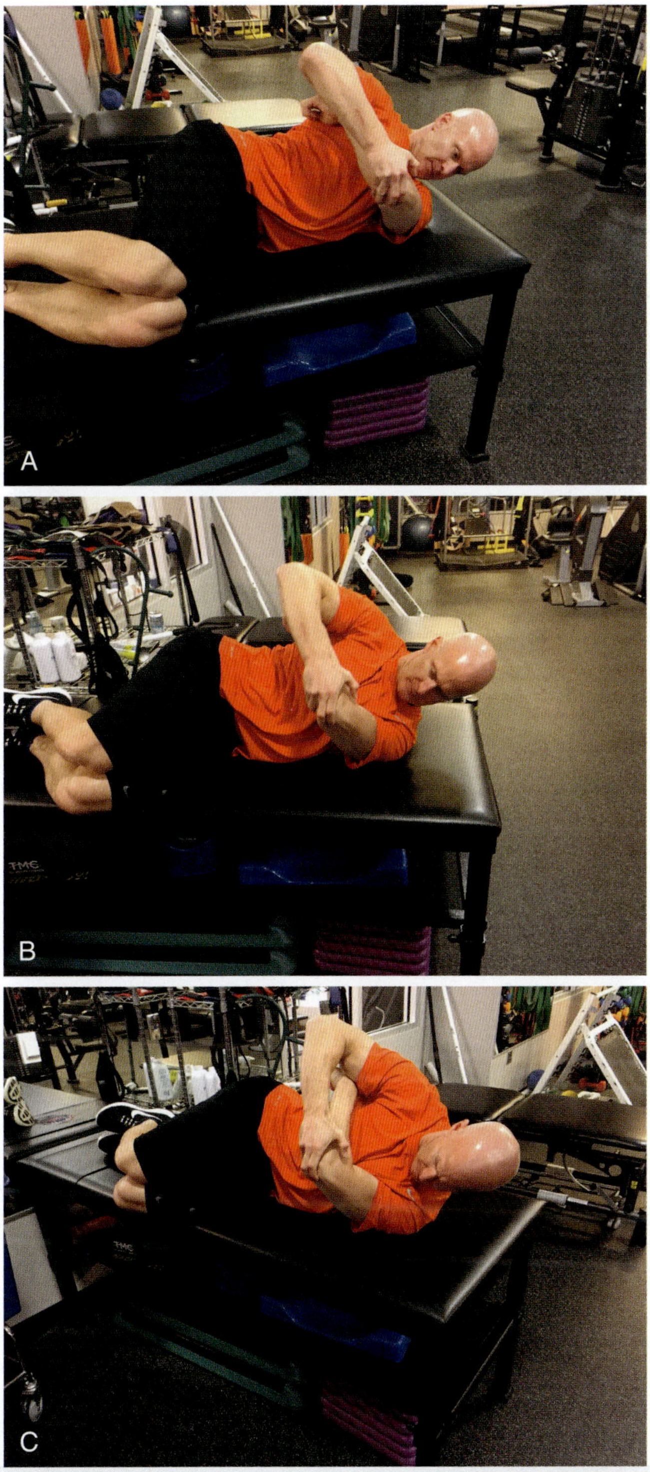

Fig. 26D.2 A to **C,** A demonstration of the modified sidelying cross-body stretch performed in the sidelying position with the affected extremity downward. The opposite hand horizontally adducts the affected shoulder, and the scapula is stabilized to resist scapular protraction.

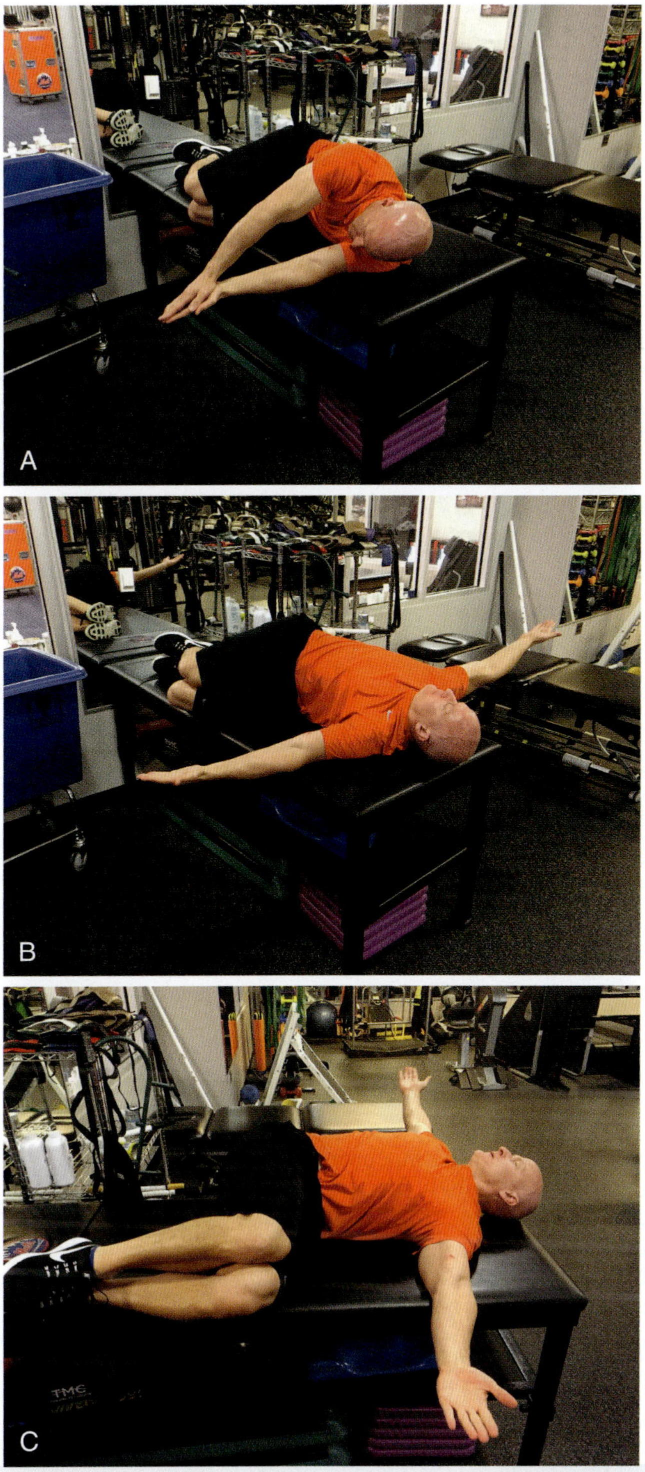

Fig. 26D.3 A to **C,** A demonstration of the open book stretch performed lying in a lateral position on the unaffected extremity with the knees and hips flexed 90 degrees and the arms stretched in front of the body. The chest is then opened, laying the affected extremity on the opposite side and looking toward it.

The intermediate phase (phase II) begins after achieving full pain-free preinjury ROM, reestablishment of neuromuscular control of the elbow complex, and improvement in muscular strength and endurance. Continued stretching and flexibility are critical, with special emphasis placed on external and internal rotation of the shoulder at 90 degrees. Adequate external rotation during overhead throwing motions can prevent excessive strain on the medial elbow structures (Fleisig et al, 1995). Internal rotation generates a protective varus force at the elbow joint (Wilk et al, 2002, 2009, 2015). Additionally, lumbopelvic and lower

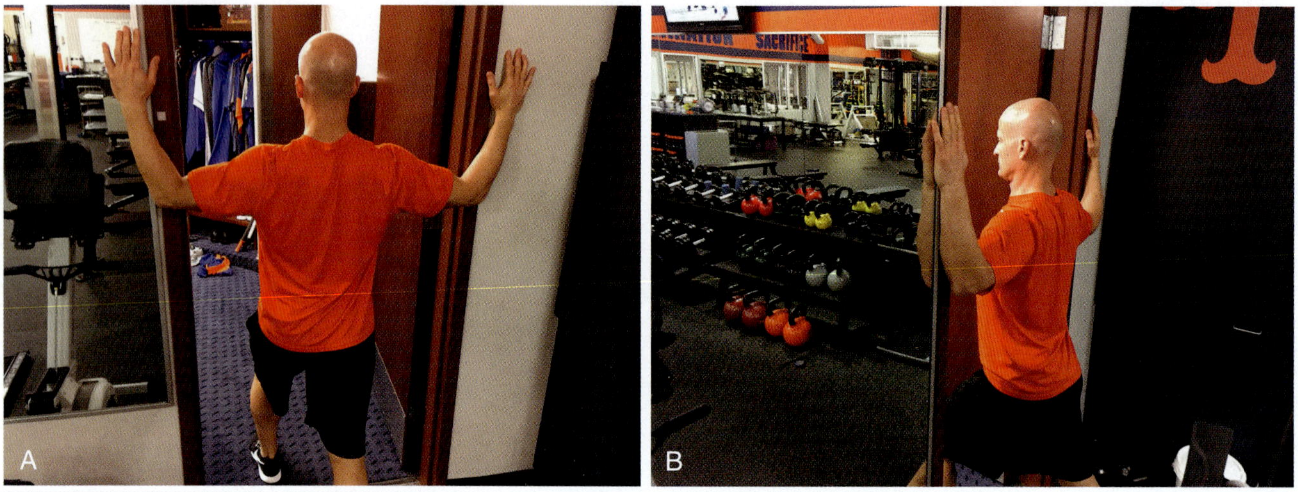

Fig. 26D.4 **A** and **B,** A demonstration of the corner stretch performed facing into a corner (or door frame) with the shoulders abducted and the elbows flexed at 90 degrees; then slowly leaning forward, the stretch is increased.

Table 26D.1 Andrews Sports Medicine Institute's Ulnar Collateral Ligament Reconstruction Rehabilitation Program

Time Period	Phase	Goal
Days 0–7	Splinted at 90 degrees flexion	Early healing of graft and fascial sling for nerve transposition
Weeks 1–5	Hinged elbow ROM brace	Protect healing tissues from valgus stress
Weeks 3–4	Light resistance isotonic exercises	Develop dynamic stabilization of the medial elbow
Week 6	Initiate Thrower's Ten Program	
Weeks 8–9	Progressive resistance exercises incorporated	
Week 12	Initiate Advanced Thrower's Ten Program Two-hand plyometric drills	
Week 14	One-hand plyometric drills	
Week 16	Interval throwing program	
Week 22 or 24	Throwing from the mound	
Months 9–12	Return to competitive throwing	

ROM, Range of motion.

extremity strengthening programs are initiated. A strengthening program such as the Thrower's Ten Program (Table 26D.4 and Video 26D.1) is instituted, focusing on complete upper extremity strengthening with special emphasis on the muscles required for overhead throwing and dynamic stability (Wilk et al, 2009, 2015).

The advanced strengthening phase (phase III) prepares for a gradual return to sport through increased strength, power, endurance, and neuromuscular control. Requirements for progression to this phase include no pain or elbow tenderness, strength at least 70% of the contralateral side, and full pain-free external and internal rotation. The athlete may progress to the Advanced Thrower's Ten Program (Table 26D.5 and Video 26D.1) designed to build on previous exercises, enhancing dynamic shoulder stabilization, muscular coactivation, strength, neuromuscular control, and endurance (Wilk et al, 2011b, 2015).

The return-to-activity phase (phase IV) involves a progressive return to competition through an interval return to throwing program. This stage requires there be no tenderness, satisfactory isokinetic testing, and full painless throwing motion. Isokinetic testing is a common method to determine if the athlete is ready to progress to an interval throwing program (Reinold et al, 1993). Interval throwing programs are sport specific based on specific stresses and motions.

Sport-Specific Rehabilitation

Although UCL injuries are typically described in pitchers, they are also described in other athletes, including javelin throwers, football quarterbacks, and softball pitchers. Each set of athletes has different throwing mechanics, imparting different unique elbow stressors. Treatment modalities and rehabilitation protocols are sport specific, accounting for the diverse requirements for each sport.

Javelin throwers throw a 2.8-m spear weighing nearly 1 kg. To account for this, they lengthen their path of acceleration by maintaining an extended elbow for as long as possible until foot strike, and during the thrust phase of a javelin throw, the elbow is flexed 40 to 60 degrees, comparable to baseball pitchers. Because of different throwing mechanics, javelin throwers undergo rapid flexion, but pitchers undergo rapid extension (O'Hagen et al,

Table 26D.2 Hospital for Special Surgery Postoperative Rehabilitation Protocol After Ulnar Collateral Ligament Reconstruction

Time Period	Treatment Strategy	Goal
Days 0–10	Splinted or hinged elbow ROM brace at 60 degrees of flexion	Promote graft healing, reduce pain and swelling
Weeks 1–4	Hinged elbow ROM brace at all times No PROM Elbow AROM in brace	Restore ROM 30 degrees-90 degrees Promote graft healing Independent home exercise
Weeks 4–6	Continue brace wear at all times Avoid PROM Avoid valgus stress Continue AROM in brace	Restore ROM 15–115 degrees Minimal pain and swelling
Weeks 6–12	Minimize valgus stress Avoid PROM by the clinician Avoid pain with exercises Continue AROM Low-intensity, long-duration stretch for extension Isotonic exercises of the scapula, shoulder, elbow, forearm, and wrist Eccentric training when strength is adequate	Restore full ROM All upper extremity strength 5/5 Begin to restore muscular endurance
Week 8	Begin ER and IR strengthening	
Weeks 12–16	Pain-free plyometric exercises Advance ER and IR to 90/90 position Neuromuscular drills Plyometric program Endurance training	Restore full strength and flexibility Prepare for return to activity
Week 16	Begin interval throwing program	
Week 16–36	Avoid pain with throwing or hitting Avoid loss of strength or flexibility Continue flexibility training Continue strengthening program	Return to activity Prevent reinjury
Week 20	Begin hitting program	

AROM, Assisted range of motion; *ER,* external rotation; *IR,* internal rotation; *PROM,* passive range of motion; *ROM,* range of motion.

Table 26D.3 Tulane/MSMOC Ulnar Collateral Ligament Repair Rehabilitation Protocol

Week 1: Physical therapy is focused on core, leg, and scapular strengthening. If no pain at elbow, shoulder and wrist isotonic exercises are added.

Brace must be worn at all times, except when showering.

Must have no pain in the elbow to perform early shoulder and wrist exercises.

Set ROM brace to pain-free arc, 60–90 degrees; increase in both directions as swelling and symptoms resolve (typically full ROM by week 4).

Weeks 4–6: Aggressive elbow and wrist rehabilitation

Weeks 6–8: Return to hit and throw program in brace

Week 12: Continue program without brace.
May return to sport when entire return-to-play program is completed

ROM, Range of motion.

Table 26D.4 Thrower's Ten Program*

1A: Diagonal pattern D2 extension—Use the involved hand to grip the tubing handle overhead and out to the side. Pull the tubing down and across the body to the opposite side of the leg.

1B: Diagonal pattern D2 flexion—Use the involved hand to grip the tubing with the arm out 45 degrees from the side, with the palm facing backward. Turn the palm forward and flex the elbow while bringing the arm up and over the involved shoulder. Turn the palm down and reverse to take the arm to the starting position.

2A: ER at 0 degrees of abduction—Stand with the involved elbow fixed at the side with the elbow at 90 degrees and the involved arm across the front of the body (the other end of tubing is fixed). Pull out with the arm, keeping the elbow at the side and return with slow, controlled motion.

2B: IR at 0 degrees of abduction—Stand with the elbow at the side, fixed at 90 degrees with the shoulder rotated out. Grip the tubing handle (the other end is fixed) and pull the arm across the body, keeping the elbow at the side. Return in a controlled manner.

2C: ER at 90 degrees of abduction—Stand with the shoulder abducted to 90 degrees and the elbow flexed to 90 degrees. Grip the tubing handle (the other end is fixed straight ahead), and keeping the shoulder abducted, rotate the shoulder back, keeping the elbow at 90 degrees. Perform both slow and fast speed sets.

2D: IR at 90 degrees of abduction—Start with the shoulder abducted to 90 degrees, externally rotated to 90 degrees, and the elbow bent at 90 degrees. Keeping the shoulder abducted, rotate the shoulder forward, keeping the elbow bent at 90 degrees. Perform both slow and fast speed sets.

3: Shoulder abduction at 90 degrees—Stand with the arm at the side, with the elbow straight and the palm against the side. Raise the arm to the side with the palm down until the arm reaches 90 degrees. Hold the position for 2 seconds and lower the arm slowly.

Continued

Table 26D.4 Thrower's Ten Program*—cont'd

4: Scaption, IR—Stand with the elbow straight and the thumb down and raise the arm to shoulder level at a 30-degree angle in front of the body not above shoulder level. Hold the position for 2 seconds and lower the arm.

5: Sidelying ER—Lie on the uninvolved side with the arm at the side of the body and the elbow bent at 90 degrees. Keeping the elbow of the involved arm fixed to the side, raise the arm. Hold for 2 seconds and lower slowly.

6A: Prone horizontal abduction (neutral)—Lie on t the able, face down with the involved arm hanging straight to the floor with the palm facing down. Raise the arm out to the side, parallel to the floor. Hold for 2 seconds and lower slowly.

6B: Prone horizontal abduction (full ER, 100 degrees of abduction)—Lie on the table, face down, with the involved arm hanging straight to the floor with the thumb rotated up (hitchhiker). Raise the arm out to the side lightly in front of the shoulder, parallel to the floor. Hold for 2 seconds and lower slowly.

6C: Prone rowing—Lie on the stomach, with the involved arm hanging over the side of the table with a dumbbell in hand and the elbow straight. Slowly raise the arm, bending the elbow and bring the dumbbell as high as possible. Hold at the top for 2 seconds and then lower.

6D: Prone rowing into ER—Lie on the stomach with the involved arm hanging over the side of the table with a dumbbell in hand and the elbow straight. Raise the arm slowly, bending the elbow and bringing the dumbbell as high as possible with the arm at 90 degrees of abduction; then rotate the arm up toward the ceiling. Hold at the top for 2 seconds and slowly lower.

7: Press-ups—Seated on a chair, place both hands on sides of the chair or table, palms down and fingers pointed outward with the hands placed equal to the shoulders. Slowly push downward through the hands and elevate the body. Hold the position for 2 seconds and lower slowly.

8: Push-ups—Start in the down position. Place the hands no more than shoulder width apart. Push up as high as possible, rolling the shoulders forward after the elbows are straight. Start with a push-up into wall and then gradually progress to a tabletop and eventually the floor as tolerable.

9A: Elbow flexion—Standing with the arm against the side and the palm facing inward, bend the elbow upward, turning the palm up while progressing. Hold 2 seconds and lower slowly.

9B: Elbow extension (abduction)—Raise the involved arm overhead. Provide support at the elbow from the uninvolved hand. Straighten the arm overhead. Hold 2 seconds and lower slowly.

10A: Wrist extension—Supporting the forearm with the palm facing downward, raise the weight in the hand as far as possible. Hold for 2 seconds and lower slowly.

10B: Wrist flexion—Supporting the forearm with the palm facing upward, lower the weight in the hand as far as possible and then curl it up as high as possible. Hold for 2 seconds and lower slowly.

10C: Wrist supination—With the forearm supported on a table and the wrist in neutral position, using a weight or hammer, roll the wrist to a palm-up position. Hold for 2 seconds and return to starting position.

10D: Wrist pronation—The forearm should be supported on a table with the wrist in neutral position. Using a weight or hammer, roll the wrist to a palm-down position. Hold for 2 seconds and return to starting position.

*This program is designed to exercise the major muscles necessary for throwing. The goal of the program is to be an organized and concise exercise program.
ER, External rotation; *IR*, internal rotation.

Table 26D.5 Advanced Thrower's Ten Program*

IR and ER tubing at 0 degrees of abduction seated on a stability ball—Sit on a stability ball with the trunk perpendicular to the floor. Retract and depress the scapula while manual resistance is applied against IR and ER. A towel roll is placed underneath the affected arm to enhance excitation of the rotator cuff.

Full can seated on a stability ball—Sit with the trunk in an upright position with the scapulae retracted and depressed. Raise both arms in the scapular plane to 90 degrees of shoulder flexion. Hold for 2 seconds and slowly lower the arms. Repeat for 10 repetitions. Next, repeat the exercise with the left arm for 10 repetitions while the right arm remains in the scapular plane at 90 degrees. Switch arms for 10 repetitions. Alternate arm repetitions with the left and right arms for 10 repetitions (30 total repetitions).

Lateral raise to 90 degrees of abduction seated on a stability ball—Raise both arms to shoulder level in a 90-degree abducted position. Hold for 2 seconds and return the arms to the side. Perform in above-stated 3-set fashion.

Sidelying ER—Performed with a dumbbell in the above-stated 3-set fashion. The unaffected arm is placed on a table with the elbow bent at 90 degrees. ER is performed for 10 repetitions or 10 seconds while preserving a neutral spine.

T-raises prone on a stability ball—Prone horizontal abduction. Position the body prone with the abdomen resting on a ball and the trunk parallel to the floor. Abduct each arm while maintaining proper positioning on the exercise ball. Perform in above-stated 3-set fashion.

Y-raises prone on a stability ball—Prone horizontal abduction at 105 degrees with full ER. Assume the same position as t-raises. Raise both arms in the scapular plane (creating a "Y" for 10 repetitions while maintaining proper positioning on the ball. Perform in above-stated 3-set fashion.

Prone row into ER seated on a stability ball—Position the body prone with the abdomen resting on a ball and the trunk parallel to the floor. Slowly raise both arms up to the level of the top of the stability ball while bending the elbows. Pause and then externally rotate the shoulders upward until the dumbbells are parallel to the floor with the elbows kept at 90 degrees. Perform in above-stated 3-set fashion.

Lower Trapezius 5 Series
Shoulder extension in ER seated on a stability ball
Shoulder extension at 45 degrees in ER seated on a stability ball
Standing wall circle slides
Standing low row
Standing table press-downs with scapular depression

Biceps curls and triceps extensions seated on a stability ball—See description in Table 26D.4 (9A and 9B) and perform while seated on a stability ball.

Wrist flexion/extension and supination/pronation—See description in Table 26D.4 (10A–10D).

*Designed for use in the advanced strengthening phase of rehabilitation of the throwing athlete's elbow. Athletes perform 2 cycles containing 3 sets of 10 repetitions of each exercise.
ER, External rotation; *IR*, internal rotation.

2015). Because of the increased weight of the javelin, recommendations for starting an interval throwing program and for return to sport are longer than for baseball players (15 months for javelin throwers compared with an average of 12 months for baseball players). Football quarterbacks have a lower incidence of UCL injury than baseball pitchers, possibly secondary to decreased maximum elbow acceleration, lower torque, abbreviated follow-through phase, and fewer overall throws per game (O'Hagen et al, 2015). Several studies demonstrate excellent return to sport in football players with nonoperative treatment (Dodson et al, 2010; Kenter et al, 2000). Softball pitcher throwing mechanics are also unique. The underhand throwing motion of softball pitchers flexes the elbow at ball release, imparting less elbow stress than an overhead throwing mechanism. Ligament repair may be a valid option in these athletes (Argo et al, 2006). UCL injuries have been reported in other sports (golf, gymnastics, tennis, wrestling, and volleyball) but with a significantly lower incidence. These athletes typically do not require UCL reconstruction for return to sport (Cain et al, 2006).

Conclusion

Although UCL rehabilitation protocols vary from institution to institution, they should include a progressive, sequential plan to achieve early motion, strength restoration, and neuromuscular control to the entire upper extremity kinetic chain before gradually incorporating sport-specific activities and return to sport. Evaluation for and treatment of factors that may contribute to valgus elbow instability should occur before initiation of rehabilitation. Deficiencies in core and leg stability, scapular dyskinesis, and the presence of GIRD should be addressed. Future studies should include validation and standardization of current rehabilitation protocols and further development of sport-specific rehabilitation treatment.

References

Argo D, Trenhaile SW, Savoie 3rd FH, Field LD. Operative treatment of ulnar collateral ligament insufficiency of the elbow in female athletes. *Am J Sports Med.* 2006;34(3):431–437.

Bernas GA, Ruberte Thiele RA, Kinnaman KA, Hughes RE, Miller BS, Carpenter JE. Defining safe rehabilitation for ulnar collateral ligament reconstruction of the elbow: a biomechanical study. *Am J Sports Med.* 2009;37(12):2392–2400.

Borstad JD. Comparison of three stretches for the pectoralis minor muscle. *J Shoulder Elbow Surg.* 2006;15(3):324–330.

Burkhart SS, Morgan CD, Kibler WB. The disabled throwing shoulder: spectrum of pathology. Part I: pathoanatomy and biomechanics. *Arthroscopy.* 2003a;19(4):404–420.

Burkhart SS, Morgan CD, Kibler WB. The disabled throwing shoulder: spectrum of pathology. Part III: the SICK scapula, scapular dyskinesis, the kinetic chain, and rehabilitation. *Arthroscopy.* 2003b;19(6):641–661.

Cain EL, Andrews JR, Dugas JR, et al. Outcomes of ulnar collateral ligament reconstruction of the elbow in 1281 athletes. Results in 743 athletes with minimum 2-year follow-up. *Am J Sports Med.* 2006;34:1594–1598.

Chow JW, Shim JH, Lim YT. Lower trunk muscle activity during the tennis serve. *J Sci Med Sport.* 2003;6(4):512–518.

Cools AMJ, Struyf F, De Mey K, Maenhout A, Castelein B, Cagnie B. Rehabilitation of scapular dyskinesis: from the office worker to the elite overhead athlete. *Br J Sports Med.* 2014;48(8):692–697.

Dodson CC, Thomas A, Dines JS, Nho SJ, Williams RJ, Altchek DW. Medial ulnar collateral ligament reconstruction of the elbow in throwing athletes. *Am J Sports Med.* 2006;34(12):1926–1932.

Dodson CC, Slenker N, Cohen SB, Ciccotti MG, DeLuca P. Ulnar collateral ligament injuries of the elbow in professional football quarterbacks. *J Shoulder Elbow Surg.* 2010;19(8):1276–1280.

Ellenbecker TS, Wilk KE, Altchek DW, Andrews JR. Current concepts in rehabilitation following ulnar collateral ligament reconstruction. *Sports Health.* 2009;1(4):301–313.

Ellenbecker TS, Wilk KE. Sport-specific rehabilitation after ulnar collateral ligament surgery. In Dines JS, Altchek DDW, eds. *Elbow Ulnar Collateral Ligament Injury.* New York: Springer Science Business Media; 2015:261–277.

Erikson BJ, Gupta AK, Harris JD, et al. Rate of return to pitching and performance after Tommy John surgery in Major League Baseball pitchers. *Am J Sports Med.* 2014;42(3):536–543.

Fleisig GS, Andrews JR. Prevention of elbow injuries in youth baseball pitchers. *Sports Health.* 2012;4(5):419–424.

Fleisig GS, Andrews JR, Dillman CJ, Escamilla RF. Kinetics of baseball pitching with implications about injury mechanisms. *Am J Sports Med.* 1995;23(2):233–239.

Fleisig GS, Andrews JR, Cutter GR, et al. Risk of serious injury for young baseball pitchers: a 10-year prospective study. *Am J Sports Med.* 2011;39(2):253–257.

Hirashima M, Kadota H, Sakurai S, et al. Sequential muscle activity and its functional role in the upper extremity and trunk during overarm throwing. *J Sports Sci.* 2002;20(4):301–310.

Kenter K, Behr CT, Warren RF, O'Brien SJ, Barnes R. Acute elbow injuries in the National Football League. *J Shoulder Elbow Surg.* 2000;9(1):1–5.

Kibler WB, Pres J, Sciascia A. The role of core stability in athletic function. *Sports Med.* 2006;36(3):189–198.

Kibler WB, Sciascia A. Rehabilitation of the athlete's shoulder. *Clin Sports Med.* 2008;27(4):821–831.

Makhni EC, Lee RW, Morrow ZS, Gualtieri AP, Gorroochurn P, Ahmad CS. Performance, return to competition, and reinjury after Tommy John surgery in major league baseball pitchers: a review of 147 cases. *Am J Sports Med.* 2014;42(6):1323–1332.

McClure P, Balaicuis J, Heiland D, Broersma ME, Thorndike CK, Wood A. A randomized controlled comparison of stretching procedures for posterior shoulder tightness. *J Orthop Sports Phys Ther.* 2007;37(3):108–114.

Mosley JB, Jobe FW, Pink M, Perry J, Tibone J. EMG analysis of the scapular muscles during a shoulder rehabilitation program. *Am J Sports Med.* 1992;20(2):128–134.

Myer GD, Chu DA, Brent JL, Hewett TE. Trunk and hip control neuromuscular training for the prevention of knee joint injury. *Clin Sports Med.* 2008;27(3):425–448.

O'Hagen T, Stucken C, Dodson CC. Sports specific outcomes for ulnar collateral ligament reconstruction, In Dines JS, Altchek DDW, eds. *Elbow Ulnar Collateral Ligament Surgery.* New York: Springer Science Business Media; 2015:219–226.

Olsen SJ, Fleisig GS, Dun S, Loftice J, Andrews JR. Risk factors for shoulder and elbow injuries in adolescent baseball pitchers. *Am J Sports Med.* 2006;34(6):905–912.

Osbahr DC, Cain EL, Raines BT, Fortenbaugh D, Dugas JR, Andrews JR. Long-term outcomes after ulnar collateral ligament reconstruction in competitive baseball players: minimum 10-year follow-up. *Am J Sports Med.* 2014;42(6):1333–1342.

Park JY, Oh KS, Bahng SC, Chung SW, Choi JH. Does well maintained graft provide consistent return to play after medial ulnar collateral ligament reconstruction of the elbow joint in elite baseball players? *Clin Orthop Surg.* 2014;6(2):190–195.

Redler LH, Degen RM, McDonald LS, Altchek DW, Dines JW. Elbow ulnar collateral ligament injuries in athletes: can we improve our outcomes? *World J Orthop.* 2016;7(4):229–243.

Reinold MM, Wilk KE, Reed J, Crenshaw K, Andrews JR. Interval sport programs: guidelines for baseball, tennis, and golf. *J Orthop Sports Phys Ther.* 1993;17:225–239.

Rohrbough JT, Altchek DW, Hyman J, Williams RJ, Botts JD. Medial collateral ligament reconstruction of the elbow using the docking technique. *Am J Sports Med.* 2002;30(4):541–548.

Savoie FH, O'Brien MJ, Field LD. Primary repair of ulnar collateral ligament injuries of the elbow. In: Dines JS, Altchek DDW, eds. *Elbow Ulnar Collateral Ligament Surgery.* New York: Springer Science Business Media; 2015:115–123.

Shaffer B, Jobe FW, Pink M, Perry J. Baseball batting. An electromyographic study. *Clin Orthop Relat Res.* 1993;292:285–293.

Watkins RG, Dennis S, Dillin WH, et al. Dynamic EMG analysis of torque transfer in professional baseball pitchers. *Spine.* 1989;14(4):404–408.

Wilk KE, Ellenbecker TS, Macrina LC. Rehabilitation of the overhead athlete's elbow. In: Dines JS, Altchek DDW, eds. *Elbow Ulnar Collateral Ligament Surgery*. New York: Springer Science Business Media; 2015:227–259.

Wilk KE, Hooks TR, Macrina LC. The modified sleeper stretch and modified cross-body stretch to increase shoulder internal rotation range of motion in the overhead throwing athlete. *J Orthop Sports Phys Ther*. 2013;43(12):891–894.

Wilk KE, Macrina LC, Fleisig GS, et al. Correlation of glenohumeral internal rotation deficit and total rotational motion to shoulder injuries in professional baseball pitchers. *Am J Sports Med*. 2011a;39(2):329–335.

Wilk KE, Meister K, Andrews JR. Current concepts in the rehabilitation of the overhead throwing athlete. *Am J Sports Med*. 2002;30(1):136–151.

Wilk KE, Obma P, Simpson CD, Cain EL, Dugas JR, Andrews JR. Shoulder injuries in the overhead athlete. *J Orthop Sports Phys Ther*. 2009;39:38–54.

Wilk KE, Yenchak AJ, Arrigo CA, Andrews JR. The Advanced Throwers Ten exercise program: a new exercise series for enhanced dynamic shoulder control in the overhead throwing athlete. *Phys Sportsmed*. 2011b;39(4):90–97.

27 Lateral: Posterolateral Rotary Instability

NATHAN WM. SKELLEY, MD and LUKE S. OH, MD, MS

Introduction

- This chapter reviews posterolateral rotary instability of the elbow.
- Elbow instability may significantly limit a patient's function and ability to perform sports and activities of daily living.
- Posterolateral rotary instability has become more frequently and accurately recognized because of improved understanding of elbow anatomy, biomechanics, diagnostic physical exam techniques, and treatment options.
- Imaging modalities are serving a more important role in the diagnosis of posterolateral elbow instability.
- Surgical reconstruction may be required in chronic or subtle posterolateral rotatory instability (PLRI) cases. Outcomes after surgery provide satisfactory results in most patients.

Epidemiology

Posterolateral rotatory instability of the elbow was originally described by O'Driscoll et al in 1991 (O'Driscoll et al, 1991). Since that time, several studies have demonstrated that the majority of posterolateral elbow instability cases result from a traumatic mechanism of injury that includes a combination of axial loading, valgus stress, and rotational force (Anakwe et al, 2001; Fedorka & Oh, 2016; Hildebrand et al, 1999; Hobgood et al, 2008; Skelley & Chamberlain, 2015). This combined loading pattern results in posterior subluxation of both the radial head and ulna from the humerus with rotation of the semilunar notch away from the trochlea (Fedorka & Oh, 2016). A recent systematic review by Anakwenze et al (2014) found that 67 of 71 (94%) patients identified a traumatic cause as the source of their lateral elbow instability. Atraumatic causes include chronic cubitus varus malunion, which has been described as an uncommon cause of chronic attenuation of stabilizing ligaments in the lateral elbow and subsequent posterolateral instability (O'Driscoll et al, 2001). Similarly, posterolateral instability may result from iatrogenic causes such as corticosteroid injections, arthroscopic procedures, or open procedures that place the primary stabilizers at risk of injury (e.g., aggressive debridement for extensor carpi radialis brevis tendinosis).

Anatomy

Appreciating elbow anatomy is very important in understanding the mechanism of injury and pathology associated with elbow instability in general as well as specifically with regard to PLRI. Elbow stability is maintained by both static and dynamic stabilizers. Static stability is provided by the bony articulations between the radiocapitellar, ulnohumeral, and proximal radioulnar joints as well as capsuloligamentous structures. The bony articulations provide stability at the extremes of motion, at either less than 20 degrees or greater than 120 degrees of elbow flexion (Fedorka & Oh, 2016). The soft tissue restraints provide primary stability throughout the remainder of the elbow's arc of motion (Fedorka & Oh, 2016).

The major soft tissue static stabilizer in the lateral elbow is the Y-shaped lateral collateral ligament (LCL) complex. This complex is composed of the radial collateral ligament, the accessory LCL, the annular ligament, and the lateral ulnar collateral ligament (LUCL) (Fig. 27.1). Some authors have suggested that these components of the LCL complex may be more accurately described to be thickenings of the capsule (similar to the glenohumeral ligaments in the shoulder) rather than discrete and separate structures (Fedorka & Oh, 2016; Mehta & Bain, 2004). The LUCL has been described to be the most important primary stabilizer against valgus stress (Anakwe et al, 2011, 2014; Ball et al, 2002; O'Driscoll et al, 1991).

The medial collateral ligament complex is composed of three bundles: the anterior bundle, posterior bundle, and transverse bundle (Fig. 27.2). The anterior bundle is the primary stabilizer to valgus stress with the elbow in extension. The anterior capsule is also important in stabilizing the elbow in extension. The posterior bundle is tight in flexion and is the main stabilizer in flexion. The transverse ligament, however, is not a significant factor in elbow stability. The role the medial collateral ligament plays in PLRI depends on the extent and mechanism of injury.

The elbow also has dynamic stabilization. Dynamic stability is provided by musculotendinous structures surrounding the elbow that function throughout elbow range of motion. This stability depends on the neuromuscular control about the joint. The biceps, triceps, and other muscles create compressive forces across the joint during flexion, extension, and rotation motion (de Haan et al, 2011).

Mechanism

Posterolateral rotatory instability injuries are commonly a result of an injury mechanism that involves a combination of axial load, valgus stress, and rotation on the outstretched upper extremity. The level of energy involved and the position of the hand, elbow, and shoulder during impact determine the type of injury sustained. PLRI is most commonly

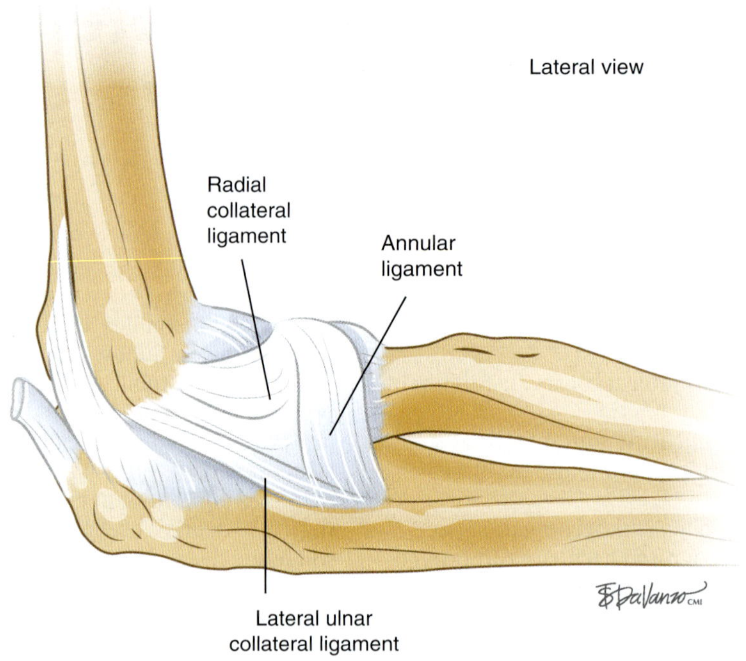

Fig. 27.1 Lateral elbow ligamentous anatomy.

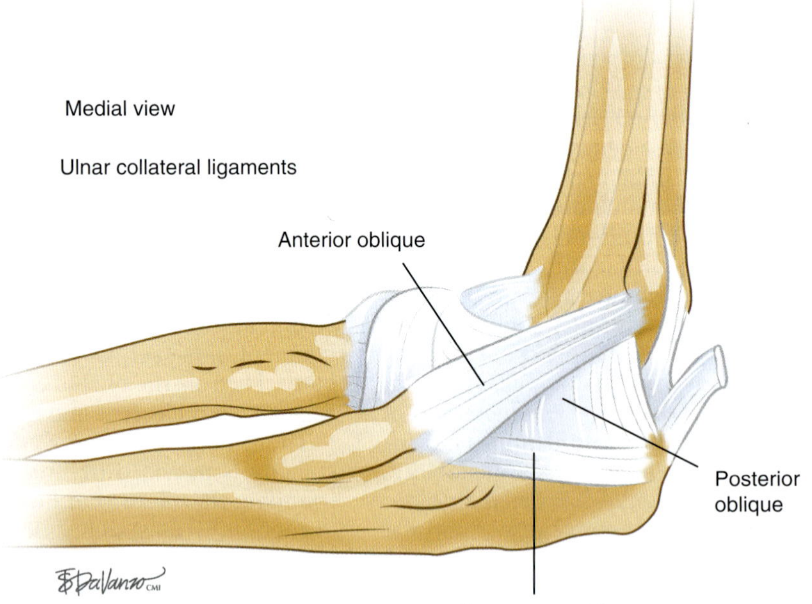

Fig. 27.2 Medial elbow ligamentous anatomy.

associated with an injury sustained while the upper extremity starts in extension and supination at the time of contact with the floor with subsequent axial load and valgus force applied to the elbow by the body weight of the falling patient (Fig. 27.3). This position places the elbow in a less stable position and more vulnerable to injury compared with a stable flexed and pronated position.

O'Driscoll et al (1992) described that the injury mechanism progresses across the elbow in a three-stage stepwise fashion from the lateral to the anterior and the anterior to the medial sides of the elbow. First, the LUCL is disrupted, then the anterior and posterior aspects of the capsule are torn, and finally the medial ulnar collateral ligament (MUCL) is disrupted. This pattern is referred to as the circle of Horii (Fig. 27.4). The primary

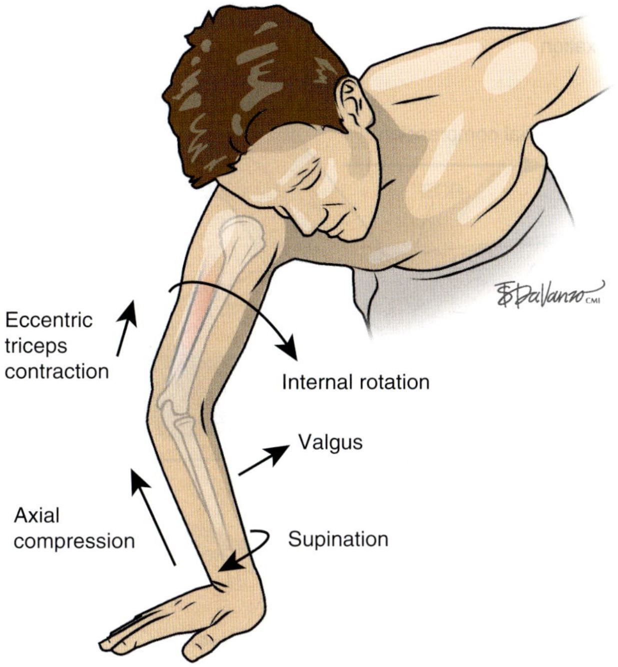

Fig. 27.3 Mechanism of elbow injury involving hyperextension, axial compression, and internal rotation.

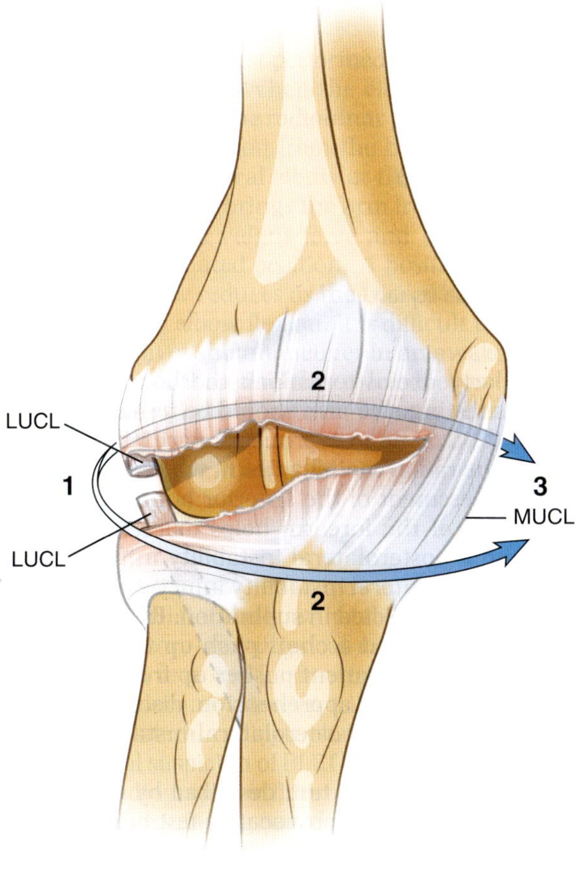

Fig. 27.4 Elbow instability progresses from lateral to medial involving the lateral ulnar collateral ligament (LUCL) capsule and medial ulnar collateral ligament (MUCL).

cause of posterolateral instability is injury to the LUCL. If the MUCL is intact, then the coronoid may not completely dislocate and may become displaced proximal to the humerus. This is a "perched" type of elbow instability injury. To have a complete posterolateral dislocation, then the combination of the LUCL, capsule, and MUCL is expected to be disrupted.

The categorization of elbow instability may be subdivided into simple or complex. Simple elbow dislocations have no associated fracture and account for approximately 60% of dislocations. Complex elbow dislocations have an associated fracture present at the time of injury (Hildebrand et al, 1999; Sheps et al, 2004; Skelley & Chamberlain, 2015). A "terrible triad" injury is a type of complex elbow dislocation involving injury of three structures: disruption of the LUCL as well as a fracture of the coronoid process and radial head or neck (Hildebrand et al, 1999; Skelley & Chamberlain, 2015).

History

Patients with posterolateral elbow rotatory instability from a traumatic cause are usually able to recall the time of injury and the specific activity that resulted in the injury (Skelley & Chamberlain, 2015). Most patients present with lateral pain as the primary symptom in association with swelling around the joint (Fedorka & Oh, 2016). Some patients may have required a reduction that was performed in the emergency department, but others may have a more subtle presentation that did not require a formal reduction. In either case, the patient may also have mechanical symptoms, including clicking, catching, snapping, and a general apprehension with elbow extension, particularly with extension and supination. Examples of activities that cause symptoms include performing a push-up and using the arms to push up from an armchair. In chronic or subtle cases of PLRI, the

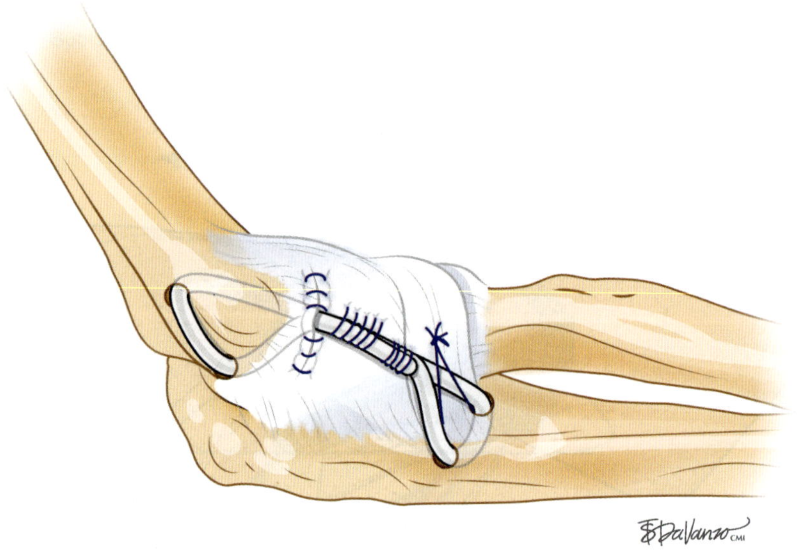

Fig. 27.7 Surgical reconstruction demonstrating the graft placement with capsular plication.

extensor carpi ulnaris and the anconeus muscle. Usually, there is a thin strip of fat and fascia between these two muscles, which helps in identifying the correct interval for the surgical approach (Mehta & Bain, 2004).

For patients with acute injury or who have adequate ligamentous and capsular tissue quality, it may be possible to perform a direct repair using transosseous sutures or suture anchors. If the LUCL is completely avulsed from the lateral epicondyle, it is referred to as "the bald eagle sign." The reattachment point is typically slightly posterior to the tip of the lateral epicondyle. The dissection should not be taken posterior to the humerus, however, and care should be taken in this area to prevent disrupting the posterior blood supply to the capitellum (Yamaguchi et al, 1997). Surgical procedures should be confined to an area anterior to the humerus to protect the posterior vascular supply (Savoie et al, 2010).

Ligament reconstruction with autograft or allograft is often required for chronic PLRI cases in which the lateral tissue may be of insufficient quality. Several different autograft sources have been used for this reconstruction, including the palmaris longus, gracilis, and triceps fascia (Charalambous & Stanley, 2008; Fedorka & Oh, 2016). The early literature on reconstruction techniques used for posterolateral instability included the overlay technique and the docking technique. Currently, there have been many modifications made to the early techniques, especially with the popularity of various types of implants.

The overlay technique described by Nestor et al (1992) uses transosseous tunnels in the humerus and ulna. Plication sutures are placed in the anterior and posterior capsule and used after the augmentation to advance and imbricate the remaining LCL complex. The reconstruction or augmentation is completed using a graft substitute such as the palmaris longus, triceps fascia, or a prosthetic ligament. Two drill holes are made through the ulna around the supinator crest and the isometry is checked with a free suture through the holes to the isometric point on the humerus. A drill hole for the tendon and two smaller holes for the sutures are created in a Y-shaped fashion in the humerus (Fig. 27.7). This allows for passing the tendon through the ulna-sided tunnel and docking the tendon in the humerus while fixing the tendon on itself at the humerus with the sutures over a bone bridge. Of their 11 study patients, they had 1 failure but obtained stability in the other 10 patients (Nestor et al, 1992).

Jones et al (2012) described the docking technique in 2012. In this technique, one limb of the graft is placed in the supinator crest of the ulna and fixed with an interference screw. The other limb of the graft is passed under the anconeus and docked into the posterior epicondyle of the humerus at the isometric point. Their study analyzed only 8 patients treated with this technique, but they had follow-up greater than 5 years on these patients. Six of the patients had complete resolution, and 2 had intermittent instability. Subjective assessment found that all patients were satisfied with their outcome (Jones et al, 2012).

Savoie et al (2010) reported on arthroscopic, open, and plication repairs in a retrospective review. They reviewed 54 patients, with an average follow-up period of 41 months (range, 12–103 months). Although several patients underwent concomitant procedures, the arthroscopic repairs improved the Andrews-Carson scores from 146 to 176 ($P = 0.0001$) and open repairs from 144 to 182 ($P < 0.001$). For both groups, subjective scores improved from 57 to 85 ($P < 0.0001$), and objective scores improved from 88 to 95 ($P = 0.008$). The study concluded that arthroscopic repair or plication (or both) of the LUCL can be successful techniques, similar to the open procedure.

Kim et al (2016) further analyzed arthroscopic LCL reconstruction in 2016 with a 13-patient study group followed for a minimum of 18 months. All patients had complete resolution of their instability; 12 rated their outcome as excellent, and 1 rated it as good. Results like these are making arthroscopic elbow stability procedures more common, but several others have noted they are technically demanding.

Anakwenze et al (2014) performed a systematic review of eight articles involving posterolateral lateral elbow instability. The studies reviewed 130 patients who underwent repair or reconstruction between 1992 and 2012. All patients had only soft tissue injuries, and the follow-up was at least 1 year. When preoperative examination data were available, the studies demonstrated that 95% of patients had a positive pivot shift test result with apprehension, subluxation, or dislocation on examination. Graft choice was recorded on 58 patients who underwent reconstruction. 30 had a triceps fascia graft, 19 had a palmaris tendon, 6 had gracilis tendons, and 1 had a semitendinosus tendon. The average Mayo Elbow Performance Score (MEPS) was 91 with 29 excellent, 14 good, 4 fair, and no poor outcomes reported. The postoperative pivot shift test was reported in only five studies, but after the surgery, the result was negative in 92% (72 of 78) of patients. Patient satisfaction was excellent with five studies reporting that 98% (50 of 51) of patients were satisfied with their final outcome. There were 8 overall complications. Six patients had recurrent episodes of elbow instability, 1 patient had a postoperative hematoma, and there was 1 superficial infection. The reoperation rate for instability was very low in these studies and recorded as only 2.6% (2 of 76 patients) (Anakwenze et al, 2014).

Outcomes from surgical repair and reconstruction of elbow instability are satisfactory to most patients and have good to excellent functional outcomes.

Rehabilitation and Return to Sport

Patients who were treated nonoperatively may return to sport when they are free from pain and instability episodes with restoration of strength and ROM compared with the contralateral side. However, patients with chronic PLRI who are unable to return to their prior level of activities are typically treated with surgery. In the postoperative period, patients are immobilized in a plaster posterior elbow splint for approximately 1 week. They are able to perform unlimited wrist and hand motion exercises. The wound is inspected at the first postoperative visit, and the patient is transitioned to a hinged elbow brace for 4 to 6 weeks. The patient may gradually increase ROM during this time starting at 30 to 90 degrees of flexion and progress as tolerated. Strengthening typically begins after restoration of full ROM and typically starts around 8 weeks postoperatively. For return to recreational activities and sports, the patient should be free from instability episodes and with similar strength and ROM to the contralateral side. Depending on the sport, full clearance to return to sports without restrictions may take 4 to 6 months after surgery.

References

Anakwe RE, Middleton SD, Jenkins PJ, McQueen MM, Court-Brown CM. Patient-reported outcomes after simple dislocation of the elbow. *J Bone Joint Surg Am*. 2001;93(13):1220–1226.

Anakwenze OA, Kwon D, O'Donnell E, Levine WN, Ahmad CS. Surgical treatment of posterolateral rotatory instability of the elbow. *Arthroscopy*. 2014;30(7):866–871.

Ball CM, Galatz LM, Yamaguchi K. Elbow instability: treatment strategies and emerging concepts. *Instr Course Lect*. 2002;51:53–61.

Camp CL, O'Driscoll SW, Wempe MK, Smith J. The sonographic posterolateral rotatory stress test for elbow instability: a cadaveric validation study. *PM R*. 2017;9(3):275–282.

Charalambous CP, Stanley JK. Posterolateral rotatory instability of the elbow. *J Bone Joint Surg Br*. 2008;90(3):272–279.

de Haan J, Schep NW, Eygendaal D, Kleinrensink GJ, Tuinebreijer WE, den Hartog D. Stability of the elbow joint: relevant anatomy and clinical implications of in vitro biomechanical studies. *Open Orthop J*. 2011;5:168–176.

Desloges W, Louati H, Papp SR, Pollock JW. Objective analysis of lateral elbow exposure with the extensor digitorum communis split compared with the Kocher interval. *J Bone Joint Surg Am*. 2014;96(5):387–393.

Fedorka CJ, Oh LS. Posterolateral rotatory instability of the elbow. *Curr Rev Muskuloskel Med*. 2016;9(2):240–246.

Hildebrand KA, Patterson SD, King GK. Acute elbow dislocations: simple and complex. *Orthop Clin North Am*. 1999;30(1):63–79.

Hobgood ER, Khan SO, Field LD. Acute dislocations of the adult elbow. *Hand Clin*. 2008;24(1):1–7.

Jones KJ, Dodson CC, Osbahr DC, et al. The docking technique for lateral ulnar collateral ligament reconstruction: surgical technique and clinical outcomes. *J Shoulder Elbow Surg*. 2012;21(3):389–395.

Kim JW, Yi Y, Kim TK, et al. Arthroscopic lateral collateral ligament repair. *J Bone Joint Surg Am*. 2016;98(15):1268–1276.

Mehta JA, Bain GI. Posterolateral rotatory instability of the elbow. *J Am Acad Orthop Surg*. 2004;12(6):405–415.

Nestor BJ, O'Driscoll SW, Morrey BF. Ligamentous reconstruction for posterolateral rotatory instability of the elbow. *J Bone Joint Surg Am*. 1992;74(8):1235–1241.

O'Driscoll SW, Bell DF, Morrey BF. Posterolateral rotatory instability of the elbow. *J Bone Joint Surg Am*. 1991;73(3):440–446.

O'Driscoll SW, Morrey BF, Korinek S, An KN. Elbow subluxation and dislocation. A spectrum of instability. *Clin Orthop Relat Res*. 1992;(280):186–197.

O'Driscoll SW, Spinner RJ, McKee MD, et al. Tardy posterolateral rotatory instability of the elbow due to cubitus varus. *J Bone Joint Surg Am*. 2001;83-A(9):1358–1369.

Regan W, Lapner PC. Prospective evaluation of two diagnostic apprehension signs for posterolateral instability of the elbow. *J Shoulder Elbow Surg*. 2006;15(3):344–346.

Savoie FH 3rd, O'Brien MJ, Field LD, Gurley DJ. Arthroscopic and open radial ulnohumeral ligament reconstruction for posterolateral rotatory instability of the elbow. *Clin Sports Med*. 2010;29(4):611–618.

Sheps DM, Hildebrand KA, Boorman RS. Simple dislocations of the elbow: evaluation and treatment. *Hand Clin*. 2004;20(4):389–404.

Skelley NW, Chamberlain A. A novel reduction technique for elbow dislocations. *Orthopedics*. 2015;38(1):42–44.

Yamaguchi K, Sweet FA, Bindra R, Morrey BF, Gelberman RH. The extraosseous and intraosseous arterial anatomy of the adult elbow. *J Bone Joint Surg Am*. 1997;79(11):1653–1662.

SECTION **X**

Elbow Tendon Injuries

SECTION OUTLINE

28 Medial: Flexor-Pronator Tendon Injury

MARK SCHICKENDANTZ, MD

Introduction

- The flexor-pronator muscle mass at the medial side of the elbow provides dynamic stability against valgus forces. Flexor-pronator tendon degeneration occurs with repetitive forced wrist extension and forearm supination during activities involving wrist flexion and forearm pronation.
- Athletes may be particularly symptomatic during the late cocking or early acceleration phases of the throwing motion.
- Nonsurgical management is the mainstay of treatment, and typically includes activity modification, nonsteroidal antiinflammatory drugs, and corticosteroid injections.
- Recent studies have investigated the impact of emerging modalities such as extracorporeal shock wave therapy and platelet-rich plasma.
- Surgical treatment via open techniques is uncommon and is typically reserved for patients with persistent symptoms.
- Progressive return to sport can be enhanced with the use of activity-specific rehabilitation and equipment modifications.

Epidemiology

Despite an overall prevalence of 1%, medial epicondylitis may affect as many as 3.8% to 8.2% of patients in occupational settings (Descatha et al, 2003; Shiri et al, 2006; Wolf et al, 2010). Medial epicondylitis typically occurs in the fourth through sixth decades of life and is a result of common flexor tendon (CFT) microtrauma and degeneration. Men and women are equally affected (Descatha et al, 2003; Shiri et al, 2006; Wolf et al, 2010).

The differential diagnoses for medial-sided elbow pain can include ulnar neuritis, tendinopathy, ligamentous instability, intraarticular pathology, and trauma. A thorough history and physical examination are critical to determine the likelihood of medial epicondylitis. In athletes, this condition is typically associated with overhead throwing, golf, or tennis; however, in the literature, it has been associated with other sports, including football, weightlifting, and bowling (Vangsness & Jobe, 1991; Wolf et al, 2010). Medial epicondylitis is also commonly found in occupational settings, especially those involving repetitive forceful grip, manual handling of loads of 44 lb (20 kg), or exposure to constant vibratory forces at the elbow (Descatha et al, 2003; Galloway et al, 1992; Shiri et al, 2006).

Anatomy

The flexor-pronator tendon is the confluence of five muscles of the forearm: the pronator teres (PT), flexor carpi radialis, palmaris longus, flexor carpi ulnaris (FCU), and flexor digitorum superficialis (Fig. 28.1). It is approximately 3 cm long and, in most elbows, crosses the ulnohumeral joint medially. The tendon attaches to the medial humeral epicondyle anteriorly and attaches proximally to the anterior bundle of the ulnar collateral ligament (UCL), with the fibers parallel to the UCL (Otoshi et al, 2014). The CFT, particularly the ulnar head of the PT, also becomes confluent with a hyperplastic section of the anteromedial joint capsule.

Mechanism of Injury

Most authors commonly accept that the principal mechanism of injury is repetitive eccentric loading of the muscles performing wrist flexion and forearm pronation, combined with valgus overload at the elbow (Ciccotti & Ramani, 2003). Strain of the medial elbow with a valgus overload moment, which occurs with overhead throwing, stimulates dynamic stabilization of the joint via eccentric contraction of the CFT. Simultaneous wrist flexion or forearm pronation during ball release may produce even greater eccentric stress on the tendon (Sisto et al, 1987). Historically, the PT has been identified as the primary dynamic stabilizer and the most likely musculotendinous unit to be injured in medial epicondylitis. Recent cadaver studies, however, have implicated every musculotendinous unit except the palmaris longus (Farber et al, 2009; Lin et al, 2007; Park & Ahmad, 2004; Udall et al, 2009).

Repetitive supraphysiologic stress on the tendon eventually results in microtrauma and degeneration. Histopathologic examination has revealed a staged process of pathologic tendon change (Regan et al, 1992). Initially, repetitive trauma results in peritendinous inflammation. Continued injury results in angiofibroblastic hyperplasia, an invasion of vascular and fibroblastic elements into the tendon. This results in structural breakdown and irreparable fibrosis or calcification. Activity causing such pathology to the CFT can eventually transfer forces deeper to the UCL, which mirrors CFT fiber orientation and histologic anatomy (Otoshi et al, 2014).

History

Patients typically present with persistent medial-sided elbow pain that is often localized to the medial epicondyle, with

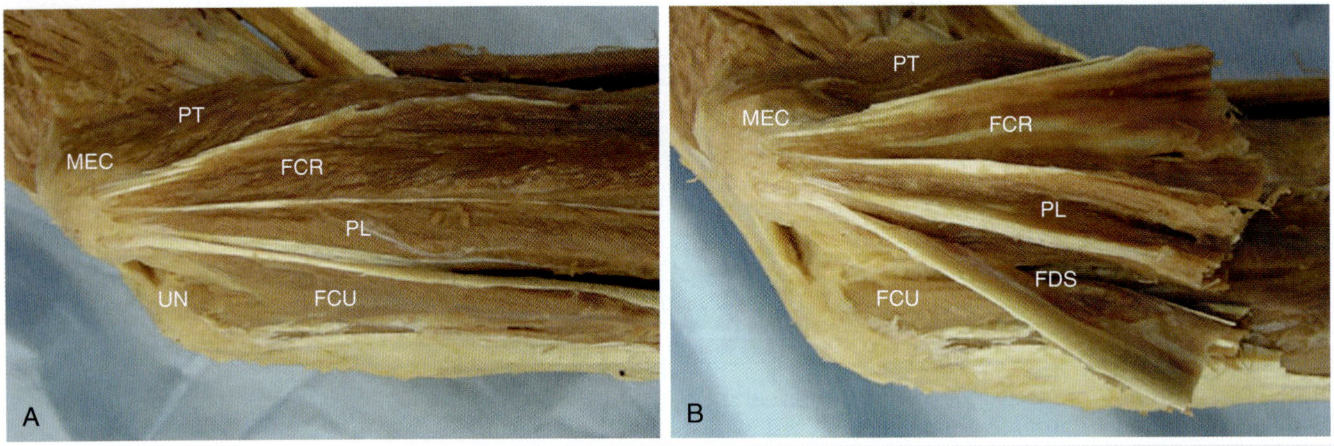

Fig. 28.1 A and **B,** Photographs of a cadaver elbow demonstrating the ulnar nerve (UN); medial epicondyle (MEC); and the anatomy of the flexor-pronator muscles, including the pronator teres (PT), flexor carpi radialis (FCR), palmaris longus (PL), flexor digitorum superficialis (FDS), and flexor carpi ulnaris (FCU). (Reproduced with permission from Otoshi K, Kikuchi SI, Shishido H, Konno SI. The proximal origins of the flexor-pronator muscles and their role in the dynamic stabilization of the elbow joint: an anatomic study. *Surg Radiol Anat.* 2014;36(3):289-294.)

radiation into the proximal forearm. Elbow pain is exacerbated by activity and is particularly bothersome during the late cocking phase in overhead throwing or during early acceleration for the thrower, tennis player, or golfer (Cain et al, 2003). Although less common, the patient history may include an acute trauma to the elbow resulting in an avulsion of the CFT. More commonly, the pain is characterized by an insidious onset, with persistence despite rest (Ciccotti & Ramani, 2003).

Physical Examination

Physical examination may detect tenderness 5 to 10 mm distal and anterior to the medial epicondyle that is accompanied by soft tissue swelling (Ciccotti & Ramani, 2003). Resisted wrist flexion, forearm pronation, or forceful grip may be weakened compared with that of the contralateral side and may exacerbate elbow pain (Pienimäki et al, 2011). Patients may present with an elbow flexion contracture secondary to pain and guarding; however, most patients present with normal passive and active range of motion (ROM) at the elbow and wrist. The neurovascular examination is typically unremarkable.

Patients suspected of having medial epicondylitis should be examined for other pathologies of the ipsilateral arm. Up to 84% of occupational patients may have concomitant work-related disorders, such as carpal tunnel syndrome, lateral epicondylitis, or rotator cuff tendinitis (Descatha et al, 2003). Overhead athletes must be examined for valgus instability secondary to an injury to the UCL. Evaluation of the UCL is performed by applying valgus stress to the elbow in 30 degrees of flexion, with the forearm pronated and the wrist flexed.

Ulnar neuritis is another common concomitant pathology. In patients with suspected ulnar neuropathy, the examination should include two-point discrimination in the ulnar sensory distribution and a comparison of the hypothenar bulk of the symptomatic and asymptomatic extremities. A positive Tinel sign can indicate compression of the ulnar nerve. Proximally, overdevelopment of the medial head of the triceps may compress the nerve against the medial intermuscular septum (Aoki et al, 2005; Gervasio & Zaccone, 2008). Distal to the medial epicondyle, the ulnar nerve travels under the arcade of Struthers and through the bifid FCU arcade distally, which may be inflamed and irritate the passing nerve (Ciccotti & Ramani, 2003). However, a positive Tinel sign may be found anywhere along the length of the nerve. Sensory changes in the ulnar hand may be reproduced by applying stress to an irritated ulnar nerve via the elbow flexion test, which is performed with maximal elbow flexion, forearm pronation, and wrist extension for 30 to 60 seconds (Ciccotti & Ramani, 2003). The presence of ulnar nerve subluxation should also be noted during examination, especially in patients who report a popping sensation during daily activities or overhead throwing. Ulnar neuritis with or without subluxation may exacerbate medial-sided elbow pain; therefore, treatment modalities specifically for medial epicondylitis provide inadequate relief. Patients with neurologic complaints or findings should also be examined for signs of cervical radiculopathy, particularly of the C6 and C7 roots, because these patients may be at increased risk of developing medial epicondylitis secondary to forearm muscle imbalance (Lee et al, 2010).

Imaging

In addition to a thorough patient history and physical examination, radiologic studies can support a diagnosis of medial epicondylitis. Although most radiographs demonstrate normal findings, up to 25% may show evidence of calcification of the CFT or UCL (Ciccotti & Ramani, 2003). Ultrasonography may be a cost-effective modality for visualizing CFT tendinosis and pathologic change. In a small series, Park et al (2008) showed that a sonogram performed by a radiologist had sensitivity, specificity, and positive and negative predictive values of 90% for diagnosis of medial epicondylitis. The authors most commonly discovered hypoechoic or anechoic areas of focal tendon degeneration on ultrasonography. This modality also allows for dynamic examination, which may improve specificity and sensitivity (Lee et al, 2011). However, the diagnostic accuracy of ultrasonography is highly dependent on the operator and may be less effective without well-trained sonographers.

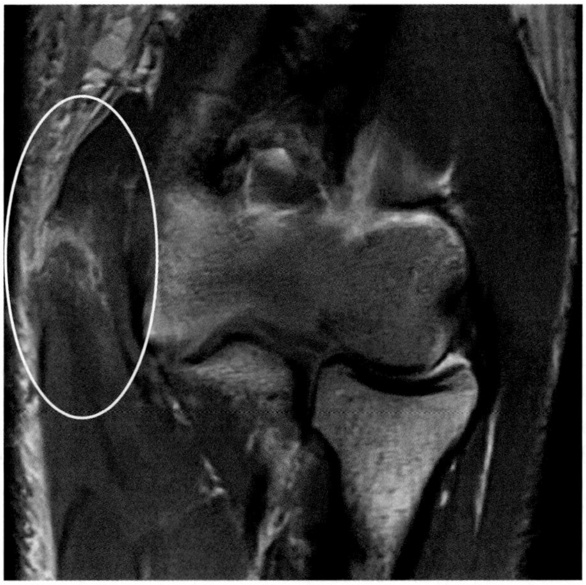

Fig. 28.2 Coronal slice of a magnetic resonance image of a minor league reliever demonstrating a tear of the flexor-pronator mass near the proximal origin *(oval).* (From Patel RM, Lynch TS, Amin NH, Calabrese G, Gryzlo SM, Schickendantz MS. The thrower's elbow. *Orthop Clin North Am.* 2014;45(3):355-376.)

Magnetic resonance imaging (MRI) remains the standard of care for radiologic detection of medial epicondylitis. Noncontrast MRI is effective for detecting pathologic change in the tendon, such as frank tendinous disruption as well as other medial elbow pathology (e.g., UCL or osteochondral injuries) (Walz et al, 2010) (Fig. 28.2). On T2-weighted sequences, intermediate to high signal intensity at the CFT, especially in the setting of peritendinous edema, is indicative of medial epicondylitis (Kijowski & De Smet, 2005). Advanced imaging is typically used when concern for concomitant pathology is high (e.g., evaluation of the UCL in an overhead thrower) or if the clinical picture is unclear regarding the source of medial elbow pain.

Nonoperative Management

As with many chronic tendinopathies, nonsurgical therapy is the mainstay of treatment. Surgical procedures are typically reserved for patients with recalcitrant or recurrent symptoms despite nonsurgical management.

The initial focus of nonsurgical supportive care is the relief of medial-sided elbow pain. Patients should refrain from activities that exacerbate symptoms, especially those that require repetitive wrist flexion, forearm pronation, and valgus stress about the elbow. Athletes with concomitant UCL injury should refrain from throwing for 6 to 12 weeks, with particular care taken to avoid valgus stress during the first 6 weeks of treatment. Periods of acute pain and swelling may be alleviated with icing, which provides both analgesic and vasoconstrictive effects (Ciccotti & Ramani, 2003). Nonsteroidal antiinflammatory drugs (NSAIDs) may also provide effective pain relief and may be used routinely for 1 to 2 weeks as tolerated by the patient. These medications are particularly effective in reducing the synovitis associated with flexor-pronator tendon degeneration (Ciccotti & Ramani, 2003; Kijowski & De Smet, 2005). Night splinting and supportive orthoses may be used simultaneously, especially extension splinting in patients with ulnar neuritis. Counterforce bracing limits the maximal contractile force generated by the flexor-pronator musculotendinous unit (Kijowski & De Smet, 2003). Chang et al (2012) demonstrated pain relief in baseball pitchers with medial epicondylitis by using forearm kinesiology taping techniques as a method of counterforce bracing. However, splinting and bracing should not involve prolonged elbow immobilization secondary to joint stiffness. In the setting of injury to the UCL, a hinged elbow brace can be used to provide varus–valgus stability and prevent full elbow extension.

Extracorporeal shockwave therapy (ESWT) may provide pain relief for a subset of patients. Electrical stimulation of the diseased tendon may promote angiogenesis, tendon healing, and short-term analgesia (Sems et al, 2006). In a study of patients with newly diagnosed epicondylitis treated with ESWT or steroid injection, Lee et al (2012) reported worse clinical pain scores at 1 and 2 weeks with ESWT but better patient satisfaction at 8 weeks. However, Krischek et al (1999) reported excellent or good clinical results with ESWT in only 7 of 30 patients at 1-year follow-up, which was notably worse than the results achieved in patients with lateral epicondylitis who underwent similar treatment. Definitive recommendations for the use of shockwave therapy for medial epicondylitis, including treatment duration and stimulation protocol, cannot be made at this point.

When noninvasive techniques prove inadequate, a corticosteroid injection is often effective in reducing medial elbow discomfort. The corticosteroid is injected into the peritendinous and synovial tissues rather than into the tendon itself (Ciccotti & Ramani, 2003). Similar to oral antiinflammatory medications, the corticosteroid may reduce the surrounding synovitis and resultant pain. Historically, direct injection deep to the flexor-pronator tendon has been the delivery technique of choice, although transcutaneous methods may be effective as well (Nirschl et al, 2003). Care should be taken to prevent iatrogenic complications such as subcutaneous atrophy, tendon weakening, or nerve injury. Local depigmentation may occur as well, especially in patients with darker skin (Ciccotti & Ramani, 2003; Stahl & Kaufman, 1997a). Needle injection also provides the benefit of tendon trephination, which may stimulate bleeding and tendon healing (Suresh, 2006). In a prospective study of 60 elbows treated with steroid injection for medial epicondylitis, Stahl and Kaufman (1997b) noted an acute improvement in pain during the 6 weeks after injection but no difference by 3 months. Lee et al (2012) demonstrated even shorter term gains after steroid injection, with acute improvement in pain scores over the first 2 weeks followed by a plateau for up to 8 weeks. Suresh et al (2006) combined needle stimulation and injection of autologous blood into the disrupted tendon, which resulted in decreased visual analog scale and Nirschl scores at 10 months.

Much attention has been devoted to platelet- rich plasma (PRP) injections in the treatment of epicondylitis, although the majority of Level I and II studies have focused on lateral epicondylitis as opposed to medial (Mishra & Pavelko, 2006; Peerbooms et al, 2010). PRP is thought to induce an acute inflammatory response with an abundance of various growth factors that may lead to healing of the damaged

Kurvers H, Verhaar J. The results of operative treatment of medial epicondylitis. *J Bone Joint Surg Am.* 1995;77(9):1374–1379.

Lee SS, Kang S, Park NK, et al. Effectiveness of initial extracorporeal shock wave therapy on the newly diagnosed lateral or medial epicondylitis. *Ann Rehabil Med.* 2012;36(5):681–687.

Lee AT, Lee-Robinson AL. The prevalence of medial epicondylitis among patients with c6 and c7 radiculopathy. *Sports Health.* 2010;2(4):334–336.

Lee MH, Cha JG, Jin W, et al. Utility of sonographic measurement of the common tensor tendon in patients with lateral epicondylitis. *AJR Am J Roentgenol.* 2011;196(6):1363–1367.

Lin F, Kohli N, Perlmutter S, Lim D, Nuber GW, Makhsous M. Muscle contribution to elbow joint valgus stability. *J Shoulder Elbow Surg.* 2007;16(6):795–802.

Mishra A, Pavelko T. Treatment of chronic elbow tendinosis with buffered platelet-rich plasma. *Am J Sports Med.* 2006;34:1774–1778.

Nirschl RP, Rodin DM, Ochiai DH, Maartmann-Moe C. DEX-AHE-01-99 Study Group. Iontophoretic administration of dexamethasone sodium phosphate for acute epicondylitis: a randomized, double-blinded, placebo-controlled study. *Am J Sports Med.* 2003;31(2):189–195.

Otoshi K, Kikuchi S, Shishido H, Konno S. The proximal origins of the flexor-pronator muscles and their role in the dynamic stabilization of the elbow joint: an anatomical study. *Surg Radiol Anat.* 2014;36(3):289–294.

Park MC, Ahmad CS. Dynamic contributions of the flexor-pronator mass to elbow valgus stability. *J Bone Joint Surg Am.* 2004;86(10):2268–2274.

Park GY, Lee SM, Lee MY. Diagnostic value of ultrasonography for clinical medial epicondylitis. *Arch Phys Med Rehabil.* 2008;89(4):738–742.

Peerbooms JC, Sluimer J, Bruijn DJ, Gosens T. Positive effect of an autologous platelet concentrate in lateral epicondylitis in a double-blind randomized controlled trial: platelet-rich plasma versus corticosteroid injection with a 1-year follow-up. *Am J Sports Med.* 2010;38:255–262.

Pienimäki T, Siira P, Vanharanta H. Widespread pain in chronic epicondylitis. *Eur J Pain.* 2011;15(9):921–927.

Regan W, Wold LE, Coonrad R, Morrey BF. Microscopic histopathology of chronic refractory lateral epicondylitis. *Am J Sports Med.* 1992;20(6):746–749.

Sems A, Dimeff R, Iannotti JP. Extracorporeal shock wave therapy in the treatment of chronic tendinopathies. *J Am Acad Orthop Surg.* 2006;14(4):195–204.

Shiri R, Viikari-Juntura E, Varonen H, Heliövaara M. Prevalence and determinants of lateral and medial epicondylitis: a population study. *Am J Epidemiol.* 2006;164(11):1065–1074.

Sisto DJ, Jobe FW, Moynes DR, Antonelli DJ. An electromyographic analysis of the elbow in pitching. *Am J Sports Med.* 1987;15(3):260–263.

Stahl S, Kaufman T. Ulnar nerve injury at the elbow after steroid injection for medial epicondylitis. *J Hand Surg Br.* 1997a;22(1):69–70.

Stahl S, Kaufman T. The efficacy of an injection of steroids for medial epicondylitis: a prospective study of sixty elbows. *J Bone Joint Surg Am.* 1997b;79(11):1648–1652.

Suresh SP, Ali KE, Jones H, Connell DA. Medial epicondylitis: is ultrasound guided autologous blood injection an effective treatment? *Br J Sports Med.* 2006;40(11):935–939. discussion 939.

Udall JH, Fitzpatrick MJ, McGarry MH, Leba TB, Lee TQ. Effects of flexor-pronator muscle loading on valgus stability of the elbow with an intact, stretched, and resected medial ulnar collateral ligament. *J Shoulder Elbow Surg.* 2009;18(5):773–778.

Unlu MC, Kesmezacar H, Akgun I, Ogut T, Uzun I. Anatomic relationship between elbow arthroscopy portals and neurovascular structures in different elbow and forearm positions. *J Shoulder Elbow Surg.* 2006;15(4):457–462.

Vangsness CT Jr, Jobe FW. Surgical treatment of medial epicondylitis: results in 35 elbows. *J Bone Joint Surg Br.* 1991;73(3):409–411.

Walz DM, Newman JS, Konin GP, Ross G. Epicondylitis: pathogenesis, imaging, and treatment. *Radiographics.* 2010;30(1):167–184.

Wolf JM, Mountcastle S, Burks R, Sturdivant RX, Owens BD. Epidemiology of lateral and medial epicondylitis in a military population. *Mil Med.* 2010;175(5):336–339.

Zonno A, Manuel J, Merrell G, Ramos P, Akelman E, DaSilva MF. Arthroscopic technique for medial epicondylitis: technique and safety analysis. *Arthroscopy.* 2010;26(5):610–616.

29 Lateral: Extensor Carpi Radialis Brevis Tendon Injury

DONOVAN W. JOHNSON, MD, MICHAEL J. O'BRIEN, MD, and FELIX H. SAVOIE III, MD

Introduction

- Lateral epicondylitis is the most common overuse disorder affecting the lateral side of the elbow.
- This syndrome typically presents with intense pain about the extensor origin (lateral aspect) of the elbow. The pathogenesis of this disease originates from the extensor carpi radialis brevis (ECRB) tendon, but other closely associated structures can cause similar pain.
- Lateral epicondylitis historically was associated with the sport of lawn tennis, but this tendon injury can occur from various activities involving repetitive wrist extension.
- Typical patients are in their 40s or 50s. Surprisingly, there is no difference in occurrence between men and women.
- *Angiofibrotic dysplasia* is the term coined for the microscopic appearance of the diseased ECRB tendon. Lateral epicondylitis is now thought to be a dysvascular degenerative-type process termed tendinosis rather than *tendonitis.*
- Eighty-five percent of patients with tennis elbow will have a resolution in symptoms after conservative treatments. These treatments include resting, antiinflammatories, bracing, and injections.
- Only 10% of patients will go on to have surgical intervention for symptom relief, and 85% to 95% will be satisfied after these interventions.
- Ultrasound ablation can be considered the currently most effective treatment of lateral epicondylitis. Most patients—as high as 95%—will be pain free after this procedure.

Lateral elbow pain is a common presentation into most sports medicine clinics. It is seen in 1% to 3% of adult patients who are aged between 35 and 50 years old (Baker et al, 2000). There are multiple causes of lateral elbow pain, including lateral epicondylitis, radial tunnel, instability, plica syndrome, annular ligament hypertrophy, radiocapitellar chondromalacia, and arthritis. Originally, lateral elbow pain was described in association with playing lawn tennis; today this complaint is less often associated with this sport. Extensive research has shown that the pathogenesis contributing to lateral epicondylitis originates from the ECRB tendon (Nirschl, 1973). The primary objective for this chapter is to describe the relationships between lateral elbow pain and the ECRB tendon. By doing so, we will summarize the most acceptable definition for the disease, lateral epicondylitis. Next, we will discuss some of the current nonsurgical options for managing patients with lateral epicondylitis as well as the surgical options when non- to minimally invasive options fail to alleviate symptoms.

Anatomy of the Extensor Carpi Radialis Brevis and Lateral Epicondyle

When trying to understand the pathogenesis of lateral epicondylitis, one must appreciate the anatomy of the lateral elbow, particularly the lateral epicondyle and its neighboring structures. The morphology of the lateral epicondyle has been described as a pyramidal bony prominence (Boyer & Hastings, 1999). Cohen et al (2008) characterized the ECRB origin as diamond shaped, beginning just anterior to the most distal aspect of the lateral supracondylar ridge. The ECRB tendon originates adjacent to the extensor digitorum communis (EDC). The ECRB footprint is located between the most proximal aspect of the capitellum and the midline of the radiocapitellar joint. Research has determined that lateral epicondylitis pathology occurs in the more superficial and the marginally deeper fibers of the ECRB tendon. The lateral collateral ligamentous complex (the radial collateral ligament, annular ligament, accessory collateral ligament, and lateral ulnar collateral ligament) lies immediately posterior to the ECRB origin, and the anconeus originates from the posterior face of the lateral epicondyle. The brachioradialis and extensor carpi radialis longus (ECRL) have their origin proximal to the ECRB along the anterior aspect of the supracondylar ridge.

Proximal to the elbow joint, the radial nerve is located between the brachialis and brachioradialis, which further divides into the two terminal branches, the superficial radial nerve and the posterior interosseous nerve (PIN). This division occurs at the level of the radial head. The PIN courses distally entering the supinator muscle. This location is sometimes termed the *radial tunnel,* and compression here has been implicated in cases of refractory lateral epicondylitis (Roles & Maudsley, 1972).

Lateral Epicondylitis

HISTORY

Lateral epicondylitis was first described in 1873 in German literature by Runge (1873). In 1883, Morris (Boyer &

Hastings, 1999) suggested an association of symptoms with the game of lawn tennis, which led to the common term *tennis elbow*. Historically, it was believed that an inflammatory process was the cause of lateral epicondylitis, proposing a partial tearing of the ECRB tendon alone, with separation of the periosteum from the lateral epicondyle to elicit this inflammatory response, resulting in symptoms. Currently, several neighboring structures to the ECRB tendon have been identified as contributing to lateral elbow pain, including the annular ligament, radial nerve, lateral capsule, and several different bands of the extensor digitorum communis. In addition, microscopic studies of excised tissue demonstrate a failure of reparative response in the ECRB tendon rather than an inflammatory response within the tissue. Nirschl is credited with redefining the pathology of damage to the ECRB as angiofibrotic dysplasia, or tendinosis, rather than tendonitis.

The clinical presentation of a patient with lateral epicondylitis is an adult individual in their fourth or fifth decade of life. There are no differences in diagnosis between men and women. It is more common in the dominant arm. Recent studies have identified several risk factors for lateral epicondylitis, including a history of manual labor with heavy tools and significant strain while performing repetitive tasks (Haahr & Andersen, 2003a). Roughly 80% of patients with newly diagnosed lateral epicondylitis improve over time, and most report symptomatic relief at one year. Most experience some residual symptoms, and only 4% to 11% of those seeking medical attention require surgical intervention (Baker et al, 2000; Boyd & McLeod, 1973; Coonrad & Hooper, 1973; Nirschl, 1979). Poor prognostic factors for successful nonsurgical treatment include participation in manual labor, dominant arm involvement, long duration of symptoms with high baseline pain levels, and poor coping mechanism (Haahr & Anderson, 2003b).

PATHOANATOMY AND HISTOLOGY

Nirschl and Pettrone (1979) and Nirschl (1992) outlined the most commonly accepted theory of the pathogenesis of this disease. Nirschl built on the previous findings of Cyriax (1936), Goldie (1964), and Coonrad and Hooper (1973), highlighting the fundamental underlying lesion was within the origin of the ECRB tendon. Overuse and repetitive motions lead to microtears in the ECRB origin. As described earlier, most microscopic studies of excised tissue demonstrate a failure of reparative response in the ECRB tendon. The normal ECRB tendon tissue is invaded by immature fibroblasts and nonfunctional vascular buds, and adjacent tissue is often disorganized and hypercellular (Faro, 2007). Nirschl and Ashman (2003) coined the term *angiofibroblastic tendinosis* because of this microscopic appearance; here there is no evidence of acute inflammation. As a result of their research, tennis elbow is now thought to be a dysvascular degenerative-type process termed *tendinosis* rather than *tendonitis*. Nirschl and colleagues have noted that 35% to 50% of patients also have degenerative changes in the EDC. These changes, as seen within the ECRB tendon, are responsible for the pain that is associated with this condition.

Box 29.1 Risk Factors in Lateral Epicondylitis: Contributing Factors in Tennis Players

- Poor technique
- Weak shoulder and wrist muscles
- Increased string tension
- Improperly sized grip
- Hitting heavy, wet, or dead balls
- Hitting "off center" on the racket

PHYSICAL EXAMINATION AND WORKUP

The typical presentation of a patient with lateral epicondylitis consists of pain at the lateral elbow worsened by active wrist extension or passive wrist flexion with the elbow extended. Patients may describe an inability to hold objects in their hand because of lateral elbow pain. Physical examination typically reveals a point of maximal tenderness 1 to 3 mm anterior and distal to the tip of the lateral epicondyle, which is reproducible by resisted wrist and finger extension. This location corresponds to the origin of the EDC and ECRB tendon. Infrequently, this pain is accompanied by warmth, swelling, or erythema. The tennis elbow stress test is performed when the examiner asks the patient to resist wrist extension from neutral while the elbow is flexed and extended, with pain isolated to the ECRB origin indicating a positive test. (Box 29.1 and Table 29.1).

IMAGING

Lateral epicondylitis is predominantly a clinical diagnosis, but several imaging modalities have been used to provide supplementary information. Plain films can occasionally show calcinosis within the mobile wad origin or intraarticular pathology (Goldie, 1964; Nirschl, 1979). Nirschl noted the findings of calcifications forecast persistent and refractory disease and were present in up to 20% of patients who required surgery (Nirschl 1973, 1979, 1992, 2003).

Magnetic resonance imaging (MRI) can be useful during the workup of lateral elbow pain. It is an excellent tool that can evaluate for intraarticular involvement, radial collateral ligament competency, and definition of the degree of tearing of the extensor origin. In 90% of symptomatic patients, MRI scans may show thickening and edema of the extensor tendon origin (Mackay et al, 2003; Potter et al, 1995; Steinborn et al, 1999). High-resolution and fine-cut scanning shows that the ECRB origin can be classified as the following: full tear of the tendon, partial tear of the tendon, thinning of the ligament, or separation away from the ulnar collateral ligament complex. However, there are some limitations when using MRI while assessing response to treatment for lateral epicondylitis. T2 signaling may persist for weeks after symptoms resolve following treatment (Savnik et al, 2004). One must correlate the findings of MRI with a clinical examination because 14% to 51% of asymptomatic elbows have edema in the common extensor origin (Mackay et al, 2003; Savnik, 2004) (Fig. 29.1).

Ultrasonography has a sensitivity of 64% to 88% when used to examine for pathology in the ECRB tendon, but specificity is variable, ranging from 36% to 100% (Levin et al, 2005; Miller et al, 2002). It can identify peritendinous fluid, thickening of the common extensor origin, intrasubstance tears, and focal hypoechoic areas. This image modality is user dependent.

Table 29.1 Differential Diagnosis of Lateral Epicondylitis

Condition	Description
Radial tunnel syndrome	Maximal tenderness is usually more distal (3–4 cm) and anterior to the lateral epicondyle, primarily deep to the brachioradialis. Resisted wrist extension may not be painful, but resisted extension of the third and fourth fingers with the wrist supported may reproduce the pain.
Cervical radiculopathy	Usually more diffuse weakness and associated numbness without point tenderness over the lateral epicondyle
Posterolateral elbow plica	Palpable band of synovium posterior to the epicondyle near the posterior radiocapitellar joint. May click and pop with extension and supination. Often associated with other elbow pathology such as lateral epicondylitis and arthritis.
Posterolateral elbow instability	May be associated with lateral epicondylitis but has more pain with supination than resisted wrist extension. Often hypersupination in 90 degrees of flexion reproduces the symptoms and increases the index of suspicion.
OCD lesion of the radiocapitellar joint	Deep posterior and lateral pain that does not diminish with cessation of activity; loss of motion. Positive findings on radiographs and usually affects a completely different age population.

OCD, osteo-chondral defect.

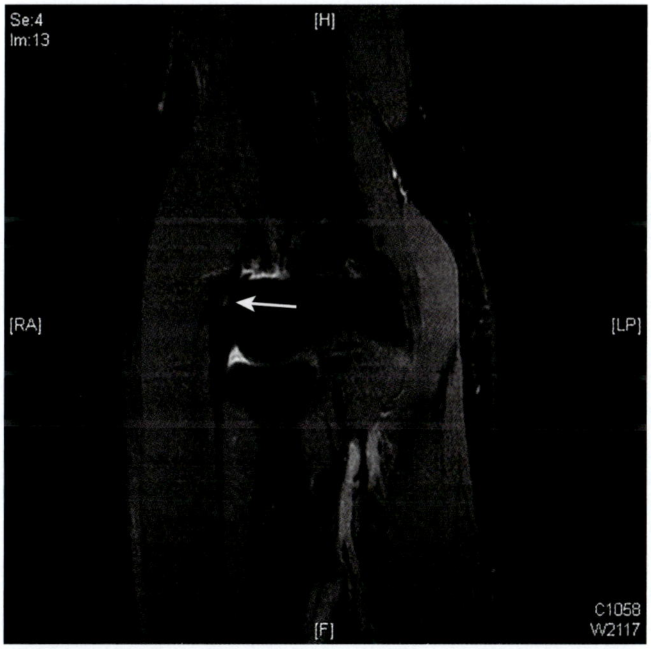

Fig. 29.1 Magnetic resonance image of extensor carpi radialis brevis damage consistent with lateral epicondylitis *(arrow)*.

Nonsurgical Treatment

Several treatment modalities have been proposed for lateral epicondylitis, and all steer to aid or enhance normal healing. Nirschl and Ashman (2003) proposed a methodical treatment program that parallels the natural healing response: (1) controlling exudation and hemorrhage; (2) promoting tissue healing; (3) encouraging general fitness; (4) control of force loading; and in a minority of patients, (5) removal of diseased tissue.

NONSTEROIDAL ANTIINFLAMMATORY DRUGS AND REST

Rest and nonsteroidal antiinflammatory drugs (NSAIDs) are the two most commonly used treatment modalities for acute lateral epicondylitis; the combination of both reduces tendon inflammation, relieves tendon strain, and provides time for tendon healing. As previously mentioned, lateral epicondylitis is described as a noninflammatory condition; NSAIDs are thought to reduce pain by reducing inflammation in the surrounding soft tissue such as the synovium, connective tissue, muscle tissue, and supportive tissue. Research has shown limited benefit in using NSAIDs for the treatment of lateral epicondylitis. Labelle and Guibert (1997) performed a multicenter, double-blinded, randomized controlled trial comparing the use of an oral NSAID (diclofenac) with placebo, and they concluded that the treatment group reported less pain. However, they did not endorse the use of NSAIDs—they found no significant benefit to overall functional ability and grip strength along with undesirable gastrointestinal side effects. To date, there is only one study comparing the use of multiple NSAIDs, and it did not find any differences between the treatment groups versus placebo (Stull & Jokl, 1986). There have been mixed reviews evaluating the effects of topical NSAIDs as well.

PHYSICAL THERAPY

Physical therapy is often prescribed to patients with lateral epicondylitis. There are no definite modes and duration of therapy plans, but the most acceptable protocol has been outlined by Nirschl (1973, 1992), Nirschl and Pettrone (1979), and Nirschl and Ashman (2003). This particular protocol consists of increasing strength, flexibility, and endurance of the forearm. It integrates stretching of the extensor origin by bringing the wrist into flexion with the elbow extended and the forearm pronated. In modern protocols, eccentric muscle training has been popular. This mode of therapy induces hypertrophy of the musculotendinous unit and increases the tensile strength of the unit, which in theory will reduce strain on the unit (Martinez-Silvestrini et al, 2005). Additionally, eccentric contractions could provide the ideal stimulus for collagen production from tendon cells and reduce the neovascularization that may contribute to the pain of lateral epicondylitis (Ohberg et al, 2004). Nirschl (1973, 1992), Nirschl and Pettrone (1979), Nirschl and Ashman (2003) also found the use of iontophoresis to be helpful in the management of lateral epicondylitis.

INJECTIONS

Steroid injections have been shown to positively correlate with improvement of lateral elbow pain. They are used for acute pain control, allowing patients to begin rehabilitation. Multiple studies have evaluated the efficacy of steroid injections versus NSAIDs and placebo. Pain relief during the first 5 days to 6 weeks are favorable for injections (Boyd & McLeod, 1973; Coonrad, 1973; Seng et al, 2015; Zhu, 2008).

However, at longer follow-up for 12 weeks to 12 months, the results of injections were the same as those in other treatment groups. There have been only a few case reports discussing common extensor tendon rupture after local steroid injection. When comparing steroid injections with platelet-rich-plasma (PRP), PRP has been shown to produce better pain relief and functionality (Peerbooms et al, 2010; Smith et al, 1999). In 2014, Mishra et al (2014) published a prospective randomized double-blinded control study evaluating the clinical usefulness of needling with PRP in patients with chronic lateral epicondylitis. This study consisted of 230 patients who had at least 3 months of symptoms and had failed conventional therapy. The study population was equally divided into a treatment group and an active control group, both of which showed no significant difference in pain at 12 weeks. However, at 24 weeks, the PRP-treated patients reported a statistically significant improvement of pain compared to the control group (Mishra et al, 2014).

ORTHOSES

The two orthotic devices usually prescribed to patients with chronic lateral epicondylitis are the proximal forearm counterforce brace and the cock-up wrist splint. Both devices are designed to reduce tension and load at the extensor origin, thus allowing time for tendon healing. Proximal forearm banding is thought to prevent extensor muscle expansion, creating a new extensor origin (Nirschl, 1973). Cock-up wrist splints are used to prevent extensor muscle contraction and, by decreasing muscle contraction, provide mechanical rest to the extensor origin (Groppel & Nirschl, 1986). Currently, there are no comparative studies between forearm bands and wrist splints that demonstrate any superiority of one device over the other (Van De Streek et al, 2004). Most physicians usually prescribe a proximal forearm brace for chronic lateral epicondylitis because it allows patients the most functional use of their upper extremity (Fig. 29.2).

AUTHORS' PREFERRED NONOPERATIVE TECHNIQUE

The authors believe in an aggressive nonoperative treatment protocol on initial presentation. The disease and natural history are discussed with the patient to improve understanding of the process. The elbow is injected, and medications, therapy, and bracing are all prescribed. The initial injection is 3 cc of 1% lidocaine without epinephrine followed immediately by a second injection of 6 cc 0.25% bupivacaine without epinephrine combined with 2 cc of preservative-free methylprednisolone. The second injection uses an 18-gauge needle, and the tip is used to "scrape" the epicondylar origin of the ECRB to improve the healing response. We also recommend massage to the ECRB origin with topical ketoprofen 10% microemulsion topical gel (with or without 2% bupivacaine) two to four times per day, a home exercise program for stretching, all exercise done with the elbow in extension and a dorsiflexion wrist brace to protect the elbow during repetitive or strenuous activity, physical therapy for phoresis treatment and patches, and deep tissue massage and eccentric exercise two times per week for 4 to 6 weeks. This program seems to be effective about 90% of the time (FHS personal data).

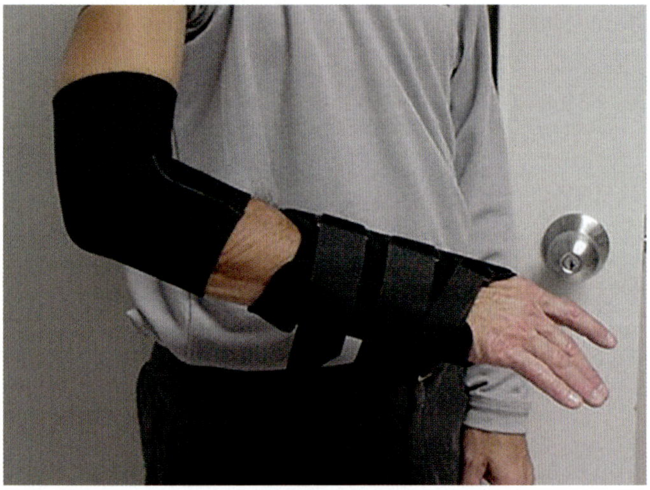

Fig. 29.2 Elbow sleeve with wrist brace.

Operative Management

The main indication for surgery for lateral epicondylitis is a failure of nonoperative management and patient frustration with the pace of recovery. Although the natural history suggests resolution within 2 years of onset, many patients may be functionally impaired or have sufficient pain to desire surgical intervention. It must be stressed that there does not seem to be any benefit to early intervention over delayed surgical treatment. Options for surgical management include ultrasound ablation, percutaneous release, open debridement with or without repair, and arthroscopic debridement or repair (Szabo et al, 2006).

ULTRASOUND ABLATION

Ultrasound ablation has proven to be a useful method of treatment for those patients who are refractory to the nonoperative treatments. Pathologic tissue of lateral epicondylitis may have calcifications and it appears hypoechoic on ultrasonography. Ultrasonography is thus a highly sensitive tool for localizing and targeting needle ablation of the diseased tissue in lateral epicondylitis (Levin et al, 2005; Zeisig et al, 2006). The TX1 (Tenex Health, Lake Forest, CA) system was developed solely for the treatment of chronic tendinopathic orthopedic conditions. This procedure is less invasive than surgical treatment and can be performed in an office setting or ambulatory surgical facility.

This novel technique is termed fasciotomy and surgical tenotomy (FAST), and the technique consists of two phases, the confirmatory phase (phase 1) and the therapeutic FAST technique (phase 2). During phase 1, a confirmatory ultrasound examination is performed identifying the hypoechoic region of the tendon. The actual ablation procedure is performed in phase 2, when local anesthesia should be introduced just distal to the site of pathology in line with the extensor fibers. Next, the local is deepened past the deep fascia toward the hypoechoic region and a small incision is made through the skin following the same direction as the injection. The TX1 needle is then passed to the hypoechoic region, particular settings are placed, and microresection of the pathologic tissue follows.

In 2013, Morrey's group published a study detailing this procedure in 20 patients. The follow-up for this study was 1 year, and 19 of 20 patients (95%) expressed satisfaction with the procedure (Koh et al, 2013). In 2015, Morrey and his colleagues published a second study evaluating the same treatment group at 3 years after the initial procedure (Seng et al, 2015). Notably, there was 100% follow-up for this study. None of the patients required further intervention for their chronic epicondylitis, and 100% continued to express their satisfaction. Ninety-four percent had resolution in their tendon hypervascularity, and tendon thickness was reduced in all patients. The hypoechoic scar was reduced in all patients, which continued up to 36 months with 20% having complete resolution of the scar (Seng et al, 2015).

PERCUTANEOUS TECHNIQUE

In-office percutaneous release was described by Turner and Yerger and popularized by Savoie et al (2010) Yerger and Turner (1985). In the technique, the origin area of the ECRB is isolated and local anesthetic injected. A #11 knife blade is then placed through the fascia to the anterior aspect of the lateral epicondyle at the site of origin of the ECRB, and the tendon is released by pivoting the blade. The patient is asked to flex and extend the wrist, confirming adequate release. The technique is relatively simple and allows for quick recovery; the main issues usually relate to excessive release or damage to the overlying ECRL or fascia. In several studies the success of the procedure was noted to be in the 80% to 90% range (Szabo et al, 2006).

OPEN TECHNIQUE

The open surgical technique (Fig. 29.3) was first described by Nirschl and Pettrone in 1979. To perform this procedure, an incision is made 3 to 4 cm in length centered just distal to the lateral epicondyle. The extensor aponeurosis should then be incised, splitting the ECRL to expose the origin of the ECRB. The lesion of the pathologic tendon should be debrided in its entirety and the lateral epicondyle bone decorticated. The degenerative tissue typically has a gray hue. The remaining tissue is either left alone and the ECRL and fascial aponeurosis closed, or else the ECRB defect can be closed and the tendon reattached to the epicondyle. An anchor may be used to reattach the ECRB tendons (Nirschl, 1979; Szabo et al, 2006). After surgery, a soft dressing should be applied, and range of motion (ROM) should be encouraged early. The arm should be placed in a splint or sling until the first postoperative appointment, usually at ten days (Rosenberg & Henderson, 2002). After the short immobilization period, ROM exercises begin, and strengthening is usually started at 6 weeks.

Excessive debridement that extends posterior to the epicondyle may compromise the lateral stability of the elbow, leading to posterolateral rotary instability. Infrequently, neuromas of the posterior cutaneous nerve of the forearm can develop, leading to persistent postoperative pain. Last, reactive bone formation after open procedures has been described (Mullett et al, 2005).

The indications for arthroscopic surgical intervention have been previously discussed. However, there are several important relative contraindications for the arthroscopic techniques, including the following: (1) previous medial elbow surgery with an ulnar nerve transposition, which will usually require localization of the nerve prior to portal placement; (2) the presence of a subluxating ulnar nerve (to note, arthroscopic surgery can occur after exposure and protection of the nerve before placing the proximal medial portal to prevent injury); (3) the presence of an active infection.

Baker et al (2000) described an arthroscopic approach with a primary goal of debridement of pathologic tissue. In their study, they reported 40 patients (42 elbows) with recalcitrant lateral epicondylitis who underwent arthroscopic surgery. A standard medial portal was used for viewing and a superior lateral portal for debriding. Many times, the lateral epicondyle was decorticated with a bur. Several reports of arthroscopic techniques have been published since this study, and all reports consistently document satisfactory results with the arthroscopic techniques (Baker et al, 2000).

Two additional tendon repair techniques can be added to the debridement procedure. A plication of the remaining ECRB to the overlying ECRL using absorbable sutures can be accomplished. Essentially, the ECRB is repaired by suturing it to the ECRL and lateral septum. A second technique uses the anterolateral portal to place an anchor into the anterior aspect of the lateral epicondyle. The sutures are then pushed into the joint and retrieved through the capsule and muscle of the ECRB. Each set is retrieved percutaneously through the tennis elbow portal and tied deep to the ECRL (Rosenberg & Henderson, 2002).

All arthroscopic surgeries are performed on an outpatient basis. The arm can be placed in a sling for comfort, and the patient should be encouraged to begin immediate active and passive ROM exercises of the elbow. Home exercises can be started after the first postoperative visit. If there is a concern for lost ROM, a prescription for physical therapy can be considered. Patients can return to light duty activities at 2 weeks and return to sports at 6 weeks after surgery.

Authors' Preferred Surgical Technique

The senior author prefers either open or arthroscopic repair of the damaged ECRB. In many cases, he has found associated damage to part of the radial ulnorhumeral ligament (RUHL) complex to be associated with both failed nonoperative and operative management. He also believes that this is an inherent observational bias of his practice, and thus believes that although the majority of patients will have successful treatment by all the various operative and nonoperative techniques listed, there will still remain a population that requires repair. The open technique used is similar to Nirschl's, with added Vicryl sutures to plicate the lateral collateral ligament (LCL) and RUHL. The arthroscopic technique is also similar to that described, with complete debridement of the angiofibrotic dysplasia (Nirschl lesion) followed by plication or repair with supplemental repair of the RUHL as indicated (Fig. 29.4).

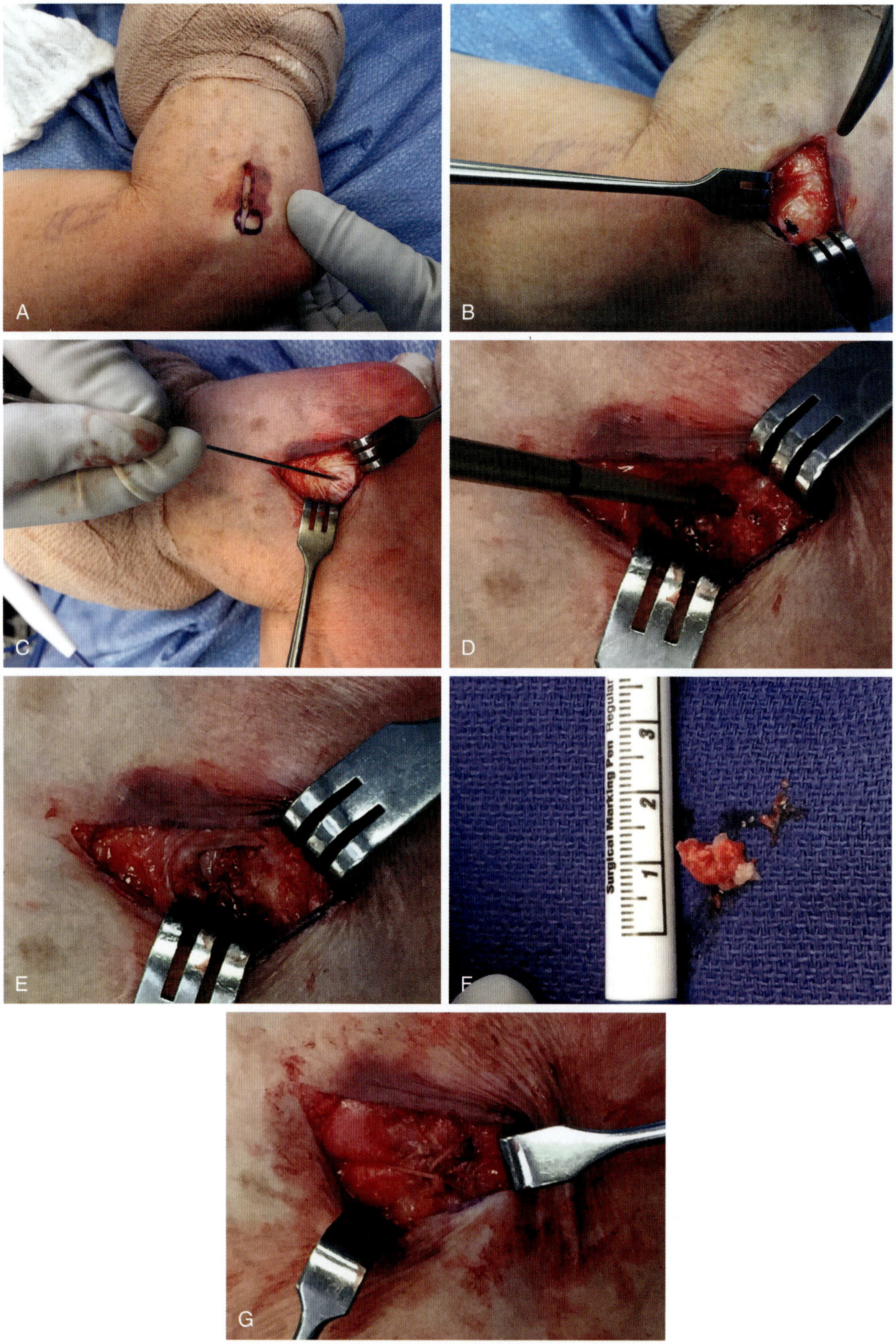

Fig. 29.3 Open treatment for lesion resection. **A,** Marked incision. **B,** Incision made and tendon exposed. **C,** Needle pointing to the Nirschl lesion's location. **D,** Nirschl lesion exposed. **E,** Completed resection. **F,** Resected tissue. **G,** Finished repair.

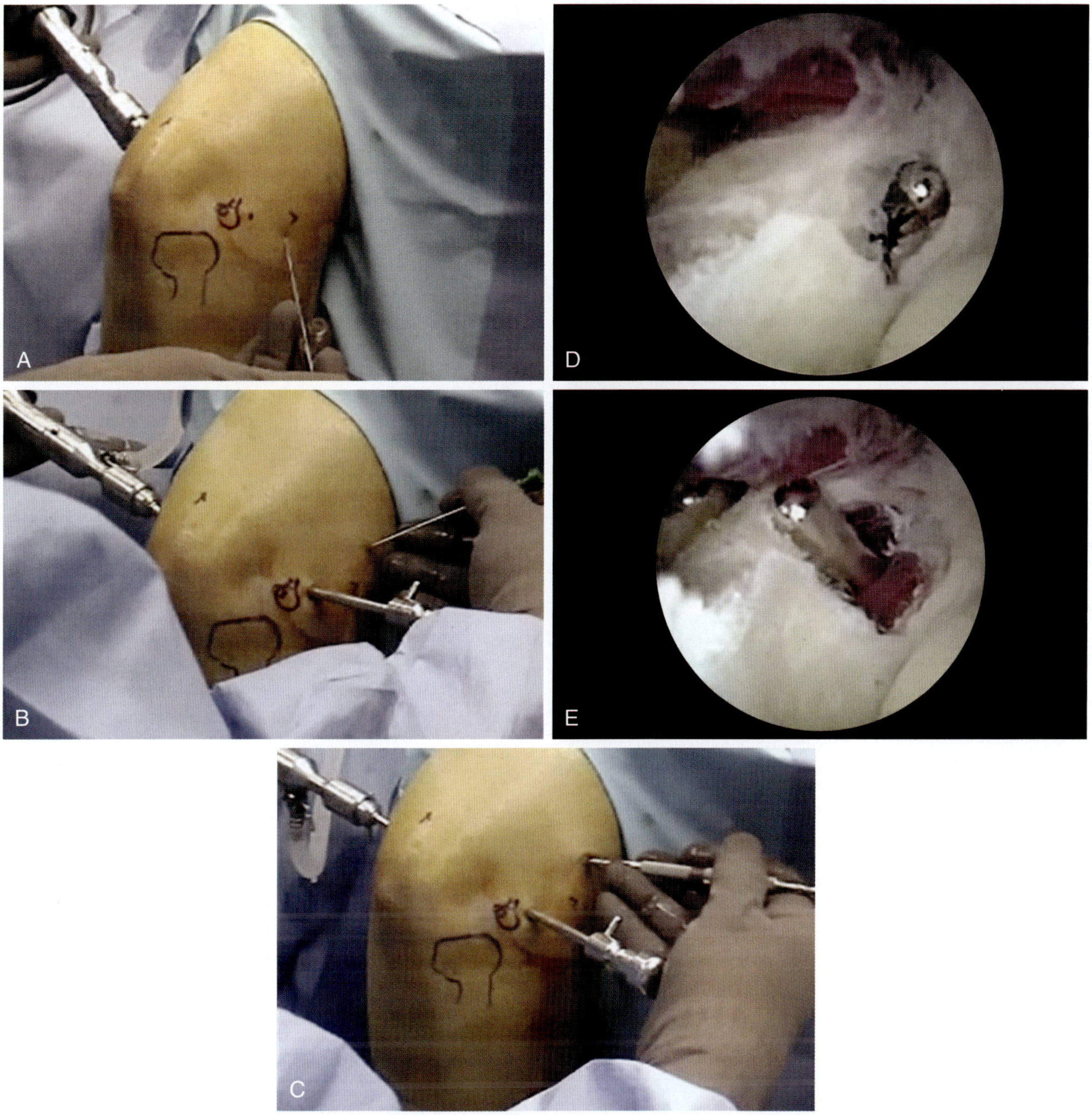

Fig. 29.4 Arthroscopic treatment for lesion resection. **A,** Setup for lateral portal placement for resection of lateral epicondylitis. **B,** Insertion of cannula for extensor carpi radialis brevis (ECRB) resection of the right elbow. **C,** Placement of superior retractor to facilitate visualization of the ECRB lesion. **D,** The beginning of the resection of the Nirschl lesion. The retractor is at the top left of the field. **E,** The lesion has been resected.

RESULTS

All forms of treatment seem to be generally successful. In general, most nonoperative management is effective 85% of the time, and most operative treatment, including ultrasound ablation, works 90% to 95% of the time.

COMPLICATIONS

The primary complications associated with lateral epicondylitis surgery seem to be either failure to recognize preexisting instability or inadvertent damage to part or all of the radial ulnohumeral ligament complex (the LCL) with subsequent instability. Radial nerve injury has been reported but appears to be relatively rare.

Conclusions

Lateral epicondylitis is a common cause of lateral elbow pain, related most often to overuse. It is usually successfully managed by nonoperative measures, with physical therapy for iontophoresis and eccentric strengthening having the most evidence of effectiveness. Surgical measures to remove the diseased tendon with or without repair have a high success rate with minimal complications

References

Baker CL Jr, Murphy KP, Gottlob CA, Curd DT. Arthroscopic classification and treatment of lateral epicondylitis: two-year clinical results. *J Shoulder Elbow Surg*. 2000;9:475–482.

Boyd HB, McLeod AC Jr. Tennis elbow. *J Bone Joint Surg Am*. 1973;55:1183–1187.

Boyer MI, Hastings H II. Lateral tennis elbow: is there any science out there? *J Shoulder Elbow Surg*. 1999;8:481–491.

Cohen MS, Romeo AA, Hennigan SP, Gordon M. Lateral epicondylitis: anatomic relationship of the extensor tendon origins and implications for arthroscopic treatment. *J Shoulder Elbow Surg*. 2008;17(6):954–960.

Coonrad RW, Hooper WR. Tennis elbow: its course, natural history, conservative and surgical management. *J Bone Joint Surg Am*. 1973;55(6):1177–1182.

Cyriax JH. The pathology and treatment of tennis elbow. *J Bone Joint Surg Am*. 1936;18:921–940.

Faro F, Wolf JM. Lateral epicondylitis: review and current concepts. *J Hand Surgery Am*. 2007;32:1271–1277.

Goldie I. Epicondylitis lateralis humeri (epicondylalgia or tennis elbow). A pathogenetical study. *Acta Chir Scand Suppl*. 1964;57(suppl 339).

Groppel JL, Nirschl RP. A mechanical and electromyographical analysis of the effects of various joint counterforce braces on the tennis player. *Am J Sports Med*. 1986;14:195–200.

Haahr JP, Andersen JH. Physical and psychosocial risk factors for lateral epicondylitis: a population based case-referent study. *Occup Environ Med*. 2003a;60:322–329.

Haahr JP, Andersen JH. Prognostic factors in lateral epicondylitis: a randomized trial with one-year follow-up in 266 new cases treated with minimal occupational intervention or the usual approach in general practice. *Rheumatology (Oxford)*. 2003b;42:1216–1225.

Koh SBJ, Mohan PC, Howe TS, et al. Fasciotomy and surgical tenotomy for recalcitrant lateral elbow tendinopathy: early clinical experience with a novel device for minimally invasive percutaneous microresection. *Am J Sports Med*. 2013;41:636–644.

Labelle H, Guibert R. Efficacy of diclofenac in lateral epicondylitis of the elbow also treated with immobilization: the University of Montreal Orthopaedic Research Group. *Arch Fam Med*. 1997;6:257–262.

Levin D, Nazarian LN, Miller TT, et al. Lateral epicondylitis of the elbow: US findings. *Radiology*. 2005;237:230–234.

Mackay D, Rangan A, Hide G, Hughes T, Latimer J. The objective diagnosis of early tennis elbow by magnetic resonance imaging. *Occup Med (Lond)*. 2003;53:309–312.

Martinez-Silvestrini JA, Newcomer KL, Gay RE, Schaefer MP, Kortebein P, Arendt KW. Chronic lateral epicondylitis: comparative effectiveness of a home exercise program including stretching alone versus stretching supplemented with eccentric or concentric strengthening. *J Hand Ther*. 2005;18:411–419.

Miller TT, Shapiro MA, Schultz E, Kalish PE. Comparison of sonography and MRI for diagnosing epicondylitis. *J Clin Ultrasound*. 2002;30:193–202.

Mishra AK, Skrepnik NV, Edwards SG, et al. Efficacy of platelet-rich plasma for chronic tennis elbow: a double-blind, prospective, multicenter, randomized controlled trial of 230 patients. *Am J Sports Med*. 2014;42(2):463–471.

Mullett H, Sprague M, Brown G, Hausman M. Arthroscopic treatment of lateral epicondylitis: clinical and cadaveric studies. *Clin Orthop Relat Res*. 2005;439:123–128.

Nirschl RP. Elbow tendinosis/tennis elbow. *Clin Sports Med*. 1992;11(4):851–870.

Nirschl RP. Tennis elbow. *Orthop Clin North Am*. 1973;4:787–800.

Nirschl RP, Ashman ES. Elbow tendinopathy: tennis elbow. *Clin Sports Med*. 2003;22:813–836.

Nirschl RP, Pettrone FA. Tennis elbow. The surgical treatment of lateral epicondylitis. *J Bone Joint Surg Am*. 1979;61:832–839.

Ohberg L, Alfredson H. Effects on neovascularisation behind the good results with eccentric training in chronic mid-portion Achilles tendinosis? *Knee Surg Sports Traumatol Arthrosc*. 2004;12:465–470.

Peerbooms JC, Sluimer J, Bruijn DJ, Gosens T. Positive effect of an autologous platelet concentrate in lateral epicondylitis in a double-blind randomized controlled trial: platelet-rich plasma versus corticosteroid injection with a 1 year followup. *Am J Sports Med*. 2010;38(2):255–262.

Potter HG, Hannafin JA, Morwessel RM, DiCarlo EF, O'Brien SJ, Altchek, DW. Lateral epicondylitis: correlation of MR imaging, surgical, and histopathologic findings. *Radiology*. 1995;196:43–46.

Roles NC, Maudsley RH. Radial tunnel syndrome: resistant tennis elbows, a nerve entrapment. *J Bone Joint Surg Br*. 1972;54:499–508.

Rosenberg N, Henderson I. Surgical treatment of resistant lateral epicondylitis: follow-up study of 19 patients after excision, release and repair of proximal common extensor tendon origin. *Arch Orthop Trauma Surg*. 2002;122:514–517.

Runge F. Zur genese und behandlung des schreibekrampfes. *Berl Klin Wochenschr*. 1873;10:245–248.

Savnik A, Jensen B, Nørregaard J, Egund N, Danneskiold-Samsøe B, Bliddal H. Magnetic resonance imaging in the evaluation of treatment response of lateral epicondylitis of the elbow. *Eur Radiol*. 2004;14:964–996.

Savoie FH, VanSice W, O'Brien MJ. Arthroscopic tennis elbow release. *J Shoulder Elbow Surg*. 2010;19:31–36.

Seng C, Mohan PC, Koh SBJ, et al. Ultrasonic percutaneous tenotomy for recalcitrant lateral elbow tendinopathy: sustainability and sonographic progression at 3 years. *Am J Sports Med*. 2015;44:504–510.

Smith AG, Kosygan K, Williams H, Newman RJ. Common extensor tendon rupture following corticosteroid injection for lateral tendinosis of the elbow. *Br J Sports Med*. 1999;33:423–425.

Steinborn M, Heuck A, Jessel C, Bonel H, Reiser M. Magnetic resonance imaging of lateral epicondylitis of the elbow with a 0.2-T dedicated system. *Eur Radiol*. 1999;9:1376–1380.

Stull PA, Jokl P. Comparison of diflunisal and naproxen in the treatment of tennis elbow. *Clin Ther*. 1986;9(suppl C):62– 66.

Szabo JS, Savoie FH, Field LD, Ramsey JR, Hosemann CD. Tenodesis of the extensor carpi radialis brevis: an evaluation of three methods of operative treatment. *J Shoulder Elbow Surg*. 2006;15:721–727.

Yerger B, Turner T. Percutaneous extensor tenotomy for chronic tennis elbow: an office procedure. *Orthopedics*. 1985;8(10):1261–1263.

Van De Streek MD, Van Der Schans CP, De Greef MH, Postema K. The effect of a forearm/hand splint compared with an elbow band as a treatment for lateral epicondylitis. *Prosthet Orthot Int*. 2004;28:183–189.

Zeisig E, Ohberg L, Alfredson H. Extensor origin vascularity related to pain in patients with tennis elbow. *Knee Surg Sports Traumatol Arthrosc*. 2006;14(7):659–663.

Zhu J, Hu B, Xing C, Li J. Ultrasound-guided, minimally invasive, percutaneous needle puncture treatment for tennis elbow. *Adv Ther*. 2008;25(10):1031–1036.

30 Distal Biceps Tendon Injury

30-30A EPIDEMIOLOGY, ETIOLOGY, ANATOMY, HISTORY, EXAMINATION, AND IMAGING

SAMUEL A. TAYLOR, MD and FRANK A. CORDASCO, MD, MS

Important Points

- Risk factors for distal biceps tendon ruptures include male gender, dominant arm, and history of contralateral distal biceps rupture, smoking, corticosteroid use, anabolic steroid use, or chronic renal disease, and increased body mass index.
- Etiology is thought to be related to a hypovascular zone, mechanical impingement, and attritional interstitial tendon weakness.
- Distal biceps insertion may include a common tendon or a bifid attachment of the short and long heads on the radial tuberosity.
- Several different physical examination maneuvers, including the hook test, have been described to identify distal biceps tendon ruptures.
- Magnetic resonance imaging (MRI) is important to evaluate for extent of injury, quality of tendons, nature of injury, and extent of retraction.

Epidemiology

One report suggested that the incidence of distal biceps tendon ruptures was 1.2 per 100,000 patients per year (Safran & Graham, 2002). A later study using the PearlDiver Technologies database, however, found an annual incidence of 2.55 per 100,000 patient-years; the average age of patients was found to be 46 years with an overwhelming (95%) male predominance (Kelly et al, 2015). Furthermore, the dominant arm is more commonly affected (86%) (Safran & Graham, 2002), and a personal history of distal biceps rupture is a significant risk factor for contralateral rupture (8%) (Green et al, 2012). Additional established risk factors include smoking, anabolic steroid use, systemic corticosteroid use, chronic renal disease, and increased body mass index. Smoking specifically has been a significant risk factor and was found in one study to impart a 7.5-fold higher risk for distal biceps rupture than nonsmoking (Green et al, 2012; Kelly et al, 2015; Safran & Graham, 2002).

Etiology

Although the exact etiology of distal biceps rupture is not yet fully elucidated, Seiler et al (1995) proposed an anatomic and mechanical rationale. Through cadaveric dissections, these investigators demonstrated a 2.1-cm hypovascular zone in the distal biceps tendon occurring between vascular contributions from the brachial artery proximally and the posterior recurrent artery distally. Furthermore, they used dynamic cross-sectional computed tomography (CT) images to show that the distance between the proximal radius and ulna was 52% shorter with the forearm in full pronation than in supination. Stated another way, the distal biceps tendon occupied nearly 85% of the space between these two bones with the arm in pronation, suggesting that some form of mechanical impingement coupled with the aforementioned vascular watershed leads to progressive tendon weakness and ultimately to tendon failure (Seiler et al, 1995).

Anatomy

The biceps muscle acts as a secondary flexor of the elbow and the primary supinator of the forearm. It has two proximal origins, or heads: the long head, which inserts on the supraglenoid tubercle, and the short head, which meshes with the coracobrachialis tendon to form the conjoined tendon on the coracoid process. Traditionally, the biceps has been thought to have a singular insertion onto the bicipital or radial tuberosity; however, later studies (discussed here) suggest otherwise. The lacertus fibrosus (bicipital aponeurosis) emanates from the biceps muscle belly at the level of the musculotendinous junction and crosses distally and medially to insert along the subcutaneous border of the ulna.

Athwal et al (2007) demonstrated that, in contrast to traditional teaching, there are normal variations among distal biceps tendons that include two distinct distal long head and short head tendon insertions. Others have reported bifurcate distal biceps tendon insertions in 25% to 60% of cadaveric specimens studied (Athwal et al, 2007; Cho et al, 2011; Dirim et al, 2008; Mazzocca et al, 2007). Voleti et al (2016) have reported on three isolated short head biceps tendon repairs (Fig. 30A.1). They found all three cases to successfully return to baseline level activity following anatomic repair of the short head component with or without the independent repair of the long head component. Other groups inserted the long head of the distal biceps tendon along the

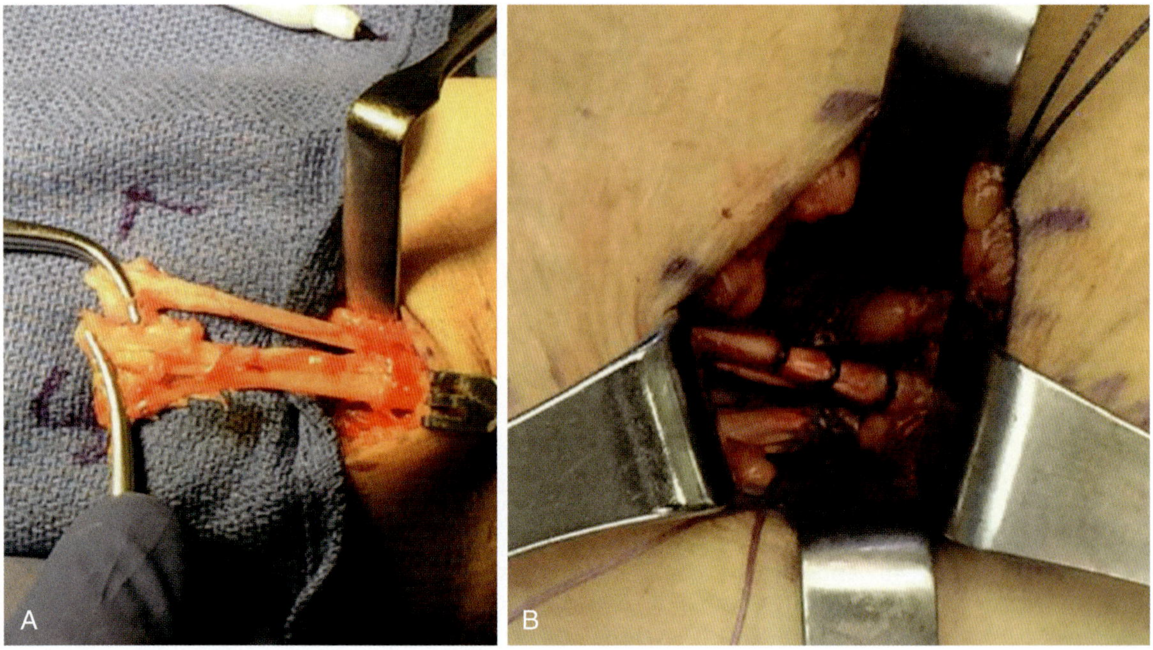

Fig. 30A.1 Intraoperative photographs demonstrating a bifurcated distal biceps tendon with separate short head and long head components before (**A**) and after (**B**) repair. (From Voleti PB, Berkowitz JL, Konin GP, Cordasco FA. Rupture of the short head component of a bifurcated distal biceps tendon. *J Shoulder Elbow Surg.* 2017;26[3]:403-408.)

proximal aspect of the bicipital tuberosity whereas the short head inserted more distally (Athwal et al, 2007; Cho et al, 2011; Forthman et al, 2008) and accounted for the majority (60%) of footprint coverage (Athwal et al, 2007; Cho et al, 2011). The bicipital tuberosity has been shown to be 21 to 22 mm in length and 7 to 15 mm in width (Athwal et al, 2007; Cho et al, 2011; Mazzocca et al, 2007). Mazzocca et al (2007), in an evaluation of 18 fresh-frozen cadaveric elbows, noted similar dimensions of the radial tuberosity as well as a ribbon-shaped distal biceps morphology.

The biceps footprint has been shown to be along the posterior/ulnar aspect of the radial tuberosity (Hutchinson et al, 2008) to maximize functional supination of the muscle tendon unit. Jarrett et al (2012) examined the biomechanical contributions of the short and long head attachments in six cadaveric specimens and found that the short head contributed the greatest to supination strength in the neutral and pronated forearm, whereas the long head attachment was more efficient with the forearm supinated.

For surgical exposure purposes, it should be noted that the radial recurrent artery most commonly crosses volar to the distal biceps tendon at an average of 4 mm proximal and 15.4 mm volar to the radial tuberosity. The radial recurrent artery bifurcates nearly half the time at an average of 9 mm from its origin (Zeltser & Strauch, 2016).

History and Physical Examination

Distal biceps tendon rupture frequently results from an acute injury in the setting of a heavy eccentric load applied with the elbow in 90 degrees of flexion. Although the most common injury pattern is avulsion of the biceps tendon from the radial tuberosity, some writers have reported intratendinous and musculotendinous locations of injury (Schamblin & Safran, 2007) as well as isolated short head biceps avulsions (Voleti et al, 2016).

History should be obtained from the patient to check for important risk factors, such as prodromal symptoms prior to the acute event, contralateral distal biceps tendon rupture, hand dominance, and tobacco and anabolic steroid use. One should elicit the patient's mechanism of injury and resulting symptoms, such as the often-described sudden, sharp, painful "pop." The sharp pain typically resolves within hours to days and may be followed by a dull ache and ecchymosis. Some describe elbow flexion and more pronounced supination weakness. This description may come in the form of newfound difficulties with activities that require these actions, such as turning a doorknob and lifting objects.

Physical examination includes inspection and palpation. Ecchymosis is often evident in the acute setting. The visible deformity resulting from unchecked retraction of the biceps muscle belly has been termed a "reverse Popeye sign" and may be considered pathognomonic for such an injury. It is critical to remember, however, that competency of the lacertus fibrosus is variable following avulsion injury. If the lacertus remains intact, it acts as a checkrein to proximal migration of the tendon and muscle belly and can masquerade as an intact tendon.

Examination of the antecubital fossa typically reveals a void where the biceps tendon inserted.

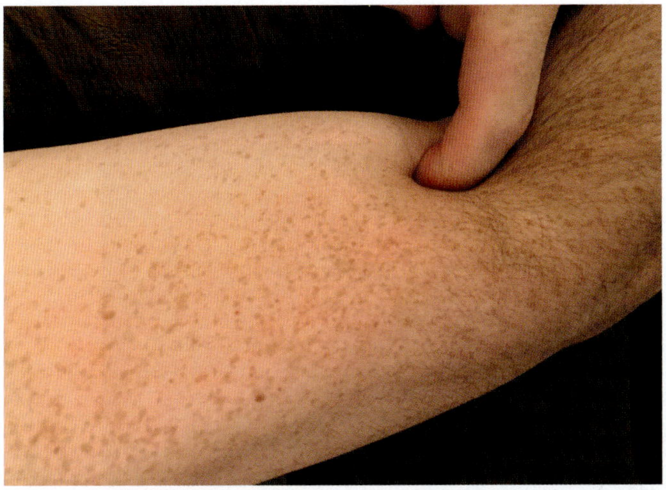

Fig. 30A.2 Hook test can be used to help determine whether the distal biceps is intact or ruptured.

Range of motion and strength testing is performed, particularly with respect to flexion and supination. Nesterenko et al (2010) compared side-to-side isokinetic elbow flexion and forearm supination strength and endurance in nine patients with untreated unilateral distal biceps ruptures and found that peak torque was nearly 50% lower in the affected arm for both flexion and supination. Results of fatigue testing in affected and normal arms, however, were not significantly different.

Several important tests have been described in the literature to improve our diagnostic capabilities in the office. The hook test, originally described by O'Driscoll et al (2007), is perhaps the most commonly employed test for distal biceps ruptures (Fig. 30A.2). Of the 45 patients in their study, 33 had complete ruptures and 12 had partial tears. Results of the hook test are positive in all complete tears and negative in all partial tears. Of the 12 patients in this group with partial tears, 9 deemed the hook test painful despite structural integrity. The investigators claimed that the hook test was more sensitive (100% vs. 92%) and specific (100% vs. 85%) than MRI for complete tears. ElMaraghy et al (2008) described the biceps crease interval test to aid in the diagnosis of distal biceps tendon ruptures. They measured the distance between the antecubital crease the elbow and the distal descent of the biceps muscle, which they called the "biceps crease interval." A biceps crease interval greater than 6 cm or a biceps crease ratio (injured to uninjured side) greater than 1.2 resulted in 96% sensitivity and 93% accuracy for distal biceps tendon ruptures. Harding (2005) described the passive forearm pronation test. Metzman and Tivener (2015) suggested the supination-pronation test in the acute setting to aid in diagnosis. With the elbow in 90 degrees of flexion, the forearm is pronated and supinated with attention to the biceps contour. In the intact distal biceps, the biceps muscle belly shortens in supination and elongates in pronation. A positive result is determined by a failure of elongation of the muscle as the forearm is actively pronated.

Devereaux and ElMaraghy (2013) evaluated the efficacy of the hook test, the passive forearm pronation test, and the biceps crease interval test in 48 patients with suspected distal biceps tendon injuries. They found 100% sensitivity and specificity when results of all three tests were all positive.

Imaging

Though often unrevealing, plain radiographs should be obtained to evaluate for osseous abnormalities such as heterotopic ossification, excrescences of the radial tuberosity, and concomitant pathologies.

MRI is an important diagnostic tool that can be particularly useful to assess the extent of injury in a partial tear and to evaluate for the degree of proximal retraction and the presence of tendinosis within the retracted tendon during preoperative planning (Fig. 30A.3). Festa et al (2010) evaluated the sensitivity and specificity of MRI to determine partial and complete distal biceps tendon ruptures by having two radiologists who were blinded to the intraoperative observation review preoperative MR images from 22 patients with partial tears, 24 patients with complete tears, and 10 asymptomatic controls. These investigators determined that MRI was 92.4% sensitive and 100% specific for distal biceps tendon tears. Sensitivity for complete tears was 100%, but specificity lagged behind at 82.8%. The sensitivity for partial tears was only 59.1% but the specificity was 100%.

Ultrasound can be a useful adjunct and has been shown to be 95% sensitive and 71% specific with 91% accuracy for complete versus partial distal biceps tendon ruptures (Lobo et al, 2013). It remains, however, a fairly user-dependent imaging modality.

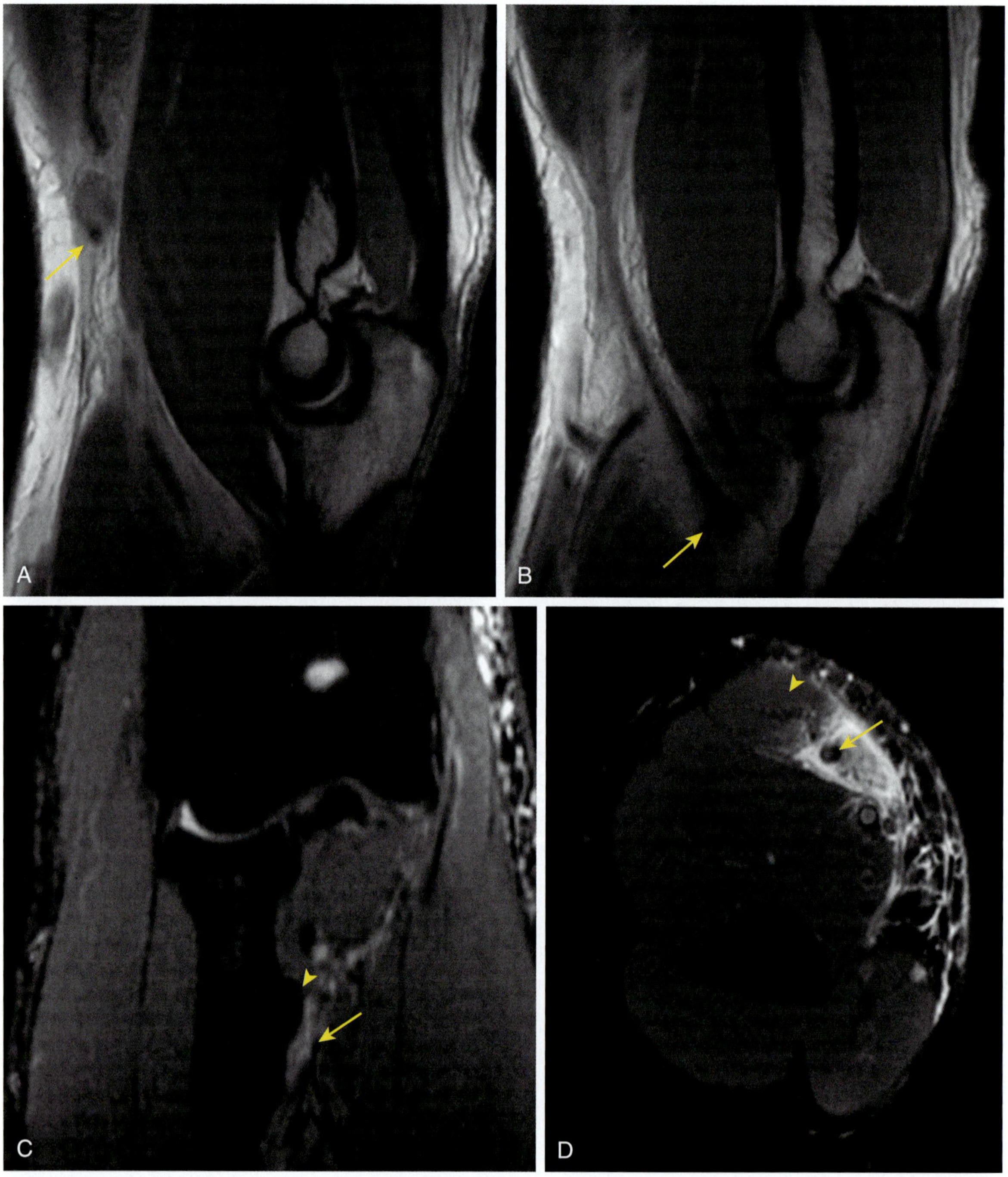

Fig. 30A.3 Sagittal fast spin echo MRI sequences demonstrating (**A**) an acute rupture of the short head distal tendon off the bicipital tuberosity with a proximally retracted and torn hyperintense tendon coiled within the distal arm *(arrow)* and (**B**) an intact long head distal tendon inserting on the proximal portion of the bicipital tuberosity *(arrow)*. (**C**) Coronal inversion recovery sequence demonstrating the long head bundle inserting normally on the proximal bicipital tuberosity *(arrowhead)* with a bare distal bicipital tuberosity *(arrow)* in the region of the normal insertion of the short head bundle. (**D**) Axial inversion recovery sequence revealing a thickened, hyperintense, and retracted torn short head distal tendon *(arrow)* with surrounding peritendinous edema and hemorrhage. Lateral to this is the muscle-tendon junction of the intact long head distal tendon *(arrowhead)*. (From Voleti PB, Berkowitz JL, Konin GP, Cordasco FA. Rupture of the short head component of a bifurcated distal biceps tendon. *J Shoulder Elbow Surg*. 2017;26[3]:403-408.)

References

Athwal GS, Steinmann SP, Rispoli DM. The distal biceps tendon: Footprint and relevant clinical anatomy. *J Hand Surg Am*. 2007;32:1225–1229. http://dx.doi.org/10.1016/j.jhsa.2007.05.027.

Cho C-H, Song K-S, Choi I-J, et al. Insertional anatomy and clinical relevance of the distal biceps tendon. *Knee Surg Sports Traumatol Arthrosc*. 2011;19:1930–1935. http://dx.doi.org/10.1007/s00167-011-1586-x.

Devereaux MW, ElMaraghy AW. Improving the rapid and reliable diagnosis of complete distal biceps tendon rupture: a nuanced approach to the clinical examination. *Am J Sports Med*. 2013;41:1998–2004. http://dx.doi.org/10.1177/0363546513493383.

Dirim B, Brouha SS, Pretterklieber ML, et al. Terminal bifurcation of the biceps brachii muscle and tendon: anatomic considerations and clinical implications. AJR. *Am J Roentgenol*. 2008;191:W248–W255. http://dx.doi.org/10.2214/AJR.08.1048.

ElMaraghy A, Devereaux M, Tsoi K. The biceps crease interval for diagnosing complete distal biceps tendon ruptures. *Clin Orthop Relat Res*.. 466:2255–2262. http://dx.doi.org/10.1007/s11999-008-0334-0.

Festa A, Mulieri PJ, Newman JS, Spitz DJ, Leslie BM. Effectiveness of magnetic resonance imaging in detecting partial and complete distal biceps tendon rupture. *J Hand Surg Am*. 2010;35:77–83. http://dx.doi.org/10.1016/j.jhsa.2009.08.016.

Forthman CL, Zimmerman RM, Sullivan MJ, Gabel GT. Cross-sectional anatomy of the bicipital tuberosity and biceps brachii tendon insertion: Relevance to anatomic tendon repair. *J Shoulder Elbow Surg*. 2008;17:522–526. http://dx.doi.org/10.1016/j.jse.2007.11.002.

Green JB, Skaife TL, Leslie BM.. Bilateral distal biceps tendon ruptures. *J Hand Surg Am*. 201;237:120–123. doi:10.1016/j.jhsa.2011.09.043

Harding WG. A new clinical test for avulsion of the insertion of the biceps tendon. *Orthopedics*. 2005;28:27–29.

Hutchinson HL, Gloystein D, Gillespie M. Distal biceps tendon insertion: An anatomic study. *J Shoulder Elbow Surg*. 2008;17:342–346. http://dx.doi.org/10.1016/j.jse.2007.05.005.

Jarrett CD, Weir DM, Stuffmann ES, Jain S, Miller MC, Schmidt CC. Anatomic and biomechanical analysis of the short and long head components of the distal biceps tendon. *J Shoulder Elbow Surg*. 2012;21:942–948. http://dx.doi.org/10.1016/j.jse.2011.04.030.

Kelly MP, Perkinson SG, Ablove RH, Tuetin JL. Distal biceps tendon ruptures: An epidemiological analysis using a large population database. *Am J Sports Med*. 2015;43:2012–2017. http://dx.doi.org/10.1177/0363546515587738.

Lobo LDG, Fessell DP, Miller BS, et al. The role of sonography in differentiating full versus partial distal biceps tendon tears: correlation with surgical findings. *AJR Am J Roentgenol*. 2013;200:158–162. http://dx.doi.org/10.2214/AJR.11.7302.

Mazzocca AD, Cohen M, Berkson E,N, et al. The anatomy of the bicipital tuberosity and distal biceps tendon. *J Shoulder Elbow Surg*. 2007;16:122–127. http://dx.doi.org/10.1016/j.jse.2006.04.012.

Metzman LS, Tivener KA. The Supination-Pronation Test for Distal Biceps Tendon Rupture. *Am J Orthop (Belle Mead, NJ)*. 2015;44:E361–E364.

Nesterenko S, Domire ZJ, Morrey BF, Sanchez-Sotelo J. Elbow strength and endurance in patients with a ruptured distal biceps tendon. *J Shoulder Elbow Surg*. 2010;19:184–189. http://dx.doi.org/10.1016/j.jse.2009.06.001.

O'Driscoll SW, Goncalves LBJ, Dietz P. The hook test for distal biceps tendon avulsion. *Am J Sports Med*. 2007;35:1865–1869. http://dx.doi.org/10.1177/0363546507305016.

Safran MR, Graham SM. Distal biceps tendon ruptures: Incidence, demographics, and the effect of smoking. *Clin Orthop Relat Res*. 2002;404:275–283.

Schamblin ML, Safran MR. Injury of the distal biceps at the musculotendinous junction. *J Shoulder Elbow Surg*. 2007;16:208–212. http://dx.doi.org/10.1016/j.jse.2006.06.009.

Seiler JG, Parker LM, Chamberland PD, Sherbourne GM, Carpenter WA. The distal biceps tendon. Two potential mechanisms involved in its rupture: arterial supply and mechanical impingement. *J Shoulder Elbow Surg*. 1995;4:149–156.

Voleti PB, Berkowitz JL, Konin GP, Cordasco FA. Rupture of the short head component of a bifurcated distal biceps tendon. *J Shoulder Elbow Surg*. 2017;26(3):403–408.

Zeltser DW, Strauch RJ. Vascular anatomy relevant to distal biceps tendon repair. *J Shoulder Elbow Surg*. 2016;25:283–288. http://dx.doi.org/10.1016/j.jse.2015.08.042.

30-30B TREATMENT, OUTCOMES, COMPLICATIONS, AND REHABILITATION

SAMUEL A. TAYLOR, MD and FRANK A. CORDASCO, MD, MS

Important Points

- Nonoperative treatment may result in persistent clinical symptoms, including pain and weakness of elbow flexion and supination.
- Two-incision repair techniques theoretically provide a more anatomic repair of the distal biceps footprint but have a relatively high incidence of postoperative heterotopic ossification and postoperative fatty infiltration of the supinator muscle.
- Single-incision techniques require less surgical dissection, may result in a biomechanically less anatomic repair location on the radial tuberosity, and have higher rates of transient neurologic complications such as lateral antebrachial cutaneous and superficial radial nerve paresthesias.
- Multiple fixation methods have been described, including cortical buttons, suture anchors, transosseous sutures, and bone tunnels.
- Although biomechanical studies suggest cortical button fixation to be strongest at the time of the repair and the single-incision and two-incision approaches have different complication profiles, there is no clinical data to suggest superiority of a specific surgical approach or method of fixation.

Surgical Treatment

Although nonoperative treatment of distal biceps tendon ruptures may produce acceptable clinical results (Freeman et al, 2009), ultimate supination strength in the unrepaired arm is decreased by nearly 40%. Nesterenko et al (2010) found peak torque to be lower for flexion and extension following distal biceps ruptures. These strength deficits, along with the patient profile (active male, fifth decade of life, and dominant side) as well as the detrimental effects of delayed surgical intervention have led surgeons to regard surgery as the conservative treatment in this population.

Once the decision has been made for a patient to undergo primary repair of an acute distal biceps tendon rupture, there are two general decisions to be made: (1) the surgical approach and (2) the method of fixation.

SINGLE-INCISION VERSUS TWO-INCISION TECHNIQUE

With regard to surgical approach, one may consider either a single-incision or a two-incision technique. Similar clinical and functional outcomes have been reported between the two approaches, but their complication profiles are somewhat different as are the purported biomechanics. The primary advantages of a single-incision approach are a less extensive surgical exposure and lower incidence of heterotopic ossification than that reported for the two-incision approach. The primary disadvantage is a higher prevalence of neurologic complications, such as lateral antebrachial cutaneous nerve and superficial radial nerve paresthesias secondary to retraction (Garon & Greenberg, 2016).

Proponents of the two-incision technique argue that the single-incision technique fails to achieve anatomic reinsertion of the distal biceps tendon, consequently decreasing footprint coverage and ultimately reducing supination strength after repair. In fact, several studies exist to support this claim. Forthman et al (2008) noted that a single-incision exposure failed to achieve anatomic restoration of the footprint in 35% of specimens they studied. The two-incision approach more accurately covers the anatomic footprint and theoretically leads to improved function. Hasan et al (2012) demonstrated in a cadaveric study that a significantly larger portion of the distal biceps footprint is covered (73.4% vs. 9.7%) after a two-incision technique than after a single-incision technique.

Biomechanical data would suggest an advantage of greater footprint coverage. Prud'homme-Foster et al (2015) observed that a more anatomic repair of the distal biceps tendon footprint on the ulnar side of the bicipital tuberosity increased supination torque by 15% in comparison with nonanatomic repairs with the arm in neutral rotation and by 40% in comparison with such repairs with the arm in 45 degrees of supination.

It should be noted, however, that the cost of the more anatomic ulnar/posterior position of the tendon repair site on the bicipital tuberosity that is gained by a two-incision approach may come in the form of increased rates of radioulnar heterotopic ossification (Garon & Greenberg, 2016). The two-incision technique has been found to result in increased supinator fat content as well (Schmidt et al, 2015). Increased risk of heterotopic ossification with the two-incision technique has led some surgeons to suggest using indomethacin as prophylaxis (Anakwenze et al, 2011). In the event that heterotopic ossification results in significant functional limitations, it may be excised. Wysocki and Cohen (2007) reported excellent results at 1-year follow-up for eight patients who were treated with heterotopic ossification excision in comparison with eight matched patients who underwent uncomplicated distal biceps tendon repairs with only 14 degrees of loss in rotation arc (151 degrees vs. 165 degrees) for forearm rotation. Ultimately, however, these patients experienced no differences in strength or outcome scores, although it would be best to avoid heterotopic ossification and the need for a second operation.

METHOD OF FIXATION

The next decision that must be made is method of fixation. Various fixation methods have been described in the literature, including transosseous tunnels, suture anchors, cortical buttons, and interference screws. Various combinations of fixation techniques have also been described. Although cadaveric biomechanical studies suggest that cortical button fixation is strongest at the time of repair, there is little clinical data to suggest the clinical relevance of this finding. In fact, the outcomes reviewed in the following discussion do not show any clinically significant differences among fixation techniques.

Pereira et al (2002), utilizing 12 matched pairs of cadaver elbows to compare suture anchor with bone tunnel repair, determined that bone tunnel fixation resulted in greater strength and stiffness. The bicipital tuberosity acts as a mechanical cam for the distal biceps tendon to improve supination strength. As a result, some writers have emphasized the importance of an anatomic repair of the distal biceps tendon to the ulnar side of the radial tuberosity and others have examined the impact of the iatrogenic effects of repair technique on tuberosity morphology and supination strength. Krueger et al (2014) examined the effect of repair technique on proximal radioulnar impingement and concluded that onlay suture anchor–type repairs resulted in the lower biceps tendon-to-ulna distances than trough or tunnel techniques in neutral rotation and pronation. They suggested that suture anchor techniques might therefore result in iatrogenic proximal impingement during pronation. Schmidt et al (2015) demonstrated the importance of preserving the normal morphology of the radial tuberosity during distal biceps tendon repair. Their cadaveric study used 10 matched specimens to compare the effect of repair technique, specifically trough repairs with onlay repairs, on supination strength. Trough repairs exhibited a 27% lower supination moment in 60 degrees of forearm supination with a reduction of tuberosity height of 3 mm.

Outcomes

Review of the literature does not demonstrate a single surgical exposure, technique, or method of fixation to be clinically superior. The complication rates are similar, but the types of complications vary (Cain et al, 2012; Cusick et al, 2014).

Grewal et al (2012) conducted a randomized trial comparing single-incision suture anchor repair with two-incision transosseous repair techniques. No significant differences were found for patient-reported outcomes. Final isometric supination strength testing was 10% greater for the two-incision group (104% vs. 94%). Shields et al (2015) compared a single-incision cortical button technique with a double-incision technique and found no differences for range of motion or strength at final follow-up. Complication rates were higher, however, for the single-incision technique, with paresthesias of the superficial radial nerve being most common. In a separate study Schmidt et al (2015) prospectively evaluated 15 patients who underwent a biceps repair using a posterior approach; this cohort was compared with a randomized selection of 17 anterior repair recipients. Quantitative MRI analysis determined the insertion site angle of the tendon, and supinator fat content and supination strength were measured in three forearm positions. The anterior approach group had a significantly higher nonanatomic insertion site angle of the tendon than the control group and the posterior group ($p < .001$). The posterior approach group had significantly greater supinator fat content ($p \leq .019$) than both the control group and the anterior approach group. After repair, the posterior approach group had significantly greater supination strength than the anterior approach group ($p = 0.027$). The researchers concluded that future studies should focus on restoring the anatomic footprint without damaging the supinator muscle.

Two systematic reviews have investigated the clinical relevance of surgical exposure and method of fixation without determining an optimal technique. Kodde et al (2016) looked at data from 1074 patients compiled from 40 articles. They compared clinical outcomes of four different fixation methods (suture anchors, bone tunnels, interference screws, and cortical buttons). Although complication rates were lower for the double-incision approach with bone tunnels, the researchers noted no significant differences for postoperative range of motion or strength of flexion or supination. Watson et al (2014) performed a systematic review comparing the complication rates for different surgical approaches and repair constructs. They studied a total of 498 elbows from 22 studies. With regard to approach, they found no significant difference between single-incision and double-incision approaches with respect to complications (33.9% vs. 25.7%). Intraosseous screw fixation had a higher complication rate (44.8%) than suture anchors (26.4%), bone tunnels (20.4%), and cortical buttons (0%). Lateral antebrachial cutaneous nerve injury was the most common complication (11.6% for single-incision approach and 5.8% for double-incision approach).

Furthermore, it can be stated that overall complication rates are quite high (36% to 52%) for primary repair of the distal biceps regardless of surgical approach or method of fixation. A wide array of complications has been reported, including neurologic problems, vascular complications, and construct failures. Cusick et al (2014) reported posterior intraosseous nerve palsy, lateral antebrachial cutaneous paresthesias, superficial radial nerve dysesthesias, brachial artery thrombosis, and failures (retear of the construct). Furthermore, Carroll et al (2014) cited an overall 42% complication rate in 50 patients who underwent single-incision repair using the Endobutton (Acufex Microsurgical, Inc, Mansfield, MA). Lateral antebrachial cutaneous nerve injury was the most common complication (36%). A posterior interosseous nerve, anterior interosseous nerve, and superficial radial nerve were each identified in 4% of patients.

Failure of fixation in the form of retear is very uncommon, occurring in approximately 1.2% to 2% of cases (Cain et al, 2012; Cusick et al, 2014; Hinchey et al, 2014). Hinchey et al (2014), reviewing a cohort of 190 patients with more than 1-year follow-up, observed a failure rate of 1.5%. Cain et al (2012) reported on 198 consecutive distal biceps repairs and found a 36% complication rate, including lateral antebrachial cutaneous nerve paresthesias (26%), superficial radial nerve paresthesias (6%), superficial infection (2%), posterior interosseous nerve injury (4%), symptomatic heterotopic ossification (3%), and rerupture (2%), with an overall reoperation rate of 3%.

On a separate note, Morrey et al (2014) suggested that significant interstitial stretch occurs in the biceps muscle in the setting of retracted distal biceps ruptures requiring repair in varying degrees of elbow flexion. In their case-control series of 188 distal biceps repairs, these investigators identified 23 cases (19 chronic and 4 acute) that required repairs in greater than 60 degrees of elbow flexion. Average end range of motion was 3 to 138 degrees. Although 3 of the 23 patients reported easy fatigability, all returned to work and reported satisfaction. One of the 23 patients was found to have rerupture through the myotendinous junction. These clinical results suggested that retracted distal biceps repairs can effectively be performed primarily without the need for allograft reconstruction.

Authors' Preferred Surgical Technique

See Video 30B.1.

REPAIR OF ACUTE BICEPS TENDON RUPTURE

The patient is placed in the supine position with a hand table after administration of regional anesthesia. In most cases we prefer a sterile tourniquet to avoid compromising the exposure during the skin preparation and draping. A transverse incision is made distal to the skin crease of the antecubital fossa. A mini–C-arm fluoroscopy unit is utilized to identify the radial tuberosity, which is usually 3 to 4 cm distal to the antecubital fossa. This maneuver facilitates minimizing the length of the transverse incision, particularly in large patients with increased subcutaneous tissue. Neurovascular structures are protected during the superficial approach. The lateral antebrachial cutaneous nerve is identified and retracted laterally with the brachioradialis muscle. The stump of the distal biceps tendon is often retracted proximally and is located superficially just under the skin and subcutaneous tissues (Fig. 30B.1). We prefer a unicortical tensioning button (Arthrex Inc., Naples, FL) for fixation. Although we have used a bicortical button technique with a socket and screw, which has some theoretical advantages, we have not found it to be clinically superior; since it requires slightly more surgical time, higher implant-associated expense, and greater potential risks, such as fracture, we have favored the unicortical technique for the past few years. The tendon is prepared by utilizing a #2 FiberLoop (Arthrex) stitch, which is then secured to the button. After the unicortical drill hole is prepared on the distal and ulnar aspect of the footprint with the forearm in maximum supination, the button is deployed and tested to confirm that it is locked on the endosteal surface of the intramedullary canal. Pulling the tendon to the footprint and thereby reducing it anatomically completes the tension slide technique. The suture limbs are tied while

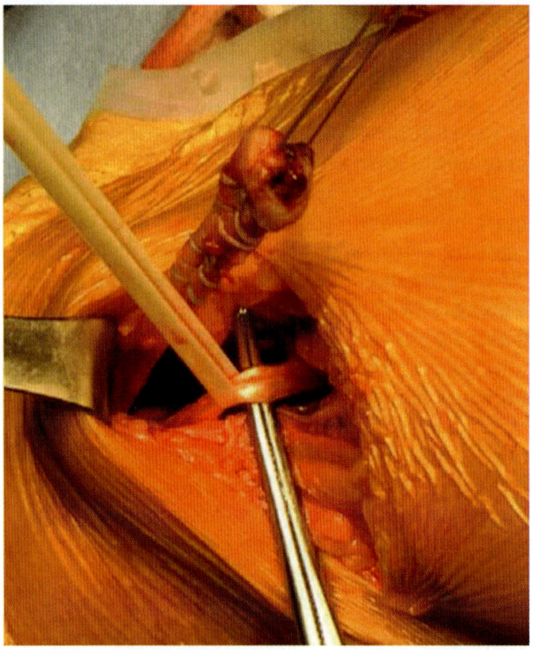

Fig. 30B.1 Intraoperative photograph demonstrating the torn short head distal tendon in the process of being repaired and the intact long head distal tendon. (From Voleti PB, Berkowitz JL, Konin GP, Cordasco FA. Rupture of the short head component of a bifurcated distal biceps tendon. *J Shoulder Elbow Surg*. 2017;26[3]:403-408.)

tension is maintained after one limb is passed through the tendon to secure the fixation. In patients with larger radial tuberosity footprints we occasionally use more than one button or augment the repair with a suture anchor. The wound is closed in layers and a subcuticular skin closure completes the repair.

REPAIR OF CHRONIC (LONGER THAN 6–8 WEEKS) BICEPS TENDON RUPTURE

If a primary repair is indicated on the basis of preoperative imaging and intraoperative findings, the technique described previously is utilized with the exception of the skin incision. A curvilinear extensile incision is utilized for improved proximal and distal exposure.

If an allograft reconstruction is anticipated, we prefer an Achilles allograft. The proximal aspect of the allograft is utilized at the biceps muscle-tendon junction. The broad-based component of the Achilles allograft is used to envelop the biceps muscle-tendon junction. It is sutured there with #2 FiberWire (Arthrex) using a modified Krackow suture technique. The calcaneus bone is removed from the Achilles allograft. The calcaneal aspect of the allograft is then attached to the radial tuberosity after myofascial sleeve tension is assessed and the allograft is shortened as necessary. It is then secured to the radial tuberosity using the same technique described for acute repairs.

Rehabilitation

Two types of rehabilitation have been described: early range of motion and delayed range of motion. More traditional rehabilitation is to restrict the range of motion for the first 6 weeks postoperatively to allow sufficient healing response. Initially the elbow is placed in a hinged elbow brace or a plaster splint, at 90 degrees of elbow flexion, until suture removal. After the wound is healed, the physical therapy guideline begins with active elbow extension and passive flexion with the goal of achieving full range of motion at 6 weeks following surgery. Passive pronation and supination of the forearm is encouraged to minimize scar formation and restore forearm rotation. In this more conservative approach, the elbow is immobilized at 90 degrees of flexion to protect the surgical repair except during physical therapy exercises.

As our fixation methods have evolved, so has the notion of early postoperative motion. Cheung et al (2005) reported on 13 patients who underwent distal biceps tendon repairs with 2 years of follow-up. Postoperative range of motion was allowed with a 60-degree extension block and opened to a 40-degree block at 2 weeks postoperatively, 20 degrees at 4 weeks, and full extension at 6 weeks. These researchers noted a 6-degree loss of terminal extension, 4-degree loss of pronation, and 8-degree loss of supination at final examination. Flexion strength was 91% and supination strength was 89% of those on the contralateral side.

In 21 patients, Cil et al (2009) allowed early postoperative range of motion following a modified two-incision distal biceps tendon repair during the first 6 weeks to include no brace for activities of daily living and a 1-lb weight restriction for elbow flexion. At 2-year follow-up, the mean isometric supination strength was 91% of that of the contralateral side and there were no reruptures.

Rose et al (2011) sought to answer the question about how much weight a patient can lift immediately postoperatively after distal biceps repair without compromising the fixation. In a cadaveric biomechanical model for distal biceps repair, they used a single incision button fixation technique and found that the construct maintained fixation for 2000 cycles with a maximum weight in the hand of 0.9 kg. Thus they concluded that early active motion with a 0.9-kg weight restriction should be well tolerated.

Our preferred rehabilitation guideline for acute repairs is detailed in Table 30B.1.

Table 30B.1 Rehabilitation Protocol

Postoperative Period	Goals	Precautions	Exercises
Weeks 0-2 HEP daily	Edema and pain control Protection of surgical repair Wrist, hand, shoulder ROM	Splint 90 degrees of flexion at all times No active supination	Gentle wrist and hand ROM Shoulder pendulum in splint Shoulder PROM exercises
Weeks 2–6 PT 2–3×/week HEP daily	Edema and pain control Protection of surgical repair ROM 15–130 degrees	Brace locked at 90 degrees Remove for shower and exercises No active elbow flexion No active supination	Gradually increase elbow ROM: Week 2: 45–100 degrees Week 4: 30–115 degrees Week 6: 0–130 degrees Active extension, passive flexion Wrist, hand, shoulder ROM continued Scapular strengthening Gripping exercises Triceps isometrics
Weeks 6–12 PT 2–3×/week HEP daily	Full ROM Protection of surgical repair	DC brace at 8 weeks No active elbow flexion	Full elbow ROM P/AA/AROM Wrist, hand, shoulder ROM continued Biceps isometrics begun Resistive strengthening cuff/deltoid Upper body ergometry (week 10)
Weeks 12–24 PT 1–2×/week HEP daily	Improvement in strength	No brace	Weeks 12–16: ROM and stretching exercises Elbow flexion resistive strengthening Weeks 16–24: Progression of strengthening as tolerated Plyometrics and sport-specific exercises
Weeks 24+ HEP daily	Return to play Unrestricted activity	Return to sport (physician directed)	Maintain ROM and strength

DC, ***, *HEP*, home exercise program; *P/AA/AROM*, passive/active assisted/active range of motion; *PT*, physical therapy; *ROM*, range of motion.

References

Anakwenze OA, Kancherla VK, Warrender W, Abboud JA. Outcomes of modified 2-incision technique with use of indomethacin in treatment of distal biceps tendon rupture. *Orthopedics*. 2011;34:e724–e729. http://dx.doi.org/10.3928/01477447-20110922-10.

Cain RA, Nydick JA, Stein MI, et al. Complications following distal biceps repair. *J Hand Surg Am*. 2012;37:2112–2117. http://dx.doi.org/10.1016/j.jhsa.2012.06.022.

Carroll MJ, DaCambra MP, Hildebrand KA. Neurologic complications of distal biceps tendon repair with 1-incision endobutton fixation. *Am J Orthop (Belle Mead. NJ)*. 2014;43:E159–E162.

Cheung EV, Lazarus M, Taranta M. Immediate range of motion after distal biceps tendon repair. *J Shoulder Elbow Surg*. 2005;14:516–518. http://dx.doi.org/10.1016/j.jse.2004.12.003.

Cil A, Merten S, Steinmann SP. Immediate active range of motion after modified 2-incision repair in acute distal biceps tendon rupture. *Am J Sports Med*. 2009;37:130–135. http://dx.doi.org/10.1177/0363546508323749.

Cusick MC, Cottrell BJ, Cain RA, Mighell MA. Low incidence of tendon rerupture after distal biceps repair by cortical button and interference screw. *J Shoulder Elbow Surg*. 2014;23:1532–1536. http://dx.doi.org/10.1016/j.jse.2014.04.013.

Forthman C, Zimmerman RM, Sullivan MJ, Gabel GT. Cross-sectional anatomy of the bicipital tuberosity and biceps brachii tendon insertion: Relevance to anatomic tendon repair. *J Shoulder Elbow Surg*. 2008;17:522–526. http://dx.doi.org/10.1016/j.jse.2007.11.002.

Freeman CR, McCormick KR, Mahone D, Baratz M, Lubahn JD. Nonoperative treatment of distal biceps tendon ruptures compared with a historical control group. *J Bone Joint Surg Am*. 2009;91:2329–2334. http://dx.doi.org/10.2106/JBJS.H.01150.

Garon MT, Greenberg JA. Complications of distal biceps repair. *Orthop Clin North Am*. 2016;47:435–444. http://dx.doi.org/10.1016/j.ocl.2015.10.003.

Grewal R, Athwal GS, MacDermid JC, et al. Single-versus double-incision technique for the repair of acute distal biceps tendon ruptures: A randomized clinical trial. *J Bone Joint Surg Am*. 2012;94:1166–1174. http://dx.doi.org/10.2106/JBJS.K.00436.

Hasan SA, Cordell CL, Rauls RB, Bailey MS, Sahu D, Suva LJ. Two-incision versus one-incision repair for distal biceps tendon rupture: A cadaveric study. *J Shoulder Elbow Surg*. 2012;21:935–941. http://dx.doi.org/10.1016/j.jse.2011.04.027.

Hinchey JW, Aronowitz JG, Sanchez-Sotelo J, Morrey BF. Re-rupture rate of primarily repaired distal biceps tendon injuries. *J Shoulder Elbow Surg*. 2014;23:850–854. http://dx.doi.org/10.1016/j.jse.2014.02.006.

Kodde IF, Baerveldt RC, Mulder PGH, Eygendaal D, van den Bekerom MPJ. Refixation techniques and approaches for distal biceps tendon ruptures: A systematic review of clinical studies. *J Shoulder Elbow Surg*. 2016;25:e29–e37. http://dx.doi.org/10.1016/j.jse.2015.09.004.

Krueger CA, Aden JK, Broughton K, Rispoli DM. Radioulnar space available at the level of the biceps tuberosity for repaired biceps tendon: A comparison of 4 techniques. *J Shoulder Elbow Surg*. 2014;23:1717–1723. http://dx.doi.org/10.1016/j.jse.2014.02.023.

Morrey ME, Abdel MP, Sanchez-Sotelo J, Morrey BF. Primary repair of retracted distal biceps tendon ruptures in extreme flexion. *J Shoulder Elbow Surg*. 2014;23:679–685. http://dx.doi.org/10.1016/j.jse.2013.12.030.

Nesterenko S, Domire ZJ, Morrey BF, Sanchez-Sotelo J. Elbow strength and endurance in patients with a ruptured distal biceps tendon. *J Shoulder Elbow Surg*. 2010;19:184–189. http://dx.doi.org/10.1016/j.jse.2009.06.001.

Pereira DS, Kvitne RS, Liang M, Giacobetti FB, Ebramzadeh E. Surgical repair of distal biceps tendon ruptures: A biomechanical comparison of two techniques. *Am J Sports Med*. 2002;30:432–436.

Prud'homme-Foster M, Louati H, Pollock JW, Papp S. Proper placement of the distal biceps tendon during repair improves supination strength—a biomechanical analysis. *J Shoulder Elbow Surg*. 2015;24:527–532. http://dx.doi.org/10.1016/j.jse.2014.09.039.

Rose DM, Archibald JD, Sutter EG, Belkoff SM, Wilckens JH. Biomechanical analysis suggests early rehabilitation is possible after single-incision EndoButton distal biceps repair with FiberWire. *Knee Surg Sports Traumatol Arthrosc*. 2011;19:1019–1022. http://dx.doi.org/10.1007/s00167-010-1348-1.

Schmidt CC, Brown BT, Williams BG, et al. The importance of preserving the radial tuberosity during distal biceps repair. *J Bone Joint Surg. Am*. 2015;97:2014–2023. http://dx.doi.org/10.2106/JBJS.N.01221.

Shields E, Olsen JR, Williams RB, Rouse L, Maloney M, Voloshin I. Distal biceps brachii tendon repairs: A single-incision technique using a cortical button with interference screw versus a double-incision technique using suture fixation through bone tunnels. *Am J Sports Med.* 2015;43:1072–1076. http://dx.doi.org/10.1177/0363546515570465.

Voleti PB, Berkowitz JL, Konin GP, Cordasco FA. Rupture of the short head component of a bifurcated distal biceps tendon. *J Shoulder Elbow Surg.* 2017;26(3):403–408.

Watson JN, Moretti VM, Schwindel L, Hutchinson MR. Repair techniques for acute distal biceps tendon ruptures: A systematic review. *J Bone Joint Surg Am.* 2014;96:2086–2090. http://dx.doi.org/10.2106/JBJS.M.00481.

Wysocki R, Cohen MS. Radioulnar heterotopic ossification after distal biceps tendon repair: Results following surgical resection. *J Hand Surg Am.* 2007;32:1230–1236. http://dx.doi.org/10.1016/j.jhsa.2007.06.018.

31 Triceps Tendon Injury

KEVIN O'DONNELL, MD, DAVID L. RUBENSTEIN, MD, and MICHAEL G. CICCOTTI, MD

Introduction

- Distal triceps tendon injuries are very rare.
- These injuries have a 2:1 male:female ratio and are most commonly seen in individuals 30 to 50 years of age.
- These injuries occur after an eccentric loading of the triceps tendon.
- Tears involving less than 50% of the tendon may be treated conservatively.
- Complete tears require operative fixation.
- Several techniques exist for fixation, each providing good to excellent outcomes.

Triceps tendon injuries are rare tendon injuries that can lead to significant dysfunction if not diagnosed and treated in a timely and appropriate fashion. These injuries can be encountered in the context of a high-energy trauma or with a low-energy mechanism in the setting of a predisposing systemic condition. This chapter reviews the common presentation, evaluation, and treatment strategies for triceps tendon injuries, focusing on both nonoperative and operative treatment options.

Epidemiology

Distal triceps tendon ruptures are uncommon injuries. Anzel et al (1959) noted that fewer than 1% of all tendon injuries involved the triceps. These occur approximately twice as often in males as in females, most commonly affecting patients between 30 and 50 years of age (Stucken & Ciccotti, 2014). In the general population, several systemic conditions may predispose a patient to triceps tendon rupture, including diabetes mellitus, hyperparathyroidism, and chronic renal disease (Tsourvakas et al, 2004). Local irritation from chronic olecranon bursitis may also increase the risk of rupture (Clayton & Thirupathi, 1984; Kachooei et al, 2015). Athletes who sustain triceps tendon rupture tend to engage in activities that require elbow extension against high loads, such as those seen in power lifting and American football (Mair et al, 2004; Sollender et al, 1998). In 1996, Mair et al (2004) reported on 21 triceps tendon ruptures occurring over the previous six seasons in professional football players. Using the National Football League (NFL) Injury Surveillance System, our institution identified 37 additional cases of triceps tendon rupture occurring between 2000 and 2009 (Finstein et al, 2015). Last, both the use of systemic anabolic steroids and repeated local corticosteroid injections have also been linked to an increased occurrence of triceps tendon rupture, particularly in weight lifters (Stannard & Bucknell, 1993; Yeh & Dodds, 2010).

Anatomy

The triceps brachii muscle is the sole muscle occupying the posterior compartment of the upper arm and is innervated by the radial nerve (C6–C8). It is composed of three tendinous origins: the long, lateral, and medial heads. The long head originates at the infraglenoid tuberosity of the scapula. The lateral head originates on the lateral intramuscular septum and posterolateral humerus proximal to the radial groove on the posterior aspect of the humerus. The medial head arises distal to the spiral groove on the posterior humerus. The confluence of the triceps heads inserts as a broad footprint along the olecranon (Fig. 31.1). The proximal aspect of the footprint begins approximately 12 mm distal to the tip of the olecranon and covers an area of 466 mm^2 (Yeh & Stephens, 2010). The medial aspect of the triceps insertion extends along the posterior crest of the ulna. Laterally, the insertion expands to blend with the fascia of the extensor carpi ulnaris and anconeus muscle. The overall width of the insertion has been found to be between 1.9 and 4.2 cm (Windisch et al, 2006).

History and Physical Examination

The diagnosis of a distal triceps tendon injury can generally be made clinically. Most commonly, the patient will report

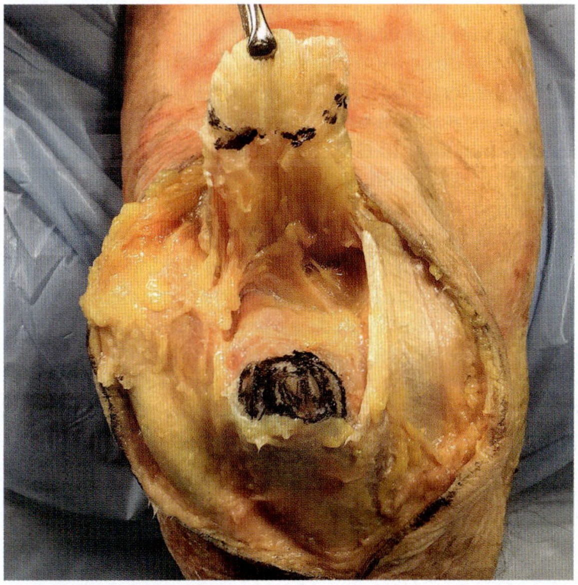

Fig. 31.1 Anteroposterior photograph of a cadaveric elbow demonstrating the broad, rectangular triceps footprint on the olecranon. Notice the footprint insertion begins approximately 12 mm distal to the tip of the olecranon and continues distally 13.4 mm on average.

a history involving an eccentric loading mechanism to the arm. This is commonly experienced during a fall onto an outstretched hand, weight lifting, or attempting to restrain oneself during a motor vehicle accident. Deep lacerations to the posterior distal aspect of the arm are also capable of completely transecting the triceps tendon. Rarely, a direct blow to the posterior arm can be responsible for a tear (van Riet et al, 2003).

Patients complain of pain localized over the posterior aspect of the elbow. On physical examination, they may exhibit swelling, tenderness, and ecchymosis. Patients with a complete rupture may have a palpable gap proximal to the tip of the olecranon; however, this is commonly masked by swelling during the acute injury period. Active extension of the elbow should be assessed in all patients with a suspected triceps tendon rupture. It is important to recognize that retention of the ability to actively extend the elbow against resistance does not rule out a triceps tendon rupture (van Riet et al, 2003). A complete tear may result in a total loss of active elbow extension. A patient with an intact lateral insertional expansion or with compensatory strength from the anconeus muscle may retain the ability to extend the triceps against gravity with the arm positioned below the shoulder. These patients should also be tested with the arm overhead and against resistance to help confirm the diagnosis (Stucken & Ciccotti, 2014).

Special tests include a modified Thompson test that is akin to the Thompson test used for Achilles tendon rupture (Viegas, 1990). During this examination, the patient is placed in a prone position with the affected arm over the edge of the table and the elbow flexed to 90 degrees. The examiner then squeezes the triceps and watches the elbow for passive extension. If there is a compete rupture of the triceps tendon, then there will likely be no motion at the elbow.

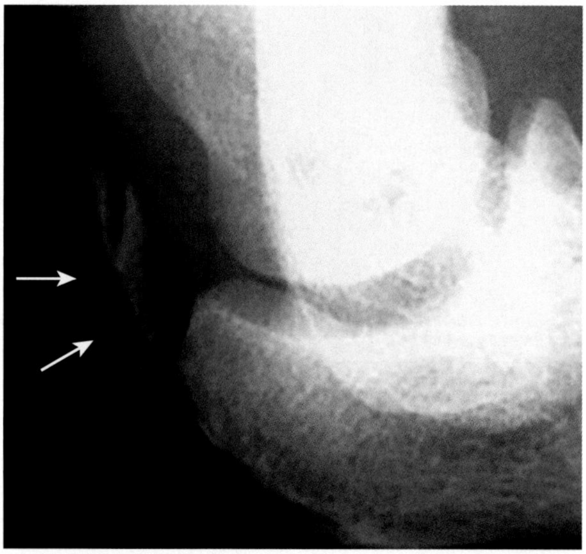

Fig. 31.2 Lateral radiograph of the elbow demonstrating an avulsion fracture at the triceps insertion *(arrows)*, also known as the "flake sign." (From Pina A, Garcia I, Sabater M. Traumatic avulsion of the triceps brachii. *J Orthop Trauma*. 2002;16:273-276.)

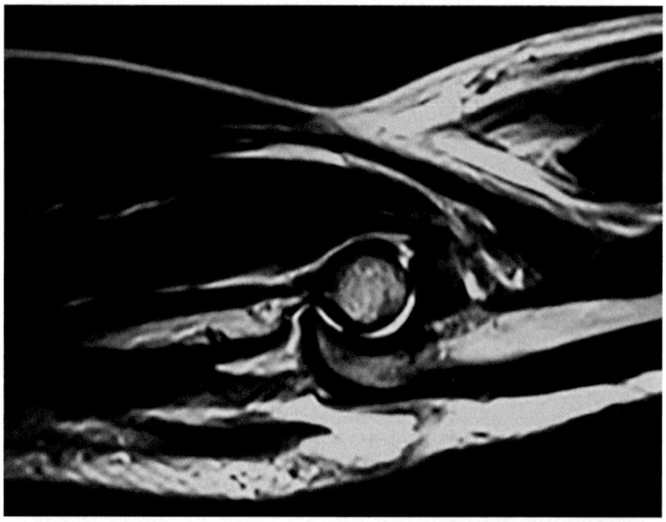

Fig. 31.3 Sagittal magnetic resonance image showing rupture of the triceps tendon. Notice the large fluid defect between the triceps stump and the olecranon insertion. (From Stucken C, Ciccotti MG. Distal biceps and triceps injuries in athletes. *Sports Med Arthrosc Rev*. 2014;22(3):153-163.)

Diagnostic Imaging

The initial evaluation should include anteroposterior and lateral radiographs of the elbow. Ruptures most commonly occur at the level of the tendon osseous insertion (Stannard & Bucknell, 1993; van Riet et al, 2003; Yeh et al, 2010). An avulsion fracture of the olecranon can be visualized on the lateral radiograph and is termed the "flake sign" (Pina et al, 2002) (Fig. 31.2). MRI is a useful imaging modality to help differentiate between a partial and complete tendon rupture if the history and physical examination are equivocal. MRI is also helpful to assess the level of tendon retraction and to evaluate for injury to adjacent structures (Tiger et al, 1993). Partial-thickness tears appear as fluid within the distal triceps tendon and surrounding swelling. Full-thickness tears show complete avulsion of the tendon with a fluid-filled gap between the distal triceps and its insertion site on the olecranon (Fig. 31.3). Sagittal cuts of T1- and T2-weighted images help to fully elucidate and characterize the injury. Ultrasound examination is also a low-cost and convenient method to further evaluate for damage to the triceps tendon and is capable of differentiating between partial and complete tears (Tagliafico et al, 2012) (Fig. 31.4).

Nonoperative Management

Treatment of triceps tears is dictated based on patient specific factors and functional deficits and the characteristics of the tear. Older, low-demand patients who retain the ability to actively extend the elbow may be treated conservatively. Partial tears, specifically tears involving less than 50% of the tendon, can be successfully treated nonoperatively (Vidal et al, 2004). Tears involving more than 50% of the tendon width most often require operative fixation, depending on the functional demand of the patient and the extension strength remaining in the arm. In older adult patients, these partial tears may be treated conservatively. In athletes or laborers, however, with high functional demands, operative intervention is most appropriate for these partial tears (Strauch, 1999; Vidal et al, 2004).

Tear characteristics also play a role in the decision for operative intervention. Proximal tears localized to the muscle belly are typically treated conservatively. Tears to the muscle belly have been reported in both a singular head of

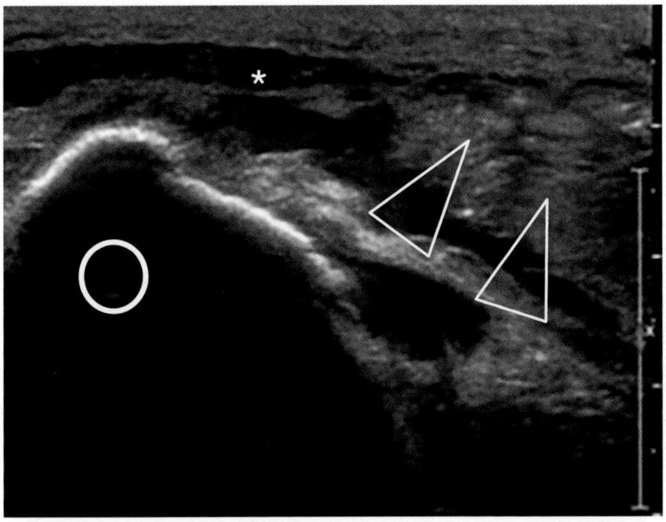

Fig. 31.4 Long-axis ultrasound image demonstrating a complete tear of the triceps tendon *(arrows)* from the olecranon *(circle)*. (From Tagliafico A, Gandolfo N, Michaud J, Perez MM, Palmieri F, Martinoli C. Ultrasound demonstration of distal triceps tendon tears. *Eur J Radiol*. 2012;81(6):1207-1210.)

the triceps as well as a complete rupture of the confluence of the heads (O'Driscoll, 1992). Both partial and complete ruptures of the triceps muscle belly heal with fibrotic scar tissue, allowing for some element of tissue apposition and return of extension strength (Aso & Torisu, 1984; O'Driscoll, 1992). There have been selected case reports of tears of the triceps muscle belly treated operatively with suture apposition; however, this is rarely performed, and most patients can be adequately managed conservatively with good outcomes (Aso & Torisu, 1984; Singh & Pooley, 2002).

High-demand athletes with partial tearing of the triceps have also been successfully managed conservatively (Mair et al, 2004). In a study of triceps tendon tears in NFL players, Mair et al (2004) reported on 10 partial tendon tears, six of which healed without surgical intervention. Three players were treated with bracing for the remainder of the season but subsequently underwent operative fixation during the offseason secondary to continuing pain and weakness. The average time missed for these players was 4.8 weeks (range, 0–9 weeks). Finally, one player progressed to a complete rupture requiring operative intervention after returning to practice in a brace 5 days after the index injury.

Nonoperative management for appropriate distal triceps tendon injuries consists of initial immobilization followed by a progressive rehabilitation program. Immobilization in a brace or splint at 30 degrees of elbow flexion is maintained for the initial 4 weeks followed by a progressive increase in elbow mobilization (Marinello et al, 2015; Yeh et al, 2010). The rate of progression is generally dictated by the patient's level of comfort. Resisted elbow extension and heavy lifting activity should be limited for 8 to 12 weeks after injury. At 3 months, most patients should be pain-free and able to perform activities of daily living without significant discomfort. Continued pain and weakness at the 3-month time mark may indicate a failure of conservative management and consideration should be given toward proceeding with operative intervention (Marinello et al, 2015).

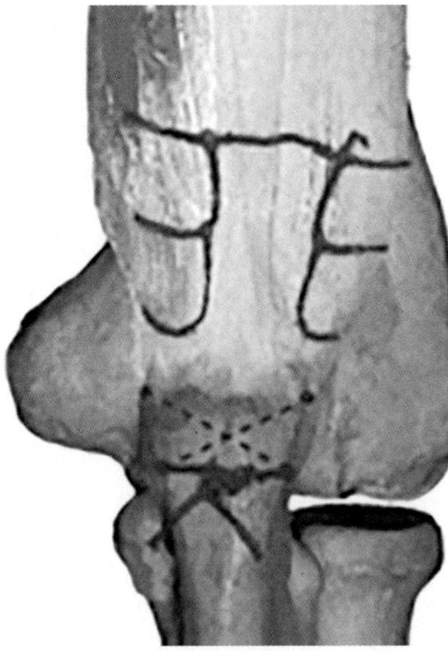

Fig. 31.5 Transosseous cruciate repair technique. Fixation is achieved through a locking Krackow stitch which is passed through crossing bone tunnels and tied over a bone bridge. (From Petre BM, Grutter PW, Rose DM, Belkoff SM, McFarland EG, Petersen SA. Triceps tendons: a biomechanical comparison of intact and repaired strength. *J Shoulder Elbow Surg*. 2011;20:213-218.)

Operative Management

Complete ruptures of the triceps tendon at the tendinous insertion with loss of strength should be treated with primary repair. Before operative intervention, all medical comorbidities need to be optimized, particularly in patients with significant systemic disease. If possible, it is ideal to repair the tendon within 2 weeks of the initial injury. Inhofe & Moneim (1996), however, have described a successful primary repair in a patient that presented in a delayed fashion 8 months after the initial injury.

The goal of operative intervention is to reduce the torn tendon and repair it securely to the tendon footprint on the olecranon. There are several methods by which this process can be achieved. Most methods use a Krackow whipstitch or Bunnell cruciate stitch to secure the tendon. Four frequently used techniques to repair the distal triceps tendon to bone are (1) transosseous cruciate drill tunnels (van Riet et al, 2003), (2) standard suture anchor repair (Bava et al, 2012; Tsourvakas et al, 2004; Viegas, 1990), (3) anatomic transosseous equivalent repair (Yeh & Stephens, 2010), and (4) knotless anatomic footprint repair (Clark et al, 2014; Paci et al, 2014). The transosseous cruciate repair technique involves securing the tendon to the footprint by passing the stitches through crossing bone tunnels in the olecranon. Typically, a 2-mm drill bit is used to place drill tunnels within the olecranon. The tunnels begin at the medial and lateral tendon footprint and extend distally to the contralateral cortical side on the dorsal ulna. A suture passer is then used to pass the stitches in the tendon distally through the bone tunnels. These stitches are then tied over a bone bridge (Fig. 31.5).

The suture anchor repair technique is performed by placing two single- or double-loaded suture anchors into the anatomic footprint. A limb of each suture is then placed in the tendon in Krackow fashion. The Krackow stitch limb is

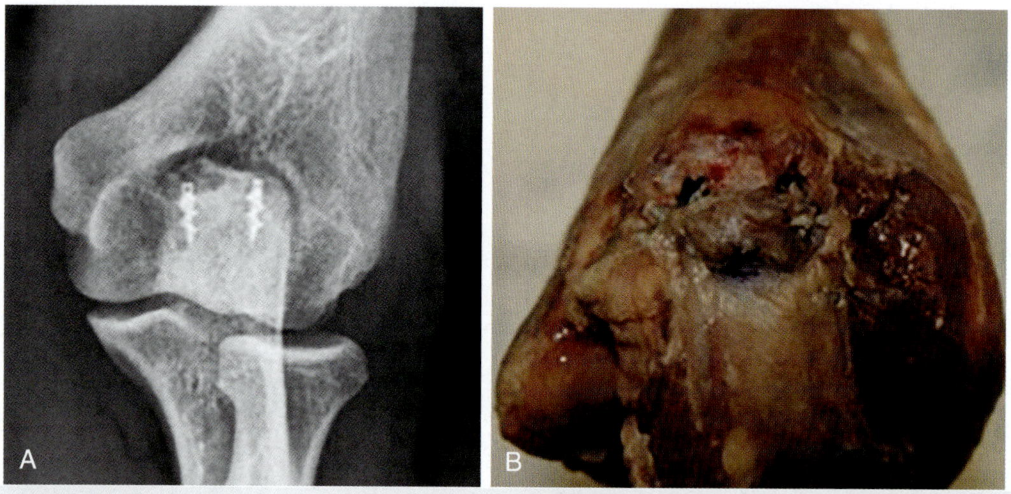

Fig. 31.6 A, Anteroposterior radiograph of the elbow demonstrating suture anchors within the tip of the olecranon providing fixation of the distal triceps tendon to bone. **B,** Cadaveric specimen demonstrating a suture anchor repair technique of a distal triceps tendon rupture. (A, From Bava ED, Barber FA, Lund ER. Clinical outcome after suture anchor repair of complete traumatic rupture of the distal triceps tendon. *Arthroscopy*. 2012;28:1058-1063. B, From Yeh PC, Stephens KT, Solovyova O, et al. The distal triceps tendon footprint and a biomechanical analysis of 3 repair techniques. *Am J Sports Med*. 2010;38:1025-1033.)

then tied down to the free suture end in the anchor, thereby reducing the tendon to the footprint (Bava et al, 2012; Viegas, 1990) (Fig. 31.6).

The anatomic transosseous equivalent technique was initially described by Yeh and Stephens (2010) and resembles a double-row rotator cuff repair. To perform the anatomic transosseous equivalent repair, a single free suture is placed in a Krackow fashion with four or five throws along the medial edge of the triceps tendon from distal to proximal, across the tendon from the medial edge to the lateral edge, and then along the lateral margin from proximal to distal. Both free ends of the Krackow stitch should exit the posterior surface of the tendon approximately 1.5 to 2 cm proximal to its distal edge (Fig. 31.7, *A*). Next, two single-loaded suture anchors are placed at the proximal margin of the anatomic tendon footprint on the olecranon (Fig. 31.7, *B*). The sutures from these anchors are passed from anterior to posterior 2 cm proximal to the tendon's distal end in a mattress fashion (Fig. 31.7, *C*). Finally, the medial limb of the Krackow stitch and a single limb from each of the suture anchors are placed into a knotless suture anchor, which is then implanted in the posteromedial olecranon 1.5 to 2 cm distal to the tendon. The lateral limb of the Krackow stitch and the remaining limbs from each of the suture anchors are then passed in a similar fashion through another knotless suture anchor which is implanted in the posterolateral aspect of the olecranon 1.5 to 2 cm distal to the tendon margin (Fig. 31.7, *D*).

The authors' preferred technique is the distal triceps knotless anatomic footprint repair described by Paci et al (2014; see also Clark et al, 2014). This technique functionally acts as a tension band construct and has demonstrated biomechanical superiority over alternative repair techniques (Paci et al, 2014).

Authors' Preferred Technique

(Video 31.1)

The patient is placed in the prone or lateral decubitus position with the elbow flexed to 90 degrees. A midline curvilinear incision is made over the posterior aspect of the elbow. The incision is curved to the radial side of the tip of the olecranon, which prevents the healed incision from being in the direct area of contact when the elbow is in a resting position on any surface. Radial and ulnar skin flaps are then developed with great care to avoid and protect the ulnar nerve. The ulnar nerve is not typically exposed. The level of the torn tendon is then identified. This is frequently located within a serous fluid collection or hematoma, which can aid in localization of the tendon stump. Often the tissue is tendinotic, forming a bulbous distal stump, which will need to be debrided to healthy tissue. Occasionally, there can be delamination between the deeper medial head insertion and the more superficial lateral head insertion.

After the entire ruptured tendon stump has been identified, mobilized, and freed of any scar or tendinotic tissue, it is then reflected superiorly. This enables the proximal aspect of the tendon footprint on the undersurface of the tendon to be identified. This area on the tendon is typically marked to aid in later identification (see Fig. 31.1) Two #2 nonabsorbable sutures, one lateral and one medial, are passed in a locking Krackow whipstitch fashion to secure the tendon. It is important to ensure that the four limbs of these two sutures all begin and end at the proximal margin of the tendon footprint exiting through the deep, anterior surface (Fig. 31.8). This allows for reconstitution of the tissue length and tension during reduction. We recommend using different color sutures or marking suture tails on the medial and lateral sides with a surgical marking pen to aid in suture management.

A free needle is then used to pass two looped nonabsorbable sutures (FiberLink; Arthrex, Naples FL), one between the medial Krackow stitch limbs and the other between the lateral Krackow stitch limbs at the proximal margin of the tendon footprint. The loops should exit out the superficial, posterior tendon surface to aid in later suture shuttling. This will result in three suture tails on the deep anterior medial side and three on the deep anterior lateral side (Fig. 31.9).

Attention is then turned to the olecranon for preparation of the triceps bony footprint. All soft tissue is debrided away

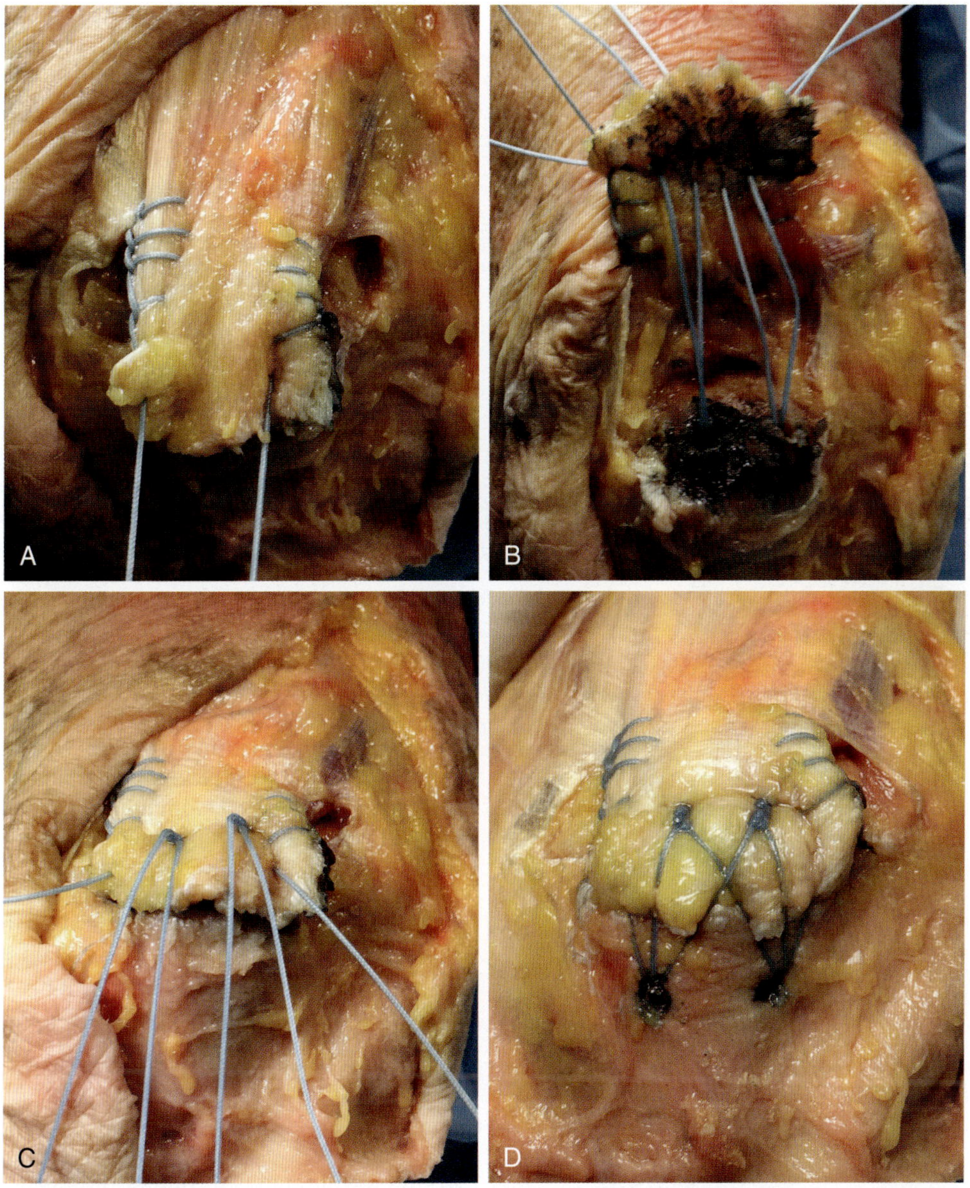

Fig. 31.7 Transosseous equivalent repair. **A,** Krackow stitch from distal to proximal on the medial side, crossing over laterally and then running from proximal to distal on the lateral side. **B,** Suture anchors are placed within the footprint, and the stitches are passed through the proximal footprint from anterior to posterior. **C,** Suture anchors are tied in mattress fashion. **D,** A suture from each mattress stitch along with the ipsilateral Krackow are placed into a knotless anchor distal to the footprint.

from the bone surface. The surface can be rasped down to promote cortical bleeding, but care should be taken not to fully decorticate the bone bed. The proximal aspect of the tendon insertion begins approximately 12 mm distal to the tip of the olecranon and will serve as the starting point for two longitudinal drill tunnels (Fig. 31.10). A 2-mm drill bit is used to create medial and lateral tunnels beginning at the proximal tendon insertion and exiting distally and dorsally on the posteromedial and posterolateral surfaces of the ulna, respectively. The authors prefer to slightly diverge the tunnels to provide room for a subsequent anchor placement. When creating these tunnels, the drill bit should be angled appropriately to avoid penetration of the sigmoid notch.

A point on the central, dorsal surface of the ulna 5 to 10 mm distal to the exit holes of the 2-mm drill tunnels is then chosen for placement of the knotless suture anchor (4.75-mm Biocomposite SwiveLock; Arthrex, Naples, FL). This location is predrilled and tapped, with care taken to angle the tunnel away from the sigmoid notch.

After all the tunnels have been drilled, then suture shuttling is begun. The three medial suture tails, two from the medial Krackow stitch and one from the medial looped suture, are then passed through the medial 2-mm drill tunnel from proximal to distal using a suture shuttling device (i.e., Hewson suture passer; Smith & Nephew, Andover, MA). This step is repeated on the lateral side with the three lateral suture tails.

The next step creates the footprint compression construct. One suture tail from the medial Krackow stitch and one tail from the lateral Krackow stitch are then passed through the loop of the lateral looped suture (Fig. 31.11). The looped suture is then pulled distally, thereby shuttling the sutures back through the tendon and lateral longitudinal drill tunnel. This step is then repeated on the medial side with the remaining tail of each Krackow stitch passed through the

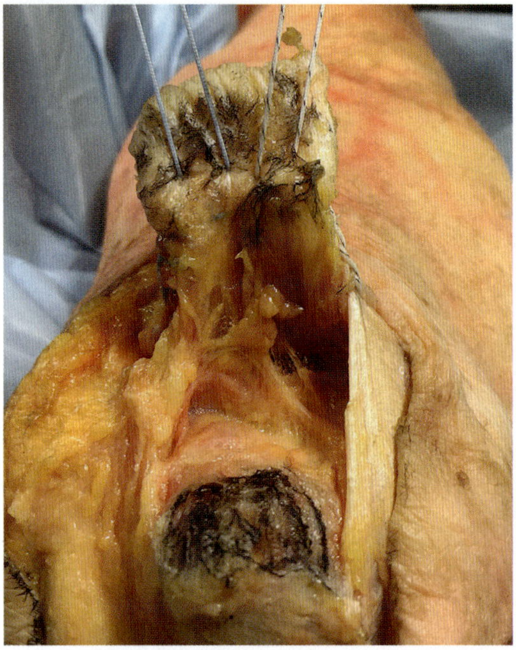

Fig. 31.8 Medial and lateral Krackow stiches exiting on the deep surface of the tendon at the level of the proximal footprint margin.

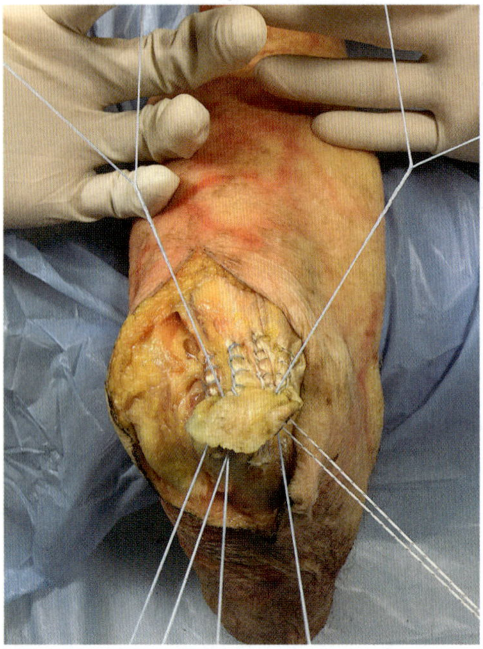

Fig. 31.9 Looped ends of suture exiting posteriorly resulting in three medial and three lateral groups of sutures exiting on the deep anterior surface.

loop of the medial looped suture, which is pulled distally, shuttling these limbs through the tendon and medial longitudinal tunnel. When this step is completed, the sutures will be in the "box-and-x" configuration to promote compression of the footprint (Paci et al, 2014) (Fig. 31.12).

All four suture limbs are then passed through the eyelet of the knotless suture anchor. To decrease bunching of the sutures, the authors recommend passing the two medial sutures from medial to lateral and the two lateral sutures from lateral to medial. The anchor is then docked within the pilot hole, and the sutures are tensioned. The elbow is then gently cycled, and the sutures are again tensioned to remove any remaining slack in the construct. The anchor is then screwed into the olecranon with tension held until the anchor is flush with the cortex of the ulna (Fig. 31.13). Any intact paratenon can then be approximated followed by routine subcutaneous and skin closures.

Postoperative Protocol

The patient is initially splinted in 60 degrees of elbow flexion for 10 to 14 days. After the initial period of immobilization, the sutures are removed, and the patient is transitioned into a hinged elbow brace. At this point, passive range of motion (ROM) is initiated from full extension to 90 degrees of flexion. This is increased by 10 degrees per week until full ROM is achieved. Active ROM is begun at 8 weeks and strengthening at 12 weeks. Return to sport or work-related activities may be up to 4 to 6 months postoperatively.

Biomechanical Comparison of Operative Techniques

The four most frequently used repair techniques are (1) transosseous cruciate drill tunnel technique, (2) the standard suture anchor repair technique, (3) the anatomic transosseous equivalent repair technique, and (4) the knotless anatomic footprint repair technique described above (Clark et al, 2014; Yeh & Stephens, 2010). The transosseous cruciate repair technique has been shown biomechanically to be weaker than the intact, uninjured tendon (Petre et al, 2011). Yeh and Stephens (2010) performed a biomechanical study comparing fixation with transosseous cruciate drill tunnels, suture anchor repair, and the anatomic transosseous equivalent. They found that with biomechanical testing, the transosseous cruciate repair experienced the greatest average displacement, and the anatomic transosseous equivalent repair experienced the least. After 1500 cycles of loading, the appearance of the repair was also markedly different among the repair constructs. In the transosseous cruciate and suture anchor repairs, the tendon was noted to pull away from the footprint, and the tendon itself showed evidence of fraying and intrasubstance tearing. In the anatomic transosseous equivalent repair, the construct was essentially unchanged after 1500 cycles of loading. The disadvantages of the anatomic transosseous equivalent repair are the expense and anatomic crowding from using four suture anchors in the tip of the olecranon. In 2014, Paci et al (2014) demonstrated the distal triceps knotless anatomic footprint repair technique. Clark et al (2014) reported a biomechanical comparison of the transosseous cruciate versus the knotless anatomic footprint repair and found superior load-to-failure, cycle-to-failure, and minimal displacement in the knotless anatomic footprint repair technique. These biomechanical data indicate that the knotless anatomic footprint construct has the added benefits of tension band compression during elbow flexion with the minimal cost and bone violation associated with use of a single suture anchor. The authors prefer the distal triceps knotless anatomic footprint repair technique described by Paci et al (2014) over the variety of alternative fixation techniques.

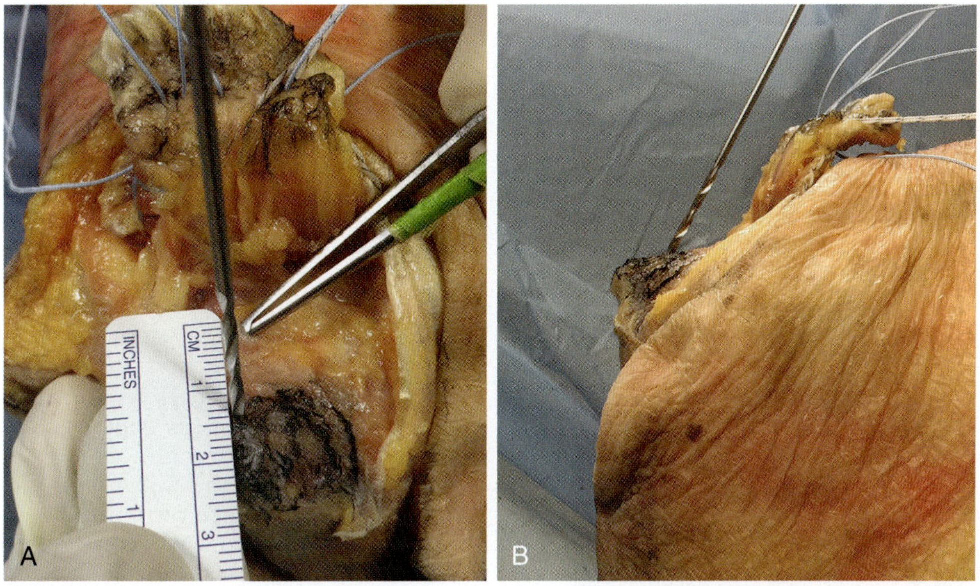

Fig. 31.10 A, Transosseous drill tunnels located at the proximal margin of the footprint approximately 12 mm distal to the tip of the olecranon. **B,** The drill should be angled away from the sigmoid notch to avoid penetrating the articular surface.

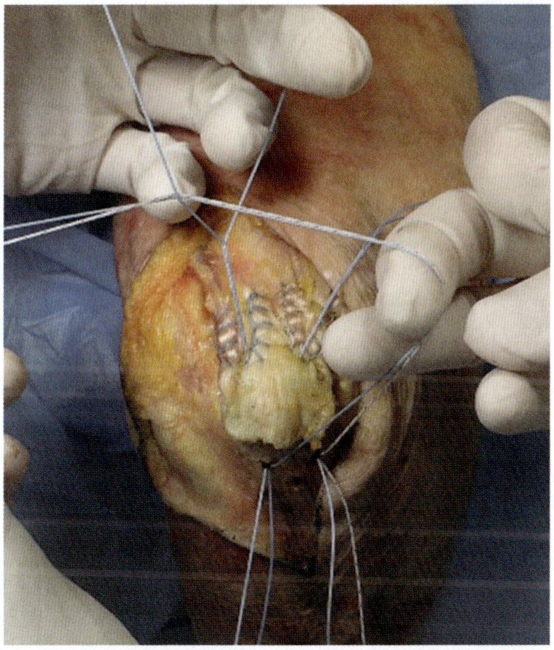

Fig. 31.11 One medial and one lateral Krackow stitch is passed through the medial looped suture. This is then repeated on the lateral side.

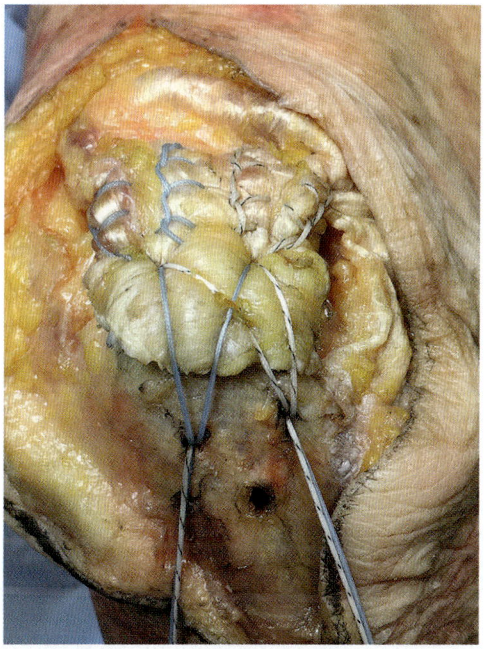

Fig. 31.12 Passage of the looped sutures distally results in the "box-and-x" configuration over the tendon footprint.

Outcomes and Return to Sport

Excellent functional results have been reported after following primary repair of distal triceps tendon rupture. In 2003, van Riet et al (2003) performed a retrospective review of 23 patients with triceps tendon rupture followed for a minimum of 1 year. Fourteen patients underwent a primary surgical repair using the transosseous cruciate technique. Of those 14 patients, 3 patients went on to rerupture after the initial repair (van Reit et al, 2003). Of note, these authors also reported that a delay in diagnosis or failure of conservative management of a partial injury led to an increased frequency of the patient requiring a reconstructive procedure versus a primary repair. Patients with a reconstructive procedure tended to have worse motion and strength than those with a primary repair. These results suggest that early surgical intervention may be beneficial in high-grade partial injuries as well as complete tears.

Bava et al (2012) reported on five patients with a 32-month follow-up after suture anchor repair. The authors noted excellent results with respect to outcome scoring (American Shoulder and Elbow Surgeons [ASES] score, 99.2; Disabilities of the Arm, Shoulder, and Hand [DASH] score, 1.4; Mayo score, 95.8). All patients were noted to obtain full elbow ROM by 6 months after the repair.

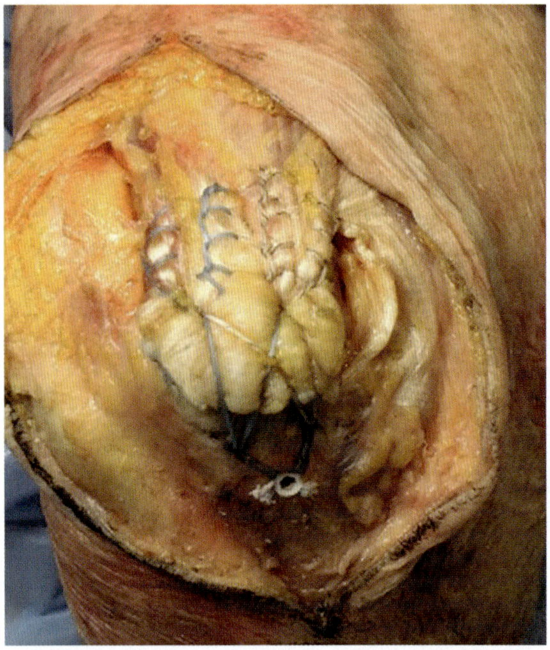

Fig. 31.13 Krackow stitch limbs are passed through the knotless anchor and cut flush.

Kokkalis et al (2013) reported on 11 patients with a complete rupture of the tendon treated with a combination transosseous cruciate and single suture anchor placed in mattress fashion in the proximal footprint. Five of the patients were engaged in weight lifting at the time of injury, and none reported anabolic steroid use or systemic disease. At an average of 23-month follow-up, 9 of the 11 patients returned to their preinjury statuses.

Kose et al (2015) reported on 8 patients who underwent transosseous suture repair of distal triceps tendon ruptures. Of the 8 patients, 3 were engaged in athletic activity at the time of injury (football, wrestling, weight lifting). The patient with the weight lifting injury reported a history of anabolic steroid use. Overall, patients were followed for a period of 18.8 months (range, 12–26). Six of the 8 reported excellent results, and 2 of the 8 reported good results on the Mayo Elbow Scoring system.

The outcomes of treatment for distal triceps tendon injuries in athletes have been documented in several studies. Consistent restoration of function and ability to return to sport have been noted. Mair et al (2004) reported on 21 professional football players in the NFL with triceps tendon injuries. Ten players sustained partial tearing that was treated with initial bracing. One player completely tore his triceps tendon after returning to practice requiring surgical fixation; 3 players finished the season with bracing and subsequently required surgery in the offseason secondary to continued pain and weakness. The 9 players who returned to play that season missed an average of 4.8 weeks of play (range, 0–9 weeks). All 10 of these players with partial tears were able to return to the NFL for at least one season. The 11 players in the study with complete ruptures were treated with immediate surgical repair. All players missed the remainder of the season, and one player retired during the offseason. The remaining 10 were able to return to play for at least 1 additional year (Mair et al, 2004). Similar outcomes were reported from our institution by Finstein et al (2015) in a study involving 37 professional football players treated with primary surgical repair. Comparison data on players treated nonoperatively were not available through the NFL Injury Surveillance System. The authors found that these injuries occurred predominantly in lineman (86%) while blocking or being blocked (78%). All 37 players were able to return to the NFL after missing an average of 165 days.

Complications

Complications after triceps tendon repair are rare. Most commonly, patients may experience a residual flexion contracture, loss of strength, and local irritation or olecranon bursitis from the underlying hardware. Rarely, a patient may experience rerupture after the initial repair, however, these patients may experience equivalent results with revision repair as those with a primary repair (van Riet et al, 2003). Kose et al (2015) reported on a case report of eight patients, two of whom developed a 5-degree flexion contraction after operative fixation. Mair et al (2004) reported on a single patient with a partial tear who sustained a complete rupture after returning to sport.

Summary

Timely diagnosis and management of distal triceps ruptures can lead to excellent outcomes in a majority of patients. Nonoperative management may be appropriate in cases of partial ruptures. In patients with complete tears, however, operative fixation remains the gold standard to return patients to their preinjury levels of strength, motion, and function. A variety of fixation constructs have been proposed, with the limited available research data suggesting that the knotless anatomic footprint repair technique may have some potential benefits. Further clinical and biomechanical research, however, is required to identify the optimal fixation technique for these injuries.

References

Anzel SH, Covey KW, Weiner AD, et al. Disruption of muscles and tendons: an analysis of 1,014 cases. *Surgery.* 1959;45:406–414.

Aso K, Torisu T. Muscle belly tear of the triceps. *Am J Sports Med.* 1984;12(6):485–487.

Bava ED, Barber FA, Lund ER. Clinical outcome after suture anchor repair of complete traumatic rupture of the distal triceps tendon. *Arthroscopy.* 2012;28:1058–1063.

Clark J, Obopilwe E, Rizzi A, et al. Distal triceps knotless anatomic footprint repair is superior to transosseous cruciate repair: a biomechanical comparison. *Arthroscopy.* 2014;30:1254–1260.

Clayton ML, Thirupathi RG. Rupture of the triceps tendon with olecranon bursitis. A case report with a new method of repair. *Clin Orthop Relat Res.* 1984;184:183–185.

Finstein J, Cohen SB, Dodson CC, et al. Triceps ruptures in National Football League Players. *Orthop J Sports Med.* 2015;3(8): 2325967115601021.

Inhofe PD, Moneim MS. Late presentation of triceps rupture. A case report and review of the literature. *Am J Orthop.* 1996;25(11):790–792.

Kachooei AR, Moradi A, Mudgal CS. Non-simultaneous bilateral closed rupture of the triceps tendon in a woman. *J Hand Microsurg.* 2015;7(1):205–207.

Kokkalis ZT, Mavrogenis AF, Spyridonos S, Papagelopoulos PJ, Weiser RW, Sotereanos DG. Triceps brachii distal tendon reattachment with a double-row technique. *Orthopedics.* 2013;36(2):110–116.

Kose O, Kilicaslan OF, Guler F, Acar B, Yuksel H. Functional outcomes and complications after surgical repair of triceps tendon rupture. *Eur J Orthop Surg Tramatol.* 2015;25:1131–1139.
Mair SD, Isbell WM, Gill TJ, et al. Triceps tendon ruptures in professional football players. *Am J Sports Med.* 2004;32:431–434.
Marinello PG, Peers S, Srai S, Evans PJ. A treat algorithm for the management of distal triceps ruptures. *Tech Hand Up Extrem Surg.* 2015;19(2):73–80.
O'Driscoll SW. Intramuscular triceps rupture. *Can J Surg.* 1992;35:203–207.
Paci JM, Clark J, Rizzi A. Distal triceps knotless anatomic footprint repair: a new technique. *Arthrosc Tech.* 2014;3(5):e621–e626.
Petre BM, Grutter PW, Rose DM, Belkoff SM, McFarland EG, Petersen SA. Triceps tendons: a biomechanical comparison of intact and repaired strength. *J Shoulder Elbow Surg.* 2011;20:213–218.
Pina A, Garcia I, Sabater M. Traumatic avulsion of the triceps brachii. *J Orthop Trauma.* 2002;16:273–276.
Singh RK, Pooley J. Complete rupture of the triceps brachii muscle. *Br J Sports Med.* 2002;36:467–469.
Sollender JL, Rayan GM, Barden GA. Triceps tendon rupture in weight lifters. *J Shoulder Elbow Surg.* 1998;7:151–153.
Stannard JP, Bucknell AL. Rupture of the triceps tendon associated with steroid injections. *Am J Sports Med.* 1993;21(3):482–485.
Strauch RJ. Biceps and triceps injuries of the elbow. *Orthop Clin North Am.* 1999;30:95–107.
Stucken C, Ciccotti MG. Distal biceps and triceps injuries in athletes. *Sports Med Arthrosc.* 2014;22(3):153–163.
Tagliafico A, Gandolfo N, Michaud J, Perez MM, Palmieri F, Martinoli C. Ultrasound demonstration of distal triceps tendon tears. *Eur J Radiol.* 2012;81(6):1207–1210.
Tiger E, Mayer DP, Glazer R. Complete avulsion of the triceps tendon: MRI diagnosis. *Comput Med Imaging Graph.* 1993;17(1):51–54.
Tsourvakas S, Gouvalas K, Gimtsas C, et al. Bilateral and simultaneous rupture of the triceps tendons in chronic renal failure and secondary hyperparathyroidism. *Arch Orthop Trauma Surg.* 2004;124:278–280.
van Riet RP, Morrey BF, Ho E, et al. Surgical treatment of distal triceps ruptures. *J Bone Joint Surg Am.* 2003;85:1961–1967.
Vidal AF, Drakos MC, Allen AA. Biceps tendon and triceps tendon injuries. *Clin Sports Med.* 2004;23:707–722.
Viegas SF. Avulsion of the triceps tendon. *Orthop Rev.* 1990;19:533–536.
Windisch G, Tesch NP, Grechenig W, Peicha G. The triceps brachii muscle and its insertion on the olecranon. *Med Sci Monit.* 2006;12:290–294.
Yeh PC, Dodds SD, Smart LR, Mazzocca AD, Sethi PM. Distal triceps rupture. *J Am Acad Orthop Surg.* 2010;18(1):31–40.
Yeh PC, Stephens KT, Solovyova O, et al. The distal triceps tendon footprint and a biomechanical analysis of 3 repair techniques. *Am J Sports Med.* 2010;38:1025–1033.

SECTION **XI**

Elbow Articular Cartilage and Bone Injuries

SECTION OUTLINE

32 Osteochondritis Dissecans of the Capitellum

CARL W. NISSEN, MD, JOSEPH MARCHESE, MD, and TAYLOR WILEY, MD

Osteochondritis dissecans (OCD) of the capitellum is a condition of the lateral elbow that often affects skeletally immature athletes, especially those who repeatedly subject the radiocapitellar joint to compressive forces. Ultimately, repetitive stress of this nature leads to disruption of a localized portion of the subchondral bone and, if allowed to progress, the overlying articular cartilage. The etiology of this disorder is multifactorial and often cannot be determined. The progression of capitellar OCD may result in significant pain, loss of motion, inability to perform weight-bearing or overhead activities, and radiocapitellar degenerative change in approximately 50% of patients (Takahara et al, 1999b). Treatment is based on lesion size and stability as well as the condition of the surrounding articular cartilage. If conservative treatment is not possible or fails, surgical options include open debridement with fragment excision, arthroscopic debridement and marrow stimulation, fragment fixation, closing wedge osteotomy of the distal humerus, osteochondral autograft, and osteochondral allograft. Each of these interventions has had variable short-term outcomes, and the ideal management strategy has yet to be determined.

Etiology/Pathology

Despite the uncertainty of its etiology, symptomatic OCD of the capitellum arises primarily from repetitive stress to the elbow (Yadao et al, 2004). Provoking compressive forces on the capitellum commonly occur in the dominant arm of overhead throwing athletes and from weight-bearing stress in gymnasts in the second decade of life. Overhead athletes place the medial elbow stabilizing complex under significant repetitive stress with consequent lateral elbow compression and shear forces. This occurs primarily during the late cocking phase of the throwing cycle as the radiocapitellar articulation, a prime secondary stabilizer to valgus stress, experiences as much as 60% of the axial compression force across the elbow (Fig. 32.1). Along the same lines, female gymnasts invoke a similar injury mechanism through repetitive loading of the radiocapitellar joint with their arms in extension (Jobe & Nuber, 1986; Indelicato et al, 1979; Singer & Roy, 1984; An & Morrey, 2000).

The pathophysiology of OCD resembles that of mechanical trauma to articular cartilage. Repetitive microtrauma in the susceptible elbow initiates fatigue fracture, resorption, and ultimately fragment separation from the underlying subchondral bone, as demonstrated by Tallqvist (1962) through rabbit models. With time, the overlying articular cartilage begins to break down and is increasingly vulnerable to shear stress because of inadequate subchondral osseous support, leading to separation, fragmentation, and loose body formation (Tallqvist, 1962). The Research in Osteochondritis of the Knee (ROCK) study group has come to define OCD as "a focal, idiopathic alteration of subchondral bone with risk of instability and disruption of adjacent articular cartilage that may result in premature osteoarthritis" (Edmonds & Shea, 2013). This same phenomenon extends to OCD of the capitellum.

In concert with traumatic insult, the vascular anatomy of the distal humerus underscores ischemia as a likely contributor to OCD of the capitellum. The blood supply to the capitellum arises primarily from posterior perforating vessels that traverse the epiphyseal articular cartilage without metaphyseal collateral circulation (Haraldsson, 1959). Through a cadaveric ink-injection study of the skeletally mature elbow, Yamaguchi et al (1997) determined that the main arterial contributors to the lateral elbow are the radial and middle collateral, radial recurrent, and interosseous recurrent arteries. Repetitive stress to and compression of this tenuous blood supply may cause ischemia of the subchondral bone within the capitellum and the characteristic osteonecrosis observed in OCD. Hence, this compromise of the subchondral support structure promotes articular cartilage fragmentation and loose body formation (Yamaguchi et al, 1997).

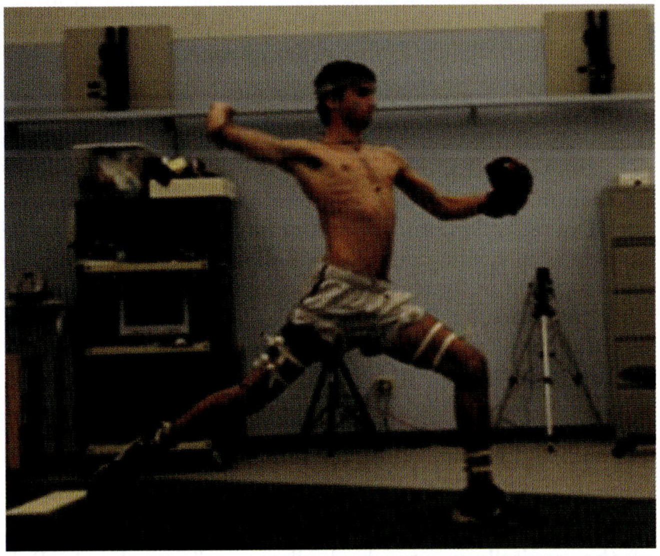

Fig. 32.1 Side view of a pitcher at the point of maximal shoulder and elbow stress. This point is defined as early acceleration with the shoulder near its point of maximal external rotation. (From Crotin RL. A collaborative approach to prevent medial elbow injuries in baseball pitchers. *Strength & Conditioning Journal.* 2011;33(5):1–24.)

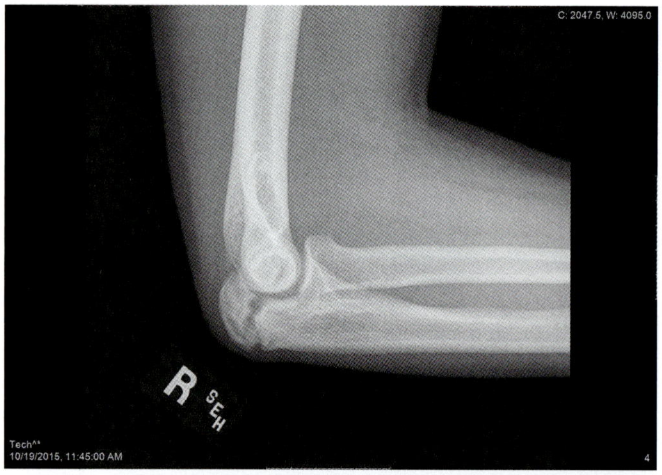

Fig. 33.6 Delayed olecranon physeal closure.

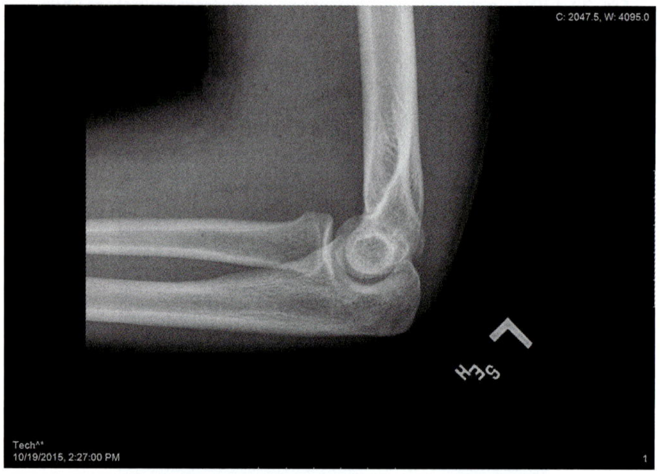

Fig. 33.7 From patient with delayed olecranon physeal closure in Fig. 33.6, the contralateral elbow for comparison.

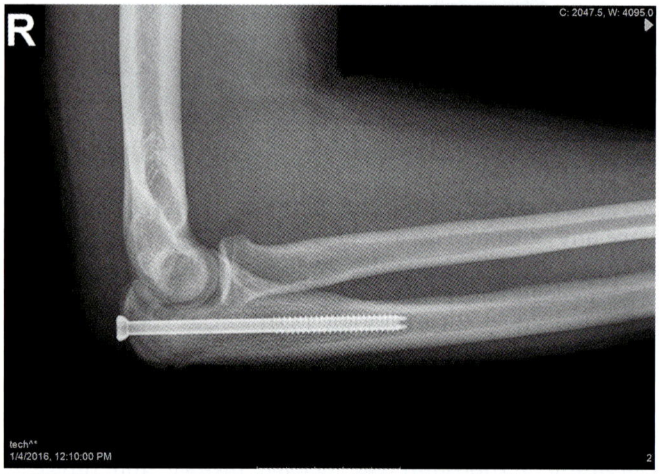

Fig. 33.8 Lateral view of the elbow after ORIF.

preceded by a period of pain or aching. Athletes should be asked whether they have increased their training intensity and to clarify any period of rest that they may have undergone (true rest versus slight decrease in intensity).

A thorough physical examination of the elbow and shoulder should be performed. It is very important to be vigilant

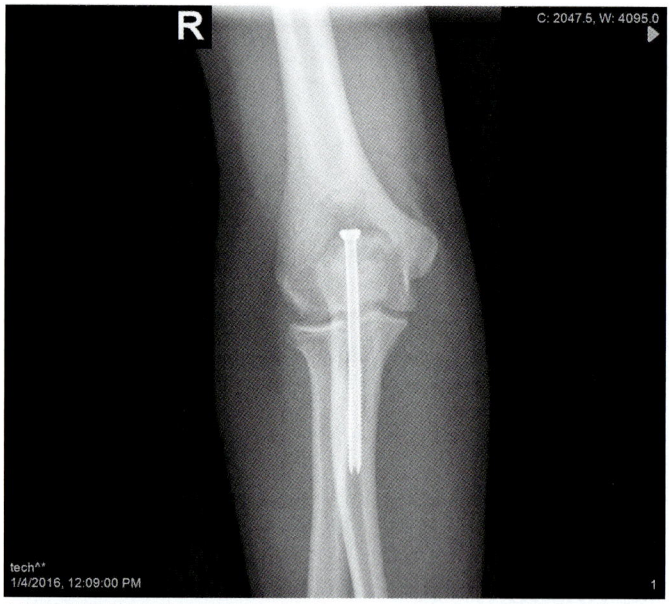

Fig. 33.9 Anteroposterior view of the elbow after ORIF.

for concomitant pathology. In the case series reported by Paci et al (2013), a concurrent procedure was performed on the elbow at the time of ORIF for the olecranon stress fracture in 44% of patients. (Patients typically report pain and soreness along the posterior elbow, with posterolateral pain being especially specific for an olecranon stress fracture in the authors' experience. However, patients may complain of posteromedial pain or direct posterior pain as well, especially if they have posteromedial impingement.

In addition to examination of the posterior compartment, the UCL, flexor-pronator mass, ulnar nerve, and radiocapitellar joint should be evaluated and a thorough examination of the shoulder should be performed.

Imaging

We routinely obtain radiographs of the affected side: anteroposterior (AP), lateral, internal and external rotation, and olecranon views. A comparison radiograph of the patient's other elbow should be obtained if delayed physeal closure is suspected. The radiographs should be examined for the presence of a stress fracture but also for any posterior osteophyte formation and signs of other injury.

Depending on the patient's physical findings and history, magnetic resonance imaging (MRI) may be obtained to evaluate for concomitant pathology. If an olecranon stress fracture is seen on radiography and the patient has no other signs of concomitant injury, MRI may not be necessary. If no stress fracture is seen on radiography, the physician may obtain MRI to look for stress reaction in the olecranon and also evaluate for other pathology, specifically UCL injury or attenuation. We do not routinely use computed tomography (CT) for these injuries unless there is concern about additional bony pathology.

Clinical Decision Making

The patient presenting with an olecranon stress fracture or delayed physeal closure is treated with a period of rest, nonsteroidal antiinflammatory drugs (NSAIDs), physical therapy and modalities, and possible use of a bone growth stimulator, followed by a progressive exercise and throwing program once the patient is asymptomatic. Schickendantz et al (2002) described the successful nonsurgical treatment of seven professional baseball players with MRI-positive olecranon osseous stress injuries. (The athletes were treated with relative rest, avoidance of throwing and valgus stress activities for at least 6 weeks, and protective bracing for 4 weeks, followed by a progressive throwing program. All seven returned to play and started their throwing programs at an average of 8 weeks after the initiation of care.

Most of the available literature on athletes with radiographic olecranon stress fractures is in the form of case series of patients in whom nonoperative treatment had failed but who did well after ORIF (Fujioka et al, 2012; Suzuki et al, 1997). In the largest series of its kind, Paci et al (2013) described the results of ORIF with a cannulated screw in 18 baseball players with radiographically positive olecranon stress fractures and an average follow-up of 6.2 years. Fracture union was achieved in all 18 patients, 17 of whom returned to baseball at or above their preinjury playing levels, although 6 of the 18 (33%) required hardware removal, for infection in 2 patients. The authors of this chapter are inclined to proceed with ORIF sooner in patients with radiographic confirmation of olecranon stress fractures rather than stress fractures visible only on MRI, but nonoperative treatment is generally attempted initially in all patients presenting with olecranon stress fractures or stress reactions. Furushima et al (2014) recommended operative treatment for any patient in whom at least 3 months of nonoperative treatment have failed.

For athletes presenting with delayed physeal closure, nonoperative treatment and rest should be initiated. When nonoperative treatment fails, ORIF with a cannulated screw is recommended. Rettig et al (2006) treated five patients who had delayed physeal closure of the olecranon with cannulated screw and washer fixation, with additional tension band wiring in four patients. Union was achieved in the five patients, all of whom returned to the same level of play at an average of 29 weeks after surgery.

Surgical Technique

Open reduction and internal fixation are performed using a cannulated, partially threaded, titanium screw. Screw size is determined by the patient's anatomy as shown by preoperative radiographs; a single titanium, cannulated, 7.3-mm or 6.5-mm screw is typically used for obliquely oriented fractures, and one or two 4.0-mm cannulated screws for transversely oriented fractures. The patient is positioned supine with the arm on a hand table. A tourniquet is placed high on the arm and out of the sterile field. After induction of anesthesia, preparation, and draping, the upper extremity is exsanguinated and the tourniquet is inflated to 250 mm Hg. A small percutaneous approach is used for screw placement, with a stab incision located over the screw insertion point. In the patient with an additional injury, a medial incision can be made to address medial-sided concomitant pathology such as an UCL injury as well as the small posterior incision for the olecranon screw. A guide pin is placed under fluoroscopic control, down the ulnar canal from proximal to distal for oblique stress fractures or perpendicular to a transversely oriented stress fracture. The guide pin is overreamed for the appropriately sized cannulated screw, which is then inserted. Radiographs are taken with the C-arm fluoroscope to confirm correct hardware position. Any additional surgical intervention is then performed, such as UCL reconstruction, elbow arthroscopy, or olecranon osteophyte excision. The tourniquet is deflated before irrigation and wound closure to avoid hematoma formation. A sterile dressing is placed, and a posterior splint applied with the elbow in 90 degrees of flexion (Paci et al, 2013).

Rehabilitation

Rehabilitation after ORIF of an olecranon stress fracture continues to be a multiphased approach (Wilk et al, 2004). Immediately after surgery, the patient's arm is placed in a posterior splint at 90 degrees of flexion, which is maintained for 7 to 10 days to allow the soft tissues to heal. The length of immobilization depends on the patient's age, osseous status, health, desired goals, and healing response. During this time, the patient is allowed to perform wrist, hand, and shoulder range-of-motion exercises. Unlimited passive motion is allowed once the splint is removed. Active pronation, supination, and flexion are allowed; however, active flexion beyond 90 degrees is avoided for 6 weeks. Achieving full range of motion in all directions by 8 weeks is expected. During this period, the patient is allowed to perform rotator cuff, scapular, and shoulder exercises. At 6 weeks, gentle active flexion greater than 90 degrees is initiated, and strengthening is started at 8 weeks. At 8 weeks after surgery, the patient starts our "thrower's ten program" designed to restore strength in the entire upper extremity, trunk, and core (Wilk et al, 2009). At 12 weeks after surgery, the patient starts the "advanced thrower's ten program" and begins plyometric exercises. Shortly thereafter, the interval throwing program is initiated, typically at 14 to 16 weeks after surgery (Reinold et al, 2002). Throwing from the mound is initiated once the patient has completed a long toss program at 120 to 145 feet without any elbow symptoms or complaints (Paci et al, 2013).

Outcomes

Both nonoperative and operative treatments have been described as treatment for olecranon stress fracture (Nuber & Diment, 1992; Schickendantz et al, 2002; Shinozaki et al, 2006). Schickendantz et al (2002) described the successful nonsurgical treatment of seven professional baseball players with MRI-positive olecranon osseous stress injuries, all of whom were able to return to play at an average of 8 weeks after the initiation of care. Isolated case reports of successful nonoperative treatment of MRI-positive olecranon stress reactions have also been published (Brucker et al, 2015).

As far as the authors are aware, there is no available literature describing successful nonoperative treatment of radiographically positive olecranon stress fractures. We believe that nonoperative treatment should be attempted initially for any stress fracture but that the physician should have a lower threshold for operating on olecranon stress fractures that are visible on radiographs. As previously described, Paci et al (2013) described the results of ORIF with a cannulated screw in 18 baseball players with oblique or transverse radiographically positive olecranon stress fractures with an average follow-up of 6.2 years. All of the patients had initially tried nonoperative treatment and rest but continued to have symptoms with throwing. Union was achieved in all 18 patients with ORIF, 17 of whom returned to baseball at or above their preinjury playing level, including two Major League Baseball (MLB) players. However, 6 of the 18 (33%) required hardware removal, for infection in 2 patients.

Fujioka et al (2012) described ORIF of olecranon stress fractures with a headless threaded screw in six patients (five baseball players and one softball player). All six patients returned to play at the same level, at an average of 4 to 6 months. Suzuki et al (1997) published their results in two baseball players who underwent ORIF of an olecranon stress fracture with a single screw and two iliac bone pegs inserted across the fracture line. Union was achieved in both players, who returned to their previous levels of pitching at 4 and 6 months, and one player who was in high school went on to play in college. Stephenson et al (2012) described a case report in a college pitcher who underwent ORIF of the olecranon with a screw for a stress fracture and in whom the stress fracture recurred 7 months after the index procedure. The patient was then treated with a revision ORIF. The initial 6.5-mm screw was removed, the canal was reamed, and a new 6.5-mm screw and a 2.7-mm medial compression screw were placed. The patient received vitamin D supplementation and used a bone stimulator postoperatively. Union was confirmed, and the athlete returned to pitching at 14 weeks after the second surgery and was able to complete the season. At 17 months of follow-up, he continued to pitch at the collegiate level and remained asymptomatic.

There is very little evidence in the literature regarding delayed olecranon physeal closures, and these injuries are typically excluded from studies of olecranon stress fracture in skeletally mature athletes. Rettig et al (2006) published a series of five patients with delayed physeal closure of the olecranon treated with cannulated screw and washer fixation. Tension band wiring was also performed in four of the patients at the time of screw insertion. Union was achieved in all five patients, who returned to preinjury levels of play at an average of 29 weeks. Of the 200 baseball players in the case series reported by Furushima et al (2014), 101 had delayed physeal closure (physeal olecranon stress fracture as described in the paper), so the actual incidence of this injury may be much higher than previously reported.

Prevention

Olecranon stress fractures and delayed physeal closure, regardless of fracture pattern or exact mechanism of injury, are inherently overuse injuries. Pitch counts should be adhered to for all athletes, not just for the game but for the season and the year. However, the injury is not isolated to pitchers and can be seen in any player at any position and in sports other than baseball (Furushima et al, 2014). Any athlete with posterior elbow pain should rest the arm and should modify his or her activities until asymptomatic; playing with arm pain should be discouraged. Special focus should be placed on the adolescent thrower, because the incidence of delayed olecranon physeal closure may be higher than previously noted (Furushima et al, 2014).

Conclusions

Olecranon stress fractures and delayed olecranon physeal closure are rare injuries typically found in baseball players but can occur in other throwing athletes such as javelin throwers and softball players. They can also be found in athletes performing repetitive upper extremity activities such as weight lifters, gymnasts, and divers. The elbow should be evaluated thoroughly and examined for any concomitant conditions such as posteromedial impingement and UCL deficiency, which may contribute to the development of an olecranon stress fracture. Nonoperative treatment should be initiated with rest, NSAIDs, possible bracing or splinting, and possible use of bone growth stimulation. For stress fractures for which nonoperative treatment fails, good results in terms of return to play and fracture union have been reported with ORIF using a single cannulated screw. A lower threshold for ORIF in radiographically positive olecranon stress fractures is recommended, and any concomitant pathology should be addressed surgically at the time of ORIF, with special emphasis on evaluation for UCL injury.

References

Ahmad CS, ElAttrache NS. Valgus extension overload syndrome and stress injury of the olecranon. *Clin Sports Med.* 2004a;23(4):665–676.

Ahmad CS, Park MC, ElAttrache NS. Elbow medial ulnar collateral ligament insufficiency alters posteromedial olecranon contact. *Am J Sports Med.* 2004b;32(7):1607–1612.

Brucker J, Sahu N, Sandella B. Olecranon stress injury in an adolescent overhand pitcher: a case report and analysis of the literature. *Sports Health.* 2015;7(4):308–311.

Cain EL Jr, Dugas JR, Wolf RS, Andrews JR. Elbow injuries in throwing athletes: a current concepts review. *Am J Sports Med.* 2003;31(4):621–635.

Fujioka H, Tsunemi K, Takagi Y, Tanaka J. Treatment of stress fracture of the olecranon in throwing athletes with internal fixation through a small incision. *Sports Med Arthrosc Rehabil Ther Technol.* 2012;4(1):49.

Furushima K, Itoh Y, Iwabu S, Yamamoto Y, Koga R, Shimizu M. Classification of olecranon stress fractures in baseball players. *Am J Sports Med.* 2014;42(6):1343–1351.

Lu CC, Chen SK, Wang CW, Chou PH. Chondromalacia of trochlear notch after healing of olecranon stress fracture: a case report. *Arch Orthop Trauma Surg.* 2006;126(4):271–274.

Nakaji N, Fujioka H, Tanaka J, et al. Stress fracture of the olecranon in an adult baseball player. *Knee Surg Sports Traumatol Arthrosc.* 2006;14(4):390–393.

Nuber GW, Diment MT. Olecranon stress fractures in throwers: a report of two cases and a review of the literature. *Clin Orthop Relat Res.* 1992;278:58–61.

Paci JM, Dugas JR, Guy JA, et al. Cannulated screw fixation of refractory olecranon stress fractures with and without associated injuries allows a return to baseball. *Am J Sports Med.* 2013;41(2):306–312.

Rao PS, Rao SK, Navadgi BC. Olecranon stress fracture in a weightlifter: a case report. *Br J Sports Med.* 2001;35(1):72–73.

Reinold MM, Wilk KE, Reed J, Crenshaw K, Andrews JR. Interval sport programs: guidelines for baseball, tennis, and golf. *J Orthop Sports Phys Ther.* 2002;32(6):293–298.

Rettig AC, Wurth TR, Mieling P. Nonunion of olecranon stress fractures in adolescent baseball pitchers: a case series of 5 athletes. *Am J Sports Med.* 2006;34(4):653–656.

Schickendantz MS, Ho CP, Koh J. Stress injury of the proximal ulna in professional baseball players. *Am J Sports Med.* 2002;30(5):737–741.

Shinozaki T, Kondo T, Takagishi K. Olecranon stress fracture in a young tower-diving swimmer. *Orthopedics.* 2006;29(8):693–694.

Stephenson DR, Love S, Garcia GG, Mair SD. Recurrence of an olecranon stress fracture in an elite pitcher after percutaneous internal fixation: a case report. *Am J Sports Med.* 2012;40(1):218–221.

Suzuki K, Minami A, Suenaga N, Kondoh M. Oblique stress fracture of the olecranon in baseball pitchers. *J Shoulder Elbow Surg.* 1997;6(5): 491–494.

Waris W. Elbow injuries of javelin-throwers. *Acta Chir Scand.* 1946;93:563–575.

Wilk KE, Obma P, Simpson CD, Cain EL, Dugas JR, Andrews JR. Shoulder injuries in the overhead athlete. *J Orthop Sports Phys Ther.* 2009;39(2):38–54.

Wilk KE, Reinold MM, Andrews JR. Rehabilitation of the thrower's elbow. *Clin Sports Med.* 2004;23(4):765–801, xii.

Wilkerson RD, Johns JC. Nonunion of an olecranon stress fracture in an adolescent gymnast: a case report. *Am J Sports Med.* 1990;18(4): 432–434.

Index

Note: Page numbers followed by "*f*" indicate figures, "*t*" indicate tables and "*b*" indicate boxes.

C

D

E

T

U